VARIANTS AND PITFALLS IN BODY IMAGING

Editor

Ali Shirkhoda, M.D., F.A.C.R.
Director, Division of Diagnostic Imaging
Department of Diagnostic Radiology
William Beaumont Hospital
Royal Oak, Michigan

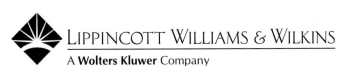
LIPPINCOTT WILLIAMS & WILKINS
A **Wolters Kluwer** Company
Philadelphia • Baltimore • New York • London
Buenos Aires • Hong Kong • Sydney • Tokyo

Acquisitions Editor: Joyce-Rachel John
Developmental Editor: Michael Standen
Production Editor: Karen G. Edmonson
Manufacturing Manager: Timothy Reynolds
Cover Designer: Patricia Gast
Compositor: Lippincott Williams & Wilkins Desktop Divison
Printer: Maple Press

© 2000 by LIPPINCOTT WILLIAMS & WILKINS
227 East Washington Square
Philadelphia, PA 19106-3780 USA
LWW.com

Printed in the USA

Library of Congress Cataloging-in-Publication Data
Variants and pitfalls in body imaging / editor. Ali Shirkhoda.
    p.   cm.
Includes bibliographical references and index.
ISBN 0-683-30058-X
1. Diagnostic imaging. I. Shirkhoda, Ali.
[DNLM: 1. Diagnostic Imaging. 2. Quality Assurance, Health Care.
3. Technology, Radiologic. WN 180 V299 1999]
RC78.7.D53V37   1999
616.07'54—dc21
DNLM/DLC
For Library of Congress   99-35193
                                                              CIP

Care has been taken to confirm the accuracy of the information presented and to describe generally accepted practices. However, the authors, editor, and publisher are not responsible for errors or omissions or for any consequences from application of the information in this book and make no warranty, expressed or implied, with respect to the currency, completeness, or accuracy of the contents of the publication. Application of this information in a particular situation remains the professional responsibility of the practitioner.

The authors, editor, and publisher have exerted every effort to ensure that drug selection and dosage set forth in this text are in accordance with current recommendations and practice at the time of publication. However, in view of ongoing research, changes in government regulations, and the constant flow of information relating to drug therapy and drug reactions, the reader is urged to check the package insert for each drug for any change in indications and dosage and for added warnings and precautions. This is particularly important when the recommended agent is a new or infrequently employed drug.

Some drugs and medical devices presented in this publication have Food and Drug Administration (FDA) clearance for limited use in restricted research settings. It is the responsibility of the health care provider to ascertain the FDA status of each drug or device planned for use in their clinical practice.

10 9 8 7 6 5 4 3 2 1

To Roxanne, Layla, and Shahrzad, who give me the love and inspiration needed for my academic ambitions.

To physicians and scientists whose research and investigations continue to shape our knowledge of body imaging.

To radiologists, physicists, and technologists who strive to create better images of the body in order to achieve a more accurate diagnosis.

Contents

Section I. Variants of Normal Anatomy and Diagnostic Pitfalls in Imaging of the Thorax and Breast

Section II. Variants of Normal Anatomy and Diagnostic Pitfalls in Imaging of the Abdomen and Pelvis

Section III. Variants of Normal Anatomy and Diagnostic Pitfalls in Imaging of the Musculoskeletal System

Section IV. Physical Aspects of Imaging Artifacts

Contributing Authors

Marco A. Amendola, M.D.
Professor
Department of Radiology
University of Miami School of Medicine
1611 Northwest 12th Avenue
Miami, Florida 33101

Arash Anavim, M.D.
Research Fellow
Department of Radiological Sciences
University of California at Irvine Medical
* Center*
101 The City Drive
Orange, California 92868

Mostafa Atri, M.D., F.R.C.P.(C)
Associate Professor
Department of Medical Imaging
University of Toronto
Chief, GU Section
Department of Medical Imaging
Princess Margaret Hospital
610 University Avenue
Toronto, Ontario M5G M9
Canada

Donovan M. Bakalyar, Ph.D.
Assistant Physicist
Department of Diagnostic Radiology
William Beaumont Hospital
3601 West Thirteen Mile Road
Royal Oak, Michigan 48073-6769

Emil J. Balthazar, M.D.
Professor
Department of Radiology
Abdominal Imaging
New York University, Tisch-Bellevue Medical
* Center*
560 First Avenue
New York, New York 10016

Jenny Bencardino, M.D.
Resident
Department of Radiology
Albert Einstein College of Medicine
1300 Morris Park Avenue
Bronx, New York 10461
Department of Radiology
Long Island Jewish Medical Center
270-05 76th Street
New Hyde Park, New York 11040

Kostaki G. Bis, M.D.
Assistant Clinical Professor
Department of Diagnostic Radiology
Wayne State University School of Medicine
Chief, Magnetic Resonance Research
Department of Diagnostic Radiology
William Beaumont Hospital
3601 West Thirteen Mile Road
Royal Oak, Michigan 48073-6769

Mark A. Brown, Ph.D.
Technical Instructor
Siemens Training and Development Center
209 Pregson Drive
Cary, North Carolina 27511

Alexander A. Cacciarelli, M.D.
Director, Division of Pediatric Radiology
Department of Diagnostic Radiology
William Beaumont Hospital
3601 West Thirteen Mile Road
Royal Oak, Michigan 48073-6769

Catherine A. D'Agostino, M.D.
Assistant Professor
Department of Radiology
New York University School of Medicine
550 First Avenue
New York, New York 10016
Associate Chief, Division US/CT/MRI
Department of Radiology
North Shore University Hospital
300 Community Drive
Manhasset, New York 11030

Abraham H. Dachman, M.D.
Associate Professor
Chief, Section of Abdominal Imaging
Department of Radiology
University of Chicago Hospital
5841 South Maryland Avenue, MC 2026
Chicago, Illinois 60637

Lilliam M. Diaz-Sola, M.D.
Postdoctoral Associate (Clinical Fellow)
Division of Body Imaging and Magnetic
  Resonance Imaging
Department of Radiology
University of Florida College of Medicine
Gainesville, Florida 32610

Georges Y. El-Khoury, M.D.
Professor
Departments of Radiology and Orthopaedics
The University of Iowa College of Medicine
Vice-Chairman
Department of Radiology
The University of Iowa Hospitals and Clinics
200 Hawkins Drive
Iowa City, Iowa 52242

Michael C. Farah, M.D.
Co-Chief, Chest Radiology
Division of Diagnostic Imaging
Department of Diagnostic Radiology
William Beaumont Hospital
3601 West Thirteen Mile Road
Royal Oak, Michigan 48073

Elliot K. Fishman, M.D.
Professor
Departments of Radiology and Oncology
Johns Hopkins University School of Medicine
601 North Wolfe Street
Baltimore, Maryland 21287

Bruno D. Fornage, M.D.
Professor
Department of Diagnostic Radiology
Chief
Section of Ultrasound
University of Texas M.D. Anderson Cancer
  Center
1515 Holcombe Boulevard
Houston, Texas 77030

Leopold Fregoli, M.D.
Fellow
Division of Diagnostic Imaging
Department of Diagnostic Radiology
William Beaumont Hospital
3601 West Thirteen Mile Road
Royal Oak, Michigan 48073

Gary G. Ghahremani, M.D.
Professor and Chairman
Department of Radiology
Evanston Hospital, Northwestern University
  Healthcare
2650 Ridge Avenue
Evanston, Illinois 60201

Donald P. Gibson, M.D.
Pediatric Radiologist
Department of Diagnostic Radiology
William Beaumont Hospital
3601 West Thirteen Mile Road
Royal Oak, Michigan 48073-6769

Dixon Gilbert, M.D.
Senior Resident
Department of Radiology
University of Chicago Hospital
5841 South Maryland Avenue, MC 2026
Chicago, Illinois 60637

Richard M. Gore, M.D.
Professor
Department of Radiology
Evanston Hospital, Northwestern University
  Healthcare
2650 Ridge Avenue
Evanston, Illinois 60201

Barry H. Gross, M.D.
Professor
Department of Diagnostic Radiology
University of Michigan Medical Center
1500 East Medical Center Drive
2910 Taubman Center
Ann Arbor, Michigan 48109

Gwen N. Harris, M.D.
Assistant Professor
Department of Radiology
New York University School of Medicine
550 First Avenue
New York, New York 10016
Physician-in-Charge, Body MRI
Department of Radiology
North Shore University Hospital
300 Community Drive
Manhasset, New York 11030

Lance V. Hefner, M.S.D.A.B.R.
Senior Physicist
Department of Diagnostic Radiology
William Beaumont Hospital
3601 West Thirteen Mile Road
Royal Oak, Michigan 48073-6769

Karen M. Horton, M.D.
Assistant Professor
Department of Radiology
Johns Hopkins Medical Institutions
600 North Wolfe Street
Baltimore, Maryland 21287

Hossein Jadvar, M.D., Ph.D.
Clinical Fellow
Joint Program in Nuclear Medicine
Harvard Medical School
330 Longwood Avenue
Boston, Massachusetts
Clinical Fellow
Division of Nuclear Medicine
Department of Radiology
Brigham & Women's Hospital and
    Massachusetts General Hospital
P.O. Box 9657
Boston, Massachusetts 02164

Zafar H. Jafri, M.D., F.A.C.R.
Clinical Associate Professor
Wayne State University School of Medicine
Chief
Section of Uroradiology
Department of Diagnostic Radiology
William Beaumont Hospital
3601 West Thirteen Mile Road
Royal Oak, Michigan 48073

Hoon Ji, M.D., Ph.D.
Assistant Professor
Department of Radiology
Ajou University
San 5 Wonchon-Dong Paldal-Gu
Suwon, Korea 442-748
Research Fellow
Department of Radiology
Brigham and Women's Hospital
Harvard Medical School
75 Francis Street
Boston, Massachusetts 02115

Dale B. Johnson, M.D.
Department of Diagnostic Radiology
Montreal General Hospital
1650 Cedar Avenue
Montreal, Quebec H3G 1A4
Canada

Ella A. Kazerooni, M.D.
Associate Professor
Department of Diagnostic Radiology
University of Michigan Medical Center
1500 East Medical Center Drive
2910 Taubman Center
Ann Arbor, Michigan 48109

John E. Kirsch, M.D.
Technical Support Physicist
Siemens Medical Systems
110 MacAlyson Court
Cary, North Carolina 27511

Andrea Laghi, M.D.
Department of Radiology
University of Rome "La Sapienza"
Policlinico Umberto I
Viale Regina Elena 324
00161 Rome, Italy

Kyung Soo Lee, M.D.
Associate Professor
Department of Radiology
Sungkyunkwan University School of Medicine
50 Ilwon-Dong, Kangnam-Ku
Seoul 135-710, South Korea
Director, Chest Radiology
Samsung Medical Centre
50 Irwon-dong, Kangnam-ku
Seoul 135-230, South Korea

Michael Macari, M.D.
Assistant Professor
Department of Radiology
Abdominal Imaging
New York University, Tisch-Bellevue Medical
    Center
560 First Avenue
New York, New York 10016

Beatrice L. Madrazo, M.D., F.A.C.R., R.U.T.
Clinical Associate Professor
Department of Diagnostic Radiology
Wayne State University School of Medicine
Chief, Ultrasound Section
Department of Diagnostic Radiology
William Beaumont Hospital
3601 West Thirteen Mile Road
Royal Oak, Michigan 48073-6769

Suzanne Marre, M.D.
Institute of Diagnostic Radiology
Inselspital
University of Berne
Freiburgstr. 12
CH-3010 Berne, Switzerland

Jose M. Mellado, M.D.
Radiologist
Rennonància Magnètica
Institut Diagnostic Per La Imaige
Hospital Joan XXIII
Doctor Mallafrè Guasch, 4
43007 Tarragona, Spain

Robert E. Mindelzun, M.D.
Associate Professor and Residency Director
Department of Radiology
Stanford University School of Medicine
300 Pasteur Drive, Rm. H-1307
Stanford, California 94305

Scott A. Mirowitz, M.D.
Associate Professor
Co-Director, Body MRI
Mallinckrodt Institute of Radiology
Washington University School of Medicine
216 South Kingshighway Boulevard
St. Louis, Missouri 63110

Paul L. Molina, M.D.
Associate Professor
Department of Diagnostic Radiology
University of North Carolina School of
*   Medicine*
Campus Box 7510
Chapel Hill, North Carolina 27599-7510
Director
Department of Computed Body Tomography
University of North Carolina Hospitals
101 Manning Drive
Chapel Hill, North Carolina 27599

Steven Morgan, D.O.
Staff Radiologist
The St. Luke Hospitals Health Alliance
85 N. Grand Avenue
Ft. Thomas, Kentucky 41075

Nestor L. Müller, M.D., Ph.D.
Professor
Department of Radiology
University of British Columbia
Deputy Chief and Associate Head, Academic
*   Affairs*
Department of Radiology
Vancouver General Hospital
855 West 12th Avenue
Vancouver, British Columbia V5Z 1M9
Canada

Vamsidhar R. Narra, M.D.
Assistant Professor
Mallinckrodt Institute of Radiology
Washington University School of Medicine
216 South Kingshighway Boulevard
St. Louis, Missouri 63110

Tara C. Noone, M.D.
Fellow
Department of Radiology
University of North Carolina Hospitals
101 Manning Drive
Chapel Hill, North Carolina 27599

Patrick O'Kane, M.D.
Assistant Professor
Department of Radiology
Temple University Medical Center
3401 North Broad Street
Philadelphia, Pennsylvania 19140

Eric K. Outwater, M.D.
Professor
Department of Radiology
University of Arizona Health Sciences Center
1501 N. Campbell Avenue, Room 1361
Tucson, Arizona 85724-5067

John S. Pellerito, M.D.
Assistant Professor
Department of Radiology
New York University School of Medicine
530 First Avenue
New York, New York 10016
Chief, Division of US, CT, and MRI
Director, Peripheral Vascular Laboratory
Department of Radiology
North Shore University Hospital
300 Community Drive
Manhasset, New York 11030-3876

Catherine W. Piccoli, M.D.
Assistant Professor and Staff Radiologist
Department of Radiology
Jefferson Medical College and Thomas
*   Jefferson University Hospital*
132 South 10th Street, 7th floor
Philadelphia, Pennsylvania 19107

Henry Pribram, M.D.
Professor
Departments of Radiological Sciences and
*   Neurology*
University of California at Irvine Medical
*   Center*
101 The City Drive
Orange, California 92868

Steven L. Primack, M.D.
Associate Professor
Department of Radiology
Oregon Health Sciences University
3181 Southwest Sam Jackson Park Road
Portland, Oregon 97201

Leslie E. Quint, M.D.
Associate Professor
Department of Diagnostic Radiology
University of Michigan Medical Center
1500 East Medical Center Drive
2910 Taubman Center
Ann Arbor, Michigan 48109

George Rappard, M.D.
Senior Resident
Department of Radiological Sciences
University of California at Irvine Medical
*   Center*
101 The City Drive
Orange, California 92868

John L. Roberts, M.D.
Staff Radiologist
Department of Diagnostic Radiology
William Beaumont Hospital
3601 West Thirteen Mile Road
Royal Oak, Michigan 48073

Pablo R. Ros, M.D., F.A.C.R.
Professor
Department of Radiology
Harvard Medical School
Executive Vice-Chairman and Associate Chief
Department of Radiology
Brigham & Women's Hospital
75 Francis Street
Boston, Massachusetts 02115

Zehava S. Rosenberg, M.D.
Associate Professor
Department of Radiology
New York University Medical School
550 First Avenue
New York, New York 10016
Attending Radiologist
Department of Radiology
Orthopedic Institute
Hospital for Joint Diseases
301 East 17th Street
New York, New York 10003

Richard C. Semelka, M.D.
Professor
Department of Radiology
University of North Carolina Hospitals
101 Manning Drive
Chapel Hill, North Carolina 27599

Anil N. Shetty, Ph.D.
Adjunct Assistant Professor
Department of Diagnostic Radiology
Wayne State University School of Medicine
Chief, MRI Physics
Department of Diagnostic Radiology
William Beaumont Hospital
3601 West Thirteen Mile Road
Royal Oak, Michigan 48073-6769

Ali Shirkhoda, M.D., F.A.C.R.
Clinical Professor
Department of Diagnostic Radiology
Wayne State University School of Medicine
Director
Division of Diagnostic Imaging
Department of Diagnostic Radiology
William Beaumont Hospital
3601 West Thirteen Mile Road
Royal Oak, Michigan 48073-6769

Jamshid Tehranzadeh, M.D.
Professor of Radiology and Orthopaedics
Chief, Section of Musculoskeletal
*   Radiology*
Department of Radiology
University of California at Irvine Medical
*   Center*
101 The City Drive, Route 140
Orange, California 92868

Michael E. Timins, M.D.
Associate Professor
Department of Diagnostic Radiology
Medical College of Wisconsin
Froedtert Memorial Lutheran Hospital
9200 West Wisconsin Avenue
Milwaukee, Wisconsin 53226

Theodore Villafana, Ph.D.
Professor
Department of Radiology
MCP-Hahnemann University
3300 Henry Avenue
Philadelphia, Pennsylvania 19129

Robin J. Warshawsky, M.D.
Department of Radiology
North Shore University Hospital
300 Community Drive
Manhasset, New York 11030

Harry G. Zegel, M.D.
Clinical Associate Professor
Department of Radiology
MCP-Hahnemann University
3300 Henry Avenue
Philadelphia, Pennsylvania 19129

Preface

During the last three decades, ultrasonography, computed tomography (CT), and magnetic resonance imaging (MRI) have had a profound impact on the practice of medicine. These modalities have undergone numerous technical upgrades with resultant exponential growth in their clinical applications. Along with these advancements, there has been an ever increasing demand for further diagnostic accuracy in complex clinical settings. Today, there continues to be a steady growth in cross-sectional imaging within virtually every medical specialty with respect to diagnosis and patient management.

Cross-sectional anatomy and pathology have been the subject of numerous texts and articles, particularly in the last two decades. With the further evolution of CT, sonography, and MRI, radiologists have been able to recognize exquisite anatomical detail allowing for ever increasing accuracy in diagnosis of pathologic conditions. However, radiologists continue to discover and recognize many variations in normal anatomy that must be distinguished from pathology. Recognition of a variety of artifacts must also be born in mind when interpreting diagnostic images so as not to confuse those with potential pathologic conditions. Clearly, the task of the radiologist is to reliably differentiate normal anatomy from pathology and both of these conditions from technical artifact. Without sufficient knowledge of normal anatomic variations and the ability to differentiate technological artifacts from pathologic conditions, it would occasionally be difficult for a radiologist to accurately and reliably interpret such images.

This book was written with the intent of providing a comprehensive knowledge of normal variations, diagnostic pitfalls, and artifacts that can occur as a result of cross-sectional imaging. It is organized by anatomic regions of the thorax, abdomen/pelvis and musculoskeletal systems and includes information on physical principles of artifacts. The goal was to provide the readers with a brief discussion of relevant anatomy or description of protocol, followed by the appropriate differential diagnosis with an attempt to point out a helpful guideline, which would allow for differentiation of normal variants and artifacts from pathology. The physical principles that apply to the generation of artifacts in CT, sonography, and MRI are provided in depth to satisfy the appetite of the beginners, as well as the more advanced individuals in physics and body imaging.

I am grateful to the many individuals whose assistance was invaluable in compiling this text. Particularly, I want to express my appreciation to the contributors without whom this book would not have become a reality.

I am deeply grateful to my wife Shahrzad and daughters Layla and Roxanne, who have patiently accepted with love and understanding the inconveniences as the result of my long preoccupation with this work. I would like to especially thank the faculty of the Division of Diagnostic Imaging at William Beaumont Hospital for their contribution and support. Special thanks goes to Mrs. Arlene Hill, for her endless hours of secretarial assistance that had become necessary to complete this project. Finally, the production of this book would not have been possible without the full support of the entire group of editors and management at Lippincott Williams & Wilkins, and in particular, Charles W. Mitchell, Joyce-Rachel John, Michael Standen, and Karen Edmonson.

Ali Shirkhoda, M.D., F.A.C.R.

SECTION I

Variants of Normal Anatomy and Diagnostic Pitfalls in Imaging of the Thorax and Breast

Variants and Pitfalls in Body Imaging,
edited by Ali Shirkhoda.
Lippincott Williams & Wilkins, Philadelphia, © 2000.

CHAPTER 1

Mediastinum: CT

Paul L. Molina

Computed tomography (CT) has become established as an excellent radiologic technique for the assessment of the mediastinum. The superior contrast resolution of CT, coupled with its cross-sectional imaging capability, generally is well suited to the depiction of mediastinal anatomy, as most major mediastinal structures are oriented perpendicular to the transaxial plane of CT imaging.

Proper interpretation of CT scans of the mediastinum requires a thorough knowledge of normal cross-sectional anatomy as well as an awareness of the wide range of anatomic variants that can exist. Familiarity with variations in the density of mediastinal structures and in the caliber and course of mediastinal vessels is also important for proper CT interpretation (1).

This chapter begins with a review of normal mediastinal anatomy to promote understanding of normal anatomic variants of the mediastinum. Proper CT protocol for performance of CT of the mediastinum is then described, along with related technical problems that may result in diagnostic pitfalls. Finally, the more commonly encountered normal anatomic variants of the mediastinum are described in detail. Ideally, increasing familiarity with the causes and appearances of these potential CT pitfalls will allow errors in diagnosis to be avoided.

NORMAL MEDIASTINAL ANATOMY

The mediastinum is the midline portion of the thorax extending from the sternum anteriorly to the vertebral bodies posteriorly. It is bounded laterally by the parietal mediastinal pleura of each lung, superiorly by the thoracic inlet, and inferiorly by the diaphragm (1). Normal mediastinal anatomic structures commonly identified on

P.L. Molina: Department of Diagnostic Radiology, University of North Carolina School of Medicine; Department of Computed Body Tomography, University of North Carolina Hospitals, Chapel Hill, North Carolina 27599.

CT include the mediastinal blood vessels, heart and pericardium, major airways, thyroid, thymus, and esophagus.

Mediastinal Blood Vessels

The aortic arch arises at the level of the upper border of the right second costosternal articulation (2) and normally has an oblique course extending posteriorly and to the left, becoming the descending aorta approximately at the level of the fourth thoracic vertebra (Fig. 1.1). The anterior portion of the arch lies in front of the trachea and is closely related to the anteromedial aspect of the superior vena cava. The midportion of the arch lies just to the left of the trachea and often causes slight indentation of the left anterolateral tracheal wall. The posterior aortic arch, at its junction with the descending aorta, lies just lateral to the esophagus.

The arch of the aorta has a general superoposterior configuration and normally gives rise to three main arterial branches in sequential fashion: the brachiocephalic artery (innominate artery), left common carotid artery, and left subclavian artery (Fig. 1.2). The brachiocephalic artery arises first at the most caudal level of the arch, followed by the left common carotid artery at a slightly higher level, and finally by the left subclavian artery, which originates from the most superoposterior portion of the arch. The brachiocephalic artery, the largest of the three arch vessels, lies directly in front or just to the right of the trachea. Its exact point of bifurcation into the right subclavian and right common carotid arteries is variable, depending on its length and degree of tortuosity (3). The left common carotid artery lies to the left and slightly posterolateral to the brachiocephalic artery; generally it has the smallest diameter of the three arch vessels. The left subclavian artery is the most posterior and lateral of the arch vessels, lying to the left and frequently adjacent to the trachea. The lateral border of the left subclavian artery often contacts the mediastinal pleural reflection of

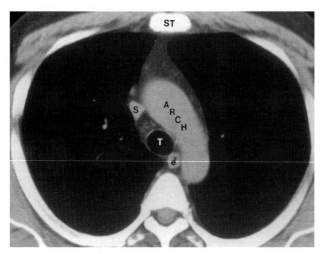

FIG. 1.1. The mediastinum. ARCH: aortic arch; S, superior vena cava; T, trachea; e, esophagus; ST, body of sternum.

the left upper lobe and sometimes indents it in a convex fashion (4).

The right and left brachiocephalic veins are located anterior to the arch vessels (see Fig. 1.2). The right brachiocephalic vein has a nearly vertical course throughout its length as it travels in a plane anterior and to the right of the trachea. The left brachiocephalic vein has a longer

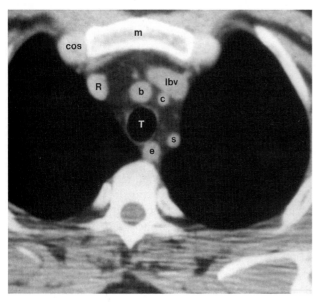

FIG. 1.2. Great vessels off the aortic arch. The brachiocephalic artery (b) is the largest of the vessels off the aortic arch; the left carotid artery (c) is the smallest, and the left subclavian artery (s), which commonly indents the left upper lobe, is intermediate in size. R, right brachiocephalic vein; lbv, left brachiocephalic vein; T, trachea; e, esophagus; m, manubrium; cos, costal cartilage of the first rib.

course and is often oriented horizontally as it crosses the anterior mediastinum from left to right to join the right brachiocephalic vein to form the superior vena cava (Fig. 1.3). The superior vena cava is located in front and to the right of the trachea, separated from it by the pretracheal space. On transaxial images, the superior vena cava has an oval, round, or elliptical configuration. Its diameter is usually one-third to two-thirds the diameter of the ascending aorta (5).

The azygous and hemiazygous veins represent cephalad continuations of the right and left ascending lumbar veins, respectively. The azygous vein begins at the level of the L1–L2 vertebral bodies and passes through the aortic hiatus into the thorax, where it lies to the right of the descending aorta. It then ascends in the right prevertebral area, usually just posterolateral to the esophagus. At the level of the T4 or T5 vertebra, the azygous vein arches forward and slightly to the right, passing over the medial aspect of the right upper lobe bronchus before draining into the posterior aspect of the superior vena cava (6) (Fig. 1.4). Just before the formation of the azygous arch, the azygous vein is joined by the right superior intercostal vein. This vein, which receives drainage from the right second through fourth intercostal veins, descends along the right anterolateral vertebral margin before emptying into the azygous vein posteriorly.

On the left side, the hemiazygous and accessory hemiazygous veins also course along the vertebral bodies, but in a more posterior plane, usually just behind the descending aorta. The hemiazygous vein generally crosses the midline prevertebrally, passing posterior to the aorta to join the azygous vein at about the T8 level; the accessory hemiazygous vein crosses the midline to join the azygous vein one or two vertebral body levels higher (7). The accessory hemiazygous vein, which collects flow from the left fourth through eighth posterior intercostal veins, may or may not communicate with the hemiazygous vein. Above the point of termination of the hemiazygous vein, the accessory hemiazygous vein ascends posterior to the descending aorta. At or just above the level of the aortic arch, the accessory hemiazygous vein is joined by the left superior intercostal vein in approximately 75% of patients (8). The left superior intercostal vein, which drains the left second to fourth intercostal veins, then forms a horizontal arch (also referred to as the arch of the hemiazygous vein) that courses anteriorly along the superolateral border of the aortic arch to join the posterior aspect of the left brachiocephalic vein. On frontal chest radiographs, the left superior intercostal vein may be seen on end, just lateral to or above the aortic knob, and has been termed the aortic nipple (9).

The main pulmonary artery lies entirely within the pericardium. It courses upward and posteriorly from its point of origin to divide into the right and left pulmonary

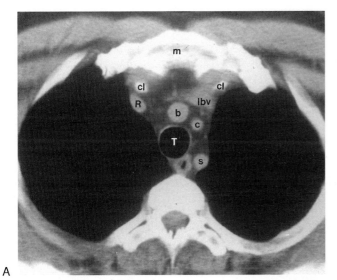
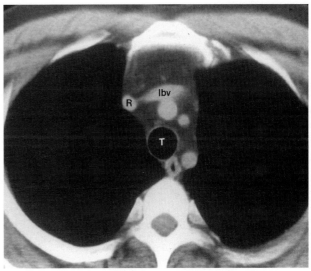

A

B

FIG. 1.3. Crossing left brachiocephalic vein. Sequential caudal scans demonstrate the left brachiocephalic vein (lbv) crossing the anterior mediastinum from left to right to join the right brachiocephalic vein (R), subsequently forming the superior vena cava. Soft tissue surrounding the inferior portion of the clavicular head (cl) should not be confused with a mass anterior to the brachiocephalic veins. b, brachiocephalic artery; c, left carotid artery; s, left subclavian artery; T, trachea; m, manubrium.

arteries behind and to the left of the ascending aorta. The normal diameter of the main pulmonary artery usually is about two-thirds that of the ascending aorta and should not exceed 28 mm (10). The right pulmonary artery extends posteriorly and to the right from the main pulmonary artery, coursing in a gentle horizontal arc behind the superior vena cava and in front of the right main and intermediate bronchus (Fig. 1.5). It exits the pericardium just after giving rise to the truncus anterior, the artery to the right upper lobe. The intrapericardial portion of the

right pulmonary artery should be visible on CT in all adult patients and normally measures 12 to 15 mm in diameter (11). The left pulmonary artery extends posteriorly from the main pulmonary artery and courses in a transverse plane 1 to 2 cm above the right pulmonary artery, at about the level of the carina. The left pulmonary artery normally measures 18 to 24 mm in diameter (10) and has a shorter intrapericardial course than the right pulmonary artery. Following its exit from the pericardium, the left pulmonary artery arches over the left

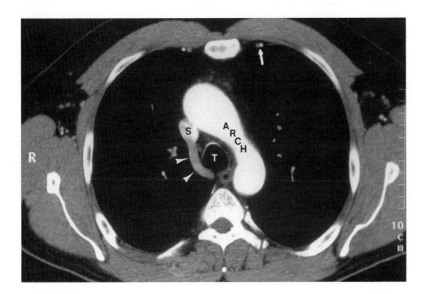

FIG. 1.4. Azygous vein arch. Computed tomogram demonstrating the azygous vein arching anteriorly to drain into the posterior aspect of the superior vena cava (S). *Arrowheads,* azygous vein arch; ARCH, aortic arch; T, trachea; e, esophagus; *arrow,* internal mammary vessels.

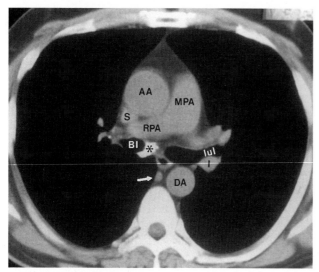

FIG. 1.5. Main and right pulmonary arteries. The right pulmonary artery (RPA) extends posteriorly and to the right of the main pulmonary artery (MPA), coursing behind the ascending aorta (AA) and the superior vena cava (S) and anterior to the bronchus intermedius (BI). Lung inserts into a notch between the left interlobar pulmonary artery (I) and the descending aorta (DA). lul, left upper lobe bronchus; *arrow*, azygous vein; *asterisk*, calcified subcarinal lymph node.

main bronchus to descend posterior to it. The right and left superior pulmonary veins generally are seen just anterior to the right pulmonary artery and the left upper lobe bronchus, respectively.

Pericardium

The pericardium is a double-layered fibroserous sac that envelopes the heart as well as the proximal portions of the great vessels (ascending aorta, main pulmonary artery, venae cavae). The thin, serous visceral layer, or epicardium, is closely applied to the surface of the heart and epicardial fat, whereas the thicker outer fibrous parietal layer covers the heart in a sac-like fashion. The two layers share a common serosal lining and between them form the pericardial cavity, which normally contains approximately 20 to 25 ml of fluid (12).

At least a portion of the normal parietal pericardium is visible on CT in almost all patients (Fig. 1.6). It appears as a thin, curvilinear, soft tissue density line, generally 1 to 2 mm in thickness (13). The anterior and caudal pericardium is commonly imaged, especially those portions where the pericardium is surrounded by fat in the mediastinum and in the subepicardial region of the heart. The posterior and cephalad portions of the pericardium are infrequently seen because of the lack of sufficient surrounding fat in these areas.

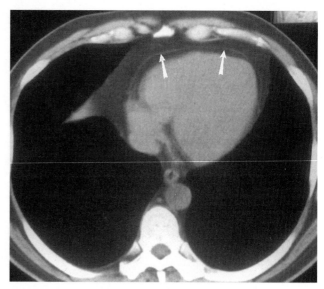

FIG. 1.6. Normal pericardium. The pericardium is seen as a thin, curvilinear soft-tissue density line *(arrows)* flanked by mediastinal and epicardial fat.

Thyroid

The thyroid gland consists of bilateral lobes that lie adjacent to the airway (Fig. 1.7). The two lobes are connected by a midline isthmus of tissue that straddles the anterior trachea (14). At about the level of the sternal notch, the inferior lobes of the thyroid gland are typically seen on both sides of the trachea and at times surround the trachea completely. On CT, the thyroid gland generally is hyperdense compared to muscle on noncontrast

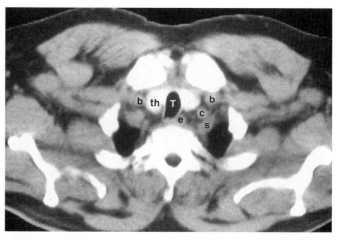

FIG. 1.7. Normal thyroid. At a level above the sternal notch, both lobes of the thyroid (th) are seen lateral to the trachea (T). The thyroid is hyperdense compared to muscle on this noncontrast image because of its iodine content. b, brachiocephalic veins; c, carotid artery; s, subclavian artery; e, esophagus.

images because of its iodine content; and following contrast administration, it often enhances homogeneously because of its marked vascularity (15,16).

Thymus

The thymus is a bilobed organ that usually lies in the anterior mediastinum at a level between the horizontal portion of the left brachiocephalic vein superiorly and the horizontal course of the right pulmonary artery inferiorly. On adult CT, its remnant may be seen on sections through the level of the aortic arch (Fig. 1.8). Usually, the left lobe is slightly larger than the right lobe and represents the main caudal extension of the organ (17,18).

Esophagus

The superior portion of the thoracic esophagus lies posterior and slightly to the left of the trachea from the level of the thoracic inlet to the carina (see Fig. 1.7). Just below the carina, the esophagus is closely related to the posterior surface of the left main bronchus, usually separated from it by a small amount of fat. More caudally, the esophagus descends behind the heart anterior and to the right of the descending aorta before passing through the esophageal hiatus (19).

On CT, small amounts of intraluminal air can be seen in the thoracic esophagus of most normal patients (19). The thickness of the esophageal wall varies with the degree of luminal distention. A wall thickness of 3 mm or more usually is abnormal when the lumen is well distended. The normal esophageal wall can be up to 5 mm

thick when the esophagus is incompletely distended (20).

COMPUTED TOMOGRAPHY TECHNIQUE

Computed tomography of the mediastinum is most commonly performed with the patient supine. The patient's arms are placed above the head to reduce beam-hardening artifact from the shoulders and upper extremities. Whenever possible, scans should be obtained with the patient breath holding. The advent of the helical (spiral) scan technique now allows imaging of the entire thorax during a single breath hold, thus eliminating the slice-to-slice variation in lung volume inherent with conventional dynamic scanning (21). For those patients who are unable to maintain a single breath hold for the entire duration of a helical scan, slowly exhaling toward the end of the scan may be acceptable (22).

Helical chest CT examinations are usually performed with 7- to 8-mm collimation, a pitch of 1, and corresponding 7- to 8-mm reconstruction intervals. In conventional CT, 8- to 10-mm slices may be obtained, with no gap between slices.

Each thoracic CT examination should be viewed with at least two sets of window settings, one for optimal display of the lung parenchyma and another for mediastinal and chest wall structures. In select cases, a third set of window settings optimized for osseous detail may be necessary. Generally, for the mediastinum, a window width between 300 and 500 Hounsfield units (HU) and a window level between 30 and 60 HU are used.

Although it is not necessary in all instances, intravenous administration of contrast material greatly facilitates the interpretation of CT scans of the mediastinum. This is particularly true in patients in whom there is a paucity of mediastinal fat, making differentiation of normal mediastinal structures from pathologic processes difficult. The use of intravenous contrast material may be necessary when a vascular abnormality is suspected, or when information regarding the particular enhancement characteristics of a mass are desired. When intravenous contrast material is utilized, it should be administered via an automated power injector using bolus injection combined with rapid scanning. A total dose of 100 to 150 ml of 60% delivered at a rate of injection between 1.5 and 3 ml per second is usually adequate.

It is important to be aware of several potential pitfalls related to the administration of intravenous contrast material. If a slow drip infusion of intravenous contrast is utilized, rather than a rapid bolus injection, the true nature of a vascular mass may be overlooked (Fig. 1.9). Such an error in diagnosis can be avoided by paying close attention to proper contrast injection technique. One should keep in mind that even when a peripheral needle site is the only available vascular access, power injection with a flow rate of 1.0 ml per second is usually still possible.

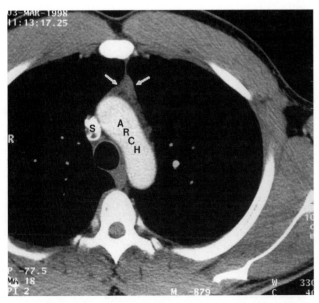

FIG. 1.8. Normal thymus. Note normal triangular-shaped thymus *(arrows)* with more prominent left lobe anterior to the aortic arch (ARCH). S, superior vena cava.

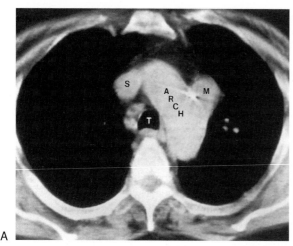
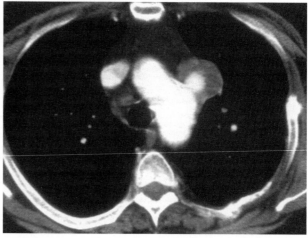

A   B

FIG. 1.9. Aortic arch aneurysm. **A:** Computed tomographic scan at the level of the aortic arch (ARCH) following slow drip infusion of contrast material demonstrates a mildly enhancing mass (M) immediately adjacent to the aortic arch. S, superior vena cava; T, trachea. **B:** Repeat CT following rapid bolus injection demonstrates the true vascular nature of the mass, found to represent a focal saccular aneurysm arising from the aortic arch. There is a moderate amount of intraluminal thrombus within the aneurysm.

At times, retrograde flow of contrast can be seen in the chest wall in side branches of the axillary and subclavian veins (Fig. 1.10). This phenomenon results from increased flow from the power injection and should not be mistaken for collateral blood flow secondary to venous obstruction. Careful analysis of contiguous CT images will demonstrate normal patency of the mediastinal venous system.

Apparent filling defects related to flow phenomena are frequently seen in the superior vena cava or other mediastinal veins following the injection of intravenous contrast (23) (Fig. 1.11). These flow artifacts are secondary to mixing of opacified and unopacified blood and typically occur at the junction of two veins at the origin of the superior vena cava, where such mixing is likely to occur. They are most frequently seen before and after the peak concentration of the bolus. Anterior filling defects are most common because the higher-density contrast layers posteriorly. The characteristic appearance and location of these filling defects, along with their tendency to become less apparent during the peak concentration of the bolus, are helpful features in distinguishing these flow-related artifacts from clot or tumor (23,24).

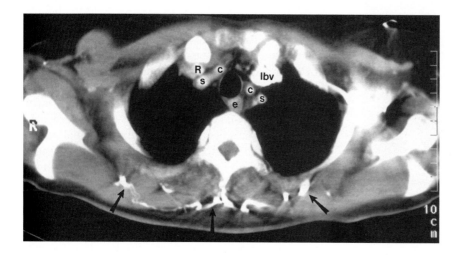

FIG. 1.10. Retrograde venous enhancement. Contrast-enhanced CT scan at the level of the sternoclavicular junction shows extensive opacification of numerous chest wall veins *(arrows)* as a result of the increased flow rate introduced by the power injector. This should not be mistaken for collateral blood flow caused by an obstruction. Sequential CT images in this patient demonstrated normal patency of the mediastinal venous system. R, right brachiocephalic vein; lbv, left brachiocephalic vein; c, carotid arteries; s, subclavian arteries; e, esophagus.

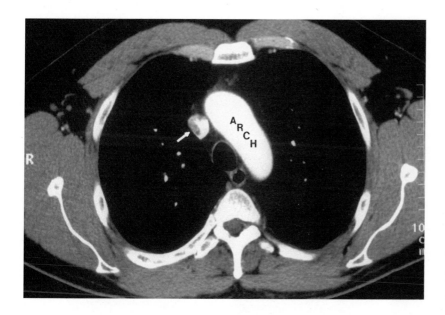

FIG. 1.11. Flow defect simulating thrombus in the superior vena cava. Computed tomographic scan at the level of the aortic arch (ARCH) following bolus intravenous administration of contrast material through a left antecubital vein demonstrates a flow-related filling defect *(arrow)* in the superior vena cava.

NORMAL ANATOMIC VARIANTS AND PITFALLS ON COMPUTED TOMOGRAPHY

Mediastinal Vascular Pitfalls

Anomalies of the mediastinal vessels, both arterial and venous, are common and can lead to potentially confusing findings on both plain film radiography and CT. In many instances, such an anomaly is detected incidentally on CT scans obtained for other reasons, and its importance lies in its proper recognition and in its not being mistaken for an enlarged lymph node or other mediastinal abnormality (25,26). In some cases, the vascular anomaly may simulate a mediastinal mass or result in mediastinal widening on plain chest radiographs, thus prompting the CT study (27). Accurate identification of these vascular anomalies or variants requires careful analysis of multiple contiguous CT sections and detailed knowledge of normal variant vascular anatomy.

Arterial Pitfalls

Tortuous Brachiocephalic Artery

Tortuosity or ectasia of the brachiocephalic artery, particularly in elderly patients with atherosclerotic vascular disease, can occasionally be mistaken for paratracheal adenopathy or mass (28) (Fig. 1.12). In such cases, the tortuous vessel often has an oval rather than a round appearance because of its more horizontal than vertical orientation. The proximal portion of the vessel appears in its usual location just in front of the trachea, whereas the

distal portion insinuates into the right paratracheal region, causing confusion with adenopathy. Evaluation of sequential CT images above the aortic arch usually allows the correct diagnosis to be made by demonstrating the proximal portion of the vessel coursing toward the distal portion, which is then seen to bifurcate into the right common carotid and subclavian arteries. Enhancement of the tortuous vessel following administration of intravenous contrast material provides more definitive evidence when needed.

Aberrant Right Subclavian Artery

An aberrant right subclavian artery originating from an otherwise normal left aortic arch is the most common congenital mediastinal arterial anomaly, occurring in approximately 1% to 2% of the population (29–32). This anomalous vessel arises as the last branch of the aortic arch rather than from the brachiocephalic artery and occurs when there is interruption of the embryologic right aortic arch between the right common carotid and right subclavian arteries. In patients with an aberrant right subclavian artery, the brachiocephalic artery (which is really the right common carotid artery) is smaller than usual, being similar in diameter to the left common carotid artery.

Symptoms related to an aberrant right subclavian artery are uncommon, and the anomaly usually is found incidentally, either by radiography or endoscopy. On CT, the aberrant right subclavian artery can be seen arising from the posteromedial portion of the distal aortic arch

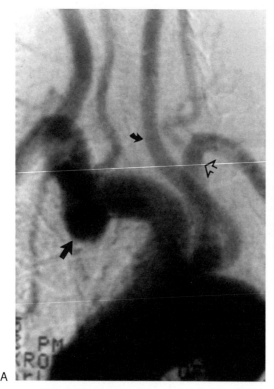
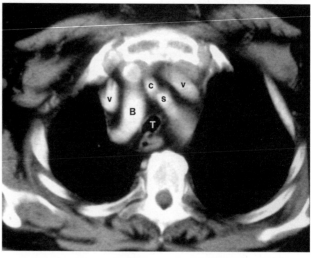

FIG. 1.12. Tortuous brachiocephalic artery. **A:** Digital aortic arch arteriogram demonstrates a tortuous right brachiocephalic artery *(straight arrow)* as well as the left common carotid *(curved arrow)* and left subclavian *(open arrow)* arteries. **B:** Scan after bolus injection of contrast material shows the tortuous brachiocephalic artery (B) coursing into the right paratracheal space, accounting for a right paratracheal mass noted on a frontal chest radiograph. v, brachiocephalic veins; c, left common carotid artery; s, left subclavian artery; T, trachea.

(Fig. 1.13). The vessel crosses the mediastinum obliquely from left to right, passing behind the esophagus and trachea on its cephalad course. The origin of the aberrant right subclavian artery is frequently widened as the diverticulum of Kommerell, representing the remnant of the distal right aortic arch, and the adjacent esophagus may be compressed or displaced to the right. Unless it is recognized as a dilated segment of an anomalous artery, the diverticulum of Kommerell can be misdiagnosed as a mediastinal mass or as an aneurysm of the arch of the aorta (33).

Aneurysms arising in an aberrant subclavian artery do occur but are rare (34) (Fig. 1.14). Such an aneurysm may or may not be associated with Kommerell's diverticulum and is believed to be the result of arteriosclerotic disease. Because of the risk of rupture, surgical resection generally is recommended (35).

Isolated Left Vertebral Artery

Normally the left vertebral artery is a branch of the left subclavian artery. In approximately 6% of patients the left vertebral artery arises directly from the aortic arch as a separate vessel, usually originating between the left common carotid and left subclavian arteries (36). In these patients, the vertebral artery will appear as an extra arch vessel on CT and should not be confused with an enlarged lymph node (Fig. 1.15).

Tortuous Aortic Arch

The caliber and the degree of tortuosity of the thoracic aorta vary, depending on age, physique, and the presence of vascular disease. In the elderly population with arteriosclerosis, the aortic arch is often tortuous and/or ectatic. Partial imaging of the top of a tortuous or dilated aortic arch on a single CT image may produce the mistaken appearance of a lung mass or an area of parenchymal consolidation (28) (Fig. 1.16). On sequential caudal CT images, the apparent mass or consolidation can be seen to be vertically aligned with, and have the same orientation in the horizontal plane as, the more readily identifiable aortic arch that produces it.

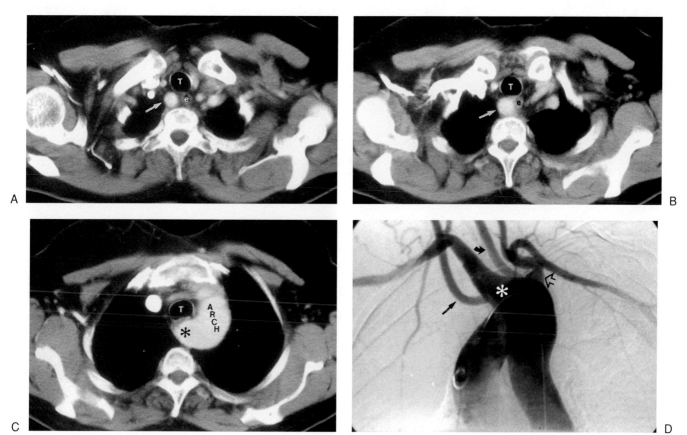

FIG. 1.13. Aberrant right subclavian artery. **A–C:** Sequential contrast-enhanced CT scans through the superior mediastinum demonstrate the normal course of an aberrant right subclavian artery. At the level of the thoracic inlet **(A)**, the aberrant vessel *(arrow)* is seen just to the right of the esophagus (e). T, trachea. More caudally **(B)**, the vessel crosses the mediastinum obliquely from left to right behind the trachea and esophagus. The wide-mouth origin of the aberrant right subclavian artery *(asterisk),* arising from the posteromedial aspect of the aortic arch (ARCH), is seen in **C.** The dilated origin of the aberrant right subclavian artery, the so-called diverticulum of Kommerell, should not be mistaken for an aneurysm of the arch of the aorta. **D:** Corresponding LAO view from a digital aortic arch arteriogram demonstrates the wide-mouth origin of the aberrant right subclavian artery *(asterisk).* Note that the aberrant right subclavian artery arises as the fourth and last branch off the aortic arch. *Straight arrow,* right common carotid artery; *curved arrow,* left common carotid artery; *open arrow,* left subclavian artery.

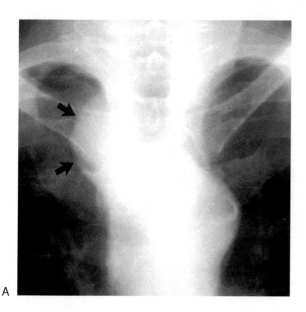

FIG. 1.14. Aberrant right subclavian artery aneurysm. **A:** Cone-down frontal posteroanterior view of the superior mediastinum demonstrates a smoothly marginated right paratracheal mass *(arrows). Continued on next page.*

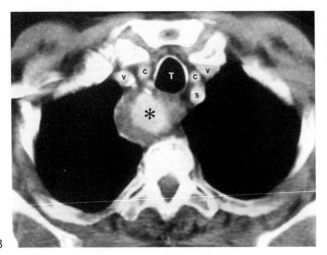

B

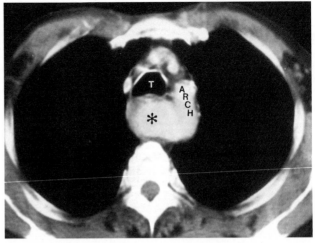

C

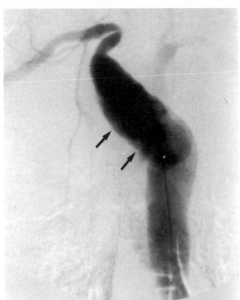

D

FIG. 1.14. *Continued.* **B,C:** Sequential contrast-enhanced CT scans demonstrate an aberrant right subclavian artery aneurysm *(asterisk)* arising from the posteromedial aspect of the aortic arch (ARCH). A moderate amount of intraluminal thrombus is present within the aneurysm. T, trachea; v, brachiocephalic veins; c, carotid arteries; s, left subclavian artery. **D:** Anteroposterior view from a digital aortic arch arteriogram following selective injection of the aberrant right subclavian artery aneurysm *(arrows)* correlates nicely with the cone-down PA chest radiograph illustrated in **A.**

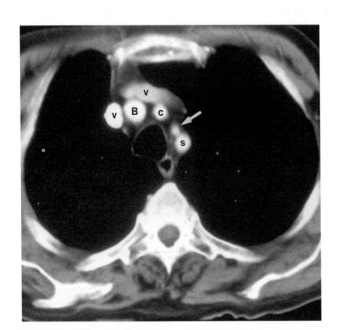

FIG. 1.15. Left vertebral artery arising directly from the aortic arch. Note the left vertebral artery *(arrow)* separate from the left subclavian artery (s). B, brachiocephalic artery; c, left common carotid artery; v, brachiocephalic veins.

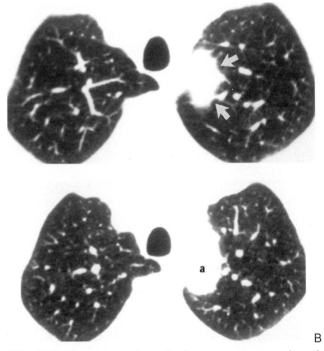

A

B

FIG. 1.16. Tortuous aortic arch. An apparent parenchymal lung mass *(arrows)* is produced by partial imaging of the top of a tortuous aortic arch. Note that the apparent mass is aligned with and has the same orientation as the aortic arch (a), which is seen 1 cm caudal to A.

Right Aortic Arch

Right aortic arch occurs in 0.02% of the population (36) and by definition passes to the right of the trachea and esophagus. The right aortic arch may descend either to the right or to the left of midline. Although five types of right aortic arch anomalies can occur, depending on the site at which the left aortic arch is embryonically interrupted, only two are relatively common: (a) right aortic arch with an aberrant left subclavian artery and (b) right aortic arch with mirror-image branching of the great vessels (37–39).

A right aortic arch with an aberrant left subclavian artery is the most common right aortic arch anomaly. This anomaly, which is infrequently associated with congenital heart disease, occurs when there is interruption of the embryologic left aortic arch between the left common carotid and left subclavian arteries (40). This results in a right aortic arch branching pattern in which the left common carotid artery arises first, followed by the right common carotid and right subclavian arteries. The aberrant left subclavian artery arises as the fourth and most distal branch of the right aortic arch.

The CT appearances of a right aortic arch with an aberrant left subclavian artery are similar to those seen with a left aortic arch with an aberrant right subclavian artery (41,42) (Fig. 1.17). The aberrant left subclavian artery crosses the mediastinum posterior to the esophagus to reach the root of the neck on the left side. Like its counterpart on the right side, the origin of the aberrant left subclavian artery is frequently widened as an aortic diverticulum, representing the remnant of the distal left aortic arch.

A right aortic arch with mirror-image branching occurs if the embryologic left aortic arch is interrupted distal to the left subclavian artery, most commonly just beyond the left ductus arteriosus (40) (Fig. 1.18). The result is a mirror image of normal, in which the left brachiocephalic artery arises as the first branch of the ascending aorta, followed by the right common carotid and right subclavian arteries. Because interruption of the embryologic left aortic arch occurs distal to the ductus arteriosus, there is no structure posterior to the trachea or esophagus. This type of right aortic arch anomaly is almost always associated with cyanotic congenital heart disease, most commonly tetralogy of Fallot and truncus arteriosus.

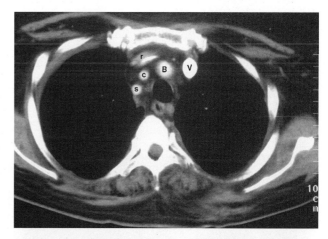
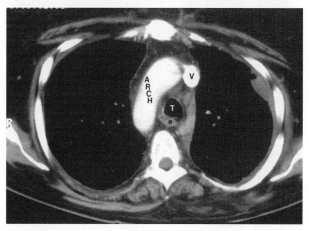

FIG. 1.18. Right aortic arch with mirror-image branching. This patient has Kartagener's syndrome and complete situs inversus. Sequential contrast-enhanced CT images through the great vessels **(A)** and aortic arch **(B).** A right-sided aortic arch (ARCH) is easily identified, lying just to the right of the trachea (T) and esophagus (e). There is mirror-image branching of the great vessels, along with a left-sided superior vena cava (V). A catheter is present in the horizontal portion of the right brachiocephalic vein (r); B, left brachiocephalic artery; c, right common carotid artery; s, right subclavian artery.

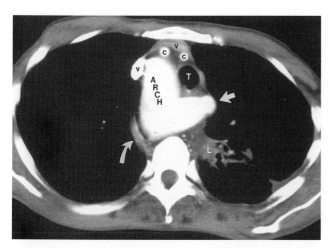

FIG. 1.17. Right aortic arch (ARCH) with aberrant left subclavian artery. The origin of the aberrant left subclavian artery *(straight arrow)* is widened as an aortic diverticulum. T, trachea; v, brachiocephalic veins; c, carotid arteries; L, left upper lobe atelectatic lung; *curved arrow,* posterior portion of azygous fissure.

Double Aortic Arch

Double aortic arch occurs less commonly than other anomalies of the aortic arch and great vessels. The double aortic arch is characterized by two separate arches arising from a single ascending aorta, both giving rise to a subclavian and carotid artery and then joining posteriorly to form a single descending aorta (43). The two arches form a vascular ring around the trachea and esophagus, and symptoms related to compression of these structures are common. Associated congenital heart disease is rare (43).

The CT findings in double aortic arch have been described in several reports (41,42) (Fig. 1.19). Usually, the right arch is larger and situated slightly more cephalad than the left arch. Each arch gives rise to two vessels, the right common carotid and subclavian arteries from the right arch, and the left common carotid and subclavian arteries from the left arch. The two arches join posterior to the esophagus and trachea and may create a mass-like density in the posterior mediastinum. If the left arch is atretic, it may be difficult or impossible to distinguish the anomaly from a right aortic arch.

Aortic Root Pseudodissection

Artifact of the proximal ascending aorta arising from motion of the aortic wall during rapid image acquisition (<2 seconds) can lead to potential false-positive diagnosis of aortic dissection (44,45) (Fig. 1.20). The artifact occurs with both conventional and helical scanning and results in a perivascular rim of low attenuation that may simulate an intimal flap or false channel of aortic dissection. Such artifacts, or apparent intimal flaps, typically occur in the aortic root and are confined to one or two contiguous CT slices (45). The findings do not extend into the aortic arch or descending aorta, and no associated mediastinal or pericardial hemorrhage is identified.

Left Pulmonary Artery

Partial volume averaging of the top of the left pulmonary artery on CT scans through the aortopulmonary window, particularly on unenhanced CT, may be mistaken for aortopulmonary window mass or adenopathy (28,46) (Fig. 1.21). The orientation of the apparent mass or adenopathy imaged within the window should be the

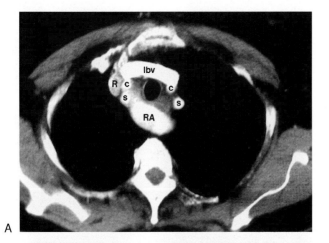

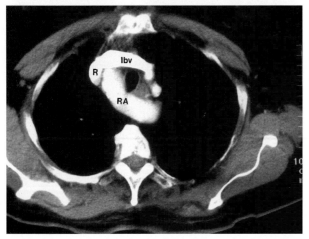

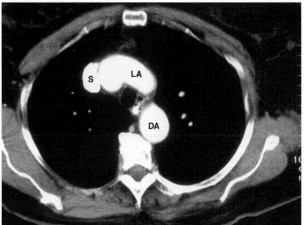

FIG. 1.19. Double aortic arch. **A–C:** Sequential contrast-enhanced CT images from the level of the horizontal portion of the left brachiocephalic vein (lbv) to the level of the proximal descending aorta (DA) in a patient with a double aortic arch status post surgical ligation of the left arch. **A:** All four arteries to the head and neck are seen. Each arch gives rise to two vessels—a carotid (c) and a subclavian (s) artery—each artery of the pair lying one in front of the other. The right aortic arch (RA) is larger and situated slightly more cephalad than the left aortic arch (LA). R, right brachiocephalic vein; S, superior vena cava.

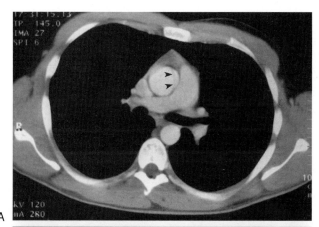

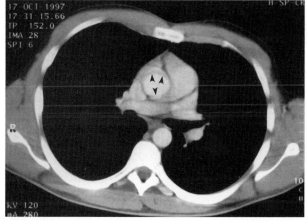

FIG. 1.20. A,B: Motion artifact simulating aortic dissection. Contiguous contrast-enhanced CT images demonstrate curvilinear artifacts *(arrowheads)* caused by motion of the aortic wall during rapid image acquisition.

same as that of the more readily identifiable left pulmonary artery on the next more caudal scan. Adenopathy tends to have a somewhat different orientation and is less homogeneous in appearance than the left pulmonary artery (Fig. 1.22).

In some patients, the top of the left and main pulmonary arteries is located more cephalad than usual, at a level alongside the aortic arch, resulting in confusion with an anterior mediastinal mass (Figs. 1.23 and 1.24). This is particularly true in patients with left upper lobe collapse or previous left upper lobectomy and elevation of the left pulmonary hilum. Review of sequential CT images will show that the apparent mass is contiguous with the main pulmonary artery anteriorly and with the left pulmonary artery posteriorly as it approaches the hilar area (46). The administration of intravenous contrast material may also help in clarifying this pitfall.

Anomalous Left Pulmonary Artery

Anomalous left pulmonary artery (pulmonary artery sling) is a developmental abnormality in which the left pulmonary artery arises from the posterior portion of the right pulmonary artery, courses posteriorly over the right main bronchus near its origin from the trachea, and then crosses the mediastinum interposed between the trachea and the esophagus to enter the left hilum. It is usually symptomatic in neonates and young infants, causing respiratory difficulties as a result of associated tracheo-

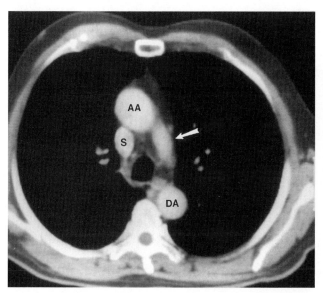

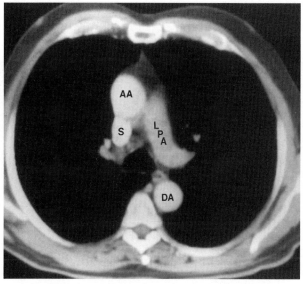

FIG. 1.21. Left pulmonary artery. On sequential CT scans through the aortopulmonary window **(A,B),** partial volume averaging of the top of the left pulmonary artery *(arrow* in **A)** may be confused with an aortopulmonary window mass. Note that the apparent mass in **A** is in perfect vertical alignment with and has the same orientation as the more readily identifiable left pulmonary artery (LPA) in **B.** AA, ascending aorta; DA, descending aorta; S, superior vena cava.

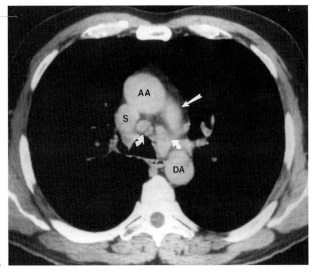
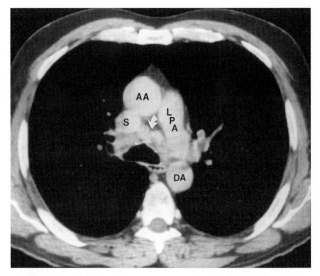

FIG. 1.22. Aortopulmonary window. **A, B;** Sequential CT scans through the aortopulmonary window demonstrate volume averaging of the top of the left pulmonary artery (straight arrow in A), as well as mediastinal lymphadenopathy (curved arrows). AA, ascending aorta; DA, descending aorta; S, superior vena cava; LPA, left pulmonary artery.

bronchial or cardiovascular anomalies (47). Rarely in adults, it may be encountered incidentally as an asymptomatic right paratracheal mass (48,49).

Contrast-enhanced CT allows delineation of the abnormal origin and course of the left pulmonary artery as well as its relationship and effect on the airway (49) (Fig. 1.25). Continuity of the anomalous left pulmonary artery at its origin from the right pulmonary artery can be seen, along with its characteristic course posterior to the trachea and anterior to the esophagus to enter the left pulmonary hilum. The main and right pulmonary arteries appear normal on CT. A noncontrast CT will often be a source of diagnostic pitfall.

Venous Pitfalls

Left Brachiocephalic Vein

There are several variable appearances of the left brachiocephalic vein that can lead to pitfalls in interpretation on CT. It can be rather prominent or dilated, leading to misinterpretation as an anterior mediastinal mass or adenopathy (Fig. 1.26). This is especially true when intravenous contrast material is administered via the right antecubital vein and the distended left brachiocephalic vein is poorly or incompletely opacified. The distended left brachiocephalic vein is usually a normal anatomic

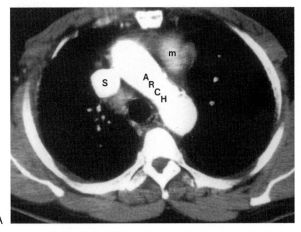
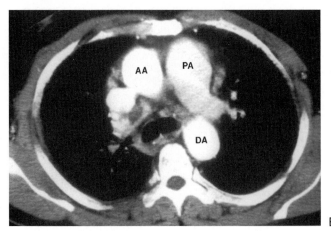

FIG. 1.23. High main and left pulmonary arteries. **A:** The appearance of a mass (m) seen lateral to the aortic arch (ARCH) is produced by partial imaging of a cephalad-positioned main and left pulmonary artery. Note that the mass blends with the main and left pulmonary artery (PA) in **B.** A 1-cm pretracheal lymph node is also present. S, superior vena cava. **B:** Note dilated main and left pulmonary artery (PA). Patient has a history of pulmonary hypertension. AA, ascending aorta; DA, descending aorta.

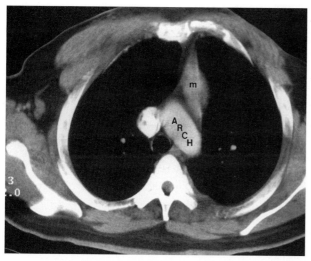
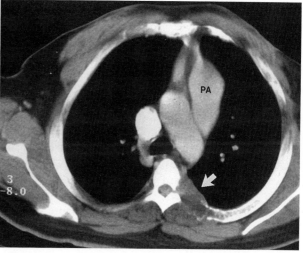

FIG. 1.24. High main and left pulmonary arteries in a patient with Hodgkin's disease and back pain. Suspicion of an anterior mediastinal mass was raised on PA and lateral chest radiographs. **A:** Apparent anterior mediastinal mass (m) located anterolateral to the aortic arch (ARCH) is produced by partial imaging of a cephalad-positioned main and left pulmonary artery. Note that the mass blends with the prominent main pulmonary artery segment (PA) in **B. B:** Note also the left paraspinal mass *(arrow)* destroying the adjacent rib and vertebra, accounting for the patient's back pain. The mass, found to represent recurrent Hodgkin's disease, extends into the spinal canal.

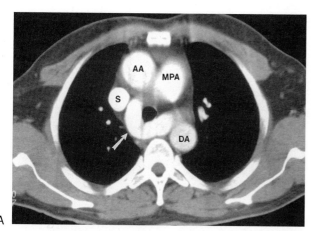
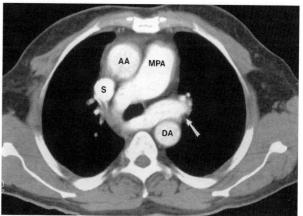

FIG. 1.25. Pulmonary artery sling. Contrast-enhanced CT scans through the distal trachea and carina demonstrate the anomalous left pulmonary artery *(arrow)* arising posteriorly from the right pulmonary artery and then crossing between the trachea and esophagus to enter the left pulmonary hilum. AA, ascending aorta; DA, descending aorta; MPA, main pulmonary artery; S, superior vena cava.

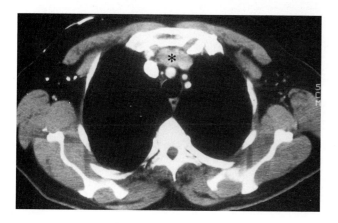

FIG. 1.26. Left brachiocephalic vein. Poorly opacified, dilated left brachiocephalic vein *(asterisk)* mimics the appearance of an anterior mediastinal mass on this contrast-enhanced CT scan following right antecubital vein injection.

variant, although it can also be seen in patients with accessory hemiazygous continuation of a left inferior vena cava or anomalous left upper lobe pulmonary venous drainage into the left brachiocephalic vein (24).

Tortuosity and variability in position of the horizontal portion of the left brachiocephalic vein is a relatively common occurrence, particularly in the elderly. Although usually seen at the level of the great vessels, the horizontal component of the left brachiocephalic vein can be found at almost any level of the superior mediastinum, including in front of the aortic arch, where it may superficially simulate the appearance of a contrast-filled false lumen of an aortic dissection (28). Careful review of contiguous CT images will demonstrate continuity of the apparent false lumen with more definitely identified portions of the vein.

At times, the left brachiocephalic vein has a more straight, vertical course as it descends in the anterior mediastinum. In such cases, it may simulate an anterior mediastinal soft-tissue nodule or mass (24). Again, careful analysis of multiple contiguous scans usually allows the correct interpretation.

Rarely, the left brachiocephalic vein has an anomalous course, descending along the left upper mediastinum lateral to and below the aortic arch, in a position similar to a persistent left superior vena cava (50,51) (Fig. 1.27). The anomalous vein then enters the aortopulmonary window and crosses the mediastinum from left to right, passing posterior to the ascending aorta and anterior to the lower trachea. It joins the right brachiocephalic vein or superior vena cava near the level of the azygous arch. This anomalously positioned vessel can mimic the appearance of mediastinal adenopathy anywhere along its course, particularly in the aortopulmonary window. Drainage into the right brachiocephalic vein or superior vena cava distinguishes this anomaly from a persistent left superior vena cava, which drains into the coronary sinus.

Persistent Left Superior Vena Cava

A persistent left superior vena cava occurs in 0.3% of normal individuals and about 5% of patients with congenital heart disease (52). This anomaly results from

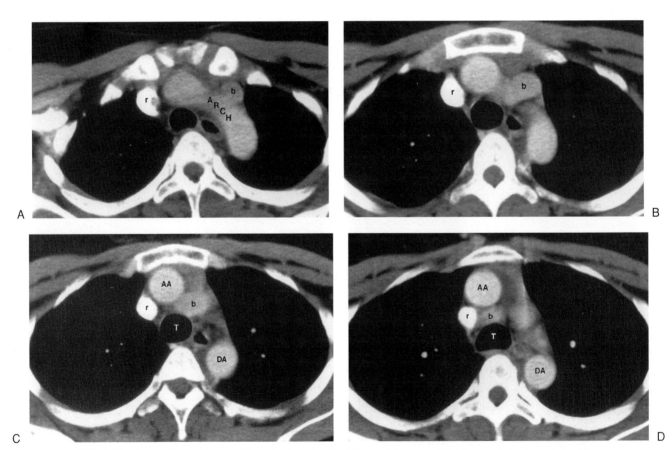

FIG. 1.27. Anomalous left brachiocephalic vein. Serial caudal scans after bolus injection of contrast material demonstrate an anomalous left brachiocephalic vein (b) coursing underneath the aortic arch (ARCH) and crossing the mediastinum from left to right to join the right brachiocephalic vein (r). The anomalous vessel passes posterior to the ascending aorta (AA) and anterior to the lower trachea (T), and may mimic the appearance of mediastinal lymphadenopathy anywhere along its course. DA, descending aorta.

embryologic failure of regression of parts of the left common and anterior cardinal veins. In 80% to 90% of cases, the right superior vena cava is also present, whereas in 65% of patients the left brachiocephalic vein is absent or small (53,54). In 20% of patients with persistent left superior vena cava, the left superior intercostal vein forms a communication between the hemiazygous vein and the cava, producing a left hemiazygous arch analogous to the right-sided azygous arch (51,54).

On CT, a persistent left superior vena cava may be confused with lymphadenopathy if the full course of the vessel is not appreciated (Fig. 1.28). The left superior vena

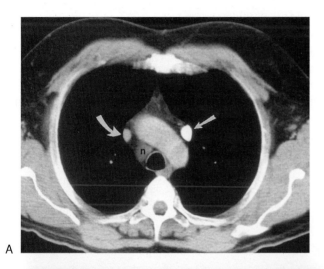

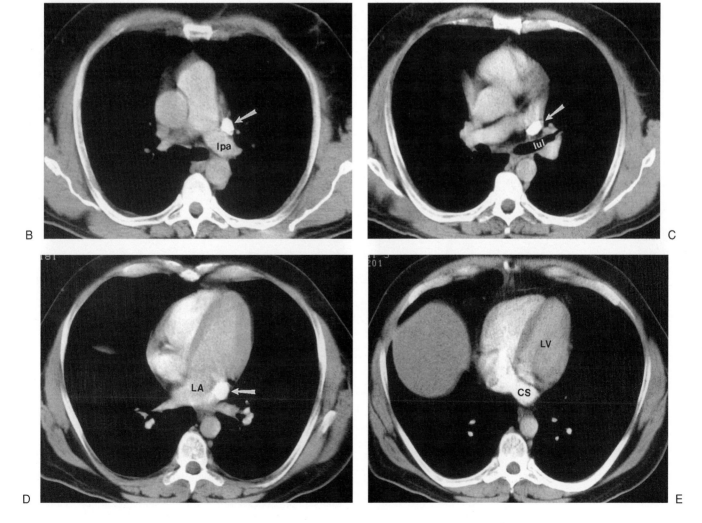

FIG. 1.28. Persistent left superior vena cava. Serial caudal scans following bolus injection of contrast material through a left antecubital vein. **A:** A persistent left superior vena cava *(straight arrow)* descends lateral to the aortic arch in the same coronal plane as the normal right superior vena cava *(curved arrow).* n, enlarged mediastinal lymph node. **B,C:** At lower levels, the left superior vena cava *(arrow)* courses anterior to the left hilum, in front of the left pulmonary artery (lpa) and the left upper lobe bronchus (lul). **D,E:** At the level of the left atrium (LA), the persistent left superior vena cava *(arrow)* is seen draining into the coronary sinus (CS) posterior to the left ventricle (LV).

cava appears on CT as a rounded, tubular soft tissue structure arising from the junction of the left subclavian and left internal jugular veins (51,55). The anomalous vessel is initially positioned lateral to the left common carotid artery and anterior to the left subclavian artery. It descends in the left mediastinum, coursing lateral to the aortic arch in approximately the same coronal plane as the normal right superior vena cava. Inferiorly, it passes lateral to the main pulmonary artery and anterior to the left hilum and typically drains into a dilated coronary sinus posterior to the left ventricle. Absence of the right superior vena cava and left brachiocephalic vein can provide additional support for the presence of a persistent left superior vena cava.

Internal Mammary Veins

The internal mammary veins frequently are well visualized on CT and asymmetry in their size is not unusual. The right and left internal mammary veins drain into the right and left brachiocephalic veins, respectively. Typically, the right internal mammary vein follows a more extensive transverse course than the left as it extends posteriorly adjacent to the anterior mediastinum to empty into the right brachiocephalic vein (Fig. 1.29). When the transverse portion of the right internal mammary vein is lengthy or prominent, it can simulate partial atelectasis of the anterior segment of the right upper lobe or be mistaken for the right lobe of the thymus gland (24,28). Proper recognition and identification of the right internal mammary vein requires following the right

internal mammary vein coursing from the right internal mammary area toward the superior vena cava on sequential transverse sections. Often, the right internal mammary vein will be seen to unite with the right brachiocephalic vein at a level just above the formation of the superior vena cava.

Superior Intercostal Veins

The right superior intercostal vein, particularly when distended, may mimic the appearance of an enlarged posterior mediastinal lymph node or a subvisceral pleural nodule bulging into the posterior segment of the right upper lobe (24,28) (Fig. 1.30). Proper recognition and

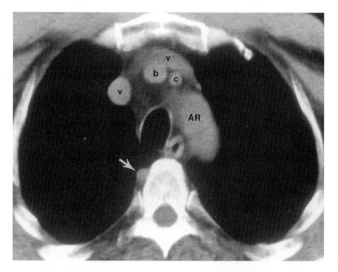

A

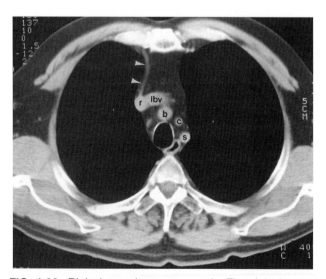

FIG. 1.29. Right internal mammary vein. The right internal mammary vein (arrowheads) is seen coursing posteriorly to empty into the right brachiocephalic vein (r). The relatively extensive horizontal course of the right internal mammary vein might be confused with residual soft tissue in the right lobe of the thymus gland. lbv, left brachiocephalic vein; b, brachiocephalic artery; c, left carotid artery; s, left subclavian artery.

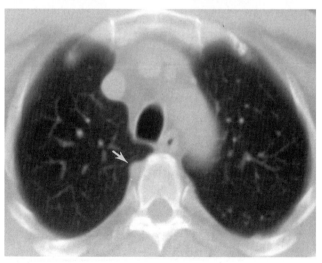

B

FIG. 1.30. Right superior intercostal vein. A,B: On a CT scan through the level of the top of the aortic arch (AR) at mediastinal (A) and lung window settings (B), the right superior intercostal vein (arrow) mimics an enlarged paraspinal lymph node or subvisceral pleural nodule. The right superior intercostal vein could be seen to drain into the posterior aspect of the azygous venous arch on sequential caudal scans. v, brachiocephalic veins; b, brachiocephalic artery; c, left carotid artery.

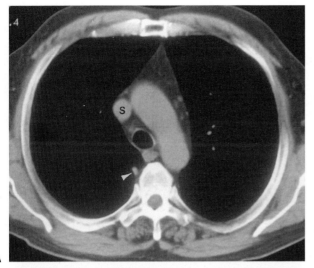

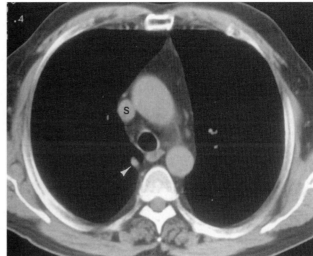

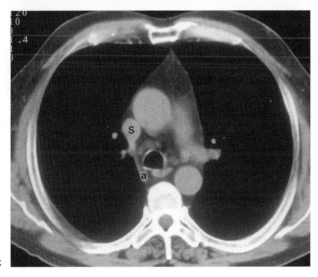

FIG. 1.31. Right superior intercostal vein. **A–C:** Sequential CT scans from cephalad to caudad show the right superior intercostal vein *(arrowhead)* moving forward along the spine to drain into the posterior aspect of the azygous vein arch (a). Distention of the vein in the supine patient should not be confused with a mass or adenopathy. S, superior vena cava.

identification of the right superior intercostal vein requires knowledge of its normal course and appearance on CT. Sequential CT scans from cephalad to caudad will show the right superior intercostal vein coursing anteriorly and inferiorly along the spine before emptying into the posterior aspect of the azygous venous arch (Fig. 1.31).

The left superior intercostal vein, which courses anteriorly alongside the aortic arch to empty into the left brachiocephalic vein, may simulate lateral aortic lymph node enlargement or, in rare instances, the false lumen of an aortic dissection (24,28) (Fig. 1.32). Again, careful review of contiguous CT slices and knowledge of the normal course of the left superior intercostal vein usually allow the correct diagnosis to be made.

Azygous Vein Arch

When the azygous vein arch is transversely oriented and seen in its entirety on a single CT slice, there usually

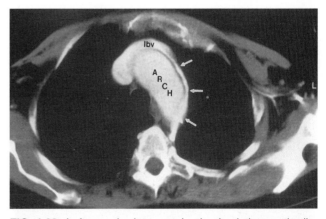

FIG. 1.32. Left superior intercostal vein simulating aortic dissection. The left superior intercostal vein *(arrows)* is seen coursing adjacent to the aortic arch (ARCH). The mediastinal fat between the arch and the intercostal vein could be confused with an intimal flap. Note continuity of the left superior intercostal vein anteriorly with the left brachiocephalic vein (lbv).

is no problem in its proper recognition and identification (Fig. 1.33). However, when the azygous vein arch is not transversely oriented, and thus not totally included within a single CT slice, its image may cause confusion (Figs. 1.34 and 1.35). In such cases, portions of the azygous vein arch from posterior to anterior on sequential transverse CT slices may simulate retrobronchial, paratracheal, or pretracheal adenopathy (28,56). Avoidance of this pitfall requires careful evaluation of multiple contiguous sections, noting continuity of the apparent "adenopathy" with other portions of the azygous arch and with the ascending azygous vein. It is also helpful to keep in mind that the azygous arch is usually imaged at the level of the aortopulmonary window, alongside the junction of the lower trachea and right main bronchus.

Azygous Lobe

An azygous lobe, the most frequent anomaly affecting the mediastinal veins, occurs in 0.4% to 1.0% of the population (57). This anomaly results from incomplete medial migration of the right posterior cardinal vein, the embryonic source of the azygous arch, during fetal development (6). Instead of migrating over the top of the medial aspect of the right upper lobe before descending to its normal position just cephalad to the origin of the right upper lobe bronchus, the right posterior cardinal vein penetrates the right upper lobe and descends through the right upper lobe parenchyma before emptying into the superior vena cava. Along its descent, the vein is accompanied by a double fold of visceral and parietal pleura, resulting in the formation of an azygous fissure. The anomaly is referred to as an azygous lobe because the medial portion of the right upper lobe appears trapped between the anomalously positioned azygous fissure and the mediastinum.

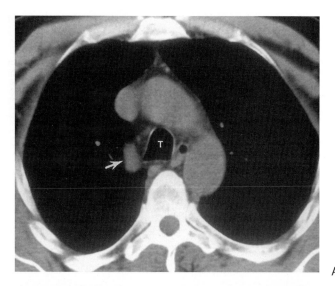

A

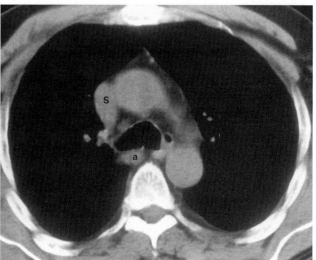

B

FIG. 1.34. Azygous vein arch simulating paratracheal adenopathy. **A,B:** On sequential noncontrast CT scans through the distal trachea (T) and carina, the midportion of the azygous vein arch *(arrow)* is seen and should not be confused with right paratracheal adenopathy. Note its continuity with the superior vena cava (S) anteriorly and with the ascending azygous vein (a) posteriorly in **B.**

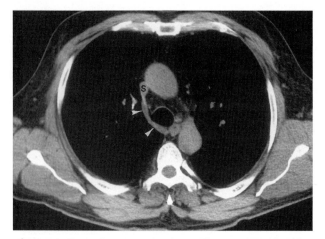

FIG. 1.33. Normal azygous vein arch. The entire azygous arch *(arrowheads)* is seen coursing from posterior to anterior to empty into the superior vena cava (S).

In patients with an azygous lobe, several alterations in mediastinal anatomy can be seen on CT (58,59). The azygous vein arch is displaced laterally and superiorly, sometimes extending as high as the level of the right brachiocephalic vein. The superior portion of the ascending azygous vein is also displaced laterally, to the right of the spine. On a single CT image, the superior portion of the ascending azygous vein or the posterior portion of the azygous vein arch may simulate a nodule in the lung, either totally surrounded by the lung or abutting its pleural surface (28,58) (Fig. 1.36). Recognition of the true nature of this apparent nodule depends on observing that an azygous lobe is present and that on sequential CT

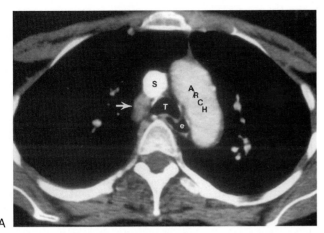
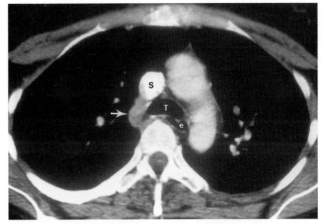

FIG. 1.35. Azygous vein arch simulating paratracheal adenopathy. A,B: On sequential contrast-enhanced CT scans through the level of the aortic arch (ARCH) and aortopulmonary window, a poorly opacified, distended azygous vein arch *(arrow)* mimics paratracheal adenopathy. S, superior vena cava; T, trachea; e, air-filled esophagus.

slices the nodule is in continuity with other definitely identified portions of the azygous arch more anteriorly.

Frequently, in patients with an azygous lobe, the superior vena cava has a somewhat elliptical shape with its longitudinal axis oriented obliquely toward the left (58). In addition, the brachiocephalic vessels tend to extend more laterally than usual, leading to a relative opacity of the medial aspect of the right upper lobe (60,61).

Azygous or Hemiazygous Continuation of the Inferior Vena Cava

When there is embryologic failure of development of the infrahepatic segment of the inferior vena cava above the renal veins, blood from the lower half of the body returns to the heart via the azygous or hemiazygous venous system, so-called azygous or hemiazygous continuation of the inferior vena cava (62). This anomaly may occur as an isolated asymptomatic condition or in association with congenital heart disease and anomalies of abdominal situs (i.e., polysplenia syndrome) (63,64).

In patients with azygous or hemiazygous continuation, the azygous and hemiazygous veins are enlarged because of increased blood flow (Figs. 1.37 and 1.38). The dilated azygous and hemiazygous veins can simulate adenopathy in the right paratracheal, posterior mediastinal, or retrocrural areas. Careful examination of serial CT scans should enable the correct diagnosis. The CT findings are diagnostic and include enlargement of the azygous arch, enlargement of the paraspinal and retrocrural portions of the azygous and hemiazygous veins, and absence of the suprarenal portion of the inferior vena cava (65–67). The most cephalad portion of the inferior vena cava may be visible because this segment draining the hepatic veins develops embryologically from the hepatic sinusoids (63,68). Dilation of the azygous and hemiazygous veins may also be seen in patients with obstruction or thrombosis of the superior or inferior vena cava.

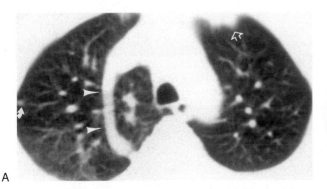
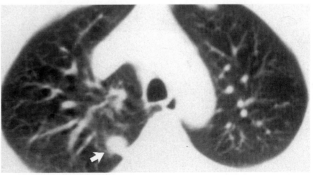

FIG. 1.36. Azygous lobe pitfall. A: Computed tomographic scan through the level of the aortic arch in a patient with an azygous lobe demonstrates an azygous fissure *(arrowheads)* and a small peripheral right pulmonary nodule *(curved arrow). Open arrow,* prominent left first rib costochondral junction. B: On a scan 1 cm caudal, the posterior portion of the azygous vein arch *(arrow)* simulates a nodule in the right upper lobe.

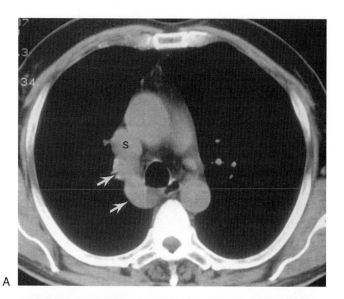

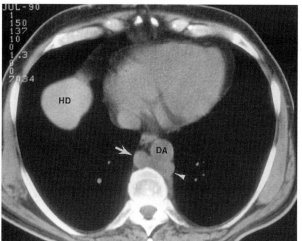

FIG. 1.37. Azygous continuation of the inferior vena cava. **A:** At the level of the aortopulmonary window, a markedly dilated azygous vein arch *(arrows)* drains into the superior vena cava (S). **B:** At the ventricular level, a dilated azygous vein *(arrow)* is seen alongside the descending thoracic aorta (DA). Anterior chest wall collateral vessels are also evident. **C:** At the level of the dome of the right hemidiaphragm (HD), a dilated hemiazygous vein *(arrowhead)* is seen crossing dorsal to the descending aorta (DA) to join the dilated azygous vein *(arrow).* The suprarenal portion of the inferior vena cava was absent on more caudal scans.

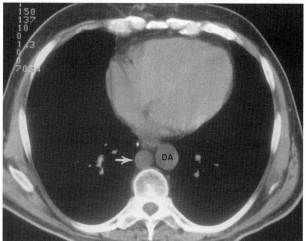

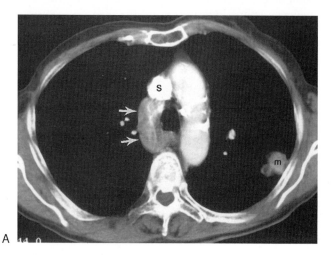

FIG. 1.38. Azygous continuation of the inferior vena cava mimicking mediastinal adenopathy in a patient with bronchogenic carcinoma. **A:** Contrast-enhanced CT scan at the level of the aortic arch demonstrates a markedly dilated azygous vein arch *(arrows)* draining into the superior vena cava (S). Note also the left upper lobe mass (m) known to represent bronchogenic carcinoma in this patient.

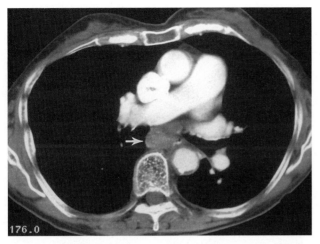
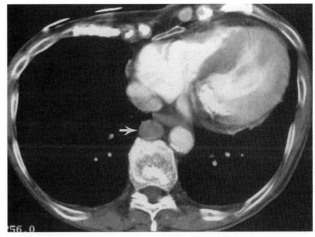

FIG. 1.38. *Continued.* **B,C:** Scans more caudally demonstrate the dilated, poorly opacified azygous vein *(arrow)* mimicking the appearance of mediastinal adenopathy. The suprarenal portion of the inferior vena cava was absent on more caudal scans.

Superior Pulmonary Veins

Portions of the right and left superior pulmonary veins can be confused with adenopathy adjacent to normal mediastinal vascular structures (69). On sequential CT slices through the mediastinum and hilum, the right and left superior pulmonary veins generally are seen to course just anterior to the right pulmonary artery and the left upper lobe bronchus, respectively, before emptying into the left atrium. Knowledge of the normal course of these vessels and, if necessary, the use of intravenous contrast medium will allow separation from enlarged lymph nodes.

Partial Anomalous Pulmonary Venous Return

Occasionally, anomalies of isolated partial pulmonary venous drainage are detected on CT. In such anomalies, blood from the anomalously drained portion of the lung is recirculated to the right side of the heart, creating a left-to-right shunt. Although it may be associated with a wide variety of cardiovascular anomalies, partial anomalous pulmonary venous drainage of one or more lobes occurs in 0.4% to 0.7% of individuals who have no other abnormalities (70–72).

In isolated anomalous pulmonary venous drainage of the left upper lobe into the left brachiocephalic vein, a vertical vein is seen coursing lateral to the aortopulmonary window and aortic arch that is similar in appearance to a persistent left superior vena cava (73,74) (Fig. 1.39). Computed tomographic analysis of the course of the left upper lobe pulmonary veins and evaluation of the number of vessels anterior to the left main bronchus should allow differentiation of these two anomalies. In partial anomalous pulmonary venous drainage of the left upper lobe, the left upper lobe pulmonary veins enter the aberrant vertical vein at the level of the aortopulmonary window. In persistent left superior vena cava, the pulmonary veins in the left upper lobe enter the normally positioned left superior pulmonary vein anterior to the left main bronchus. With persistent left superior vena cava, two vessels (the left cava and the left superior pulmonary vein) will be seen in the left hilar region anterior to the left main bronchus, whereas in anomalous pulmonary venous drainage of the left upper lobe, only one vessel will be found in this location (the anomalous vertical vein, which connects the left superior pulmonary vein to the left brachiocephalic vein). In the case of persistent left superior vena cava, blood flow is caudal, into the coronary sinus, whereas with anomalous pulmonary venous drainage of the left upper lobe, blood flow in the vertical vein is in a cranial direction.

Other anomalies of pulmonary venous drainage that may be recognized on CT include that from the right inferior pulmonary vein cephalad into the azygous vein (72) or caudad into an anomalous scimitar vein in patients with the scimitar syndrome (75) (Fig. 1.40). Usual manifestations of the scimitar syndrome are hypoplasia of the

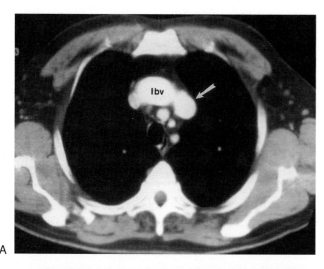

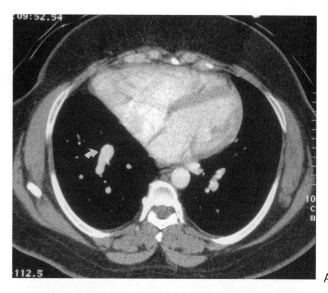

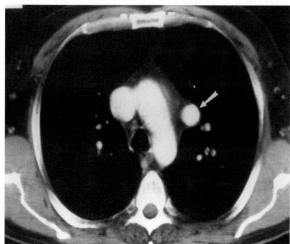

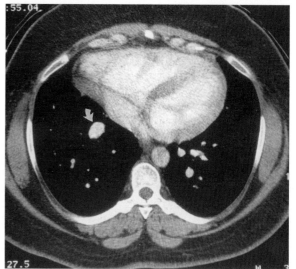

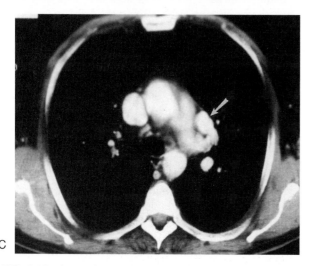

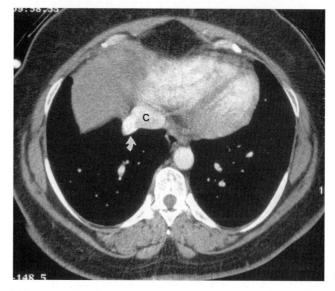

FIG. 1.39. Anomalous pulmonary venous drainage of the left upper lobe. **A–C:** Sequential, selected contrast-enhanced CT scans demonstrate anomalous drainage of the left upper lobe pulmonary veins into an aberrant vertical vein *(arrow)*, which courses cephalad to drain into the left brachiocephalic vein (lbv).

FIG. 1.40. Scimitar syndrome. **A–C:** Sequential contrast-enhanced CT scans through the lung bases demonstrate an enlarged, anomalous right lower lobe pulmonary vein *(curved arrow)* draining into the inferior vena cava (C).

right lung and right pulmonary artery, anomalies of lobation and bronchial distribution, partial or total anomalous arterial supply from the systemic circulation, and anomalous pulmonary venous drainage from all or most of the right lobes into an anomalous scimitar vein. The anomalous scimitar vein can be seen on CT coursing through the right lower lobe parallel to the right heart border before draining into the inferior vena cava, either below the diaphragm or at the junction of the inferior vena cava and right atrium.

Pericardial Recesses

The pericardial cavity contains several recesses around the heart and great vessels where small physiologic amounts of fluid can normally collect (76–78) (Fig. 1.41). These include the retroaortic recess (transverse sinus) posterior to the ascending aorta, the preaortic recess in front of the main pulmonary artery and the aorta, the oblique recess along the posterior aspect of the left atrium and the left ventricle, and the right and left lateral recesses. The right lateral recess extends along the superior vena cava and the

right pulmonary artery. The left lateral recess surrounds the left pulmonary artery. Knowledge of the location and appearance of these recesses is important in order not to confuse fluid within them with a mediastinal mass or an enlarged mediastinal lymph node.

On CT, the pericardial recesses usually appear as crescentic, triangular, or curvilinear structures of near-water density, but they may be difficult to distinguish from soft tissue because of their small size. The most commonly identified recess, seen in about 50% of adult patients undergoing CT examination of the mediastinum, is the retroaortic recess or transverse sinus of the pericardium (76) (Fig. 1.42). The retroaortic recess appears on CT as a crescentic or triangular shaped near-water-density structure posterior to the ascending aorta at or slightly above the level of the left pulmonary artery. Its characteristic homogeneous near-water-density appearance, coupled with its location in immediate apposition to the posterior aspect of the ascending aorta, should allow differentiation from an enlarged mediastinal lymph node or mass (28,76) (Fig. 1.43).

At times, the superior pericardial recesses may simulate the appearance of aortic dissection on CT (79). Again, recognition of their characteristic location, shape, and appearance should allow the correct interpretation.

Small amounts of fluid may also collect in the caudal portions of the pericardial cavity, simulating a short segment of pericardial thickening or a small pericardial effusion (77). The most distal portion of the pericardium, just before its insertion into the central tendon of the diaphragm, in front of the inferior surface of the right

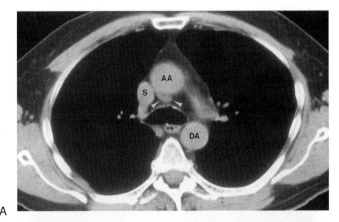
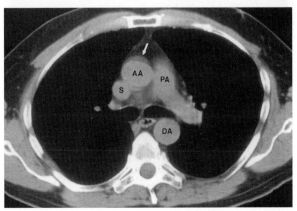

FIG. 1.41. Normal pericardial recesses. **A,B:** Sequential CT scans demonstrate the retroaortic *(arrowheads)* and preaortic *(arrow)* recesses. AA, ascending aorta; DA, descending aorta; S, superior vena cava; PA, pulmonary artery.

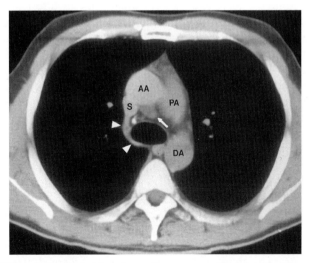

FIG. 1.42. Normal retroaortic recess. Computed tomographic scan at the level of the azygous vein arch *(arrowheads)* demonstrates the triangular-shaped near-water density retroaortic recess *(arrow)* posterior to the ascending aorta (AA). DA, descending aorta; S, superior vena cava; PA, pulmonary artery.

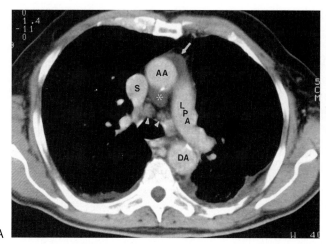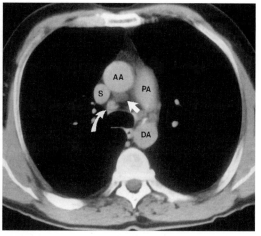

A   B

FIG. 1.43. Retroaortic recess versus mediastinal lymphadenopathy. **A:** Computed tomographic scan at the level of the left pulmonary artery (LPA) shows homogeneous near-water density preaortic *(arrow)* and retroaortic *(asterisk)* recesses. Note also the more heterogeneous-appearing soft-tissue density mediastinal lymph nodes *(arrowheads).* AA, ascending aorta; DA, descending aorta; S, superior vena cava. **B:** In another patient, the near-water-density retroaortic recess *(straight arrow)* has a more rounded configuration. The retroaortic recess abuts the posterior wall of the ascending aorta (AA). DA, descending aorta; S, superior vena cava; PA, pulmonary artery; *curved arrow,* enlarged mediastinal lymph node.

ventricle, may measure up to 3 to 4 mm in thickness because of accumulation of small physiologic amounts of pericardial fluid (13) (Fig. 1.44). The normal fluid should be seen on only one or two scan levels near the diaphragm.

Phrenic Bundle

Occasionally, the normal phrenic bundle, consisting of the phrenic nerve and the pericardiacophrenic artery and vein, may be identified on CT as a 1- to 3-mm rounded or linear structure adjacent to the posterolateral surface of the pericardium (28,80) (Fig. 1.45). The small protuberance of the phrenic bundle should not be mistaken for a pulmonary, pleural, or pericardial nodule. It is most often seen along the lower cardiac borders, at the level of the inferior pulmonary veins and below, with the right phrenic bundle tending to be located more posteriorly (along the right atrium or inferior vena cava) than the left phrenic bundle (along the cardiac apex) (28).

Atrial Appendages

The right atrial appendage, particularly when prominent, may simulate a thymic mass or an enlarged mediastinal lymph node (24,28). The right atrial appendage extends cephalad from the right atrium and typically appears as a curved triangular structure located lateral and sometimes anterior to the proximal ascending aorta,

with the superior vena cava slightly posterior to it. Contiguity of the appendage with the right atrium will be seen on sequential CT scans.

The left atrial appendage, which can also be confused with mediastinal lymphadenopathy, is seen as a rounded structure anterior to the left superior pulmonary vein and posterior to the right ventricular outflow tract and the left coronary artery (24,28). Review of sequential CT images

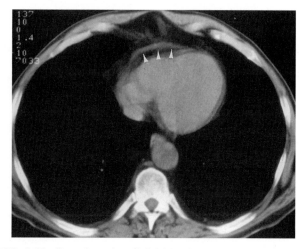

FIG. 1.44. Pseudopericardial thickening. Just before its caudal insertion into the central tendon of the diaphragm, there may be apparent anterior thickening of the pericardium *(arrowheads),* where small physiologic amounts of pericardial fluid accumulate and where the transaxial CT scan images the pericardial sac tangentially.

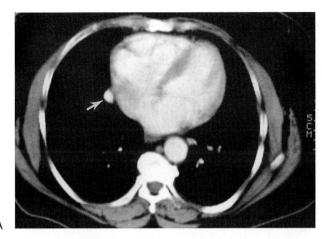 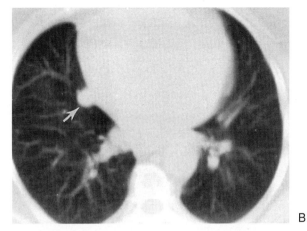

FIG. 1.45. Right phrenic bundle. Contrast-enhanced CT scan through the lung bases at mediastinal **(A)** and lung window settings **(B)** in a patient with metastatic melanoma. A prominent right phrenic bundle *(arrow)* adjacent to the posterolateral surface of the right atrium mimics the appearance of a pulmonary nodule. Note enhancement of vessels within the phrenic bundle in **A.**

will demonstrate contiguity of the appendage with the left atrium.

Intrathoracic Thyroid

Imaging of the inferior pole of one or both lobes of the thyroid gland may produce the appearance of a paratracheal mass or adenopathy (28) (Fig. 1.46).The apparent mass or adenopathy will be seen to blend with the more definitely identified thyroid gland on sequential cranial scans. In addition, if intravenous contrast material has not been administered, the mass may appear slightly more dense than the surrounding mediastinal vascular structures, presumably because of the increased iodine content of the normal thyroid gland.

An enlarged intrathoracic thyroid gland, an intrathoracic goiter, usually is located in the anterior mediastinum, but occasionally it can extend posterior to the great vessels and be confused with paratracheal adenopathy (Fig. 1.47). Knowledge of the typical CT appearance of an intrathoracic goiter generally allows its proper recognition and identification (81,82). Intrathoracic goiters usually are well defined and often demonstrate marked, prolonged contrast enhancement following administration of intravenous contrast material. They may contain areas of focal calcification as well as areas of relatively low attenuation secondary to cystic degeneration or colloid formation (Fig. 1.48). Most importantly, contiguous scans will show contiguity of the goitrous mass with the cervical thyroid.

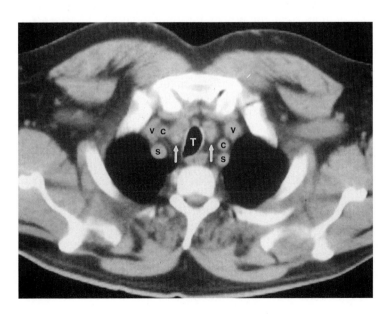

FIG. 1.46. Intrathoracic thyroid. The inferior lobes of the thyroid *(arrows)* are seen lateral to the trachea (T) and mimic the appearance of paratracheal adenopathy. Continuity with the remainder of the thyroid gland could be seen on sequential cranial scans. v, brachiocephalic veins; c, carotid arteries; s, subclavian arteries.

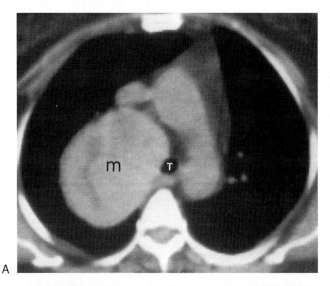

A

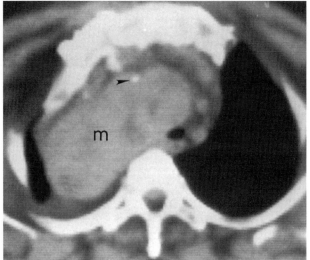

B

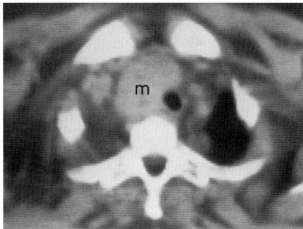

C

FIG. 1.47. Intrathoracic goiter. **A:** Computed tomographic scan at the level of the aortic arch shows a large right paratracheal mass (m). T, trachea. **B:** The mass (m) enlarges at a higher level and contains calcification *(arrowhead)*. **C:** The mass (m) extends up into the thoracic inlet and is contiguous with an enlarged right lobe of the thyroid.

Thymus

The normal thymus usually lies in the anterior mediastinum at a level between the horizontal portion of the left brachiocephalic vein superiorly and the horizontal course of the right pulmonary artery inferiorly. On occasion, particularly in infants and young children, it may extend into the superior mediastinum above the level of the left brachiocephalic vein or into the posterior mediastinum between the superior vena cava and the trachea (83–86). Proper recognition of such an ectopically positioned thymus is important so that it is not mistaken for a pathologic mass. On CT, the diagnosis of superior or posterior thymic extension is suggested by the direct continuity of the ectopic thymus with anterior mediastinal thymic tissue, and by the identical attenuation values of the normal and ectopic thymus (87, 88). Although adjacent mediastinal structures are generally unaffected by the ectopic thymus (86, 89), brachiocephalic artery and tracheal compression can occur (90).

There is considerable age-related variation in the size, shape, and density of the normal thymus on CT, and knowledge of these normal variant appearances is important for proper CT interpretation (17,18,91,92). In infants and young children, the thymus often has a quadrilateral shape and convex lateral margins (Fig. 1.49). If its outer contour is lobular in appearance, it can be confused with an abnormal mediastinal mass. In older children and young adults, the thymus is usually triangular or bilobed with a more prominent left lobe (Fig. 1.50). Throughout the first decade of life and until puberty, the thymus is homogeneous in appearance and has a density similar to that of chest wall musculature. After puberty, areas of inhomogeneity and diminished density may be seen, reflecting normal fatty infiltration of the thymus (Fig. 1.51). This fatty involution is usually gradual and progressive but can be quite variable. Considerable fat can be seen in the thymus of some patients under age 20, whereas others have very little thymic fat even at age 30 (Fig. 1.52). Over the age of 30, small linear or nodular densities of

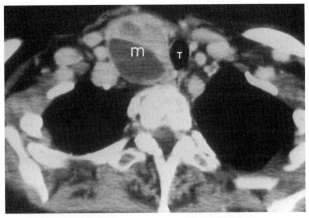
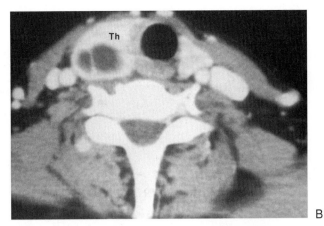

A   B

FIG. 1.48. Intrathoracic goiter. **A,B:** A large heterogeneously enhancing mass (m) containing areas of low attenuation displaces the trachea (T) to the left and is contiguous with an enlarged right lobe of the thyroid (Th).

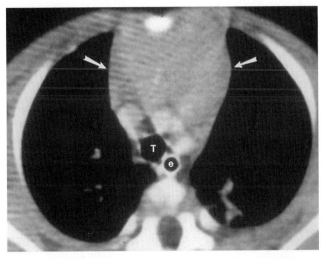

FIG. 1.49. Normal thymus, 5-month-old boy. The thymus *(arrows)* is quadrilateral in shape with slightly convex lateral borders and a wide retrosternal component. The density of thymus is equal to that of chest wall musculature. T, trachea; e, esophagus.

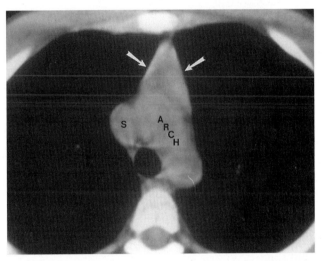

FIG. 1.50. Normal thymus, 14-year-old boy. The thymus *(arrows)* has assumed a triangular, bilobed configuration with a more prominent left lobe. It still has a density equal to that of chest wall musculature. S, superior vena cava; ARCH, aortic arch.

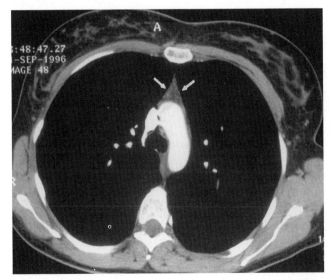

FIG. 1.51. Normal thymus, 30-year-old woman. The thymus *(arrows)* maintains its triangular shape but has decreased in density, reflecting normal fatty infiltration of the thymic parenchyma.

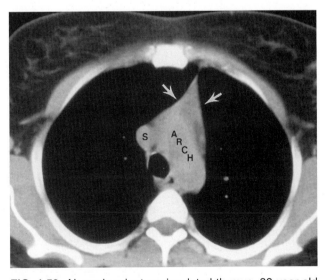

FIG. 1.52. Normal variant noninvoluted thymus, 38-year-old woman. There is minimal fatty infiltration of the thymus *(arrows)*. S, superior vena cava; ARCH, aortic arch.

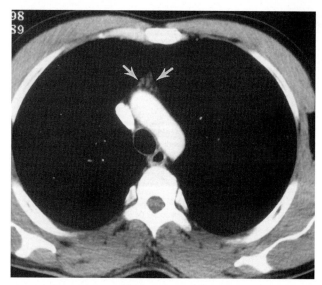

FIG. 1.53. Normal thymic remnants in a 40-year-old man. Small nodular remnants of normal thymic tissue are seen within surrounding fat in the thymus *(arrows)*. The thymic remnants should not be mistaken for anterior mediastinal lymph nodes.

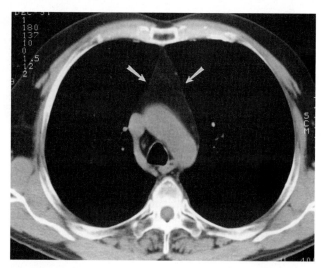

FIG. 1.54. Normal thymus, 50-year-old man. The anterior mediastinum is almost totally composed of fat within the thymic remnant *(arrows)*.

residual thymic parenchyma may be seen within a background of more abundant fat and should not be mistaken for anterior mediastinal lymph nodes (Fig. 1.53). In older patients, only a thin fibrous remnant of the thymus is present, and the anterior mediastinum is almost totally composed of fat within the thymic remnant (Fig. 1.54).

In addition to the aforementioned changes in thymic morphology and density, thymic dimensions also vary with age. The most reliable and meaningful measurement of the thymus is its thickness (largest distance across the long axis of each lobe), which normally decreases with advancing age (91,92). Before the age of 20 when the thymus is most prominent, the maximum thickness of either lobe is 1.8 cm. Thereafter, the maximum thickness is 1.3 cm.

Rebound Thymic Hyperplasia

Rebound thymic hyperplasia, a phenomenon in which the atrophic thymus gland grows back to an even larger size than normal, has been reported after recovery from a wide variety of stresses, including burns (93), cardiac surgery (94), treatment of Cushing's syndrome (95), and chemotherapy (96–98). The phenomenon is most fre-

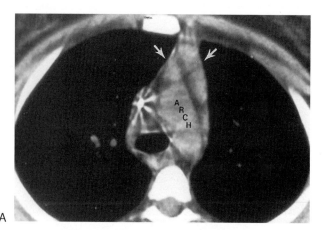

A

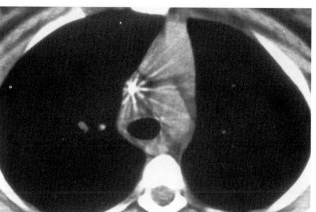

B

FIG. 1.55. Rebound thymic hyperplasia. A 14-year-old girl receiving chemotherapy for Hodgkin disease. **A:** Computed tomographic scan at the time of diagnosis shows a normal bilobed thymus *(arrows)* anterior to the aortic arch (ARCH). Considerable streak artifact emanates from a central venous catheter in the superior vena cava. **B:** Computed tomographic scan 3 months later shows symmetric enlargement of both lobes of the thymus. The patient was doing well clinically. A follow-up CT study 4 months later showed reduction in size of the thymus.

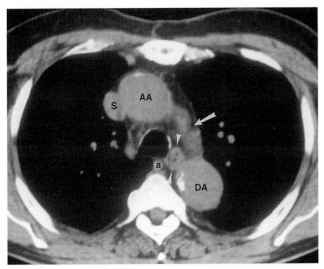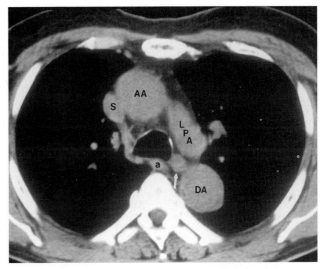

FIG. 1.56. Tortuous esophagus. **A:** The esophagus *(arrowheads)* insinuates into the posteromedial aspect of the aortopulmonary window. There is a small amount of intraluminal air within the esophagus. Note volume averaging of the top of the left pulmonary artery *(arrow)* mimicking adenopathy in the aortopulmonary window. AA, ascending aorta; DA, descending aorta; S, superior vena cava; a, azygous vein. **B:** On a scan 5 mm caudal, the collapsed esophagus *(arrow)* mimics an enlarged mediastinal lymph node. LPA, left pulmonary artery.

quent in children and young adults, in whom the incidence is approximately 25% (96). On CT, diffuse enlargement of the thymus is seen, especially in its thickness, and the normal shape of the thymus gland is preserved (Fig. 1.55).

Rebound thymic hyperplasia after chemotherapy presents a diagnostic problem because it may simulate a primary neoplasm or recurrent disease. The diagnosis depends on the absence of clinical or other features indicating tumor recurrence in a patient with a reason for thymic rebound. If the patient is doing well clinically, and no recurrent or residual disease is evident elsewhere in the body, the patient can be followed up with serial scanning

(96,97). A gradual reduction in size of the thymus corroborates the diagnosis of benign rebound thymic hyperplasia.

Esophagus

The esophagus, which frequently contains a small amount of air, usually descends through the mediastinum in a nearly midline position. At times, however, it may have a somewhat tortuous descent, coursing into the posteromedial aspect of the aortopulmonary window (Fig. 1.56), into the azygoesophageal recess, or along the lower thoracic paraspinal regions (Fig. 1.57). When the esophagus is fluid-filled or collapsed in these

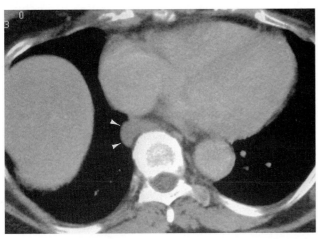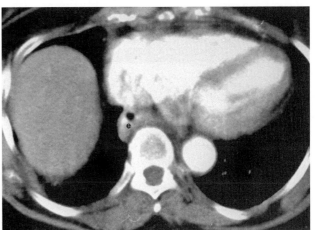

FIG. 1.57. Tortuous esophagus. **A:** Computed tomographic scan at the level of the cardiac ventricles demonstrates an apparent paraspinal mass *(arrowheads)*. **B:** Repeat CT scan following administration of oral and intravenous contrast material shows that the apparent mass represents a tortuous esophagus (e). Note the presence of air and contrast material within the esophageal lumen.

regions, it may be mistaken for a mediastinal mass or an enlarged mediastinal lymph node (24,28). Establishing continuity of the apparent mass with other more definitely identified portions of air-containing esophagus on sequential scan levels and, if necessary, the administration of oral contrast material should permit distinction on CT.

REFERENCES

1. Gamsu G. The mediastinum. In: Moss AA, Gamsu G, Genant HK, eds. *Computed tomography of the body with magnetic resonance imaging, 2nd ed.* Philadelphia, WB Saunders, 1992;43–118.
2. Warwick R, Williams PL. Angiology. In: *Gray's anatomy, 35th ed.* Philadelphia: WB Saunders, 1973;619–626.
3. Gutierrez FR, Woodard PK, Fleishman MJ, Semenkovich JW, Anderson DC. Thorax: Techniques and normal anatomy. In: Lee JKT, Sagel SS, Stanley RJ, Heiken JP, eds. *Computed body tomography with MRI correlation, 3rd ed.* Philadelphia: Lippincott-Raven, 1998;183–259.
4. Naidich DP, Zerhouni EA, Siegelman SS. *Computed tomography and magnetic resonance of the thorax, 2nd ed.* New York: Raven Press, 1991;35–148.
5. Guthaner DF, Wexler L, Harell G. CT demonstration of cardiac structures. *Am J Roentgenol* 1979;133:75–81.
6. Heitzman ER. *The mediastinum, 2nd ed.* Berlin: Springer-Verlag, 1988; 215–269.
7. Takasugi JE, Godwin JD. CT appearance of the retroaortic anastomoses of the azygous system. *Am J Roentgenol* 1990;154:41–44.
8. Ball JB, Proto AV. The variable appearance of the left superior intercostal vein. *Radiology* 1982;144:445–452.
9. McDonald CJ, Castellino RA, Blank N. The aortic nipple: The left superior intercostal vein. *Radiology* 1970;96:533–536.
10. Kuriyama K, Gamsu G, Stern RG, et al. CT-determined pulmonary artery diameters in predicting pulmonary hypertension. *Invest Radiol* 1984;19:16–22.
11. O'Callaghan JP, Heitzman ER, Somogyi JW, Spirt BA. CT evaluation of pulmonary artery size. *J Comput Assist Tomogr* 1982;6:101–104.
12. Moncada R, Baker M, Salinas M, et al. Diagnostic role of computed tomography in pericardial heart disease: Congenital defects, thickening, neoplasms and effusions. *Am Heart J* 1982;103:263–280.
13. Silverman PM, Harell GS. Computed tomography of the normal pericardium. *Invest Radiol* 1983;18:141–144.
14. Price DC. Radioisotopic evaluation of the thyroid and the parathyroids. *Radiol Clin North Am* 1993;31:991–1015.
15. Iida Y, Konishi J, Harioka T, et al. Thyroid CT number and its relationship to iodine concentration. *Radiology* 1983;147:793–795.
16. Gayler BW, Kashima HK, Martinez CR. Computed tomography of the neck. *CRC Crit Rev Diag Imag* 1985;23:319–376.
17. Baron RL, Lee JKT, Sagel SS, Peterson RR. Computed tomography of the normal thymus. *Radiology* 1982;142: 121–125.
18. deGeer G, Webb WR, Gamsu G. Normal thymus: assessment with MR and CT. *Radiology* 1986;158:313–317.
19. Halber MD, Daffner RH, Thompson WM. CT of the esophagus: Normal appearance. *Am J Roentgenol* 1979;133:1047–1050.
20. Desai RK, Tagliabue JR, Wegryn SA, Einstein DM. CT evaluation of wall thickening in the alimentary tract. *RadioGraphics* 1991;11: 771–783.
21. Vock P, Soucek M, Daepp M, Kalender W. Lung: Spiral volumetric CT with single-breath-hold technique. *Radiology* 1990;176:864–867.
22. Touliopoulos P, Costello P. Helical (spiral) CT of the thorax. *Radiol Clin North Am* 1995;33:843–861.
23. Godwin JD, Webb WR. Contrast-related flow phenomena mimicking pathology on thoracic computed tomography. *J Comput Assist Tomogr* 1982;6:460–464.
24. Glazer HS, Aronberg DJ, Sagel SS. *Monograph issue: Pitfalls in mediastinal computed tomography. Diagnostic considerations in computerized tomography.* Mallinckrodt, Inc., St. Louis, Missouri, 1986;1–18.
25. Glazer HS, Aronberg DJ, Sagel SS. Pitfalls in CT recognition of mediastinal lymphadenopathy. *Am J Roentgenol* 1985;144:267–274.
26. Jasinski RW, Yang CF, Rubin JM. Vena cava anomalies simulating adenopathy on computed tomography. *J Comput Assist Tomogr* 1981;5: 921–924.
27. Baron RL, Levitt RG, Sagel SS, Stanley RJ. Computed tomography in the evaluation of mediastinal widening. *Radiology* 1981;138:107–113.
28. Proto AV, Rost RC. CT of the thorax: Pitfalls in interpretation. *RadioGraphics* 1985;5:699–812.
29. Felson B, Cohen S, Courter SR, McGuire J. Anomalous right subclavian artery. *Radiology* 1950;54:340–349.
30. Klinkhamer AC. Aberrant right subclavian artery: clinical and roentgenologic aspects. *Am J Roentgenol* 1966;97:438–446.
31. Proto AV, Cuthbert NW, Raider L. Aberrant right subclavian artery: Further observations. *Am J Roentgenol* 1987;148:253–257.
32. Freed K, Low VHS. The aberrant subclavian artery. *Am J Roentgenol* 1997;168:481–484.
33. Walker TG, Geller SC. Aberrant right subclavian artery with a large diverticulum of Kommerell: A potential for misdiagnosis. *Am J Roentgenol* 1987;149:477–478.
34. Austin EH, Wolfe WG. Aneurysm of aberrant subclavian artery with a review of the literature. *J Vasc Surg* 1985;2:571–577.
35. Akers DL, Fowl RJ, Plettner J, Kempczinski RF. Complications of anomalous origin of the right subclavian artery: Case report and review of the literature. *Ann Vasc Surg* 1991;5:385–388.
36. Haughton VM, Rosenbaum AE. The normal and anomalous aortic arch and brachiocephalic arteries. In: Newton TH, Potts DG, eds. *Radiology of the skull and brain: Angiography.* St Louis: CV Mosby, 1974;1145–1163.
37. Shuford WH, Sybers RG. *The aortic arch and its malformations.* Springfield, IL: Charles C Thomas, 1974;41–92.
38. Taber P, Chang LWM, Campion GM. Diagnosis of retroesophageal right aortic arch by computed tomography. *J Comput Assist Tomogr* 1979;3:684–685.
39. Glanz S, Gordon DH. Right aortic arch with left descent. *J Comput Assist Tomogr* 1981;5:256–258.
40. Shuford WH, Sybers RG, Edwards FK. The three types of right aortic arch. *Am J Roentgenol* 1970;109:67–74.
41. McLoughlin MJ, Weisbrod G, Wise DJ, Yeung HPH. Computed tomography in congenital anomalies of the aortic arch and great vessels. *Radiology* 1981;138:399–403.
42. Webb WR, Gamsu G, Speckman JM, et al. CT demonstration of mediastinal aortic arch anomalies. *J Comput Assist Tomogr* 1982;6:445–451.
43. Shuford WH, Sybers RG, Weens HS. The angiographic features of double aortic arch. *Am J Roentgenol* 1972;116:125–140.
44. Silverman PM, Cooper CJ, Weltman DI, Zeman RK. Helical CT: Practical considerations and potential pitfalls. *RadioGraphics* 1995;15: 25–36.
45. Burns MA, Molina PL, Gutierrez FR, Sagel SS. Motion artifact simulating aortic dissection on CT. *Am J Roentgenol* 1991;157:465–467.
46. Mencini RA, Proto AV. The high left and main pulmonary arteries: A CT pitfall. *J Comput Assist Tomogr* 1982;6:452–459.
47. Capitanio MA, Ramos R, Kirkpatrick JA. Pulmonary sling: Roentgen observations. *Am J Roentgenol* 1971;112:28–31.
48. Hatten HP, Lorman JG, Rosenbaum HD. Pulmonary sling in the adult. *Am J Roentgenol* 1977;128:919–921.
49. Stone DN, Bein ME, Garris JB. Anomalous left pulmonary artery: Two new adult cases. *Am J Roentgenol* 1980;135:1259–1263.
50. Takada Y, Narimatsu A, Kohno A, et al. Anomalous left brachiocephalic vein: CT findings. *J Comput Assist Tomogr* 1992;16:893–896.
51. Webb WR, Gamsu G, Speckman JM, Kaiser JA, Federle MP, et al. Computed tomographic demonstration of mediastinal venous anomalies. *Am J Roentgenol* 1982;139:157–161.
52. Cha EM, Khoury GH. Persistent left superior vena cava: Radiologic and clinical significance. *Radiology* 1972;103:375–381.
53. Campbell M, Deuchar DC. The left-sided superior vena cava. *Br Heart J* 1954;16:423–439.
54. Winters FS. Persistent left superior vena cava. Survey of the world literature and report of thirty additional cases. *Angiology* 1954;5:90–132.
55. Huggins TJ, Lesar ML, Friedman AC, Pyatt RS, Thane TT. CT appearance of persistent left superior vena cava. *J Comput Assist Tomogr* 1982;6:294–297.
56. Smathers RL, Buschi AJ, Pope TL, Brenbridge AN, Williamson BR. The azygous arch: Normal and pathologic CT appearance. *Am J Roentgenol* 1982;139:477–483.
57. Boyden EA. The distribution of bronchi in gross anomalies of the right upper lobe, particularly lobes subdivided by the azygous vein and those containing pre-eparterial bronchi. *Radiology* 1952;58:797–807.

58. Speckman JM, Gamsu G, Webb WR. Alterations in CT mediastinal anatomy produced by an azygous lobe. *Am J Roentgenol* 1981;137:47–50.

59. Mata J, Caceres J, Alegret X, Coscojuela P, DeMarcos JA. Imaging of the azygous lobe: Normal anatomy and variations. *Am J Roentgenol* 1991;156:931–937.

60. Caceres J, Mata JM, Alegret X, Palmer J, Franquet T. Increased density of the azygous lobe on frontal chest radiographs simulating disease: CT findings in seven patients. *Am J Roentgenol* 1993;160:245–248.

61. Akan H. Cause of an opaque azygous lobe on frontal chest radiographs. *Am J Roentgenol* 1995;164:510–511.

62. Floyd GD, Nelson WP. Developmental interruption of the inferior vena cava with azygous and hemiazygous substitution. *Radiology* 1976;119: 55–57.

63. Chuang VP, Mena CE, Hoskins PA. Congenital anomalies of the inferior vena cava: Review of embryogenesis and presentation of a simplified classification. *Br J Radiol* 1974;47: 206–213.

64. Mayo J, Gray R, St Louis E, et al. Anomalies of the inferior vena cava. *Am J Roentgenol* 1983;140:339–345.

65. Breckenridge JW, Kinlaw WB. Azygous continuation of the inferior vena cava: CT appearance. *J Comput Assist Tomogr* 1980;4:392–397.

66. Churchill RJ, Wesby G, Marsan RE, et al. Computed tomographic demonstration of anomalous inferior vena cava with azygous continuation. *J Comput Assist Tomogr* 1980;4:398–402.

67. Ginaldi S, Chuang VP, Wallace S. Absence of hepatic segment of the inferior vena cava with azygous continuation. *J Comput Assist Tomogr* 1980;4:112–114.

68. Berdon WE, Baker DH. Plain film findings in azygous continuation of the inferior vena cava. *Am J Roentgenol* 1968;104:452–457.

69. Naidich DP, Khouri NF, Scott WW, Wang KP, Siegelman SS. Computed tomography of the pulmonary hila: 1. Normal anatomy. *J Comput Assist Tomogr* 1981;5:459–467.

70. Healey JE. An anatomic survey of anomalous pulmonary veins. *J Thorac Cardiovasc Surg* 1952;23:433–444.

71. Adler SL, Silverman JF. Anomalous venous drainage of the left upper lobe. *Radiology* 1973;108:563–565.

72. Schatz SL, Ryvicker MJ, Deutsch AM, Cohen HR. Partial anomalous pulmonary venous drainage of the right lower lobe shown by CT scans. *Radiology* 1986;159:21–22.

73. Pennes DR, Ellis JH. Anomalous pulmonary venous drainage of the left upper lobe shown by CT scans. *Radiology* 1986;159:23–24.

74. Dillon EH, Camputaro C. Partial anomalous pulmonary venous drainage of the left upper lobe vs duplication of the superior vena cava: Distinction based on CT findings. *Am J Roentgenol* 1993;160:375–379.

75. Olson MA, Becker GJ. The scimitar syndrome: CT findings in partial anomalous pulmonary venous return. *Radiology* 1986;159:25–26.

76. Aronberg DJ, Peterson RR, Glazer HS, Sagel SS. The superior sinus of the pericardium: CT appearance. *Radiology* 1984;153:489–492.

77. Levy-Ravetch M, Auh YH, Rubenstein WA, Whalen JP, Kazam E. CT of the pericardial recesses. *Am J Roentgenol* 1985;144:707–714.

78. Vesely TM, Cahill DR. Cross-sectional anatomy of the pericardial sinuses, recesses, and adjacent structures. *Surg Radiol Anat* 1986;8: 221–227.

79. Chiles C, Baker ME, Silverman PM. Superior pericardial recess simulating aortic dissection on computed tomography. *J Comput Assist Tomogr* 1986;10:421–423.

80. Taylor GA, Fishman EK, Kramer SS, Siegelman SS. CT demonstration of the phrenic nerve. *J Comput Assist Tomogr* 1983;7:411–414.

81. Bashist B, Ellis K, Gold RP. Computed tomography of intrathoracic goiters. *Am J Roentgenol* 1983;140:455–460.

82. Glazer GM, Axel L, Moss AA. CT diagnosis of mediastinal thyroid. *Am J Roentgenol* 1982;138:495–498.

83. Cory DA, Cohen MD, Smith JA. Thymus in the superior mediastinum simulating adenopathy: appearance on CT. *Radiology* 1987;162:457–459.

84. Rollins NK, Currarino G. MR imaging of posterior mediastinal thymus. *J Comput Assist Tomogr* 1988;12: 518–520.

85. Shackleford GD, McCallister WH. The aberrantly positioned thymus: a cause of mediastinal or neck masses in children. *Am J Roentgenol* 1974;120:291–296.

86. Siegel MJ, Glazer HS, Wiener JI, Molina PL. Normal and abnormal thymus in childhood: MR imaging. *Radiology* 1989;172:367–371.

87. Cohen MD, Weber TR, Sequeria FW, Vane DW, King H. The diagnostic dilemma of the posterior mediastinal thymus: CT manifestations. *Radiology* 1983;146:691–693.

88. Heiberg E, Wolverson MK, Sundaram M, Nouri S. Normal thymus: CT characteristics in subjects under age 20. *Am J Roentgenol* 1982;138: 491–494.

89. Swischuk LE, John SD. Normal thymus extending between the right brachiocephalic vein and the innominate artery. *Am J Roentgenol* 1996;166:1462–1464.

90. Hennington MH, Detterbeck FC, Molina PL, Wood RE. Innominate artery and tracheal compression due to aberrant position of the thymus. *Ann Thorac Surg* 1995;59:526–528.

91. Francis IR, Glazer GM, Bookstein FL, Gross BH. The thymus: Reexamination of age-related changes in size and shape. *Am J Roentgenol* 1985;145:249–254.

92. St Amour TE, Siegel MJ, Glazer HS, Nadel SN. CT appearances of the normal and abnormal thymus in childhood. *J Comput Assist Tomogr* 1987;11:645–650.

93. Gelfand DW, Goldman AS, Law EJ. Thymic hyperplasia in children recovering from thermal burns. *J Trauma* 1972;12:813–817.

94. Risk G, Cuteo L, Amplatz K. Rebound enlargement of the thymus after successful corrective surgery for transposition of the great vessels. *Am J Roentgenol* 1972;116:528–530.

95. Doppman JL, Oldfield EH, Chrousos GP, et al. Rebound thymic hyperplasia after treatment of Cushing's syndrome. *Am J Roentgenol* 1986; 147:1145–1147.

96. Choyke PL, Zeman RK, Gootenburg JE, et al. Thymic atrophy and regrowth in response to chemotherapy: CT evaluation. *Am J Roentgenol* 1987;149:269–272.

97. Cohen M, Hill CA, Cangir A, Sullivan MP. Thymic rebound after treatment of childhood tumors. *Am J Roentgenol* 1980;135:151–156.

98. Kissin CM, Husband JE, Nicholas D, Eversman W. Benign thymic enlargement in adults after chemotherapy: CT demonstration. *Radiology* 1987;163:67–70.

Variants and Pitfalls in Body Imaging,
edited by Ali Shirkhoda.
Lippincott Williams & Wilkins, Philadelphia, © 2000.

CHAPTER 2

The Heart and the Great Thoracic Vessels: MRI

Kostaki G. Bis and Anil N. Shetty

Magnetic resonance imaging (MRI) of the cardiovascular system is assuming an increasing role in the evaluation of cardiovascular disease. With the development of a multitude of sequences for evaluating the cardiovascular system, MRI and magnetic resonance angiography (MRA) have great potential as the single modality of choice for providing a noninvasive comprehensive examination of the cardiovascular system. To this end, the normal anatomy is briefly reviewed, followed by discussion of technical considerations and related artifacts and pitfalls in performing cardiovascular MRI and MRA. Pertinent anatomic variations and diagnostic pitfalls on MRI/MRA of the heart and great vessels are then reviewed for the following categories: congenital heart disease, tumors/masses, pericardial disease, valvular and myocardial disease, and, finally, pulmonary artery and thoracic aortic disease.

ANATOMY

The flexibility in magnetic field gradients allows one to image the cardiovascular system in various orthogonal and specialized cardiac planes. The transaxial plane (Fig. 2.1) is routinely used for most cardiovascular examinations. This is frequently supplemented with the other orthogonal, coronal, and sagittal planes of imaging. For the specialized cardiac planes, the axial image is used as a scout to prescribe the vertical long-axis (two-chamber) view. An imaginary line is drawn from the mid–mitral valve to the left ventricular apex; imaging parallel to this line yields the two-chamber or vertical long-axis view. An imaginary line is then placed from the mid–mitral valve

to the apex on the vertical long-axis view; the horizontal long axis plane is prescribed parallel to this line and the short axis plane is prescribed perpendicular to this line or perpendicular to the interventricular septum on the horizontal long axis view.

As a brief review, the cross-sectional anatomy of the heart and great vessels is demonstrated in the axial and short-axis planes using breath-hold turbo (FAST) spin-echo imaging and breath-hold segmented gradient echo sequences (see Figs. 2.1 and 2.2). Coronary and coronary artery bypass graft anatomy (Fig. 2.3) is also shown.

TECHNICAL CONSIDERATIONS, RELATED ARTIFACTS, AND DIAGNOSTIC PITFALLS

As with other MR examinations, patients must be screened for contraindications such as various metallic implants and pacemakers. In addition to the selection of appropriate receiver coils, proper placement of ECG leads (Fig. 2.4) and selection of appropriate pulse sequences and parameters, full cooperation of the patient is needed. Irregular breathing, coughing, and frequent swallowing all have adverse effects on image quality. Younger children and claustrophobic patients require sedation and appropriate constant monitoring of the vital signs by a nurse or a physician. A monitor is required for assessment of oxygen saturation (oximetry), expired Pco_2 (capnography), heart rate, and respiratory rate.

Receiver Coils

The image quality and signal in each pixel depend strongly on the type of receiver coil that is utilized. For infants and small children, the extremity coil or circular

K. G. Bis and A. N. Shetty: Department of Diagnostic Radiology, Wayne State University School of Medicine, Detroit, Michigan; and William Beaumont Hospital, Royal Oak, Michigan 48073-6769.

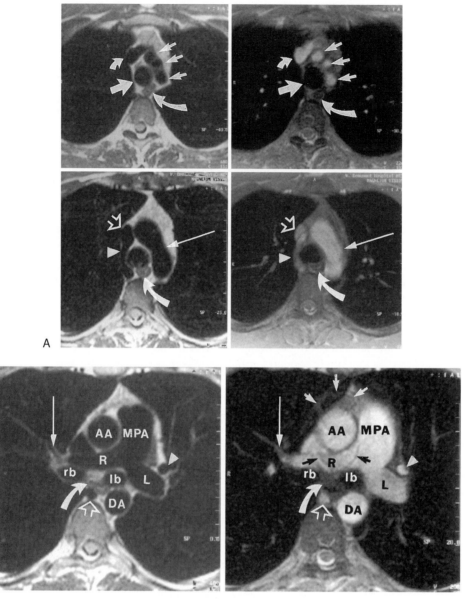

FIG. 2.1. Axial anatomy. Serial black blood (turbo spin-echo) and corresponding white **(A,B)** blood breath-hold cine MR images from above the aortic arch down to the liver dome. **A:** Innominate vein confluence *(short curved arrow)*, innominate artery *(upper short arrow)*, left common carotid artery *(middle short arrow)*, left subclavian artery *(lower short arrow)*, trachea *(thick arrow)*, esophagus *(curved arrow)*, superior vena cava *(open arrow)*, azygous arch *(arrowhead)*, aortic arch *(long thin arrow)*. **B:** Main pulmonary artery (MPA), right pulmonary artery (R), left pulmonary artery (L), ascending aorta (AA), descending aorta (DA), right main stem bronchus (rb), left main stem bronchus (lb), esophagus *(curved arrow)*, azygous vein *(open arrow)*, truncus anterior *(straight thin arrow)*, left upper lobe pulmonary vein *(arrowhead)*, and pulsation artifacts from the ascending and descending aorta *(short thick black and white arrows)*.

polarized (CP) head coil is used for optimizing resolution and signal-to-noise (S/N) ratio. For older children and adults, the Helmholtz body coil and quadrature body coil are used, respectively. Currently, however, body phased-array coils are becoming implemented to significantly improve spatial resolution and S/N ratios on newer updated MR units. The typical array coil has

four individual elements, two posteriorly and two anteriorly. Each element receives signal and noise from only a small portion of the body, resulting in higher S/N ratios. The use of body phased-array coils is, therefore, highly encouraged for adults, and to optimize their use, certain features have to be considered. First, when the individual coil elements are activated, the data will be

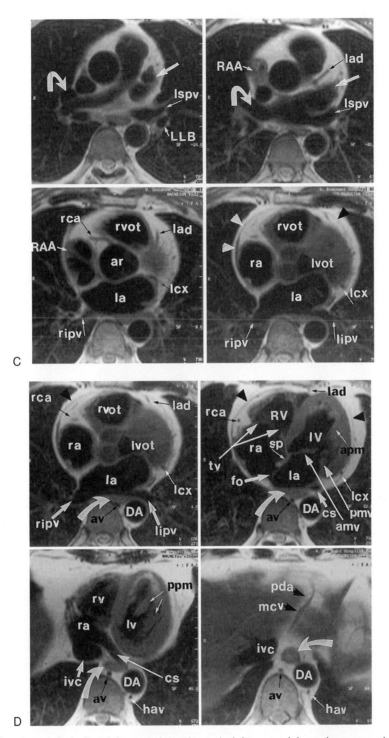

FIG. 2.1. *Continued.* **C:** Left atrial appendage *(arrow),* right upper lobe pulmonary vein *(curved arrow),* left lower lobe bronchus (LLB), right atrial appendage (RAA), left anterior descending coronary artery (lad), right ventricular outflow tract (rvot), right coronary artery (rca), left atrium (la), left superior pulmonary vein (lspv), right atrium (ra), right inferior pulmonary vein (ripv), left inferior pulmonary vein (lipv), pericardium *(arrowheads),* left circumflex coronary artery (lcx), left ventricular outflow tract (lvot). **D:** Septum primum (sp), fossa ovalis (fo), left ventricle (lv), right ventricle (rv), tricuspid valve (tv), anterior mitral valve leaflet (amv), posterior mitral valve leaflet (pmv), anterolateral papillary muscle (apm), posteromedial papillary muscle (ppm), coronary sinus (cs), azygous vein (av), inferior vena cava (ivc), middle cardiac vein (mcv), posterior descending coronary artery (pda), hemiazygous vein (hav) and esophagus *(curved arrows).*

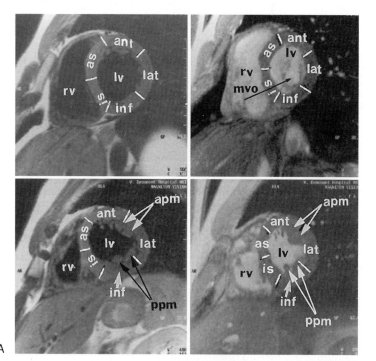

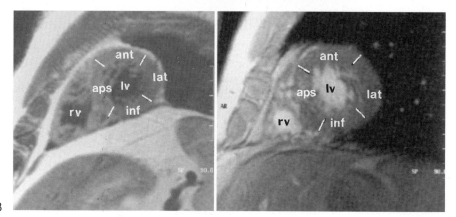

FIG. 2.2. Short-axis anatomy. Serial black blood turbo spin-echo and corresponding white blood breath-hold cine MR images in the short-axis plane are demonstrated at the base of the heart (upper two images in **A)**, at the middle third (lower two images in **A)** of the heart, and at the apical third **(B)** of the heart. Left ventricle (lv), right ventricle (rv), anterior myocardium (ant), lateral myocardium (lat), inferior myocardium (inf), anterior septal myocardium (as), inferior septal myocardium (is), apical septum (aps), anterolateral papillary muscles (apm), posteromedial papillary muscles (ppm), and mitral valve orifice (mvo).

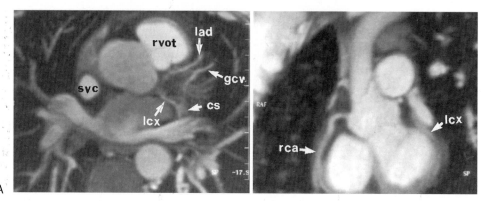

FIG. 2.3. Coronary artery and coronary artery bypass graft anatomy. **A:** Coronary artery anatomy. The axial maximum-intensity projection image on the left obtained with a three-dimensional navigator technique without intravenous contrast demonstrates the following anatomic structures: left anterior descending artery (lad), great cardiac vein draining (gcv) into the coronary sinus (cs), and left circumflex coronary artery (lcx). The oblique sagittal maximum-intensity projection image on the right obtained with breath-hold two-dimensional time-of-flight technique demonstrates the proximal mid- and distal right coronary artery (rca) as well as portions of the left circumflex coronary artery (lcx). Increased signal is noted in areas where there is more through-plane flow. Right ventricular outflow tract (rvot), superior vena cava (svc). Saturation effects may be decreased by narrowing the three-dimensional slab thickness or through the implementation of variable flip angles during the three-dimensional acquisition. Alternatively, contrast infusion may be employed when extracellular fluid or blood pool contrast agents are used.

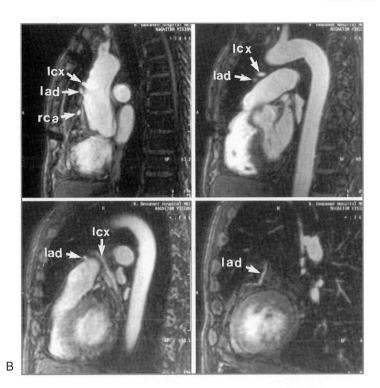

B

FIG. 2.3. *Continued.* **B:** Coronary artery bypass graft anatomy. Left circumflex (lcx), left anterior descending (lad), and right coronary artery (rca) vein grafts at and just beyond their aortotomy sites are shown in the upper left-hand image. The left circumflex and left anterior descending vein grafts over the main pulmonary artery are shown in the upper right-hand and the lower left-hand images. The left anterior descending vein graft as it approaches its target site is demonstrated in the lower right-hand image.

combined automatically to produce one image. Alternatively, one can view individual images from each activated coil. If one element is deactivated or not working, there is local signal loss in the resultant image from the anatomy under that element. Second, because of the surface characteristics of array coil elements, the body parts closest to the coil appear brightest. To create a more uniform signal intensity distribution over the field of view, a normalization filter can be used during image reconstruction.

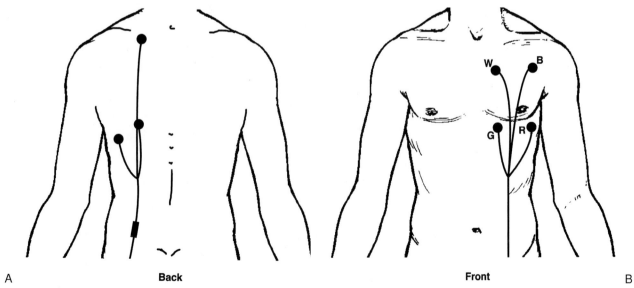

A   **Back**   **Front**   B

FIG. 2.4. Electrocardiogram (ECG) lead placement on the chest and back. **A:** ECG placement on the back with a three-lead system. To enhance the R wave amplitude in some instances, the lower left lead may be placed more anteriorly. The three-lead system is suboptimal and requires frequent maneuvering of the ECG electrodes to maximize the R wave amplitude. The back is chosen with the three-lead approach because there are fewer motion artifacts in this location. **B:** A four-lead ECG technique is demonstrated with the two upper leads at the second intercostal space just to the left of the sternum and the lower two leads at the fourth intercostal space just below the breast line. With this approach, one has the option of choosing one of six different leads (I, II, III, AVR, AVL, AVF). In a patient with large breasts, the breasts must be lifted to place the inferior leads.

Cardiac Gating/Triggering

Prospective and retrospective methods are available for cardiac imaging. The majority of cardiac examinations performed are prospectively triggered. However, to fully evaluate the diastolic phase of the cardiac cycle in instances where diastolic dysfunction is of concern or when accurate flow volume quantification is desired, retrospective gating is suggested (1). Regardless of the method, it is essential to have a reliable, consistent, and noise-free ECG tracing (Fig. 2.5). With MR imaging, motion artifacts result in image blurring, and this is especially true in imaging the cardiovascular system (Fig. 2.6). For example, the periodic motion of the heart results in periodic modulation of the signal with periodic ghosts along the phase-encode direction (see Fig. 2.1B). To suppress these artifacts from periodic motion, data acquisition is synchronized with the car-

diac cycle. Most commonly, cardiac triggering techniques use a trigger pulse that is generated by the R wave of the QRS complex in the electrocardiogram amplifier. Triggered MR pulse sequences are initiated either at the rise of this trigger pulse (for cine sequences) or following a predetermined delay time (50 to 100 milliseconds for spin-echo sequences). A major source of interference in most cardiac studies is the pick-up noise generated in the ECG leads by RF and gradient pulse switching. The actual ECG tracing, therefore, has superimposed artifacts from these induced potentials, which can lead to inappropriate triggering or gating (see Fig. 2.5).

Four leads are usually placed over the anterior chest (See Fig. 2.4) when utilizing an external triggering device such as the *in vivo* patient monitor system (Invivo Company, Research Parkway, FL). With this four-lead system and monitor, there is an option to choose whichever of the

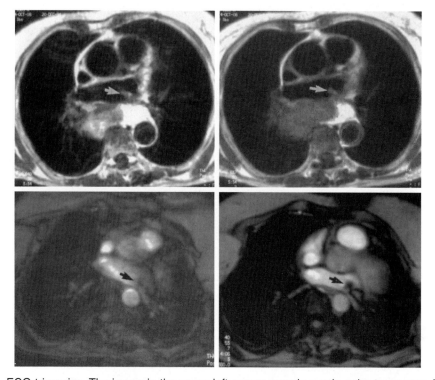

FIG. 2.5. ECG triggering. The image in the upper left corner reveals a spin-echo transverse ECG-triggered image with mild to moderate pulsation artifacts. This image was acquired in a multislice, multiphase spin-echo acquisition with an ECG tracing that exhibited a weak R wave amplitude and superimposed noise. The ECG leads were on the patient's back. A transverse spin echo image in the upper right corner reveals a significant decrease of pulsation artifacts. Reduction of artifacts was achieved after appropriate placement of the ECG leads on the anterior chest and use of an external monitor for acquisition of a noise-free ECG signal. Lead II was selected to maximize the R wave amplitude. Transverse cine MR image in the lower left corner reveals moderate pulsation artifacts. This study was acquired with the ECG leads placed on the back, which resulted in a weak R wave amplitude and superimposed noise. A transverse cine MR image in the lower right corner demonstrates a significant improvement in the reduction of pulsation artifacts after the ECG leads were placed on the anterior chest and triggering was performed via lead II, which yielded the maximum R wave amplitude with no superimposed noise. These images demonstrate a pitfall within the left atrium near the inflow of the inferior left pulmonary vein *(arrow)*. The spin-echo images reveal a focal area of intermediate signal that can be of low signal on cine MR. Findings can mimic a small mass such as a thrombus in this location. This is a normal anatomic variant in this location and should not be mistaken for a mass.

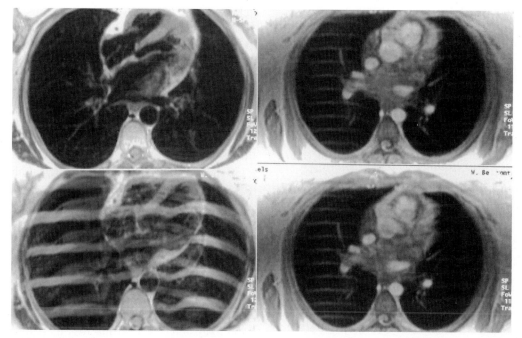

FIG. 2.6. Respiratory motion artifact. Marked respiratory motion artifact on breath-hold turbo spin-echo imaging is demonstrated in the lower left image and on the cine images demonstrated on the right. These ghost artifacts from the anterior chest wall are noted in the phase-encode direction. With appropriate breath-hold, no respiratory motion artifacts are noted in the upper left image.

six combinations among four ECG leads (I, II, III, AVR, AVL, or AVF) exhibits the maximum R wave amplitude free of underlying noise and magnetic field distortion. The need for selecting a different lead for triggering or gating arises when there is underlying pathology altering the electrical axis of the heart. Without this approach (i.e., when three ECG leads are used, typically on the patient's back), one may have to repeatedly reposition the electrodes to achieve congruence with the electrical axis of the heart. Of utmost importance, these leads are fully extended and shielded, avoiding any coiling configuration and possible burning of the patient's skin. Before lead placement, the intended positions over the chest are scrubbed with an alcohol swab and shaved, if needed. Nonmetallic radiotranslucent (Vermont Medical Inc., Bellows Falls, VT) graphite leads are placed at the appropriate sites with intervening built in conductive jelly.

Morphologic Evaluation

Conventional spin-echo sequences (2) are the work horses on most scanners for imaging the cardiovascular system with a multislice/multiphase technique. T_1-weighted images are obtained by prospectively triggering to every R wave (T_R up to 800 milliseconds and 80% of R-R interval) with a short T_E of 12 to 30 milliseconds. T_2-weighted conventional spin-echo images are obtained by triggering to every other or every third R wave (T_R of 1,800 to 3,000 milliseconds) with echo times of 20 to 30 and 60 to 90 milliseconds. Both T_1- and T_2-weighted

spin-echo techniques can be coupled with fat saturation. Most commonly, contrast-enhanced T_1-weighted fat saturation and T_2-weighted fat saturation sequences are used in patients with myocardial infarction. T_2-weighted bright blood sequences can be flow compensated to reduce pulsation artifacts. In addition, pulsation artifacts can be reduced with an associated increase in contrast to noise by improving the flow void phenomenon in the blood pool with black blood sequences.

Technically, there are three ways to achieve dark or black blood imaging with spin-echo sequences. The first method is the washout effect, which is based on the change in amplitude of the spin magnetization because of flow. The second method is based on dephasing the phase of the spin magnetization using gradients. The third is through the use of a double-inversion pulse-pair dark blood preparation scheme (3). Although the dark blood preparation scheme significantly reduces blood pool signal, increased signal is frequently demonstrated, especially in areas of sluggish flow typically seen at the cardiac apex (Fig. 2.7) and within atrial appendages.

The saturation bands can be placed above and below the area being imaged to reduce the blood signal and resultant artifacts on spin-echo sequences. This results in saturation of spins flowing into the area being imaged. A parallel pair of saturation bands are routinely placed when imaging the cardiovascular system in the transverse plane.

Currently, faster means of spin-echo imaging are available through ECG-triggered breath-hold or non-breath-

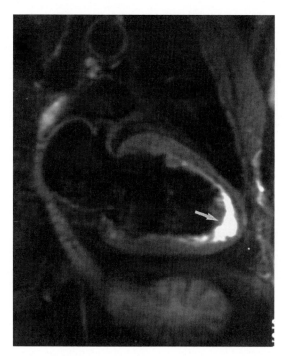

FIG. 2.7. Sluggish intracardiac flow. Vertical long-axis short-tau inversion recovery image employing a dark blood preparation reveals a significant decrease of the blood pool signal. The apical region reveals increased signal *(arrow)* as a result of very sluggish flow. The apex and atrial appendages are typical sites where one may encounter increased signal as a result of slower flow.

hold turbo (FAST) spin-echo and half-Fourier single-shot turbo spin-echo (HASTE) imaging schemes. With these sequences, black blood is achieved with a double-inversion pulse pair (nonselective and selective) scheme. When performing non-breath-hold turbo (FAST) spin-echo acquisitions, one obtains approximately five signal averages (acquisitions or Nex) on turbo T_1-weighted sequences (FAST) to average out motion artifacts, especially when the body array coil is used. T_2-weighted images are currently performed with either a breath-hold turbo (FAST) spin-echo (one acquisition or Nex) or preferably with a breath-hold turbo (FAST) short-tau (STIR) inversion recovery sequence (3). With these latter two sequences, one imaging slice is obtained during the breath-hold period.

The T_R on breath-hold T_1-weighted turbo (FAST) spin-echo sequences is typically set to approximately 100 milliseconds less than the R-R interval and should be below 750 milliseconds. If there is insufficient blood nulling or myocardial motion artifacts, it can be adjusted to reduce them. For breath-hold T_2-weighted turbo (FAST) and segmented HASTE sequences, the T_R is set to be approximately equal to the R-R interval, but no greater than 900 milliseconds. This avoids systolic motion-induced artifacts for these and other black blood sequences (Fig. 2.8). Although triggering is to every second heart beat, the T_2-weighted images are considered to have weak T_2 contrast. The T_R is also set not greater than 900 milliseconds and approximately equal to the RR interval for breath-hold short-T-turbo (FAST) inversion recovery (STIR) and inversion recovery segmented HASTE sequences. Due to the larger effective T_E, there is a strong T_2-contrast for pathologic evaluation, especially for the turbo (FAST) STIR sequence.

Functional Assessment

The physiologic variations of myocardial and valvular motion and blood flow dynamics can be studied using bright blood techniques in which low-flip-angle gradient-echo pulse sequences are commonly employed (4–6). Using gradient-echo pulse sequences in a cine mode allows one to assess physiologic variations during the cardiac cycle. Gradient-echo pulse sequences are flow compensated along the readout and slice directions to improve overall flow-related enhancement and are

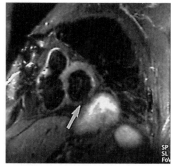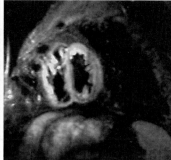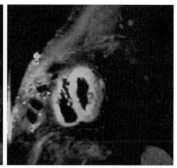

FIG. 2.8. Appropriate inversion time on black blood preparation sequences. Serial short-axis black blood turbo STIR images obtained at the base of the heart **(left)**, middle of the heart **(middle)**, and apex of the heart **(right)** with a fixed trigger delay and black blood inversion time. Because of the greater amount of motion at the base of the heart, there is signal loss in the myocardium, especially inferiorly *(arrow)*. As a result, one may need to vary the trigger delay and inversion time and try to drive the acquisition window in this region of the heart more toward diastole to avoid myocardial signal loss.

employed with echo times as short as 5 to 7 milliseconds and as high as 10 to 12 milliseconds. The shorter echo time is used to minimize the phase dispersion effects from signal loss in areas of turbulent flow. They are routinely used for imaging the aorta for dissection and heart for myocardial function and tumors. The longer echo time is required to allow for more spin dephasing and subsequent signal loss in areas of flow disturbance. The longer echo time accentuates signal void in areas of turbulent flow from valvular or vascular stenosis, valvular insufficiency, and intracardiac shunting. Thus, depending on the clinical situation and indication for scanning, it is important to choose the echo time appropriately for cine examinations. When multislice non-breath-hold cine acquisitions are done, to reduce blood pool saturation effects, imaging slices are separated in space by one to three slice positions. The gaps are subsequently filled in by shifting the entire set of slices by the appropriate shift distance. For prospective triggered acquisitions, the number of phases is adjusted such that the product of T_R and the number of phases is about 10% less than the average R-R interval. The number of phases is reduced if there is inconsistent triggering. For retrospective gating, the number of phases exceeds the maximum expected R-R interval. This will allow one to visualize the full cardiac cycle, including late diastole.

In a conventional nonsegmented cardiac cine pulse sequence, each phase-encode line (Fourier line) is acquired per heartbeat. This not only prolongs the scan time but also allows for more artifacts of respiratory and involuntary motion. However, k space can be subdivided into individual segments with several lines in each. The segmented flash sequences with flow compensation along the readout and slice select directions are ideal for this type of imaging. Segmented sequences can be applied in either a multislice (five-slice acquisitions) sequential non-breath-hold or single-slice breath-hold mode. With prospective triggered non-breath-hold sequential studies, the number of phases is adjusted such that the product of T_R and the number of phases is about 10% less than the average R-R interval as with conventional nonsegmented gradient-echo sequences. For faster heart rates (R-R interval <750 milliseconds), use the shorter-T_R (30 or 40 milliseconds) sequence. For slower heart rates (R-R interval >750 milliseconds), the larger-T_R (50 or 60 milliseconds) sequences are used. In the case of single slice breath hold cine studies, the number of phases is calculated as above. A shorter-T_R (40 milliseconds) sequence is used for faster heart rates (>75 beats/min), and the larger-T_R (50 milliseconds) sequence is applied if the heart rate is less than 75 beats/min. A single phase can be acquired in a 30- to 60-millisecond window. Multiple phases (12 to 20) can be acquired depending on the heart rate. The best blood/myocardial contrast with cine sequences is achieved with thorough-plane flow. These sequences are, therefore, routinely used for

assessing the aorta in the transverse plane for presence of aortic dissection and the left ventricle in the short-axis plane for global and regional myocardial function. For long-axis-oriented cine acquisitions, the flip angle is reduced by approximately 5 degrees, and the T_R is increased to reduce the spin saturation effects.

Cine MRI with spatial modulation of magnetization (7,8) employs the use of thin saturation bands in the horizontal and vertical orientation or, alternatively, in a radial spoke-wheel or two-dimensional stripe distribution. These are placed onto the imaging slice immediately before systole at the onset of the R wave. The displacement and deformation of myocardial tags is followed over time with cine MRI utilizing non-breath-hold conventional or breath-hold segmented gradient-echo sequences employing nine to 20 frames per cardiac cycle and a 5- to 8-mm tag spacing. These sequences highlight underlying wall motion abnormalities and can be used in patients with ischemic heart disease to highlight regional myocardial dysfunction. It should be noted that when intravenous MR contrast is employed, there is a more rapid dissipation of the tag in the blood pool and in the myocardium. Thus, one may need to perform these sequences before administering IV contrast, especially when quantitative analysis is to be performed. Also, a grid spacing of at least 5 pixels is recommended for good tag definition and persistence. Finally, within areas of stagnant blood flow (aneurysms of the heart), there is a lack of tag dissipation, and this may lead to the error of overestimating the myocardial thickness.

Flow Quantification

The principle of these techniques is based on the phase shift acquired by moving spins along a magnetic field gradient (9). Because the net phase shift of moving spins is directly proportional to spin velocity as well as signal intensity, flow velocities are easily obtained by measuring the signal intensity of the blood pool at an area of interest. Typically, 30 time frames are obtained per cardiac cycle in which both magnitude and phase images are obtained. Flow quantification sequences can be applied in the plane of flow (in-plane sequences) or perpendicular to the flow direction (through-plane sequences). The velocity encoding (venc) values are as follows: 40 to 50 cm/sec (venous flow), 75 to 150 cm/sec (coronary arteries), 150 cm/sec (pulmonary artery), 250 cm/sec (aorta), 400 to 500 cm/sec (coarctation, vascular stenoses, valvular stenoses). The short-T_E (4 milliseconds) sequences are applied for very fast flow to decrease intravoxel dephasing effects. For flow quantification and assessment of flow volumes (i.e., stroke volume), through-plane sequences are employed. The volume of blood flow is subsequently obtained via the product of mean velocity through the entire cross section of a blood vessel and the cross-sectional area. Through-plane or in-plane sequences are used at the site of suspected vascular stenosis for measurement of peak velocity (m/sec) and subsequent pressure gradient (mm Hg), where pressure gradient $= 4V^2$ (modified Bernoulli equation).

Velocity-encoded or dynamic phase-contrast sequences are currently performed with segmented gradient-echo sequences allowing for breath-hold acquisitions (10). Both in-plane and through-plane schemes can be employed. Pitfalls of dynamic phase-contrast techniques arise when the appropriate velocity encoded (venc) value is not chosen. For instance, if the actual flow velocity is greater than the venc value, aliasing effects (Fig. 2.9) are demonstrated. On the other hand, if the venc value is much greater than the actual velocity to be measured, not enough signal on the phase image is obtained. Both scenarios will yield inaccurate velocity information. Finally, one needs to accurately adjust the ROI on the magnitude image when performing flow volume quantification. The cross-sectional area may vary with the cardiac cycle, and the region of interest (ROI) must be corrected for this variation because the flow volume is the product of mean velocity and cross-sectional area.

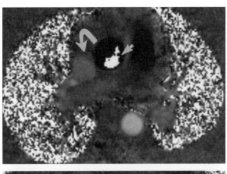

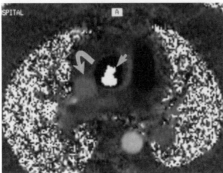

FIG. 2.9. Aliasing effect within the blood pool. Transverse dynamic phase-contrast images reveal aliasing of flow velocities within the ascending aorta, resulting in this irregular patchy area of white signal *(arrow)*. This changes over the cardiac cycle. Aliasing effects are noted, given the very high flow velocities within the ascending aorta relative to the lower velocity-encoding (venc) value that was employed for evaluating slower flow within the superior vena cava *(curved arrow)*. A velocity-encoding value of 75 cm/sec was used in this case for systemic venous flow assessment. Stroke volume assessment of the ascending aorta is performed with a venc value of 250 cm/sec.

Perfusion

The turbo flash sequence (11,12) is a magnetization-prepared gradient-echo sequence that employs a preparatory 180-degree RF pulse. An appropriate delay time is chosen for achieving T_1 contrast in which signal intensity of the myocardium is low, as is that of the underlying blood pool. Typically, one image is obtained in a given plane every cardiac cycle. Imaging is performed with a total number of measurements equal to 60 to 90. After ten heartbeats or images, the patient is instructed to hold his or her breath for as long as tolerated. At that time, MR contrast is injected as a bolus over 5 seconds (0.04 to 0.1 mmol/kg contrast dose).

Currently, imaging artifacts have been significantly reduced with the introduction of saturation recovery flash sequences. In the past, dark (low-signal) bands within the subendocardial region were typically found anteriorly and posteriorly on short-axis turbo flash images. This would result in erroneous diagnoses of subendocardial ischemia. When saturation recovery flash is implemented on high-gradient performance units (25 mT/m, 300- to 600-second rise times), three slices can be obtained in one heartbeat with either similar or different planes for extending the area of myocardium that is imaged. The parameters for the saturation recovery flash sequence are as follows: bw 780 Hz/px, 8-mm slice thickness, T_E 1.2 milliseconds. Currently, first-pass myocardial perfusion studies are performed at rest, and up to three slices per heartbeat may be obtained. However, with exercise or pharmacologically induced (dipyridamole or adenosine) stress, the increase in heart rate will reduce the number of slices per heartbeat. Furthermore, dyspnea may decrease the breath-holding capabilities. Thus, there are several technical difficulties that are encountered with stress-induced first-pass perfusion imaging and that render these studies suboptimal, requiring further technological improvements of MR hardware and software for clinical implementation.

Coronary Angiography

For imaging of the coronary arteries with a two-dimensional approach, segmented gradient echo pulse sequences with flow compensation along the readout and slice directions together with fat saturation are used (13–15). The sequence employs multiple-line acquisition per segment in a single breath-hold. The number of lines per segment varies from five to 11. The five-line-per-segment sequence has the shortest acquisition window, making it least sensitive to cardiac motion. However, the disadvantage of acquiring fewer lines per heartbeat is that more heartbeats are required to fill *k* space. As a rule of thumb, for higher patient heart rate (low R-R interval), use lower-line-per-segment sequences. As the R-R interval increases, use higher-line-per-segment sequences. Although the preliminary results of these breath-hold fat saturation sequences were promising, the misregistration between consecutive breath-holds results in suboptimal maximum-intensity projection (MIP). Thus, these single-slice/breath-hold sequences are becoming replaced with non-breath-hold three-dimensional fat saturation sequences that are respiratory compensated (16) using navigator echoes that detect diaphragm position. However, because of the three-dimensional slab acquisition, there are frequent saturation effects on the blood pool. Variable flip angle implementation, however, can increase blood pool signal. The future implementation of blood pool agents, however, should further increase the blood pool signal on these three-dimensional MRA studies. It should be noted that when two- or three-dimensional fat saturation coronary MRA is performed, adequate shimming is also essential for optimized fat suppression (Fig. 2.10).

Three-Dimensional Contrast-Enhanced Magnetic Resonance Angiography

Recently, ECG-triggered three-dimensional contrast-enhanced MRA employing a breath-held three-dimensional contrast-enhanced technique in a single breath hold was reported for evaluating coronary artery bypass graft (CABG) patency (17). This is a sequence that can also be applied for performing contrast-enhanced MRA of the thoracic aorta, pulmonary arteries, and thoracic systemic veins. Optimized results are obtained with implementation of body phased-array coils. A three-dimensional flash sequence is used. Artifacts related to breathing are eliminated with breath holding, and sensitivity to cardiac motion and vascular pulsation is minimized with ECG triggering. The parameters are as follows: T_R/T_E, 5/2 milliseconds, flip angle 14 degrees, matrix 256×96 to 124×256, slab thickness 100 to 110 mm, 20 to 24 partitions, and partition thickness of 2.5 to 3.5 mm. Triggering is to every R wave, and all lines of any given partition are filled in one R-R interval. There-

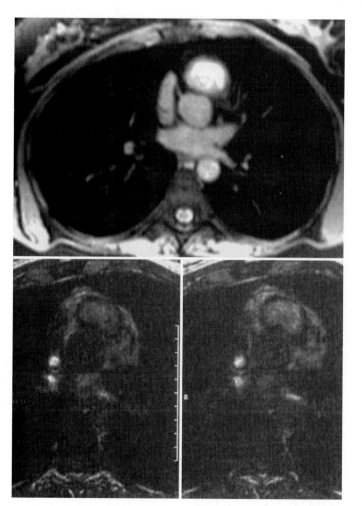

FIG. 2.10. Inappropriate shimming. The axial breath-hold fat saturation two-dimensional time-of-flight MR coronary angiogram in the upper image reveals the cardiac and coronary artery anatomy with appropriate suppression of fat and appropriate bright signal from the blood pool. This was obtained after appropriate shimming. With inadequate shimming and magnetic field inhomogeneity, the fat saturation pulse may be centered over the resonant frequency of water, and as a consequence, there will be suppression of blood pool signal with inadequate suppression of fat signal, as demonstrated in the lower images.

fore, the number of partitions dictates the number of heartbeats required to complete the acquisition. A triggered time delay of 50 to 250 milliseconds is used to drive the acquisition toward diastole. This further decreases artifacts related to cardiac motion and vascular pulsation because the acquisition is obtained during the quiescent phase of the cardiac cycle. The sum of the time delay and the number of lines multiplied by the T_R should always be kept slightly less than one R-R interval to avoid missing a heartbeat. Noncontrast imaging always precedes the contrast-enhanced sequence. The patient is hyperventilated, and subsequently, 0.1 to 0.2 mmol/kg of MR contrast is injected at a rate of 2 to 3 cc/sec. Scanning commences approximately 10 seconds after the start of the injection through an antecubital vein when thoracic aortic MRA is needed. For pulmonary angiography, scanning commences approximately 5 seconds after the onset of injection. Back-to-back measurements can be performed with interscan delays of 8 seconds, during which the patient exhales and then inhales and holds the breath for a second and third or fourth time. Delayed imaging is required for thoracic systemic venous visualization. Given the three-dimensional data set, multiplanar reformations can also be performed.

The ECG-triggered flash sequence described above is certainly a robust technique for imaging the intrathoracic vasculature with very few pulsation artifacts. However, with improved gradient performance where gradient rise times of 300 μsec can be achieved, the repetition time (T_R) and echo-time (T_E) can be decreased to 3.2 and 1.2 milliseconds, respectively. Furthermore, when the data in the Fourier domain are sync interpolated, the number of partitions is doubled, whereby individual three-dimensional partitions are reconstructed with a 50% overlap. This slice interpolation process significantly improves the MIP resolution in all projections. Furthermore, the reduction of T_R allows for a reduction in the imaging time for one three-dimensional acquisition. This is important in reducing the amount of contrast while preserving high vascular-to-background contrast. Finally, the short echo time of 1.2 milliseconds results in a moderate reduction of pulsation artifacts. Thus, the acquisition is not ECG triggered, allowing for a simple and more rapid protocol for MRA imaging than with ECG triggered acquisitions. For optimal contrast-to-noise, the flip angle at a T_R of 3.2 milliseconds was optimized with the Bloch equation at 25 to 30 degrees. If high-gradient performance (≤300 msec rise time gradients) is not available, the same sync interpolated sequence can be performed with slightly longer T_R/T_E values of 4.8 and 1.8 milliseconds, respectively, using 600-μsecond rise time gradients.

Additional General Artifacts

Metallic

Magnetic susceptibility artifact with resulting signal loss and distortion from underlying metallic implants is seen when the heart and great vessels are imaged with MRI and MRA techniques (Fig. 2.11). The artifacts are most prominent on gradient-echo and long-T_E sequences.

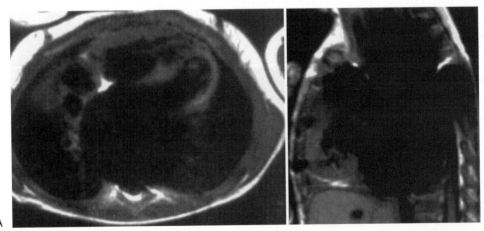

A

FIG. 2.11. Magnetic susceptibility artifacts. **A:** From Gianturco coils, transverse (left) and sagittal (right) images reveal a significant loss of signal in the posterior anatomy in this patient with tetralogy of Fallot who had the bronchial arterial vessels embolized with Gianturco coils. These coils are extremely ferromagnetic and result in significant signal loss, as demonstrated. **B:** From sutures, valve, or pacing wire, axial cine (upper two images) and black blood turbo spin-echo images (lower two images) reveal significant signal loss on the white blood cine images where the mitral valve prosthesis *(arrow),* sternal wire sutures *(curved arrow),* and epicardial pacing wire *(arrowhead)* were noted. Very little in the way of signal loss is noted on the turbo spin-echo images. **C:** From wire and clips, white blood axial cine and black blood HASTE images reveal significant focal signal loss from sternal wire sutures *(arrow)* and coronary artery bypass graft clips *(curved arrow)* on the cine images. Signal loss is absent on the black blood HASTE images. HASTE sequences routinely display the underlying anatomy with little in the way of signal loss from magnetic susceptibility artifact caused by metal hardware. This is related to the very long echo-train length.

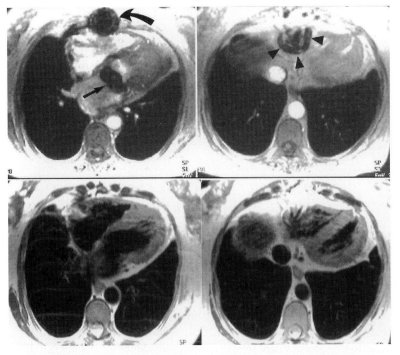

B

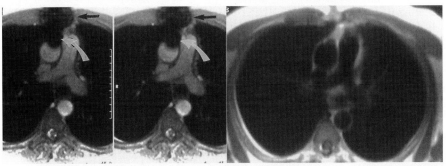

C

FIG. 2.11. *Continued.* **D:** From coronary stent, axial images (above) and short-axis (below) white blood cine images reveal a focal area of signal loss *(arrows)* along the course of the left anterior descending coronary artery. This focal signal loss results from the magnetic susceptibility artifact from a coronary artery stent. **E:** From wire and sutures, transverse breath-hold cine images in a patient following ascending aortic graft placement for type A dissection reveals focal signal loss from sternal wire sutures *(arrows).* The dissection flap *(curved arrow)* is noted to persist above the distal ascending aortic anastomosis **(upper image).** At the level of anastomosis, there is focal irregular signal loss surrounding the circumference of the aortic lumen as a result of suture artifact *(arrowheads)* **(lower image).** This should not be mistaken for pathology. This may be seen on white blood cine and on contrast-enhanced MRA sequences.

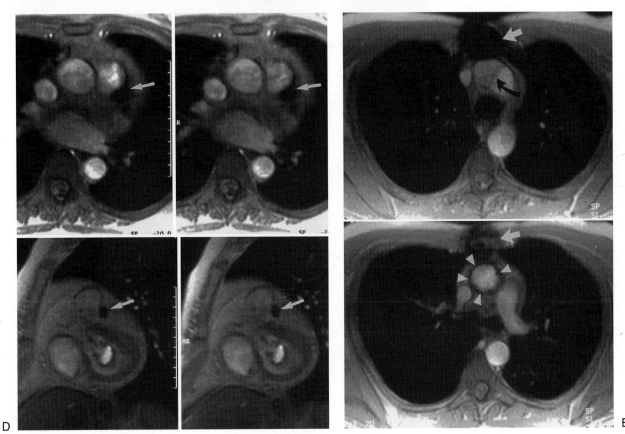

D

E

They are minimized by using turbo (FAST) spin-echo rather than conventional spin-echo sequences, by reducing the minimum T_E on T_1 and cine as well as in contrast-enhanced MRA sequences, and increasing the matrix and decreasing the slice thickness. It should be noted that HASTE sequences have the minimum signal loss among the variety of spin-echo sequences.

Respiratory

Respiratory motion artifacts (see Fig. 2.6) are seen with breath-hold sequences when either the data acquisition is begun before the patient began to breath-hold or when the patient terminates the breath-hold period during scan acquisition. With an external video camera, monitoring of the patient's ventilation can be achieved. Alternatively, a cup may be placed or taped on the patient's chest or abdomen for monitoring respiration. One can then monitor the onset of breath-hold for subsequent onset of a breath-hold sequence. If a patient is unable to hold his or her breath for the entire scan time of a breath-hold sequence, one can use rectangular field-of-view, reduce the number of phase-encode steps, or decrease the number of partitions in a three-dimensional slab. Real-time cine acquisitions in the future will require no breath-hold and may be used in patients who cannot hold the breath. Turbo spin-echo T_1-weighted sequences can also be employed with a higher number of acquisitions (five or six) to average out motion artifacts with signal averaging.

Aliasing

Oversampling techniques are used in the phase-encode direction to reduce the wraparound or aliasing artifacts of the extremities when performing thoracic MRI and MRA. Alternatively, one can increase the field-of-view or wrap the upper extremities with a radio frequency blanket.

ANATOMIC VARIATIONS AND DIAGNOSTIC PITFALLS

Congenital Heart Disease

Because of the high spatial resolution of spin-echo imaging, the anatomy and pathoanatomy of congenital heart defects (18,19) are routinely depicted. Following diagnosis of intracardiac shunts, MRI can accurately assess both pulmonic and aortic flow volumes, rendering effective right and left ventricular stroke volumes (20) for assessment of QP/QS and, subsequently, degree of intracardiac shunting. Finally, the postoperative status (21–23) of conduits, shunts and intra- and extracardiac anastomoses are routinely assessed throughout the patient's lifetime without the exposure to ionizing radiation. It is not the scope of this chapter to show the various congenital variations of the heart and great vessels because they are not normal variations. Variations in the appearance of the interatrial (Fig. 2.12) and interventricular (Fig. 2.13) septum are demonstrated. Diagnostic pitfalls related to intracardial shunts (Fig. 2.14) arise when, inappropri-

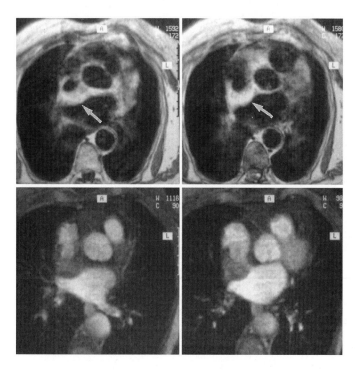

FIG. 2.12. Lipomatous hypertrophy or infiltration of the interatrial septum. Axial T_1-weighted images **(top)** reveal thickening of the interatrial septum *(arrows)* with high signal, which suppresses on the fat saturation breath-hold images demonstrated in lower two images. This is a frequent variation in the appearance of the interatrial septum and usually has no clinical significance.

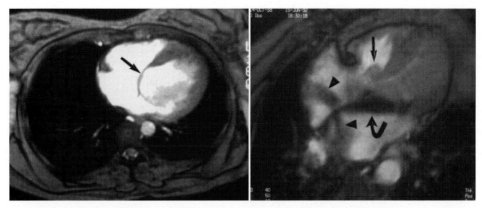

FIG. 2.13. Interventricular septal aneurysms. White blood transverse cine images in two different patients reveal diffuse large **(left image)** and small focal **(right image)** interventricular aneurysms *(arrows)* as a result of spontaneous closure of perimembranous intraventricular septal defects. Bulging is typically noted during the systolic phase, as demonstrated in these two patients. Incidentally noted in the **right image** is mitral insufficiency *(curved arrow)* and a bidirectional atrial septal defect *(arrowheads).*

ately, a lower T_E cine sequence is chosen. Figure 2.15 demonstrates the potential pitfall of confusing cases of pulmonary atresia for truncus arteriosus. Figure 2.16 shows a case of potentially misdiagnosing the presence of a pulmonary sling on sagittal imaging.

Tumors/Thrombi

Cardiac tumors and thrombi are more readily evaluated with MRI than with other modalities. MRI is not only accurate for the diagnosis of tumors (24–27) and thrombi (28) but it remains as one of the better modalities for differentiation of the two (29). A contrast-enhanced ECG-triggered

three-dimensional gradient-echo sequence is faster and more robust than cine imaging and eliminates spin saturation effects that are problematic with cine MRI (Fig. 2.17). Additional variations and diagnostic pitfalls when assessing the heart for underlying mass lesions are illustrated in Figs. 2.18 through 2.20.

Pericardial Disease

The findings of constrictive physiology following cardiac catheterization are frequently nonspecific, and the differential diagnosis of constrictive pericarditis versus restrictive cardiomyopathy is frequently raised. Abnormally thickened pericardium can be diagnosed with MRI in

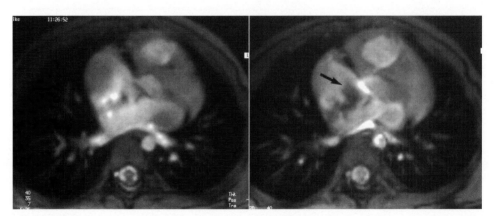

FIG. 2.14. Turbulent flow. Transverse cine images in a patient with a secundum atrial septal defect reveal very little signal loss in the left image, which was obtained with an echo time of 6 milliseconds. The signal loss *(arrow)* is better appreciated in the **right image** when an echo time of 12 milliseconds was employed. The longer echo time allows for more time for spin-dephasing effects to take place and is required to consistently detect intracardiac shunts or turbulent flow from stenosis.

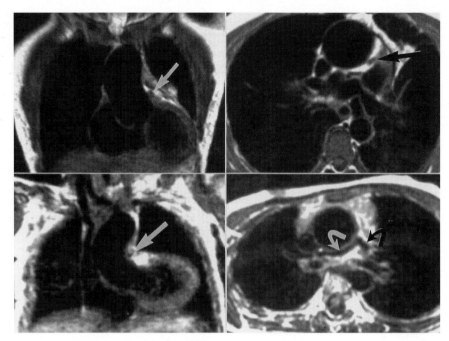

FIG. 2.15. Differentiation of pulmonary atresia from truncus arteriosus. Coronal and axial images demonstrated in two different patients, both with pulmonary atresia, could be mistaken for truncus arteriosus if one does not closely inspect for the presence of the atretic main and central pulmonary arteries. Both cases reveal the very diminutive main pulmonary artery *(arrows).*

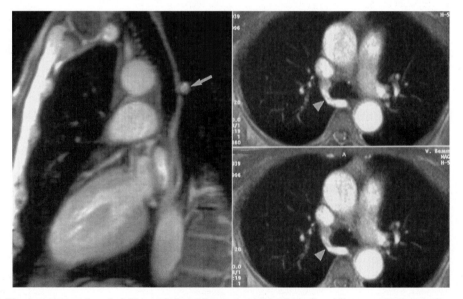

FIG. 2.16. Azygous vein mimicking a left pulmonary artery sling. An oblique sagittal two-dimensional time-of-flight breath-hold image in the chest reveals a vascular structure *(arrow)* posterior to the trachea. This is a typical location for a pulmonary artery sling; however, axial imaging reveals continuity of this with the azygous arch *(arrowheads).*

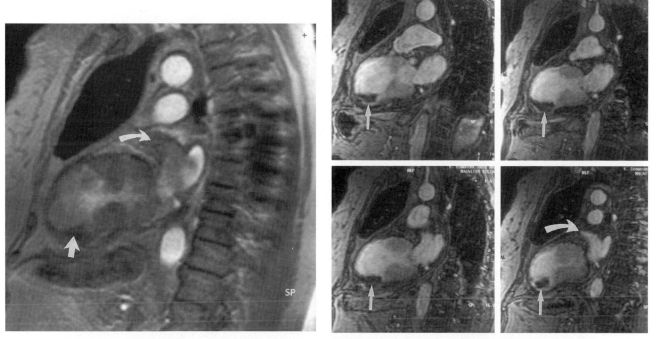

A   B

FIG. 2.17. Pitfalls of cine MRI in evaluation of mass lesions. **A:** Vertical long-axis cine image demonstrates significant blood pool saturation effects resulting in obscuration of thrombus in the apical left ventricular aneurysm *(arrow)*. In addition, saturation of blood pool signal in the left atrial appendage *(curved arrow)* leads to a false impression of underlying thrombus. **B:** Contrast-enhanced three-dimensional ECG-triggered flash results in a significant enhancement of the blood pool and clear visualization of a left ventricular thrombus *(arrows)* and normal left atrial appendage *(curved arrow)*.

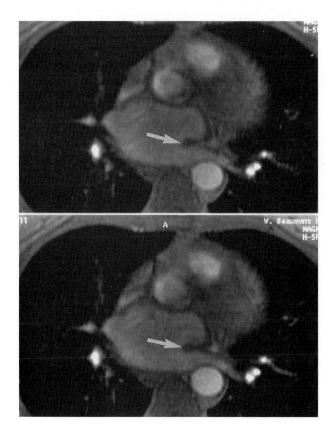

FIG. 2.18. Left inferior pulmonary vein inflow pseudomass. Two axial cine images reveal prominence of the left atrial wall *(arrows)* at the inflow of the inferior pulmonary vein on the left. This may at times be more prominent and present as a small mass-like lesion. It should not be confused with a tumor or thrombus. This is also demonstrated in Fig. 2.5.

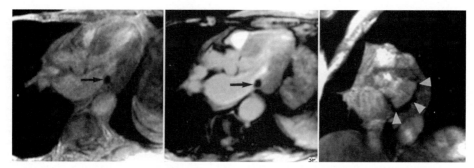

FIG. 2.19. Calcified mitral annulus simulating a thrombus. Horizontal long-axis cine **(left)** and contrast-enhanced MRA **(middle)** demonstrate a low signal intensity rounded focal area *(arrows)* near the posterior mitral valve leaflet that can be mistaken for a small thrombus. This, however, can be identified on multiple images extending from the heart superiorly toward the inferior aspect of the heart and is best appreciated *(arrowheads)* as a calcified mitral annulus on short-axis imaging **(right).**

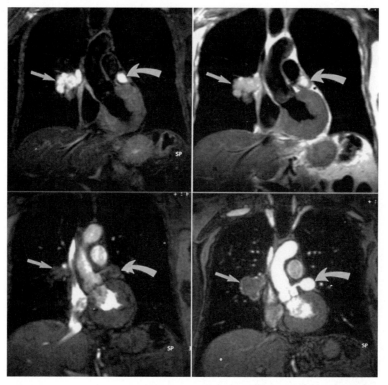

FIG. 2.20. Slow flow mimicking a mass. Coronal turbo STIR **(left)** and T$_2$-weighted turbo spin-echo **(upper right)** reveal a right middle lobe carcinoma *(arrows)* with mediastinal invasion. Both images also reveal a high-signal-intensity lesion inferior and lateral to the main pulmonary artery, which was initially interpreted as a contralateral metastasis *(curved arrows)*. The coronal cine image **(lower left)** revealed low signal and, therefore, the possibility of a mass *(curved arrow)*. This, however, represents slow flow within a left coronary aneurysm. The slow flow presents as high signal on STIR and T$_2$ turbo spin-echo sequences and low signal on the cine sequences. It is confirmed as a coronary aneurysm *(curved arrow)* following a three-dimensional contrast-enhanced MRA **(lower right).**

patients with constrictive pericarditis (30). In addition, MRI is useful in the diagnosis and differentiation of pericardial tumors and cysts (31). Diagnostic pitfalls usually arise when the pericardium is calcified and of normal thickness (<3 mm) on MRI (Fig. 2.21). Pericardial fluid spin saturation can mimic hemorrhage on cine MRI (Fig. 2.22).

Valvular Disease

Cine MRI consistently displays the signal void in areas of turbulent flow related to either valvular stenosis or insufficiency (32,33). The size of signal loss is dependent on the degree of turbulent flow and on the echo time that is chosen (Fig. 2.23). Following diagnosis of valvular stenosis or insufficiency, velocity-encoded cine MRI (34) can be performed for measurement of peak velocities through areas of stenosis. The effective right and left ventricular stroke volumes are also obtained by measuring flow volumes in the pulmonary artery and aorta, respectively. This technique allows one to calculate regurgitant fractions in patients with single-valve insufficiency. Alternatively, retrograde flow in the aorta can be assessed

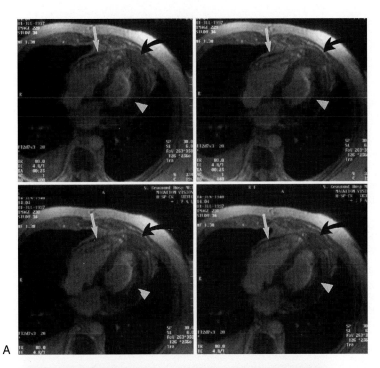

A

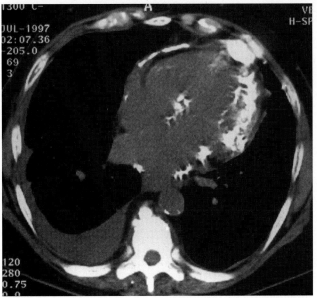

B

FIG. 2.21. Pericardial and myocardial calcification pitfall on MRI. **A:** Transverse cine images reveal slight thickening of the anterior pericardium *(arrows),* which has low signal, as well as an intermediate elliptical mass *(curved arrows)* at the apex of the heart. Vague ill-defined low signal *(arrowheads)* is also noted in the myocardium. **B:** Although, constrictive pericarditis was suspected on the MRI study, the extent of pericardial disease was better appreciated on the non-contrast-enhanced CT. In addition, there is extensive myocardial calcification, which was undetected on MRI.

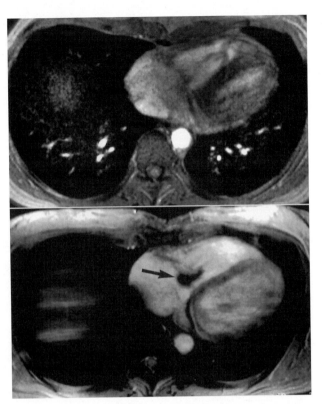

FIG. 2.23. Valve insufficiency and appropriate echo time implementation. The breath-hold transverse cine MR image **(upper image)** was acquired with an echo time of 6 milliseconds, and the non-breath-hold conventional cine MR image **(lower image)** was acquired with an echo time of 12 milliseconds. Turbulent flow as a result of tricuspid insufficiency *(arrow)* results in a loss of signal because of spin-dephasing effects, and this will be more prevalent with a longer echo time. Such abnormal flow turbulence may go undetected with the implementation of shorter echo time breath-hold cine studies. The other factor in nonvisualization of the signal loss from turbulent flow in the upper image is the flow compensation used in the read and slice directions.

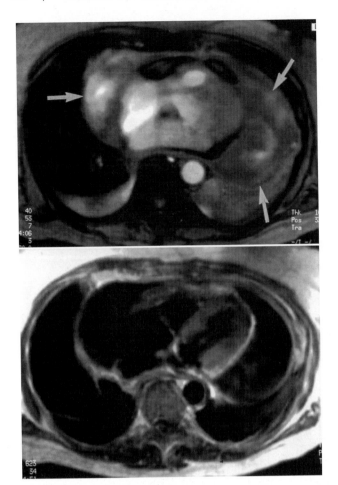

FIG. 2.22. Pericardial fluid spin saturation mimicking hemorrhagic effusion on cine MRI. A transverse cine MR image **(upper image)** reveals a gross pericardial effusion *(arrows)*. Much of the effusion, especially on the left, is of low signal; however, this is not from the magnetic susceptibility artifacts of hemorrhage, but rather, it is from spin saturation effects of this fluid on gradient-echo cine imaging. The fluid demonstrates dark signal on T_1-weighted sequences **(lower image)**.

with a through-plane velocity-encoded sequence for measurement of aortic insufficiency. Breath-hold cine and breath-hold turbo (FAST) spin-echo sequences are currently providing exquisite detail of leaflet anatomy. Variations and pitfalls related to valvular disease are shown in Figs. 2.24 and 2.25.

Myocardial Disease

There are a number of myocardial disorders (35–39) that have been evaluated with MRI, and applications are rapidly expanding. In the evaluation of patients with ischemic heart disease, one needs to assess global and regional myocardial function, and this is performed with conventional or breath-hold cine sequences. Cine

sequences with myocardial tagging (7,8,40–43) further delineate areas of wall motion abnormality. This is followed by tissue characterization with T_2-weighted images to denote the presence of myocardial edema and injury from either ischemic or reperfusion insult. However, the depiction of increased signal on T_2-weighted and/or contrast-enhanced T_1-weighted sequences does not imply irreversible injury or myocardial necrosis (Fig. 2.26). The issue of tissue viability (44) can be further pursued with first-pass myocardial perfusion (32,33) imaging using gadolinium chelate contrast agents. Myocardial infarction (irreversible myocardial injury) and chronic scar will lack first-pass perfusion whereas viable (reversible injury) myocardium will have preserved or only mildly decreased perfusion. Complications of myocardial infarction such as true and false aneurysms and underlying thrombi are also routinely assessed. A number of diag-

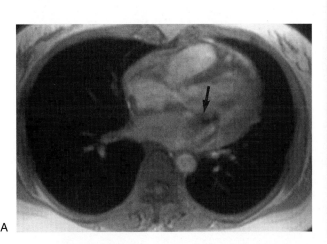
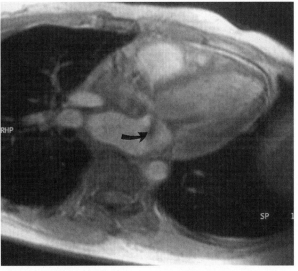

A   B

FIG. 2.24. Double-orifice mitral valve mimicking mitral insufficiency. **A:** An axial cine MR image demon-strates apparent mitral insufficiency *(arrow)*. **B:** The valve leaflets are further interrogated with the hor-izontal long-axis cine image and reveal a defect in the anteromitral valve leaflet representing a hole-type double-orifice mitral valve. The insufficiency *(curved arrow)* was not through the mitral valve orifice. It was through the defect in the anterior mitral valve leaflet.

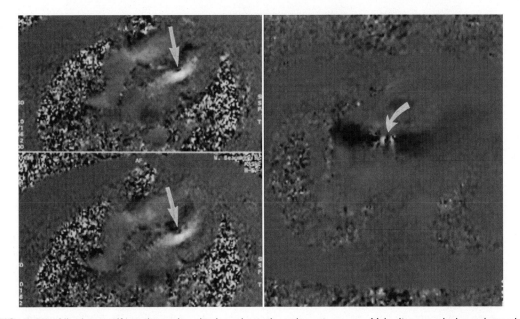

FIG. 2.25. Aliasing artifact through mitral and aortic valve stenoses. Velocity-encoded or dynamic phase-contrast cine MRI **(left images)** through an area of mitral stenosis *(arrows)* as well as through an area of aortic valve stenosis *(curved arrow)* **(right)** reveal a speckled appearance to the signal on the phase images because of aliasing artifact as a result of choosing a velocity-encoding value much lower than the actual flow velocity that was interrogated.

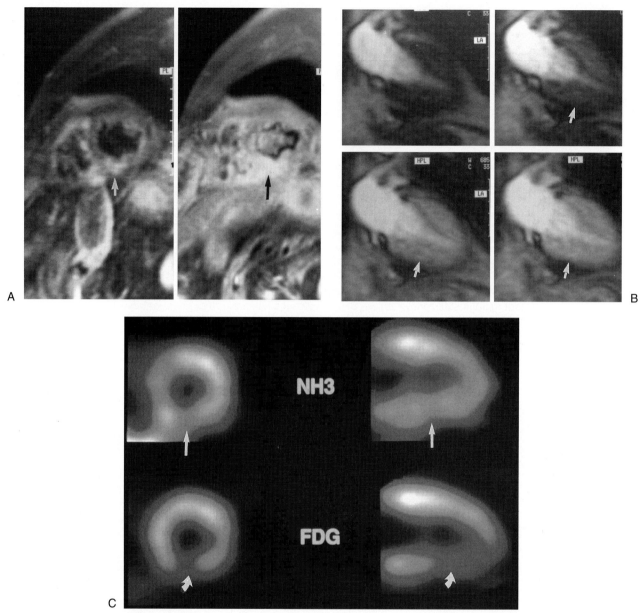

FIG. 2.26. Stunned myocardium, not myocardial infarction. **A:** Short-axis T$_2$- **(left)** and contrast-enhanced T$_1$-weighted **(right)** images were obtained after early reperfusion of an occluded right coronary artery. A focal area of increased signal is seen in the inferior wall *(arrows),* which denotes the region of myocardial injury from ischemia and reperfusion injury. This, however, does not correspond to the zone of myocardial infarction (necrosis). **B:** On first-pass perfusion, there is preserved perfusion indicative of intact microvasculature. **C:** The ^{13}N-ammonia and ^{18}F-FDG scan demonstrate discordant areas of diminished uptake compatible with a pattern of myocardial stunning (decreased metabolism on the ^{18}F-FDG image with preserved perfusion on the ^{13}N perfusion image). A follow-up cine study demonstrated improvement of regional function, confirming the diagnosis of myocardial stunning. This diagnosis is made with MRI by denoting the presence of intact perfusion despite increased signal on T$_2$-weighted or contrast-enhanced T$_1$-weighted images.

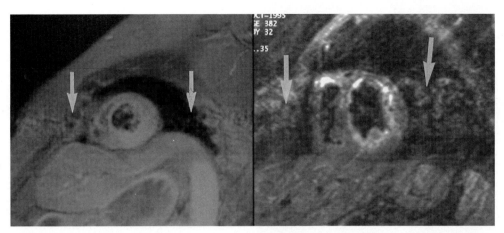

FIG. 2.27. Cardiac pulsation artifacts. Short-axis contrast-enhanced T$_1$- **(left)** and T$_2$-weighted ECG-triggered short-axis spin-echo images with fat saturation **(right)** reveal a moderate amount of pulsation artifact *(arrows)* in the phase-encode direction. These pulsation artifacts can significantly degrade image quality and visualization of underlying myocardial infarction. The breath-hold black blood preparation sequences described in the text currently have markedly reduced the blood pool signal and corresponding phase-encoded ghost artifacts.

nostic pitfalls such as cardiac perfusion artifacts, pitfalls related to turbo-flash perfusion, etc., are shown in Figs. 2.27 through 2.30.

Coronary and Coronary Artery Bypass Graft Angiography

Multiple institutions are currently active in developing MR coronary angiography (13–15,45). Preliminary results are promising for depicting the proximal and even distal anatomy. With phase-modulation techniques, coronary blood flow velocities can be assessed during rest and under adenosine stress. This may allow for a physiologic quantification of the degree of coronary stenosis. Currently, coronary imaging and flow mapping require further improvement of signal-to-noise, temporal, and spatial resolution, because there are frequent pitfalls such as partial volume average phenomenon as a vessel courses

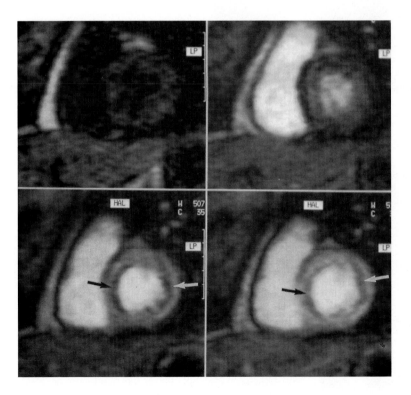

FIG. 2.28. Turbo-flash perfusion pitfall. Short-axis turbo-flash images at the same slice position following intravenous contrast administration reveal subendocardial dark zones *(arrows)* anteriorly and posteriorly within the myocardium. These, however, do not represent subendocardial ischemia or infarction in this patient, who had a normal cardiac catheterization, normal sestamibi perfusion scintigraphy, and normal PET perfusion examination. This phenomenon is related to the rapid changes of T$_1$ relaxation and also to motion, as it is seen anteriorly and posteriorly in the phase-encode direction. The development of saturation recovery flash sequences has virtually eliminated this artifact.

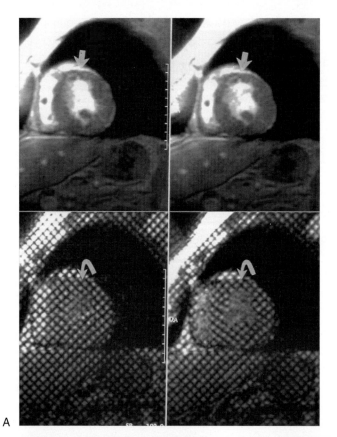

A

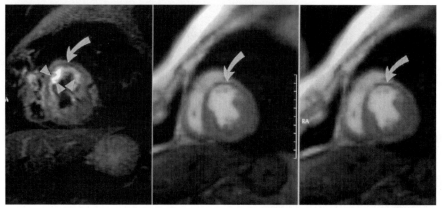

B

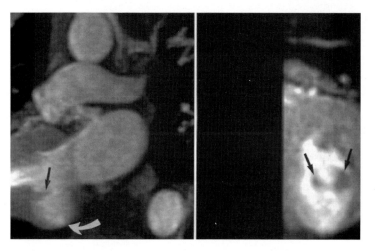

FIG. 2.29. Slow flow resulting in overestimation of wall thickness on myocardial tagging (SPAMM). **A:** Short-axis systolic cine MR images **(top two)** reveal the true thickness of the anterior wall *(arrows)* of the myocardium. Because of sluggish flow in the subendocardial region of the anteromyocardium as a result of a chronic anteromyocardial infarction, the myocardial tag *(curved arrows)* does not dissipate on the systolic time frames on the myocardial tag study **(bottom two).** Consequently, this can lead to overestimation of wall thickness on myocardial tag studies, and one needs to carefully evaluate the cine, STIR, and first-pass perfusion examination. **B:** Short-axis STIR **(left)** and short-axis first-pass perfusion images **(middle and right)** reveal marked thinning of the anterior wall *(curved arrows)*. The high signal *(arrowheads)* noted on the STIR image represents sluggish flow. This area enhances on the perfusion images postcontrast, indicating lumen and not anterior myocardial wall.

FIG. 2.30. False impression of pseudoaneurysm of the heart. Vertical long-axis contrast-enhanced MRA of the heart **(left)** reveals an aneurysm at the base of the heart *(curved arrow)*. This is a classic location for false or pseudoaneurysms related to periinfarction rupture of myocardium. These require surgical treatment, and the diagnosis is suspected because of the apparent narrow neck leading into this aneurysm compared to the widest diameter of the aneurysm. This case, in fact, is giving a false impression of a pseudoaneurysm and is related to the overlying posteromedial papillary muscle *(arrow)*. A short-axis multiplanar reformation **(right)** through the three-dimensional data set reveals the true size of the aneurysm neck, which is quite wide and, therefore, renders the diagnosis of a true aneurysm, which does not require surgical treatment. This was confirmed at cardiac catheterization. It should be noted that it was not detected on spin-echo images because of the slow flow within the aneurysm, resulting in increased signal. In addition, because of the sluggish flow and spin-saturation effects, it was not readily identified on cine MRI. Posterior papillary muscles *(arrows)*.

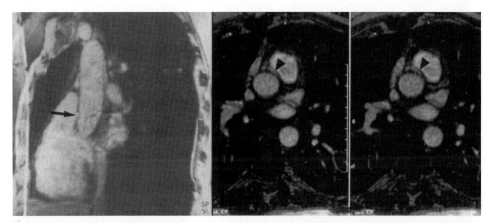

FIG. 2.31. Slow flow in anomalous left main coronary artery. A sagittal breath-hold two-dimensional time-of-flight fat saturation image reveals the anomalous left coronary artery *(arrow)* as it courses between the main pulmonary artery and the ascending aorta. It was only seen on this two-dimensional time-of-flight technique when the imaging plane was perpendicular to the anomalous vessel. Axial imaging did not show the anomalous coronary artery. Likewise, axial three-dimensional time-of-flight navigator coronary MRA with fat suppression did not demonstrate the anomalous coronary artery. It is seen on axial imaging **(two right images)** *(arrowheads)* when a three-dimensional contrast-enhanced MRA sequence is employed. The diagnosis was made only with the contrast-enhanced sequence. Ordinarily, two- and three-dimensional time-of-flight coronary MRA techniques depict the proximal course of anomalous coronary arteries; however, in this case, only the three-dimensional contrast-enhanced MRA sequence made the diagnosis.

in and out of the section plane. Although MR coronary angiography is not performed clinically for ischemic heart disease, it is considered the gold standard for depicting the proximal course of anomalous left coronary arteries. One should be careful with two- and three-dimensional-TOF techniques since with slow and/or in-plane flow, signal can become saturated (Fig. 2.31). Also, fluid in the pericardial space may be mistaken for epicardial coronary vessels (Fig. 2.32). A variety of diagnostic pitfalls related to coronary artery disease (Figs. 2.33 and 2.34), and coronary artery bypass graft imaging (Fig. 2.35 and 2.36) are illustrated here.

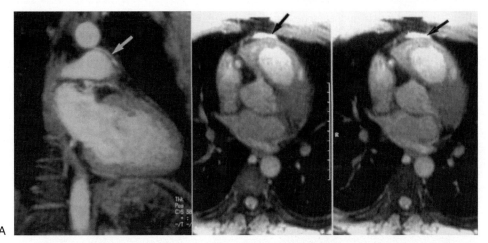

FIG. 2.32. Pericardial fluid mimicking epicardial coronary vasculature. **A:** Vertical long-axis **(left)** and axial two-dimensional time-of-flight fat saturation breath-hold **(middle and right)** coronary MRA images reveal several areas of increased signal overlying the heart and great vessels that are related to small amounts of pericardial fluid *(arrows)*. This should not be mistaken for epicardial or anomalous coronary arteries. *Continued on next page.*

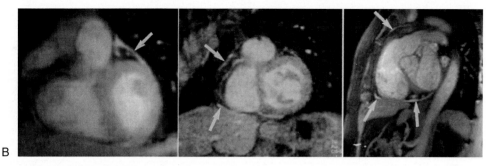

B

FIG. 2.32. *Continued.* **B:** Similar pericardial fluid *(arrows)* is denoted on various planes of short-axis MRA images.

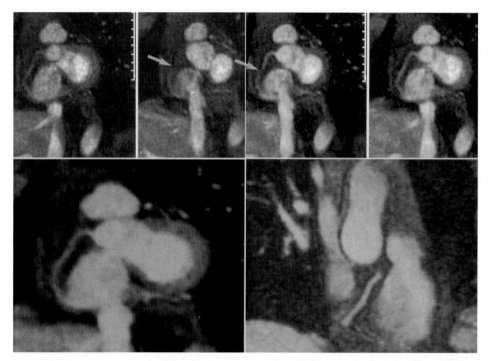

FIG. 2.33. Coronary artery pseudostenoses on single breath-hold two-dimensional coronary MRA. Serial breath-hold two-dimensional fat saturation coronary MRA images through the right coronary artery depict areas of signal loss *(arrows)* as a result of the course of the vessel out of the plane of imaging. When viewed on cine mode, this is more apparent. Likewise, if there is no misregistration between the breath-hold slices, maximum-intensity projection **(lower left)** reveals a normal course and caliber of the coronary artery. In addition, oblique imaging parallel with the vessel **(lower right)** reveals the normal caliber of the coronary artery. The coronary arteries are frequently tortuous and will course in and out of an imaging plane, and this pitfall is, therefore, quite frequent, requiring additional postprocessing and/or imaging planes.

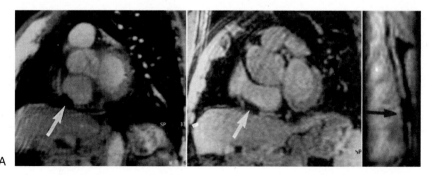

A

FIG. 2.34. Coronary artery MRA pitfalls. **A:** Pseudostenosis as a result of coronary artery stent. Two- **(left)** and three-dimensional **(middle)** coronary MRA images reveal focal signal loss *(arrows)* in the distal right coronary artery. This is also noted on the oblique multiplanar reformation **(right).** The patient has a history of a distal right coronary stent, and this represents signal loss from the magnetic susceptibility artifact of the stent. It should not be confused with a focal stenosis. *Continued on next page.*

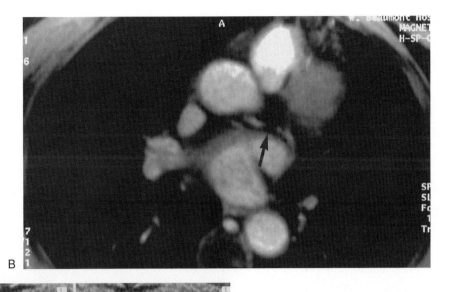

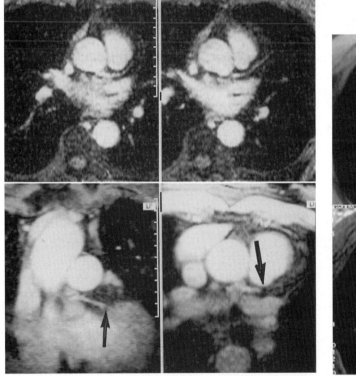

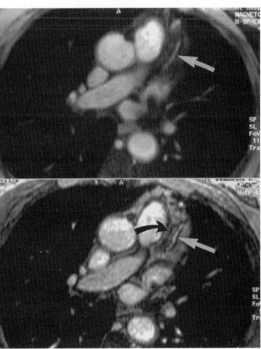

FIG. 2.34. *Continued.* **B:** Disease overgrading. An axial two-dimensional fat-suppressed coronary artery MRA image reveals focal signal loss *(arrow)* in the left circumflex coronary artery. The complete signal loss would suggest occlusion; however, on cardiac catheterization, this represented a severe to critical stenosis. This results in spin dephasing on this time-of-flight technique and overestimation of disease severity. **C:** Overgrading of coronary stenosis. Axial breath-hold two-dimensional coronary artery fat-suppressed MRA **(upper images)** reveal a normal left anterior descending (LAD) coronary artery following angioplasty of a critical stenosis of the LAD. The coronal and axial coronary artery MRA **(lower images)** obtained before the angioplasty reveal abrupt cutoff *(arrows)* of the left anterior descending coronary artery with loss of signal beyond this site. The MRA diagnosis of occlusion was prospectively made. Because of the critical stenosis, there was an extremely sluggish flow beyond the lesion resulting in spin saturation effects on this time-of-flight technique and nonvisualization of the lumen. Perhaps a contrast-enhanced MRA study would obviate this pitfall. **D:** False-positive impression of coronary artery patency. An axial fat-suppressed two-dimensional coronary artery MRA (upper image) reveals apparent patency of the left anterior descending coronary artery. This, however, represents the patent great cardiac vein *(arrows)* and the adjacent LAD as seen on three-dimensional contrast-enhanced MRA without fat suppression is actually occluded *(curved arrow)* **(lower image).**

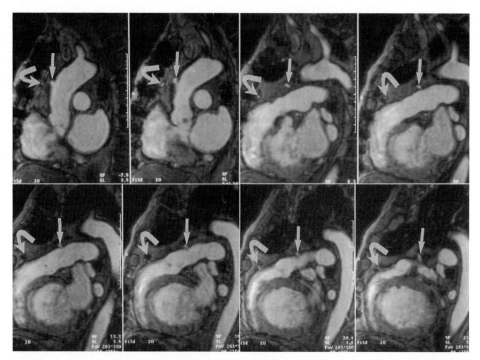

FIG. 2.35. Coronary artery bypass graft metallic clip artifacts obscuring vein graft anatomy. Serial three-dimensional contrast-enhanced partitions reveal a vein graft to the left circumflex coronary artery *(arrows)* and an internal mammary artery graft *(curved arrows)* to the LAD. The LAD mammary graft is obscured in multiple images by the overlying metal clip artifact. This should not be mistaken for focal stenosis. The reappearance of the graft on subsequent partitions indicates patency. Certainly, it is difficult to differentiate true stenoses from metallic clip artifacts; however, metallic clip artifacts usually are larger than the lumen of the graft because of the blooming effects of the magnetic susceptibility artifact. The artifacts, however, are greatly diminished on current sequences, which employ shorter echo times. This study was performed with a T_E of 2 milliseconds, and even the metallic artifact can be further reduced with the reduction of the T_E values to 1.2 milliseconds.

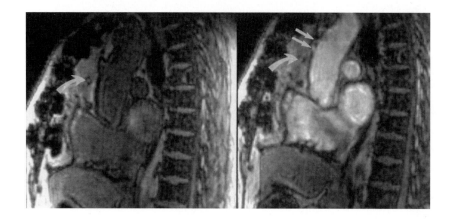

FIG. 2.36. False-positive diagnosis of patent vein graft. The contrast-enhanced three-dimensional MRA partition on the right reveals enhancing vein grafts *(arrows)*. The LAD vein graft *(curved arrow)* also shows high signal intensity; however, this is of high signal on the precontrast image and did not increase in signal-to-noise ratio following postcontrast. It represents an occluded vein graft that was misdiagnosed as a patent vein graft. One should, therefore, pay particular attention to the precontrast studies to avoid this pitfall.

Thoracic Aorta

The most common applications of MR imaging of the thoracic aorta involve work-up of congenital and acquired abnormalities. Congenital anomalies such as interruption of the aorta, double aortic arch, and coarctation are routinely assessed. The site of coarctation is depicted with exquisite detail utilizing spin-echo and cine MR imaging and the pressure gradient can be assessed by measuring peak velocity through the area of stenosis utilizing velocity-encoded cine MRI. However, with the development of significant collateral flow, one may not detect a pressure gradient through a severe stenosis (Fig. 2.37). The combination of spin-echo and cine MRI for evaluating thoracic aortic dissection virtually has a 100% accuracy (46,47). Currently, evaluation of aortic dissection is rendered faster with breath hold cine sequences. Diagnostic pitfalls for aortic dissection are shown in Figs. 2.38 through 2.42.

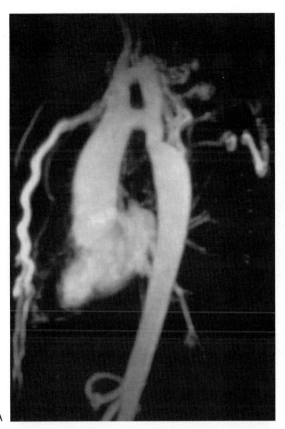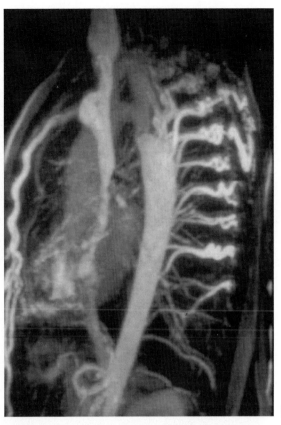

A

B

FIG. 2.37. Significant coarctation lacking pressure gradient because of collaterals. **A,B:** Sagittal three-dimensional contrast-enhanced MRA images during early and late phase reveal a significant coarctation of the aorta with enlarged internal mammary arteries and intercostal collateral arteries. The significant collateral circulation is noted on the late contrast-enhanced MRA, which reconstitutes the descending thoracic aorta beyond the coarctation. The ascending aorta has washed out, but the descending aorta remains enhanced with more prominent collateral circulation identified. As a result of the reconstitution from significant collateralization, a pressure gradient could not be measured with very careful interrogation of the coarctation site. Velocity-encoded cine MRI was performed in plane and through plane, and flow velocities were not significantly elevated. This should not denote an insignificant coarctation. These collateral vessels are currently identified with exquisite vascular-to-background contrast, given the subtraction technique of the time-resolved turbo MRA sequences.

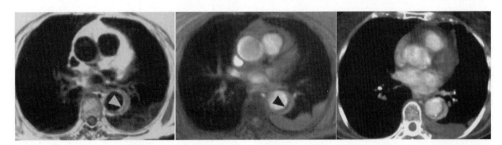

FIG. 2.38. Subtle aortic wall hematoma (atypical dissection) and pseudo-aortic wall thickening from atelectasis. Transverse T_1 **(left)** and cine MRI **(middle)** reveal moderate thickening of the aortic wall that is crescentic in nature. There is a left-sided pleural effusion. The T_1-weighted sequences reveal a subtle area of increased signal near the intima *(arrowhead)* on T_1 that is part of the dark signal on the cine image. The possibility of a very small aortic wall hematoma was raised, rendering a possible diagnosis of atypical dissection. The contrast-enhanced CT study **(right)**, however, demonstrates that the bulk of this aortic wall thickening represents enhancing subjacent atelectasis, and the atypical dissection with intramural hematoma is actually quite thin in nature. The proof of atypical dissection was made on a follow-up MRI examination, which revealed conversion into a communicating and more classic-appearing dissection.

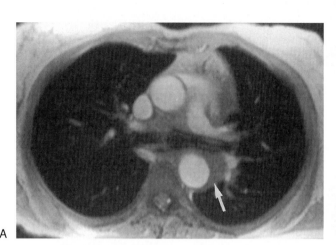
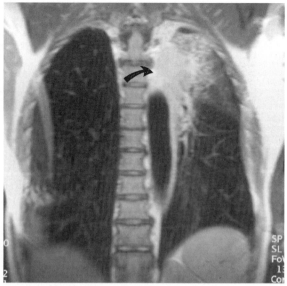

FIG. 2.39. Pseudodissection from mediastinal lymphoma. **A:** The axial cine MR image reveals moderate crescentic thickening *(arrow)* of the descending thoracic aorta, which has the appearance of aortic wall hematoma mimicking atypical/noncommunicating aortic dissection. **B:** Multiplanar imaging and more careful examination of the extent of this apparent aortic wall thickening reveals a large supra-aortic mass *(curved arrow)* related to non-Hodgkin's lymphoma. The differential diagnosis for aortic wall thickening also includes Takayasu's arteritis and thrombus from aneurysm.

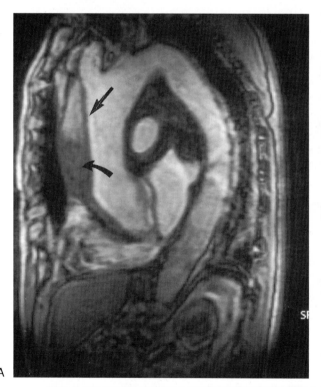
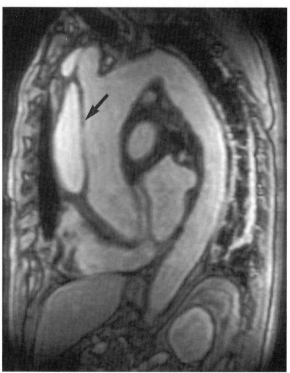

FIG. 2.40. Pseudothrombosis of false channel. Contrast-enhanced three-dimensional sagittal MRA partitions in a patient with type A dissection involving the ascending aorta reveals an intimal flap *(arrows)*. **A:** On the early contrast-enhanced MRA study performed approximately 10 to 15 seconds after onset of injection, decreased signal *(curved arrow)* was noted in the anterior false channel, which could be misdiagnosed as thrombosis of the false channel. For this reason, it is routine to repeat a breath-hold acquisition after the early immediate postcontrast acquisition to avoid this pitfall. **B:** The later contrast-enhanced MRA study reveals early washout of the true channel and persistent more intense enhancement of the false channel.

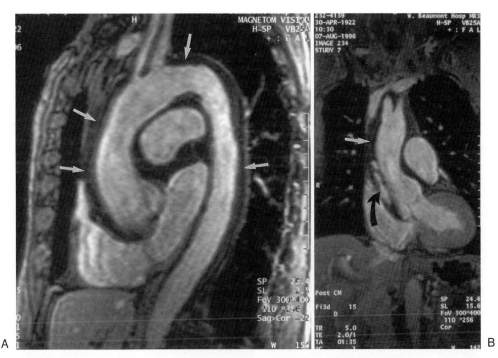

FIG. 2.41. Pseudothrombosis of false channel. Sagittal **(A)** and coronal **(B)** contrast-enhanced three-dimensional MRA of the thoracic aorta shows near-complete thrombosis of the false channel *(arrows)*. The residual patent false lumen *(curved arrow)* is seen only on the coronal acquisition. For this reason, it is routine to image the aorta with coronal as well as sagittal three-dimensional MRA. Alternatively, axial multiplanar reformations can be performed to evaluate the aortic lumen in a second plane.

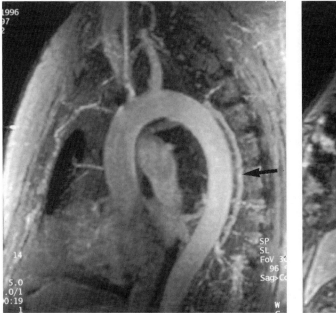
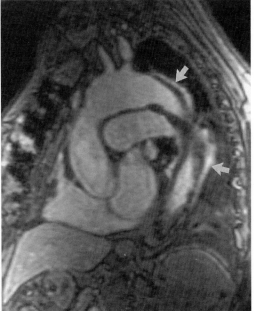

FIG. 2.42. Pseudodissection. **A:** Because of the azygous vein, sagittal three-dimensional contrast-enhanced MRA in this patient with a right aortic arch and right descent of the descending aorta reveals the appearance of a dissection related to the adjacent azygous vein *(arrow)*. Axial imaging revealed the right aortic arch and descent and avoided this potential pitfall of aortic dissection. **B:** As a result of enhancing atelectasis, sagittal contrast-enhanced three-dimensional MRA partition reveals apparent true and false lumina. The apparent false lumen is an effect of contrast enhancement of adjacent atelectasis *(arrows),* and careful examination of all partitions in various planes is required to avoid this potential pitfall.

The MRI is also accurate for assessing the size, location, and relationships of thoracic aortic aneurysms and penetrating atherosclerotic ulcers; however, with slow flow, ulcers may go undetected on spin-echo and cine sequences because of higher blood pool signal and spin saturation effects, respectively. Furthermore, it is imperative to evaluate the source data of contrast-enhanced MRA studies because the MIP process can obscure dissection flaps (Fig. 2.43) or underlying thrombus (Fig. 2.44) within aneurysms.

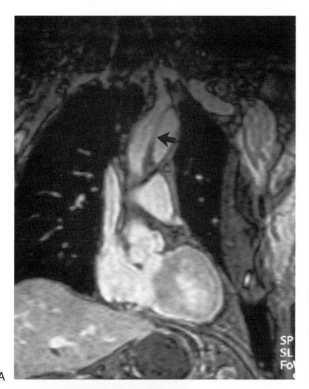

A

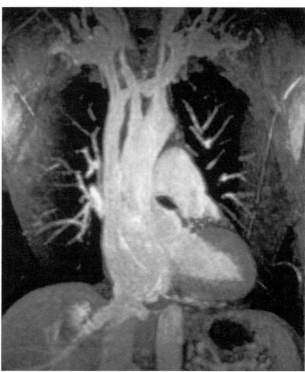

B

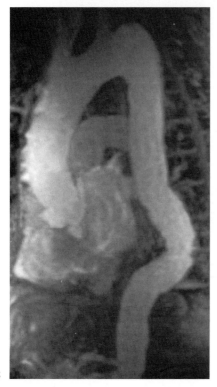

C

FIG. 2.43. False-negative impression of dissection on maximum-intensity projection and sagittal three-dimensional MRA. Coronal three-dimensional contrast-enhanced MRA **(A)** reveals a dissection flap in the ascending aorta *(arrow)* that is obscured on the MIP image shown in **B. C:** The sagittal three-dimensional contrast-enhanced MRA study does not reveal the intimal flap because the plane of acquisition was parallel with the intimal flap. It is for this reason that coronal MRI and/or three-dimensional contrast-enhanced MRA sequences are needed to avoid missing a dissection. The intimal flap in this patient was identified only on the coronal acquisition. Furthermore, it is important to review the source data for diagnosing the presence of a dissection.

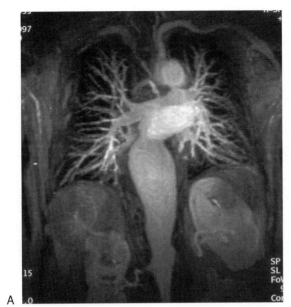 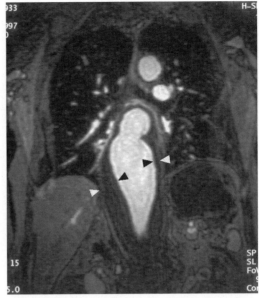

FIG. 2.44. Aneurysm underestimation on maximum-intensity projection. **A:** A coronal maximum-intensity projection image in a patient with a thoracoabdominal aortic aneurysm underestimates the size of the aneurysm because the thrombus does not project on the maximum-intensity projection process. **B:** It is imperative in aneurysm evaluations with contrast-enhanced MRA to also evaluate the source data for accurate measurement of aortic aneurysm size and extent. The thrombosed (arrowheads) part of the aneurysm is best depicted in **B.**

Pulmonary Artery

Both MRI and MRA of the pulmonary arterial circulation have been described in the evaluation of congenital abnormalities, thromboembolic pulmonary disease, hypertensive pulmonary arterial disease and neoplastic disease. Variations of signal on spin-echo sequences are noted to occur, especially when multislice-multiphase imaging is performed. As noted, increased signal within the blood pool can be identified if the phase-encode steps for a particular slice are obtained during the diastolic phase of the cardiac cycle. This increased signal could be mistaken for intraluminal thrombus. Cine MRI could be performed along with contrast-enhanced MRA to confirm the presence of underlying thromboembolic disease. With respect to congenital pulmonary arterial abnormalities, certain pitfalls arise, especially when the central pulmonary arteries cannot be detected. The differential would include pulmonary atresia/pulmonary stenosis versus truncus arteriosus, and careful attention is needed to identify the atretic pulmonary arteries in cases of pulmonary atresia (see Fig. 2.22). With contrast-enhanced MRA using centric reordering, if the data acquisition is not appropriately timed, central low-signal artifact is noted. With respect to thromboembolic pulmonary disease evaluation, it is imperative to evaluate the individual partitions of a three-dimensional data set for underlying nonocclusive thrombi. Nonocclusive thrombi will in many instances be obscured on the maximum-intensity projection processing (Fig. 2.45). In addition, when there is significant atelectasis and/or pleural disease, restriction of ventilation will lead to reflex hypoxic vasoconstriction. In these instances, the segmental and subsegmental pulmonary arteries are barely visualized (Fig. 2.46) and, therefore, cannot be evaluated for the presence of underlying thromboembolic disease. In the diagnosis of occlusive thrombus, the vascular cut off sign can also be seen with pneumonectomy (Fig. 2.47). Occasionally, hilar nodes may mimic chronic organized (endothelialized) thrombus, and careful analysis is required (Fig. 2.48).

CONCLUSIONS

Significant developments of cardiovascular magnetic resonance imaging have been made since the 1980s. Spin-echo sequences that depict morphology and allow for tissue characterization were developed initially. In the future, these sequences will be universally replaced with faster pulse sequences such as FAST (turbo) spin-echo imaging. Gradient-echo sequences that have been developed for cine MRI are also being replaced in many centers with segmented gradient-echo sequences, allowing for breath-hold imaging. Magnetization prepared gradient-echo sequences (TURBO flash) that allow for myocardial perfusion over one slice position will likely be replaced in the future with other techniques allowing for whole-heart perfusion studies. Phase-modulation techniques, which provide information regarding flow velocities and volumes, will be replaced with faster breath-hold sequences or non-

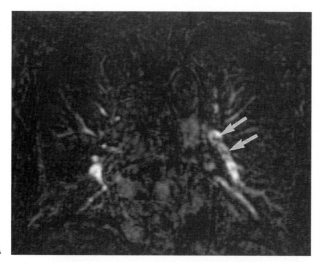

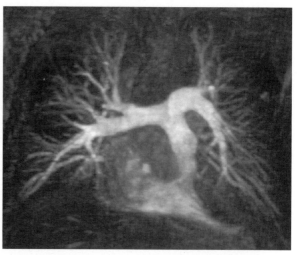

A

B

FIG. 2.45. Obscuration of nonocclusive thrombus on maximum-intensity projection. Coronal three-dimensional contrast-enhanced MRA partition **(A)** and coronal maximum-intensity projection image **(B)** reveal central filling defects *(arrows)* related to nonocclusive thrombus in the left pulmonary artery. These are most readily appreciated on the source data and are frequently obscured on maximum-intensity projection because of the overlying blood pool signal. It is imperative to evaluate the source data when evaluating cases of suspected thromboembolic pulmonary disease.

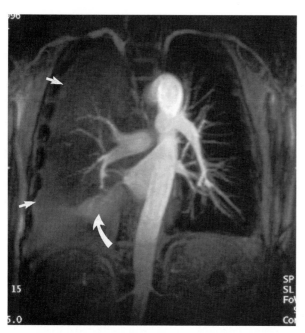

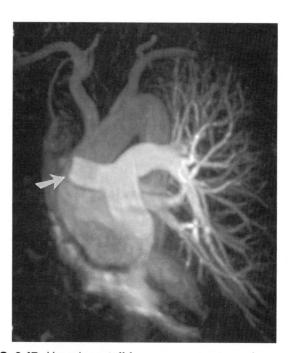

FIG. 2.46. Hypoxic vasoconstriction pitfall. A three-dimensional coronal contrast-enhanced MRA maximum-intensity projection image reveals a large right-sided pleural effusion *(arrows)*. This resulted in hypoxic vasoconstriction. In addition, there is enhancing atelectasis *(curved arrow)* at the right lung base. The vasculature on the right is markedly attenuated compared to the pulmonary vasculature on the left. In such an instance, it is difficult to evaluate the subsegmental vessels for underlying thromboembolic disease, and one should realize limitations on such examinations.

FIG. 2.47. Vascular cutoff from pneumonectomy. A coronal three-dimensional contrast-enhanced MRA maximum-intensity projection image reveals a vascular cutoff sign *(arrow)* of the right pulmonary artery in this patient who has a history of pneumonectomy. It is also important to evaluate T_1-weighted spin-echo images in central vascular cutoff signs. The differential diagnosis also includes pulmonary atresia or hypoplasia. Presence of abundant fat in and around the obstructed pulmonary artery would indicate the presence of atresia/hypoplasia.

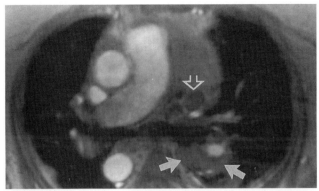

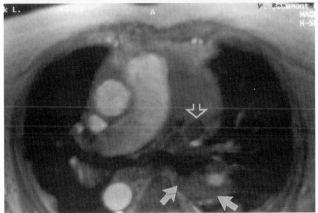

FIG. 2.48. Hilar nodes mimicking pulmonary embolus. Axial cine MR images reveal areas with low signal *(arrows)* in the vicinity of the left pulmonary artery. Additional low-signal nodes *(open arrows)* are noted within the mediastinum. Hilar nodes can frequently mimic the presence of underlying pulmonary embolus, and the multiplanar imaging capabilities of MRI or multiplanar reformation capabilities of MRI and/or CT are required to avoid this pitfall. This patient has a history of sarcoidosis and associated lymphadenopathy, which should not be confused with underlying chronic endothelialized pulmonary embolus.

breath-hold navigator sequences. Coronary angiography with single-slice breath-hold fat saturation sequences will be replaced with either breath-hold echoplanar (48) or spiral MR acquisitions of the entire coronary bed. Because of the development of faster pulse sequences, higher gradient performance, and improved coils, a comprehensive cardiovascular examination will become feasible with MRI in the near future. With these improvements, artifacts and diagnostic pitfalls should be reduced with significant improvements in image quality.

REFERENCES

1. Lenz G, Haack EM, White RD, et al. Retrospective cardiac gating: a review of technical aspects and future directions. *Magn Reson* 1989; 7:445–455.
2. Johnston DL. Myocardial tissue characterization with magnetic resonance imaging techniques. *Am J Card Imag* 1994;8:140–150.
3. Simonetti OP, Finn JP, White RD, et al. Black blood T_2-weighted inversion-recovery MR imaging of the heart. *Radiology* 1996;199:49–57.
4. White RD, Holt WW, Cheitlin MD, et al. Estimation of the functional and anatomic extent of myocardial infarction using magnetic resonance imaging. *Am Heart J* 1988;115:740–748.
5. Pflugfelder PW, Sechtem U, White RD, et al. Quantification of regional myocardial function by rapid cine MR imaging. *Am J Roentgenol* 1988; 150:523–529.
6. Pattynama PMT, deRoos A, van der Walle E, et al. Evaluation of cardiac function with magnetic resonance imaging. *Am Heart J* 1994;128: 595–607.
7. Axel L, Dougherty L. Heart wall motion: improved method of spatial modulation for MR imaging. *Radiology* 1989;172:349–350.
8. McVeigh ER, Atalar E. Cardiac tagging with breath-hold MRI. *Magn Reson Med* 1992;28:317–327.
9. Haacke EM, Smith AS, Lin W, et al. Velocity quantification in magnetic resonance imaging. *Topics Magn Reson Imaging* 1991;3:34–49.
10. Edelman RR, Manning WJ, Gervino E, et al. Flow velocity quantification in human coronary arteries with fast breath-hold MR-angiography. *J Magn Reson Imag* 1993;3:699–703.
11. Manning WJ, Atkinson DJ, Grossman W, et al. First-pass MR imaging studies using gadolinium DTPA in patients with coronary artery disease. *J Am Coll Cardiol* 1991;18:959–965.
12. Wilke N, Jerosch-Herold M, Stillman AE, et al. Concepts of myocardial perfusion imaging in magnetic resonance imaging. *Magn Reson Q* 1994;10:249–286.
13. Edelman RR, Manning WJ, Burstein D, et al. Coronary arteries: breath-hold MR-angiography. *Radiology* 1991;181:641–643
14. Manning WJ, Li W, Edelman RR. Fat suppressed breath-hold magnetic resonance coronary angiography. *Circulation* 1993;87:94–104.
15. Manning WJ, Li W, Edelman RR. A preliminary report comparing magnetic resonance coronary angiograph with conventional angiography. *N Engl J Med* 1993;328:828–832.
16. Hofman MBM, Paschal CB, Li D, et al. MRI of coronary arteries, 2D breath-hold versus 3D respiratory gated acquisition. *J Comput Assist Tomogr* 1995;19:56–62.
17. Vrachliotis TG, Bis KG, Aliabadi D, et al. Three-dimensional breath-held ECG-triggered contrast enhanced MR angiography for evaluation of coronary artery bypass graft patency. *Am J Roentgenol* 1997;168: 1073–1080.
18. Higgins CB, Byrd BF, Farmer DW, et al. Magnetic resonance imaging in patients with congenital heart disease. *Circulation* 1984;70(5): 851–860.
19. Didier D, Higgins CB, Fisher MR, et al. Congenital heart disease: Gated MR imaging in 72 patients. *Radiology* 1986;158:227–235.
20. Kondo C, Caputo GR, Semelka R, et al. Right and left ventricular stroke volume measurements with velocity encoded cine MR imaging: *In vitro* and *in vivo* validation. *Am J Roentgenol* 1991;157:9–16.
21. Soulen RL, Donner RM, Capitanio M. Post operative evaluation of complex congenital heart disease by MRI. *RadioGraphics* 1987;7(5): 975–1000.
22. Kersting-Sommerhoff BA, Seelos KC, Hardy C, et al. Evaluation of

surgical procedures for cyanotic congenital heart disease by using MR imaging. *Am J Roentgenol* 1990;155:259–266.

23. Fellows KE, Weinberg PM, Baffa JM, et al. Evaluation of congenital heart disease with MR imaging: Current and coming attractions. *Am J Roentgenol* 192;159:925–931.

24. Amparo EG, Higgins CB, Farmer D, et al. Gated MRI of cardiac and paracardiac masses: Initial experience. *Am J Roentgenol* 1984;143:1151–1156.

25. Winkler M, Higgins CB. Suspected intracardiac masses: Evaluation with MR imaging. *Radiology* 1987;165:117–122.

26. Rienmuller R, Louis L, Loret J, et al. MR imaging of pediatric cardiac tumors previously diagnosed by echocardiography. *J Comput Assist Tomogr* 1989;13(14):621–626.

27. Lund JT, Ehman RL, Julsrud PR, et al. Cardiac masses: Assessment by MR imaging. *Am J Roentgenol* 1989;152:469–473.

28. Dooms GC, Higgins CB. MR imaging of cardiac thrombi. *J Comput Assist Tomogr* 1986;10(3):415–420.

29. Seelos KC, Caputo GR, Carrol CL, et al. Cine gradient refocussed echo (GRE) imaging of intravascular masses: Differentiation between tumor and non-tumor thrombus. *J Comput Assist Tomogr* 1992;16(2):169–175.

30. Soulen RL, Stark DD, Higgins CB. Magnetic resonance imaging of constrictive pericardial disease. *Am J Cardiol* 1985;55:480–484.

31. Olson MC, Posniak HV, MacDonald V, et al. Computed tomography and magnetic resonance imaging of the pericardium. *RadioGraphics* 1989;9(4):633–649.

32. Suzuki J, Caputo GR, Kondo C, et al. Cine MR imaging of valvular heart disease: display and imaging parameters affect the size of the signal void caused by valvular regurgitation. *Am J Roentgenol* 1990;155:723–727.

33. Sechten U, Pflugfelder PW, White RD, et al. Cine MR imaging: Potential for the evaluation of cardiovascular function. *Am J Roentgenol* 1987;148:239–246.

34. Mostbeck GH, Caputo GR, Higgins CB. MR measurement of blood flow in the cardiovascular system. *Am J Roentgenol* 1992;159:453–461.

35. Sakuma H, Fujita N, Foo TKF, et al. Evaluation of left ventricular volume and mass with breath hold cine MR imaging. *Radiology* 1993;188:377–380.

36. deRoos A, Matheijssen NAA, Doornbos J, et al. Myocardial infarct size after reperfusion therapy: Assessment with Gd-DTPA-enhanced MR imaging. *Radiology* 1990;176:517–521.

37. Higgins CB, Saeed M, Wendland M. MR in ischemic heart disease: Expansion of the current capabilities with MR contrast. *Am J Card Imag* 1991;5(1):38–50.

38. Masui T, Saeed M, Wendland MF, et al. Occlusive and reperfused myocardial infarcts: MRI differentiation with nonionic Gd-DTPA-BMA. *Radiology* 1991;181:77–83.

39. Dulce MC, Duerinckx AJ, Hartiala J, et al. MR imaging of the myocardium using nonionic contrast media: Single intensity changes in patients with subacute myocardial infarction. *Am J Roentgenol* 1993;160:963–970.

40. Wagner S, Buser P, Auffermann W, et al. Cine MRI: Tomographic analysis of left ventricular function. *Cardiol Clin* 1989;7(3):651–659.

41. Buchalter MB, Simms C, Dickson AK, et al. Measurement of regional left ventricular function using labeled magnetic resonance imaging. *Br J Radiol* 1991;64:953–958.

42. Axel L, Goncalves RC, Bloomgarden D. Regional heart wall motion: Two dimensional analysis and functional imaging with MR imaging. *Radiology* 1992;183:745–750.

43. Thomsen C. "Chess-board pattern" spatial modulation of magnetization. *Acta Radiol* 1992;33:16–23.

44. Bis KG, Shetty AN, Juni JE, et al. Assessment of tissue viability with contrast (Gadoteridol) enhanced magnetic resonance imaging in patients with ischemic heart disease: Correlation with positron emission tomography. *Am J Roentgenol* 1994;162(3):177.

45. Edelman RR, Manning WJ, Pearlman J, et al. Human coronary arteries: Projection angiograms reconstructed from breath hold two dimensional MR images. *Radiology* 1993;187:719–722.

46. Nienaber CA, Spielman RP, Kodolitsch Y, et al. Diagnosis of thoracic aortic dissection: Magnetic resonance imaging vs. transesophageal echocardiography. *Circulation* 1992;85:434–447.

47. Bis KG, Farah M. Precise evaluation crucial in aortic dissection. *Diag Imag* 1993;Feb:88–97.

48. Wendland MF, Saeed M, Masui T, et al. Echoplanar MR imaging of normal and ischemic myocardium with gadodiamide injection. *Radiology* 1993;186:535–542.

Variants and Pitfalls in Body Imaging,
edited by Ali Shirkhoda.
Lippincott Williams & Wilkins, Philadelphia, © 2000.

CHAPTER 3

The Lungs and the Pleura

High-Resolution and Conventional (or Spiral) CT

Steven L. Primack, Kyung Soo Lee, and Nestor L. Müller

Normal anatomic variants of the bronchi, pulmonary vessels, visceral and parietal pleura are common and may mimic disease on conventional, spiral, and high-resolution CT. Furthermore, a number of technical and patient-related artifacts may cause potential pitfalls in the interpretation of the CT images. Awareness of anatomic variants and of the various image artifacts is essential for optimal assessment of the CT images and reliable distinction of normal from abnormal lung and pleura.

OPTIMAL COMPUTED TOMOGRAPHIC TECHNIQUES

There is no universal agreement as to what constitutes the optimal CT study. Spiral CT using relatively thick sections (7- to 10-mm collimation) allows assessment of the entire lung volume during a single breath-hold. However, this results in volume averaging within the plane of section with consequent decrease in spatial resolution. Thinner sections (1- to 1.5-mm collimation) allow optimal assessment of fine parenchymal detail but do not allow assessment of the entire volume of the lungs. The technique used in any given case therefore represents a compromise between imaging of the entire volume of the lungs or imaging for assessment of fine parenchymal detail. Assessment of the entire lung volume is obviously required when one is

S. L. Primack: Department of Radiology, Oregon Health Sciences University, Portland, Oregon 97201.

K. S. Lee: Department of Radiology, Sungkyunkwan University School of Medicine, and Samsung Medical Centre, Seoul 135-230, South Korea.

N. L. Müller: Department of Radiology, University of British Columbia, and Vancouver General Hospital, Vancouver, British Columbia V5Z 1M9, Canada.

investigating a patient with suspected primary or metastatic pulmonary neoplasms, whereas examination of fine parenchymal detail is essential in the evaluation of interstitial lung disease. The following are the CT scan techniques that we currently use in our department.

Assessment of Patients with Suspected Interstitial Lung Disease or Bronchiectasis

Computed tomographic scans in these patients are obtained using the thinnest available collimation (1 mm) and a high spatial frequency reconstruction algorithm ("lung" or "bone" algorithm). The scans are usually performed at the end of inspiration at 10-mm intervals through the chest and photographed at lung windows (window level of -600 to -700 HU, window width of 1,000 to 1,500 HU) and soft tissue windows (window level 30 to 50 HU, window width 300 to 500 HU).

In some patients, prone scans may be required to distinguish dependent atelectasis from irreversible parenchymal disease. Some investigators routinely recommend prone CT scans in patients who are being assessed for suspected interstitial lung disease who have normal chest radiographs. Prone scans are not required in patients who have abnormal radiographs because the abnormalities in these patients are diffuse and not limited to the dependent lung regions.

Assessment for the Presence of Primary Bronchogenic Carcinoma

The CT scans in these patients are usually performed using 5- to 7-mm collimation CT scans through the chest

73

using spiral technique. The images are photographed at both lung windows (window level −600 to −700 HU, window width 1,000 to 1,500 HU), and mediastinal or soft tissue windows (window level 30 to 50 HU, window width 300 to 500 HU). We routinely perform thin-section CT scans (1-mm collimation) through the lung nodules in these patients to assess for the presence of calcification (helpful in the diagnosis of granulomas) and fat (diagnostic of hamartomas).

Metastatic Disease

Assessment for nodules in patients with suspected metastatic disease should be performed using relatively thin collimation (such as 5 mm) and overlapping reconstructions (3 mm) in order to most easily distinguish small nodules from pulmonary vessels.

NORMAL ANATOMIC VARIANTS

Bronchi

Tracheal Bronchus

Tracheal bronchus refers to an anomalous bronchus arising from the right lateral wall of the trachea at the proximity of the carina (Fig. 3.1). Tracheal bronchus can be described as either displaced or supernumerary. In most cases, the right upper lobe bronchus bifurcates, and the tracheal bronchus is regarded as displaced (1). If it trifurcates, the bronchus is regarded as supernumerary.

Tracheal bronchus occurs in 0.1% of adults and may be associated with postobstructive pneumonia, abscess, and bronchiectasis (1,2). Bronchogenic carcinoma may involve the bronchus (Fig. 3.2).

An ectopic bronchus may arise from the right main bronchus rather than from the lateral wall of the trachea. The site of ectopic bronchus depends on the embryonic period in which the abnormal diverticulum arises. A tracheal bronchus arises earlier in the embryonic period than an ectopic bronchus from the right main bronchus (2).

Accessory Cardiac Bronchus

Accessory cardiac bronchus is a supernumerary anomalous bronchus (3). The bronchus arises from the medial wall of the bronchus intermedius proximal to the origin of the right lower lobe superior segmental bronchus and usually before the origin of the middle lobe bronchus (3–6) (Fig. 3.3). The bronchus is then directed inferiorly toward the mediastinum. The length

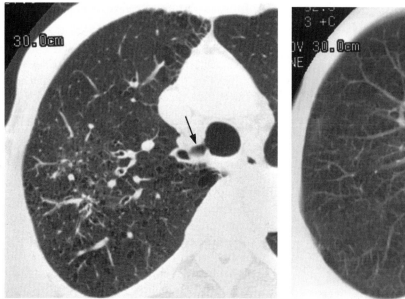
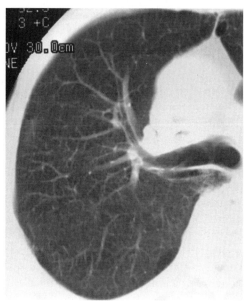

FIG. 3.1. Tracheal bronchus. **A:** High-resolution (1.0-mm collimation) CT scan obtained at distal tracheal level shows tracheal bronchus *(arrow)* budding laterally from the distal trachea. **B:** Conventional (10-mm collimation) CT scan obtained at level of main bronchi 25 mm caudad to A shows anterior and posterior segmental bronchi of right upper lobe arising from upper lobar bronchus.

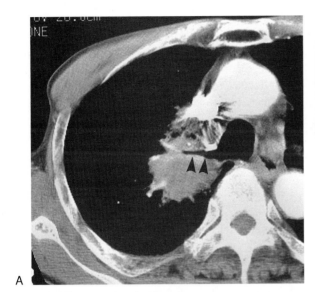 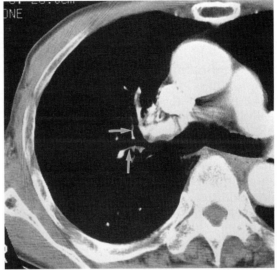

FIG. 3.2. Bronchogenic carcinoma arising from tracheal bronchus. **A:** Mediastinal window of conventional CT (10-mm collimation) scan obtained at distal tracheal level shows soft tissue mass arising from tracheal bronchus *(arrowheads)*. **B:** Computer tomographic scan obtained 18 mm caudad to **A** shows anterior and posterior segmental bronchi *(arrows)* arising from right upper lobar bronchus.

of the bronchus is variable. The short type is usually a simple bronchial stump without associated alveolar tissue, whereas the longer subtype occurs with or without associated rudimentary alveolar tissue. The bronchus is lined by endobronchial mucosa and has cartilaginous rings within its walls.

The prevalence of the cardiac bronchus ranges from 0.1% to 0.5% in the general population and is greater in men (3). Cardiac bronchus can be a source of infection as a result of retained secretions and resultant inflammation.

Among six cases of cardiac bronchus reported by McGuinness et al. (6), four were associated with lung parenchymal tissue on CT. Three cases were associated with discrete soft tissue mass, presumably representing vascularized bronchial or vestigial parenchymal tissue.

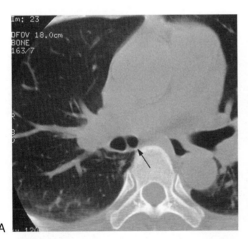 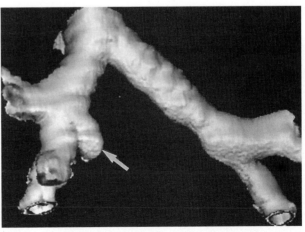

FIG. 3.3. Cardiac bronchus. **A:** Thin-section (3.0-mm collimation) CT scan obtained at subcarinal level shows air-filled cystic structure *(arrow)* medial to distal bronchus intermedius. **B:** Three-dimensional reconstruction image with shaded-surface display technique reveals cardiac bronchus *(arrow)* medial to distal bronchus intermedius.

Vessels

Nodule in the Posterior Wall of the Bronchus Intermedius

A focal nodular opacity in the posterior wall of the bronchus intermedius is occasionally seen on normal HRCT scans (Fig. 3.4). This focal nodularity is caused by a pulmonary vein—either by a branch of the vein from the posterior segment of the right upper lobe (71%) or by a branch of the vein from the superior segment of the right lower lobe (29%)—and it is observed in 5% of normal adults (7). This nodular opacity can be followed on multiple sections, indicating that it is a vessel and should be easily differentiated from thickening caused by tumor.

Interlobar Fissures

The interlobar fissures are formed by a double layer of visceral pleura and represent extensions of the pleural space between lobes of the lungs. On conventional CT scans, the fissures usually appear as avascular bands and less often as lines or high-attenuation bands. On thin-section CT, the fissures are seen as lines. Various forms of the right minor fissure as well as variant fissures are reviewed and illustrated.

The Right Minor Fissure

On thin-section CT scans, the right minor fissure is identified in 80% to 92% of patients (8,9). The dome of the right middle lobe, delineated by the minor fissure, can be medially high (Fig. 3.5), laterally high (Fig. 3.6), domed centrally, or posterocentrally high. However, the dome of the right middle lobe is mostly either medial or lateral. The anterior portion of the minor fissure may have a sagittal orientation (10). In this variant, the anterior segment of the right upper lobe occupies a paracardiac location and can abut the right hemidiaphragm, delineated by the laterally located sagittal anterior minor fissure (Fig. 3.7).

The Left Minor Fissure

As a counterpart of the right minor fissure, the left minor fissure separates the lingula from the anterior segment of the left upper lobe. The left minor fissure has been reported in 6% to 18% of autopsies (11) and can be seen in approximately 2% of chest radiographs (12).

Berkmen et al. (13) analyzed CT findings of 18 accessory fissures of the left upper lobe in 17 adults. The fissures separated the anterior segment of the left upper lobe from the superior lingular segment (left minor fissure) in 13 cases (72%) (Fig. 3.8), the superior from the inferior segment of the lingula in three cases (17%), and the apicoposterior from the anterior segment in two cases (11%). Eleven (61%) of the accessory fissures were incomplete.

Azygos Lobe Fissure

Azygos lobe fissure consists of four layers of pleura and contains the azygos vein within its lower margin. The fissure separates the right upper lobe into the azygos lobe medially and remaining right upper lobe laterally. The azygos lobe is ventilated by the apical or posterior segmental bronchus of the right upper lobe and is perfused by the corresponding pulmonary artery branch (14). The azygos lobe

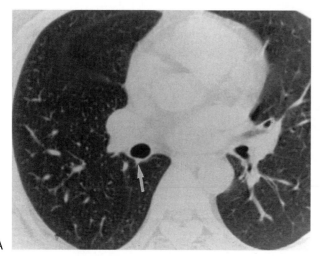
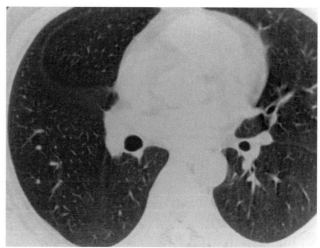

A B

FIG. 3.4. Pulmonary vein with nodular appearance of the posterior wall of bronchus intermedius. **A:** High-resolution (1.0-mm collimation) CT scan obtained at the level of bronchus intermedius shows nodule *(arrow)* at the posterior wall of bronchus intermedius. **B:** Computed tomographic scan obtained 5 mm caudad to **A** demonstrates medial shift of nodule. This vessel continues to the right inferior pulmonary vein.

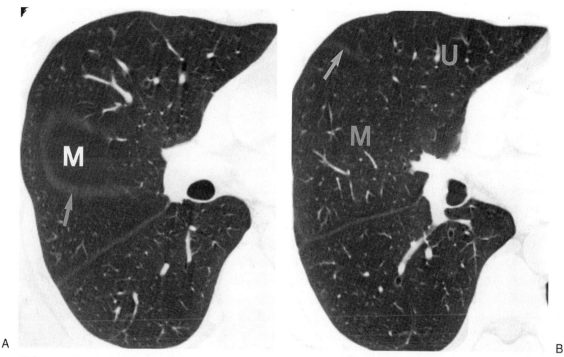

A

B

FIG. 3.5. Right minor fissure with medially high right middle lobe. **A:** High-resolution (1.5-mm collimation) CT scan obtained at the level of proximal bronchus intermedius shows incomplete right minor fissure *(arrow)* with medially located dome of right middle lobe (M). **B:** Computed tomographic scan obtained 15 mm caudal to **A** shows incomplete minor fissure *(arrow)* between expanded right middle lobe (M) and right upper lobe (U).

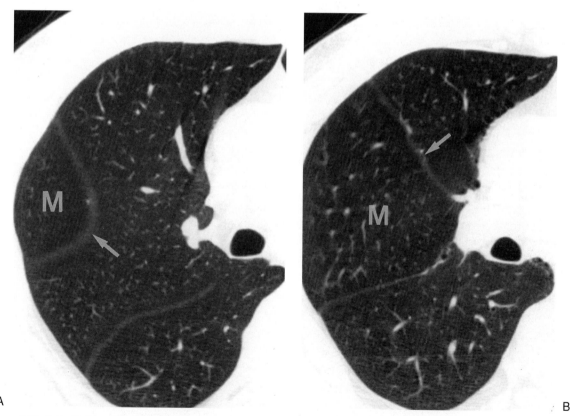

A

B

FIG. 3.6. Right minor fissure with laterally high right middle lobe. **A:** High-resolution (1.5-mm collimation) CT scan obtained at the level of proximal bronchus intermedius shows right minor fissure *(arrow)* with laterally located dome of right middle lobe (M). **B:** Computed tomographic scan obtained 15 mm caudad to **A** shows right minor fissure *(arrow)* bordering right middle lobe (M) and right upper lobe.

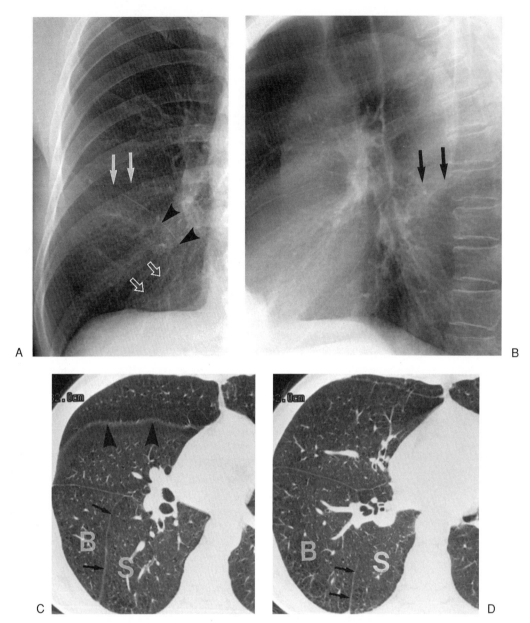

FIG. 3.7. Sagittal orientation of anterior right minor fissure and superior and inferior accessory fissures. **A:** Chest radiograph shows right superior accessory fissure *(arrows)*, inferior accessory fissure *(open arrows),* and sagittally oriented anterior right minor fissure *(arrowheads).* **B:** Lateral radiograph shows superior accessory fissure *(arrows)* located inferior to superior portion of major fissure. **C:** High-resolution (1.0-mm collimation) CT scan shows right superior accessory fissure *(arrows)* between superior (S) and basal segments (B) of right lower lobe. Also note right minor *(arrowheads)* and major fissures. **D:** Computed tomographic scan obtained 20 mm caudad to **C** demonstrates medially oriented superior accessory fissure (arrows).

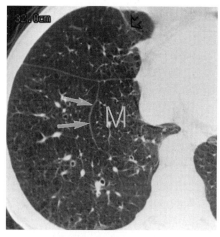
E

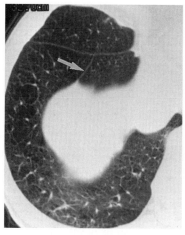
F

FIG. 3.7. *Continued.* **E:** Computed tomographic scan obtained 40 mm caudad to **D** shows right inferior accessory fissure *(arrows)* behind the right major fissure and between medial basal segment (M) and other basal segments. At this level, right minor fissure *(open arrow)* is still seen with sagittal orientation. **F:** Computed tomographic scan obtained 20 mm caudad to **E** demonstrates inferior accessory fissure *(arrow)* limited anteriorly by right major fissure.

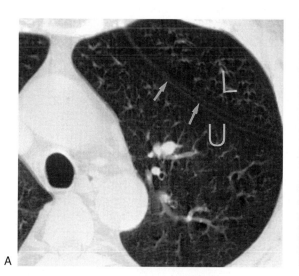
A

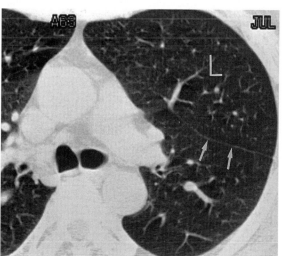
B

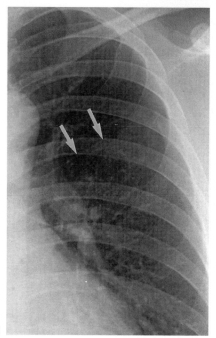
C

FIG. 3.8. Left minor fissure. **A:** High-resolution (1.0-mm collimation) CT scan obtained at level of distal trachea shows left minor fissure *(arrows)* between superior lingular segment (L) and anterior segment of left upper lobe (u). Note double fissure sign caused by respiratory motion. **B:** Computed tomographic scan obtained 20 mm caudad to **A** demonstrates lingula (L) anterior to left minor fissure (arrows). **C:** Chest radiograph shows fissure *(arrows)* in left upper lung zone.

extends into the pretracheal and retrotracheal mediastinum, contacting the anterior wall of the trachea, the medial wall of the superior vena cava, and the posterior wall of the trachea in the majority of patients (14,15) (Fig. 3.9).

Inferior Accessory Fissure

The inferior accessory fissure separates the medial basal segment of the lower lobe from the other basilar segments. On the diaphragmatic surface of the lung, the fissure extends laterally from near the pulmonary ligament and then makes a convex arc forward to join the major fissure. The fissure is present in 40% to 50% of autopsy specimens (16). However, its depth and prominence are variable. When fully developed, the fissure forms a cleft that is only 0.5 to 2.0 cm in depth. In some cases, the fissure continues medially and superiorly toward the hilum. However, in most cases the fissure remains as only a subpleural groove on the diaphragmatic surface of the lung without definite cleft (16).

On CT scans, the fissure appears at the lung bases as a thin arc extending from the mediastinum near the esophagus (inferior pulmonary ligament) to the major fissure anteriorly (see Fig. 3.7). The line may be thicker anteriorly, where the cleft is often deeper on anatomic specimens. The fissure is not usually seen at higher levels. When it is visible at higher levels, its circumference is smaller, as expected from the tapering, pyramidal shape of the medial basal segment. The fissure appears as a band on conventional 10-mm collimation CT and as a thin line on high-resolution CT (16). Juxtaphrenic peak refers to a small sharply defined radiographic shadow projecting upward from the medial half of the hemidiaphragm at or near the highest point of the dome in association with atelectasis of the upper lobe or combined upper and middle lobe atelectasis (17). The peak is most commonly related to an inferior accessory fissure, although occasionally it may be secondary to a medial septum or an accessory fissure other than the inferior accessory fissure (18).

Superior Accessory Fissure

The superior accessory fissure separates the superior segment of the lower lobe from the basal segments. It varies from a complete fissure to a subtle notch. It is seen in anatomic specimens in 14% of left lungs and 30% of right lungs (16). On frontal radiographs, the fissure resembles a minor fissure on the right or left, except that it is usually lower. On lateral radiograph, the fissure extends posteriorly from the major fissure.

On conventional 10-mm collimation CT scans, the fissure is visible only as an area devoid of major pulmonary vessels at the lower edge of the superior segment because the fissure is horizontal. However, on high-resolution (1- to 2-mm collimation) CT, the fissure is seen as a thin line (see Fig. 3.7).

Inferior Pulmonary Ligament

The inferior pulmonary ligament is a double layer of pleura that drapes caudally from the lung root and loosely tethers the medial aspect of the lower lobe of the lung to the mediastinum (19–21). The ligament extends downward and posteriorly for a variable distance and often extends to the diaphragm. The ligament, rarely visible on normal chest radiographs, is identified on conventional CT only on

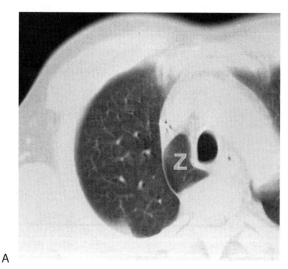
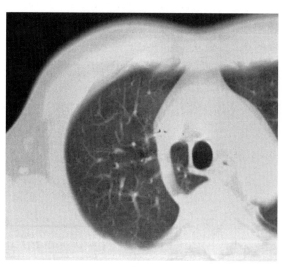

A
B

FIG. 3.9. Azygos fissure. **A:** Conventional (7-mm collimation) CT scan obtained at level of aortic arch shows azygos fissure between azygos lobe (Z) and remaining right upper lobe. **B:** Computed tomographic scan obtained 10 mm caudal to **A** shows thickened azygos fissure containing azygos vein.

the left in 30%, only on the right in 26%, on both sides in 32%, and is not identified in 12% (19). It is seen on CT as a soft tissue beak or point oriented laterally from the mediastinum. It is usually continuous with the intersubsegmental septum (19,22) (Fig. 3.10). Because there is no clear boundary between the tissue of the ligament and that of the septum, ligament and septum can be considered as an anatomic unit (20,21). The septum is seen as a thin intraparenchymal band on CT (19,22). The ligament may be continuous with an inferior accessory fissure in some patients, forming a cardiac lobe (medial basal segment) of the lung (23) (see Fig. 3.10).

Intersegmental (Intersublobar) Septum of the Lower Lobe

Intersegmental or intersublobar septum refers to a thin horizontal line that extends laterally from the mediastinal surface of the lung within the area between the inferior pulmonary vein and the diaphragm (16,22). The linear attenuation seen on CT scan is a septum of thin, loose intraparenchymal connective tissue that is bounded medially by the base of the pulmonary ligament, where the two sleeves of the visceral pleura appose each another, and laterally by a vertically oriented vein (Fig. 3.11). The septum is seen in 78% (39/50) of normal CT scans (22). The septum separates the medial basal segment from the posterior basal segment of the lower lobe.

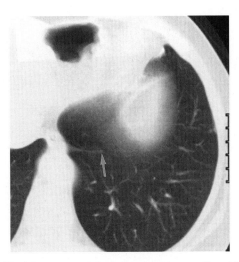

FIG. 3.11. Intersegmental septum in a conventional (10-mm collimation) CT scan obtained at level of liver dome shows linear attenuation that is bound medially by the base of the pulmonary ligament and laterally by branch of pulmonary vein (arrow).

Pleura

Transverse Thoracic and Subcostal Muscles Simulating Pleural Thickening

The visceral and parietal pleura along with the endothoracic fascia and the innermost intercostal muscle appear as a 1- to 2-mm-thick line on high-resolution CT between lung and chest wall. In the paravertebral location, the innermost intercostal muscle is lacking. Therefore, a thin line in this area represents the pleura and endothoracic fascia. Transverse thoracic and subcostal muscles can be seen as soft tissue attenuation internal to a rib and may simulate pleural thickening (Fig. 3.12). However, in pleural thickening, the thickened pleura is visible at least focally as a discrete, thin, irregular or smooth line separated from the underlying rib, intercostal muscle, or subcostal muscle in most locations by a 1- to 4-mm-thick fat layer (see Fig. 3.12). This layer represents the extrapleural fat layer that is normally present (24).

Extrapleural Fat Simulating Pleural Plaque

Intrathoracic fat is usually extrapleural, located outside the parietal pleura in the chest wall or mediastinum. An appreciable amount of extrapleural fat is noted in 15% of persons at autopsy (25). Extrapleural fat tends to accumulate posterolaterally in the region of the fourth to eighth ribs. Because of this location, it may mimic pleural thickening on the chest radiograph (26). Sargent et al. (27) studied 30 patients with known asbestos exposure who underwent CT scans to clarify apparent pleural abnormalities observed on chest radiograph. They demon-

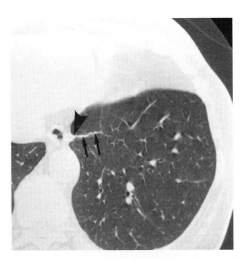

FIG. 3.10. Inferior pulmonary ligament and incomplete inferior accessory fissure. High-resolution (1.0-mm collimation) CT scan obtained at level of liver dome demonstrates inferior pulmonary ligament (arrowhead) appearing as a small soft-tissue beak oriented laterally from the esophageal wall. Ligament is continuous with intersegmental septum (arrows).

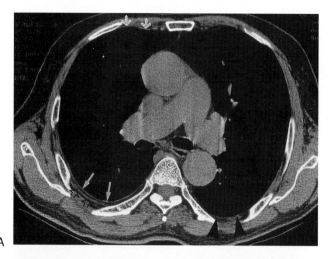

A

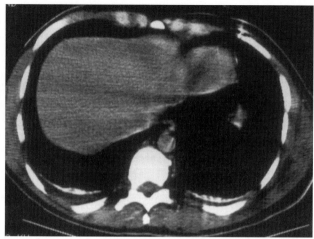

C

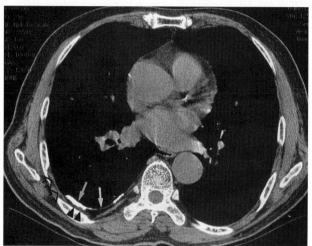

B

FIG. 3.12. Normal pleura versus pleural thickening. **A:** High-resolution (1.0-mm collimation) CT scan obtained at subcarinal level shows pleural thickening *(arrows)* anterior to innermost intercostal muscle *(open arrows)*. Also note normal pleura *(arrowheads)* in left posterior hemithorax and transverse thoracic muscle *(small arrows)* anteriorly in the right. **B:** Computed tomographic scan obtained at level of left atrium shows pleural thickening and calcification *(arrows)* anterior to innermost intercostal muscle *(open arrows)* and subcostal muscle *(arrowheads)*. **C:** Computed tomographic scan 1 week after bipedal lymphangiogram. Bilateral subpleural densities depict lymphangiographic contrast in periphery of dependent lungs, probably representing contrast emboli. (**C,** courtesy of A. Shirkhoda, M.D., William Beaumont Hospital.)

strated that the changes were caused by extrapleural fat rather than pleural plaques in 14 (48%).

Pleural plaques can be confidently diagnosed on chest radiographs only in the presence of calcification or when the plaques involve the diaphragmatic surface. When the apparent pleural thickening involves only the lateral or posterolateral aspect of the chest wall, the differentiation cannot be confidently made on chest radiographs. Chest radiographic features that suggest extrapleural fat include bilateral location along the midlateral chest wall and a symmetric appearance. Pleural plaques are most commonly asymmetric (28).

High-resolution CT is superior to chest radiograph and conventional CT in detecting pleural plaques. Pleural plaques and extrapleural fat should be easily distinguished on HRCT (26,28).

Apicolateral Pleural Tenting Simulating Pleural Thickening

Although extrapleural fat is most abundant in the region of the fourth to eighth ribs, it can also be found at the apicolateral portions of the hemithoraces. Muscular tissue (innermost intercostal or subcostal muscle) is also found in a similar location. When the contact between the lung and apicolateral extrapleural fat or muscular tissue is tangent to the x-ray beam, the radiographic soft tissue shadow produced is easily confused with true pleural thickening (29) and is called apicolateral pleural tenting (30). Computed tomography demonstrates that the apicolateral pleural tenting is caused by apicolateral extrapleural fat or muscle (Fig. 3.13).

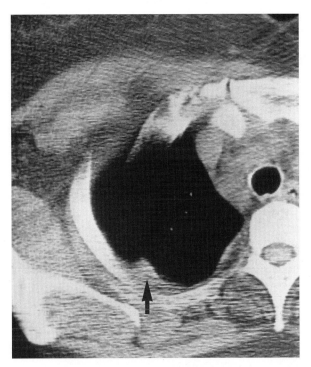

FIG. 3.13. Apicolateral pleural tenting simulating pleural thickening. Conventional CT (7-mm collimation) scan obtained at thoracic inlet shows right apicolateral muscle and fat *(arrow)*. Because extrapleural muscle and fat are tangent to the x-ray beam, they simulated pleural thickening on chest radiograph (not shown here).

PITFALLS

Technical Pitfalls

Volume averaging within the plane of section with 7- to 10-mm-thick conventional or spiral scans limits the

identification of abnormal lung attenuation or early pulmonary fibrosis. Although ground-glass attenuation may be suspected on thicker sections, it can be confidently diagnosed only on high-resolution CT (31). In cases where thicker sections demonstrate nonspecific abnormal lung attenuation, HRCT may show more specific abnormalities (Fig. 3.14).

Window Width and Level

There are no standardized lung window widths or levels for photographing HRCT images. Although opinions vary, most authors recommend window widths between 1,000 HU and 2,000 HU. Most authors recommend a lung window level between -500 and -700 HU. Reducing the window level to a more negative number or reducing the window width magnifies parenchymal structures. This is particularly evident in small structures such as interlobular septa and bronchial walls (Fig. 3.15). Reducing the window width or level may also result in a pattern of ground-glass attenuation (see Fig. 3.15). We recommend lung window widths of 1,000 to 1,500 HU and window levels of -700 HU.

Tube Current

Adequate HRCT images can be obtained in the majority of patients by using lower tube current (mA) (32) (Fig. 3.16). However, lowering the current increases image noise on HRCT scans because noise is inversely proportional to the square root of the current. Thus, in large patients, images taken with low current may prove suboptimal, and current may need to be increased in these patients (Fig. 3.17).

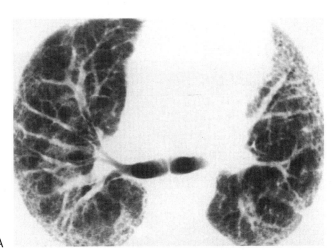
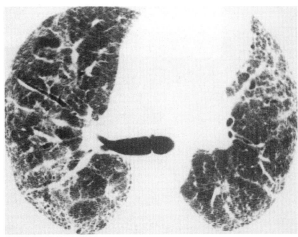

A   B

FIG. 3.14. Effect of slice thickness in a patient with idiopathic pulmonary fibrosis. **A:** Conventional (10-mm collimation) CT scan shows poorly defined areas of increased attenuation in the lung periphery. It is unclear whether this represents active disease or fibrosis. **B:** High-resolution CT (1-mm collimation) demonstrates peripheral honeycombing and architectural distortion consistent with end-stage fibrosis.

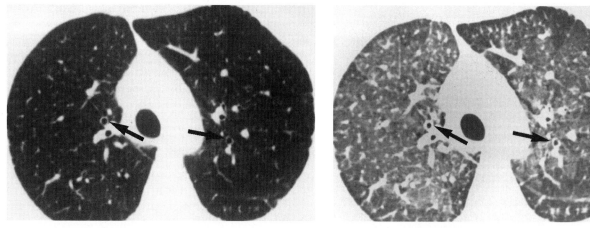

A   B

FIG. 3.15. Effect of window level and width. **A:** High-resolution CT scan filmed at appropriate window level of -700 HU and width of 1,500 HU shows patchy emphysema. **B:** High-resolution CT scan filmed at window level of -900 HU and width of 600 HU demonstrates patchy areas of ground-glass attenuation and apparent interlobular septal thickening. Note increased thickness of bronchial wall *(arrows)* when compared to **A.**

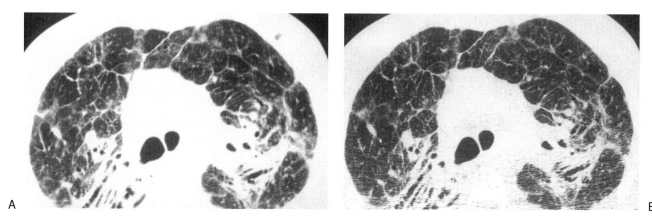

A   B

FIG. 3.16. Conventional-dose HRCT compared with low-dose HRCT scan in a patient with sarcoidosis. **A:** The HRCT scan obtained with 340 mA shows perihilar fibrosis. **B:** The HRCT scan obtained with 40 mA demonstrates increased noise, but the pattern and extent of abnormalities are seen as well as in **A.** (From *Am J Roentgenol* 1996;167:413–418, with permission.)

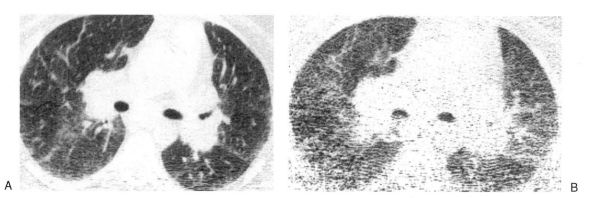

A   B

FIG. 3.17. Low-dose HRCT in a large patient with extrinsic allergic alveolitis. **A:** The HRCT scan obtained with 400 mA demonstrates patchy areas of ground-glass attenuation. **B:** The HRCT scan obtained with 80 mA is uninterpretable. (Primack SL, Remy-Jardin M, Remy J, Müller NL. High resolution CT of the lung: pitfalls in the diagnosis of infiltrative lung disease. *AJR* 1996;167:413–418.)

Reconstruction Algorithm

Using the appropriate reconstruction algorithm is critical in performing HRCT scans. High-resolution CT is obtained by using a high-spatial-frequency reconstruction algorithm. The high-spatial-frequency algorithm reduces image smoothing and increases spatial resolution. Structures such as vessels, bronchi, interlobular septa, and cystic air spaces appear sharper (33) (Fig. 3.18). The high-resolution reconstruction algorithm increases image noise, which is usually not a factor on lung windows, but may cause perceptible noise on mediastinal windows. Therefore, if a chest CT scan is obtained to evaluate the aorta or pulmonary arteries, a standard (soft tissue) reconstruction algorithm should be used.

Beam-Hardening Artifact

Beam hardening occurs when the CT x-ray beam passes through a high-density structure such as a vertebral body or contrast-enhanced vessel. Lower-energy components of the x-ray beam are preferentially absorbed, leaving higher-energy photons in the transmitted beam. Lung tissue exposed to the higher energy will appear to have lower attenuation, potentially mimicking emphysema or a pneumothorax (Fig. 3.19).

Patient-Related Artifacts

Cardiac and Respiratory Motion

Motion during acquisition of an HRCT image may cause appearances that are potential pitfalls in interpretation. Breathing during an HRCT scan acquisition may cause a double image of a pulmonary vessel, which simulates bronchiectasis (Fig. 3.20). The presence of other associated findings of motion such as blurring of vessels or double image of a major fissure are helpful in distinguishing pseudobronchiectasis from true bronchiectasis. Inadequate breath holding during acquisition of an HRCT image causes areas of ground-glass attenuation, which may mimic a diffuse infiltrative process. Ground-glass attenuation caused by respiratory motion usually has associated blurring of pulmonary vessels and double images of fissures and pulmonary vessels. Repeat scanning may be helpful in differentiating ground-glass attenuation caused by respiratory motion from an infiltrative process (Fig. 3.21). Cardiac pulsation produces move-

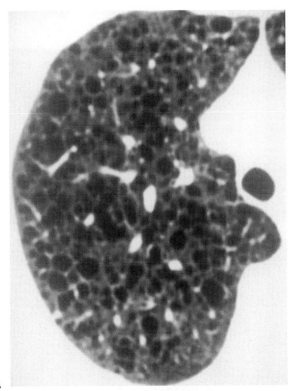 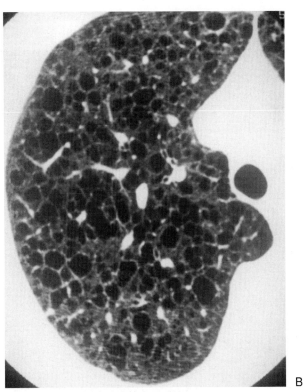

A   B

FIG. 3.18. Effect of reconstruction algorithm in patient with lymphangioleiomyomatosis. **A:** A 1.5-mm scan using standard reconstruction algorithm shows areas of low attenuation with poorly defined walls. **B:** A 1.5-mm scan using high-spatial-frequency reconstruction algorithm (high-resolution CT) demonstrates much better definition of the walls. Note that vessels are also much better defined. (Primack SL, Remy-Jardin M, Remy J, Müller NL. High resolution CT of the lung: pitfalls in the diagnosis of infiltrative lung disease. *AJR* 1996;167:413–418.)

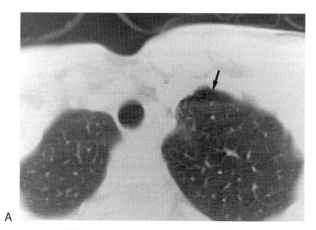

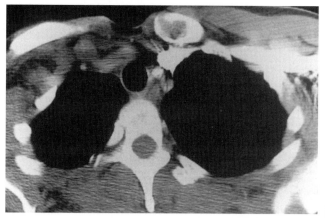

A

B

FIG. 3.19. Beam-hardening artifact mimicking pneumothorax. Computed tomographic scan filmed at lung windows **(A)** demonstrates a linear band of low attenuation anteriorly on the left *(arrow)*. This lucent band is caused by beam-hardening artifact from the contrast-enhanced left brachiocephalic vein **(B).**

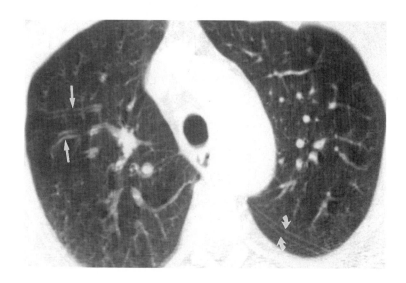

FIG. 3.20. Pseudobronchiectasis caused by respiratory motion. High-resolution CT with respiratory motion shows multiple double images of pulmonary vessels, mimicking bronchiectasis *(straight arrows).* Note blurring of vascular markings and double image of the left major fissure *(curved arrows).* (Primack SL, Remy-Jardin M, Remy J, Müller NL. High resolution CT of the lung: pitfalls in the diagnosis of infiltrative lung disease. *AJR* 1996;167: 413–418.)

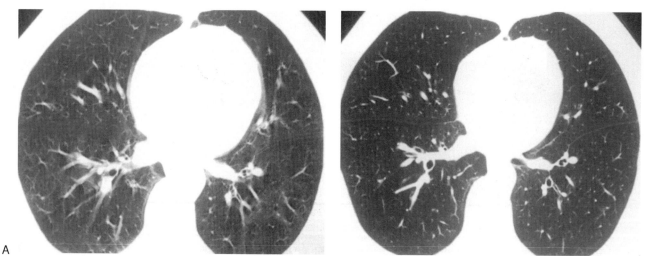

A

B

FIG. 3.21. Ground-glass attenuation caused by respiratory motion. **A:** High-resolution CT scan shows patchy bilateral areas of ground-glass attenuation. Note double image of left major fissure, suggesting respiratory motion. **B:** Repeat HRCT scan with good breath holding demonstrates clear lungs. Note that there is no longer a double image of the major fissure.

ment of pulmonary vessels adjacent to the left ventricle, which may result in an appearance resembling bronchiectasis (34) (Fig. 3.22).

Depth of Inspiration

High-resolution CT scans are routinely obtained at suspended full inspiration. Scans obtained with poor inspiratory effort or in expiration result in areas of ground-glass attenuation (35,36). These areas of ground-glass attenuation may be diffuse or patchy in distribution and mimic the presence of parenchymal lung disease (Fig. 3.23).

Body Position

Atelectasis commonly occurs in the dependent lung regions and may result in dependent density or subpleural lines (37). A band of increased attenuation in the most gravity-dependent lung occurs from decreased ventilation of dependent alveoli and increased blood flow from the effect of gravity (Fig. 3.24). Subpleural dependent density is usually not a diagnostic problem; however, in selected cases, scanning in both supine and prone positions may be required to distinguish depen-

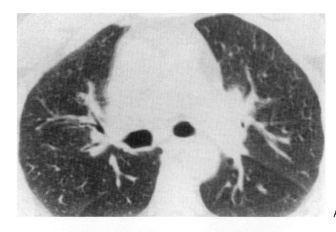

A

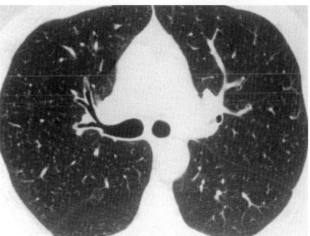

B

FIG. 3.23. Ground-glass attenuation caused by low lung volumes. **A:** High-resolution CT scan obtained at end-expiration shows hazy areas of increased attenuation bilaterally. **B:** High-resolution CT scan obtained at deep inspiration shows clear lungs.

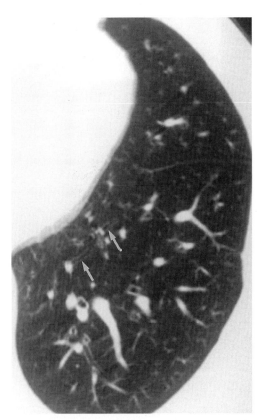

FIG. 3.22. Pseudobronchiectasis caused by cardiac motion. The HRCT scan with good breath holding shows double images of pulmonary vessels adjacent to the left ventricle, mimicking bronchiectasis (arrows).

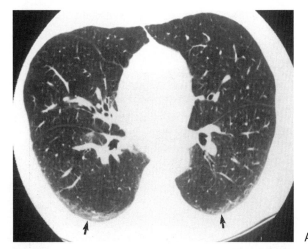

A

FIG. 3.24. Subpleural dependent density. **A:** High-resolution CT scan with patient supine shows a band of increased attenuation posteriorly (arrows) in both lower lobes. (Continued on next page).

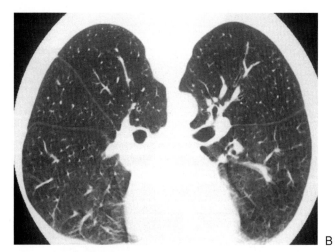

B

FIG. 3.24. *(Continued).* **B:** Prone HRCT scan demonstrates resolution of the posterior ground-glass attenuation, indicating that it is dependent on gravity and not fixed.

dent density (Fig. 3.24) from infiltrative lung disease (Fig. 3.25).

Parenchymal Abnormalities of Vascular Origin

Abnormalities of vascular origin may produce patterns on HRCT that mimic infiltrative lung disease. A pattern of mosaic perfusion has been described in patients with pulmonary arterial hypertension (38,39). Occlusion or constriction of peripheral pulmonary arterial branches leads to an increase in blood flow in the remaining normal vessels. If there is significant redistribution of blood flow away from the abnormal regions, it may result in patchy areas of ground-glass attenuation in the relatively normal lung. The areas of ground-glass attenuation caused by blood flow redistribution are associated with enlarged vessels and therefore can be distinguished from ground-glass attenuation related to parenchymal disease (Fig. 3.26).

Patients with intrinsic airway disease or emphysema may also have a pattern of mosaic perfusion on HRCT. Decreased ventilation in the abnormal areas causes reflex vasoconstriction secondary to hypoxia. Redistribution of blood flow away from these areas produces ground-glass attenuation in less severely involved lung (40). The ground-glass attenuation is associated with larger vessels and represents the relatively normal lung with increased blood flow (Fig. 3.27).

Pulmonary vessels perpendicular to the plane of section may be difficult to distinguish from small nodules on HRCT (Fig. 3.28). This is because of the thin-section technique and lack of continuity of sections. On conventional or spiral 7- to 10-mm collimation CT scans,

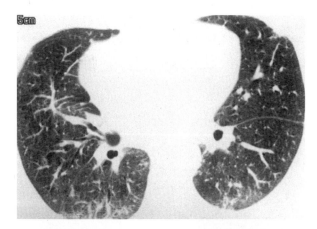

A

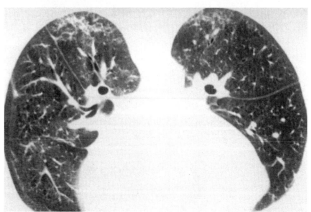

B

FIG. 3.25. Methotrexate toxicity **A:** Supine HRCT scan shows areas of ground-glass attenuation posteriorly in both lower lobes. **B:** Prone HRCT scan demonstrates that the ground-glass attenuation is unchanged, thereby indicating the presence of infiltrative lung disease.

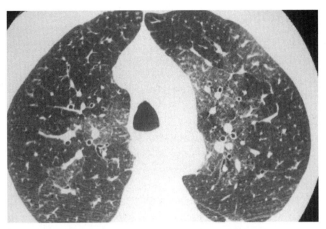

FIG. 3.26. Mosaic perfusion in a patient with recurrent pulmonary emboli. The HRCT scan demonstrates a mosaic pattern of sharply demarcated areas of ground-glass attenuation. Note that the areas of increased attenuation are associated with larger vessels than the low-attenuation areas and represent the relatively normal lung with increased blood flow as a result of blood flow redistribution away from areas with pulmonary artery occlusion.

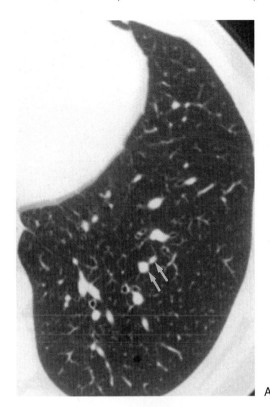

A

volume averaging within the plane of section allows for confident identification of pulmonary vessels.

Another potential pitfall is enhancing atelectasis adjacent to the descending thoracic aorta, which may mimic an acute aortic dissection (Fig. 3.29).

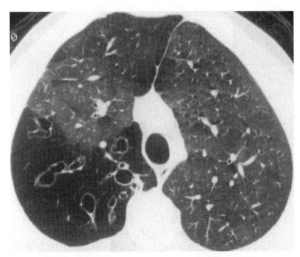

FIG. 3.27. Redistribution of blood flow as a result of airway disease. High-resolution CT scan in a patient with bronchiolitis obliterans shows bronchiectasis and decreased attenuation throughout the right lower lobe. Ground-glass attenuation and larger pulmonary vessels are present throughout the left lung because of redistribution of blood flow. (Primack SL, Remy-Jardin M, Remy J, Müller NL. High resolution CT of the lung: pitfalls in the diagnosis of infiltrative lung disease. *AJR* 1996; 167:413–418.)

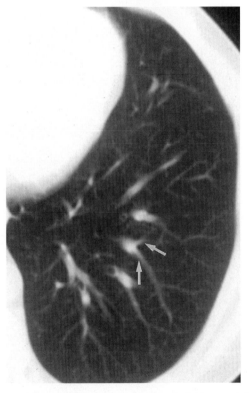

B

FIG. 3.28. Normal pulmonary vessels mimicking nodules. **A:** A 1-mm collimation HRCT scan shows nodular opacities *(arrows)* not definitely associated with bronchi. **B:** Conventional 10-mm collimation CT scan at the same level clearly demonstrates that these opacities are linear, branching structures and represent pulmonary vessels (arrows).

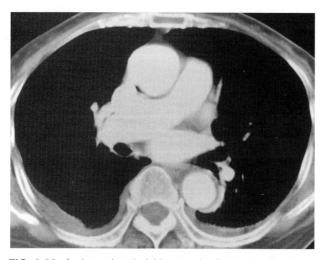

FIG. 3.29. Atelectasis mimicking aortic dissection. Contrast-enhanced CT scan demonstrates enhancing atelectasis adjacent to the descending aorta. This should not be confused with an enhancing false lumen of an aortic dissection.

PSEUDONODULES

The articulation of the first rib and manubrium may mimic a pulmonary nodule in the upper lobes (Fig. 3.30). Evaluation of mediastinal windows and adjacent CT sections can clarify the nature of this pseudonodule. Another potential pitfall is the presence of localized fluid collections within the interlobar fissures (Fig. 3.31) or extension of fat into the fissure (Fig. 3.32), which can mimic lung nodules on the radiograph and CT.

Previous Procedures

Computed tomographic scans performed shortly after bronchoalveolar lavage often demonstrate areas of ground-glass attenuation in the segments that were lavaged (Fig. 3.33). Transbronchial lung biopsy may result in focal nodules or cysts with or without surrounding ground-glass attenuation (41) (Fig. 3.34). In addition, CT scans done during several days after pedal lymphangiogram may show enhancement in dependent portions of the lungs near the pleural surface (Fig. 3.35). This is probably caused by contrast emboli.

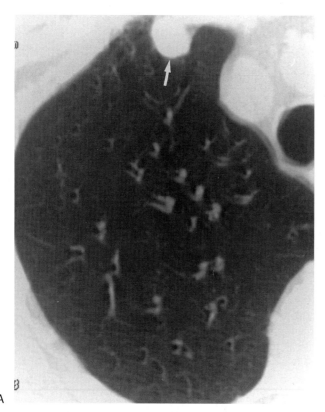

A

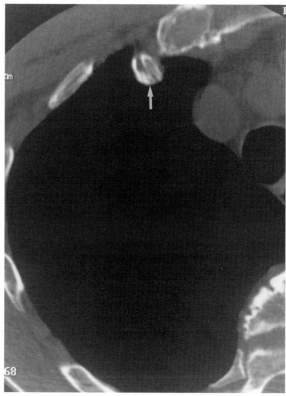

B

FIG. 3.30. Costomanubrial junction mimicking a pulmonary nodule. **A:** Computed tomographic scan filmed at lung windows shows a focal nodular opacity *(arrow)* anteriorly. **B:** Computed tomographic scan filmed at mediastinal windows demonstrates that this nodule is the articulation of the first rib and manubrium (arrow).

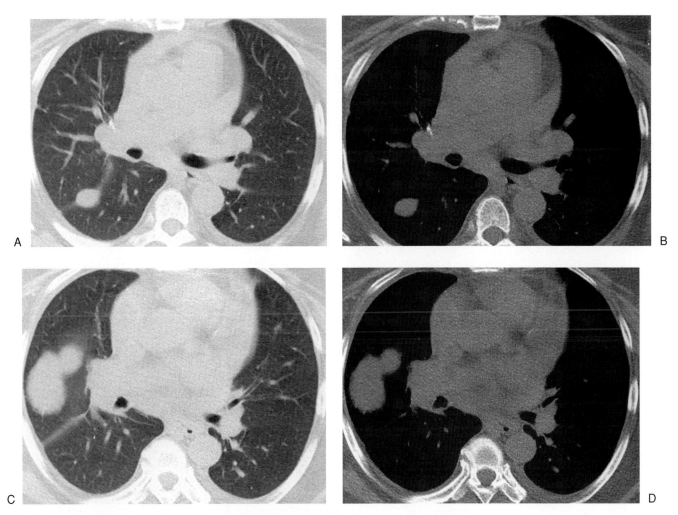

FIG. 3.31. Loculated fluid in interlobar fissures mimicking pulmonary nodules. Lung **(A)** and mediastinal windows **(B)** show fluid in the major interlobar fissure; lung **(C)** and mediastinal windows **(D)** demonstrate fluid in the minor fissure. The focal fluid collections within the interlobular fissures can mimic the appearance of pulmonary nodules on mediastinal windows.

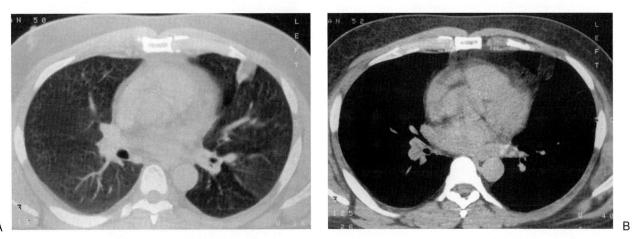

FIG. 3.32. Extension of fat into the fissure mimicking pulmonary nodule. Lung window **(A)** shows soft tissue density adjacent to the pleura extending into the fissure in the left side. The mediastinal window **(B)** demonstrates the fatty nature of the soft tissue mass.

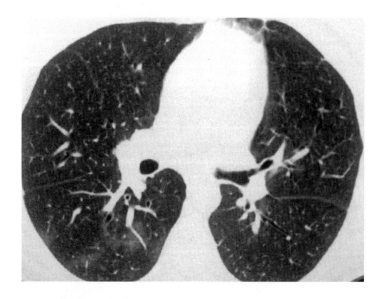

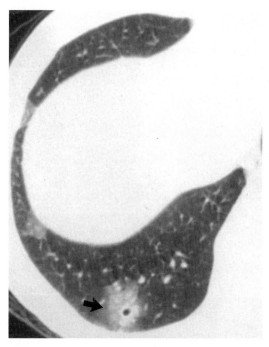

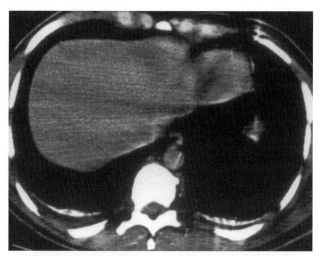

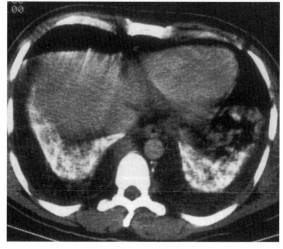

FIG. 3.33. Bronchoalveolar lavage. High-resolution CT scan performed following bronchoalveolar lavage of the superior segment of the right lower lobe shows patchy areas of ground-glass attenuation in the lavaged segment. (Primack SL, Remy-Jardin M, Remy J, Müller NL. High resolution CT of the lung: pitfalls in the diagnosis of infiltrative lung disease. *AJR* 1996; 167:413–418.)

FIG. 3.34. Transbronchial lung biopsy. High-resolution CT through the right lung base obtained shortly after transbronchial lung biopsy shows a focal lucency and surrounding ground-glass attenuation at the site of biopsy *(arrow).* (Primack SL, Remy-Jardin M, Remy J, Müller NL. High resolution CT of the lung: pitfalls in the diagnosis of infiltrative lung disease. *AJR* 1996;167:413–418.)

FIG. 3.35. Chest CT one week after lymphangiogram. **A:** The mediastinal window in this 23-year-old man with germ cell tumor reveals curvilinear high density adjacent to the pleura in the dependent portion of the lungs. **B:** Within 24 hours, the patient's shortness of breath prompted a repeat CT, which reveals bilateral pleural effusion and high-density material in the dependent portion of the atelectatic lungs. Notice prominent azygos vein. The patient had developed congestive heart failure. *(Continued on next page)*

A

B

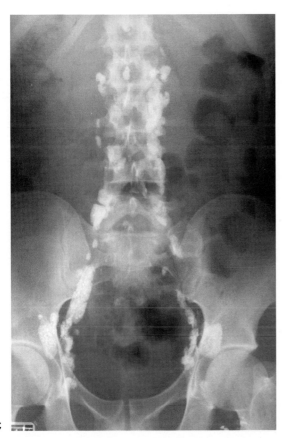

C

FIG. 3.35. *Continued.* **C:** The key to the diagnosis is the history of the patient and the fact that 1 week earlier he had a bipedal lymphangiogram in a search for adenopathy from his underlying germ cell tumor. The CT findings are probably related to embolization of the lungs from lymphangiographic contrast material. (Case courtesy of A. Shirkhoda, M.D., William Beaumont Hospital.)

CONCLUSION

A number of anatomic variants and technical and patient-related artifacts can mimic pleural and parenchymal lung disease on conventional and high-resolution CT. Awareness of these potential pitfalls is essential for optimal assessment of the CT images.

REFERENCES

1. Middleton RM, Littleton JT, Brickey DA, Picone AL. Obstructed tracheal bronchus as a cause of post-obstructive pneumonia. *J Thorac Imag* 1995;10:223–224.
2. Ritsema GH. Ectopic right bronchus: indications for bronchography. *Am J Roentgenol* 1983;140:671–674.
3. Mangiula VG, Razvzn VS. The accessory cardiac bronchus: bronchologic aspect and review of the literature. *Chest* 1968;54:35–38.
4. Atwell SW. Major anomalies of the tracheobronchial tree with a list of minor anomalies. *Chest* 1967;52:611–615.
5. Sotile SC, Brady MB, Brogdon BG. Accessory cardiac bronchus: demonstration by computed tomography. *J Comput Assist Tomogr* 1988;12:144–146.
6. McGuinness G, Naidich DP, Garay SM, et al. Accessory cardiac bronchus: CT features and clinical significance. *Radiology* 1983;189:563–566.
7. Kim JS, Choi D, Lee KS. CT of the bronchus intermedius: frequency and cause of a nodule in the posterior wall on normal scans. *Am J Roentgenol* 1995;165:1349–1352.
8. Berkmen YM, Auh YH, Davis SD, Kazam E. Anatomy of the minor fissure: evaluation with thin-section CT. *Radiology* 1989;170:647–651.
9. Lee KS, Kim PN, Kim IY, Bae WK, Lee BH. The fissural complex of the lung: anatomy and variations on thin-section CT. *J Kor Radiol Soc* 1994;30:481–488.
10. Gross BH, Spizarny DL, Granke DS. Sagittal orientation of the anterior minor fissure: radiography and CT. *Radiology* 1988;166:717–719.
11. Boyden EA. *Segmental anatomy of the lungs.* New York: McGraw-Hill, 1955;95:99–102.
12. Austin JHM. The left minor fissure. *Radiology* 1986;161:433–436.
13. Berkmen T, Berkmen YM, Austin JHM. Accessory fissures of the upper lobe of the left lung: CT and plain film appearance. *Am J Roentgenol* 1994;162:1287–1293.
14. Kolbenstredt A, Kolmannskog F, Aakhus T. The appearance of an anomalous azygos vein on computed tomography of the chest. *Radiology* 1979;130:386.
15. Speckman JM, Gamsu G, Webb WR. Alterations in CT mediastinal anatomy produced by an azygos lobe. *Am J Roentgenol* 1981;137:47–50.
16. Godwin JD, Tarver RD. Accessory fissures of the lung. *Am J Roentgenol* 1985;144:39–47.
17. Kattan KR, Eyler WR, Felson B. The juxtaphrenic peak in upper lobe collapse. *Semin Roentgenol* 1980;15:187–193.
18. Davis SD, Yankelevitz DF, Wand A, Chiarella DA. Juxtaphrenic peak in upper and middle lobe volume loss: assessment with CT. *Radiology* 1996;198:143–149.
19. Godwin JD, Vock P, Osborne DR. CT of the pulmonary ligament. *Am J Roentgenol* 1983;141:231–236.
20. Cooper C, Moss AA, Buy J-N, Stark DD. CT appearance of the normal inferior pulmonary ligament. *Am J Roentgenol* 1983;141:237–240.
21. Rost RC, Proto AV. Inferior pulmonary ligament: computed tomographic appearance. *Radiology* 1983;148:479–483.
22. Berkmen YM, Drossman SR, Marboe CC. Intersegmental (intersublobar) septum of the lower lobe in relation to the pulmonary ligament: anatomic, histologic, and CT correlations. *Radiology* 1992;185:389–393.
23. Hanke R. Das ligamentum pulmonale (bzw. Ligamentum pulmodiaphragmale) im Rontgenbild. *ROFO* 1978;129:1–12.
24. Im J-G, Webb WR, Rosen A, Gamsu G. Costal pleura: appearances at high-resolution CT. *Radiology* 1989;171:125–131.
25. Vix VA. Extrapleural costal fat. *Radiology* 1974;112:563–565.
26. Lee KS, Müller NL. How to distinguish between pleural plaques and pleural fat. *J Respir Dis* 1993;14:1319.
27. Sargent EN, Boswell WD, Ralls PW, et al. Subpleural fat pad in patients exposed to asbestos: distinction from non-calcified pleural plaques. *Radiology* 1984;152:297–309.
28. Müller NL. Imaging of the pleura. *Radiology* 1993;186:297–309.
29. Proto AV. Conventional chest radiographs: anatomic understanding of newer observations. *Radiology* 1992;183:593–603.
30. Sung DW, Yoon Y, Jeong YM, et al. Apical pleural tenting formed by the upper border of the subcostal muscle: CT findings. *Radiology* 1996;201(p):363.
31. Webb WR, Müller NL, Naidich DP. *High-resolution CT of the lung,* 2nd ed. Philadelphia: Lippincott-Raven, 1996.
32. Lee KS, Primack SL, Staples CA, Mayo JR, Aldrich JE, et al. Chronic infiltrative lung disease: comparison of diagnostic accuracies of radiography and low- and conventional-dose thin-section CT. *Radiology* 1994;191:669–673.
33. Murata K, Khan A, Rojas KA, Herman PG. Optimization of computed tomography technique to demonstrate the fine structure of the lung. *Invest Radiol* 1988;23:170–175.
34. Tarver RD, Conces DJ, Godwin JD. Motion artifacts on CT simulate bronchiectasis. *Am J Roentgenol* 1988;151:1117–1119.
35. Robinson PJ, Kreel L. Pulmonary tissue attenuation with computed tomography: comparison of inspiration and expiration scans. *J Comput Assist Tomogr* 1979;3:740–748.
36. Webb WR, Stern EJ, Kanth N, Gamsu G. Dynamic pulmonary CT: findings in normal adult men. *Radiology* 1993;186:117–124.
37. Aberle DR, Gamsu G, Ray SC, Feurstein IM. Asbestos-related pleural and parenchymal fibrosis: detection with high-resolution CT. *Radiology* 1988;166:729–734.

38. Martin KW, Sagel SS, Siegal BA. Mosaic oligemia simulating pulmonary infiltrates on CT. *Am J Roentgenol* 1986;147:670–673.

39. Engeler CE, Kuni CC, Tashjian JH, Engeler CM, du Cret RP. Regional alterations in lung ventilation in end-stage primary pulmonary hypertension: correlation between CT and scintigraphy. *Am J Roentgenol* 1995;164:831–835.

40. Hansell DM, Wells AV, Rubens MB, Cole PJ. Bronchiectasis: functional significance of areas of decreased attenuation at expiratory CT. *Radiology* 1994;193:369–374.

41. Root JD, Molina PL, Anderson DJ, Sagel SS. Pulmonary nodular opacities after transbronchial biopsy in patients with lung transplants. *Radiology* 1992;184:435–436.

Variants and Pitfalls in Body Imaging,
edited by Ali Shirkhoda.
Lippincott Williams & Wilkins, Philadelphia, © 2000.

CHAPTER 4

The Thorax: Postoperative and Postradiation Changes

Ella A. Kazerooni, Barry H. Gross, and Leslie E. Quint

Thoracic surgery, endoscopic procedures, percutaneous interventions, and radiation therapy of the chest alter the normal appearance of the thorax and its contents. Although some radiologic manifestations of these procedures are expected, others may mimic ongoing or recurrent thoracic pathology. It is important to be familiar with the typical appearance of these procedures on cross-sectional imaging and to recognize what variations should raise the suspicion of active disease states, particularly recurrent malignancy. An extensive presentation of all open, reconstructive, and percutaneous procedures is beyond the scope of this chapter. What follows is a presentation of the characteristic postoperative, postprocedural, and postradiation changes that occur after the more commonly performed thoracic surgeries in addition to atypical appearances and radiologic findings that can mimic ongoing disease states.

POSTOPERATIVE AND POSTPROCEDURAL CHANGES

Lung Resection: Lobectomy, Pneumonectomy, and Wedge Resection

Following a lobectomy, many of the same alterations of the thoracic anatomy seen with lobar collapse occur, minus the soft tissue opacity or enhancing atelectasis of the collapsed lobe (1). In fact, many of the signs of volume loss after lobectomy are more accentuated than with lobar collapse, as the volume occupied by the collapsed lobe is absent. In addition to decrease in size of the hemithorax and rib cage on the side of resected lung, mediastinal structures, the diaphragm and abdominal contents, pleural fissures, and the opposite lung are displaced and rotated

toward the resected lobe (Fig. 4.1). Recognition of the repositioning is important to avoid confusion with a soft tissue mass that could represent recurrent malignancy. The reorientation of the remaining pleural fissure after a right lobectomy creates newly formed fissures or neofissures (1). Bronchial orientation is altered. The lobe or lobes remaining after a lobectomy may hyperinflate and expand, resulting in an appearance of fewer pulmonary artery and vein branches compared to the contralateral lung, which should not be confused with hypoperfusion secondary to pulmonary thromboembolism or air trapping secondary to an endobronchial obstructing lesion (see Figs. 4.1–4.3). A thoracotomy defect caused by rib resection and the presence of surgical clips are telltale signs of lung resection. Advances in video-assisted thoracoscopic surgery (VATS) make wedge resection, lobectomy, and even pneumonectomy possible through a thoracoscope. After a VATS resection, no rib defect or surgical clips may be present to indicate that surgery has occurred. If the remaining lobes hyperexpand to fill the surgical space with little rearrangement of other anatomic structures, there may be little volume loss, particularly with resection of the smallest lobe of the lung, the right middle lobe. The combination of this with a VATS resection makes it easy to overlook that there has been lung resection when interpreting computed tomography (CT) examinations in these patients.

After an uncomplicated lobectomy or pneumonectomy, the postsurgical space gradually fills with fluid, while the pleural air in the surgical bed is resorbed. Over time, the space decreases in size, and scar tissue or fibrothorax develops, which may appear as smooth pleural thickening; less commonly pleural calcification may be seen (1–3). Once these changes occur, any subsequent enlargement of the postresection space should raise the possibility of recurrent malignancy or pleural infection (Figs. 4.4 and 4.5). Similarly, the later appearance of air in the sur-

E. A. Kazerooni, B. H. Gross, and L. E. Quint: Department of Diagnostic Radiology, University of Michigan Medical Center, Ann Arbor, Michigan 48109.

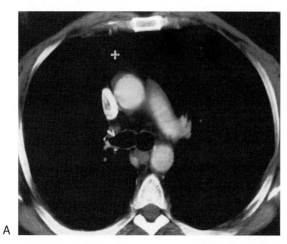
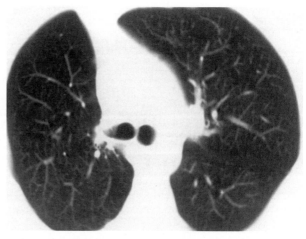

A

B

FIG. 4.1. Right middle lobectomy. Computed tomographic scan of the chest at the level of the carina in a 58-year-old man 1 year following right middle lobectomy for bronchogenic carcinoma demonstrates **(A)** surgical clips at the right hilum on soft-issue windows, with displacement of the anterior mediastinal fat (+) and vascular structures to the right, and **(B)** relative oligemia of the remaining right lung, which is lower in attenuation and has a greater distance between pulmonary vessels than the left lung. This could be confused with true oligemia secondary to pulmonary embolism or air trapping with secondary redistribution of blood flow to normal lung.

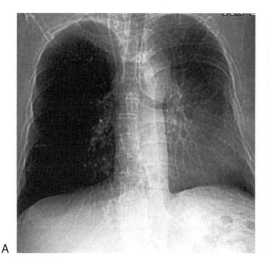
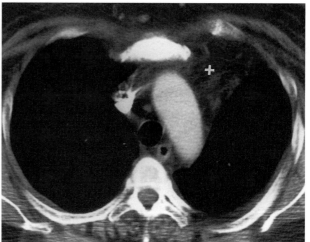

A

B

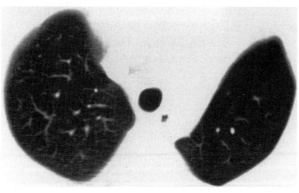

C

FIG. 4.2. Left upper lobectomy. Images of the chest in a 56-year-old woman 5 years following a left upper lobectomy for stage II (T2N1) bronchogenic carcinoma. **A:** The CT scout topogram demonstrates an ill-defined left heart border and shift of mediastinal structures to the left, similar findings to left upper lobe collapse, with additional findings of a rib thoracotomy defect and left hilar surgical clips. **B:** Axial CT images demonstrate displacement of the mediastinum, including the anterior mediastinal fat (+), to the left on soft tissue windows. **C:** There is reduced attenuation and a paucity of blood vessels in the hyperexpanded left lower lobe compared to the normal right upper lobe; the interface of the left lower lobe with the mediastinal fat could be mistaken for the major fissure bordering a collapsed upper lobe on the lung windows.

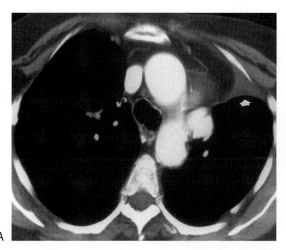
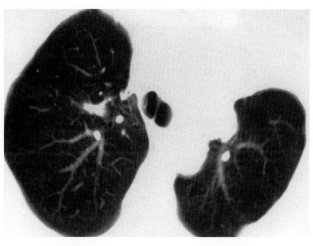

A

B

FIG. 4.3. Bilateral upper lobectomies. Computed tomographic scan of the chest in a 73-year-old woman 4 years following left upper lobectomy and 6 years following right upper lobectomy, both for bronchogenic carcinoma. There is slight shift of mediastinal structures to the left, as the volume of the resected left upper lobe and lingula is greater than the volume of the resected right upper lobe. **A:** A small amount of fluid *(arrow)* in the resection space seen on soft tissue windows was unchanged on CT for several years. Any increase in the fluid or development of pleural thickening or nodularity should raise the suspicion of infection or recurrent malignancy. **B:** The pulmonary vessel branching pattern is distorted, the carina rotated and anteriorly displaced, and the central bronchovascular structures displaced anteriorly, as demonstrated on lung windows.

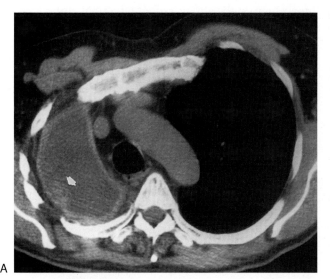
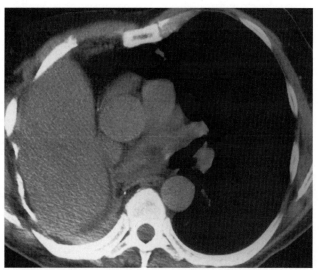

A

B

FIG. 4.4. Right pneumonectomy. Computed tomographic scan of the chest in a 66-year-old man 5 years following completion of a pneumonectomy for bronchoalveolar cell carcinoma; he had undergone a right upper lobectomy 14 years ago and right middle lobectomy 6 years ago. **A:** Image at the level of the aortic arch demonstrates fluid in the resection space and displacement of mediastinal structures to the right, as typically seen after pneumonectomy. There is also a pleural soft tissue nodule *(arrow)* representing recurrent malignancy, subsequently proven by thoracentesis. Smooth pleural thickening representing fibrous tissue or fibrothorax may be seen after a pneumonectomy but should not become thicker after the postsurgical changes have stabilized. In this case, the circumferential pleural thickening had been stable for several years; only the nodule was new. **B:** Image at the level of the main pulmonary artery demonstrates a soft tissue mass in the right midthorax, representing the right lobe of the liver, displaced into the right hemithorax.

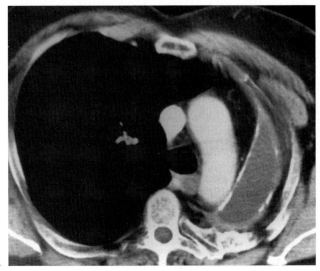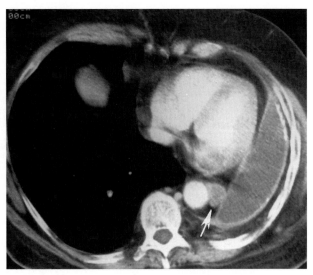

A

B

FIG. 4.5. Left pneumonectomy. CT scan of the chest in a 65-year-old man 10 years following a left pneumonectomy for bronchogenic carcinoma demonstrates **(A)** fluid in the resection space, smooth pleural thickening, pleural calcification, and leftward displacement of the mediastinum on this image taken at the level of the aortic arch. **B:** Similar findings are seen on this image at the level of the dome of the right hemidiaphragm. Note also the repositioning of the esophagus *(arrow)* lateral to the descending thoracic aorta that could mimic a soft tissue mass. Both of these findings could potentially be mistaken for a soft-tissue mass.

gical space strongly suggests the presence of a bronchopleural fistula, usually secondary to recurrent malignancy or pleural infection (1–4).

Following a right pneumonectomy, the left main bronchus may become compressed between the thoracic spine and aorta posteriorly and the pulmonary artery anteriorly. This is referred to as postpneumonectomy syndrome (Fig. 4.6) (5). This is rare following left pneumonectomy in the absence of either a right aortic arch or mediastinal anomaly (6). Treatment consists of placing a prosthesis in the pleural space to reduce the severity of mediastinal shift or, more recently, placement of an endobronchial stent (5,6).

Wedge resections of lung are commonly performed for focal pulmonary lesions, often using VATS. Although a solitary lung lesion not yet known to be malignant or

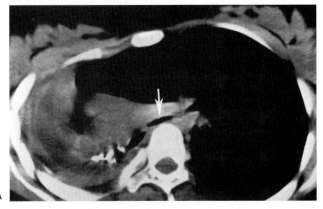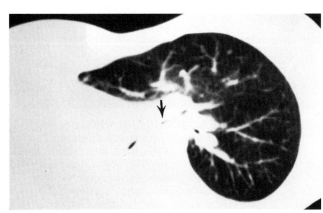

A

B

FIG. 4.6. Postpneumonectomy syndrome and treatment with prosthesis. Computed tomographic images of the chest following a right pneumonectomy. **A:** There is typical fluid and smooth pleural thickening in the resection space, surgical clips at the right hilum, displacement of mediastinal structures to the right, and herniation of the left lung across midline on soft tissue windows. There is also compression of the left main bronchus between the pulmonary artery and the spine *(arrow)*. **B:** Near complete occlusion of the left main bronchus is seen on lung windows *(arrow)*. At fluoroscopy there was complete collapse of the left main bronchus during expiration or with coughing.

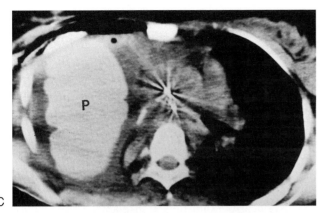

C

FIG. 4.6. *Continued.* **C:** Treatment consisted of placing a prosthesis in the resection space (P), returning mediastinal structures to midline. The left main bronchus is returned to a normal position, relieving the bronchial compression. (This figure submitted courtesy of Jo-Anne Shepard, M.D., Massachusetts General Hospital, Boston, MA.)

benign may be resected, followed by an immediate lobectomy if shown to be malignant at frozen section, patients with poor pulmonary reserve may also undergo wedge resection of a bronchogenic carcinoma as a lung-sparing procedure (7). Multiple nodules may undergo wedge resection, particularly in patients with sarcoma metastases to the lung (8). A small amount of soft tissue representing fibrous scar may be seen adjacent to a staple line

(Fig. 4.7A). Nodular soft tissue at a staple line is highly suspicious for recurrent malignancy (Fig. 4.7B).

Bronchoscopy and Transbronchial Biopsy

Chest radiographs performed to evaluate for the possibility of postprocedure pneumothorax after bronchoscopy often demonstrate areas of alveolar or air-space opacity as a result of hemorrhage or residual bronchoalveolar lavage fluid. Small nodules, either solid or cavitary, may also be seen following transbronchial biopsy on chest radiographs (9). These findings may also be seen on CT images (10). Transbronchial biopsy-related lung injury is seen on CT up to 1 month after the procedure (Fig. 4.8). The injury is thought to be related to the large-gauge alligator forceps used to obtain pieces of lung parenchyma, usually measuring 1 to 2 mm in diameter, sometimes as large as 5 mm. Several specimens are taken from the same location, leaving lung lacerations that measure up to 15 mm on CT (10). Lung transplant recipients commonly undergo surveillance bronchoscopy at regular intervals in search of subclinical allograft rejection and similarly may undergo surveillance CT scanning (11,12). Transbronchial biopsies are usually taken from several lobes of the transplanted lung, with as few as two or three or as many as 15 biopsy specimens taken during the procedure (11). Computed tomographic images after these procedures may demonstrate multiple solid and/or cavitary nodules throughout the lung (Figs. 4.9 and 4.10).

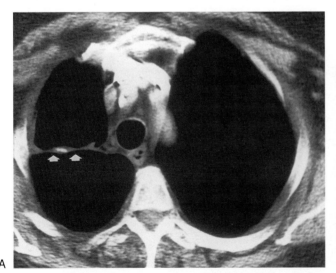

A

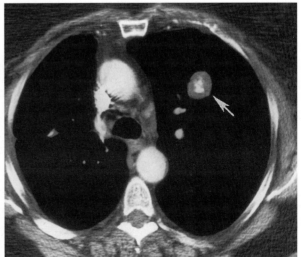

B

FIG. 4.7. Bilateral wedge resections with and without recurrent malignancy. Computed tomographic scan of the chest in a 74-year-old woman following bilateral apical wedge resections for bilateral stage I bronchogenic carcinomas. **A:** Image at the level of the aortic arch demonstrates a right upper lobe staple line with thin rim of soft tissue attenuation *(arrows)* consistent with fibrous scar. **B:** Image at the level of aortopulmonary window demonstrates a soft tissue attenuation nodule centered on a wedge resection staple line *(arrow)* consistent with recurrent malignancy.

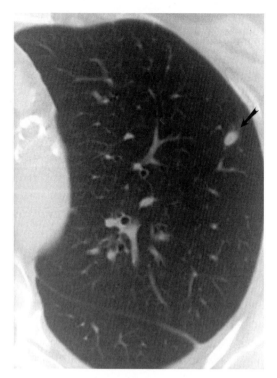

FIG. 4.8. Solitary solid lung nodule after transbronchial biopsy. Computed tomographic image of a 53-year-old woman after bilateral lung transplantation, 19 days after transbronchial biopsy demonstrates a solid 8-mm lung nodule *(arrow)* with minimal adjacent ground-glass attenuation. The radiologic differential diagnosis for this noncalcified nodule is otherwise nonspecific and includes infection, malignancy, and rejection in a lung transplant recipient. (Reproduced from reference 10 with permission from the Radiological Society of North America and Ella A. Kazerooni, M.D.)

These nodules are often surrounded by a halo of ground-glass attenuation, a finding commonly seen with invasive aspergillosis. Failure to recognize the temporal relationship of these lesions to bronchoscopy can lead to the misdiagnosis of infection or malignancy (Fig. 4.11).

Lung Transplantation

Lung transplantation is performed most commonly for emphysema, idiopathic pulmonary fibrosis (IPF), and cystic fibrosis in adults (13). The Registry of the International Society for Heart and Lung Transplantation lists nearly 9,000 lung transplantation procedures performed in the last 14 years, either as single lung transplant, double lung transplant, or combined heart-lung transplant procedures (13). With the improvements and refinements in patient selection, surgical technique, perioperative care, and immunosuppressant regimens, the 3-year survival for all lung transplant recipients combined is nearly 60%, and the 5-year survival 40%. The growing population of living lung transplant patients often undergo chest CT for surveillance in search of clinically occult allograft rejection or infection, in hopes that early intervention may spare lung function (12).

Bronchial dilation is the hallmark of obliterative bronchiolitis (OB) or chronic rejection (Fig. 4.12). High-resolution CT (HRCT) images should be obtained in this patient population, as bronchial dilation may be missed on conventional CT images performed with 5- to 10-mm collimation. Diminution of peripheral vascular structures,

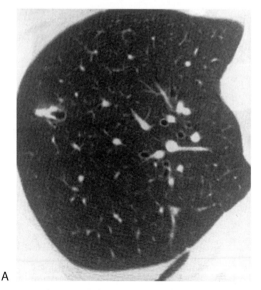

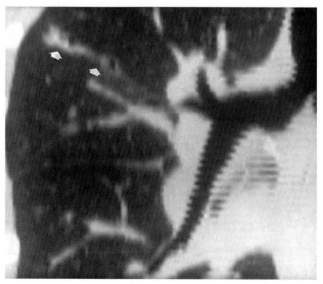

A   B

FIG. 4.9. Solitary cavitary lung nodule after transbronchial biopsy. Computed tomographic scan of the chest in a 55-year-old lung transplant recipient 13 days following transbronchial biopsy. **A:** There is a 10 × 10 × 5 mm oval-shaped cavitary nodule with a faint halo of ground-glass attenuation that raises the suspicion of infection, particularly invasive aspergillosis in this patient on immunosuppressant medications. **B:** Computed tomographic scan reconstructed in the coronal plane shows that the abnormality radiates outward from the hilum along the course of a segmental/subsegmental bronchus *(arrows).* (Reproduced from reference 10 with permission from the Radiological Society of North America and Ella A. Kazerooni, M.D.)

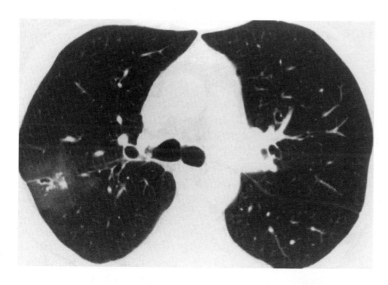

FIG. 4.10. Cavitary and solid lung nodules with hemorrhage after transbronchial biopsy. Computed tomographic image of a 43-year-old man after bilateral lung transplantation, 8 days after transbronchial biopsy demonstrates a cluster of solid and cavitary lung nodules with adjacent ground-glass attenuation consistent with pulmonary laceration and hemorrhage. These lesions mimic infection, particularly fungal and mycobacterial infections.

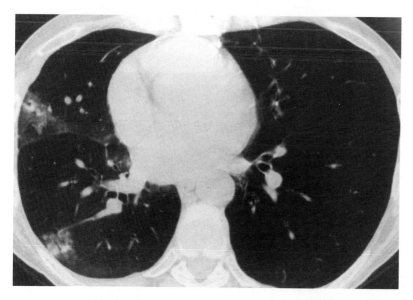

FIG. 4.11. Multilobar solitary and cavitary lung nodules after transbronchial biopsy. Computed tomographic image of a 58-year-old woman after right lung transplant, 6 hours after transbronchial biopsy. Clusters of solid and cavitary nodules are present in both the right middle and lower lobes, with adjacent ground-glass attenuation consistent with lung lacerations and hemorrhage. These lesions mimic infection, particularly fungal and mycobacterial infections.

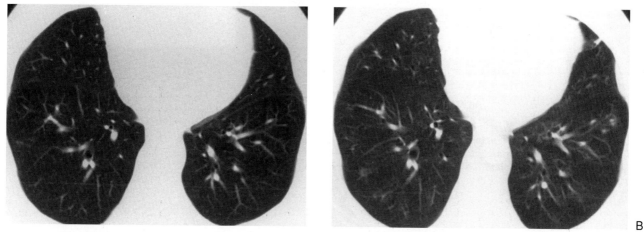

A

B

FIG. 4.12. Obliterative bronchiolitis (chronic allograft rejection) in a bilateral lung transplant recipient. Computed tomographic images of a 46-year-old man demonstrate **(A)** normal lungs 4 years after lung transplantation at a time when pulmonary function was stable and the patient was asymptomatic. **B:** Five years after transplantation, there is diffuse cylindrical bronchiectasis on this 5-mm collimation CT image consistent with obliterative bronchiolitis. *Continued on next page.*

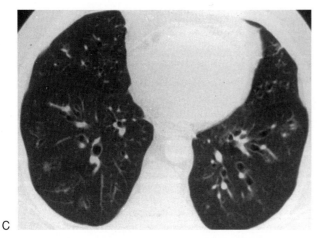

C

FIG. 4.12. *Continued.* **C:** The findings are better seen on a 1-mm collimation HRCT image. At this time there was a reduction in pulmonary function, and the patient was short of breath.

septal thickening, and volume reduction are seen on CT with OB and may precede the clinical diagnosis (12,14). Normal CT findings can mimic significant disease in these patients. Airway anastomotic complications are less frequent now than in the early years of lung transplantation and include bronchial stenosis and dehiscence (14). However, a mild narrowing of the bronchial anastomosis is common (referred to as a bronchial "shelf") and is without clinical significance (Figs. 4.13 and 4.14). This appears on CT as a mild narrowing of the main bronchus. When there is doubt, expiratory CT images for the evaluation of air trapping within the transplanted lung or collapse of the airway may be useful. Also, mismatch of the donor and recipient atrial cuff may appear as an outpouching from the left atrial wall, mimicking an aneurysm (Fig. 4.15). Solitary and cavitary pulmonary nodules with adjacent ground-glass attenuation on CT may be seen up to 1 month following the commonly per-

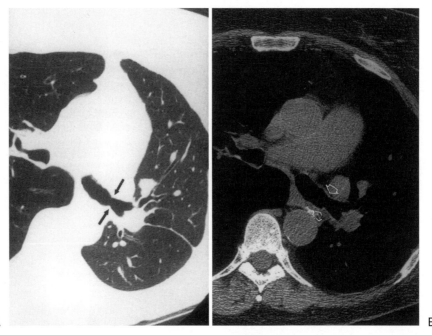

A   B

FIG. 4.13. Anastomotic shelf. Computed tomographic image of a 52-year-old woman 5 years following left lung transplant for emphysema demonstrates mild narrowing of the left main bronchus anastomosis *(arrows)* on both **(A)** lung and **(B)** soft tissue windows. At the time the patient had stable pulmonary function without shortness of breath, wheezing, or cough. Hyperinflation of the native emphysematous right lung is demonstrated with displacement of the mediastinum to the left and extension of the right lung anteriorly into the left hemithorax. These findings have remained stable for 6 years.

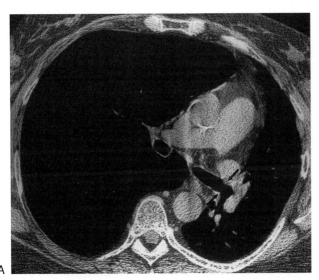
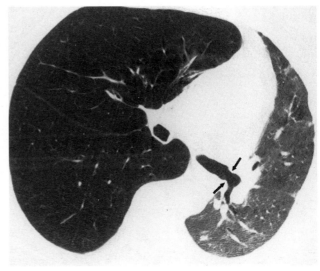

A

B

FIG. 4.14. Anastomotic shelf. Computed tomographic image of a 53-year-old woman 4 years following left lung transplant for emphysema demonstrates mild narrowing of the left main bronchus anastomosis *(arrows)* on both **(A)** soft tissue and **(B)** lung windows. At the time the patient had stable pulmonary function without shortness of breath, wheezing, or cough. Hyperinflation of the native emphysematous right lung is demonstrated with displacement of the mediastinum to the left and extension of the right lung anteriorly into the left hemithorax. These findings have remained stable for 8 years.

formed transbronchial biopsies in this population, mimicking infection (see Figs. 4.8–4.11).

Chest Wall Resection, Reconstruction, and Transthoracic Procedures

Chest wall malignancy (including primary chest wall sarcomas (Figs. 4.16 and 4.17; see Fig. 4.44), metastases to the chest wall (and chest wall invasion by bronchogenic carcinoma), and non-malignant conditions (including traumatic injury, lung herniation into the chest wall, chronic infection and congenital anomalies) are indications for chest wall resection and reconstruction (15). In cases of malignancy, a wide margin of normal tissue is necessary to provide the best chance for disease-free survival, so even small lesions require a large resection of the chest wall (Fig. 4.16).

Herniation of the lung may occur after chest wall trauma, thoracotomy, thoracoscopy, or tube thoracostomy; rarely it is congenital (17,18). Small lung hernias are more commonly recognized today, with the use of CT, than in the era before CT scanning of the chest (19,20). During expiration, the amount of lung within the chest wall increases, and visible focal chest wall deformity may be demonstrated. A lung hernia may be an incidental finding in an asymptomatic patient and require no surgical repair. When symptoms occur they may include vague discomfort or pain (17, 21). Confusion with other chest wall or extrapulmonary air collections can be reduced by recognizing the contiguity of the chest wall air collection with lung or extension of pulmonary vessels into the air

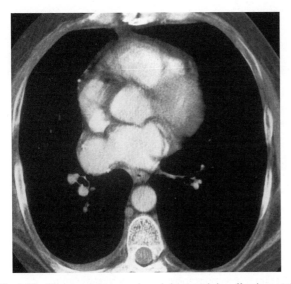

FIG. 4.15. Donor atrium and recipient atrial cuff mismatch. Intravenous contrast-enhanced CT image of a 51-year-old man 6 weeks after right lung transplantation. There is a contrast-enhanced convex outward deformity of the right posterolateral wall of the left atrium with adjacent surgical clips, which tapered into the normal-sized right inferior pulmonary vein. The donor left atrium was noted to be large at the time of surgery and was trimmed to better match the recipient atrial cuff. This deformity mimics a varix or aneurysm of the pulmonary vein or left atrium.

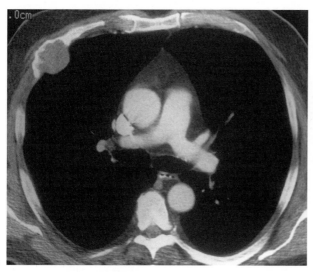
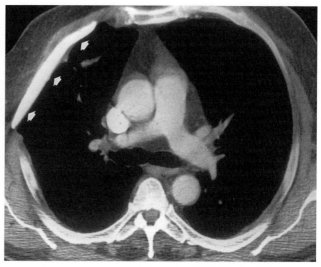

FIG. 4.16. Chest wall resection and reconstruction. Computed tomographic images of the chest in a 54-year-old man with a Ewing's sarcoma of the right fourth rib, before and after chest wall resection and reconstruction. The entire fourth rib and 5-cm portions of both the third and fifth ribs were resected. In addition, the mass invaded the adjacent right upper and middle lobes, requiring lung resection. **A:** Pre-operative CT image demonstrates a 2.8-cm soft tissue mass destroying the anterior aspect of the right fourth rib. **B:** Computed tomographic image 6 months after surgery demonstrates a chest wall prosthesis *(arrows)* fashioned to match the defect at the time of surgery. The right and left anterior chest wall contours are relatively symmetric. The prosthesis is high in attenuation, which may mimic sclerotic bone.

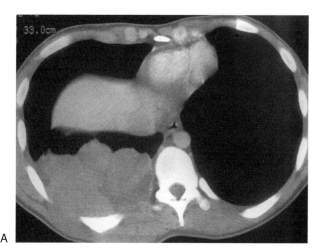
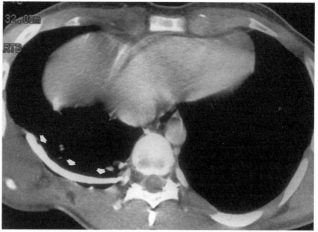

FIG. 4.17. Chest wall resection and reconstruction. Computed tomographic images of the chest in an 18-year-old man with a primitive neuroectodermal tumor of the right chest wall, before and after chest wall resection and reconstruction. The patient underwent *en-bloc* resection of the chest wall tumor with wedge resection of the right lower lobe and partial resection of the right hemidiaphragm and the eighth, ninth, and tenth ribs. **A:** Preoperative CT image demonstrates a large soft tissue mass in the posterior right hemithorax surrounding the posterior ribs and deforming the contour of the chest. There is a large component of the mass inside the rib cage, with an irregular border with the adjacent lung, consistent with right lower lobe of lung invasion by the tumor. **B:** Computed tomographic image 5 months after surgery demonstrates a chest wall prosthesis *(arrows)* fashioned from methylmethacrylate between two layers of propylene mesh that was formed to match the defect at the time of surgery. The triangular shaped 10 × 9 × 7 cm prosthesis was sewn into place to the adjacent musculature and to ribs through holes drilled in the ribs. The prosthesis is high in attenuation, which may mimic sclerotic bone.

collection (Figs. 4.18 and 4.19). In difficult cases, an expiratory image showing enlargement of the lung hernia compared to the inspiratory images can confirm the diagnosis. Chest wall muscles can also be injured by a tube thoracostomy, creating a soft tissue mass that mimics a tumor (Fig. 4.20).

Following thoracic surgery, postoperative atrophy of the chest wall musculature may occur ipsilateral to the surgery (22). Atrophy is thought to be secondary to denervation injury caused by the surgical incision. On CT, this is most recognizable among the larger posterolateral chest wall muscles, including the latissimus dorsi and serratus anterior muscles (Figs. 4.21 and 4.22) (22). Diffuse ipsilateral chest wall atrophy may otherwise suggest the possibility of disuse atrophy, as occurs following a large cerebrovascular accident.

Thoracoplasty, commonly performed for the treatment of tuberculosis in decades past, creates recognizable deformity of the chest wall on chest radiographs. The CT appearance of this procedure is not well known (23). In addition to volume loss and pleural thickening, the ribs are crowded and become realigned within the axial CT

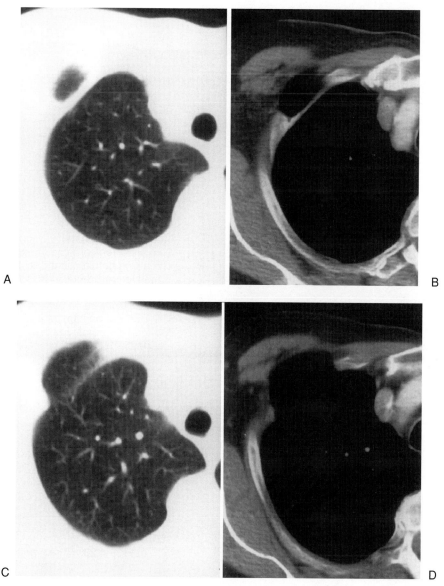

FIG. 4.18. Lung hernia secondary to right thoracotomy. Computed tomographic images of a 70-year-old woman with a lung hernia secondary to an exploratory right thoracotomy. Consecutive CT images displayed on both **(A,C)** lung and **(B,D)** soft tissue windows demonstrate air in the right anterior chest wall, elevating the pectoralis major and minor muscles. Pulmonary vessels extend from the lung directly into the air collection.

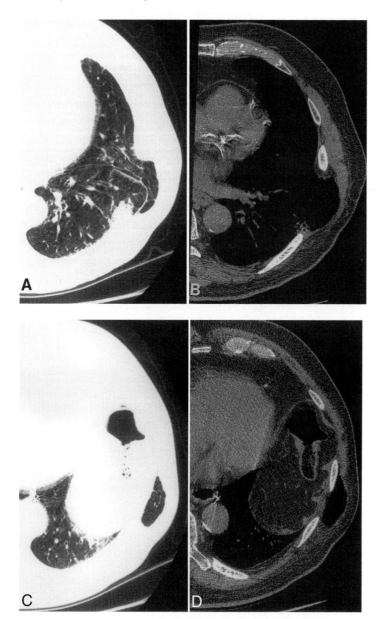

FIG. 4.19. Lung hernia secondary to left thoracotomy. Computed tomographic images of a 76-year-old man with a lung hernia secondary to a left thoracotomy performed for transthoracic Nissen fundoplication repair of a paraesophageal hernia. Computed tomographic images displayed on both **(A,C)** lung and **(B,D)** soft tissue windows demonstrate air extending from the lung into the left lateral chest wall, elevating the intercostal muscles. Pulmonary vessels extend from the lung directly into the air collection.

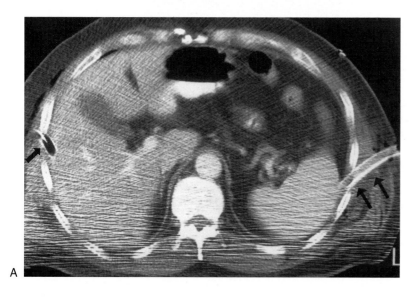

FIG. 4.20. Chest wall muscle injury following tube thoracostomy. Computed tomographic images of a 47-year-old man injured during a motor vehicle accident, requiring bilateral tube thoracostomies. **A:** Computed tomographic image immediately following trauma demonstrates bilateral tube thoracostomies *(arrows)*. The left tube passes through the serratus anterior and external abdominal oblique muscles.

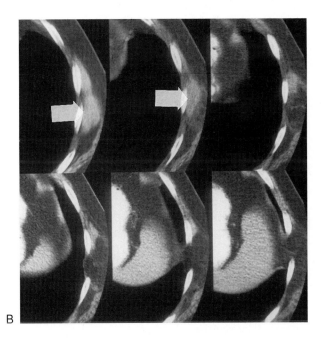

B

FIG. 4.20. *Continued.* **B:** Consecutive CT images obtained 17 months later demonstrate a soft tissue mass in the left chest wall *(arrow),* representing the injured and contracted serratus anterior muscle.

plane: in some places they become more perpendicular, and in other places more parallel and in-plane (Fig. 4.23). Scoliosis convex to the side of the thoracoplasty is typically seen (23). The ribs may have a sclerotic appearance, mimicking chronic infection of bone, osteonecrosis, or metastases (see Fig. 4.23).

An Eloesser procedure or open-window thoracostomy is performed for the treatment of a chronic pleural empyema that has failed thoracostomy or empyema tube drainage. A U-shaped incision is made through the skin, subcutaneous

tissue and chest wall muscle down to the ribs, creating a soft tissue flap. A portion of the adjacent two or three ribs is resected, creating an opening into which the soft tissue flap is folded and sutured to the parietal pleura and empyema lining. The opening in the chest wall permits long-term drainage without chest tubes (24). The thick empyema peel prevents herniation of the lung through the opening. On CT, there is an air-filled cavity in the pleural space that communicates with the air outside the body wall. The cavity has a soft tissue attenuation lining, representing the thickened

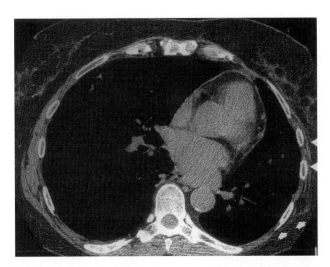

FIG. 4.21. Chest wall muscle atrophy following left thoracotomy. Computed tomographic image of a 52-year-old woman 5 years following left lung transplantation through a left thoracotomy. Atrophy of the left latissimus dorsi *(solid arrows)* and serratus anterior *(arrowheads)* muscles is demonstrated relative to the right chest wall muscles. The intercostal muscles and deep back muscles are spared.

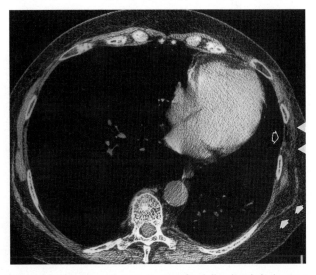

FIG. 4.22. Chest wall muscle atrophy following left thoracotomy. Computed tomographic image of a 53-year-old woman 4 years following left lung transplantation through a left thoracotomy demonstrates atrophy of the left latissimus dorsi *(solid arrows)* and serratus anterior *(arrowheads)* muscles, compared to the right chest wall muscles. An intercostal muscle is also atrophied *(open arrow).*

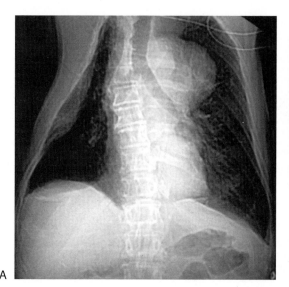
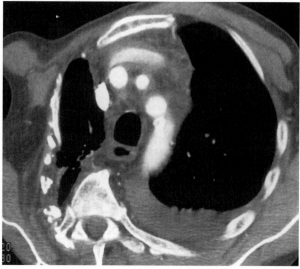

A

B

FIG. 4.23. Right thoracoplasty. Computed tomographic images of a 76-year-old man 47 years following a thoracoplasty for tuberculosis with partial resection of seven ribs. **A:** Scout topogram demonstrates characteristic deformity of the upper right chest, with convex inward deformity, designed to decrease the volume of right apical lung. Incidentally, there is a 7-cm aneurysm of the proximal descending thoracic aorta. Note the right convex scoliosis. **B:** Computed tomographic image just above the aortic arch demonstrates deformity and decrease in volume of the right chest wall, with reorientation of the ribs, many of which appear sclerotic and smaller than the corresponding left ribs.

pleura. The infolded skin flap is contiguous with the skin and subcutaneous tissue of the chest wall, with a fat attenuation component wrapped around the rib, covered by a thin, soft tissue attenuation band of the overlying skin (Fig. 4.24). Over time, the window decreases in size as granulation tissue forms. The opening may become obliterated, or a small opening may persist, particularly if there is ongoing infection requiring drainage (24,25). Familiarity with this procedure is necessary to avoid confusion with a large chest wall fistula or chest wall destruction.

Surgical Flaps

Soft tissue flaps may be transposed into the chest to promote healing or to reinforce surgical anastomoses or resection margins. The native vascular supply of the flap

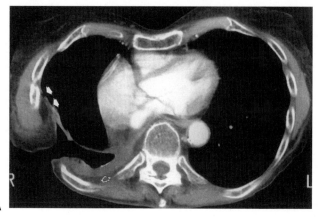
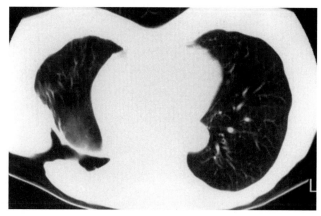

A

B

FIG. 4.24. Eloesser flap. Computed tomographic images of a 72-year-old woman 6 months after an Eloesser flap performed for a chronic empyema and bronchopleural fistula that developed following a lower lobectomy. **A:** Computed tomographic image at soft tissue windows demonstrates an air-filled space within the right hemithorax posterolaterally, which extends through the chest wall to the body surface. The fat attenuation representing the subcutaneous fat of the infolded flap wraps around the rib *(arrow).* Soft tissue attenuation pleural thickening is seen posteriorly *(open arrow).* **B:** The thickening of the visceral pleura covering the lung is better appreciated on lung windows.

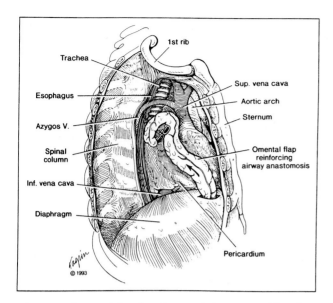

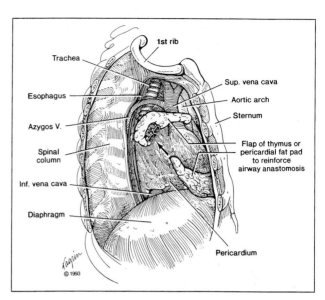

FIG. 4.25. Omental flap for airway reinforcement. Line drawing of the mediastinum presented from the right side demonstrates a pedicle of greater omentum extending through an opening in the diaphragm, wrapping around the central airway. (Reproduced from reference 26 with permission from the Radiological Society of North America and Jo-Anne Shepard, M.D.)

FIG. 4.26. Pericardial fat pad flap and thymic flap for airway reinforcement. Line drawing of the mediastinum presented from the right side demonstrates the use of the pericardial fat pad and thymus to reinforce the central airway. (Reproduced from reference 26 with permission from the Radiological Society of North America and Jo-Anne Shepard, M.D.)

is maintained by preserving the vascular pedicle of the transposed tissue (17, 26, 27). Adipose tissue from a pericardial fat pad or omentum (Figs. 4.25–4.27), or muscle tissue, such as intercostal muscles (Fig. 4.28), the serratus anterior, latissimus dorsi, pectoralis, and rectus abdo-

minis muscles are most commonly used. Flaps may also be formed from the thymus (Fig. 4.29), pleura, and mediastinal fat. A flap may be used to reinforce an airway anastomosis (see Figs. 4.25, 4.26, and 4.29) or cover a bronchial resection stump. An esophageal anastomosis or

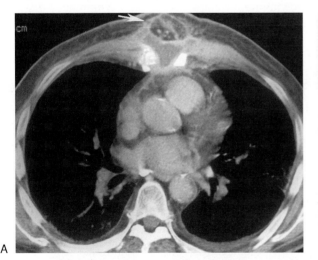

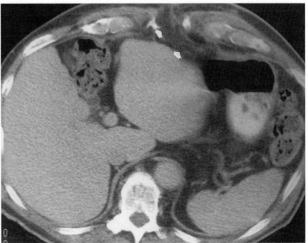

A

B

FIG. 4.27. Omental flap for treatment of an infected sternotomy incision. Computed tomographic images of the chest in a 78-year-old man 2 months following exploration and debridement of an infected sternal wound and wound closure with an omental flap. The initial sternotomy was performed 1 month earlier for coronary artery bypass graft surgery complicated by wound infection and mediastinitis. **A:** Computed tomographic image at the level of the midsternal body demonstrates fluid in the osseous sternal defect, with an ovoid fat attenuation structure with a thin soft tissue rim *(arrow)*, representing the transposed flap of greater omentum. **B:** Computed tomographic image of the upper abdomen demonstrates extension of the fat attenuation greater omental flap *(arrows)* from its native location in the upper abdomen, through the anterior abdominal wall.

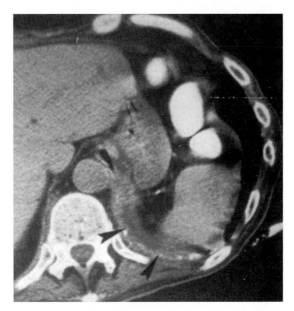

FIG. 4.28. Intercostal muscle flap for reinforcement of an esophageal tear. Computed tomographic image through the lower chest demonstrates a partially calcified or ossified intercostal muscle flap extending from the esophagus posteriorly into the left paraspinal location *(arrowheads).* (Reproduced from reference 26 with permission from the Radiological Society of North America and Jo-Anne Shepard, M.D.)

tear may be reinforced with a flap to promote healing (see Fig. 4.28), or a flap may be used to obliterate a persistent space after lung resection (26,27). Persistent chest wall incisions complicated by infection, such as a median sternotomy, may be filled with a pedicle flap that maintains

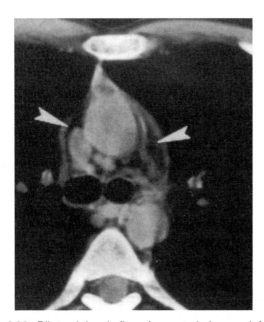

FIG. 4.29. Bilateral thymic flaps for central airway reinforcement. Computed tomographic image demonstrates bilateral fat attenuation thymic flaps *(arrowheads)* used to reinforce the airway during bilateral lung transplantation. (Reproduced from reference 26 with permission from the Radiological Society of North America and Jo-Anne Shepard, M.D.)

the vascular supply of the flap to promote healing (see Fig. 4.27) (16). Knowledge of the anatomy of these flaps is necessary to prevent confusion with fat and soft tissue attenuation masses. The adipose tissue flaps from the pericardial fat pad or omentum are fat in attenuation on CT and could be confused with lipomatosis or lipomatous tumor. Muscle flaps are soft tissue in attenuation and may be confused with a soft tissue mass. Muscle flaps usually atrophy over time because of denervation and/or disuse and may even calcify or ossify (Fig. 4.28).

Mastectomy, Lumpectomy, and Axillary Lymph Node Dissection

The CT appearance following a mastectomy depends on the type of mastectomy: radical, modified radical or simple. A simple mastectomy involves complete resection of only the breast tissue. Correspondingly, the breast tissue is absent on CT (see Fig. 4.44). During a radical mastectomy, the breast tissue and pectoralis major and minor muscles are resected, and an extensive axillary lymph node dissection is performed. On CT, the pectoralis muscles and breast tissue are absent. A modified radical mastectomy includes complete resection of the breast tissue and usually resection of the pectoralis major muscle (Fig. 4.30). One variation of the modified radical mastectomy is resection of the pectoralis muscle fascia without the pectoralis muscle, sometime referred to as a total mastectomy. Another variation includes partial resection of the pectoralis major muscle as well. The CT appearance is dependent on the tissues resected (28).

Postoperative changes occur in the surgical bed following lumpectomy and axillary lymph node dissection (Figs. 4.31 and 4.32). The appearance of these changes

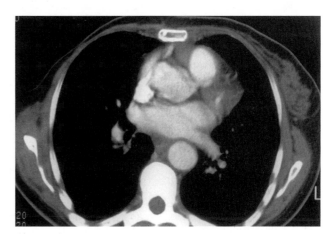

FIG. 4.30. Right mastectomy. Computed tomographic image of the chest in a 62-year-old woman, 5.5 years following a modified radical mastectomy. Right breast tissue is absent, consistent with either a radical, modified radical, total, or simple mastectomy. The appearance of the pectoralis muscles can be used to determine the type of mastectomy performed.

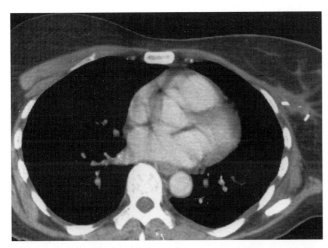

FIG. 4.31. Left breast lumpectomy scar. Computed tomographic image of the chest in a 56-year-old woman 5 months following a left breast lumpectomy for invasive ductal carcinoma. Abnormal soft tissue is present in the surgical bed with straight borders, adjacent to surgical clips. On a single examination alone, the presence of residual or recurrent breast cancer cannot be excluded. However, stability or decrease in size of the abnormality over time, especially stability on breast physical examination and mammography, can be used to assess the significance of this finding.

depends on the temporal relationship to the surgical procedure. Acutely, there is skin thickening over the surgical site, with streaky soft tissue attenuation or edema, often accompanied by fluid collections representing postoperative seromas or hematomas; these usually do not persist beyond a few weeks. These are often seen on radiation therapy planning scans performed in the perioperative period. As the hematoma organizes, the fluid attenuation on CT may change to soft tissue attenuation, mimicking a soft tissue mass of recurrent or residual breast cancer. Eventually, stellate and streaky soft tissue abnormality may remain, representing fibrous scar.

Sometimes this has a nodular appearance, particularly centrally. In one study, the severity of postoperative scar formation was shown to correlate with the severity of postoperative hematoma formation and not with tumor size (29). These postsurgical changes are often, but not always, adjacent to high-attenuation surgical clips. It is important for the radiologist to be aware of the temporal relationship between the CT examination being interpreted and the surgical procedure in determining the significance of the appearance of the operative bed. Last, stability of the postoperative findings over time supports that the findings represent postoperative fibrosis and scar.

Breast Implants

Between 1.5 and 2 million women in the United States have breast implants, with approximately 80% placed for cosmetic reasons (30,31). Therefore, breast implants are not uncommonly seen as incidental findings on CT examinations of the chest obtained for other reasons. Knowledge of their typical and atypical appearances is important to avoid confusion with infection or a soft tissue mass that may mimic malignancy. The CT appearance of breast implants depends on the composition of the implant, usually silicone gel, saline or both. Regardless of the internal composition, most implants are elliptical in shape and have a semipermeable, smooth or textured, silicone elastomer shell that appears as a high-attenuation line bordering the implant on CT (30–32). A fibrous capsule forms around the implant as the body responds to a foreign object. The capsule may calcify over time, with a reported prevalence of 24% on mammography in a large series of 350 patients who had undergone placement of a breast implant (32). Calcification is seen more commonly on CT, with a reported prevalence of 30% in a series of 27 implants (32).

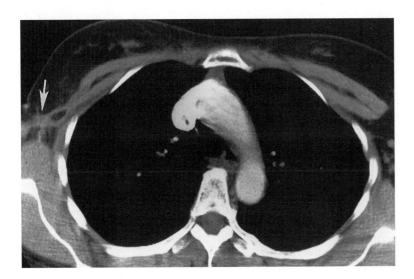

FIG. 4.32. Right axillary lymph node dissection scar. Computed tomographic image of the chest in a 57-year-old woman 4.5 months following a right breast lumpectomy and axillary lymph node dissection for infiltrating ductal carcinoma. Stellate-appearing soft tissue in the right axilla *(arrow)* is consistent with postoperative scar. Correlation with the physical examination and stability over time are important in determining the significance of this finding.

Saline implants are filled with normal saline through a valve at the time of surgery. On CT they are water attenuation (Figs. 4.33 and 4.34). Single-lumen silicone implants are filled with silicone gel. Double-lumen implants have an inner silicone prosthesis surrounded by saline. Infolding or invagination of the higher-attenuation silicone component may be seen but does not necessarily represent implant rupture (Figs. 4.35 and 4.36) (32,34). Implants are placed either in a retromuscular location, underneath the pectoralis major and minor muscles, or in a retroglandular location between the glandular tissue of the breast and the pectoralis muscles. Implant location can usually be determined by identifying the pectoralis muscles on CT. Atrophy of these muscles can make this determination difficult.

Capsular contracture is a late complication and may result in a rounded shape to the implant, rather than the normal elliptical shape. It is diagnosed clinically using the Baker four-grade classification scheme, which ranges from normal to a hard, tender, cold, and painful distorted breast (Fig. 4.37) (30). This is seen less often with retromuscular implants than with retroglandular implants. High-attenuation bands within an implant on CT represent the CT equivalent of the "linguine sign" on MRI and are evidence of intracapsular implant rupture (see Fig. 4.37) (35).

Occasionally an external breast prosthesis worn as part of a patient's clothing is seen on CT (Fig. 4.38). These are usually soft tissue in attenuation and parallel the shape of

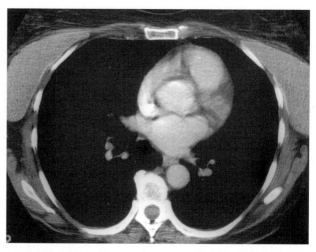

FIG. 4.34. Bilateral retroglandular drooping saline breast implants. Computed tomographic image of the chest in a 61-year-old woman with bilateral cosmetic breast implants. Breast glandular tissue can be seen anterior to the implants, indicating that the implants are retroglandular in location.

the anterior chest wall. An air gap can be seen between the skin and prosthesis.

A nodule near an implant could represent extracted silicone gel, scar tissue, or recurrent breast cancer and would require further evaluation (Figs. 4.39 and 4.40).

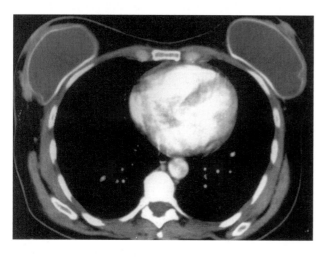

FIG. 4.33. Bilateral retroglandular saline breast implants. Computed tomographic image of the chest in a 52-year-old woman with bilateral cosmetic breast implants. The implants are water in attenuation, and the capsule surrounding both implants is partially calcified. The nodular soft tissue anterior and anterolateral to the breast implants represents compressed breast glandular tissue and should not be confused with soft tissue masses.

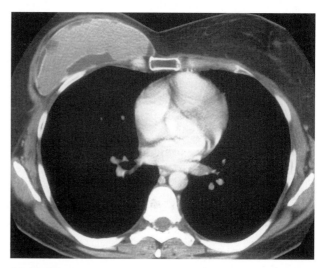

FIG. 4.35. Double-lumen silicone and saline subpectoral implant. Computed tomographic image of the chest in a 35-year-old woman who had undergone a modified radical right mastectomy for breast cancer. The CT demonstrates an implant of water attenuation peripherally, representing normal saline, and higher attenuation centrally, representing silicone gel. Note the irregular contour of the silicone component, which does not indicate implant rupture. Note the fat attenuation of the left breast and absence of glandular tissue, representing a transabdominal rectus abdominis musculocutaneous (TRAM) flap performed for reconstruction of the breast following a left mastectomy. This is discussed further in the next section of the chapter.

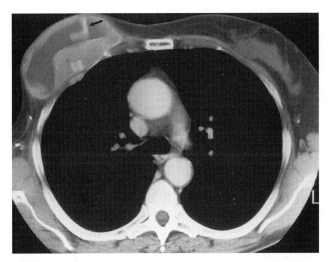

FIG. 4.36. Becker expander mammary prosthesis. Computed tomographic image of the chest in a 67-year-old woman after right modified radical mastectomy for breast carcinoma and placement of a Becker prosthesis 7 years earlier. The CT demonstrates an outer silicone component surrounding the water-attenuation saline component of the implant. The high-attenuation L-shaped structure *(arrow)* within the implant represents a portion of the tube used to fill the saline component of the prosthesis.

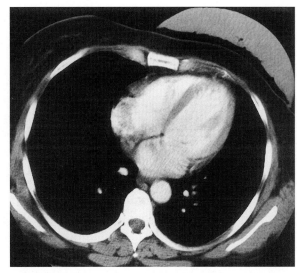

FIG. 4.38. External prosthesis. Computed tomographic image of a 47-year-old woman following a left mastectomy demonstrates a soft tissue attenuation external prosthesis worn within the clothing. There is an air gap between the skin and the prosthesis.

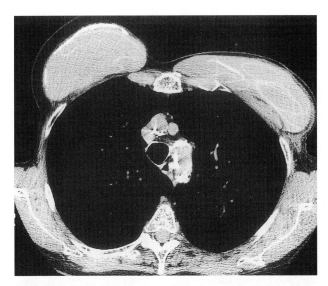

FIG. 4.37. Bilateral silicone single-lumen breast implants with capsular contracture on the right, and bilateral intracapsular implant rupture. Computed tomographic image of the chest in a 67-year-old woman 19 years following bilateral mastectomies and breast implants, demonstrates a rounded shape of the right breast with a calcified capsule, consistent with capsular contracture. Note the high-attenuation bands running throughout both implants, representing the CT linguine sign of bilateral intracapsular implant rupture, similar to findings described on MRI.

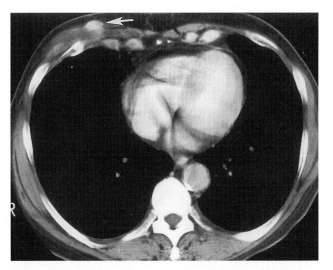

FIG. 4.39. Nodule adjacent to a breast implant. Computed tomographic image of the same patient illustrated in Fig. 4.35 demonstrates a 1-cm-diameter soft tissue nodule *(arrow)* adjacent to the inferomedial aspect of the implant 7 years following mastectomy for breast cancer. Differential diagnosis includes ruptured silicone gel and recurrent breast cancer. Magnetic resonance imaging may be useful to determine whether the nodule does or does not represent extruded silicon, based on the signal characteristics of the nodule and contrast enhancement. A nodule adjacent to an implant should not be assumed to represent scar tissue or extruded silicone gel. Surgical excision demonstrated recurrent breast cancer.

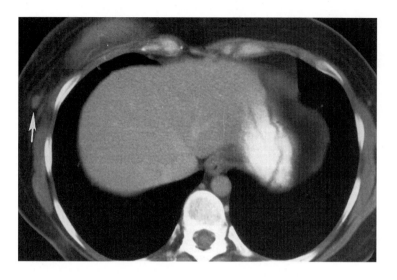

FIG. 4.40. Nodule adjacent to a breast implant. Computed tomographic image of the same patient illustrated in Fig. 4.36 demonstrates an 8-mm-diameter soft tissue nodule *(arrow)* adjacent to the outer and inferior aspect of the implant. Surgical resection revealed a lymph node with obstructive changes and no malignancy.

Breast Reconstruction

Musculocutaneous flaps taken from the chest or abdominal wall are an alternative to breast implants for reconstruction of the breast following mastectomy (28,36,37). Latissimus dorsi musculocutaneous flaps often also require the use of a breast implant to preserve the volume of the breast. Use of an implant is avoided with the transabdominal rectus abdominis musculocutaneous flap, more commonly referred to as a TRAM flap, as a larger amount of tissue can be transferred. The TRAM

flap procedure has gained popularity following reports of local and systemic complications secondary to silicone implants (38). This is a major surgical procedure in which the skin, subcutaneous fat and rectus abdominis muscle are incised, rotated (usually to the contralateral side) and transferred to the chest wall (37,38). A pedicle TRAM flap preserves the blood supply of the rectus abdominis muscle from the superior epigastric artery. For a free TRAM flap, these vessels are ligated, necessitating revascularization.

On CT, a portion or all of the rectus abdominis muscle may be absent from the abdominal wall (Figs. 4.41–4.43).

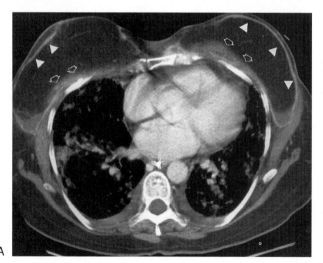

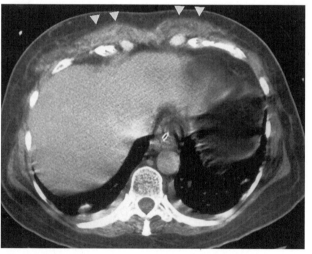

A   B

FIG. 4.41. Bilateral ipsilateral pedicle TRAM flap breast reconstruction: immediate postoperative appearance. Computed tomographic images of the chest and abdomen in a 60-year-old woman 12 days following bilateral TRAM flap breast reconstruction. Previously the patient had undergone bilateral mastectomies and implants. The intact implants were removed at the time of the TRAM procedure. At the time of this CT examination, the patient was suffering from acute respiratory distress syndrome (ARDS). **A:** Computed tomographic image through the midchest demonstrates fat attenuation of the reconstructed breasts, with a thin curvilinear soft tissue band *(solid arrowheads)* representing the skin of the musculocutaneous flap, and the superficial tissues representing the native skin and subcutaneous fat from this location and the deeper fat from the flap. The muscular portion of the flap lies immediately on top of the anterior ribs *(open arrows)*. Note postsurgical fluid in the dependent portion of the flap, which later resolved. Small bilateral pleural effusions and pulmonary consolidation are secondary to ARDS and fluid status. **B:** Computed tomographic image at the level of the seventh costochondral cartilage junction demonstrates 10-mm-thick rectus abdominis muscles *(arrowheads)* extending in the cephalad direction from the abdominal wall.

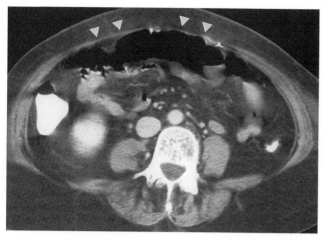

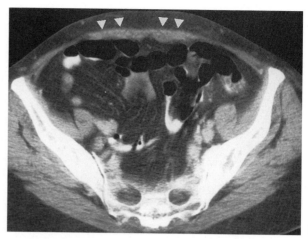

FIG. 4.41. *Continued.* **C:** Computed tomographic image of the abdomen 3 cm above the umbilicus demonstrates the empty rectus abdominis muscle fascia *(arrowheads)* where the muscle was removed and surgical clips in the anterior abdominal wall. **D:** Computed tomographic image at the level of the iliac crests demonstrates intact lower portion of the rectus abdominis muscles *(arrowheads).*

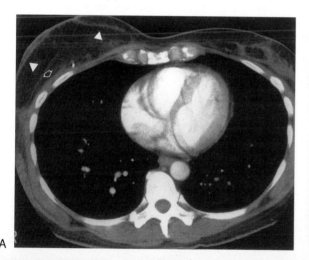

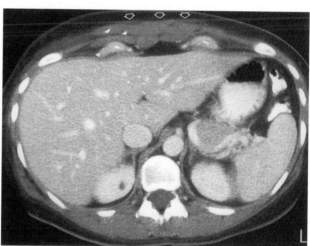

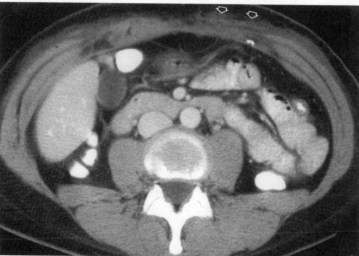

FIG. 4.42. Right unilateral contralateral pedicle TRAM flap breast reconstruction 1 month after surgery. Computed tomographic images of a 46-year-old woman following combined modified radical right mastectomy and TRAM reconstruction. **A:** Computed tomographic image through the midchest demonstrates fat attenuation of the reconstructed right breast, with a thin curvilinear soft tissue band *(arrowheads)* representing the skin of the musculocutaneous flap. The more superficial tissues represent the native skin and subcutaneous fat from this location, and the deeper fat is from the flap. The muscular portion of the flap lies immediately on top of the anterior ribs *(open arrows)*. There is a surgical clip adjacent to the transferred muscle. **B:** Computed tomographic image at the level of the seventh costochondral cartilage junction demonstrates 12-mm-thick rectus abdominis muscles *(open arrows)* crossing from the left abdominal wall obliquely to the right chest wall. **C:** Computed tomographic image of the midabdomen demonstrates the empty left rectus abdominis muscle fascia *(open arrows)* where the muscle was removed, surgical clips in the anterior abdominal wall, and streaky postoperative changes in the remaining abdominal wall fat.

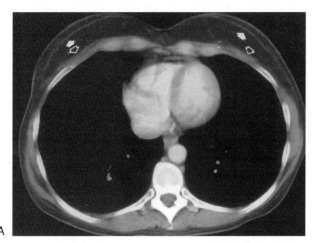

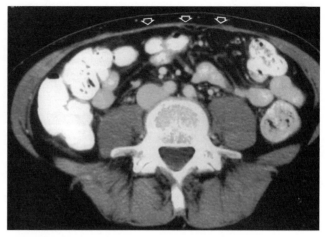

A

B

FIG. 4.43. Bilateral pedicle TRAM flap breast reconstruction 3 years after surgery. **A:** Computed tomographic images of a 47-year-old woman 3 years following bilateral mastectomies and TRAM reconstruction. Computed tomographic image through the midchest demonstrates fat attenuation of the reconstructed right breast, with a thin curvilinear soft tissue band *(solid arrows)* representing the skin of the musculocutaneous flap. The more superficial tissues represent the native skin and subcutaneous fat from this location, and the deeper fat is from the flap. The muscular portion of the flap lies immediately on top of the anterior ribs and is barely recognizable because of atrophy *(open arrows).* **B:** Computed tomographic image of the midabdomen demonstrates the empty rectus abdominis muscle fascia *(open arrows)* where the muscle was removed.

The soft tissue attenuation muscle can be seen crossing the midline at approximately the sixth or seventh anterior costochondral junction level (see Figs. 4.41 and 4.42). More cephalad, the rectus muscle is a soft tissue attenuation band that lies immediately on top of the ribs, covered by the subcutaneous fat from the flap. The thickness of the transferred rectus muscle will decrease over time because of denervation. Before denervation atrophy occurs, the rectus abdominis muscle may mimic a soft tissue mass (Fig. 4.44). A thin soft tissue attenuation line may parallel the skin surface, representing the skin of the flap, on top of which sits the native subcutaneous fat and skin (see Fig. 4.41). In some cases the remaining rectus abdominis muscle is reinforced with a Teflon mesh, which appears high attenuation on CT. Many patients undergo several breast resection and reconstruction procedures (Fig. 4.45), as described in the figure legends, depending on the patient's chest and abdominal wall musculocutaneous tissues, development of scar tissue, implants, and radiation therapy-related changes in the chest wall.

Esophagectomy, Esophageal Stents, and Fundoplication

Transhiatal esophagectomy with gastric interposition (THE) is usually performed for the treatment of esophageal carcinoma, often in combination with preoperative radiation therapy and/or chemotherapy (39,40). Less commonly, benign esophageal conditions such as radiation or lye-related strictures are treated by THE.

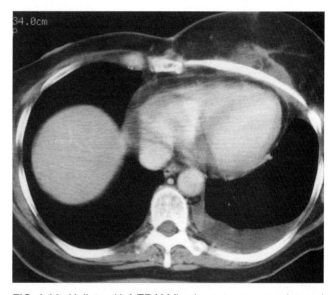

FIG. 4.44. Unilateral left TRAM flap breast reconstruction and chest wall reconstruction with a soft tissue mass. Computed tomographic image of the chest in a 66-year-old woman 1 month following left TRAM flap and chest wall resection for recurrent left chest wall breast carcinoma. Eleven years previously, the patient had undergone a modified left radical mastectomy for breast cancer and a prophylactic simple right mastectomy. There is a soft tissue mass immediately anterior to the high-attenuation methylmethacrylate chest wall prosthesis in the expected location of the TRAM flap muscular portion. This represents lack of denervation atrophy of the muscle and not recurrent cancer.

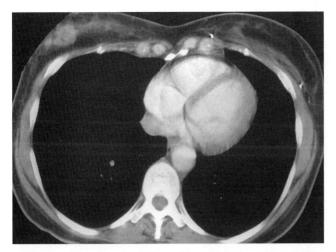

FIG. 4.45. Bilateral TRAM flap breast reconstruction and soft tissue mass. Computed tomographic image of the chest in a 50-year-old woman. Twenty months earlier the patient underwent a right modified radical mastectomy with ipsilateral right free TRAM flap and left simple mastectomy with ipsilateral pedicle TRAM flap for right diffuse ductal carcinoma *in situ.* There is a soft tissue mass in the middle of the right flap, representing recurrent breast cancer.

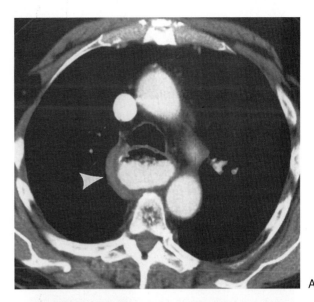

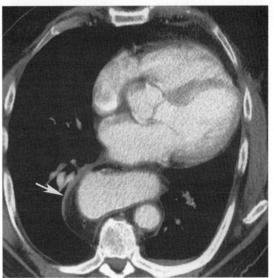

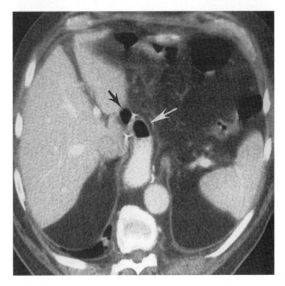

Through upper abdominal and lower cervical incisions, and using blunt dissection, the thoracic esophagus is mobilized, and the stomach is placed into the middle mediastinum. The cervical esophagus is anastomosed to the stomach through the incision in the lower left side of the neck. By avoiding a thoracotomy incision and a mediastinal anastomosis, procedure-related morbidity and mortality are reduced (39).

On CT, air, fluid, food, and/or contrast fill the intrathoracic stomach, which occupies the prior location of the esophagus (Figs. 4.46 and 4.47). As with the stomach in its normal abdominal location, incomplete distention of the intrathoracic stomach on CT may mimic gastric disease. The arch of the azygous vein may lie against the intrathoracic stomach, mimicking focal gastric wall thickening (see Fig. 4.46A). Similarly, compressive atelectasis may be seen adjacent to the distended stomach, mimicking pleural thickening (see Fig. 4.46B). Within the upper abdomen, the reoriented pylorus and duodenal bulb may appear as double bubbles of gas,

FIG. 4.46. Normal transhiatal esophagectomy. Computed tomographic scan of the chest in a 74-year-old man 2 months following surgery for esophageal adenocarcinoma. **A:** The arch of the azygous vein *(arrowhead)* lies along the right border of the air- and oral contrast-filled intrathoracic stomach, mimicking gastric wall or pleural thickening. **B:** Compressive atelectasis *(arrow)* adjacent to the intrathoracic stomach may mimic pleural thickening. **C:** Double-bubble appearance of the distal gastric antrum near the pylorus *(white arrow)* and duodenal bulb *(black arrow).*

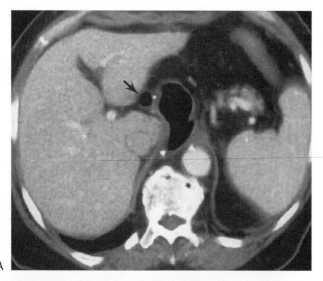

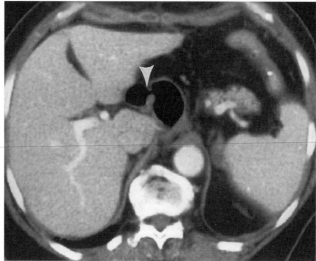

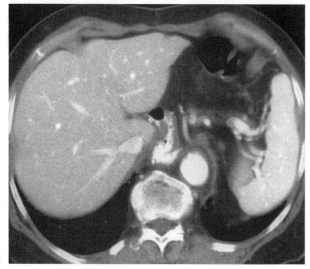

FIG. 4.47. Normal transhiatal esophagectomy: pyloroduodenal junction. Computed tomographic images of the upper abdomen in an 82-year-old woman 5 weeks following surgery for esophageal squamous cell carcinoma. **A:** Air collection in the duodenal bulb *(arrow)* adjacent to the pylorus may mimic extraluminal air. **B:** Identifying the contiguity of this structure with pylorus *(arrowhead)* can be useful in avoiding this pitfall. **C:** A CT image with oral contrast can also better delineate the relationship of the air collection to the duodenum.

mimicking extraluminal gas (see Fig. 4.46C and 4.47). Food within the stomach may mimic a soft tissue mass (Fig. 4.48), simulating recurrent esophageal carcinoma (Fig. 4.49) (40).

Colonic interposition is a less commonly performed procedure for the treatment of esophageal carcinoma and benign esophageal conditions, often used when both an esophagectomy and gastrectomy are required (41,42). A portion of either the left or right colon is resected and interposed between the cervical esophagus and either the gastroesophageal junction, gastric fundus, or jejunum, maintaining the integrity of the vascular pedicle. Postoperative complications, such as strictures, are usually related to inadequate vascular supply to the interposed colon. The colon is usually positioned posterior to the sternum in the anterior mediastinum (Fig. 4.50), and less often in the native esophageal bed (Fig. 4.51).

Gastroesophageal reflux may require an antireflux procedure, including many variations of the fundoplication procedure. A one-way gastric valve or reconstituted lower esophageal sphincter is created to prevent reflux by wrapping the gastric fundus around the lower esophagus at the gastroesophageal junction. These patients are not uncommonly encountered when being evaluated for unrelated conditions. On CT, the wrap may appear as a soft tissue mass at the gastric fundus or have a target appearance, similar to an intussusception (Fig.4.52) (43).

Esophageal stents may be used for palliative treatment of patients with unresectable esophageal carcinoma or patients who are not surgical candidates for other reasons, such as poor cardiac or pulmonary function. Other indications include extrinsic esophageal compression, such as fibrosing mediastinitis, tracheoesophageal fistula, or recurrent esophageal stricture (44). There are many types of esophageal stents. Those in use today include several expandable, pliable metal stents in addition to earlier rigid plastic stents (44). On CT, the rim of the stent is high attenuation, with a round shape in cross section (Figs. 4.53 and 4.54).

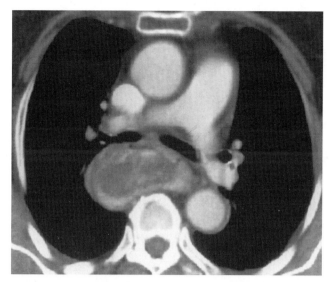

FIG. 4.48. Mass within the intrathoracic stomach following transhiatal esophagectomy: ingested food. Computed tomographic image of the chest in the same 82-year-old woman as in Fig. 4.47 5 weeks following surgery for esophageal squamous cell carcinoma. The soft tissue attenuation mass centered in the intrathoracic stomach filled more than two-thirds of the stomach in craniocaudal dimension, representing recently ingested food. Gastric outlet obstruction by an incomplete pyloromyotomy or recurrent cancer may promote the formation of a bezoar that may have a similar appearance.

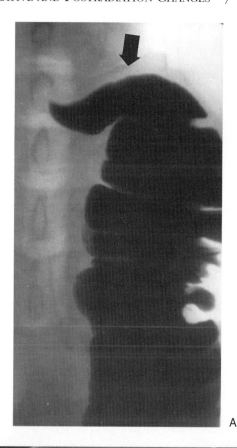

A

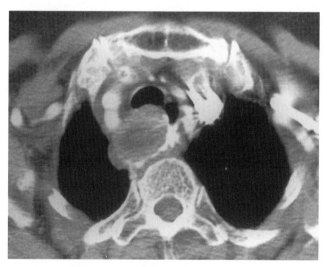

FIG. 4.49. Mass within the intrathoracic stomach following transhiatal esophagectomy: recurrent cancer. Computed tomographic image of the same patient illustrated in Figs. 4.47 and 4.48 18 months after THE demonstrates a soft tissue mass within the stomach near the cervical esophagogastric anastomosis, deforming the posterior wall of the trachea. Bronchoscopy with transtracheal biopsy confirmed recurrent esophageal cancer.

B

FIG. 4.50. Colonic interposition in the anterior mediastinum. Images of a 64-year-old man 7 years following surgery for Barrett's esophagus and high-grade esophageal dysplasia. **A:** Barium swallow demonstrates anastomosis of the proximal esophagus *(arrow)* and colon. **B:** Computed tomographic image of the lower chest demonstrates the air- and contrast-filled colon (+) in the anterior mediastinum.

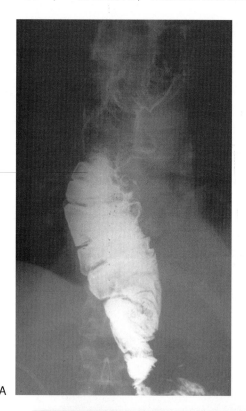

A

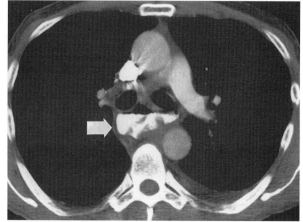

FIG. 4.51. Colonic interposition in the middle mediastinum. Images of a 57-year-old man 21 months following surgery for esophageal carcinoma with an extensive gastric component requiring esophagogastrectomy. **A:** Barium swallow demonstrates the intrathoracic colon and colojejunal anastomosis. **B:** Computed tomographic images of the midchest and **(C)** lower chest demonstrate the air- and contrast-filled interposed colon *(arrows)* located in the esophageal bed. Normal haustra are outlined by the contrast.

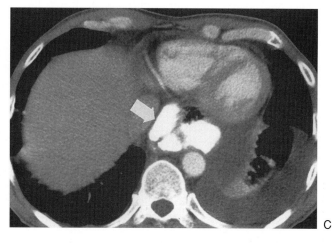

B

C

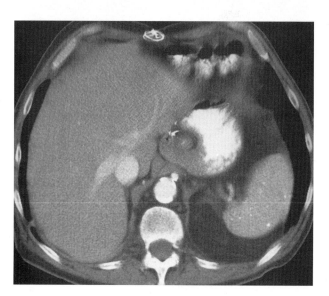

FIG. 4.52. Nissen fundoplication. Computed tomographic image of a 73-year-old man 4 years following surgery for gastroesophageal reflux demonstrates a target appearance to the gastroesophageal junction, similar in appearance to intussusception of the large or small bowel.

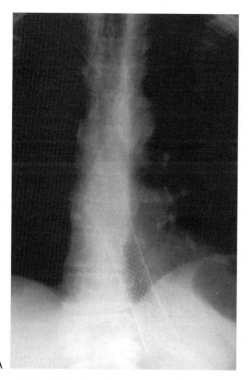

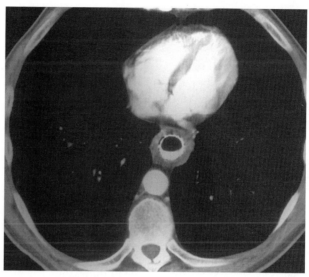

FIG. 4.53. Esophageal stent. Images of a 55-year-old man 3 months following placement of an esophageal stent for dysphagia and weight loss secondary to esophageal adenocarcinoma. **A:** Coned-down radiograph demonstrates the obliquely oriented flexible metallic stent extending from the distal esophagus into the gastric fundus. **B:** Computed tomographic image of the midchest demonstrates the round high-attenuation stent filled with air and oral contrast and thickening of the esophageal wall, representing the known esophageal carcinoma.

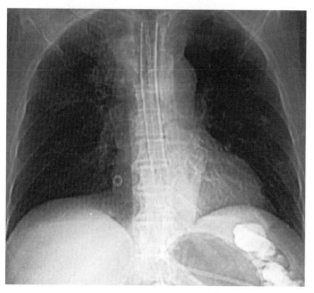

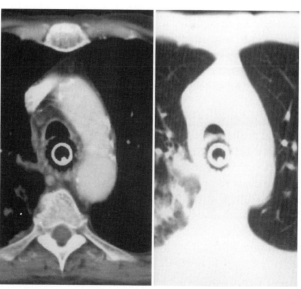

FIG. 4.54. Esophageal stent, esophageal cancer, and tracheoesophageal fistula. Images of a 76-year-old man 1 year following placement of a Wilson-Cook esophageal stent for a tracheoesophageal fistula secondary to esophageal carcinoma. **A:** Computed tomographic scout topogram demonstrates the 14-cm-long esophageal stent extending from the thoracic inlet to 5 cm above the gastrojejunal junction. A feeding tube passes through the stent into the stomach. **B,C:** Computed tomographic images at the level of the aortic arch at **(B)** soft tissue and **(C)** lung windows demonstrate the round high-attenuation stent in cross section. The round structure within the stent is the feeding tube in cross section. Note that on soft tissue windows there appears to be a tracheoesophageal fistula at this level that is not present on the lung window image. Failure to recognize the tracheal wall on lung windows may either lead to the erroneous diagnosis of a fistula or overestimate the size of a fistula. *Continued on next page.*

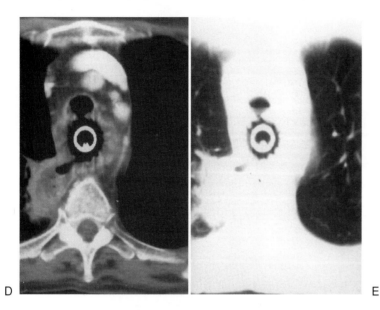

D   E

FIG. 4.54. *Continued.* **D,E:** Computed tomographic images 2 cm above the aortic arch at **(D)** soft tissue and **(E)** lung windows demonstrate the actual location of the tracheoesophageal fistula. In addition, there is a posterior esophageal fistula extending into the mediastinum and pleural space.

Aortic Reconstruction

Patients who have undergone surgical repair of the thoracic aorta often undergo CT examinations for follow-up of a residual dissection or aneurysm, evaluation of potential postoperative complications, new chest pain or in the evaluation of unrelated conditions. It is important to understand the normal appearance of the thoracic aorta after surgical repair in order to avoid misidentifying normal postoperative structures as aortic pathology and to avoid overlooking significant complications. These surgical procedures are complex, and a detailed discussion is beyond the scope of the chapter. Portions of the aorta may be resected or opened, grafts may be sewn end to end or end to side, and branch vessels may be reimplanted or grafted (45–47).

Felt pledgets are often used to repair a bypass cannulation site in the native aorta or an air evacuation needle site in the graft. Felt strips may be used to reinforce the anastomosis. On CT, felt appears as high-attenuation material bordering the wall of the aorta or graft (Fig. 4.55). High-attenuation felt could be confused with extravascular contrast material secondary to a leaking graft (Fig. 4.56). Sometimes there is kinking of the graft or puckering at the anastomosis, usually without hemodynamic significance (Figs. 4.57 and 4.58). Occasionally this creates the appearance of a transverse low-attenuation band traversing the aorta on axial images, mimicking a dissection flap; this pitfall can be avoided in questionable cases using multiplanar reconstructions of the CT data.

When a composite graft is used to repair the aortic valve and the ascending thoracic aorta, the coronary arteries must be reimplanted to preserve cardiac blood

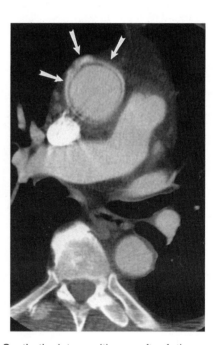

FIG. 4.55. Synthetic interposition graft of the ascending aorta: normal appearance 14 months after surgery. Computed tomographic image demonstrates a circumferential high-attenuation felt reinforcing ring *(arrows)* around the distal anastomosis of an ascending aortic graft. (Reprinted from reference 45, with permission from the Radiological Society of North America.)

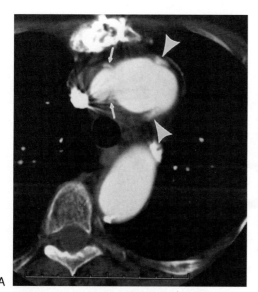
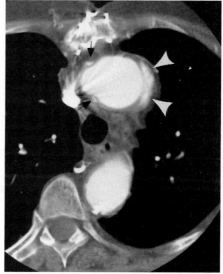

FIG. 4.56. Synthetic interposition graft of the ascending aorta and aortic arch: normal appearance 4 months after surgery. **A:** Felt reinforcing ring at the distal anastomosis *(arrowheads).* **B:** This ring may be mistaken for a pseudoaneurysm on a contiguous image *(arrowheads).* The circumferential nature of the ring on adjacent CT sections establishes the correct diagnosis. Note also portions of felt ring surrounding an innominate artery island implanted into the arch graft *(arrows)* **(A,B).** (Reprinted from reference 45, with permission from the Radiological Society of North America.)

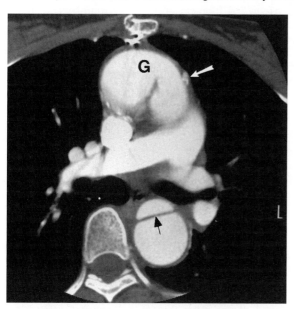

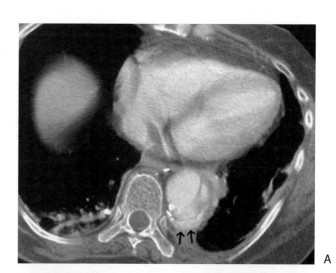

FIG. 4.57. Composite graft of the aortic root and arch 15 months after surgery for aortic dissection repair. The CT demonstrates kinking and tortuosity of the graft (G) and a high-density felt pledget *(white arrow)* in the graft. The dissection flap *(black arrow)* is present in the native descending thoracic aorta. (Reprinted from reference 45, with permission from the Radiological Society of North America.)

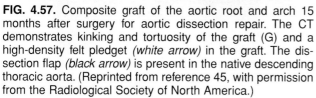

FIG. 4.58. Puckering of the native aorta at a graft anastomosis simulating a pseudoaneurysm and/or dissection flap. Computed tomographic images 4 months after reconstruction of the descending aorta. **A:** Axial image demonstrates a low-attenuation band traversing the lumen of the aorta, mimicking an aortic dissection. **B:** Puckering of the aorta at the distal graft anastomosis creates a pseudoflap *(open arrow).* The anatomic relationships are more clearly displayed on the parasagittal reconstruction. *Arrows,* felt rings; G, graft. (Reprinted from reference 45, with permission from the Radiological Society of North America.)

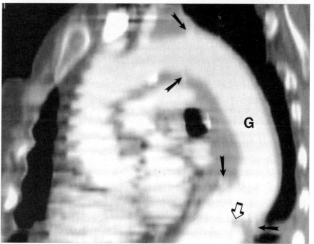

flow and myocardial viability. One method is to take a small portion of the native aorta around the coronary artery ostium, referred to as a coronary button, and implant this on the graft; felt may be used to reinforce the anastomoses (Fig. 4.59). Failure to recognize the coronary artery button may lead to the incorrect diagnosis of a pseudoaneurysm (Fig. 4.60). Circumferential low-attenuation and/or soft tissue attenuation material is often noted adjacent to the reconstructed aorta, particularly in the weeks after surgery; this is usually attributed to postoperative fluid and/or hematoma and often decreases in size over time. The abnormality may persist for months to years after surgery and may mimic an infected surgical bed or leaking aorta (see Figs. 4.60 and 4.61). This appearance differs from that of a true postoperative pseudoaneurysm (Fig. 4.62), which is usually focal and eccentric, containing contrast material. Other mimics of pathology include the collapsed native aorta adjacent to a graft (Fig. 4.63) and reinforcement of a graft with bovine pericardium (Fig. 4.64).

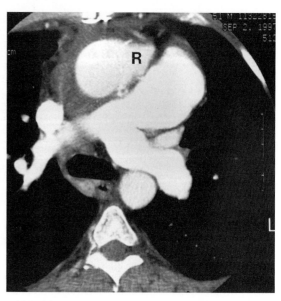

FIG. 4.60. Right coronary artery button simulating a pseudoaneurysm. Computed tomographic image demonstrates a contrast-enhanced, triangular-shaped outpouching (R) from the ascending thoracic aortic graft, representing the right coronary artery button (R). This may simulate a pseudoaneurysm. Low-attenuation material adjacent to the graft 4 months after composite root replacement is consistent with hematoma. (Reprinted from reference 45, with permission from the Radiological Society of North America.)

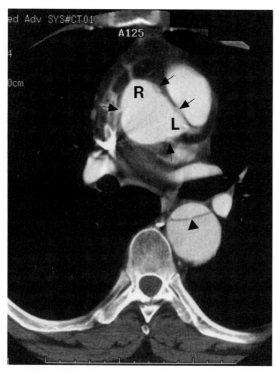

FIG. 4.59. Composite aortic root graft with right and left coronary artery buttons 14 months after surgery for aortic dissection repair. The CT demonstrates small outpouchings of the ascending aortic graft, distorting the normal rounded appearance of the graft in cross section. These outpouchings are the right (R) and (L) coronary artery buttons, representing reimplantation of the coronary arteries and aortic wall onto the graft. Portions of the felt rings *(arrows)* surrounding the coronary artery buttons are visible. A dissection flap is present in descending aorta *(arrowhead).* (Reprinted from reference 45, with permission from the Radiological Society of North America.)

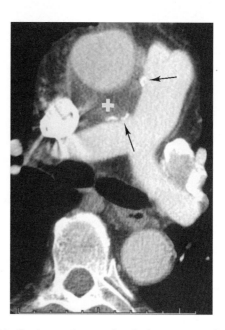

FIG. 4.61. Postoperative perigraft hematoma. Computed tomograph demonstrates low-attenuation material (+) adjacent to a composite graft 30 months after surgery. Felt strips are seen surrounding a pulmonary artery patch *(arrows).* (Reprinted from reference 45, with permission from the Radiological Society of North America.)

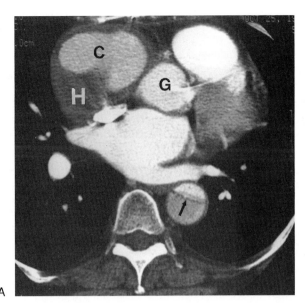
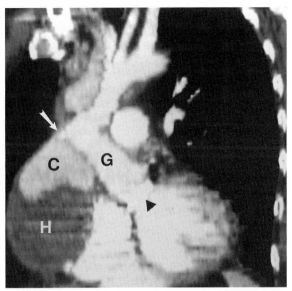

FIG. 4.62. Large pseudoaneurysm 4 months after composite root grafting. **A:** Axial CT image and **(B)** parasagittal reconstruction demonstrate low-attenuation material, consistent with hematoma (H), and extravasated contrast material (C) adjacent to the distal graft anastomosis *(white arrow)*, representing a pseudoaneurysm. A dissection flap is noted in the descending thoracic aorta *(black arrow)*. G, graft; *arrowhead*, prosthetic aortic valve. (Part **B** reprinted from reference 45, with permission from the Radiological Society of North America.)

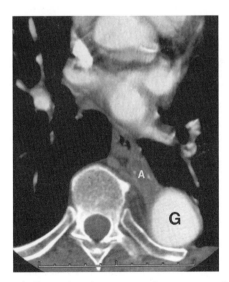

FIG. 4.63. Collapsed native aorta adjacent to an interposition graft. Computed tomographic image 27 months following reconstruction of the descending thoracic aorta. There is a low-attenuation structure with peripheral calcification (A) anteromedial to the aortic graft (G), representing the collapsed native aorta. This could potentially mimic a mediastinal fluid collection such as an abscess or pseudoaneurysm.

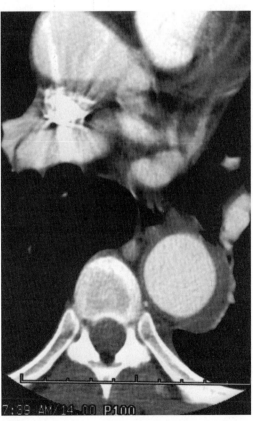

FIG. 4.64. Bovine pericardial wrap. Computed tomographic image 29 months following reconstruction of the descending thoracic aorta demonstrates low-attenuation material along the left side of the aorta representing a bovine pericardial wrap. This could potentially mimic thrombus within the false lumen of an aortic dissection.

RADIATION THERAPY

Radiation therapy to the thorax may induce changes in the structures within the radiation portal, including the lung, esophagus, skin, chest wall, pleura, and pericardium (48). Acute lung injury is referred to as radiation pneumonitis, whereas the persistent abnormality is referred to as radiation fibrosis (49). Clinically symptomatic radiation pneumonitis occurs in 7% to 8% of patients. Radiologic changes are seen in up to 80% of patients on chest radiographs and in a greater percentage of patients on CT (50,51). Clinical symptoms include cough, fever, and shortness of breath (50). A relationship has been demonstrated between the radiation dose and the frequency of lung injury (52). The threshold for lung injury is 3 to 4 Gy (49). Changes on CT may be seen within 3 to 4 weeks after radiation therapy (49). Recognition of the patterns of lung injury is necessary to avoid confusion with malignancy and infection.

The lung abnormalities on CT induced by radiation therapy include minimal ground-glass attenuation (Figs. 4.65–4.67) and consolidation acutely (Figs. 4.68 and 4.69), which may progress to honeycombing and bronchiectasis (Figs. 4.70 and 4.71). The border of the radiation-induced lung injury may be straight or oblique, representing the border of the radiation portal (see Fig. 4.67), or may be curved, as seen with the newer technique of conformal radiation therapy (see Fig. 4.71). Sometimes the injury is mass-like, mimicking tumor recurrence; stability over time and temporal relationship to radiation therapy are important in avoiding this mistake (see Figs. 4.68 and 4.69). Tangential beam radiation therapy for breast carcinoma to the chest wall and axilla may cause injury to the periphery of the lung, sometimes referred to loosely as the "axillary" segment of the lung, even though it is not a true anatomic segment (Fig. 4.72). Patchy and diffuse radiation injury may be seen throughout an entire lung if radiation therapy is given for the treatment of diffuse pleural metastases and

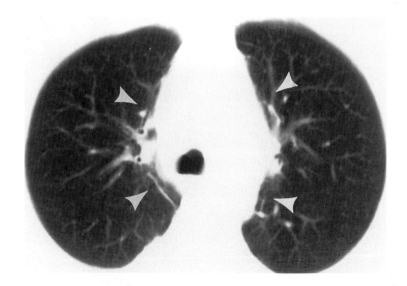

FIG. 4.65. Radiation lung injury: minimal ground-glass attenuation. Computed tomographic image of a 39-year-old woman 8 months following mediastinal radiation therapy and chemotherapy for stage IIa Hodgkin's lymphoma. There is faint ground-glass attenuation in the paramediastinal portion of both lungs *(arrowheads),* with retraction of the upper lobe bronchovascular bundles toward the mediastinum.

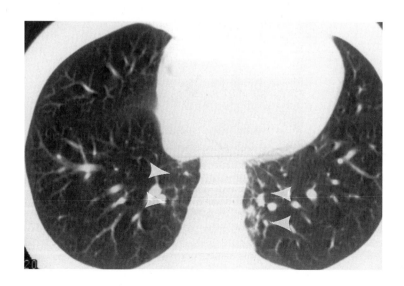

FIG. 4.66. Radiation lung injury: minimal ground-glass attenuation. Computed tomographic image of a 33-year-old woman 9 months following palliative radiation therapy to the thoracic spine for metastatic breast carcinoma. There is faint ground-glass attenuation in the paramediastinal portion of both lower lobes *(arrowheads).* The left lower lobe bronchovascular bundles are retracted toward the mediastinum.

includes the entire lung in the treatment field. Less common CT manifestations include decreased vascularity (Fig. 4.73) and spontaneous pneumothorax (49). The CT findings may resolve, consistent with radiation pneumonitis (see Fig. 4.72), or persist, consistent with fibrosis (see Fig. 4.70). Occasionally lung abnormality may be seen outside of the radiation field, and even in the contralateral lung (53,54) (see Fig. 4.70). This may be secondary to an immunologically mediated hypersensitivity pneumonitis or lymphocytic alveolitis (53,54).

Pleural and pericardial effusions may also be seen following radiation therapy, mimicking metastatic disease (Figs. 4.74 and 4.75) (48). These effusions are often small or loculated and are recognized with greater frequency on CT than chest radiography. Criteria for radiation pleuritis include an effusion that develops within 6 months after the completion of radiation therapy, resolves spontaneously and is associated with radiation pneumonitis. Pericardial injury may be acute in nature and resolve or progress to chronic pericarditis with thickening and fibrosis of the parietal pericardium, including symptomatic constrictive pericarditis or a loculated pericardial fluid collection. In one large series, 60% of pericardial changes were identified within 4 to 12 months of com-

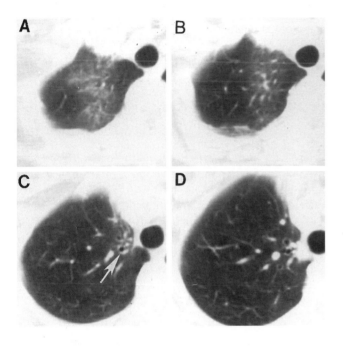

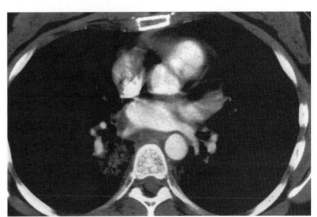

FIG. 4.67. Radiation lung injury: minimal ground-glass attenuation. Consecutive CT images of a 53-year-old woman 7 months following radiation therapy for metastatic breast carcinoma to the supraclavicular region. There is ground-glass attenuation in the right upper lobe, with a straight lateral border representing the border of the radiation portal. The bronchovascular bundles are retracted toward the mediastinum, and there is mild bronchial dilation *(arrow)*.

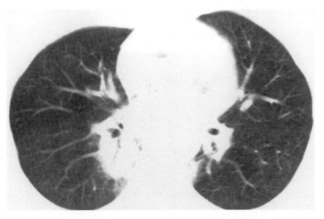

FIG. 4.68. Radiation lung injury: mass-like consolidation. Computed tomographic images of a 37-year-old woman 5 months following radiation therapy for small-cell lung cancer. **A:** Lung windows demonstrate mass-like, round consolidated lung in the right lower lobe, consistent with radiation lung injury. **B:** Air-bronchograms are seen on soft tissue windows. This finding has been stable on CT for 2 years. Unless the primary lung cancer was bronchoalveolar cell carcinoma, the air bronchograms throughout this rounded consolidation would be unusual for recurrent malignancy.

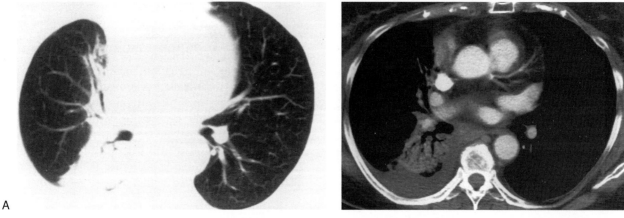

A

B

FIG. 4.69. Radiation lung injury: mass-like consolidation. Computed tomographic images of a 71-year-old man 4 months following radiation therapy for non-small-cell lung cancer. **A:** Lung windows demonstrate mass-like, round consolidated lung in the superior segment of the right lower lobe in addition to the more characteristic consolidation with a straight lateral border more anteriorly in the right middle lobe. **B:** Air-bronchograms are better appreciated on soft tissue windows. This finding has been stable on CT for almost 2 years. There is also volume loss of the right lung compared to the left lung, and a right pleural effusion, thought to be secondary to radiation therapy. Unless the primary lung cancer was bronchoalveolar cell carcinoma, the air-bronchograms throughout this rounded consolidation would be unusual for recurrent malignancy.

pleting radiation therapy, 20% between 12 and 24 months, and 20% were seen more than 2 years following radiation therapy (55).

Radiation esophagitis may appear on CT as esophageal wall thickening, usually within 1 to 3 months after the completion of therapy, typically following 4.5 to 6 Gy given over 6 to 8 weeks (Fig. 4.76) (56). The motility changes seen during the fluoroscopic portion of espho-grams are not appreciated readily on CT, but mild esophageal dilation or retained oral contrast in the esophagus may be indicators of this (56). Strictures may develop 4 to 8 months after therapy and are not readily visible on CT. Less commonly, fistulas or pseudodiverticula may develop (56). Radiation sclerosis or lysis of bone may mimic sclerotic and lytic bone metastases or infection (Figs. 4.77 and 4.78) (48,57).

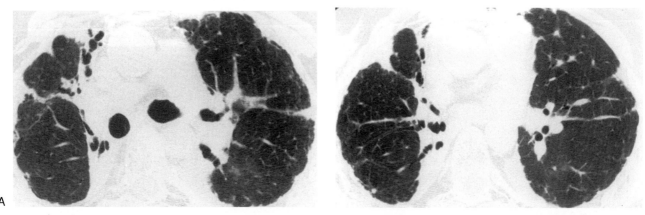

A

B

FIG. 4.70. Radiation lung injury: fibrosis and bronchiectasis. Computed tomographic images of a 46-year-old woman 13 years following radiation therapy for Hodgkin's lymphoma. Lung windows at the level of the carina and 5 cm below the carina demonstrate bilateral paramediastinal consolidated lung parenchyma with straight borders, retraction of the bronchovascular bundles toward the mediastinum, and extensive bronchiectasis, particularly in the right lung. The patient complained of nonproductive cough and shortness of breath, attributed to the radiation lung injury. The peripheral changes in both lungs were felt to represent radiation lung injury outside the radiation field.

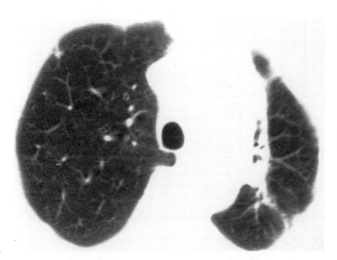
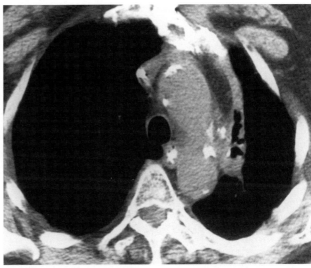

A

B

FIG. 4.71. Radiation lung injury: round contour. Computed tomographic images of a 72-year-old woman 6 years following left upper lobectomy for non-small-cell lung cancer and 4 years following radiation therapy for recurrent disease at the aortopulmonary window. **A:** Lung windows demonstrate consolidated paramediastinal left lung with a rounded contour, often seen with conformal radiation therapy. **B:** Air-bronchograms and dilated bronchi are also appreciated on soft tissue windows.

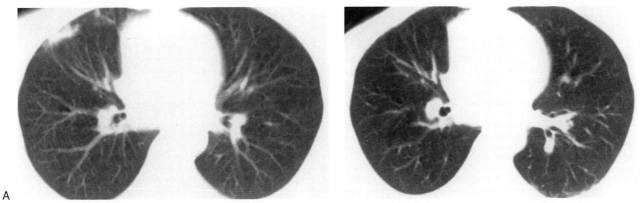

A

B

FIG. 4.72. Radiation lung injury: axillary. Computed tomographic images of a 39-year-old woman following modified radical mastectomy for invasive and infiltrating adenocarcinoma of the breast with 13/17 positive lymph nodes and postoperative tangential beam radiation therapy. **A:** Computed tomogram 8 months after the completion of radiation therapy demonstrates consolidation along the periphery of the right middle lobe, with the radiation portal used for chest wall and axillary radiation therapy. This is sometimes referred to as the axillary segment of the lung. **B:** Computed tomogram 24 months after the completion of radiation therapy demonstrates complete resolution of the earlier radiation pneumonitis.

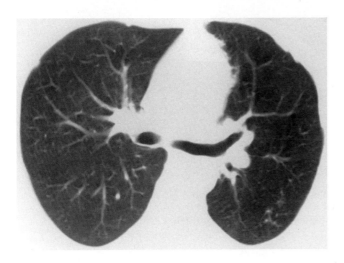

FIG. 4.73. Radiation lung injury: decreased vascularity. Computed tomographic image of a 52-year-old man 8 months following radiation therapy for unresectable poorly differentiated adenocarcinoma of the left upper lobe demonstrates decreased vascularity in the left lung compared to the right lung.

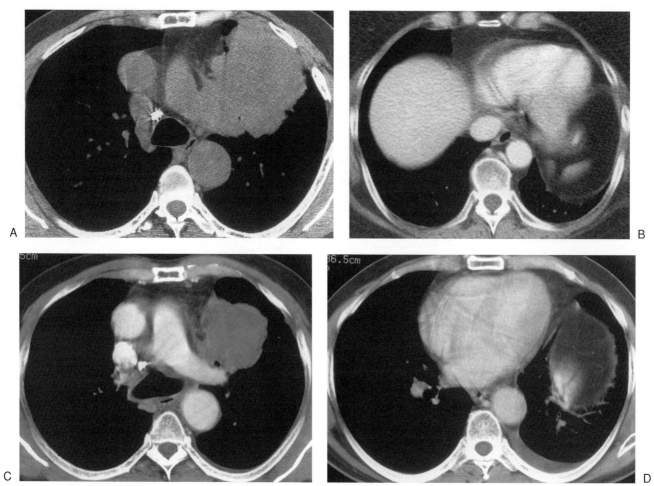

FIG. 4.74. Radiation pleuritis. Computed tomographic images of the chest in a 59-year-old man immediately before and 3 months following radiation therapy for unresectable bronchogenic carcinoma. Computed tomographic images before radiation therapy demonstrate **(A)** a large left upper lobe mass invading the mediastinum and **(B)** no pleural effusion. Computed tomographic images after radiation therapy demonstrate **(C)** marked decrease in size of the mass and **(D)** a new small left pleural effusion that later resolved spontaneously. This could be confused with a malignant pleural effusion if the temporal relationship to radiation therapy is not recognized.

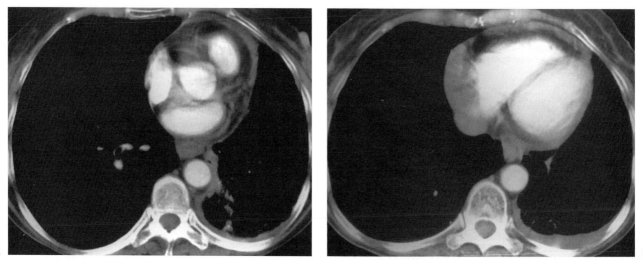

FIG. 4.75. Radiation pericarditis. Computed tomographic images of the chest in a 66-year-old woman 6 months following radiation therapy for squamous cell carcinoma of the lung demonstrate a small left pleural effusion before radiation therapy, new **(A)** mild pericardial thickening and **(B)** a pericardial effusion after radiation therapy. This could be confused with a malignant pericardial effusion if the temporal relationship to radiation therapy is not recognized.

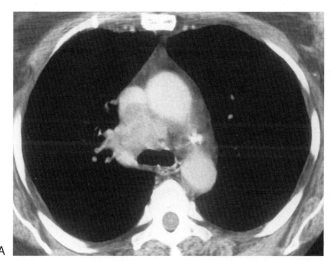 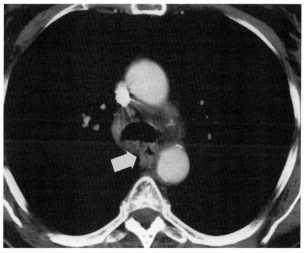

A

B

FIG. 4.76. Radiation esophagitis. Computed tomographic images of the chest in a 71-year-old woman 6 weeks following radiation therapy for small-cell carcinoma demonstrate **(A)** enlarged right paratracheal lymph nodes and normal esophagus before radiation therapy and **(B)** marked decrease in size of the mediastinal lymph node mass and new circumferential esophageal wall thickening *(arrow)* 6 weeks after the completion of radiation therapy. The patient was experiencing odynophagia at the time of this CT scan.

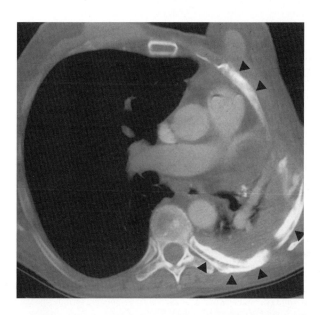

FIG. 4.77. Radiation osteosclerosis. Computed tomographic image of the chest in a 63-year-old man 3.5 years following left upper lobectomy, chest wall resection, and radiation therapy for stage IIIA adenocarcinoma of the lung demonstrates sclerosis of several left ribs *(arrowheads)*. He is without evidence of malignancy 5 years after surgery.

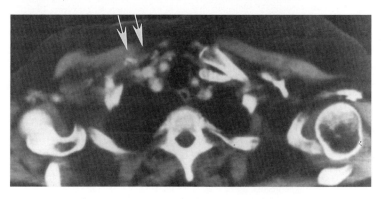

FIG. 4.78. Radiation osteolysis. Computed tomographic image of the chest in a 52-year-old woman 18 months following modified radical mastectomy and 40-Gy radiation therapy to the supraclavicular and internal mammary regions for breast cancer. There is almost complete absence of the medial right clavicle *(arrows)* 5 months following a traumatic fracture of the medial third of the clavicle that could be confused with a lytic metastasis. (Reproduced from reference 57 with permission from Aman Buzdar, M.D. and the American Medical Association.)

REFERENCES

1. Holbert JM, Libshitz HE, Chasen MH, Mountain CF. The postlobectomy chest: anatomic considerations. *RadioGraphics* 1987;7:889–911.
2. Silver AW, Espinoso EE, Byron FX. The fate of the post-resection space. *Ann Thorac Surg* 1966;2:311–327.
3. Biondetti PR, Fiore D, Sartori F, Colognato A, Ravasini R, Romani S. Evaluation of the post-pneumonectomy space by computed-tomography. *J Comput Assist Tomogr* 1982;6:238–242.
4. Laissy JP, Rebibo G, Trotot PN, Zizen MT, Cabanis EA, Benozio M. Post-pneumonectomy evaluation of the chest: a prospective comparative study of MRI with CT. *Magn Res Imag* 1989;7:55–60.
5. Shepard JA, Grillo HC, McLoud TC, Dedrick CG, Spizarny DL. Right-pneumonectomy syndrome: radiologic findings and CT correlation. *Radiology* 1986;61:661–664.
6. Cordova FC, Travaline JM, O'Brien GM, Ball DS, Lippmann M. Treatment of left pneumonectomy syndrome with an expandable endobronchial stent. *Chest* 1996;109:567–570.
7. Landreneau RJ, Mack MJ, Dowling RD, et al. The role of thoracoscopy in lung cancer management. *Chest* 1998;113:6S–12S.
8. Ferson PF, Keenan RJ, Luketich JD. The role of video-assisted thoracic surgery in pulmonary metastases. *Chest Surg Clin North Am* 1998;8(1):59–76.
9. Root JD, Molina PL, Anderson DJ, Sagel SS. Pulmonary nodular opacities after transbronchial biopsy in patients with transplanted lungs. *Radiology* 1992;184:435–436.
10. Kazeroni EA, Cascade PN, Gross BH. Transplanted lungs: nodules following transbronchial biopsy. *Radiology* 1995;194:209–212.
11. Kukafka DS, O'Brien GM, Furukawa S, Criner GJ. Surveillance bronchoscopy in lung transplant recipients. *Chest* 1997;111:377–381.
12. Iko T, Kivisaari L, Taskinen E, Piilonen A, Harjula AL. High-resolution CT in long term follow-up after lung transplantation. *Chest* 1997;111:370–376.
13. Hosenpud JD, Bennett LE, Keck BM, Fiol B, Novick RJ. The registry of the international society for heart and lung transplantation: fourteenth official report 1997. *J Heart Lung Transplant* 1997;7:691–712.
14. Herman SJ. Radiologic assessment after lung transplantation. *Radiol Clin North Am* 1994;32:663–678.
15. Evans KG, Miller RR, Muller NL, Nelems B. Chest-wall tumours. *Can J Surg* 1990;33:229–232.
16. Maddern IR, Goodman LR, Almassi GH, Haasler GB, McManus RP, Olinger GN. CT after reconstructive repair of the sternum and chest wall. *Radiology* 1993;186:665–670.
17. Minai OA, Hammond G, Curtis A. Hernia of the lung: a case report and review of literature. *Connecticut Med* 1997;61:77–81.
18. van den Brink WA, Meek JC, Boelhouwer RU. Herniation of the lung following video-assisted minithoracotomy. *Surg Endosc* 1995;9:706–708.
19. Seibel DG, Hopper KD, Ghaed N. Mammographic and CT detection of extrathoracic lung herniation. *J Comput Assist Tomogr* 1987;11:537–538.
20. Sadler MA, Shapiro RS, Wagreich J, Halton K, Hecht A. CT diagnosis of acquired intercostal lung herniation. *Clin Imag* 1997;21:104–106.
21. Scullion DA, Negus R, al-Kutoubi A. Case report: extrathoracic herniation of the lung with a review of the literature. *Br J Radiol* 1994;67:94–96.
22. Goodman P, Balachandran S, Guinto FC. Postoperative atrophy of posterolateral chest wall musculature: CT demonstration. *J Comput Assist Tomogr* 1992;17:63–65.
23. Moore NR, Phillips MS, Shneerson JM, Smith ML, Flower CD, Dixon AK. Appearances on computed tomography following thoracoplasty for pulmonary tuberculosis. *Br J Radiol* 1988;61:573–578.
24. Shapiro MP, Gale ME, Daly BD. Eloesser window thoracostomy for treatment of empyema: radiographic appearance. *Am J Roentgenol* 1988;150:549–552.
25. Adebo OA, Osinowa O. Management of empyema and bronchopleural fistula, experience with Eloesser window. *Trop Doct* 1987;17:26–29.
26. Bhalla M, Wain JC, Shepard JO, McLoud TC. Surgical flaps in the chest: anatomic considerations, applications and radiologic appearance. *Radiology* 1994;192:825–830.
27. Bhalla M. Noncardiac thoracic surgical procedures: definitions, indications and postoperative radiology. *Radiol Clin North Am* 1996;34:137–155.
28. Shea WJ Jr, de Geer G, Webb WR. Chest wall after mastectomy. Part I. CT appearance of normal postoperative anatomy, postirradiation changes, and optimal scanning techniques. *Radiology* 1987;162:157–161.
29. Orford JE, Ingram DM, Kaard AO, Sheiner HJ. Scar formation after breast-conserving surgery for cancer. Sir Charles Gairdner Hospital Breast Cancer Group. *Br J Surg* 1996;80:1003–1004.
30. Steinbach BG, Hardt NS, Abbitt PL. Mammography: breast implants types, complications, and adjacent breast pathology. *Curr Probl Diagn Radiol* 1993;22:39–86.
31. Steinbach BG, Hardt NS, Abbitt P, Lanier L, Caffee HH. Breast implants, common complications, and concurrent breast disease. *RadioGraphics* 1993:13:95–118.
32. O'Boyle MK, Wechsler RJ, Concant EF, Lev-Toaff As, Sagerman J. Breast implants: incidental findings on CT. *Am J Roentgenol* 1994;162:311–313.
33. Destouet JM, Monsees BS, Oser RF, Nemecek JR, Young VL, Pilgram TK. Screening mammography in 350 women with breast implants: prevalence and findings of implant complications. *Am J Roentgenol* 1992;159:973–978.
34. O'Mara EM, Pennes DR, Argenta LA. Combination gel-inflatable mammary prosthesis: appearance at CT. *Radiology* 1989;170:78.
35. Ahn CY, DeBruhl ND, Gorczyca DP, Bassett LW, Shaw WW. Silicone implant rupture diagnosis using computed tomography: a case report and experience with 22 surgically removed implants. *Ann Plast Surg* 1994;33:624–628.
36. Loyer EM, Kroll SS, David CL, DuBrow RA, Libshitz HI. Mammographic and CT findings after breast reconstruction with a rectus abdominis musculoskeletal flap. *Am J Roentgenol* 1991;156:1159–1162.
37. Lejour M, Dome M. Abdominal wall function after rectus abdominis transfer. *Plast Reconstr Surg* 87:1054–1068.
38. Lejour M. Reconstructive options after cancer surgery of the breast. *Eur J Surg Oncol* 1989;15:496–503.
39. Gross BH, Agha FP, Glazer GM, Orringer MB. Gastric interposition following transhiatal esophagectomy: CT evaluation. *Radiology* 1985;155:177–179.
40. Carlisle JG, Quint LE, Francis IR, Orringer MB, Smick JF, Gross BH. Recurrent esophageal carcinoma: CT evaluation after esophagectomy. *Radiology* 1993;189:271–275.
41. Seltzer SE, Herman PG, Sagel SS. Differential diagnosis of mediastinal fluid levels visualized on computed tomography. *J Comput Assist Tomogr* 1984;8:244–246.
42. Larson TC, Shuman LS, Libshitz HI, McMurtrey MJ. Complications of colonic interposition. *Cancer* 1985;56:681–690.
43. Pavone P, Laghi A, Catalano G, et al. CT of Nissen's fundoplication. *Abdom Imag* 1997;22:457–460.
44. Gollub MJ, Gerdes H, Bains MS. Radiographic appearances of esophageal stents. *RadioGraphics* 1997;17:1169–1182.
45. Quint LE, Francis IR, Williams DM, Monaghan HM, Deeb DM. Synthetic interposition grafts of the thoracic aorta: postoperative appearance on serial CT studies. *Radiology* 1999;221:317–324.
46. Quint L, Francis I, Williams D, et al. Evaluation of thoracic aortic disease with the use of helical CT with multiplanar reconstructions: comparison with surgical findings. *Radiology* 1996;201:37–41.
47. Rofsky N, Weinreb J, Grossi E, et al. Aortic aneurysm and dissection: normal MR imaging and CT findings after surgical repair with the continuous-suture graft-inclusion technique. *Radiology* 1993;186:195–201.
48. Libshitz HI, Southard ME. Complications of radiation therapy: the thorax. *Semin Roentgenol* 1974;9:41–49.
49. Libshitz HI. Radiation changes in the lung. *Semin Roentgenol* 1993;28:303–320.
50. Movasa B, Raffin TA, Epstein AH, Link CJ. Pulmonary radiation injury. *Chest* 1997;111:1061–1076.
51. Libshitz HI, Shurman LS. Radiation-induced pulmonary changes: CT findings. *J Comput Assist Tomogr* 1984;8:15–19.
52. Mah K, Van Dyke J, Keane T, et al. Acute radiation-induced pulmonary damage: a clinical study on the response to fractionated radiation therapy. *Int J Radiat Oncol Biol Phys* 1986;13:179–188.
53. Movasa B, Raffin TA, Epsein AH, Link CJ. Pulmonary radiation injury. *Chest* 1997;111:1061–1076.
54. Van Haecke P, Vansteenkiste J, Paridaens R, Van der Schueren E, Demedts M. Chronic lymphocytic alveolitis with migrating pulmonary infiltrates after localized chest wall irradiation. *Acta Clin Belg* 1998;53:39–43.
55. Stewart JR, Fajardo LF. Radiation-induced heart disease: clinical and experimental aspects. *Radiol Clin North Am* 1971;9:511–531.
56. Lepke RA, Libshitz HI. Radiation-induced injury of the esophagus. *Radiology* 1983;148:375–378.
57. Skinner WL, Buzdar AU, Libshitz HI. Massive osteolysis of the right clavicle developing after radiation therapy. *JAMA* 1988;260:375–376.

Variants and Pitfalls in Body Imaging,
edited by Ali Shirkhoda.
Lippincott Williams & Wilkins, Philadelphia, © 2000.

CHAPTER 5

The Diaphragm

Michael C. Farah and Ali Shirkhoda

The diaphragm is a dynamic barrier separating the abdominal and thoracic cavities and performs most of the work of inspiration. It is routinely included in CT or MRI of the abdomen and chest and often changes its appearance depending on the phase of respiration. Knowledge of the spectrum of its normal anatomic variances will allow one to avoid misinterpreting such variances as pathology and, therefore, to avoid diagnostic pitfalls.

ANATOMIC CONSIDERATIONS

The diaphragm is a musculotendinous structure that is approximately 5 mm thick and is covered by pleura on its thoracic side and by the peritoneum on its abdominal side. It has two distinct anatomic parts: a central tendinous portion and a peripheral muscular portion. The central tendinous portion is thin yet strong and is called the central tendon (Fig. 5.1). It is incompletely divided into three leaflets and has a trifoliate appearance (1). The middle leaflet of the central tendon fuses with the inferior surface of the fibrous pericardium. The right and left leaflets form the domes of the diaphragm (2).

The peripheral muscular portion is composed of closely applied band-like strips of muscle (slips) that attach the central tendon to the thoracic wall. The peripheral attachment of the muscular diaphragm can be divided into the sternal, costal, and lumbar portions. The sternal portion is the smallest component of the muscular diaphragm and is composed of two small slips that attach to the xiphoid process. The costal portion arises from the lower six ribs and attaches to the central tendon. The lum-

bar portion arises from the lumbar spine and includes the crura and arcuate ligaments (1,3).

The Arcuate Ligaments

These ligaments represent areas of fascial thickening overlying the superior aspects of the psoas muscles (medial arcuate ligament) and quadratus lumborum muscles (lateral arcuate ligament). The medial arcuate ligament extends from the lateral aspect of the L1 vertebral body, arches over the psoas muscle, and attaches to the transverse process of L1. The lateral arcuate ligament extends from the transverse process of L1, arches over the quadratus lumborum muscle, and attaches to the midportion of the 12th rib (see Fig. 5.1) (1,3). Because of the curved nature of the arcuate ligaments, they may appear nodular or band-like when imaged in the axial plane. Adjacent to the lateral arcuate ligament lies a triangular area of muscular deficiency called the vertebrocostal triangle. This thin areolar membrane is a site for hernias or eventration (see Fig. 5.1) (1).

Diaphragmatic Crura

For the most part, the crura are oriented along the axis of the spine and merge with the anterior longitudinal ligament (Fig. 5.2). The right crus usually is broader than the left and arises from the anterolateral surface of L1 through L3. Superiorly, it surrounds the esophageal hiatus (see Fig. 5.1), and inferiorly, it lies posterior and medial to the infrahepatic portion of the inferior vena cava and right renal artery (Fig. 5.3). This relationship is important to keep in mind to avoid potential pitfalls. The left crus is shorter and arises from the anterior surface of L1 and L2 and joins the right crus anteriorly over the abdominal aorta via the median arcuate ligament. On axial plane, the crura have a band-like appearance superiorly as they course over the

M. C. Farah and A. Shirkhoda: Department of Diagnostic Radiology, William Beaumont Hospital, Royal Oak, Michigan 48073.

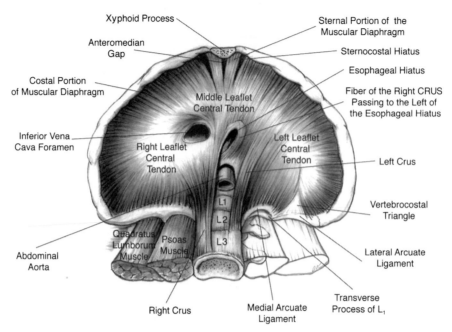

FIG. 5.1. Anatomy of the diaphragm. Drawing of the anatomic detail of muscular and tendinous components of the diaphragm as well as foramina and attachments. (Courtesy of Alexander Cacciarelli, William Beaumont Hospital.)

esophagus and abdominal aorta, but inferiorly they may appear nodular (see Fig. 5.2).

Diaphragmatic Openings

There are three major openings in the diaphragm: the aortic hiatus, esophageal hiatus, and inferior vena cava foramen. The aortic hiatus corresponds to the T12 vertebral level and is the most posterior and inferior of the three openings (1,3). The azygos vein, hemiazygous vein, and thoracic duct accompany the aorta in the retrocrural space. The esophageal hiatus lies within the muscular portion of the diaphragm at the level of T10. It is surrounded by the fibers of the right crus and lies anterior and slightly to the

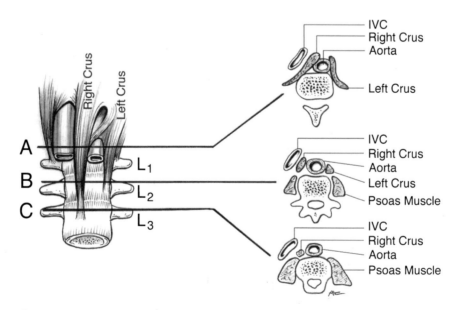

FIG. 5.2. Anatomy of the diaphragmatic crura. Drawing of the diaphragmatic crura illustrating their attachment sites and the variable thicknesses in the right and left on sectional imaging. Note the asymmetry of the crura, the right being thicker and longer than the left. At level **C,** the right crus can mimic a node (Courtesy of Alexander Cacciarelli, William Beaumont Hospital.)

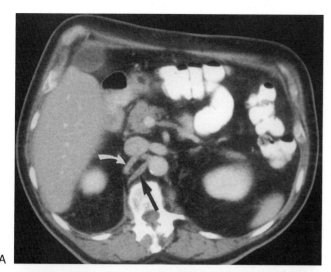

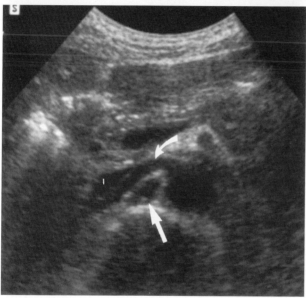

FIG. 5.3. Right crus. Both CT **(A)** and ultrasound **(B)** show the relationship of the right crus *(straight arrow)* posterior to the IVC (I) and right renal artery *(curved arrow)*. It is important not to mistake the right crus for retrocaval adenopathy on ultrasound.

left of the abdominal aorta (see Fig. 5.1). This anatomic relationship is a useful landmark when imaging by ultrasound or MRI in the sagittal plane. The vagus nerve and esophageal branches of the left gastric artery and vein course though the esophageal hiatus. The inferior vena cava foramen is the most anterior and superior opening and lies within the central tendon at the level of T8-9 (see Fig. 5.1). Branches of the right phrenic nerve accompany the inferior vena cava through the hiatus (1,3).

Another clinically significant opening is the sternocostal hiatus (see Fig. 5.1). This is also known as the foramen of Morgagni and lies between the small muscular slips that attach to the xiphoid process (sternal portion of the diaphragm) and the adjacent costal portion of the

muscular diaphragm. This is the site where Morgagni hernias occur (1). The superior epigastric vessels pass through the sternocostal foramen (3). Aside from these openings, the diaphragm may contain holes or areas of discontinuity through which fluid can pass from the peritoneal cavity into the pleural space. This may also occur through transdiaphragmatic lymphatics (2).

IMAGING OF THE DIAPHRAGM

The diaphragm, as seen on chest radiographs, is convex upward. When it is imaged with CT in the axial plane, the lung and pleura are peripheral to the diaphragm, whereas the abdominal viscera, fat, and the retroperitoneum are central. Knowledge of this relationship is important because much of the diaphragm is not visualized adjacent to the liver or spleen on CT unless there is interposed fat (4).

On abdominal ultrasound, the diaphragm is routinely seen as an echogenic line adjacent to the liver. The echogenicity is produced by a strong sound wave reflection from the interface between the diaphragm and the air-filled lung above it (Fig. 5.4). Occasionally, on high-resolution ultrasound, it has a three-line appearance; the inner hyperechoic line from the diaphragm–liver capsule interface, the middle hypoechoic line from the diaphragmatic muscle, and the outer hyperechoic line from the diaphragm–lung interface (see Fig. 5.4). A fourth line can sometimes be seen on the thoracic side that is echogenic and is a mirror-image artifact of the diaphragm–lung interface (5).

During routine spiral (or helical) scanning of the chest or abdomen, diagnostic questions may arise as a result of diaphragmatic or peridiaphragmatic abnormalities. Many of these questions may be answered with reconstruction of the original data at closer intervals in the sagittal or coronal plane. Some questions may be answered by imaging with thinner slices or in different phases of respiration (i.e., inspiration/expiration).

Imaging of the diaphragm usually occurs when a peridiaphragmatic abnormality has been identified that needs further evaluation or in the setting of traumatic rupture. In a traumatized patient, one may opt not to use oral contrast if the patient is going to surgery. However, oral contrast is helpful, particularly in evaluating diaphragmatic hernias. Intravenous contrast facilitates the evaluation of pleural abnormalities, atelectasis, and in distinguishing thoracic abnormalities from those in the liver and spleen. Breath-hold spiral scanning is the technique of choice in which respiratory artifacts can be eliminated. A targeted study to the peridiaphragmatic abnormality can be performed with 2- to 5-mm slice thickness and a table increment of 2 to 8 mm. The data are then reconstructed at 1 to 2 mm to obtain sagittal and coronal images. One hundred twenty milliliters of intravenous contrast (low osmolality 280 to 320 mg I/ml, high osmolality 282 mg I/ml of 60% solution) is injected at 3 ml/sec in the antecubital vein through a 20-gauge angiocath.

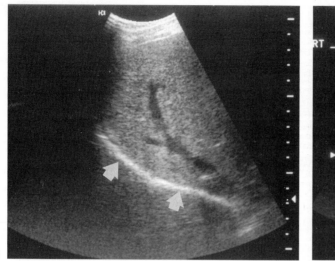
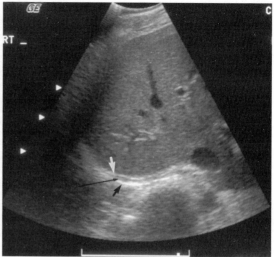

FIG. 5.4. Normal diaphragm on ultrasound. A: The diaphragm can be seen as a single echogenic line *(arrows)*. B: It may also have a normal three-line appearance. The inner hyperechoic line *(white arrow* in B) is from the diaphragm–liver capsule interface. The middle hypoechoic line is from diaphragmatic muscle *(thin black arrow)*. The outer hyperechoic line is from the diaphragm–lung interface *(black arrow)*.

Spiral scanning is begun at 30 seconds following the start of IV contrast if the abnormality is in the lung and at 60 to 80 seconds if the suspected abnormality is in the abdomen (8). The patient is hyperventilated and then asked to take a deep breath in before scanning begins.

Imaging in the direct sagittal and coronal plane makes MRI an attractive modality for evaluation of the diaphragm. The use of phased-array body coils and breath-hold gradient sequences has improved resolution and reduced motion artifact from respiration. Although T_2^* gradient-echo pulse-sequence images are rapidly acquired, the inherent suppression of fat signal impairs visualization of the diaphragm and adds no additional information. Also, depending on the T_E and the strength of the magnetic field, there is a potential for a pseudo-diaphragm to arise from a circumferential chemical shift artifact when a gradient-echo sequence is used (6). T_1-weighted imaging has the advantage of excellent contrast between the peridiaphragmatic fat and the diaphragm. Despite these advantages, portions of the diaphragm are not always visualized, particularly the central tendon (6,7).

On MRI, the diaphragm is seen as a low-signal-intensity band on T_1 and gradient-echo sequences (Fig. 5.5).

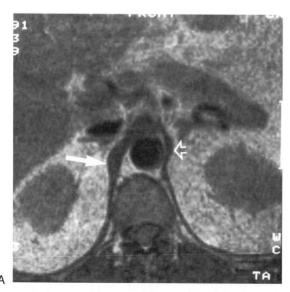
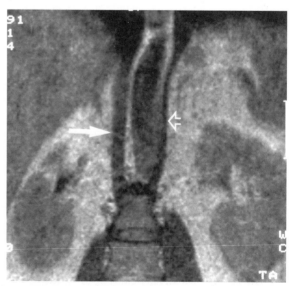

FIG. 5.5. Normal variation in the thickness in the crus. T_2-weighted MRIs in the axial (A) and coronal (B) planes demonstrate the normal thicker right crus *(arrow)* compared to the left *(open arrow)*.

The high signal intensity of abdominal and mediastinal fat as well as the intermediate higher signal intensity of the abdominal viscera on T_1-weighted images allow optimal visualization of the diaphragm (6). This is best demonstrated in sagittal and coronal planes. However, Kanematsu and colleagues studied the diaphragm using gadolinium-enhanced single-slice, breath-hold, dynamic spoiled gradient echo (SPGRE) imaging at 1.5 T and found that the diaphragm was partially depicted in 92% and not depicted in 7.5% (7). The muscular portion of the diaphragm was best visualized on the sagittal images, whereas the dome, where the thin fibers of the central tendon are located, may not be identified. They also noted an enhancing thin layer between the diaphragm and the liver on delayed enhanced MR images, probably indicating enhancing vessels.

ANATOMIC VARIATIONS AND DIAGNOSTIC PITFALLS

Variable Appearances of the Crus

Variation in the Normal Thickness of the Right and Left Crura

The right crus is thicker than the left crus in 91% of patients (see Figs. 5.2 and 5.5). There are a small percentage of cases in which the left crus will be larger than the right, and these should not be mistaken for adenopathy (9). This pitfall can be avoided by noting continuity of the apparent nodule with the crus superiorly and demonstrating a decrease in thickness on expiration. Another situation in which the left crus can be larger than the right is situs inversus (Fig. 5.6). There is no correlation between the thickness of the crura and age or sex (10,11).

Respiratory Variation of the Thickness of the Crura

The thickness of the crura also changes with respiration. During inspiration, the muscles of the diaphragm contract, which causes the crura to thicken and even appear nodular. During expiration, the diaphragm relaxes, and the crura decrease in thickness (9). Patients being followed with serial CT or MRI do not always take in the same breath for a scan. This can lead to apparent increasing in thickness and nodularity of the crura on a follow-up study. Awareness of the change in thickness and nodularity, depending on the degree of inspiration, will help to avoid misdiagnosing the crura as abnormal or as adenopathy (Fig. 5.7). Other findings that help confirm the crura to be normal include homogeneous density with the remainder of the crus, no alteration in contrast enhancement with the remainder of the crus, and concomitant change in thickness of the peripheral muscular slips of the diaphragm. One can also look

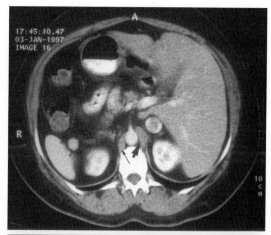

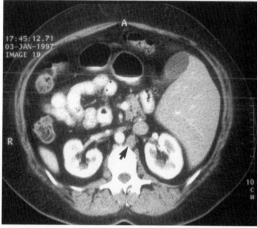

FIG. 5.6. Situs inversus with increased thickness of the left crus. Note the larger left crus *(thick arrow)* compared to the right *(thin arrow)*.

for other findings that could indicate differences in inspiration, such as a lower position of the liver, spleen, and kidneys in relation to a fixed structure such as the celiac axis or the superior mesenteric artery and widened intercostal spaces on deeper inspiration (see Fig. 5.7). If there is still a question, one can repeat the scan in expiration, which will show a decrease in the thickness of the crus.

Discontinuity of the Crura

Discontinuity or defects in the diaphragm are usually seen in the posterior aspect of the diaphragm in the region of the crus (Fig. 5.8). They are more common in older individuals, affecting approximately 56% of patients in the seventh and eighth decades. There appears to be no correlation with the status of skeletal muscle or obesity and diaphragmatic defects. However, there is a strong association of diaphragmatic defects and emphysema (10).

Caskey and colleagues have described three types of diaphragmatic defects. Type 1 defects demonstrate a focal

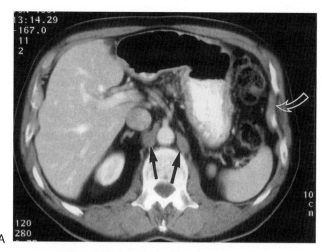

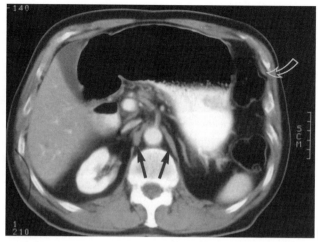

FIG. 5.7. Variation in the thickness of the crura with respiration. **A:** Nodular appearing crura *(arrows)* in deep inspiration. **B:** The same patient with a lesser inspiration demonstrates the decrease in thickness and nodularity of the crura *(arrows)*. Note the concomitant decrease in thickness of the muscular slips of the diaphragm *(open curved arrows)* from **A** to **B.** The two images were obtained at the level of the celiac axis.

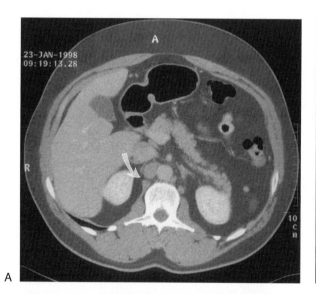

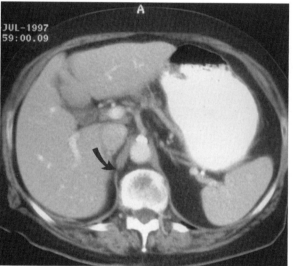

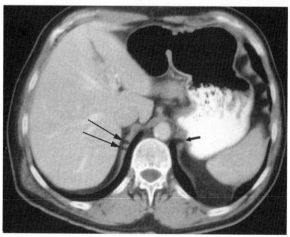

FIG. 5.8. A, B and **C:** Discontinuity in the crura. Small defects in the right and left crura *(arrows)* are seen as a normal variant in these two different patients.

area of decreased thickness but still maintain continuity with the remaining diaphragm. Type 2 defects demonstrate separation of the muscle fibers into parallel layers. Type 3 defects exist when a portion of the diaphragm is absent and there is loss of continuity with the remaining diaphragm. Herniation of intraabdominal fat is a feature of type 3 defects (10).

When discontinuity of the diaphragm is seen in close proximity to the adrenal gland, it can mimic an adrenal nodule (Fig. 5.9). This pitfall can be avoided by following the discontinuous portion above and below on multiple slices, where it becomes continuous with the crus. If there

is still uncertainty, repeat scans using thin slices or during inspiration and expiration may be useful.

It is important to keep in mind that defects in the crura are not uncommon in routine abdominal CT and should be carefully evaluated in a traumatized patient and not misinterpreted as a diaphragmatic rupture. Factors to consider in this setting include the following: (a) most diaphragmatic ruptures occur posterolaterally on the left side, not in the crura (12); (b) defects in the diaphragm are not common in the third and fourth decades (10); (c) presence of herniation of abdominal viscera with a colar sign (constriction of the viscera at the point of herniation) is seen in diaphragmatic rupture; and (d) other signs such as location of abdominal contents peripheral to the lung or diaphragm, blood in the pleural space or peritoneal cavity, or pneumothorax and pneumomediastinum would be more indicative of diaphragmatic rupture (12). Magnetic resonance imaging can be useful in helping to diagnose diaphragmatic rupture (6).

Lumpy, Bumpy Crus

Nodularity of the crus is thought to result from age-related laxity in the connective tissues that bind the muscular fibers of the diaphragm (13). During inspiration, infolding and redundancy develop as the muscle fibers contract.

Localized nodularity of the crus is not an uncommon finding, particularly in older patients. Nodularity may be single or multiple, giving a lumpy, bumpy appearance to the crus (Fig. 5.10). In some cases the focal bulge appears as a perpendicular polypoid projection from the crus. This may even project laterally, producing an apparent retrocaval nodule (Fig. 5.11). When a nodular-appearing crus is associated with the discontinuity of the diaphragm, it can mimic an adrenal nodule (see Fig. 5.9).

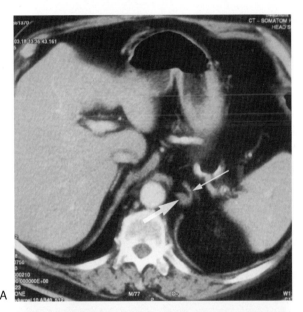

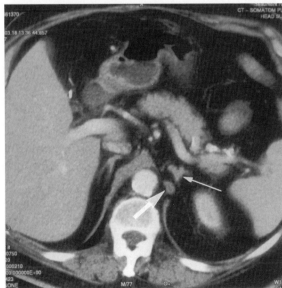

FIG. 5.9. Discontinuity in the left crus mimicking a left adrenal nodule. **A:** Focal discontinuous area of the left crus *(thick arrow)* comes into contact with the crural limb of the left adrenal gland *(thin arrow)*, mimicking a nodule. **B:** On the lower image, the normal left adrenal gland *(thin arrow)* is seen.

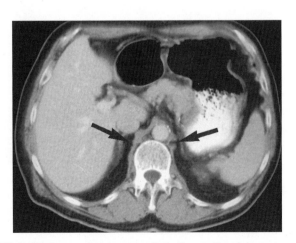

FIG. 5.10. Lumpy, bumpy crus. Note the multinodular appearance of the right and left crura *(arrows)*.

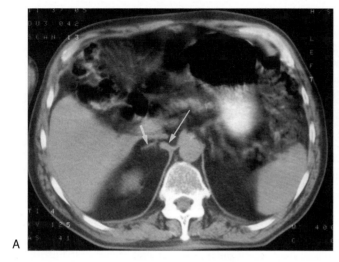
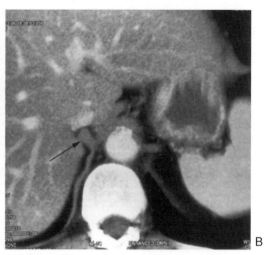

FIG. 5.11. Perpendicular polypoid projection of the crus. **A:** Note the projection of the right crus *(long arrow)* into the suprarenal area adjacent to the right adrenal gland *(short arrow)*. **B:** The nodular right crus *(arrow)* projecting into the liver mimics a retrocaval nodule.

Bulges or pseudotumors of the crus should not be mistaken for metastasis. Bulges in the diaphragm enhance homogeneously with the rest of the diaphragm following intravenous contrast. They markedly decrease in size and number on expiratory scans (13).

The caudal aspect of the crus is also a source of pitfalls. The right crus is not only thicker but also longer than the left crus. Its inferior aspect lies posterior to the inferior vena cava and can mimic retrocaval adenopathy (Fig. 5.12) (14). This can also occur on the left side and

mimic left para-aortic adenopathy. This pitfall can be avoided by showing contiguity with the crus on more superior images. As was described previously, one should be aware that the crus can change in thickness depending on the degree of inspiration and not misdiagnose that as an enlarging lymph node. Remember that the crus, like the rest of the muscular diaphragm, increases in size with inspiration and decreases in size on expiration (see Fig. 5.7). This observation is particularly helpful when ultrasound is used.

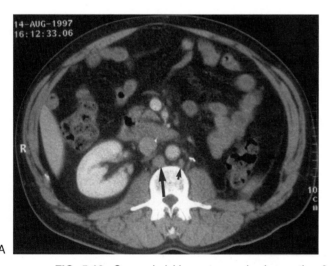
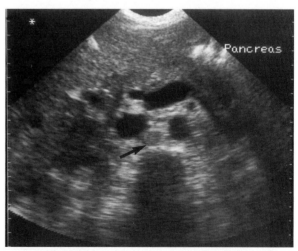

FIG. 5.12. Crus mimicking retrocaval adenopathy. **A:** Computed tomogram demonstrates the larger right crus *(large arrow)* as a retrocaval nodule and the smaller left crus *(small arrow)* as a left paraaortic nodule. **B:** On ultrasound, the right crus *(arrow)* is seen mimicking retrocaval adenopathy. Real-time change in thickness may be observed during expiration.

Variable Appearance of the Arcuate Ligament

Nodular or Band-like Appearance Mimicking Posterior Pararenal Disease

The lateral arcuate ligament extends from the transverse process of L1 and arches over the quadratus lumborum to insert on the 12th rib. It represents an area of fascial thickening (see Fig. 5.1). Occasionally, the lateral

arcuate ligament appears nodular or band-like and mimics metastasis in the posterior pararenal space (Fig. 5.13) (2,15). In the same area but lateral to the arcuate ligament, a similar finding can be seen secondary to redundancy in the muscular diaphragm (16). In both cases, demonstrating contiguity with the diaphragm helps distinguish this from pathology.

On proton density- or T_1-weighted images, the band-like area of intermediate or low signal intensity of the fibrous arcuate ligament can mimic perirenal fluid or nodule (Fig. 5.14). However, unlike fluid that is bright on T_2-weighted images, the arcuate ligament maintains its low signal intensity (Fig. 5.15).

Variable Appearance of the Muscular Diaphragm

Anterior Muscular Diaphragm

Gale has described three appearances of the anterior diaphragm on CT (17). The most common is a curved anterior band that is concave posteriorly and smoothly continuous with the anterolateral fibers. In the second type, the anterior muscle fibers are oriented at an angle to the lateral fibers and therefore appear discontinuous. The third appearance is that of a broad muscular band with irregular or poorly defined margins (Fig. 5.16). In some patients, the anterior component of the diaphragm is not identifiable.

Scalloped or Nodular Appearance of the Muscular Insertions (Slips) of the Diaphragm

The scalloped or nodular appearance of the muscular diaphragm increases in frequency with age and occurs

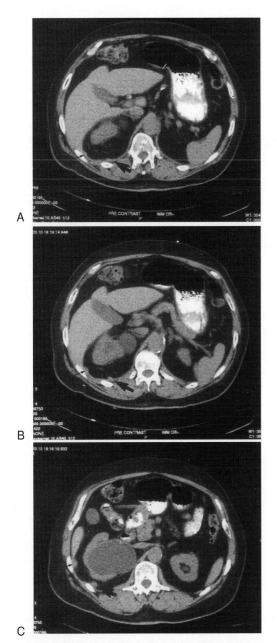

FIG. 5.13. Lateral arcuate ligament mimicking perirenal pathology on CT. Consecutive noncontrast axial images **(A–C)** show a nodular density adjacent to the 12th rib representing the arcuate ligament *(large arrow)* with its associated muscular diaphragmatic component inserting on the 12th rib. Note the continuity with the diaphragm over multiple images. More laterally is a muscular slip inserting on the 11th rib *(small arrow),* producing a nodular density next to the 11th rib.

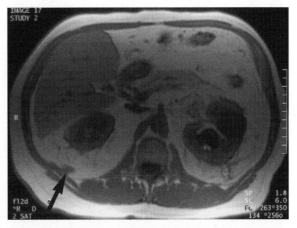

FIG. 5.14. Lateral arcuate ligament mimicking perirenal nodule. Axial breath-hold T_1-gradient echo image demonstrates a nodular structure of intermediate signal intensity in the posterior pararenal fat *(arrow)*. This lies adjacent to the region of the 12th rib and could be followed over multiple images (not shown) and represents the lateral arcuate ligament. Note that ribs are difficult to visualize on MRI.

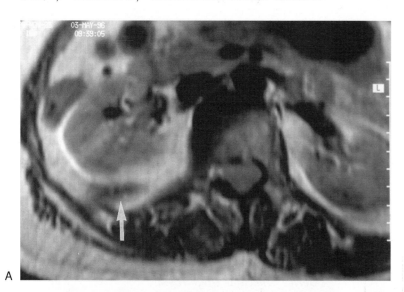

A

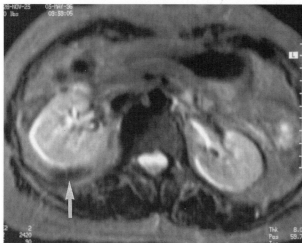

B

FIG. 5.15. Band-like lateral arcuate ligament mimicking perirenal pathology. **A:** An axial proton-density image demonstrates a band-like area of decreased signal intensity posterior to the right kidney (arrow). **B:** On T_2 it remains low in signal intensity and therefore does not represent perirenal fluid (arrow). **C:** Contrast-enhanced CT in the same patient shows that this structure represents the lateral arcuate ligament (arrow) adjacent to the 12th rib.

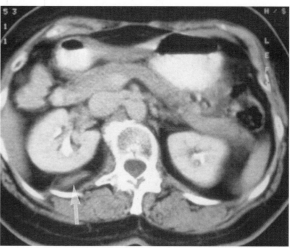

C

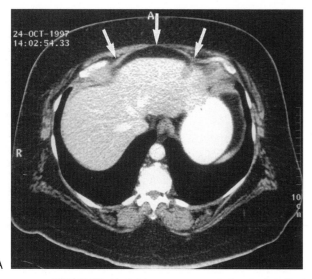

A

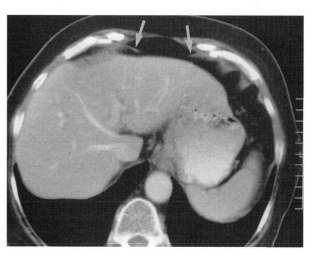

B

FIG. 5.16. Variable appearance of anterior diaphragm. **A:** The smoothly curved anterior diaphragm (arrows) becomes continuous with the more lateral fibers. **B:** The anterior diaphragm appears discontinuous (arrows).

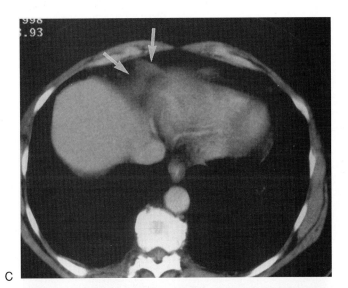

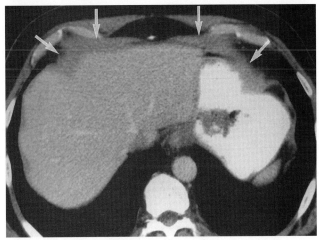

FIG. 5.16. *Continued.* **C:** Broad band is poorly defined anterior diaphragm *(arrows).* **D:** The anterior diaphragm can look quite thick as it becomes continuous with the anterolateral diaphragm.

most commonly in the elderly population. This is also the population of patients who are more likely to have malignancy with potential for peritoneal metastasis. Therefore, familiarity with this appearance of the diaphragm will allow one to distinguish it from neoplastic condition.

The scalloped appearance of the diaphragm has an easily recognizable appearance on CT. It is seen as a series of arcs, nodules, or linear densities at the periphery of the upper intra-abdominal fat (Fig. 5.17) and may invaginate into the liver. When ascites is present, these diaphragmatic projections can become displaced from the invaginations. This results in the typical appearance of the V-shaped diaphragmatic peaks lying opposite to the corresponding defects on the liver surface (Figs. 5.18 and 5.19).

Nodular invaginations occur most commonly over the costal portion of the muscular diaphragm from the seventh through the 11th ribs, particularly on the left side

(10,13). With aging, laxity develops in the connective tissue that binds the diaphragmatic fibers together, and that plus decreased muscle tone lead to redundancy in the periphery of the diaphragm (13). During inspiration, the diaphragm contracts, and areas of nodular redundancy bulge inward and thus enlarge. In cases where distinguishing between nodular muscular insertions and metastasis is difficult, several observations may be helpful.

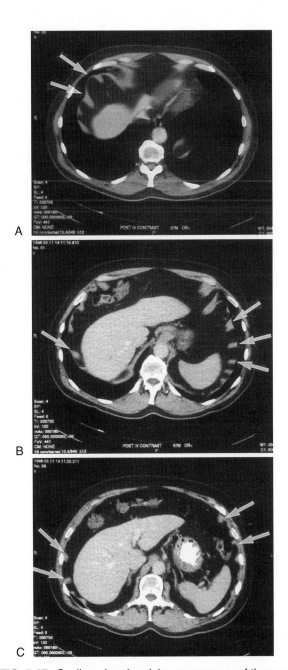

FIG. 5.17. Scalloped and nodular appearance of the muscular insertions (slips) of the diaphragm. Three consecutive contrast-enhanced CT scans of the same patient show the typical scalloped and nodular appearance *(arrows)* of the diaphragm on both sides.

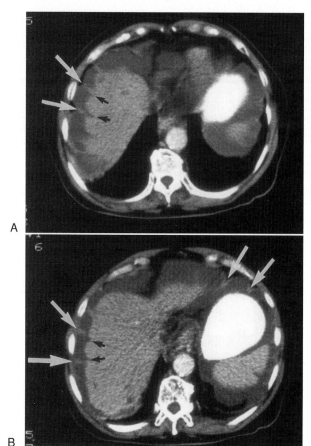

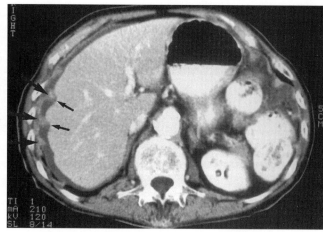

FIG. 5.18. Scalloped appearance in a patient with ascites. Non-contrast scans of the upper abdomen demonstrate the V-shaped peripheral projections on the muscular diaphragm *(arrows)* outlined by peritoneal fluid in **A** and **B.** Notice that opposite to invaginations are accessory fissures in the liver *(small black arrows)*, where they have been delineated by ascites. **C:** This is also seen in another patient on contrast-enhanced CT.

Metastatic nodules abruptly change size on multiple contiguous scans, whereas the diaphragm-related nodular invaginations can be followed (see Fig. 5.17). At the periphery of a nodular bulge of the diaphragm, the nodule typically widens or has a linear extension peripherally (see Fig. 5.19). If a question still remains, expiratory images may be obtained. On expiration the nodular invaginations of the diaphragm typically decrease in size.

Accessory Hepatic Fissures and Pseudolesions

Accessory hepatic fissures, unlike the major fissures, are limited to the superior aspect of the liver near the diaphragmatic dome. They are formed by the invagination of the muscular diaphragm into the liver. This occurs most commonly in the superior aspect of the right lobe of the liver and is common in elderly patients (18). Accessory hepatic fissures can be single or multiple, giving a scalloped appearance to the liver (Fig. 5.20). Subdiaphragmatic fat and the peritoneum accompany the muscular diaphragm in the accessory fissure (19), and, there-

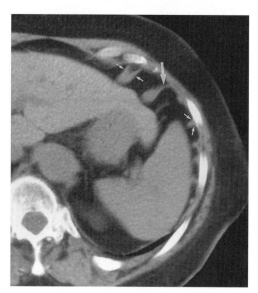

FIG. 5.19. Nodular peripheral diaphragm. Noncontrast CT demonstrates the nodular appearance of the slips of the diaphragm. Note the peripheral linear extension *(large arrow)* and peripheral widening *(small arrows)* helping distinguish the apparent nodules as part of the diaphragm.

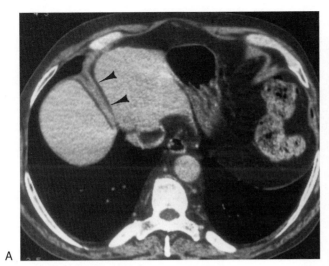

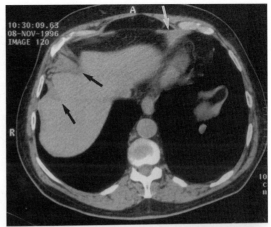

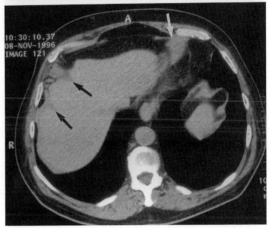

FIG. 5.20. Accessory hepatic fissures. **A:** Contrast-enhanced CT demonstrates a single accessory fissure secondary to invagination of the diaphragm and subdiaphragmatic fat *(arrowheads)*. **B,C:** Multiple hepatic accessory fissures *(black arrows)* giving a scalloped appearance. Note the triangular-shaped muscular diaphragm on the left *(white arrow)*. (**A** from Shirkhoda A. Diagnostic pitfalls in abdominal CT. *RadioGraphics* 1991;11:969–1002, with permission.)

fore, when ascites is present, it can extend into the accessory fissures (see Fig. 5.18).

On ultrasound, the accessory fissures are seen as single or multiple thin lines of increased echogenicity projecting inward from the periphery of the liver. They may be associated with indentation of the peripheral hepatic contour (Fig. 5.21).

Hepatic pseudolesions occur when the diaphragmatic invaginations are shorter, oriented more in the cranial–caudal plane, and the indentation of the liver surface is less pronounced or located more cephalad to the pseudolesion (Figs. 5.22 and 5.23). This can also occur when the diaphragmatic invagination next to the indentation in the liver is round (Fig. 5.24). In this situation, rescanning the patient in expiration is helpful. On expiration, the pseudolesion will decrease in size.

Hepatic pseudolesions secondary to diaphragmatic invagination also occur on ultrasound. They have a variety of appearances on transverse images such as peripherally located wedge-shaped, round, oval, lobulate, or irregular structures (19,20). They usually mimic hemangiomas. This pitfall can be avoided by rotating the probe

along the long axis of the lesion, which will cause it to elongate. One can also look for the characteristic indentation of the liver surface.

Gastric and Perigastric Pseudolesions

In some instances a nodular diaphragmatic invagination lies adjacent to or even protrudes into the stomach, mimicking a gastric lesion (Fig. 5.25). Several observations are helpful in distinguishing this from a true gastric lesion: (a) look for a thin peripheral curvilinear muscular strand connecting the nodule to the diaphragm; (b) look for intraabdominal fat separating the stomach from the nodule; (c) repeat the images without gastric distention and scan in expiration. The diaphragmatic nodule will decrease in size on expiration (13).

Muscular Diaphragm Mimicking Pararenal Disease

Like the arcuate ligament discussed earlier, nodular or band-like invaginations of the muscular diaphragm can produce findings in the fat surrounding the kidney that can be mistaken as abnormal (16). The key to recognizing

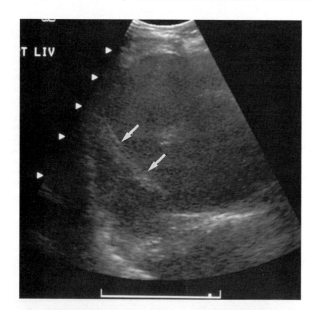

A

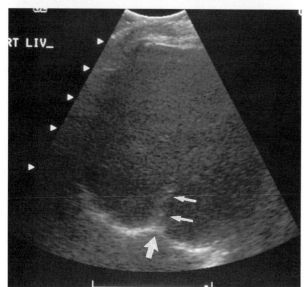

B

FIG. 5.21. Accessory hepatic fissure on ultrasound. **A:** Transverse image of the liver demonstrates the echogenic line of the accessory hepatic fissure *(arrows)*. **B:** Sagittal scan shows the typical indentation of the hepatic contour *(fat arrow)* associated with the accessory fissure *(arrows)*.

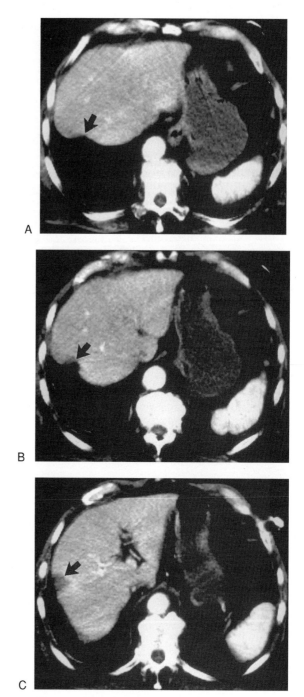

A

B

C

FIG. 5.22. Hepatic pseudolesion secondary to diaphragmatic invagination. Three consecutive CT images reveal the pseudolesion *(arrow)* with no appreciable indentation in the adjacent liver surface in the lower image **(C)** but one that becomes broader at the liver surface *(arrow)* in the higher levels **(B,A)**.

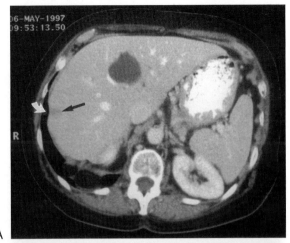

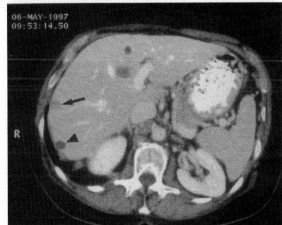

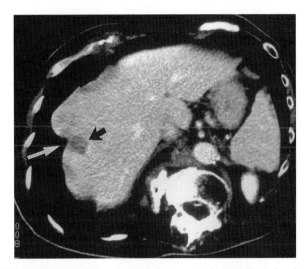

FIG. 5.23. Hepatic pseudolesion secondary to diaphragmatic invagination. Two consecutive contrast-enhanced CT scans show a pseudolesion in **A** and **B** *(arrow)* and a hepatic cyst in **B** *(arrowhead)* in the right lobe of the liver The pseudolesion was also seen on the scan above **(A)** with the associated indentation of the liver surface *(curved arrow)*. Note the lack of indentation of the liver surface adjacent to the cyst in **B.**

FIG. 5.24. Hepatic pseudolesion secondary to invagination of the diaphragm. Contrast-enhanced CT with liver windows demonstrates the nodular appearance of this pseudolesion *(black arrow)* on a scan taken on full inspiration. Note the characteristic adjacent indentation on the liver surface *(white arrow)* as a result of diaphragmatic invagination. The right crus is also prominent.

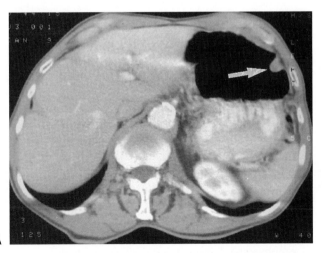

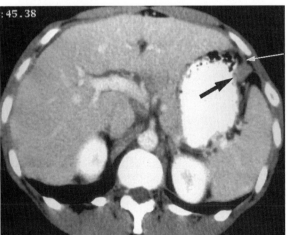

FIG. 5.25. Gastric and perigastric pseudolesion secondary to a nodular diaphragmatic invagination. **A:** The lack of subdiaphragmatic fat makes this diaphragmatic invagination *(arrow)* difficult to distinguish from a gastric polyp or mural lesion. **B:** In another patient, one can identify the peripheral linear extension *(white arrow)* from the nodule *(black arrow)* to the diaphragm and surrounding subdiaphragmatic fat, helping to identify this as diaphragm and not a perigastric lesion.

the structure as diaphragm is to demonstrate continuity with the diaphragm. This can be done by identifying a thin linear peripheral connection to the diaphragm and/or showing continuity on adjacent scans (Fig. 5.26 and 5.27).

Discontinuity in the Muscular Diaphragm

Discontinuities in the diaphragm increase in number and severity with age, particularly in the seventh and

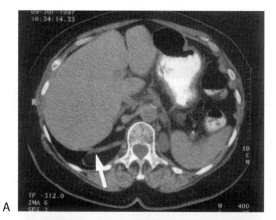

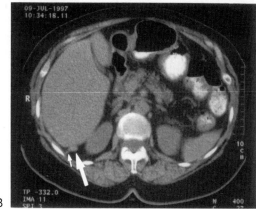

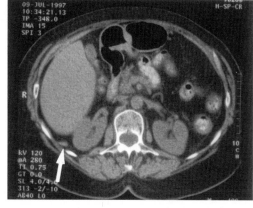

FIG. 5.26. Nodular muscular diaphragm mimicking pararenal disease. Three consecutive noncontrast CT images of the abdomen demonstrate a nodular density in the right pararenal space *(large arrow)*. If this is followed over three scans, continuity with the diaphragm is appreciated. Also note the peripheral linear projection from the nodule in **(B)** *(small arrow)*. This is characteristic of the nodular diaphragm.

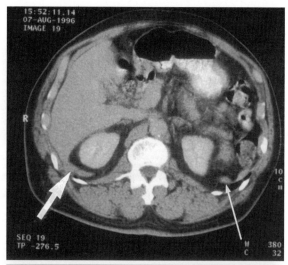

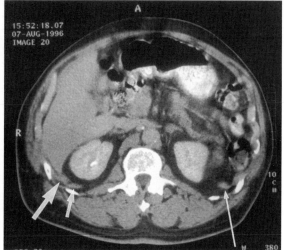

FIG. 5.27. Band-like muscular diaphragm mimicking pararenal disease. Two consecutive contrast-enhanced CT images show a band-like appearance of the diaphragm in the right posterior pararenal space *(large arrows)*. In **A** it appears to be an extension of the right lobe of the liver. However, in **B** one can see the nodular appearance of the diaphragm. The more medial component *(small arrow)* is probably related to the arcuate ligament. Note a similar appearance on the left side *(thin arrows)*.

eighth decades of life. They are more common on the left side and are associated with emphysema (10). Diaphragmatic defects are typically asymptomatic and are discovered as an incidental finding on imaging studies (12). They may be associated with herniation of intra-abdominal fat or viscera (Fig. 5.28). Caskey and colleagues postulate that many asymptomatic diaphragmatic defects are acquired because, in their experience, such defects were nonexistent in the third and fourth decades and increased in number and severity to affect 56% of patients in the 7th and 8th decades. Interestingly, 84% of patients with emphysema demonstrated diaphragmatic defects (10).

Bochdalek hernias are considered congenital abnormalities secondary to patency of the pleuroperitoneal canal (21). When large, they present in the neonatal period. However, small Bochdalek hernias remain asymptomatic and are

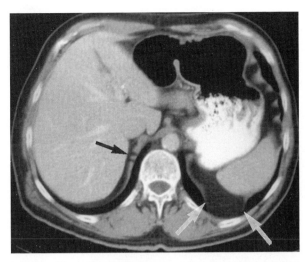

FIG. 5.28. Discontinuity of the muscular diaphragm with herniation of intra-abdominal fat. Abdominal CT shows discontinuity of the posterior left hemidiaphragm *(white arrows)* with herniation of intra-abdominal fat. Note focal discontinuity is also present in the right crus *(black arrow)*.

incidentally discovered on imaging studies. They are seen twice as often on the left side as they are on the right (Fig. 5.29) (21). Small bulges, when imaged in the axial plane, can mimic a pulmonary nodule (Figs. 5.30 and 5.31).

As discussed earlier, one should be aware of asymptomatic defects when considering the diagnosis of diaphragmatic rupture. Despite a diaphragmatic defect being the most sensitive sign of rupture, according to Murray and colleagues (12), diagnosis based solely on the presence of a defect should be made with caution.

Miscellaneous

Pseudodiaphragm from Lower Lobe Atelectasis

Atelectasis of the lower lobe associated with a pleural effusion can mimic the diaphragm surrounded by fluid. Subpulmonic fluid and pleural fluid surrounding the inferolateral tip of atelectatic lung may produce a thin linear structure mimicking the diaphragm when imaged in cross section (Fig. 5.32) (22).

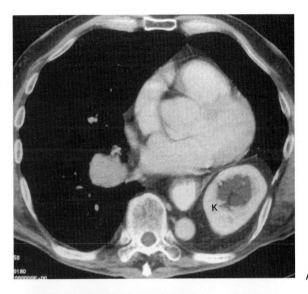

A

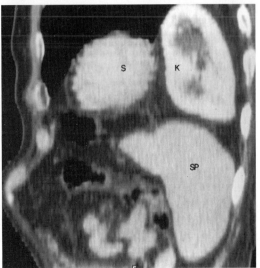

B

FIG. 5.29. Bochdalek hernia containing the left kidney and retroperitoneal fat. Contrast-enhanced abdominal CT **(A)** and sagittal reconstruction **(B)** demonstrate the left kidney (k) and retroperitoneal fat in a Bochdalek hernia. Note the typical posterior location on the left. Stomach (s), spleen (sp).

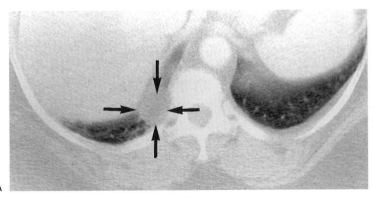

A

FIG. 5.30. Focal herniation of subdiaphragmatic fat mimicking a pulmonary nodule. **A:** Computed tomogram of the posterior costophrenic sulcus shows a nodule *(arrows)* on lung windows. *Continued on next page.*

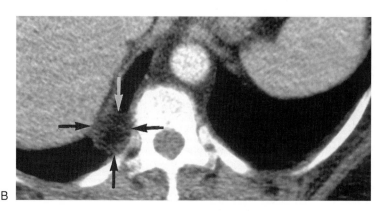

B

FIG. 5.30. *Continued.* B: Mediastinal windows reveal focal herniation of subdiaphragmatic fat (arrows).

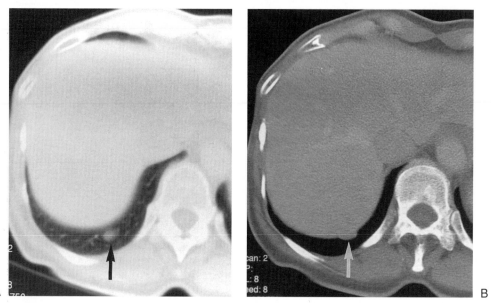

A

B

FIG. 5.31. Focal herniation of the liver mimicking a pulmonary nodule. A: A small pseudonodule *(arrow)* is seen on lung windows. B: Mediastinal windows demonstrate the focal herniation of the liver *(arrow)* causing the pseudonodule.

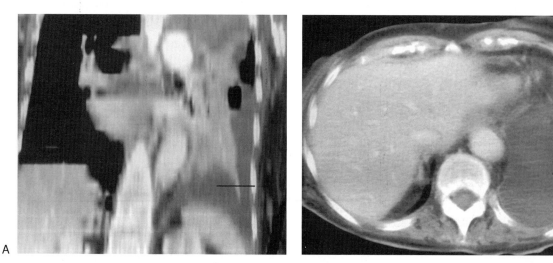

A

B

FIG. 5.32. Pseudodiaphragm. Left lower lobe atelectasis associated with pleural fluid mimicking the diaphragm surrounded by fluid. A: Coronal reconstruction CT demonstrates pleural fluid surrounding the atelectatic left lower lobe. An axial scan through the inferior aspect of the atelectatic lung *(line)* demonstrates the pseudodiaphragm *(arrow)* in B.

Mirror-Image Artifact

When ultrasound is used to scan through the upper abdomen, the curving diaphragm–lung interface acts as a specular (mirror-like) reflector. This results in an artifactual mirror image of the liver or spleen above the diaphragm and should not be confused with lung pathology (23).

REFERENCES

1. Williams PL, Warwick R, eds. *Gray's anatomy, 38th ed.* New York: Churchill Livingston, 1995;815–819.
2. Panicek DM, Benson CB, Gottleib RH, et al. The diaphragm: Anatomic, pathologic and radiologic considerations. *RadioGraphics* 1988;8:385–425.
3. Moore KL. The diaphragm. In: *Clinically oriented anatomy, 2nd ed.* Baltimore: Williams & Wilkins, 1985;268–275.
4. Naidich DP, Megibow AJ, Ross CR, et al. Computed tomography of the diaphragm: Normal anatomy and variants. *J Comput Assist Tomogr* 1983;7(4):633–640.
5. Verschakelen JA, Marchal G, Verbeken E, et al. Sonographic appearance of the diaphragm: a cadaver study. *J Clin Ultrasound* 1989;17:222.
6. Shanmuganathan K, Mirvis SE, White CS, et al. MR imaging evaluation of hemidiaphragms in acute blunt trauma: Experience with 16 patients. *Am J Roentgenol* 1996;167:397–402.
7. Kanematsu M, Imaeda T, Mochizuki R, et al. Dynamic MRI of the diaphragm. *J Comput Assist Tomogr* 1995;19:67–72.
8. Brink J, Heiken J, Semenkovich J, et al. Abnormalities of the diaphragm and adjacent structures; findings on multiplanar spiral CT scans. *Am J Roentgenol* 1994;163:307–310.
9. Williamson BRJ, Gouse JC, Rohrer D, et al. Variation in the thickness of the diaphragmatic crura with respiration. *Radiology* 1987;163:683–684.
10. Caskey CL, Zerhouni EA, Fishman EK, et al. Aging of the diaphragm: A CT study. *Radiology* 1989;171:385–389.
11. Dovgan DJ, Lenchik L, Kaye AD. Computed tomographic of maximal crural thickness. *Conn Med* 1994;58:203–206.
12. Murray JG, Caoili E, Gruden JF, et al. Acute rupture of the diaphragm due to blunt trauma: Diagnostic sensitivity and specificity of CT. *Am J Roentgenol* 1996;166:1035–1039.
13. Rosen A, Auh YH, Rubinstein WA, et al. CT appearance of diaphragmatic pseudotumors. *J Comput Assist Tomogr* 1983;7:995–999.
14. Callen PW, Filly RA, Korobkin M. Computed tomographic evaluation of the diaphragmatic crura. *Radiology* 1978;129:413–416.
15. Silverman PM, Cooper C, Zeman RK. Lateral arcuate ligaments of the diaphragm: Anatomic variations at abdominal CT. *Radiology* 1992;185:105–108.
16. Parienty RA, Marichez M, Pradel J, et al. Pararenal pseudotumors of the diaphragm: Computed tomographic features. *Gastrointest Radiol* 1987;12:131–133.
17. Gale ME. Anterior diaphragm: Variation in the CT appearance. *Radiology* 1986;161:635–639.
18. Auh YH, Rubenstein WA, Zirinski K, et al. Accessory fissures of the liver: CT and sonographic appearance. *Am J Roentgenol* 1984;143:565–572.
19. Hawkins SP, Hine AL. Diaphragmatic muscle bundles (SLIPS): Ultrasound evaluation of incidence and appearance. *Clin Radiol* 1991;44:154–157.
20. Yeh H-C, Halton KP, Gary CE. Anatomic variations and abnormalities in the diaphragm seen with ultrasound. *RadioGraphics* 1990;10:1019–1030.
21. Gale ME. Bochdalek hernia: Prevalence and CT characteristics. *Radiology* 1985;156:449–452.
22. Federle MP, Mark AS, Guillaumin ES. CT of subpulmonic pleural effusions and atelectasis: Criteria for differentiation from subphrenic fluid. *Am J Roentgenol* 1986;146:685–689.
23. Brant WE. Chest. In: McGahan JP, Goldberg BB, eds. *Diagnostic ultrasound. A logical approach.* Philadelphia: Lippincott-Raven, 1998;1063–1086.

Variants and Pitfalls in Body Imaging,
edited by Ali Shirkhoda.
Lippincott Williams & Wilkins, Philadelphia, © 2000.

CHAPTER 6

Breast Sonography

Bruno D. Fornage

Artifacts may aid in diagnosis or induce pitfalls, so their proper identification represents a significant step in the interpretation of sonograms (1–10). In this chapter, we review the most common and most significant artifacts and pitfalls encountered during sonographic examination of the breast and regional lymph nodes.

Artifacts can be related to the equipment used, technique applied, normal anatomic structures, pathologic processes, and/or foreign bodies. Whenever a sonogram exhibits an unusual or unexpected appearance, every effort should be made to first rule out an artifact. Also, normal variants can mimic pathology, and they must be known and identified as such to avoid significant diagnostic errors.

ARTIFACTS AND PITFALLS RESULTING FROM INADEQUATE EQUIPMENT, IMPROPER SETTINGS, AND POOR SCANNING TECHNIQUE

Sector transducers have a poor near-field resolution. In addition, the diverging beam on the lateral portions of the scan is oblique to most interfaces, which usually results in scattering of the beam that significantly degrades the quality of the sonograms to an unacceptable level, except in a narrow central portion. For those reasons, flat, linear-array transducers with the highest frequency possible compatible with the thickness of the breast tissue to be examined should be used.

If the overall gain chosen is too low, it may result in failure to display real echoes of minimal amplitude (e.g., low-level echoes representing inspissated material or debris within cysts). An improper setting of the time-gain-compensation curve may also result in artifactual bright or dark bands at certain depths in the sonogram.

B. D. Fornage: Department of Diagnostic Radiology, Section of Ultrasound, University of Texas M. D. Anderson Cancer Center, Houston, Texas 77030.

Great care must be taken to adjust the focus of electronic transducers to the region of interest, especially when lesions are very small (11,12). For example, the ultrasound energy passing on the sides of a very small calcification or cyst that does not lie in the focal zone of the transducer may prevent the formation of a typical shadow or enhancement, respectively. Minute calcifications and cysts will be better demonstrated if they lie in the focal zone of the transducer, where the scan plane is thinnest. The thickness of the scan plane also explains volume-averaging artifacts such as display of echoes within small cysts (see below) (2).

Examination of the skin and very superficial subcutaneous tissues is best done by using a thin standoff pad. However, artifacts reverberating from the strong interface between the pad and the skin are often noticed within the breast. They project at a distance that is twice the distance between the transducer's footprint and the reflector that causes the artifact. These reverberation (or repetition) artifacts can be easily identified by the fact that they are displaced when the distance between the transducer and the reflector is altered by either increasing or decreasing the pressure on the transducer (Fig. 6.1) (13). Air-filled cracks in the pad create bright echoes within the pad, sometimes associated with shadowing. Any loss of contact between the transducer and the surface of the breast, such as at the site of retracted scars, around the nipple, in the axilla, or between the standoff pad and the skin, will also result in shadows.

ARTIFACTS AND PITFALLS ASSOCIATED WITH NORMAL ANATOMIC STRUCTURES

Cooper's Ligaments

Cooper's ligaments course through the subcutaneous fat from the surface of the breast parenchyma up to the

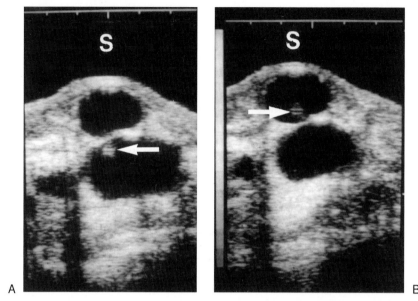

FIG. 6.1. Reverberation artifacts projecting in cysts and mimicking intracystic lesions. Sonograms have been obtained with the use of a standoff pad. **A:** A strong reverberation echo duplicating the interface between the standoff pad (S) and the skin projects at the anterior aspect of the deeper of two cysts and mimics an intracystic mass *(arrow)*. **B:** Increased pressure with the transducer has decreased the distance between the transducer's footprint and the surface of the skin. Accordingly, the distance between the skin and the reverberation echo has also decreased, and the artifact now projects within the lumen of the more superficial of the two cysts *(arrow)*. Reverberation echoes can be identified by their displacement as the distance between the transducer and the original reflector is altered. (Reprinted from reference 13 with permission.)

skin. Ligaments that are steeply oblique in relation to the ultrasound beam scatter the beam significantly, which results in shadowing. Firm compression with the transducer usually flattens out the spiking ligament and clears (or at least significantly reduces) the shadow, confirming the absence of a real lesion (Fig. 6.2).

Nipple

The nipple is hypoechoic and shows significant individual variations in size and shape (Figs. 6.3–6.5). The nipple–areola complex has been described as a source of shadowing that can impair the study of underlying breast

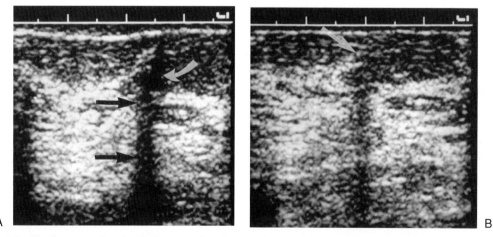

FIG. 6.2. Shadow associated with Cooper's ligament. **A:** Sonogram shows a marked shadow *(arrows)* distal to a questionable hypoechoic area *(curved arrow)* mimicking a mass. **B:** Firm compression with the transducer flattens the ligament *(arrow)* and dramatically reduces the amount of shadowing associated with it.

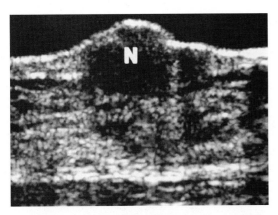

FIG. 6.3. Normal nipple. Sonogram of the nipple–areola complex shows a normal nipple (N), the echogenicity of which is decreased. The retroareolar region remains well demonstrated.

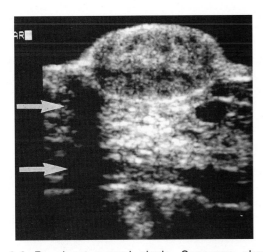

FIG. 6.4. Prominent normal nipple. Sonogram shows a prominent nipple with medium to high echogenicity. Note the moderate distal sound enhancement and refraction shadowing from the edge of the nipple in the left portion of the scan *(arrows).*

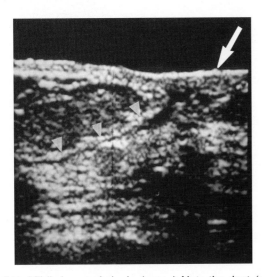

FIG. 6.5. Mildly inverted nipple *(arrow).* Note the duct *(arrowheads)* coursing toward the nipple.

tissue. Such a situation has been rare in our experience. The use of a standoff pad and/or a liberal amount of coupling gel to avoid the presence of any residual air around the nipple usually allows satisfactory study of the nipple–areola complex and underlying breast tissue.

Costal Cartilages

The costal cartilages appear on parasternal sagittal scans as well-defined oval to round markedly hypoechoic structures that should not be confused with a true breast mass such as a cyst or a fibroadenoma (Fig. 6.6). With advancing age, coarse internal calcifications develop centrally in the costal cartilage and are associated with acoustic shadowing (Fig. 6.7). On transverse oblique sonograms along the axis of a rib, it is possible to visualize the junction between the hypoechoic cartilage (without distal shadowing) and the highly reflective rib (with marked distal shadowing and reverberations).

Fat Lobules

Probably the most common pitfall in breast sonography is misdiagnosis of a prominent fatty lobule as a hypoechoic solid tumor (usually a fibroadenoma) (13). Indeed, some fat lobules have the same low echogenicity, echo texture, and smooth margins as fibroadenomas (Fig. 6.8). The correct diagnosis is established by swiveling the transducer over the hypoechoic fatty lobule until the hypoechoic area blends with the surrounding fat (Fig. 6.9).

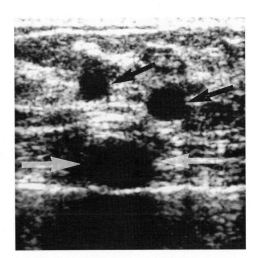

FIG. 6.6. Pitfall associated with a costal cartilage. Longitudinal parasternal sonogram shows the anechoic cross section of the cartilage *(white arrows).* Note the two minute cysts located more superficially in the breast tissue *(black arrows).* The anechoic cartilage can be differentiated from breast cysts in that it lies in the chest wall, not in the breast tissue.

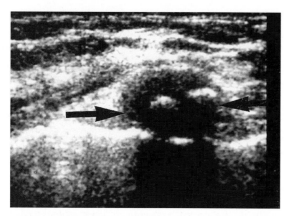

FIG. 6.7. Calcified costal cartilage. Longitudinal parasternal sonogram shows the cross section of a hypoechoic costal cartilage with internal calcifications *(arrows).* Note the distal shadow posterior to each of the two calcifications, interrupting the brightly echogenic pleural interface. The cartilage, which lies within the chest wall, should not be mistaken for a calcified fibroadenoma.

Intramammary Lymph Nodes

Intramammary lymph nodes are usually located in the outer quadrants, although rare cases of intramammary lymph nodes in the inner breast have been reported. They appear typically as small, well-defined round or oval lobulated hypoechoic masses with a characteristic echogenic fatty hilum, which correlates with the fatty hilar radiolucency seen on mammograms (Fig. 6.10). However, an echogenic hilum is not always present, and intramammary nodes undergoing inflammatory changes

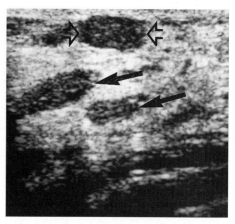

FIG. 6.8. Fat lobules and fibroadenoma. The biopsy-proven fibroadenoma *(open arrows)* has the same echogenicity as the fat lobules *(arrows).*

may appear completely hypoechoic. In such a case, the differential diagnosis is much broader, and fine-needle aspiration (FNA) is usually required to rule out malignancy.

Arterial Calcifications

Arterial calcifications in the breast are relatively common in elderly women. The cross section of a calcified artery gives rise to a narrow shadow, and the walls of the calcified artery *per se* are difficult to identify (Fig. 6.11).

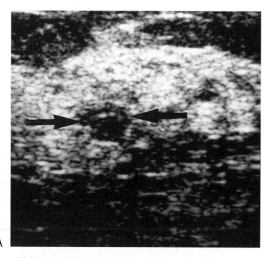

A

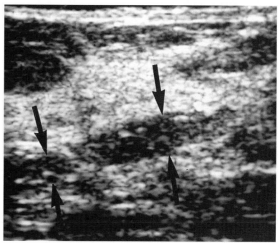

B

FIG. 6.9. Fat lobule. **A:** Sonogram shows a small, oval, hypoechoic area *(arrows)* embedded in the echogenic breast parenchyma. **B:** Sonogram obtained after swiveling the transducer approximately 90 degrees from **A** shows that the pseudolesion seen in **A** is in fact the transverse cross section of an elongated fat lobule *(arrows).*

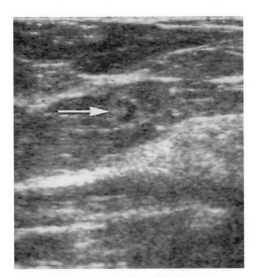

FIG. 6.10. Intramammary lymph node. Sonogram shows a typical very small (0.4-cm) intramammary lymph node *(arrow)* with the characteristic echogenic fatty hilum. However, a reactive intramammary node may be completely hypoechoic, possibly mimicking a small carcinoma.

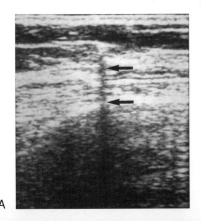

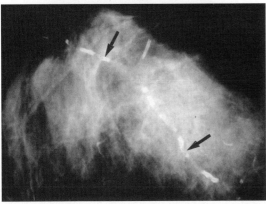

FIG. 6.11. Calcified mammary artery. **A:** Sonogram shows a narrow shadow *(arrows)* with no evidence of a mass that would be responsible for it. **B:** Mammogram shows markedly calcified mammary arteries *(arrows)*.

Pitfalls in the Axilla

Normally, axillary nodes are progressively replaced by echogenic fat that is difficult to distinguish from the surrounding axillary fat. There is, however, a thin characteristic residual hypoechoic rim at the periphery of the node. Not rarely, the central fat is hypoechoic, and the appearance of the node is reversed: the central portion is hypoechoic and is surrounded by a hyperechoic rim (Fig. 6.12). On occasion, a second thin outer hypoechoic rim results in a target-like appearance. However, a closer look at the echogenicity of the lymph node indicates that the central fat has the same low-level echogenicity as the subcutaneous fat; this echogenicity is usually higher than that of lymph node metastases.

Malformations of axillary and subclavian veins are rare and can mimic lymph nodes adjacent to those veins. For example, a small sacciform aneurysm or varix of the subclavian vein can mimic a small infraclavicular lymph node, and care should be taken not to attempt to perform ultrasound-guided FNA in such a case. The clues to proper identification of such a venous malformation include the demonstration of swirling echoes inside the lesion on close inspection of gray-scale real-time images; the possible demonstration of color Doppler signals inside the lesion, although this is unlikely because of the slow venous flow inside the lesion; and, most important, the change in size (including the complete disappearance) of the abnormality during compression (Fig. 6.13).

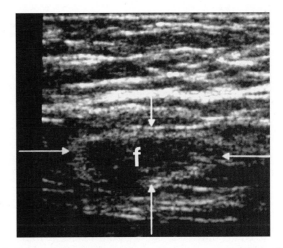

FIG. 6.12. Normal axillary node with a reversed pattern. The node *(arrows)* has a thin hyperechoic rim and is replaced by hypoechoic fat (f). The vast majority of fat-replaced lymph nodes have a thin hypoechoic rim and are echogenic.

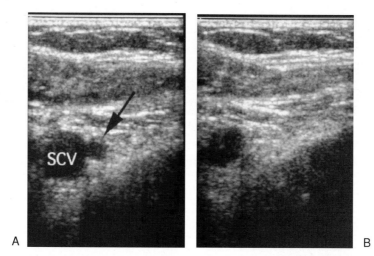

FIG. 6.13. Varix of the subclavian vein mimicking an abnormal infraclavicular lymph node in a patient who was followed up for breast cancer. **A:** Longitudinal sonogram of the infraclavicular region shows a very small hypoechoic and questionable mass *(arrow)* adjacent to the subclavian vein (SCV). **B:** Sonogram obtained during compression of the infraclavicular region shows the pseudomass has collapsed completely, which confirms its venous nature.

Pitfalls in the Region of the Internal Mammary Vessels

Mirror Images of Internal Mammary Vessels

Because of the marked mismatch of acoustic impedance between the chest wall and the lung, the highly reflective pleura acts as an acoustic mirror, and mirror color Doppler images of the internal mammary vessels can be seen projecting in the lung (Fig. 6.14).

Branches of the Internal Mammary Artery

Branches of the internal mammary artery perforate the pectoralis major muscle. The site of perforation of the muscle by the vessel may appear as a focal hypoechoic area, possibly mimicking a small mass. Color Doppler imaging confirms the vascular nature of the hypoechoic area and the absence of a lesion (Fig. 6.15).

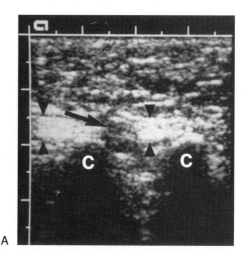

FIG. 6.14. Mirror Doppler images of the internal mammary vessels on the other side of the pleural interface. Transverse Doppler scan of a right intercostal space shows the internal mammary vessels *(arrows)* and their mirror images projecting beneath the pleura *(open arrows)*. L, lung; S, sternum.

FIG. 6.15. Branch of the internal mammary artery perforating the pectoralis major muscle and mimicking a hypoechoic mass. **A:** Longitudinal parasternal sonogram shows a small, irregular hypoechoic area *(arrow)* interrupting the echogenic pectoralis major muscle *(arrowheads)*.

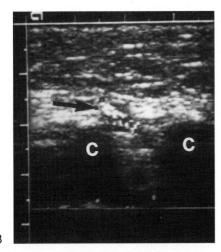

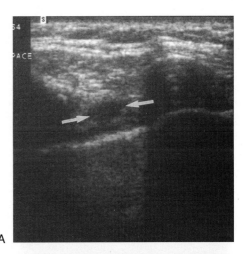

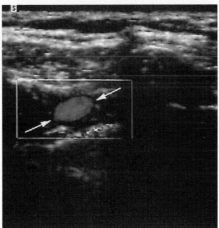

FIG. 6.15. *Continued.* **B:** Doppler scan confirms the vascular nature of the hypoechoic defect *(arrow)*. c, costal cartilages.

Pseudomasses Related to the Internal Mammary Vein and Its Branches

A prominent internal mammary vein may mimic an enlarged lymph node on gray-scale images (Fig. 6.16). This can be seen in particular in patients with inflammatory breast cancer. On occasion, the cross section of the slightly oblique internal mammary vein in the first intercostal space may result in an oval hypoechoic area mimicking a lymph node. After a slight change in the scan plane orientation, the vein is demonstrated in its full length (Fig. 6.17).

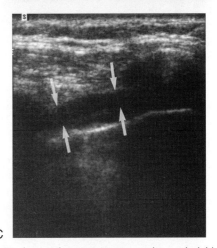

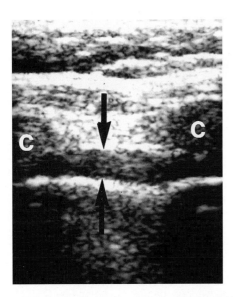

FIG. 6.16. Enlarged internal mammary vein mimicking lymphadenopathy in a patient with inflammatory breast cancer. Longitudinal parasternal sonogram of the second intercostal space shows the enlarged internal mammary vein *(arrows)*, which should not be misdiagnosed as a flattened, enlarged lymph node. c, costal cartilages.

FIG. 6.17. Internal mammary vein mimicking lymphadenopathy. **A:** Strict longitudinal parasternal sonogram of the first intercostal space shows an elliptical hypoechoic area *(arrows)*, possibly representing an abnormal lymph node. **B:** Doppler scan shows that the hypoechoic area seen in **A** is in fact the oblique cross section of the internal mammary vein *(arrows)*. **C:** Oblique parasternal sonogram of the first intercostal space displays the entire vein *(arrows)*.

Rarely, focal dilatation of a vein (varix) can also mimic a small focal lesion. Unlike the arterial branches described above, color Doppler sonography may be useless in confirming the varix because blood flow inside the lesion is too slow to be detected. However, swirling echoes may be seen on standard gray-scale real-time examination, and compression with the transducer will confirm the disappearance of the pseudolesion (Fig. 6.18).

Fat Lobules Mimicking a Lymph Node

The fat that surrounds the internal mammary vessels is usually of medium to high echogenicity. On occasion, however, a small lobule of fat may appear hypoechoic, and in a breast cancer patient, the question may be raised whether this represents an early and small lymph node metastasis. Fat lobules usually retain an elongated shape, and their hypoechogenicity remains moderate; in contrast, lymph node metastases tend to be more round and more hypoechoic.

ARTIFACTS AND PITFALLS ASSOCIATED WITH COMMON PATHOLOGIC CONDITIONS IN THE BREAST

Cysts

Not all cysts display a typical sonographic appearance. Small cysts may lack the typical distal sound enhancement (Fig. 6.19), and inflammatory cysts may exhibit a thickened wall with increased vascularity on color Doppler imaging (Fig. 6.20). However, the major problem in the sonographic diagnosis of cysts is the not-so-rare presence of intracystic echoes, which may be real or artifactual (12,14,15). Artifactual echoes projecting in a cyst can be due to reverberation from interposed reflectors, side-lobe artifacts from echogenic structures located adjacent to the cyst wall, or volume averaging (slice-thickness artifact) (Figs. 6.21 and 6.22) (2,4,7). Real echoes can be due to proteinaceous debris or cholesterol crystals (Fig. 6.23). Internal echoes may represent sediment in the dependent portion of the cyst and move with

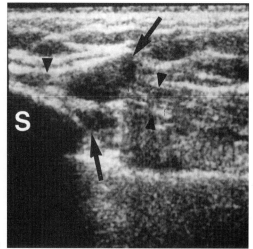

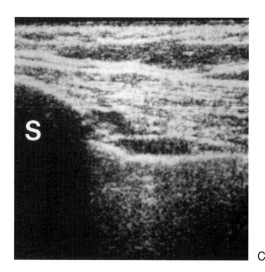

FIG. 6.18. Ectasia of a branch of the internal mammary vein mimicking a hypoechoic mass. **A:** Transverse sonogram of a left intercostal space shows an oval hypoechoic mass *(arrows)* interrupting the pectoralis major muscle *(arrowheads).* **B:** Doppler scan obtained in the same orientation confirms the venous nature of the mass. **C:** Transverse sonogram obtained in the same orientation during firm compression shows the disappearance of the pseudolesion. S, sternum.

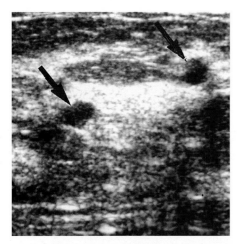

FIG. 6.19. Atypical cysts. Sonogram shows two small cysts *(arrows)* with irregular margins and a few low-level internal echoes. Note the absence of sound enhancement because of the small size of the cysts.

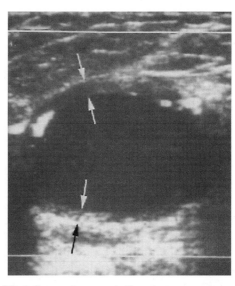

FIG. 6.20. Inflammatory cyst. Doppler sonogram shows a thick wall *(arrows)* with increased vascularity. Note that the vessels drape at the surface of the cyst.

gravity as the patient changes position (Fig. 6.24). Inspissated cysts contain viscid material responsible for uniformly distributed low-level internal echoes and may mimic a solid mass. Most often, there is a distinctive two-tone pattern in inspissated cysts with a totally anechoic component and a mildly echogenic component, the two being separated by a flat or undulating interface (Fig. 6.25). Color Doppler examination of intracystic calcifications often reveals a typical "comet-tail" color artifact distal to the calcifications (Fig. 6.26).

Fibroadenomas

A refraction artifact (edge shadowing) is often noted at each lateral margin of smoothly marginated fibroadenomas. Contours of fibroadenomas are irregular in about 25% of cases, and in a small number of cases, marked shadowing makes the hypoechoic mass suspicious for malignancy.

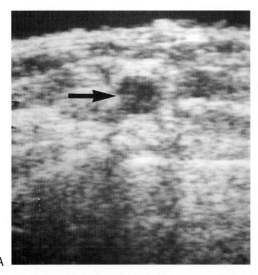
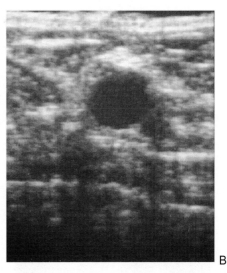

A   B

FIG. 6.21. Spurious echoes in a small cyst attributable to volume averaging. **A:** Very small cyst *(arrow)* examined with a 5-MHz transducer contains some artifactual echoes caused by volume averaging (slice-thickness artifact). **B:** Examination of the same cyst with a 7.5-MHz transducer (and therefore a thinner scan plane) shows the cyst with an anechoic lumen.

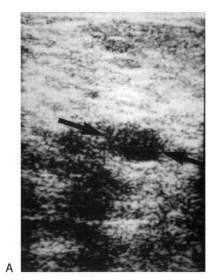
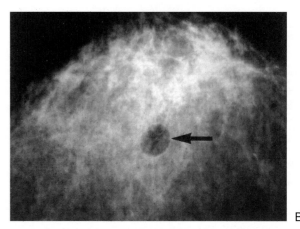

A B

FIG. 6.22. Artifactual echoes in a small cyst attributable to volume averaging. **A:** Sonogram shows an ill-defined hypoechoic mass *(arrows)* with some internal echoes in a dense breast. Ultrasound-guided FNA confirmed a cyst, which was completely drained and insufflated. **B:** Pneumocystogram confirms the smooth internal wall of the cyst *(arrow).*

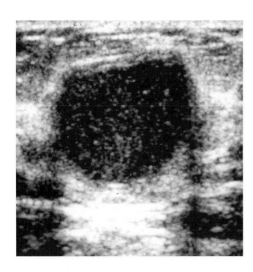

FIG. 6.23. Atypical cyst with thickened wall and internal echoes. Sonogram shows a cyst with an irregular, thickened wall. Note the presence of multiple specular echoes in the lumen. These echoes were seen to move when the patient changed from a supine to a sitting position, when motion was applied to the breast with the transducer, and when the Doppler was turned on.

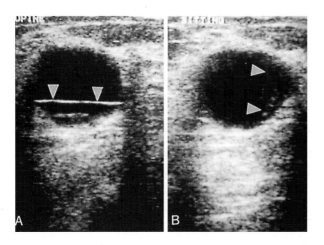

A B

FIG. 6.24. Cyst with layering sediment. **A:** Sonogram obtained with the patient in a supine position shows moderately echogenic sediment in the dependent portion of the cyst and an echogenic interface *(arrowheads).* **B:** Examination performed with the patient in a sitting position. The sediment has moved in the dependent portion of the cyst (which is now in the right part of the scan). Because the interface between the fluid and the sediment is now parallel to the ultrasound beam, it is not clearly depicted *(arrowheads).*

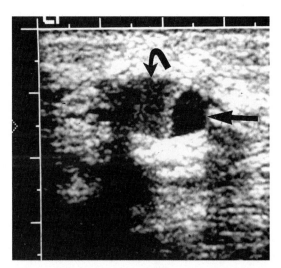

FIG. 6.25. Inspissated cyst. Sonogram shows the typical "two-tone" appearance of an inspissated cyst with an anechoic component *(straight arrow)* and a more echogenic component *(curved arrow),* separated by a flat interface. The two different components of the cyst may move inside the lumen according to changes in the patient's position, depending on their relative viscosity.

Very rarely, a fibroadenoma has the same hypoechogenicity as the surrounding fat, and the fibroadenoma's demonstration may require a number of maneuvers, including scanning from various angles with various degrees of compression (Fig. 6.27). At the other end of the spectrum, massively calcified fibroadenomas are detected only through their pronounced associated shadow.

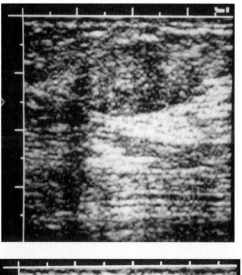
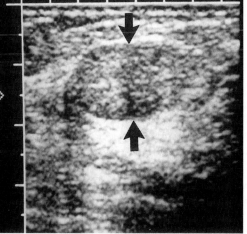

FIG. 6.27. Fibroadenoma isoechoic relative to the surrounding fat. **A:** Sonogram cannot clearly delineate the lesion. **B:** Sonogram obtained with a different angulation of the transducer and a different amount of compression shows the lesion better *(arrows).*

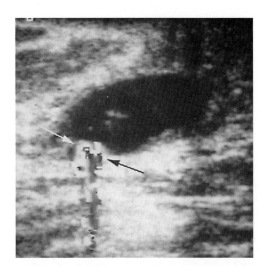

FIG. 6.26. Doppler artifacts associated with calcifications. Doppler scan of a cyst containing small calcifications shows a typical "comet-tail" artifact distal to a collection of intracystic microcalcifications *(arrows).*

Carcinomas

Initially reported as pathognomonic for carcinoma, shadowing is associated only with carcinomas that have a significant amount of fibrosis (about 50% of cases in our experience). The partial shadowing seen with some carcinomas may be the result of beam scattering by jagged margins. However, all the masses that shadow are not carcinoma. In fact, a number of benign lesions are associated with shadowing, including fat necrosis, granulomatous mastitis, granular cell tumor, fibroadenomas, and scars (12).

Ten to fifteen percent of carcinomas appear as a well-circumscribed mass. These include the so-called soft carcinomas such as medullary and mucinous carcinomas.

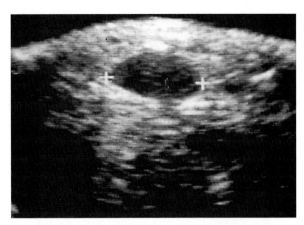

FIG. 6.28. Benign-appearing breast carcinoma. Sonogram shows a well-defined, smoothly marginated, elongated, hypoechoic mass *(calipers),* the appearance of which is suggestive of fibroadenoma. Needle biopsy diagnosed medullary carcinoma.

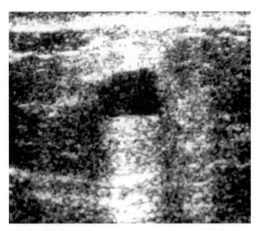

FIG. 6.29. Medullary carcinoma with a cystic appearance. Sonogram shows a slightly irregular, markedly hypoechoic tumor with marked sound-through transmission.

Some of them have a fibroadenoma-like appearance (Fig. 6.28), whereas others (especially medullary cancers) have a cystic appearance (Fig. 6.29) (16).

Some large or fast-growing cancers are massively necrotic. By demonstrating flow within the markedly hypoechoic mass, color Doppler imaging can differentiate between the fluid and the solid components of the tumor (Fig. 6.30).

Postoperative Changes

Changes in the breast after excisional biopsy may result in misleading appearances. Prominent fibrous scar tissue may cause shadowing and mimic a recurrent tumor after breast-conserving surgery for breast cancer. The change in shape of the scar under compression is the key to the diagnosis (Fig. 6.31).

Hematomas do not always appear as fluid collections and may at times mimic solid masses. The color Doppler demonstration of vessels coursing through the mass virtually rules out a hematoma and reinforces the suspicion for residual or recurrent disease, but the absence of flow does not eliminate cancer (17).

The breast that has been reconstructed with a transverse rectus abdominis myocutaneous flap is characterized by a lack of glandular breast tissue and the presence of abdominal subcutaneous fat. The most common lesion found in such a reconstructed breast is fat necrosis.

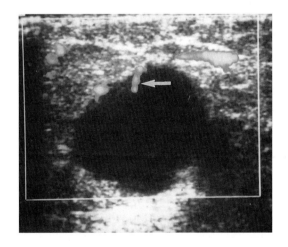

FIG. 6.30. Necrotic carcinoma mimicking a cyst. The entirely necrotic carcinoma appears as a fluid collection. However, the margins are slightly irregular, and Doppler shows vessels *(arrow)* coursing at the periphery of the anechoic lesion. The vessels are located in a rim of moderately hypoechoic tissue, which was not visible on this scan but was demonstrated at higher gain. Note the difference between the direction of these vessels *(arrow)* and those seen in the thickened wall of the inflammatory cyst in Fig. 6.20.

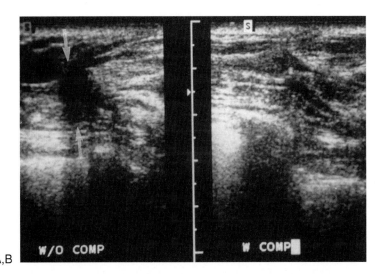

A,B

FIG. 6.31. Postbiopsy scarring mimicking carcinoma. **A:** An irregular hypoechoic area *(arrows)* is seen at the site of a previous lumpectomy, raising the possibility of recurrent disease. **B:** Examination done under firm compression shows the nearly complete disappearance of the abnormality.

ARTIFACTS AND PITFALLS ASSOCIATED WITH FOREIGN BODIES

Traumatic foreign bodies are rarely found in the breast, but iatrogenic foreign bodies are less rare. Plastic bodies (e.g., catheters) are usually associated with some degree of shadowing. A case of retained surgical gauze causing marked shadowing has been reported (Fig. 6.32) (18).

Metallic bodies are associated with a typical comet-tail artifact—long, continuous, echogenic, reverberating trail (3,5,9,19). Metallic bodies found in the breast include surgical clips, transected localizing hook wires, iridium-therapy wires, Port-a-cath reservoirs (Fig. 6.33), biopsy needles, and metallic markers placed in carcinomas during preoperative chemotherapy to tag the tumor bed before lumpectomy in case the cancer responds com-

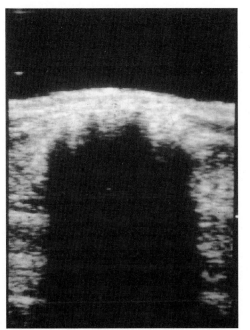

A

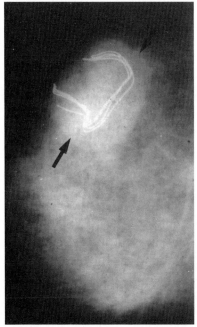

B

FIG. 6.32. Retained surgical gauze. The patient returned 3 months following lumpectomy for breast cancer with a suspicion of recurrent disease. **A:** Sonogram shows a massive clean shadow. **B:** Mammogram confirms the retained gauze *(arrows).* (Reprinted from reference 18 with permission.)

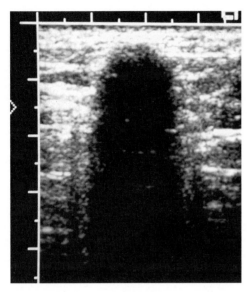

FIG. 6.33. Port-a-cath. Sonogram shows a marked shadow in the infraclavicular area, corresponding to a Port-a-cath reservoir.

pletely to such treatment (Fig. 6.34). Because of the difference in sound velocity between the surrounding fat and most fibroadenomas and carcinomas, there is an apparent bayonet deformity of the biopsy needle (especially large-core cutting needles inserted nearly horizontally) when it enters the lesion (Fig. 6.35) (20). This artifact indicates that the needle has successfully penetrated a medium of different acoustic impedance from that of the surrounding fat.

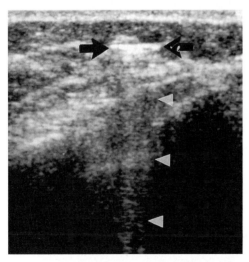

FIG. 6.34. Metallic markers inserted during preoperative chemotherapy for breast cancer. Sonogram done before surgery identifies one of four 5-mm-long metallic rods *(arrows)* that were placed in the shrinking tumor. After completion of chemotherapy, the tumor has completely regressed. Because the tumor bed was tagged by the metallic markers, it could be excised without difficulty by the surgeon. Note the characteristic comet-tail artifact *(arrowheads)* of the marker.

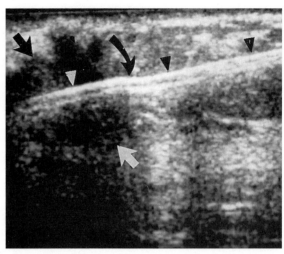

FIG. 6.35. Bayonet artifact affecting the cutting needle during large-core needle biopsy of a breast cancer. Postfiring longitudinal sonogram shows the echogenic needle *(arrowheads)* traversing the hypoechoic solid tumor *(arrows)*. The step-like deformity of the needle *(curved arrow)* results from the faster sound velocity in the tumor than in the surrounding fat. Therefore, the segment of the needle's shaft traversing the tumor is plotted closer to the transducer's footprint than the rest of the needle is.

A significant pitfall associated with needle biopsy is volume averaging. This artifact may result in the display of the biopsy needle inside the lesion on longitudinal scans when the needle is in fact at the periphery of or even outside the lesion (Fig. 6.36). Checking the position

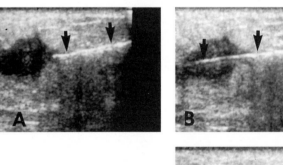

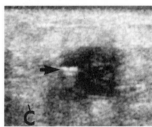

FIG. 6.36. Pitfall associated with volume averaging during large-core needle biopsy of a breast tumor. **A:** Prefiring longitudinal sonogram shows the echogenic needle *(arrows)* in contact with the tumor. **B:** Postfiring longitudinal sonogram shows the echogenic needle *(arrows)* apparently penetrating the central portion of the tumor. **C:** Postfiring transverse sonogram shows that the echogenic cross section of the needle *(arrow)* is at the edge of the mass, not in its center. The misleading appearance in **B** sonogram was caused by volume averaging between the tumor and the biopsy needle.

of the needle on transverse sonograms, which show the cross sections of the tumor and of the needle, is mandatory for the biopsy of small lesions.

ARTIFACTS AND PITFALLS ASSOCIATED WITH BREAST IMPLANTS

A thorough discussion of the artifacts and pitfalls associated with the numerous types of breast implants is beyond the scope of this chapter. The two common types of breast implants, saline-filled and silicone-gel-filled, have significantly different appearances on sonograms. An implant filled with saline solution appears on sonograms as a flat fluid-filled collection without any apparent deformity of its shape. In contrast, sound propagates in silicone at a markedly reduced velocity (1,000 m/sec)

compared with soft tissues (1,540 m/sec). However, because the ultrasound scanner assumes the same propagation speed (1,540 m/sec) for all returning echoes, it plots the echoes from the deep wall of the prosthesis at 1.5 times its actual distance from the anterior wall, with a resulting 50% increase in the apparent thickness of the silicone-gel-filled prosthesis (Fig. 6.37) and, as a corollary, an apparent deformity of the underlying chest wall (Fig. 6.38).

Reverberation echoes from the anterior wall of a prosthesis project over the lumen of the implant and form a moderately echogenic band underneath the wall of the prosthesis, whether it is filled with saline or silicone.

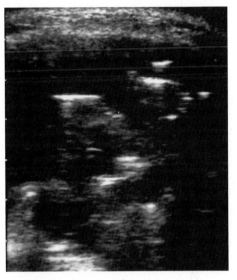

FIG. 6.39. Dual-chamber prosthesis. Sonogram shows multiple internal echoes resulting from folds, not to be confused with a contained rupture.

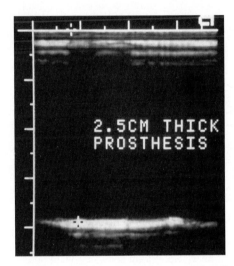

FIG. 6.37. Speed propagation artifact associated with silicone-gel-filled prosthesis. *Ex vivo* sonogram of a 2.5-cm-thick prosthesis shows that the apparent thickness of the prosthesis is 3.8 cm. This 50% increase in the apparent thickness of the prosthesis is caused by the slower sound speed in silicone (1,000 m/sec) than in soft tissues (1,540 m/sec).

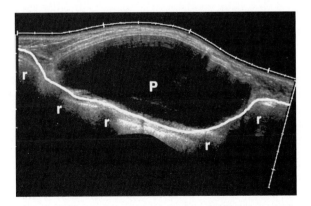

FIG. 6.38. Silicone-gel-filled prosthesis. Sonogram obtained using extended-field-of-view (SieScape™ imaging) technology shows the falsely thickened prosthesis (P) and the apparent excavation of the underlying chest wall *(white line)*. r, rib.

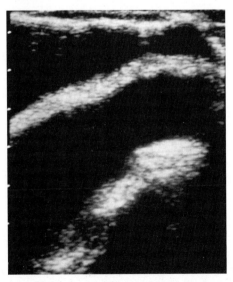

FIG. 6.40. Unusual sonographic appearance of a breast in which two prostheses have been inserted, one on top of the other.

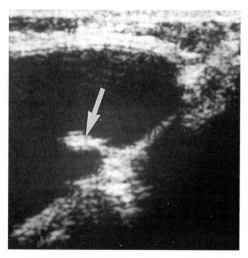

FIG. 6.41. Silicone-gel-filled prosthesis. Sonogram shows an internal fold *(arrow)*.

Double-chamber prostheses usually consist of an outer saline-filled chamber and an inner silicone-filled chamber. Numerous folds may result from this configuration and should not be mistaken for a contained rupture (Fig. 6.39). Under rare circumstances, a plastic surgeon may have inserted two prostheses, one on top of the other (Fig. 6.40).

In the case of a contained rupture of a silicone-gel prosthesis, the abnormally echogenic silicone may be difficult to differentiate from reverberation echoes. The echogenic floating fragments of the ruptured bag are known as the "linguini" sign and are usually readily

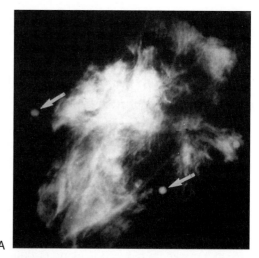

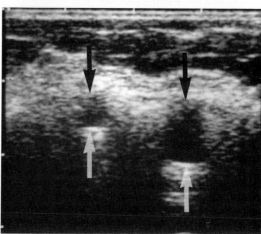

FIG. 6.43. Free residual silicone in a breast following removal of a silicone-gel-filled prosthesis. **A:** Mammography shows several perfectly round densities *(arrows)* representing blobs of free silicone. **B:** Sonogram shows cystic structures *(arrows)* that are 1.5 times taller than wide. This is characteristic of free silicone (see also Fig. 6.37).

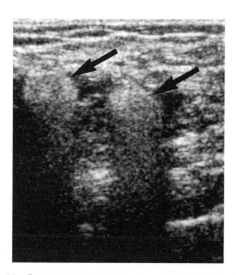

FIG. 6.42. Snowstorm artifact associated with silicone-induced granulomas in axillary lymph nodes in a patient with a history of a ruptured silicone-gel-filled prosthesis. Sonogram of the axilla shows two echogenic nodes *(arrows)* with a combination of shadowing and trail of reverberation characteristic of silicone-induced granulomas.

identified and differentiated from folds in the prosthesis (Fig. 6.41).

In extracapsular ruptures, silicone-induced granulomas appear as brightly echogenic areas with a combination of shadowing and reverberation trail, known as the "snowstorm" appearance (Fig. 6.42). This pattern is unique and easily recognized. In contrast, collections of free silicone appear as cysts with a taller-than-wide shape caused by the markedly reduced speed of sound in silicone compared with the surrounding soft tissues (Fig. 6.43).

CONCLUSIONS

Artifacts are present in most sonograms. They may become prominent and interfere with the formation and interpretation of the images. The operator should "think artifact" whenever he or she is confronted with unusual images. Most artifacts in the breast can be identified by verifying the correct settings of the equipment, by switching to a different transducer, by changing the probe's position and tilt, by increasing (or decreasing) the pressure on the transducer, and by changing the patient's position.

REFERENCES

1. Robinson DE, Wilson LS, Kossoff G. Shadowing and enhancement in ultrasonic echograms by reflection and refraction. *J Clin Ultrasound* 1981;9:181–188.
2. Goldstein A, Madrazo BL. Slice-thickness artifacts in gray-scale ultrasound. *J Clin Ultrasound* 1981;9:365–375.
3. Wendell BA, Athey PA. Ultrasonic appearance of metallic foreign bodies in parenchymal organs. *J Clin Ultrasound* 1981;9:133–135.
4. Fiske CE, Filly RA. Pseudo-sludge: A spurious ultrasound appearance within the gallbladder. *Radiology* 1982;144:631–632.
5. Ziskin MC, Thickman DI, Goldenberg NJ, et al. The comet tail artifact. *J Ultrasound Med* 1982;1:1–7.
6. Pierce G, Golding RH, Cooperberg PL. The effects of tissue velocity changes on acoustical interfaces. *J Ultrasound Med* 1982;1:185–187.
7. Laing FC, Kurtz AB. The importance of ultrasonic side-lobe artifacts. *Radiology* 1982;145:763–768.
8. Laing FC. Commonly encountered artifacts in clinical ultrasound. *Semin Ultrasound CT MR* 1983;4:27–43.
9. Thickman DI, Ziskin MC, Goldenberg NJ, et al. Clinical manifestations of the comet tail artifact. *J Ultrasound Med* 1983;2:225–230.
10. Kremkau FW, Taylor KJW. Artifacts in ultrasound imaging. *J Ultrasound Med* 1986;5:227–237.
11. Kimme-Smith C, Hansen M, Bassett L, Sarti D, King W III. Ultrasound mammography: effects of focal zone placement. *RadioGraphics* 1985; 5:955–969.
12. Kimme-Smith C, Rothschild PA, Bassett LW, Gold RH, Westbrook D. Ultrasound artifacts affecting the diagnosis of breast masses. *Ultrasound Med Biol* 1988;1:203–210.
13. Fornage BD. Ultrasound of the breast. *Ultrasound Q* 1993;11:1–39.
14. Bassett LW, Kimme-Smith C. Breast sonography. *Am J Roentgenol* 1991; 156:449–455.
15. Khaleghian R. Breast cysts: pitfalls in sonographic diagnosis. *Australas Radiol* 1993;37:192–194.
16. Heywang SH, Dunner PS, Lipsit ER, Glassman LM. Advantages and pitfalls of ultrasound in the diagnosis of breast cancer. *J Clin Ultrasound* 1985;13:525–532.
17. Fornage BD. Role of color Doppler imaging in differentiating between pseudocystic malignant tumors and fluid collections. *J Ultrasound Med* 1995;14:125–128.
18. Fornage BD. Sonographic diagnosis of a retained surgical sponge in the breast. *J Clin Ultrasound* 1987;15:285–288.
19. Fornage BD, Schernberg FL. Sonographic diagnosis of foreign bodies of the distal extremities. *Am J Roentgenol* 1986;147:567–569.
20. Fornage BD. US-guided core needle biopsy of breast masses: the "bayonet artifact." *Am J Roentgenol* 1995;164:1022–1023.

Variants and Pitfalls in Body Imaging,
edited by Ali Shirkhoda.
Lippincott Williams & Wilkins, Philadelphia, © 2000.

CHAPTER 7

Breast MRI

Catherine W. Piccoli

The two primary applications of breast MRI are the detection and characterization of parenchymal lesions and the assessment of silicone implant integrity. Contrast-enhanced breast MRI (CE-MRI) is recognized as the most sensitive method for detection of invasive breast cancer. However, problems affecting sensitivity and, particularly, specificity have prevented widespread, routine use of this powerful diagnostic modality.

In this chapter, after a brief review of anatomy and physiology, there is a discussion regarding the CE-MRI factors contributing to these problems, and then a summary of difficulties encountered with MRI implant evaluation is presented. Although MRI is the most accurate method for assessment of silicone gel implant integrity, certain ambiguous findings such as redundant infoldings of the implant shell may lead to erroneous diagnoses.

OVERVIEW OF BREAST ANATOMY AND PHYSIOLOGY

The breast is variably composed of glandular tissue and stromal structures including fat and supportive fibrous tissue. The glandular elements are arranged in 15 to 25 lobes, each of which is drained by a collecting duct that opens onto the nipple. From the nipple to the acinar tissue, the collecting duct branches sequentially into numerous segmental, subsegmental, and terminal ducts. The ductal system is enveloped by fibroadipose tissue, which constitutes much of the bulk of the breast tissue in the nonpregnant, nonlactating woman.

There is tremendous variation in the architecture of the breast among individuals as well as variation with age and hormonal status in the same person. Proliferative changes of the breast parenchyma occur over the course of the menstrual cycle and include ductal proliferation during the follicular phase and lobular enlargement as a result of alveolar dilation, hyperemia, and edema during the luteal phase (1). With pregnancy, there is a marked change in the parenchymal structures with proliferation of the ducts and acini and concomitant regression of the interlobular stroma and the fatty lobules of the subcutaneous and submammary layer (2). Postmenopausal involution occurs gradually with regression of the lobular and ductal tissues and a variable proliferation of the stroma. The parenchyma is variably replaced by fatty tissue containing atrophic ducts and thin fibrous septa or by coalescent dense connective tissue (2).

CONTRAST-ENHANCED MAGNETIC RESONANCE IMAGING

Various indications have been offered as potentially appropriate for CE-MRI. These include benign/malignant differentiation of palpable or mammographically evident masses, staging of known cancers, evaluation of lumpectomy sites for tumor recurrence, identification of occult tumor in a patient with metastatic lymphadenopathy, and screening of high-risk patients or those with radiographically dense breast tissue. Reported accuracies using variations of this method have differed greatly. Although most sensitivity values for invasive disease are greater than 90%, specificity has differed markedly among investigators, ranging from 28% to 97% (3–16). Overall accuracy is dependent on a number of variables, which include technical protocol, composition of study population, diagnostic criteria, and biological variability.

Technical Considerations

The variables in technique include system field strength, dose of contrast agent, bolus administration of

C. W. Piccoli: Department of Radiology, Jefferson Medical College and Thomas Jefferson University Hospital, Philadelphia, Pennsylvania 19107.

contrast agent versus slow infusion, timing of contrast administration with imaging and acquisition times, type of breast coil, imaging parameters, slice thickness, fat suppression versus image subtraction, and use of other postprocessing techniques.

The majority of investigations have been carried out on 1.0-T or 1.5-T magnets. The efficacy of lower-field-strength magnets for breast evaluation has not been substantiated. However, early investigations suggest that medium-field-strength (0.5-T) units are capable of producing similar, if not superior, results (17,18). Virtually all investigators have utilized either commercially available or modified surface coils for breast imaging.

Gadopentetate dimeglumine (Gd-DTPA) has been used in the majority of investigations in dosages ranging from 0.1 to 0.2 mmol/kg, but newer gadolinium chelates are also appropriate for breast imaging. The dosage of contrast has been addressed by few investigators, with only one published study suggesting an optimum dose of 0.16 mmol/kg of Gd-DTPA for three-dimensional (3-D) fast low-angle shot (FLASH) imaging (19). Optimum dosages for other protocols and other contrast agents remain undetermined.

Technical factors of the MR imaging protocol will affect detectability of some malignancies. If immediate postcontrast images are not available, or if image acquisition is prolonged (over 3 to 5 minutes), enhancement of parenchymal tissue may obscure significant disease (Fig. 7.1). On the other hand, because some tumors enhance slowly, extending the imaging time to approximately 10 minutes may result in identification of otherwise occult disease. Technical mishaps must also be recognized before diagnostic conclusions are made, such as contrast administration difficulty, improper sequence or slice selection, and MR unit malfunction including inadvertent water saturation (20) (Fig. 7.2).

Fat suppression improves lesion conspicuity but can be problematic because of field inhomogeneities. Nevertheless, various forms of fat suppression are in use (3,13,21). Subtraction for elimination of fat signal increases conspicuity, but patient motion between pre- and postcontrast acquisitions may result in interpretative errors with or without fat suppression or subtraction (22). Although most commercial breast surface coils image the noncompressed pendant breast, it has been suggested that immobilization of the breast would eliminate motion and allow a reduction in the slice number (23). However, strong compression of the breast interferes with lesion enhancement to the degree that cancers may not be detectable (24).

Slice thickness affects the minimum detectable lesion size. A slice thickness greater than 5 mm is considered unacceptable because early, very small malignancies may be obscured as a result of volume averaging. A 1- to 2-mm slice thickness is encouraged and can be achieved using a three-dimensional (3-D) technique with no interslice gap. Small enhancing lesions also may be obscured

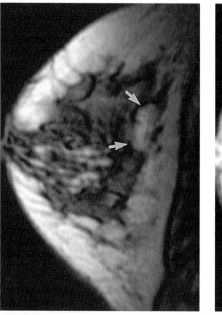 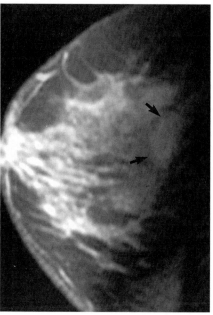

A B

FIG. 7.1. Rapidly enhancing invasive ductal carcinoma with early washout. **A:** Immediate postcontrast image shows a rapidly enhancing carcinoma *(arrows)* [sagittal, T_1-weighted multiplanar spoiled gradient echo (MPSPGR), T_R 120/T_E 2.9]. **B:** The tumor is obscured on an 8-minute delayed acquisition because of enhancement of surrounding tissue and washout of contrast from the tumor [sagittal, T_1-weighted spin echo (SE) with fat saturation, T_R 450/T_E 14].

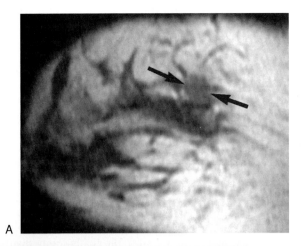

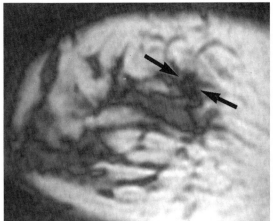

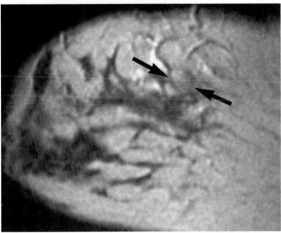

FIG. 7.2. False-negative study because of equipment malfunction. This patient has a mass *(arrows)* that, on conventional mammography and sonography, was highly suspicious for malignancy. **A:** The tumor exhibits moderate signal intensity on sagittal T_1-weighted SE (T_R 416/T_E 11). **B:** It also displays high signal on sagittal T_2-weighted fast spin echo (T_R 6,500/T_E 85). Fat suppression was attempted on dynamic and delayed postcontrast acquisitions. Although it was noted that fat suppression failed, inadvertent water suppression was not recognized. **C:** Because of a combination of water suppression and out-of-phase imaging, a paradoxic decrease in tumor signal occurred on the postcontrast acquisitions (sagittal, postcontrast, T_1-weighted SE, T_R 550/T_E 14).

by chemical shift artifact with out-of-phase imaging. Therefore, in-phase T_1-weighted pre- and postcontrast sequences are advised. It should be noted that the degree of T_1 weighting will affect measurable signal intensity on any individual MR unit (25). Similarly, on comparison of scanners from different manufacturers, it has been shown that different measurements of signal intensity are obtained for the same lesion despite the use of the same sequences and imaging parameters (26). Therefore, if enhancement thresholds are utilized for diagnosis, care must be taken to use criteria developed using the same imaging parameters and the same MR unit.

Factors Affecting Specificity

Patient Preselection

Many breast MR investigators have recommended MRI of the breast in patients scheduled for biopsy of breast masses discovered by conventional clinical or imaging techniques. However, others have focused on problem solving for patients with ambiguous or difficult physical or imaging examinations, and still others have exclusively examined patients with known malignancy.

The accuracy of MRI diagnosis of these different populations depends in large part on the pretest probability of disease, which is related to patient preselection.

This concept of preselection is illustrated by review of investigators who compared two patient populations evaluated with the same MR technique and diagnostic criteria (27). Group I patients had suspicious discrete lesions on traditional breast work-up and were scheduled for biopsy before MRI. Group II had questionable clinical or mammographic abnormalities. The two groups showed similar high sensitivity on CE-MRI, but only group II showed significantly improved specificity compared to mammography. This difference resulted from the inability of MRI to substantially increase specificity in a population with a high number of malignancies relative to benign lesions (group I: 131 cancers vs. 119 benign lesions). In the diagnostically difficult group II, there were relatively few malignancies among many benign findings (group II: 34 cancers vs. 158 benign lesions), and MRI was able to exclude malignancy in a greater proportion of these patients, thereby improving specificity. On the other hand, the pretest difference in malignant to benign ratios between the two groups accounts, in part, for the fact that the positive predictive value (PPV) of group I was twice that of group II (60% vs. 31%).

Biological Variabilities

The variation of breast tissue composition during the menstrual cycle has been studied with plain and contrast MR imaging (28–32). With progression of the menstrual cycle, significant glandular changes occur affecting parenchymal volume and T_1, but not T_2, values (28,29). Parity and oral contraceptive use have varying effects on the parenchyma and water content (30). In one study in which women in all age groups were involved, the investigators used CE-MRI and found parenchymal enhancement to be significantly lower between cycle days 7 and 20, and overall parenchymal enhancement was greatest in women aged 35 to 50 (31). Another study involving weekly CE-MRI examinations over a menstrual cycle or over a 4-month interval among patients 21 to 41 years of age revealed both diffuse and nodular foci of enhancement, particularly during weeks 1 and 4, 73% of which resolved on follow-up. Interestingly, 43% of the enhancing foci that resolved had met defined malignancy criteria (32) (Fig. 7.3).

Normal parenchymal tissue in postmenopausal patients enhances minimally, and generally uniformly, leaving a homogeneous background for detection of enhancing lesions. Studies examining the mammograms of women treated with estrogens or a combination of estrogens and progesterone have shown a marked increase in fibroglandular tissue in 17% to 25% (33–35). Although the effect of exogenous hormones on MR imaging of the postmenopausal breast is not well established, anecdotal evidence suggests specificity dilemmas similar to those encountered in premenopausal patients (Figs. 7.4 and 7.5).

Benign Conditions

Benign Proliferative Breast Disease

Benign breast disease occasionally shows significant contrast enhancement, which is often a source of false-positive MRI findings (36–38). The term "proliferative dysplasia" may be applied to a variety of conditions, including that of moderate intraductal or extraductal proliferation, associated with minimally increased risk of malignancy or high-grade proliferation considered precancerous or markers of high risk. Such benign disease includes sclerosing adenosis, apocrine metaplasia, epithelial hyperplasia, lobular neoplasia, and atypical ductal hyperplasia. The MRI appearance of these proliferative changes seems to parallel the pathologic distribution when enhancement occurs (37) (Fig. 7.6).

Benign Enhancing Breast Masses

Fibroadenomas are composed of fibrous stroma, proliferating ducts, and acinar tissue and evolve from proliferation of multiple lobules, which coalesce into nodules (39). These enlarge centrally with continued epithelial and stromal proliferation and peripherally with recruitment of hyperplastic lobules. The percentage of epithelial and stromal components varies; some are predominantly adenomatous, and others show stromal hypercellularity (fibrous) or extensive myxoid change. The nonenhancing septations

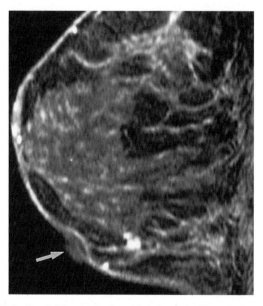

FIG. 7.4. Ductal hyperplasia without atypia. Postmenopausal patient on exogenous hormone therapy presented with a palpable focus in the lower breast but had negative mammography. Sagittal postcontrast imaging [fat suppressed, T_1-weighted fast gradient echo (FGR)] shows diffusely scattered enhancing foci and one intensely enhancing focus in the lower breast corresponding to the palpable focus (note skin marker, *arrow*), which was surgically proven to be benign ductal hyperplasia.

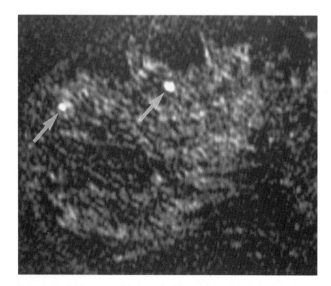

FIG. 7.3. Diffuse, nonspecific pattern of enhancement in a premenopausal patient. Multiple rapidly enhancing nodules (two of which are identified with *arrows*) appeared on a background of diffuse parenchymal enhancement [sagittal, immediate postcontrast subtraction image, 3-D spoiled gradient echo (SPGR), T_R 12.8/T_E 4.2].

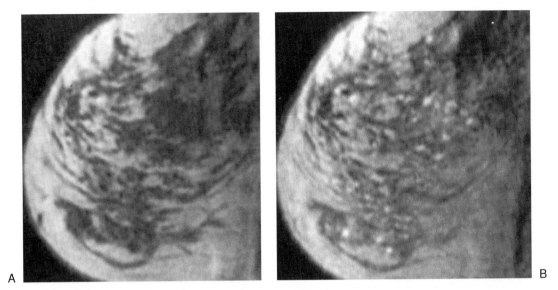

FIG. 7.5. Diffuse, nonspecific enhancement in a postmenopausal patient on exogenous hormone therapy. Sagittal precontrast **(A)** and immediate postcontrast **(B)** T_1-weighted fast gradient echo (FGRE) (T_R 13/T_E 4).

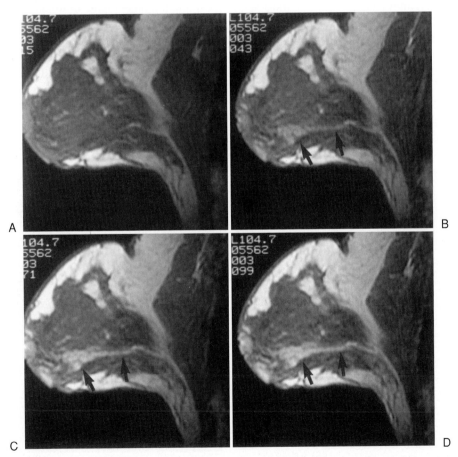

FIG. 7.6. Benign fibrocystic change. Serial images from a dynamic contrast-enhanced sequence shows **(A)** the precontrast appearance, **(B)** immediate enhancement, and **(C,D)** increasing enhancement of a wedge of tissue with apparent ductal enhancement extending posteriorly *(arrows)*. This enhancing area corresponded to a segmental distribution of microcalcifications visible mammographically (sagittal, 3-D SPGR, T_R 22/T_E 5).

described within enhancing fibroadenomas on MRI (40) may correlate with the margins of adjacent proliferating lobules. Enhancement patterns vary among the histologic subtypes (37). Myxoid tumors show rapid and strong enhancement, similar to carcinoma. Predominantly glandular fibroadenomas are intermediate in speed and amplitude of enhancement. Fibrous fibroadenomas enhance very little. Fibroadenomas in premenopausal patients tend to exhibit significant enhancement, presumably because of continued biological activity of the tumor, whereas those in older women exhibit minimal enhancement. Approximately 80% of fibroadenomas enhance continuously and gradually without washout or ring enhancement, but 20% of fibroadenomas enhance in a pattern indistinguishable from malignant lesions (41) (Fig. 7.7).

Papillomas are epithelial fronds supported by a fibrovascular stroma, generally located in the subareolar region or major ducts (42). Serous or serosanguinous nipple discharge is commonly the presenting complaint. The involved duct is dilated and occasionally cystic. Papillomas are not associated with a significant risk for development of breast cancer, although multiple papillomas or papillomatosis involving multiple terminal duct–lobular units are associated with an increased risk. The morphologic characteristics, amplitude, and speed of contrast enhancement on MR imaging have been found to be similar for benign and malignant solitary papillomas, other malignancies, and some fibroadenomas (37) (Fig. 7.8). The use of MRI in the evaluation of papillomatosis for determining disease extent has been described (43).

Phyllodes tumor is an uncommon lesion composed of benign epithelial elements and a spindle-cell stroma and are morphologically lobulated and well circumscribed (44). Patients tend to present with a rapidly enlarging breast mass, which may be massive in size. Approximately 16% of low-grade tumors recur following excision, and 7% of high-grade lesions metastasize (44). The accurate prediction of the biological behavior and prognosis of phyllodes tumors is difficult on histopathologic evaluation as well as on imaging. Even low-grade phyllodes tumors display rapid contrast enhancement and inhomogeneous but high signal intensity (37,45). In cases of large, rapidly growing breast masses, MRI should not be used for diagnostic purposes, as biopsy is necessary, although determination of disease extent for purposes of preoperative planning may be useful.

Breast hamartomas are mammographically characteristic as an encapsulated inhomogeneous mass containing fat. However, if detectable fat is absent, both the mammographic and MRI diagnoses are difficult (46). Enhancement hamartomas on CE-MRI are variable and inhomogeneous, depending on the amount of adenomatous change (37).

Fibrosing lesions may mimic malignancy on both clinical and mammographic examination. On MRI evaluation, fibrosing masses exhibit variable enhancement patterns that are dependent on the biological activity of the fibrosing process. Fibrosis generally produces a gradual enhancement pattern but may display signal intensity that is less than, equal to, or slightly greater than parenchymal tissue (Figs. 7.9 and 7.10). In the postoperative or trauma-

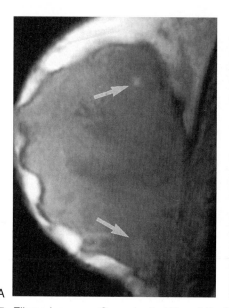 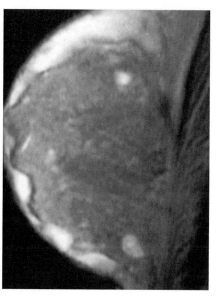

A   B

FIG. 7.7. Fibroadenomas. One-minute **(A)** and 2-minute **(B)** postcontrast sagittal images showing two enhancing fibroadenomas *(arrows)* [T_1-weighted, fast multiplanar spoiled gradient echo (FMSPGR), T_R 132.5/T_E 3.4]. On comparison of **A** with **B,** the central portion of the superior mass is noted to enhance before its periphery, a benign characteristic. Although more heterogeneous, the inferior mass does not exhibit centripetal enhancement and enhances with less intensity.

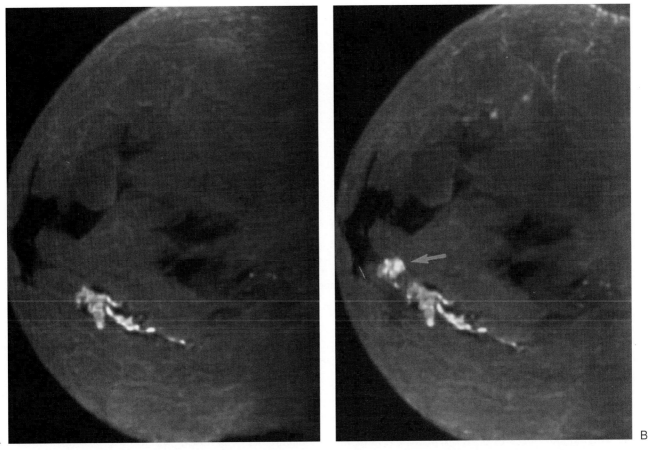

A

B

FIG. 7.8. Benign papilloma. Precontrast **(A)** and immediate postcontrast **(B)** images of a heterogeneously and strongly enhancing mass in the retroareolar region *(arrow)*. The bright serpiginous signal
on the precontrast image represents inspissated debris in an obstructed duct. Although the enhancement pattern did not allow differentiation between benign and malignant, the location and lobulated margination of the mass suggested the correct diagnosis (sagittal, inversion recovery prepared gradient
echo, T_R 19.1/T_E 5.9/T_I 150).

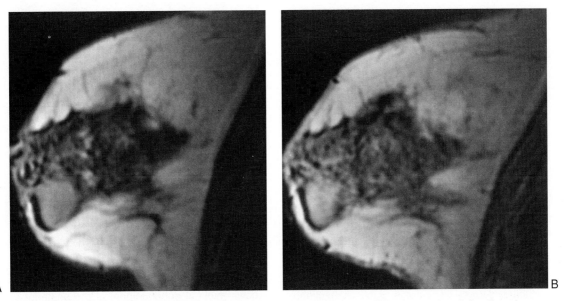

A

B

FIG. 7.9. Stromal fibrosis. Precontrast **(A)** and 4-minute postcontrast **(B)** images of a minimally enhancing focus of tumoral fibrosis (sagittal, T_1-weighted, MPSPGR, T_R 130/T_E 2.9).

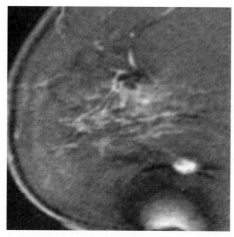
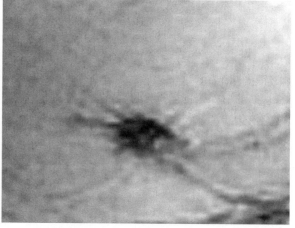

A   B

FIG. 7.10. Fibrosis. This patient had undergone neoadjuvant chemotherapy for a breast carcinoma that was no longer identifiable by clinical or imaging examinations. **A:** At a site distant from the tumor, an intensely enhancing focus of enhancement was noted [sagittal, T_1-weighted, enhanced fast gradient echo (EFGRE), T_R 8/T_E 3/T_I 24]. **B:** The mass appeared spiculated (sagittal, FSE, T_R 6,000/T_E 195). Fibrosis was found at surgery.

tized breast, early fat necrosis may clinically simulate carcinoma by presenting as a palpable mass and may be visible mammographically as a new mass, architectural distortion, calcium deposition, or "oil cyst" (47). Microscopically, damaged fat cells dissolve and fuse and are surrounded by histiocytes and giant cells with or without acute inflammatory cells (44). In the acute stages of fat necrosis, significant enhancement may be seen on CE-MRI (37) (Fig. 7.11). Fibroblasts gradually deposit colla-

gen, with the resulting fibrosis occasionally producing architectural change (Fig. 7.12). In patients treated for breast cancer, MRI is useful for differentiating recurrent disease from postsurgical/postradiation changes (48,49). However, it has been shown that MRI is inaccurate because of false-positive enhancement of scar if performed earlier than 6 months following surgical excision alone or 9 to 18 months following radiation therapy (50,51) (Fig. 7.13). In patients who have undergone radiation therapy for breast cancer, aggressive fibrosis may develop at sites distant from the original tumor, mimicking malignancy in its morphology and enhancement pattern (Fig. 7.14).

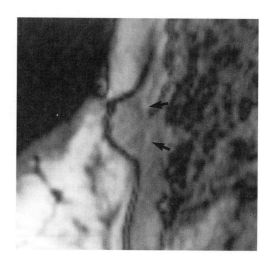

FIG. 7.11. Postbiopsy fat necrosis and scarring. Sagittal, T_1-weighted, fat-suppressed SE (T_R 550/T_E 12) image showing enhancement at a biopsy site 4 months after surgery. Reexcision histopathology showed fat necrosis, giant cell reaction, and scarring. A focus of ductal carcinoma *in situ* identified at reexcision was not identifiable on MRI.

FIG. 7.12. Fibrosis at the lumpectomy site in a breast after radiation therapy. A palpable mass corresponded to a spiculated density on mammography but was visualized incompletely because of its deep location. This postcontrast image shows minimal enhancement at the posterior aspect of an otherwise nonenhancing mass *(arrows)*, prospectively diagnosed as scar (sagittal, SPGR, T_R 119.6/T_E 2.9).

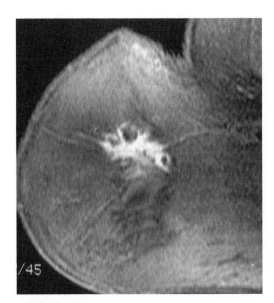

FIG. 7.13. Postlumpectomy, postradiation scarring. Six months after final radiation therapy treatment, MRI was performed to evaluate a questioned abnormality on mammography, distant from the lumpectomy site. Note the intense, irregular enhancement at the lumpectomy site on this post-contrast image (sagittal, T_1-weighted, fat-suppressed, 3-D FSPGR, T_R 27.4/T_E 3.5).

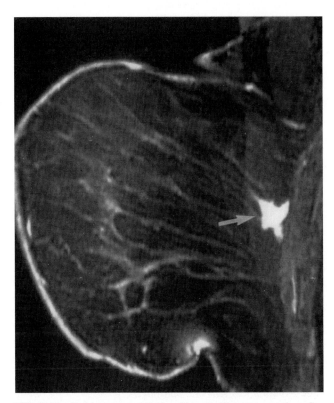

FIG. 7.14. Benign postradiation fibrosis. Twenty months after radiation therapy for invasive lobular carcinoma, an enhancing mass with marked irregularity of shape and margins (arrow) was incorrectly diagnosed as malignant (sagittal, fast gradient echo). This focus of fibrosis was 10 cm remote from the lumpectomy site.

Contrast-Enhanced Magnetic Resonance Protocols

Dynamic Imaging Protocols

Magnetic resonance imaging of the breast has exploited the greater vascularity of tumors relative to normal breast parenchyma as the major factor in lesion detection and differentiation. Gadolinium chelates administered intravenously are nonspecific extracellular contrast agents that diffuse rapidly from the intravascular to interstitial space and will affect T_1 relaxation with resultant increase in signal. Such contrast agents will accumulate most rapidly and in greatest concentration in tissues with increased vascularity and permeability relative to normal tissue, a condition that describes most invasive malignancies. With dynamic technique, initial imaging is completed within a few seconds to approximately 1 minute after rapid bolus administration of contrast with subsequent repetitive imaging for several minutes (5–14,52). This approach allows analysis of rise and fall in signal intensity over time within a given lesion and surrounding parenchyma.

Dynamic technique as a means of obtaining optimal specificity has been advocated primarily by European investigators. In 1989, Kaiser reported results on 1,000 examinations with sensitivity 98.3%, specificity 97.0%, positive predictive value (PPV) 82.1%, and accuracy 97.2% (5). As these results represented a significant improvement over the PPV for mammographically identified lesions, which is not greater than about 30% in the United States (53), the hope that MRI could improve the false-positive biopsy rate for lesions detected mammographically prompted numerous dynamic contrast investigations. Imaging protocols have differed greatly. For example, acquisition times have ranged from 2.3 to 90 seconds (5–12,14,52,54). Diagnostic criteria have varied as well, and although sensitivity for cancer detection has been generally 95% to 100%, specificity values have ranged between 53% and 89.5% (5–12,14,54).

For diagnostic protocols dependent on dynamically acquired time–intensity curves, definition and placement of the user-defined range-of-interest area (ROI) is critical for accurate diagnosis (55). Malignant tumors can show internal variation in enhancement amplitudes. Therefore, the ROI must be placed over foci of maximal enhancement and should not encompass the entire lesion that is frequently heterogeneous in contrast uptake.

Avoiding ROI measurements, a few investigators of dynamic technique have used time of lesion enhancement relative to vascular enhancement. In one study, positive lesion enhancement was defined as occurring simultaneously with blood vessel enhancement in the breast, which resulted in a 95% sensitivity and 53% specificity (54). In another study, the internal enhancement pattern of the lesion and time of enhancement relative to the aorta were considered for diagnosis (11); although three false negatives occurred, specificity was improved by noting the presence of a "benign" pattern of enhancement that began centrally and progressed peripherally in four of ten rapidly enhancing fibroadenomas.

Static Imaging Protocols

For whole-breast CE-MRI, higher resolution may be obtained with 3-D imaging, which has the theoretical advantage of improved small lesion detection because this technique allows for smaller slice thickness, minimizing volume averaging. These advantages have been offset by prolonged acquisition times. Notable is the fact that longer acquisition times may allow detection of the occasional carcinoma that does not enhance in the typical rapid, intense pattern (56).

One well-publicized breast-imaging protocol, utilizing rotating delivery of excitation off resonance (RODEO; acquisition time >5 minutes), was initially described as producing a specificity of only 37% (3). This low specificity may partly be explained by the experimental diagnostic criteria, which designated any focus of enhancement as positive, without consideration of other potentially diagnostic findings. Morphologic characteristics appear to be of benefit for diagnostic interpretation. Consideration of mass margination on MRI (56) is analogous to assessment based on mammography (57) or ultrasound (58). Orel et al. abandoned dynamic imaging because of substantial overlap between benign and malignant lesions, and utilizing

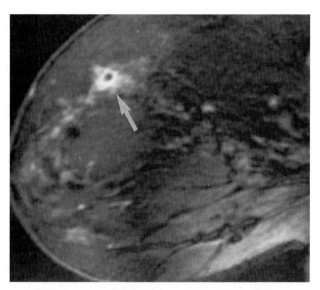

FIG. 7.16. Atypical hyperplasia with rim enhancement; MRI performed in a patient with axillary lymph nodes positive for malignancy. This strongly enhancing focus with lack of central enhancement *(arrow)* was suspicious for the primary tumor (sagittal, 3-D FGRE, T_R 7.7/T_E 2.6). MRI-guided needle localization was performed for histopathologic diagnosis.

high-resolution 3-D imaging with a 256×512 matrix requiring 3- to 5-minute imaging times, described certain characteristic architectural patterns: nonenhancing internal septations within some fibroadenomas and intense early rim enhancement within some carcinomas (21,59) (Fig. 7.15). Although more typically delayed, peripheral enhancement of benign lesions may occur (20) (Fig. 7.16).

Factors Affecting Sensitivity

Biological Factors

It is universally accepted that after intravenous contrast injection, the majority of invasive carcinomas enhance rapidly. If imaging is continued for 8 to 12 minutes following bolus contrast injection, a malignant pattern of early enhancement with washout or biphasic enhancement is commonly encountered (60). Unfortunately, a small number of invasive tumors do not enhance in a recognizable pattern, enhancing either late or minimally or not at all (20,51,61) (Fig. 7.17). There is a positive correlation between microvessel density of malignant tumors and their enhancement behavior (62). However, other factors correlate with tumoral enhancement patterns, including mitotic index and interstitial space (63). Therefore, intrinsic histopathologic differences of individual invasive tumors may account for differences in enhancement rate and intensity.

Ductal carcinoma *in situ* (DCIS) may be recognized on CE-MRI by patterns of dendritic or clumped enhancement, although mass-like or regional enhancement may occur (64,65) (Figs. 7.18 and 7.19). The enhancement of DCIS tends to differ from that of invasive tumors with a

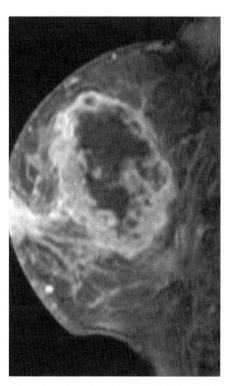

FIG. 7.15. Invasive ductal carcinoma with rim enhancement. Large ductal carcinoma with central necrosis displays rim enhancement (sagittal, 3-D SPGR, T_R 27.1/T_E 5.5).

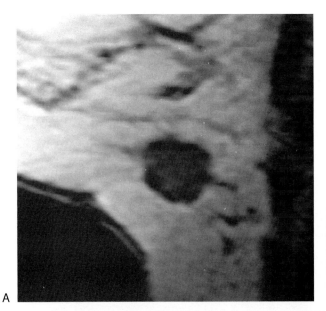 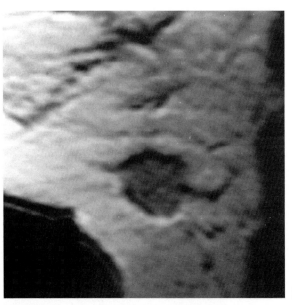

A   B

FIG. 7.17. Invasive ductal carcinoma. Precontrast **(A)** and postcontrast **(B)** images of a high-grade carcinoma that enhances minimally (sagittal, 3-D SPGR, T_R 23/T_E 5). Morphologically, this mass is suspicious for malignancy because of its irregular margination.

lower enhancement velocity and a steadily increasing intensity without a washout phase, similar to benign findings (65). Enhancement associated with DCIS appears to be secondary to tumor angiogenesis in the stroma surrounding the affected duct, and lack of angiogenesis correlates with lack of enhancement (66). Therefore, DCIS without invasion is not reliably detectable by CE-MRI based on enhancement alone. Sensitivity for DCIS is reportedly as low as 60% to 72% (21,67).

A proposed indication for CE-MRI is as a monitoring device for chemotherapeutic treatments (Fig. 7.20). In one report, lesions in eight patients who responded to chemotherapy showed a flattening of the contrast uptake curve after the first drug cycle or complete absence of uptake after the fourth cycle (68). However, the change in contrast uptake led to an underestimation of tumor extent in two and to false-negative diagnoses in four patients.

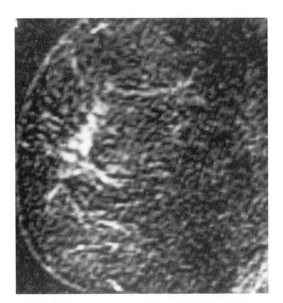 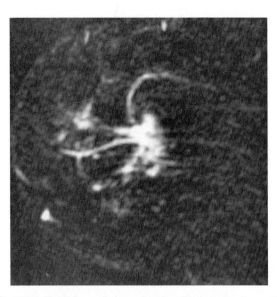

FIG. 7.18. Ductal carcinoma *in situ.* Postcontrast, sagittal, fat-nulled EFGRE (T_R 8/T_E 3/T_I 24) image shows a combination of clumped and dendritic enhancement.

FIG. 7.19. Ductal carcinoma *in situ.* Postcontrast, sagittal, fat-nulled EFGRE (T_R 7/T_E 2/T_I 24) image shows mass-like enhancement with radiating linear structures.

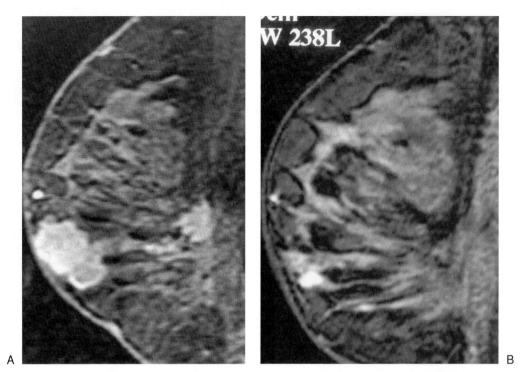

FIG. 7.20. Tumor response to chemotherapy. Postcontrast images showing a large anterior invasive ductal carcinoma and a posterior focus of ductal carcinoma *in situ* **(A)** before and **(B)** 8 weeks following induction of chemotherapy. In **A**, note marked enhancement of the invasive ductal carcinoma anteriorly with posterior ductal extension reaching a focus of segmental enhancement (sagittal, 3-D FGRE, T_R 19.7/T_E 1.5). The posterior disease was unsuspected on prior mammographic and sonographic work-up. In **B**, the anterior tumor mass showed a marked decrease in size, and the posterior tumor mass is no longer identifiable (sagittal, 3-D FGRE, T_R 7.3/T_E 2.4). However, on subsequent surgical excision, the area in the posterior breast that had shown substantial enhancement on the prechemotherapy MRI but not on the posttherapy MRI contained viable and extensive ductal carcinoma *in situ*.

SILICONE GEL IMPLANT EVALUATION

Background

Interest in accurate imaging of silicone gel implants for evaluation of their integrity emerged with the intense media coverage and subsequent legal ramifications surrounding the FDA ban of these devices in the early 1990s. Mammography, xeromammography, ultrasound, CT, and MRI have been utilized for implant imaging (69–71). Screen-film mammography is of limited use in the evaluation of implants because portions of the implant are never imaged, and the internal structure is obscured by the radiodense silicone. Ultrasound is most accurate if extracapsular silicone or a collapsed implant shell is present (70). Magnetic resonance imaging has been shown to be both highly sensitive and specific for evaluation of both intracapsular and extracapsular rupture (72).

Structure and Complications of Breast Implants

The structure and manufacture of implants is diverse. Implants may be single lumen (containing silicone or saline), double lumen (generally with an inner core of sil-

icone and outer lumen of saline) (Fig. 7.21), or triple lumen. Generally filled with saline, some expandable implants contain valves for augmenting implant volume. The implant shells are composed of a silicone elastomer, which may be smooth, textured, or coated with polyurethane. Fibrous encapsulation, occurring in virtually all patients, may result in capsular contracture. The degree of encapsulation differs between patients and may differ between breasts of an individual patient. Infolding of the implant shell is common and is affected by the thickness of the shell, the amount of silicone gel filling the implant, as well as the extent of fibrous encapsulation.

The goal of imaging is primarily to evaluate the implant for rupture, but other complications of augmentation may be identified, such as hematoma, abscess, extensive scarring, and implant displacement. The two main categories of implant dysfunction include intracapsular and extracapsular ruptures. There is a third, ambiguous category referred to in this chapter as "bleed." An intracapsular rupture occurs when the implant shell tears or disintegrates but the silicone gel is contained by an intact fibrous capsule. An extracapsular rupture is the extrusion of silicone through tears in both the implant and

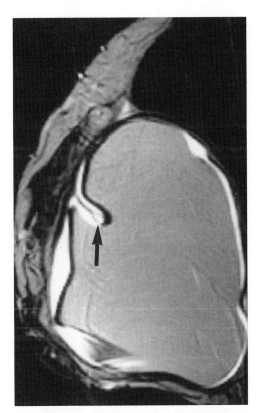

FIG. 7.21. Double-lumen breast implant. Sagittal image of the breast shows a "bag within a bag" appearance. Saline filling the outer lumen has the brightest signal on this strongly T_2-weighted image [fast spin echo (FSE), T_R 5,200/T_E 180]. The silicone gel in the inner lumen is slightly more intense than breast fat. Note the fold *(arrow)* in the outer lumen. There is a "keyhole" or "teardrop" appearance suggesting fluid lying between the outer surface of the opposed casing, which most likely represents a small amount of serous fluid deep to the fibrous capsule, bathing the implant, but that could be the result of a focal leak of saline.

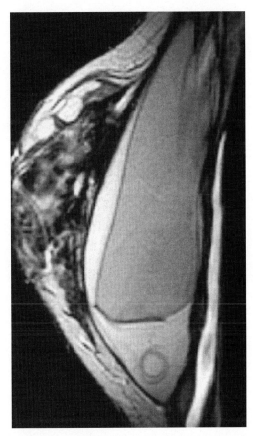

FIG. 7.22. Stacked implants. On first review of this examination, a diagnosis was made of rupture of the outer casing of a double-lumen implant. However, the surgical history was not initially known. This patient has a posterior solid silicone implant and an anterior single-lumen silicone gel implant. The anterior implant displays a collapsed casing without extrusion of silicone into the breast tissue, consistent with an intracapsular rupture (sagittal, FSE, T_R 9,633/T_E 1,700).

overlying fibrous capsule. "Bleed" refers to the passage of silicone fluid (which bathes the silicone polymers of the gel) through a porous, though intact, implant shell (73). In the recent past, "gel bleed" has been considered to be a "normal" occurrence in which sticky gel is found on the outer surface of an uncollapsed, seemingly intact implant shell at surgical revision or in which a thin rim of silicone along the outer margin of an uncollapsed implant is detected on imaging. This finding may actually represent an intracapsular rupture in which a small amount of silicone gel has leaked through a tiny hole in the implant shell and spread around the surface of the implant (73). Nevertheless, it is feasible that extensive silicone fluid bleed may be confused with an uncollapsed rupture associated with a small amount of gel leak.

Knowledge of the patient's implant history is extremely valuable because findings considered abnormal in the evaluation of one type of implant or surgical technique may be normal for another (Fig. 7.22). Important facts for diagnostic consideration are the type of implant and the surgical history, including incidence of prior rupture and implant revision (Fig. 7.23).

Technical Considerations

Technical factors can affect conspicuity of small extracapsular silicone collections or internal membranous abnormalities. Marked T_2-weighting allows visual differentiation of fat, silicone, and water in many cases, although addition of a fat-suppressed sequence can be beneficial in identification of extra-implant silicone deposits (Fig. 7.24). Chemical-shift-based fat or silicone suppression can be troublesome because small inhomogeneities in the magnetic field will cause inadvertent suppression of one or another entity (Fig. 7.25). This is because of the small difference in resonance frequencies between fat and silicone (1.5 ppm). Comparatively, the water–silicone resonance difference (5 ppm) is approxi-

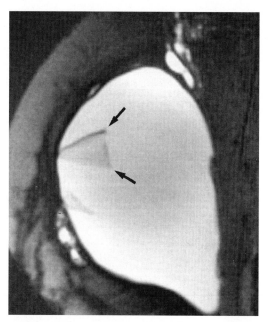

FIG. 7.23. Residual silicone in parenchyma from a prior extracapsular rupture. Sagittal image (FSE, water suppression, T_R 6,000/T_E 36) shows an intact implant (revised) containing a broad fold *(arrows)*, as well as silicone in breast parenchyma from prior rupture.

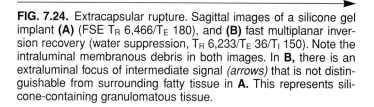

FIG. 7.24. Extracapsular rupture. Sagittal images of a silicone gel implant **(A)** (FSE T_R 6,466/T_E 180), and **(B)** fast multiplanar inversion recovery (water suppression, T_R 6,233/T_E 36/T_I 150). Note the intraluminal membranous debris in both images. In **B,** there is an extraluminal focus of intermediate signal *(arrows)* that is not distinguishable from surrounding fatty tissue in **A.** This represents silicone-containing granulomatous tissue.

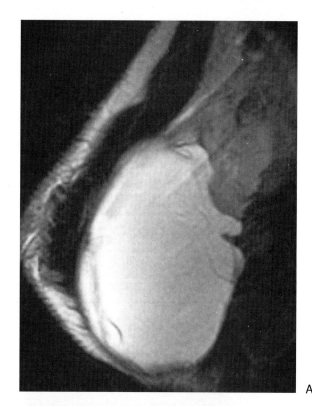

A

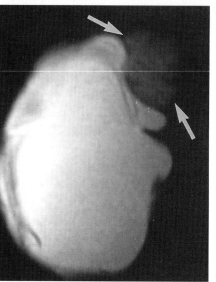

B

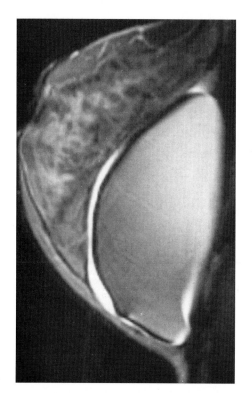

FIG. 7.25. Intact polyurethane-coated implant. Sagittal image of a single-lumen polyurethane-coated silicone gel implant (FSE, fat suppression, T_R 7,000/T_E 85). This type of implant is frequently associated with a surrounding seroma and may have the appearance of a double-lumen implant. Note that there is focal suppression of silicone signal and inhomogeneous fat suppression as a result of magnetic field inhomogeneities.

mately twice that of the chemical shift between fat and water. An inversion recovery technique to null the signal intensity of fat is suggested rather than chemical-shift-based saturation. Motion artifact near the chest wall may be aggravated by long T_E on conventional T_2-weighted SE. This artifact is greatly reduced on fast SE imaging.

Magnetic Resonance Imaging Evaluation of Breast Implants

A variety of diagnostic pitfalls of MRI implant evaluation have been reported. A collapsed intracapsular rupture may be identified by the presence of low-intensity curvilinear or linear debris within the silicone gel bed, a finding known as the "linguine sign" (74). Normal prominent infoldings of the intact shell may be confused with the linguine sign (74) (Figs. 7.26–7.28). Nearly all

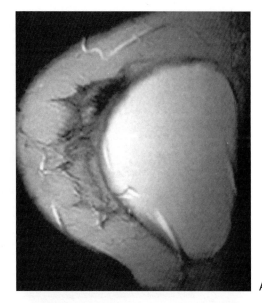

A

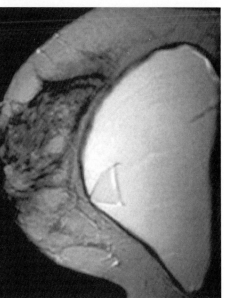

B

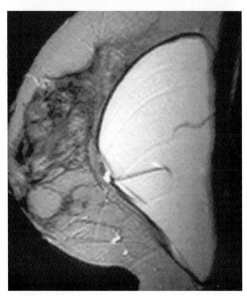

C

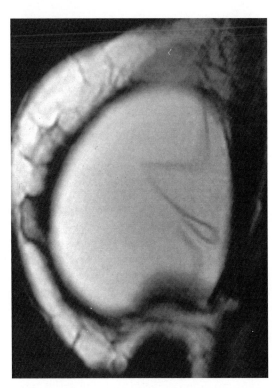

FIG. 7.26. Intact implant with prominent fold. Sagittal image of a single-lumen silicone gel implant containing a curvilinear membranous structure representing a normal, prominent fold (FSE, water suppression, T_R 4,600/T_E 90).

FIG. 7.27. Intact implant with folds. Sagittal images of a single-lumen silicone gel implant containing curvilinear membranous structures representing normal folds. Note the chemical shift artifact visible along the more vertically oriented folds (parallel with the frequency-encoding gradient) in **A** and **B**. Chemical shift artifact is not seen along the more horizontal folds in **B** or **C**. Chemical shift artifact is thought to be a consequence of a small amount of fluid caught between the outer surface of the folds (FSE, T_R 5,200/T_E 180).

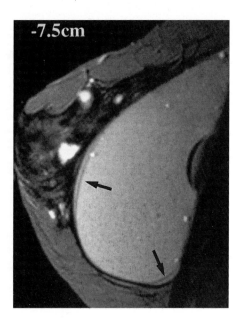

FIG. 7.28. Early intracapsular rupture. Sagittal image of silicone gel implant shows the casing to be pulling away from the capsule *(arrows)*. Silicone signal is present on both sides of the casing. High-signal water droplets within the implant presumably entered the lumen through tears in the casing. (FSE, T_R 6,500/T_E 171).

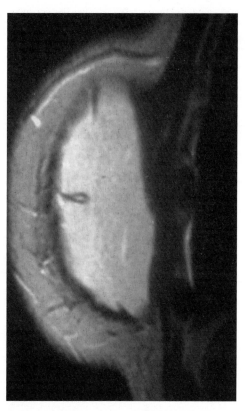

FIG. 7.29. Intracapsular rupture. Sagittal image of a silicone gel implant shows a fold with silicone on both its outer and inner surfaces. This is an example of the teardrop or noose sign (FSE, T_R 6,500/T_E 180).

implants are associated with some infolding (75). Infolding of an intact casing appears on T_2-weighted imaging as a hypointense line extending into the lumen from the implant margin. Short folds will appear on several slices and may have the appearance of freely floating membranous debris on any given slice. Intraluminal linear foci must be followed carefully from slice to slice to determine the relationship to the implant margin.

We have noted the presence of linear chemical shift artifact following at least portions of the folds of many intact single-lumen implants (76). Our hypothesis for this phenomenon is that a small amount of serous fluid bathes the outer aspect of the implant within the capsule, and some fluid may get trapped between the two layers of a fold. Consequently, because of the differences in the NMR spectra of the silicone-containing elastomer shell and water, linear chemical shift artifact will occur, most visibly when the fold runs perpendicular to the frequency-encoding plane. We have found the presence of linear chemical shift artifact to be a reliable sign that the fold in question is normal and, in most cases, that the implant is intact (see Fig. 7.27). The exception is the implant with focal rupture that has not progressed to affect the remainder of the implant; therefore, signs of rupture take precedence in diagnosis. With rupture, silicone gel migrates along the outer surface of the elastomer casing. Subtle signs of rupture include subcapsular lines where the casing is separated from the capsule by a rim of silicone (75) or the teardrop (noose) sign, which describes the appearance of small amounts of silicone between fold layers (71,73,74) (see Figs. 7.28 and 7.29).

Plastic surgeons have been known to inject such materials as antibiotics and steroids to decrease capsular contraction and saline to augment implant size. Fluid injected into silicone gel implants may mimic a failed internal shell of a double-lumen implant (77). Seromas are commonly present around polyurethane-coated or textured-surface implants and may appear similar to double-lumen devices (78) (see Fig. 7.25).

Silicone in the soft tissues will induce a fibrous reaction, encapsulating the rupture. If extruded silicone remains in continuity with silicone gel in the implant bed, fibrous encapsulation of the extruded material may cause difficulty for both imaging and surgical differentiation of an extracapsular from an intracapsular rupture. This differentiation may be important for surgical planning, as some surgeons will not remove a contained rupture if the cosmetic result is good and the patient is not symptomatic. Additionally, exuberant fibrosis may cause contour abnormality of the implant, which may be mistaken for silicone gel extrusion (20) (Fig. 7.30). Although unusual contour may suggest rupture, contour abnormality alone could be due to compression and should not be used as a sole indicator of rupture (Figs. 17.31 and 17.32).

In conclusion, in evaluating the breast for parenchymal disease or implant dysfunction, it is important to weigh all

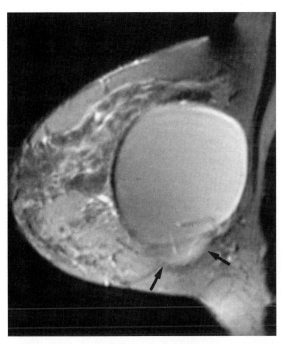

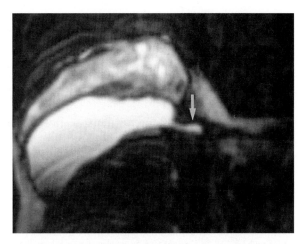

FIG. 7.32. Intact implant. Axial image of a retropectoral silicone gel implant with a tongue of silicone *(arrow)* extending medially, deep to the pectoralis muscle (FSE T$_R$ 6,000/T$_E$ 48). This appearance was prospectively thought to represent rupture but is caused by compression of the intact implant by the overlying muscle.

FIG. 7.30. Intact implant with focal capsular fibrosis. Sagittal image of a single-lumen silicone gel implant (FSE, fat suppression, T$_R$ 7,000/T$_E$ 85). There is an appearance of outpouching of silicone gel at the posterior aspect of the implant *(arrows)*, prospectively thought to represent extrusion of silicone gel into the soft tissues. In retrospect, normal folds are present adjacent to the contour abnormality. At implant removal, exuberant fibrosis was found, deforming the implant focally. The fibrosis was also the source of pain that prompted the surgery.

information available when formulating a diagnosis and offering recommendations for management. This information includes patient history and findings at physical examination, mammography, and sonography. Because of the problems with both sensitivity and specificity of MRI examination, factors other than the MRI result will sometimes take precedence in patient management planning.

REFERENCES

1. Vogel PM, Georgiade NG, Fetter BF, Vogel FS, McCarty KS Jr. The correlation of histologic changes in the human breast with the menstrual cycle. *Am J Pathol* 1981;104:23–34.
2. Cole-Beuglet CM, Goldberg BB, Patchefsky AS, et al. Normal breast structure and its ultrasound characteristics. In: Telles NC, ed. *Atlas of breast ultrasound.* Philadelphia: Thomas Jefferson University Hospital, 1980;38–78.
3. Harms SE, Flaming DP, Hesley KL, et al. MR imaging of the breast with rotating delivery of excitation off resonance: clinical experience with pathologic correlation. *Radiology* 1993;187:493–501.
4. Hachiya J, Seki T, Okada M, et al. MR imaging of the breast with Gd-DTPA enhancement: comparison with mammography and ultrasonography. *Radiat Med* 1991;9:232–240.
5. Kaiser WA, Zeitler E. MR imaging of the breast: fast imaging sequences with and without Gd-DTPA. Preliminary observations. *Radiology* 1989; 170:681–686.
6. Kaiser WA, Reiser M. False positive cases in dynamic MR mammography. *Radiology* 1992;185(P):245.
7. Fischer U, von Heyden D, Vosshenrich R, Viewig I, Grabbe E. Signal characteristics of malignant and benign lesions in dynamic 2-D-MRT of the breast. *Rofo Fortschr geb Rontgenstr Neuen Bildgeb Verfahr* 1993; 158:287–292.
8. Kelcz F, Santyr GE, Mongin SJ, Fairbanks EJ. *Reducing false positive gadolinium-enhanced breast MRI results through parameter analysis of the enhancement profile.* Paper presented at the 12th Annual Meeting, Society of Magnetic Resonance in Medicine, New York, 1993;121.
9. Kelcz F, Santyr GE, Fairbanks EJ, Mongin SJ. Gadolinium-enhanced breast MR for characterization of suspicious breast lesions. *J Magn Reson Imag* 1993;3(P):47.
10. Flickinger FW, Allison JD, Sherry RM, Wright JC. Differentiation of benign from malignant breast masses by tine-intensity evaluation of contrast enhanced MRI. *Magn Reson Imag* 1993;11:617–620.

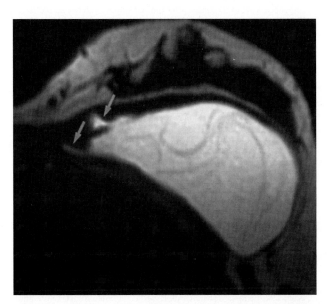

FIG. 7.31. Intracapsular rupture. Axial image of a retropectoral silicone gel implant with unusual contour suggesting extrusion of silicone into and around the medial aspect of the pectoralis muscle *(arrows)* (axial, T$_2$-weighted spin echo, water suppression, T$_R$ 3,000/T$_E$ 80). Note also the intraluminal membranous debris indicative of intracapsular rupture. In this case, the abnormal contour may be caused by lack of a containing membrane.

11. Boetes C, Barentsz JO, Mus RD, et al. MR characterization of suspicious breast lesions with a gadolinium-enhanced turbo-flash subtraction technique. *Radiology* 1994;193:777–781.

12. Turkat TJ, Klein BD, Polan RL, Richman RH. Dynamic MR mammography: a technique for potentially reducing the biopsy rate for benign breast disease. *J Magn Reson Imag* 1994;4:563–568.

13. Hulka CA, Smith BL, Sgroi DC, et al Benign and malignant breast lesions: differentiation with echo-planar MR imaging. *Radiology* 1995;197:33–38.

14. Stomper PC, Herman S, Klippenstein DL, et al. Suspect breast lesions: findings at dynamic gadolinium-enhanced MR imaging correlated with mammographic and pathologic features. *Radiology* 1995;197:387–395.

15. Boné B, Aspelin P, Bronge L, et al. Sensitivity and specificity of MR mammography with histopathological correlation in 250 breasts. *Acta Radiol* 1996;37:208–213.

16. Heywang-Koebrunner SH. Diagnosis of breast cancer with MR—review after 1250 patient examinations. *Electromedica* 1993;61:43–52.

17. Kuhl CK, Kreft BP, Hauswirth A, et al. MR mammography at 0.5 tesla. I. Comparison of image quality and sensitivity of MR mammography at 0.5 and 1.5 T. *Rofo Fortschr Geb Rontgenstr Neuen Bildgeb Verfahr* 1995;162:381–389.

18. Kuhl CK, Kreft BP, Hauswirth A, et al. MR mammography at 0.5 tesla. II. The capacity to differentiate malignant and benign lesions in MR mammography at 0.5 and 1.5T. *Rofo Fortschr Geb Rontgenstr Neuen Bildgeb Verfahr* 1995;162:482–491.

19. Heywang-Koebrunner SH, Haustein J, Pohl C, et al. Contrast-enhanced MRI of the breast: comparison of two different doses of gadopentetate dimeglumine. *Radiology* 1994;191:639–646.

20. Piccoli CW, Greer JG, Mitchell DG. Breast MR imaging for cancer detection and implant evaluation: potential pitfalls. *RadioGraphics* 1996;16:63–75.

21. Orel SG, Schnall MD, Powell CM, et al. Staging of suspected breast cancer: effect of MR imaging and MR-guided biopsy. *Radiology* 1995;196:115–122.

22. Zuo CS, Jiang A, Buff BL, Mahon TG, Wong TZ. Automatic motion correction for breast MR imaging. *Radiology* 1996;198:903–906.

23. Schorn C, Fischer U, Doler W, Funke M, Grabbe E. Compression device to reduce motion artifacts at contrast-enhanced MR imaging in the breast. *Radiology* 1998;206:279–282.

24. Kuhl CK, Leutner C, Mielcarek P, Gieseke J, Schild HH. Breast compression interferes with lesion enhancement in contrast-enhanced breast MR imaging. *Radiology* 1997;205P:538.

25. Kenney PH, Sobol WT, Smith JK, Morgan DE. Computed model of gadolinium enhanced MRI of breast disease. *Eur J Radiol* 1997;24:109–119.

26. Pabst T, Kenn W, Kaiser WA, Hahn D. The necessity of a calibration phantom for comparison in dynamic contrast-enhanced MR mammography. *Radiology* 1997;205(P):163.

27. Heywang-Koebrunner SH. Appearance of various tissues and lesions. In: *Contrast-enhanced MRI of the breast.* Basel: Karger, 1990;177–179.

28. Martin B, El Yousef SJ. Transverse relaxation time values in MR imaging of normal breast during menstrual cycle. *J Comput Assist Tomogr* 1986;10:924–927.

29. Nelson TR, Pretorius DH, Schiffer LM. Menstrual variation of normal breast NMR relaxation parameters. *J Comput Assist Tomogr* 1985;9:875–879.

30. Fowler PA, Casey CE, Cameron GG, Foster MA, Knight CH. Cyclic changes in composition and volume of the breast during the menstrual cycle, measured by magnetic resonance imaging. *Br J Obstet Gynaecol* 1990;97:595–602.

31. Mueller-Schimpfle M, Ohmenhèuser K, Stoll P, Dietz K, Clausser DC. Menstrual cycle and age: influence on parenchymal contrast medium enhancement in MR imaging of the breast. *Radiology* 1997;203:145–149.

32. Kuhl CK, Bieling HB, Gieseke J, et al. Healthy premenopausal breast parenchyma in dynamic contrast-enhanced MR imaging of the breast: normal contrast medium enhancement and cyclical-phase dependency. *Radiology* 1997;203:137–144.

33. Berkowitz JE, Gatewood OM, Goldblum LE, Gayler BW. Hormonal replacement therapy: mammographic manifestations. *Radiology* 1990;174:199–201.

34. Marugg RC, Hendriks JH, Ruijs JH. Effects of hormonal replacement therapy on the mammographic breast pattern in postmenopausal women. *Radiology* 1993;189(P):405.

35. Stomper PC, Van Voorhis BJ, Ravnikar VA, Meyer JE. Mammographic changes associated with postmenopausal hormone replacement therapy: a longitudinal study. *Radiology* 1990;174:487–490.

36. Barth V, Prechtel K. Mastopathy. In: *Atlas of breast disease.* Philadelphia: DC Decker, 1991;76–100.

37. Heywang-Koebrunner SH. Appearance of various tissues and lesions. In: *Contrast-enhanced MRI of the breast.* Basel: Karger, 1990;46–176.

38. Kaiser WA, Mittelmeier O. MR mammography in patients at risk. *Rofo Fortschr geb Rontgenstr Neuen Bildgeb Verfahr* 1992;156:576–581.

39. Tavassoli FA. Intraductal hyperplasias, ordinary and atypical. In: *Pathology of the breast.* Norwalk, CT: Appleton & Lange, 1992;155–192.

40. Orel SB, Schnall MD, Livolsi VA, Troupin RH. High-resolution MR imaging of breast carcinomas and fibroadenomas with radiologic–pathologic correlation. *Radiology* 1993;189(P):106.

41. Brinck U, Fischer U, Korabiowska M, et al. The variability of fibroadenoma in contrast-enhanced dynamic MR mammography. *Am J Roentgenol* 1997;168:1331–1334.

42. Tavassoli FA. Papillary Lesions. In: *Pathology of the breast.* Norwalk, CT: Appleton & Lange, 1992;193–228.

43. Merchant TE, Kievit HC, Beijerink D, van der Putte SC, de Graaf PW. MRI appearance of multiple papilloma of the breast. *Breast Cancer Res Treat* 1991;19:63–67.

44. Tavassoli FA. Biphasic tumors. In: *Pathology of the breast.* Norwalk, CT: Appleton & Lange, 1992;425–482.

45. Grebe P, Wilhelm K, Brunier A, Mitze M. MR tomography of cystosarcoma phylloides. A case report. *Akt Radiol* 1992;2:376–378.

46. Kievit HCE, Sikkenk AC, Thelissen GRP, Merchant TE. Magnetic resonance image appearance of hamartoma of the breast. *Magn Reson Imag* 1992;11:293–298.

47. Kopans DB. Pathologic, mammographic, and sonographic correlation. In: *Breast imaging.* Philadelphia: JB Lippincott, 1989;260–311.

48. Dao TH, Rahmouni A, Campana F, et al. Tumor recurrence versus fibrosis in the irradiated breast: differentiation with dynamic gadolinium-enhanced MR imaging. *Radiology* 1993;187:751–755.

49. Gilles R, Guinebretiere JM, Shapeero LG, et al. Assessment of breast cancer recurrence with contrast-enhanced subtraction MR imaging: preliminary results in 26 patients. *Radiology* 1993;188:473–478.

50. Heywang SH, Hilbertz T, Beck R, et al. Gd-DTPA enhanced MR imaging of the breast in patients with postoperative scarring and silicon implants. *J Comput Assist Tomogr* 1990;14:348–356.

51. Heywang-Koebrunner SH, Schlegel A, Beck R, et al. Contrast-enhanced MRI of the breast after limited surgery and radiation therapy. *J Comput Assist Tomogr* 1993;17:891–900.

52. Stack JP, Redmond OM, Codd MB, Dervan PA, Ennis JT. Breast disease: tissue characterization with Gd-DTPA enhancement profiles. *Radiology* 1990;174:491–494.

53. Rosenberg AL, Schwartz GF, Feig SA, Patchefsky AS. Clinically occult breast lesions: localization and significance. *Radiology* 1987;162:167–170.

54. Gilles R, Guinebretiere J-M, Lucidarme O, et al. Nonpalpable breast tumors: diagnosis with contrast-enhanced subtraction MR imaging. *Radiology* 1994;191:625–631.

55. Gribbestad IS, Nilsen G, Fjøsne HE, et al. Comparative signal intensity measurements in dynamic gadolinium-enhanced MR mammography. *J Magn Reson Imag* 1994;4:477–480.

56. Heywang-Koebrunner SH. Contrast-enhanced magnetic resonance imaging of the breast. *Invest Radiol* 1994;29:94–104.

57. Sickles EA. Management of probably benign lesions of the breast. *Radiology* 1994;193:582–586.

58. Stavros AT, Thickman D, Rapp CL, et al. Solid breast nodules: use of sonography to distinguish between benign and malignant lesions. *Radiology* 1995;196:123–134.

59. Orel SB, Schnall MD, Livolsi VA, Troupin RH. Suspicious breast lesions: MR imaging with radiologic–pathologic correlation. *Radiology* 1994;190:485–493.

60. Kuhl CK, Leutner C, Mielcarek P, Seibert C, Schild HH. Cycle phase dependency of fibroadenoma enhancement in dynamic breast MR imaging. *Radiology* 1997;205P:235.

61. Boetes C, Strijk SP, Holland R, et al. False-negative MR imaging of malignant breast tumors. *Eur Radiol* 1997;7:1231–1234.

62. Buadu LD, Murakami J, Murayama S, et al. Breast lesions: correlation of contrast medium enhancement patterns on MR images with histopathologic findings and tumor angiogenesis. *Radiology* 1996;200:639–649.

63. Mueller-Schimpfle MP, Noack F, Oettling G, et al. Correlation of cap-

illary density, proliferation, and interstitial space with enhancement parameters in MR imaging of the breast. *Radiology* 1997;205(P):235.

64. Soderstrom CE, Harms SE, Copit DS, et al. Three-dimensional RODEO breast MR imaging of lesions containing ductal carcioma *in situ. Radiology* 1996;201:427–432.

65. Kuhl CK, Mielcarek P, Leutner C, Schild HH. Diagnostic criteria of DCIS versus invasive breast cancer in dynamic breast MR imaging. *Radiology* 1997;205P:235.

66. Gilles R, Zafrani B, Guinebretiere J-M, et al. Ductal carcinoma in situ: MR imaging-histopathologic correlation. *Radiology* 1995;196:415–419.

67. Fischer U, Westerhof JP, Brinck U, et al. Das duktale In-situ-Karzinom in der dynamischen MR-Mammographie bei 1,5 T. *Rofo Fortschr Geb Rontgenstr Neuen Bildgeb Verfahr* 1996;164:290–294.

68. Rieber A, Zeitler H, Rosenthal H, et al. MRI of breast cancer—influence of chemotherapy on sensitivity. *Br J Radiol* 997;70:452–458.

69. Steinbach BG, Hardt NS, Abbitt PL, Lanier L, Caffee HH. Breast implants, common complications, and concurrent breast disease. *RadioGraphics* 1993;13:95–118.

70. DeBruhl ND, Gorczyca S, Ahn CY, Shaw WW, Bassett LW. Silicone breast implants: US evaluation. *Radiology* 1993;189:95–98.

71. O'Boyle MK, Wechsler RJ, Conant EF, Lev-Toaff AS, Sagerman J. Breast implants: incidental findings on CT. *Am J Roentgenol* 1994;162:311–313.

72. Everson LI, Parantainen H, Detlie T, et al. Diagnosis of breast implant rupture: imaging findings and relative efficacies of imaging techniques. *Am J Roentgenol* 1994;163:57–60.

73. Middleton MS. MR Evaluation of breast implants and soft tissue silicone. *Top Magn Reson Imag* 1998;9:92–137.

74. Gorczyca DP, Sinha S, Ahn CY, et al. Silicone breast implants *in vivo: MR imaging.* Radiology 1992;185:407–410.

75. Soo MS, Kornguth PJ, Walsh R, Elenberger CD, Georgiade GS. Complex radial folds versus subtle signs of intracapsular rupture of breast implants: MR findings with surgical correlation. *Am J Roentgenol* 1996;166:1421–1427.

76. Murphy TJ, Piccoli CW. Correlation of single lumen silicone implant integrity with chemical shift artifact on T_2-weighted MR images. *Radiology* 1997;205(P):540.

77. Berg WA, Anderson ND, Zerhouni EA, Chang BW, Kuhlman JE. MR imaging of the breast in patients with silicone breast implants: normal postoperative variants and diagnostic pitfalls. *Am J Roentgenol* 1994;163:575–578.

78. Berg WA, Caskey CI, Hamper UM, Kuhlman JE, Anderson ND. Diagnosing breast implant rupture with magnetic resonance imaging, ultrasound, and mammography. *RadioGraphics* 1993;13:1323–1336.

Variants of Normal Anatomy and Diagnostic Pitfalls in Imaging of the Abdomen and Pelvis

Variants and Pitfalls in Body Imaging,
edited by Ali Shirkhoda.
Lippincott Williams & Wilkins, Philadelphia, © 2000.

CHAPTER 8

The Liver: Helical (Spiral) and Conventional CT

Karen M. Horton and Elliot K. Fishman

Computed tomography (CT) has been the study of choice for nearly two decades in the evaluation of hepatic pathology. Whether the study is performed for the assessment of parenchymal liver disease or for the detection of metastases or primary hepatic tumors, CT has been shown to have high sensitivity and specificity. However, CT scanning of the liver has resulted in significant debate regarding optimal injection rates, contrast volumes, and data acquisition. Much of this controversy has revolved around the recognized technical limitations of conventional CT.

Over the years, the capabilities of CT scanners have evolved significantly. Even the best conventional dynamic studies could only obtain up to 10 scans per minute and required a 3- to 5-minute examination, even with 5-mm scan collimation. This lengthy acquisition time made it impossible to obtain arterial-phase imaging of the liver, or even portal-phase images, in a timely fashion.

In the early 1990s, spiral (or helical) CT was introduced and provided many of the capabilities that were lacking with traditional dynamic scanners. First, spiral technique allows rapid second or subsecond scanning, thus permitting scanning during different phases of hepatic enhancement (i.e., arterial vs. portal vs. delayed). Second, partial volume averaging through liver lesions is reduced, as axial reconstructions can be performed at user-selected intervals, and overlapping reconstructions can be obtained. Third, respiratory misregistration can be eliminated when the liver is scanned

during a single breath-hold. Finally, spiral CT data sets form the basis for three-dimensional (3-D) imaging and CT angiography.

Although CT offers distinct advantages over other modalities for liver imaging, there are many factors on both conventional and spiral CT that can result in potential difficulties in diagnosis or even misdiagnosis. Inadequate technique, misinterpretation of normal anatomy, and variations, artifacts, and changes related to phase of enhancement, are only some of the potential pitfalls in liver imaging.

This chapter reviews and illustrates normal anatomy and common anatomic variants of the liver, portal vein, hepatic arteries, hepatic veins, and bile ducts as well as potential pitfalls in diagnosis related to technique and artifacts. Specific emphasis is placed on those findings that can simulate disease and lead to misdiagnosis.

LIVER

Normal Anatomy

The liver occupies the right upper quadrant of the abdomen and extends to a variable degree across the midline into the left upper quadrant. It is divided by fissures/ligaments into lobes. The interlobar fissure separates the right and left hepatic lobes and extends from the gallbladder fossa and IVC to the middle hepatic vein. The right lobe of the liver is divided into its anterior and posterior segments by the right intersegmental fissure. It is not well visualized on imaging studies but can be approximated by a line along the plane of the right hepatic vein (Fig. 8.1).

The left intersegmental fissure or falciform ligament is also known as the fissure for the ligamentum teres and separates the medial and lateral segments of the left

K. M. Horton: Department of Radiology, Johns Hopkins Medical Institutions, Baltimore, Maryland 21287.

E. K. Fishman: Departments of Radiology and Oncology, Johns Hopkins University School of Medicine, Baltimore, Maryland 21287.

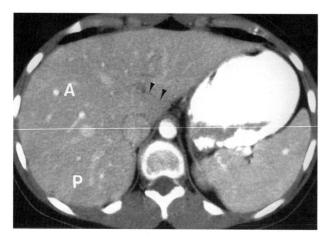

FIG. 8.1. Contrast-enhanced spiral CT demonstrates normal liver anatomy. The right hepatic lobe is divided into anterior (A) and posterior (P) segments. This division is approximated by a line along the plane of the right hepatic vein. *Arrowhead,* fissure for ligamentum venosum.

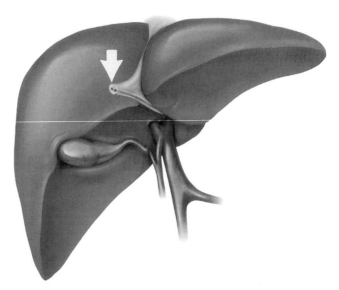

FIG. 8.3. Illustration showing the ligamentum teres and small paraumbilical veins *(arrow),* located in the inferior portion of the falciform ligament.

hepatic lobe (Fig. 8.2). Its inferior portion contains the ligamentum teres, which represents the atrophied umbilical vein (Fig. 8.3). The ligamentum teres extends from the liver to the anterior abdominal wall and contains a few small collapsed paraumbilical veins, which may enlarge in patients with portal hypertension (Fig. 8.4).

The fissure for the ligamentum venosum (see Fig. 8.1) separates the caudate from the left hepatic lobe (1). It

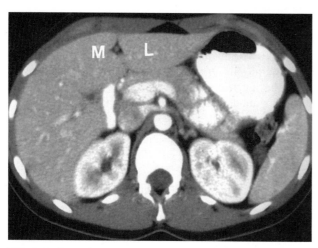

FIG. 8.2. Contrast-enhanced spiral CT demonstrates normal liver anatomy. The left hepatic lobe is divided into medial (M) and lateral (L) segments by the falciform ligament.

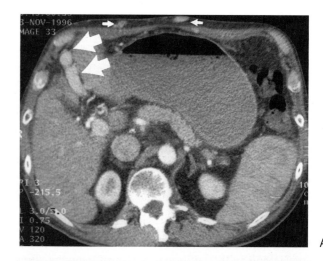

A

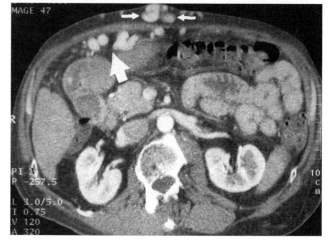

B

FIG. 8.4. A,B: A 63-year-old man with a history of cirrhosis and portal hypertension from alcohol abuse. Axial images from a contrast-enhanced spiral CT demonstrate a dilated enhancing paraumbilical vein in the falciform ligament *(large arrows).* Dilated enhancing epigastric veins *(small arrows)* are demonstrated in the anterior abdominal wall.

contains the gastrohepatic ligament, which contains the left gastric artery and vein and lymph nodes. It courses from the lesser curve of the stomach to the inferior margin of the liver, where it attaches to the ligamentum venosum and right crus of the diaphragm. The gastrohepatic ligament is an important site to look for adenopathy, as it receives drainage from both the esophagus and stomach. It is also a common site for varices in patients with portal hypertension.

The inferior process of the caudate lobe is divided into a medial papillary process and a lateral caudate process. A fatty cleft can sometimes be seen separating the two processes (1). If prominent, the papillary process can

mimic periportal adenopathy or a mass in the head of the pancreas (Fig. 8.5) (2,3).

Accessory fissures are common. They are formed by reflections of the diaphragm and are located along the superior aspect of the liver, often resulting in a lobular appearance (Fig. 8.6). Supernumerary fissures are rare and are caused by infolding of the peritoneum on the undersurface of the liver (1).

The liver is covered with peritoneum except for the gallbladder fossa, the porta, a small area surrounding the IVC, and a small area to the right of the IVC called the bare area of the liver. This bare area comes in contact with the right adrenal gland and kidney. Fluid adjacent to

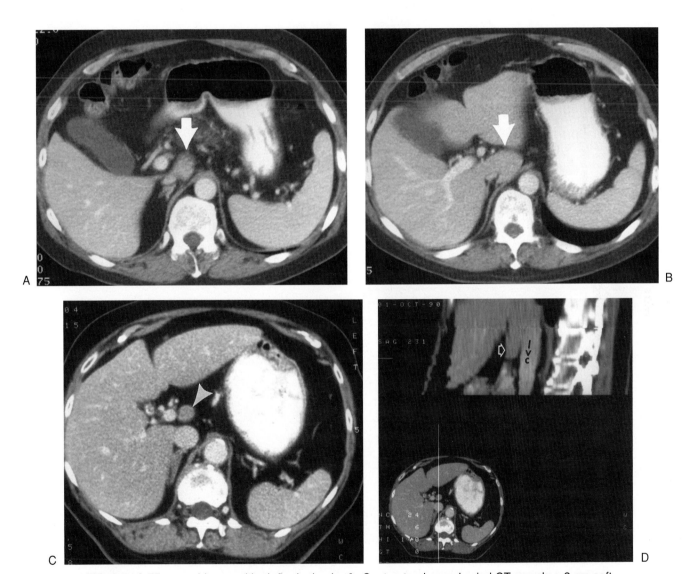

FIG. 8.5. A 55-year-old man with abdominal pain. **A:** Contrast-enhanced spiral CT reveals a 2-cm soft tissue mass in the portocaval region *(arrow)*, presumed to be adenopathy. **B:** A scan performed superior to **A** demonstrates that this is actually an extension to the papillary process of the caudate lobe mimicking an enlarged portocaval node. **C,D:** In another patient, its axial image suggests a node *(arrowhead)* at the porta hepatis **(C).** The sagittal reformatted image **(D)** proves the extension of caudate lobe *(arrow)* in front of IVC. (**C** and **D** courtesy of A. Shirkhoda, M.D., William Beaumont Hospital.)

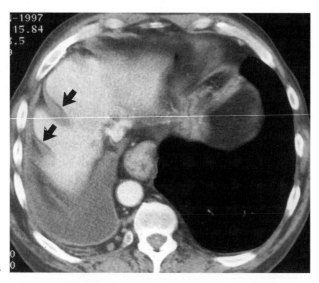
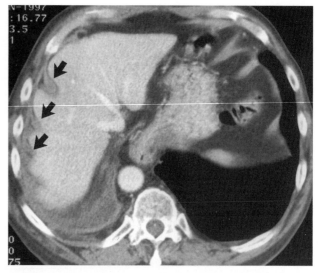

FIG. 8.6. A 73-year-old man with lung cancer. Contrast-enhanced spiral CT demonstrates prominent diaphragmatic slips *(arrows)*. A moderate right pleural effusion, right hemidiaphragm elevation, and small hiatal hernia are also present.

the bare area of the liver is in the pleural space and should not be mistaken for ascites (Fig. 8.7).

Subsegmental Anatomy

Over the past decade there has been a trend to adopt a subsegmental approach for liver anatomy. The description of the subsegmental anatomy of the liver that is commonly used today was first described in 1957 by Couinard (4) and later modified by Bismuth (5). This now serves as a system for localizing hepatic lesions and is therefore useful in preoperative planning.

In this system, the liver is divided into segments based on the distribution of portal vein branches and hepatic veins (Fig. 8.8). The caudate lobe is segment 1. There are eight segments and subsegments (2, 3, 4a, 4b, 5, 6,

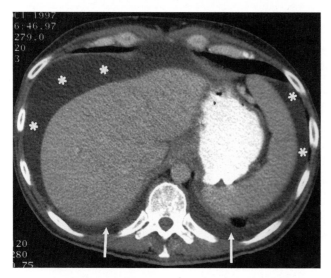

FIG. 8.7. A 47-year-old man with pancreatitis. The CT demonstrates ascites *(asterisks)* and small bilateral pleural effusions *(arrows)*. This case nicely demonstrates the CT appearance of ascites versus pleural fluid. Ascites will not extend to involve the bare area of the liver. If fluid is present adjacent to the bare area, it must be pleural.

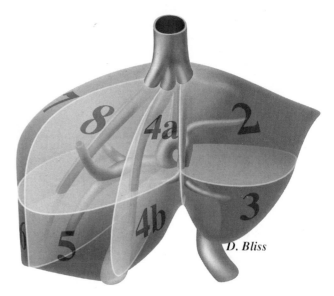

FIG. 8.8. Frontal view of subsegmental anatomy of the liver. (Soyer P, et al. Surgical Segmental Anatomy of the Liver. *Am J Roentgenol* 1994;163:99–103.)

7, and 8), which are defined by three vertical planes and one horizontal plane. The first vertical plane contains the middle hepatic vein and divides the liver into the right and left lobes. The second vertical plane contains the right hepatic vein and divides the right hepatic lobe into anterior and posterior segments. The third vertical plane contains the left hepatic vein and separates the left hepatic lobe into the medial and lateral segments. The segments are then divided into subsegments by a transverse plane, which is drawn through the main right and left portal vein branches.

Application of this hepatic subsegmental terminology to standard axial CT slices can been difficult. However, computer-based tools for teaching the segmental anatomy of the liver have been developed and appear to be an effective interactive method to teach three-dimensional subsegmental liver anatomy and how to apply this to standard axial CT slices (6).

Anatomic Variants/Anatomic Anomalies

Agenesis/Hypoplasia

The size and shape of the liver vary in normal individuals. Both agenesis and hypoplasia can affect the right or left hepatic lobes. Congenital absence of the left lobe of the liver is a rare anomaly that is defined as the absence of liver tissue to the left of the gallbladder fossa. It is typically associated with hyperplasia of the right hepatic lobe (7), an accessory lobe (8), or hyperplasia of the caudate lobe (9). Agenesis of the right lobe of the liver has also been reported but is very rare. It is thought to be a developmental anomaly and may be associated with absence of the right hemidiaphragm. These entities are distinct from atrophy of the hepatic lobes, which may occur in cirrhosis or after radiation (Fig. 8.9).

Riedel's Lobe

Riedel's lobe is a common anatomic anomaly in which an accessory lobe extends inferiorly from the right hepatic lobe along the paracolic gutter into the iliac fossa (1). This occurs more commonly in asthenic women and is usually asymptomatic but may be mistaken for hepatomegaly on physical exam (Fig. 8.10).

Left Lobe Variations

There is significant variation in the size and configuration of the left hepatic lobe. It may be quite large and extend into the left upper quadrant, abutting the spleen and mimicking splenomegaly, splenic mass, splenic laceration, or perisplenic pathology. It may also rarely extend inferiorly to the level of the pelvic brim, similar to Riedel's lobe on the right (1).

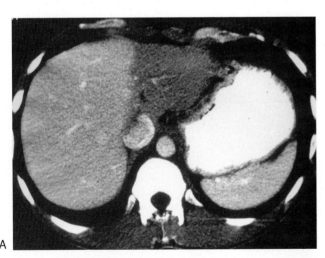 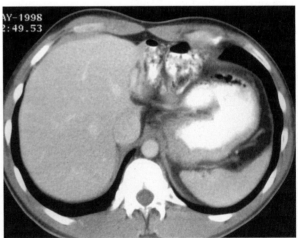

FIG. 8.9. A 30-year-old man following radiation therapy for Hodgkin's lymphoma. **A:** There is diffuse decreased attenuation noted in the left hepatic lobe without evidence of mass effect. Normal vessels can be seen within this area, compatible with fatty infiltration as a result of radiation. **B:** Repeat CT obtained 19 months after **A** demonstrates marked atrophy of the left lobe, also a result of the radiation. (Courtesy of A. Shirkhoda, M.D., William Beaumont Hospital).

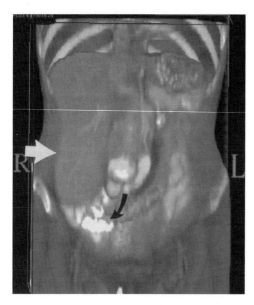

FIG. 8.10. A 64-year-old thin woman with a palpable mass in the right lower quadrant. Enhanced spiral CT with 3-D volume rendering in the coronal plane shows a prominent right hepatic lobe *(straight arrow)* extending below the right iliac crest and displacing the right kidney *(curved arrow)* inferiorly. Liver function tests were normal. This is an example of a prominent Riedel's lobe.

Diaphragmatic Slips

The diaphragm typically has a smooth surface. If there are abnormalities in the diaphragmatic muscles such as eventration, scalloping, or tenting, it can indent the liver surface or create furrows (10,11). Diaphragmatic inden-

tation of the liver increases with age and can be seen in 71% of patients over age 80. These have a characteristic appearance on CT and should not be mistaken for hepatic pathology (Fig. 8.6). Diaphragmatic slips may be especially prominent in patients with hyperinflation of the lungs secondary to emphysema. (See Chapter 5)

Chilaiditi's Syndrome

Hepatodiaphragmatic interposition (Chilaiditi's syndrome) is an anomaly in which a portion of the colon is interposed between the liver and the right hemidiaphragm. Although this is typically an incidental finding and of no clinical significance, it may occasionally be associated with nonspecific gastrointestinal symptoms (12). Rarely, surgical intervention has been necessary for volvulus (13). Bowel loops may also be interposed between the anterior liver and the abdominal wall, simulating free peritoneal air (Fig. 8.11).

Accessory Hepatic Lobes

Accessory lobes of the liver are usually attached to the inferior liver surface and are comprised of normal liver parenchyma with blood vessels and bile ducts. They are asymptomatic and usually an incidental finding but, if pedunculated, can mimic a mass or adenopathy (11,14, 15) (Fig. 8.12). There is an increased incidence of accessory hepatic lobes in patients with congenital defects in the anterior abdominal wall (i.e., omphalocele) (16).

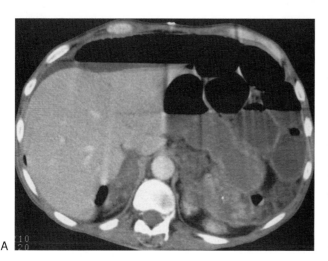
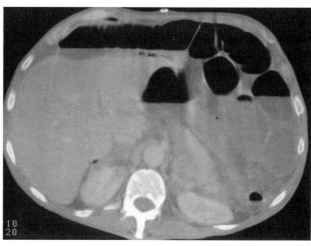

FIG. 8.11. A 64-year-old man with abdominal pain 2 days after splenectomy for polycythemia vera. Enhanced spiral CT demonstrates ascites and moderate dilation of fluid-filled small bowel loops. There is interposition of a bowel loop anterior to the liver. **A:** This can simulate pneumoperitoneum on the soft tissue windows. **B:** Images obtained with lung windows demonstrate that the air is actually within a bowel loop.

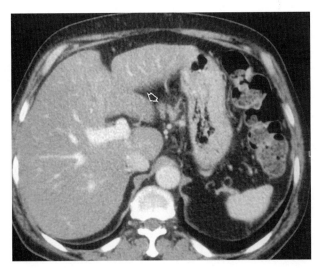

FIG. 8.12. Helical CT with intravenous and oral contrast demonstrates a small accessory lobe from the left hepatic lobe *(arrow)*. Accessory lobes are rare. (Courtesy of A. Shirkhoda, M.D., William Beaumont Hospital.)

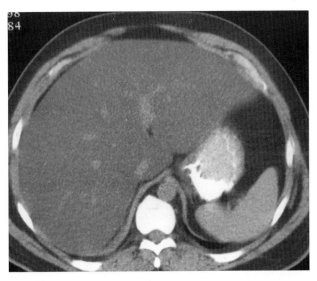

FIG. 8.13. A 33-year-old diabetic man with abdominal pain. Spiral CT with oral contrast only demonstrates diffuse low attenuation of the liver, compatible with fatty infiltration. The intrahepatic vessels are well visualized and appear high attenuation relative to the fatty infiltrated liver.

Spiral Computed Tomography and Normal Enhancement of the Liver

Technique

Spiral CT of the liver is usually performed after the administration of intravenous contrast. Typically, 120 cc of Omnipaque 350 is injected at a rate of 2 to 3 cc/sec. It is important to note that CT technique differs for a screening study of the liver as compared to a scan performed to characterize a known lesion. For evaluation of a possible liver mass, a dedicated multiple-phase spiral CT can be performed through the liver with additional delayed scans as needed. A 3- to 5-mm slice thickness is used with a pitch of 1 to 1.5 and a reconstruction interval of 3 mm. In situations where there is a known liver mass that requires further characterization of enhancement patterns (i.e., hemangioma or FNH), sequentially timed CT images are obtained over the lesion for a period of 3 to 10 minutes after the administration of intravenous contrast. This technique allows close observation of the dynamic enhancement pattern of the lesion, which frequently allows a specific diagnosis to be made.

Noncontrast Scans

On noncontrast scans, the attenuation of normal liver ranges between 40 and 60 HU. The attenuation of the liver is typically 10 to 15 HU greater than that of the spleen. If the attenuation is less than that of the spleen, fatty infiltration should be suspected (Fig. 8.13). If liver attenuation is increased, conditions such as hemochromatosis, hemosiderosis, or prior Thoratrast administration should be considered (Fig. 8.14). The presence of calcification can easily be recognized on the noncontrast

study and is usually related to granulomatous diseases such as TB or histoplasmosis. However, a variety of other entities can result in liver calcification, including infarct, abscess, and tumors (Fig. 8.15).

Normal intrahepatic vessels are typically visible on noncontrast scans and should not be mistaken for liver masses (1). These will enhance after IV contrast.

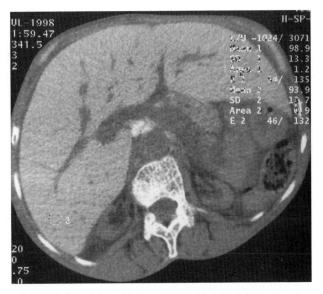

FIG. 8.14. A 46-year-old woman with sickle cell disease and renal failure. The liver demonstrates increased attenuation (94 to 99 HU) on this noncontrast scan, as a result of iron deposition from multiple transfusions. The native kidneys are small, compatible with renal failure.

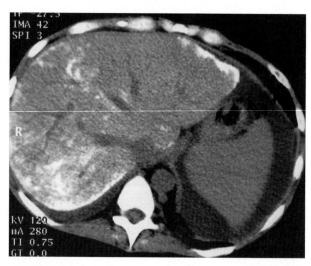

FIG. 8.15. A 42-year-old woman with a history of multiple hepatic infarcts after liver transplant. Noncontrast CT demonstrates extensive calcification in the periphery of the liver.

Enhanced Scans

Arterial Phase

The development of faster scanners now allows imaging during the arterial phase of liver enhancement. This typically occurs at a scan delay of 25 to 30 seconds and reflects enhancement of the liver by the hepatic artery. Imaging of the liver during the hepatic arterial phase will result in little enhancement of the liver parenchyma, as only 25% of its blood is supplied by the hepatic artery. Therefore, there will be minimal enhancement of the liver parenchyma, but the hepatic artery and its branches will appear enhanced. At this time, the portal and hepatic veins are often unopacified and can be mistaken for lesions unless additional scans are performed (Fig. 8.16). Conversely, small hypovascular liver lesions may not be appreciated on arterial-phase scans. Thus, hepatic-arterial phase imaging is usually performed with imaging in the portal venous phase, which allows better evaluation of the liver vasculature and other intraabdominal organs (17).

Imaging during the arterial phase is especially useful for hypervascular tumors that receive their blood supply from the hepatic artery (hepatocellular carcinomas, metastases from renal carcinoma, etc.). These hypervascular tumors will enhance against a minimally enhancing background. Numerous articles have carefully defined the specific advantages of CT scanning in arterial phase. For example, in the evaluation of suspected hepatoma, Hwang et al. noted that in 81 hepatocellular carcinomas, the arterial-phase images detected a statistically significant larger number of tumors compared with portal-phase and delayed-phase images (18). Arterial-phase imaging is also crucial when evaluating the liver for vascular metastases from primaries such as renal cell carcinoma, carcinoid, or islet cell tumors (Fig. 8.17). One potential pitfall in arterial-phase imaging, however, is that small hemangiomas may "fill in" quickly and simulate a vascular metastasis (Fig. 8.18). Our experience is that this is rare and only occurs with hemangiomas in the 1-cm size range. Similarly, small hepatic artery aneurysms may simulate vascular metastases on arterial-phase imaging (Fig. 8.19).

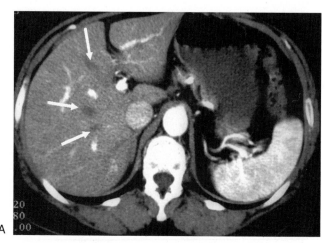

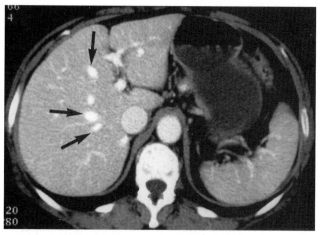

A   B

FIG. 8.16. A 58-year-old woman with colon cancer. Contrast-enhanced spiral CT performed during the arterial phase demonstrates multiple low-attenuation lesions in the liver *(arrows)*, which represent unopacified hepatic veins. These should not be mistaken for metastases. If there is concern, additional scans should be performed in the portal phase to confirm that these lesions are definitely vascular structures.

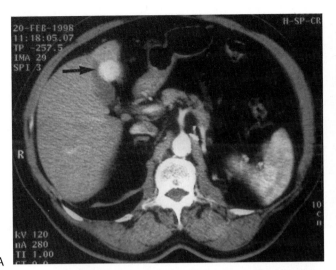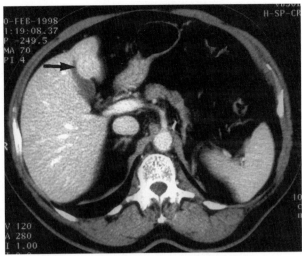

A
B

FIG. 8.17. A 72-year-old man after a left nephrectomy for renal cell carcinoma. Enhanced spiral CT performed in the arterial phase demonstrates a densely enhancing mass in the left hepatic lobe compatible with metastasis. The mass is barely visible in the portal phase.

In scanning during the arterial phase of liver enhancement, foci of liver can demonstrate hyperenhancement. This is referred to as transient hepatic attenuation differences (THAD) (19). It has been described in many conditions that alter the balance of hepatic arterial and portal venous blood flow to a portion of the liver—arterioportal shunts, hypervascular tumors, gallbladder inflammation, hepatic congestion, systemic portal shunts, portal vein obstruction, etc. (19–22). These attenuation differences may be anatomic and follow a lobar, segmental, or subsegmental distribution or, alternatively, in cases such as hepatic congestion, the defect may not follow any obvious anatomic distribution. Occasionally, THAD may appear very focal and can mimic a hypervascular tumor.

On enhanced spiral CT, THAD appears as an area of increased enhancement of the liver on arterial scans that often persists in the portal phase (Fig. 8.20). This may not be as apparent on noncontrast or delayed scans.

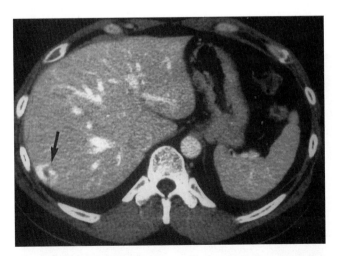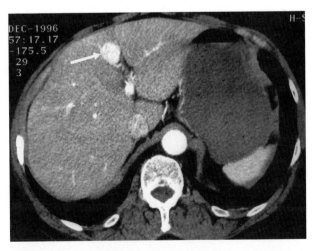

FIG. 8.18. A 45-year-old woman. Early-phase imaging after intravenous contrast demonstrates a vascular mass in the posterior segment of the right hepatic lobe *(arrow)*. This was proven to be a hemangioma. Small hemangiomas may enhance quickly, mimicking a small hepatoma or vascular metastasis.

FIG. 8.19. A 66-year-old man with abdominal pain. Early-phase spiral CT after intravenous contrast demonstrates a 2-cm densely enhancing mass *(arrow)* adjacent to a branch of the left hepatic artery. Three-dimensional reformatting (not shown) confirmed this to be an aneurysm.

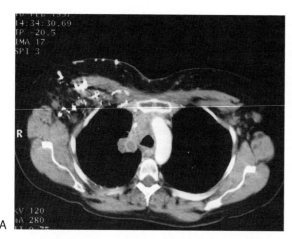
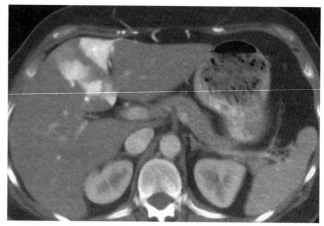

FIG. 8.20. A 47-year-old woman with lung cancer. **A:** Contrast-enhanced spiral CT of the chest demonstrates a 2×3-cm mass in the medial right upper lobe with bulky adenopathy in the right peritracheal and pretracheal regions. The mass encases the superior vena cava, resulting in numerous small chest wall collaterals. **B:** Contrast-enhanced spiral CT of the abdomen reveals dense enhancement of the medial segment of the left hepatic lobe and numerous collateral vessels in the abdominal mass, compatible with collateral venous drainage secondary to the superior vena cava obstruction.

Portal Phase

Conventional contrast-enhanced CT is performed during the portal venous phase of hepatic enhancement, which allows good detection of hypovascular liver tumors and metastases (Fig. 8.21). At this time, the liver parenchyma is enhanced significantly, as 75% to 80% of its blood is supplied by the portal vein. The portal and hepatic veins will be opacified. This is not the optimal phase to image vascular tumors, as both the tumors and the liver parenchyma will be enhanced. Several recent articles have addressed the potential pitfalls of imaging during the portal phase. Hwang et al. found that in 81 cases of hepatoma, 35% would be missed if imaging were performed only in the portal phase (18). Paulson et al. found that 28 (13.6%) of 206 metastases from carcinoid tumor were identified only on the arterial-phase scans (23). Also, Kuszyk et al. reported than although portal-phase imaging was sensitive for detecting hepatic tumors (primary tumors and metastases) greater than 1 cm, it is relatively insensitive for tumors less than 1 cm (24). Therefore, in cases of vascular primary tumors or vascular metastases, portal-phase imaging alone is inadequate.

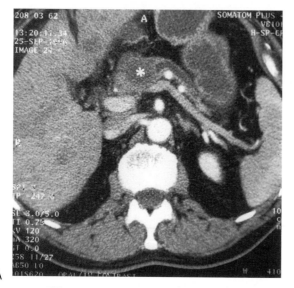
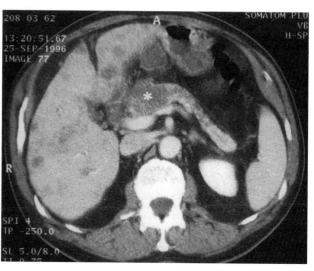

FIG. 8.21. A 70-year-old man with metastatic pancreatic cancer. Enhanced spiral CT was performed in the arterial **(A)** and portal **(B)** phases. There are numerous low-attenuation lesions in the liver compatible with metastases. Notice that the lesions are much easier to detect on the portal-phase images. A 3-cm mass is also noted in the pancreas *(asterisk),* causing ductal dilation.

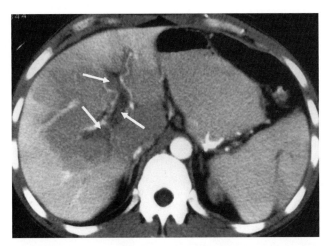

FIG. 8.22. A 44-year-old man with a history of pancreatitis presents with abdominal pain. Contrast-enhanced spiral CT demonstrates portal vein thrombosis involving both the right and left branches *(arrows)*. There is decreased enhancement of the central region of the liver as a result of the portal vein thrombosis. The superior mesenteric and splenic veins were also thrombosed (not shown).

During the portal phase, the liver should enhance homogeneously. If there is an obstruction to blood flow to the liver (e.g., portal vein thrombosis) or away from the liver (e.g., Budd-Chiari, severe heart failure), the liver may demonstrate mottled enhancement or perfusion defects that can mimic infiltrating tumor (Fig. 8.22). Delayed scans may be helpful in these cases.

Delayed Phase

If specific liver pathology is suspected or for better characterization of a liver mass (e.g., hemangioma),

delayed scans through the liver can be obtained. Delayed images may be valuable in detecting intrahepatic or hilar cholangiocarcinomas, which may demonstrate delayed enhancement on CT scans (Fig. 8.23). Keogan et al. found that this delayed enhancement was optimally detected if the patient was scanned 10 to 20 minutes after injection (25).

Imaging Pitfalls

Fatty Infiltration

Fatty infiltration of the liver is associated with obesity, alcohol use, diabetes, steroid use, hyperalimentation, and malnutrition. On early-phase spiral CT, the density of the liver may appear low in attenuation because of incomplete liver enhancement. It may be difficult in these cases to compare the liver/spleen attenuation, and therefore, comparison with muscle as an internal standard is necessary. On CT, fatty liver will appear homogeneously or heterogeneously low in attenuation (see Fig. 8.13). Lesion detection in a fatty liver may be challenging because the contrast between the low-attenuation lesions and liver is often decreased.

Because of differences in perfusion, fatty infiltration of the liver may occasionally appear regional or focal (Figs. 8.24 and 8.25). This should not be mistaken for a liver mass or infarction (Fig 8.26). In cases of fatty infiltration, the normal vessels can be seen coursing through the affected area, and there should be no mass effect. However, when focal fat appears as a small nodule, it can be confused with a hepatic mass or metastases (26,27). Focal fatty changes commonly occur adjacent to the falciform ligament, a watershed area of the arterial blood supply (Fig. 8.27) (27,28).

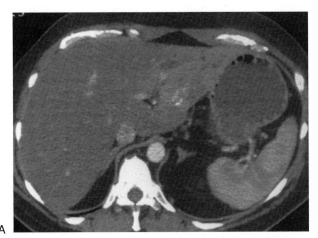 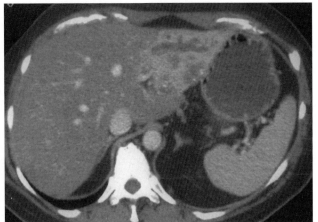

A B

FIG. 8.23. A 57-year-old woman with cholangiocarcinoma. Enhanced spiral CT was performed in the arterial and portal phases **(A,B)**. A 4-cm enhancing mass was detected near the left portal vein (not shown). The central mass results in left intrahepatic ductal dilation and a transient hyperattenuation defect in the lateral segment of the left hepatic lobe. This is more striking on portal or delayed scans **(B)**.

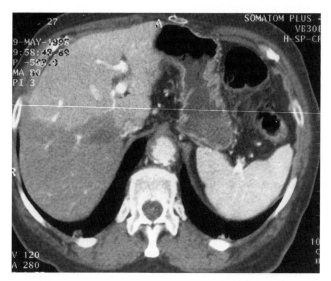

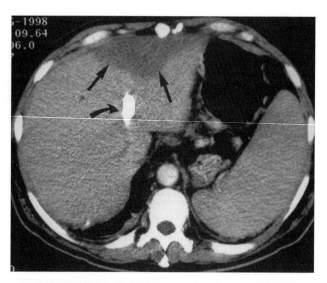

FIG. 8.24. A 78-year-old woman with uncontrollable hypertension. The study was performed to evaluate for possible aortic dissection. There is diffuse decreased attenuation noted in the posterior segment of the right hepatic lobe without evidence of mass effect. Normal vessels can be seen within this area compatible with fatty infiltration. Moderate atherosclerotic plaque with ulceration is present in the aorta.

FIG. 8.26. A 45-year-old man with cirrhosis and portal hypertension, 2 days after placement of TIPS catheter. There is a peripheral wedged-shaped region of decreased attenuation in the left lobe of the liver *(arrows),* compatible with infarct. No vessels can be seen within this area. The TIPS catheter *(curved arrow)* is also identified.

Occasionally, nonuniform fatty infiltration of the liver may simulate a space-occupying mass because of focal areas of fat sparing (Fig. 8.28), which are especially common in the periportal region. When further radiologic imaging is necessary to distinguish focal fat or fat sparing from a mass lesion, ultrasound or MRI can be helpful. Occasionally, percutaneous biopsy may be needed.

Radiation Injury to the Liver

The liver may be included in the radiation field during therapy for a primary hepatic mass (e.g., hepatoma) or tumors in adjacent organs (e.g., mass of the lower lung or pancreas). One potential pitfall in these cases can occur. On early-phase imaging, enhancement of the portion of the liver in the radiation field may be less than the adjacent nonirradiated liver and may, therefore, simulate focal fatty replacement or mass. If noncontrast images or equilibrium-phase (delayed) images are obtained, this attenuation difference will not be appreciated. In patients with mild radiation-induced hepatic injury, there may be minimal elevation of the liver enzymes. Chronic changes from radiation therapy include fat infiltration and atrophy (see Fig. 8.9).

Fluid Collections

Loculated fluid in the hepatic fissures or recesses and periportal edema (Fig. 8.29) can be mistaken for intrahepatic lesions. The radiologist must be aware of these potential pitfalls. The fissure for the ligamentum teres is in communication with the greater sac and occasionally may contain fluid. Fluid may also accumulate in the fissure for the ligamentum venosum, which is in communication with the lesser and greater sac. Fluid can accumulate in the fissure for the gallbladder as a complication of cholecystectomy, and intraperitoneal fluid can accumulate in the potential space created by the transverse fissure. The radiologist must be careful not to mistake these for focal intrahepatic tumors or abscesses (29).

Fluid that accumulates near the right lobe of the liver can potentially be in three distinct spaces: pleural, sub-

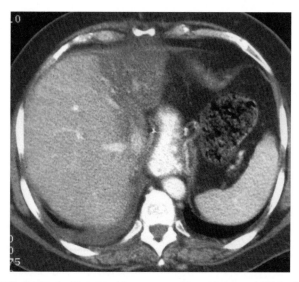

FIG. 8.25. A 48-year-old woman with a history of Whipple surgery and radiation therapy for pancreatic cancer. The medial portion of the liver appears shrunken with decreased attenuation, compatible with fatty infiltration caused by radiation injury. Normal vessels are identified coursing through the region.

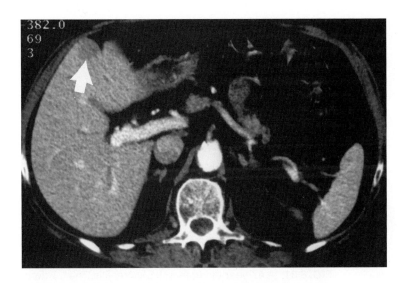

FIG. 8.27. A 55-year-old man with colon cancer. Enhanced spiral CT demonstrates a focal area of decreased attenuation *(arrow)* in the liver adjacent to the falciform ligament. This is a result of focal fat deposition and should not be mistaken for a primary or metastatic mass.

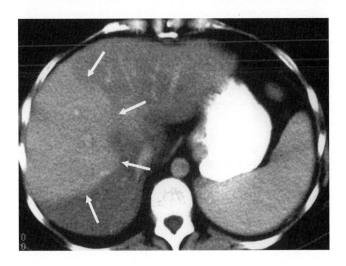

FIG. 8.28. A 34-year-old man with colon cancer. Contrast-enhanced spiral CT demonstrates fatty infiltration of the liver with relative sparing of the anterior segment of the right hepatic lobe *(arrows).* Surgical clips are present in the porta compatible with cholecystectomy. There is also moderate splenomegaly.

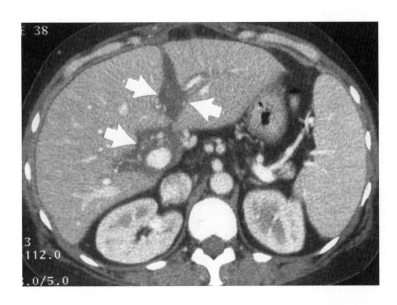

FIG. 8.29. A 45-year-old woman after liver transplant. Contrast-enhanced spiral CT reveals moderate periportal edema *(arrows).* This should not be mistaken for biliary ductal dilation. Unlike ductal dilation, periportal edema will be present on both sides of the portal vein.

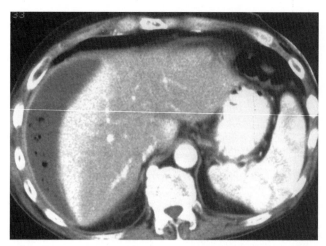

FIG. 8.30. A 57-year-old man with fever after laparoscopic cholecystectomy. There is a large subcapsular hepatic fluid collection containing air. This is consistent with a subcapsular abscess, which is compressing the adjacent parenchyma, resulting in increased attenuation.

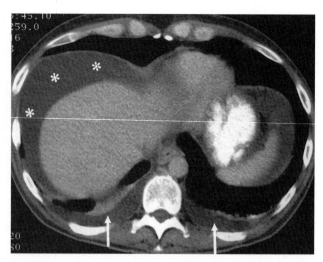

FIG. 8.31. A 47-year-old man with pancreatitis. The CT demonstrates ascites *(asterisks),* small bilateral pleural effusions *(arrows),* and minimal atelectasis at the right lung base. Perihepatic ascites will form a crescent shape and will not compress the parenchyma.

capsular, or perihepatic. Fluid in the right pleural space will layer posteriorly when the patient is supine and will accumulate in the posterior costophrenic angle. On an abdominal scan, fluid will be seen in the bare area of the liver, which identifies it as being in the right pleural space, and ascites can not accumulate here (see Fig. 8.7). Subcapsular fluid is fluid that is under the liver capsule and will compress the adjacent liver parenchyma (Fig. 8.30). Perihepatic fluid is often seen in patients with ascites and simply represents free fluid that is located near the liver.

It will often assume a crescent configuration and should not exert mass effect on the liver (Fig. 8.31).

Artifacts

Partial Volume Effects

Partial volume artifacts can occur anywhere in the body when two adjacent tissues differ significantly in attenuation because each CT pixel value is a function of

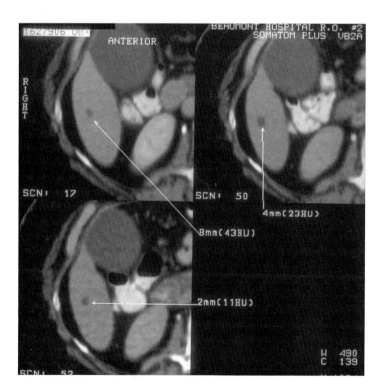

FIG. 8.32. There is a 1-cm cyst in the posterior segment of the right hepatic lobe. This figure illustrates the principle of volume averaging. Volume averaging may be reduced by decreasing the slice thickness to a point at which the real attenuation value is obtained. (Courtesy of A. Shirkhoda, M.D., William Beaumont Hospital).

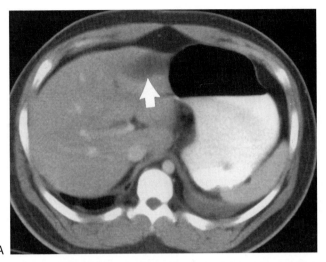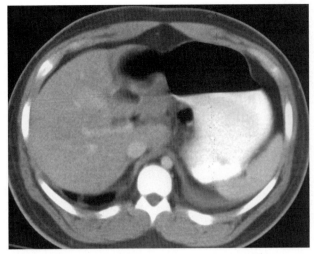

A

B

FIG. 8.33. A 16-year-old boy after a motor vehicle accident. **A:** Spiral CT demonstrates ill-defined low attenuation in the lateral segment of the left hepatic lobe. **B:** Another scan obtained 4 mm inferior to **A** demonstrates air distention of the gastric antrum. This is an example of how adjacent extrahepatic organs may appear as intrahepatic lesions secondary to partial volume effect.

the average density of the corresponding voxel. If a voxel includes tissues of differing attenuation coefficients, the resultant pixel has an intermediate attenuation value, blurring the border between the different tissues. On conventional CT, partial volume artifact can be reduced or avoided by decreasing slice thickness (Fig. 8.32). Although partial volume effects are greater with spiral CT than with conventional CT, they can be reduced by overlapping reconstructed slices. Studies have shown that the detection of a focal hepatic lesion with spiral CT can be improved by decreasing

the interscan spacing (overlapping slices) (30). Spiral CT allows extra images to be generated through the area of interest without additional radiation dose to the patient. This can essentially eliminate partial volume averaging.

Partial volume artifacts also result in the misdiagnosis of extrahepatic structures as intrahepatic lesions (Fig. 8.33). Common problem areas include confusion of large right adrenal, renal masses (Fig. 8.34) or periportal nodes with primary hepatic tumors. This problem is especially common in children or thin adults with little intra-

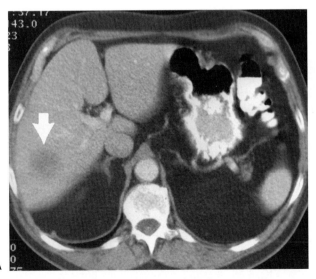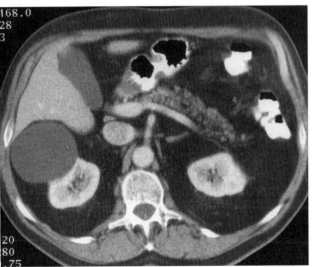

A

B

FIG. 8.34. A 70-year-old man with abdominal pain. **A:** Contrast-enhanced spiral CT demonstrates an ill-defined low-density lesion in the posterior segment of the right hepatic lobe. **B:** Scan performed inferior to **A** reveals a large right renal cyst. This is an example of how extrahepatic structures can mimic intrahepatic pathology secondary to partial volume averaging.

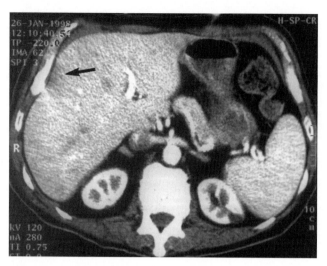

FIG. 8.35. A 70-year-old man with abdominal pain. Enhanced spiral CT reveals an ill-defined low-attenuation region *(arrow)* in the periphery of the liver, near a rib. This is an example of beam-hardening artifact and should not be mistaken for a mass.

abdominal fat. Decreasing the slice thickness or 3-D reformatting can be helpful in difficult cases.

Beam-Hardening Artifacts

Beam-hardening artifact occurs when the polychromatic x-ray beams penetrate bone and hardens (shifts to a higher mean energy). This can occur in the liver near the ribs, resulting in ill-defined low attenuation in the liver parenchyma adjacent to the lower right ribs (Fig. 8.35) or near high-density catheters or surgical clips. This artifact should not be mistaken for intrahepatic masses or lacerations. In select cases, delayed or repeat

CT scans with a higher current value can be useful in overcoming this pitfall.

PORTAL VEIN

Normal Anatomy

The portal vein receives venous drainage from the gut and delivers this blood to the liver. It is formed by the confluence of the superior mesenteric vein and splenic vein and normally supplies 70% to 75% of incoming blood to the liver. As the portal vein enters the porta hepatis, it divides into the right and left portal veins. The right portal vein subsequently divides to supply the anterior and posterior segments of the right hepatic lobe. The left portal vein has an initial horizontal segment before it divides to supply the medial and lateral segments of the left hepatic lobe. While in the porta hepatis, the portal vein lies posterior to the hepatic artery and common duct (Fig. 8.36).

Anatomic Variants

Several variations in portal venous anatomy have been described on ultrasound (US), CT, and MR. The site of the portal vein bifurcation is variable. In a study by Schultz of 31 cadavers, the bifurcation was intrahepatic in 25.8%, at the liver capsule in 25.8%, and extrahepatic in 48.4% (31). The site of bifurcation may be important for placement of intrahepatic portosystemic shunt placement, as it is an optimal site for portal vein puncture.

Trifurcation of the portal vein is the most common intrahepatic variant seen at autopsy. After entering the porta hepatis, the main portal vein immediately divides into the left, right anterior, and right posterior branches (Fig. 8.37).

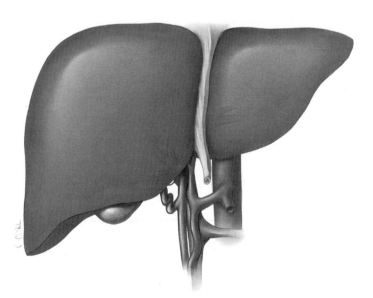

FIG. 8.36. Illustration depicting the posterior location of the portal vein in relation to hepatic artery and bile duct in the porta hepatis. Note the splenic vein crossing in front of the aorta.

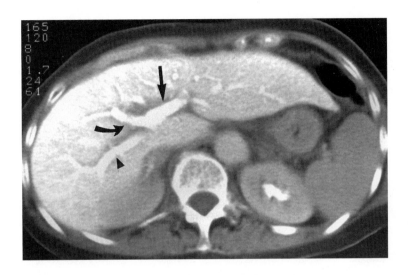

FIG. 8.37. Helical CT obtained after arterial portography at the level of the porta hepatis demonstrates trifurcation of the portal vein into the left portal vein *(straight arrow)*, right anterior portal branch *(curved arrow)*, and right posterior portal branch *(arrowhead)*. (From reference 33, with permission.)

Another anatomic variant described on US (32) and CT during arterial portography (CTAP) (33) is the absence of the horizontal segment of the left portal vein. In this variant, blood flow to the left hepatic lobe is supplied from an aberrant vessel arising from the anterior branch of the right portal vein (Fig. 8.38). This then becomes the vertical segment of the left portal vein and divides normally.

Other variants described on US and MR include origin of either the anterior or posterior segments of the right portal vein from the left portal vein and absence of the entire right portal vein, resulting in a small-appearing right lobe that receives its blood supply from multiple aberrant vessels originating from the left portal vein.

In summary, variations in portal venous anatomy are not uncommon, and identification of these variants may help to better localize lesions and aid surgical planning for tumor resection.

Imaging Pitfalls

Portal Vein Thrombosis

There are many causes of portal vein thrombosis, including cirrhosis and portal hypertension, malignancies, trauma, blood dyscrasias, sepsis, pancreatitis, appendicitis, diverticulitis, and inflammatory bowel disease. Portal vein thrombosis is also a recognized complication of liver transplant, occurring in up to 10% of orthotopic liver transplant patients.

Acute thrombus will have high attenuation (60 to 80 HU) on nonenhanced scans because of the acute clotted blood. On contrast-enhanced CT, low-attenuation intramural thrombus can be identified as a filling defect within the main portal vein and/or its branches (see Figs. 8.22 and 8.39) (34). The portal vein may appear enlarged and expanded by the thrombus. One advantage to CT, in addition to its ability to detect portal vein thrombosis, is

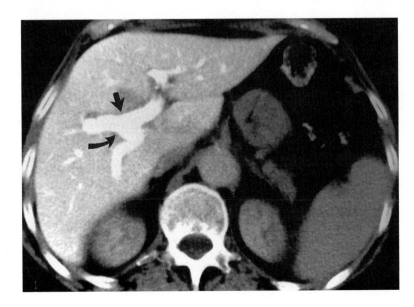

FIG. 8.38. Helical CT obtained after arterial portography shows that the left main portal vein *(straight arrow)* arises from the anterior branch of the right portal vein *(curved arrow)*. (From reference 33, with permission.)

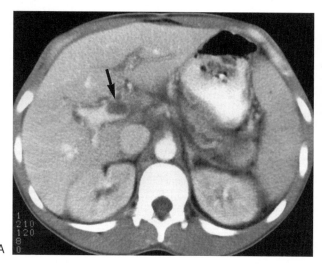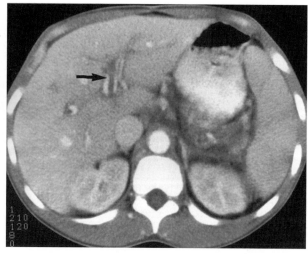

FIG. 8.39. A 32-year-old man with AIDS. Contrast-enhanced spiral CT demonstrates clot in the main portal vein that extends into the main right and left branches. The spleen is minimally enlarged.

its ability to determine the cause of the thrombosis in many instances.

The mixing of contrast-enhanced and nonenhanced blood in the portal vein during an early arterial-phase scan should not be confused with portal venous thrombus. Also, in early scanning, the hepatic artery will be enhanced, but the portal vein is not, simulating a thrombus (Fig. 8.40). Repeat, slightly delayed, images can be obtained if this is a concern. Because the portal vein is surrounded by low-attenuation fat, the appearance of portal vein clot can also be created by partial-volume effects. In these cases, overlapping scans can be reconstructed to minimize partial-volume effects.

Occasionally dilation of the hepatic artery will occur as a result of portal vein thrombus and should not be mistaken for a patent portal vein.

Cavernous Transformation

Cavernous transformation occurs when many small preexisting periportal venous collaterals form secondary to occlusion of the portal vein. This may occur in as little as 6 to 20 days postobstruction.

On contrast-enhanced CT, cavernous transformation appears as a tangle of small vessels in the porta hepatis replacing the normal architecture of the obliterated portal

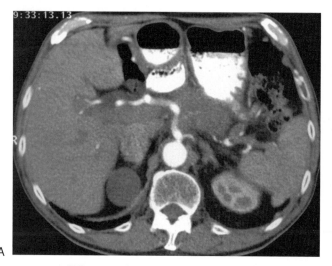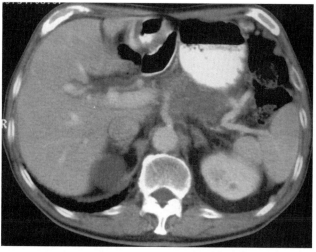

FIG. 8.40. Contrast-enhanced spiral CT performed in the arterial phase nicely demonstrates the opacified hepatic artery. Unopacified blood in the portal vein can simulate portal vein thrombus or periportal adenopathy in early-phase imaging. Scan obtained at the same level during the portal phase demonstrates normal opacification of the portal vein. A right renal cyst is also identified. (Courtesy of A. Shirkhoda, M.D., William Beaumont Hospital.)

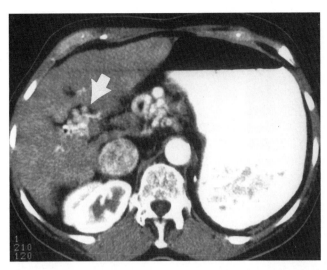

FIG. 8.41. A 55-year-old man with cirrhosis and portal hypertension. A tangle of vessels *(arrow)* are at the porta hepatis compatible with cavernous transformation. Varices are also noted in the gastrohepatic ligament. The stomach is distended.

vein (Fig. 8.41) (34). On noncontrast CT, cavernous transformation can mimic adenopathy or a mass in the porta hepatis or pancreatic head. In patients with chronic portal vein thrombosis, the portal vein may not be visualized, and only the collateral vessels can be defined.

HEPATIC ARTERY

Normal Anatomy

The hepatic artery usually lies medial to the common bile duct and anterior to the portal vein (see Fig. 8.36). It is rarely located anterior to the common duct or posterior to the portal vein.

The celiac axis branches into the common hepatic artery and the splenic artery (Fig. 8.42). The common

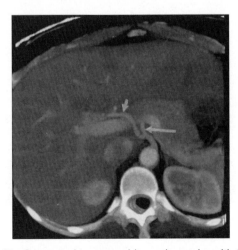

FIG. 8.42. Computed tomographic angiography with 3-D volume rendering nicely demonstrates the normal branching of the celiac axis into the hepatic artery *(short arrow)* and splenic artery *(long arrow).*

hepatic artery divides into the gastroduodenal artery and proper hepatic artery. The proper hepatic artery then bifurcates into the right and left hepatic branches, which also subdivide into segmental and subsegmental branches. However, this classic anatomy occurs in only 55% of the population (35).

Normal Variants

At least ten anatomic variations of the hepatic artery have been described at autopsy (36). With the development of spiral CT and CT angiography, it is now possible to routinely image the hepatic artery and variants (37). Therefore, the radiologist should be familiar with these variants, as variant anatomy may be clinically relevant in patients being evaluated for liver transplantation.

One variant involves the middle hepatic artery, which usually arises from the right or left hepatic artery and supplies the medial segment of the left hepatic lobe (segment 4). In approximately 10% of cases, the proper hepatic artery will trifurcate into the right, middle, and left hepatic arteries (36). Another common variant occurs when the right hepatic artery arises from the superior mesenteric artery (Fig. 8.43). Accessory hepatic arteries can arise in addition to the normal hepatic artery origin. These accessory arteries include an accessory left hepatic artery arising from the left gastric artery and an accessory right hepatic artery arising from the superior mesenteric artery. Accessory arteries are the sole blood supply to their specific areas. Combinations of replaced and accessory arteries can occur. Rarely, no hepatic arteries will arise from the celiac axis, and the hepatic trunk will arise from the superior mesenteric artery (Fig. 8.44) or left gastric artery (36). The hepatic artery may also arise directly from the aorta, adjacent to the origin of the splenic artery (Fig. 8.45).

Imaging Pitfalls

In order to optimize visualization of the hepatic artery, scanning must be performed in the arterial phase. The exam is optimized by avoiding positive oral contrast agents and using thin sections (3 mm) and narrow (1- to 3-mm) interscan spacing. Three-dimensional CT angiography is very helpful in evaluating the hepatic artery and its variants.

Hepatic Artery Thrombosis

Thrombosis of the hepatic artery may result in heterogeneous liver enhancement or discrete infarcts (see Fig. 8.26). This is most commonly a complication of surgery, including laparoscopic cholecystectomy, but may also occur in trauma.

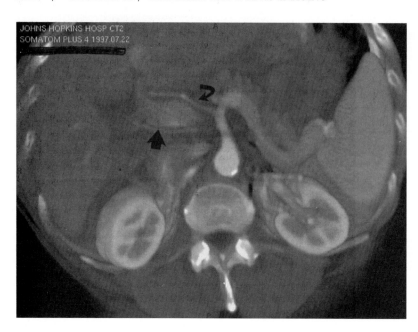

FIG. 8.43. Computed tomographic angiography with 3-D volume rendering demonstrates a small vessel *(straight arrow)* coursing behind the portal vein compatible with replaced right hepatic artery. The left hepatic artery *(curved arrow)* arises from the celiac axis and courses anterior to the portal vein.

Aneurysms

Hepatic artery aneurysm is rare and usually is a result of atherosclerotic disease. The vessel may be calcified, which aids in the diagnosis. Hepatic artery aneurysms may also occur in intravenous drug abusers or secondary to trauma. These aneurysms are typically small (<2 cm) and appear on CT as a hypervascular lesion, simulating a vascular tumor (see Fig. 8.19). Care must be taken to identify the course of the vessel to avoid a serious interpretive error. Pseudoaneurysms may appear identical to true aneurysms but are usually the result of biopsy, prior biliary catheter placement, or intra-arterial chemotherapy. Also, rarely, arterioportal fistulas may occur, usually secondary to trauma, biopsy, or surgery, and require arterial-phase imaging to optimize visualization (Fig. 8.46).

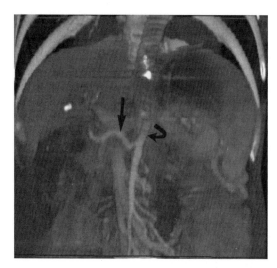

FIG. 8.44. Computed tomographic angiography with 3-D volume rendering demonstrates the common hepatic artery *(straight arrow)* arising from the superior mesenteric artery *(curved arrow)*.

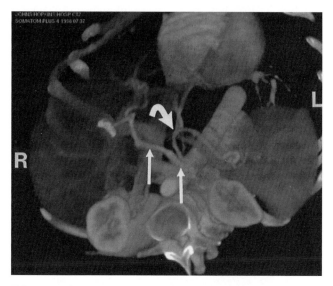

FIG. 8.45. Computed tomographic angiography with 3-D volume rendering (viewed from below) demonstrates the common hepatic artery *(straight arrows)* arising directly from the aorta. The splenic artery *(curved arrow)* has its origin from the aorta, immediately inferior to the hepatic artery origin.

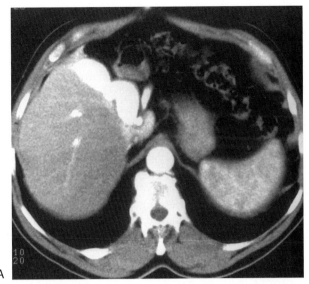
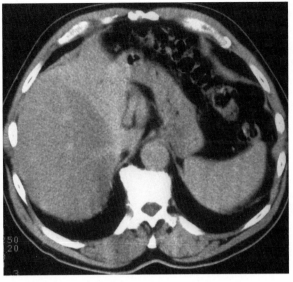

FIG. 8.46. A 66-year-old man with arterioportal fistula. Contrast-enhanced spiral CT was performed in the arterial and portal phases of liver enhancement. The vascular nature of the lesion is easily identified on the arterial-phase images. On the portal-phase images, there is minimal increased enhancement of the region, but the fistula is not visualized.

HEPATIC VEINS

Normal Anatomy

The hepatic veins constitute the venous drainage from the liver into the inferior vena cava. Classically there are three main hepatic veins (right, middle, and left), which converge and enter the IVC. This forms a "W" configuration, which can commonly be visualized on axial CT slices.

Anatomic Variants

Variations in intrahepatic portions of the hepatic veins are occasionally seen on CTAP and US (38) and are being recognized more frequently on spiral CT (33). The classic anatomy is usually present in only approximately 70% of patients. The most frequently encountered variant at CTAP is the presence of an additional inferior hepatic vein that drains segments 5 and 6 and enters the IVC caudal to the level of the three main hepatic veins (Fig. 8.47) (33). Other variants can occur such as common hepatic vein trunks (Figs. 8.48 and 8.49). Recognition of these variants is important in preoperative evaluation and surgical planning of patients with liver tumors.

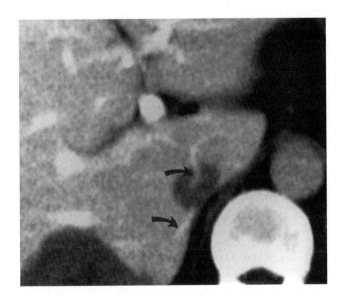

FIG. 8.47. Computed tomogram obtained after arterial portography demonstrates two small-caliber hepatic veins *(curved arrows)* joining the inferior vena cava. (From reference 33, with permission.)

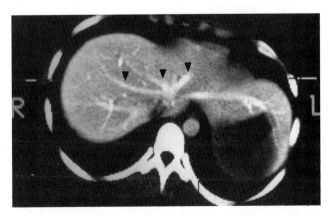

FIG. 8.48. Helical CT obtained during arterial portography demonstrates three middle hepatic veins *(arrows)* joining a common trunk as they empty into the inferior vena cava. (From reference 33, with permission.)

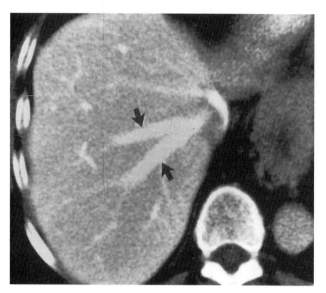

FIG. 8.49. Helical CT during arterial portography demonstrates two right hepatic veins *(arrows)* joining to form a common trunk before emptying into the inferior vena cava. (From reference 33, with permission.)

Imaging Pitfalls

Congestive Heart Failure/Passive Congestion of the Liver

During the arterial phase of liver enhancement, the hepatic veins and inferior vena cava are normally not opacified. However, in patients with cardiac dysfunction, contrast can reflux from the right atrium into the intrahepatic IVC and hepatic veins (Fig. 8.50).

Increased right-sided pressures in the heart caused by congestive heart failure or constrictive pericarditis can result in passive congestion of the liver by causing a functional obstruction to hepatic venous outflow. This condition is typically reversible with improvement of cardiac function but, in severe, prolonged cases, may result in permanent liver injury, called cardiac cirrhosis.

In cases of passive congestion, the liver will demonstrate a mottled parenchymal enhancement after intravenous contrast. The inferior vena cava and hepatic veins typically appear distended, with reflux of contrast from the right atrium into the IVC and hepatic veins (Fig. 8.51) (39). Periportal edema may also be seen in these cases. In addition to congestive heart failure, constrictive pericarditis may also result in a similar appearance because of passive congestion of liver.

Budd-Chiari Syndrome

Patients with obstruction of venous outflow from the liver, or Budd-Chiari syndrome, present with abdominal pain, hepatomegaly, and ascites. Etiologies include hepatic vein thrombosis caused by hypercoagulable states, medications, radiation, vascular webs, and invasion by tumor. The caudate lobe drains directly into the inferior vena cava and therefore may be spared in Budd-Chiari syndrome. The caudate may appear enlarged with dense enhancement (Fig. 8.52).

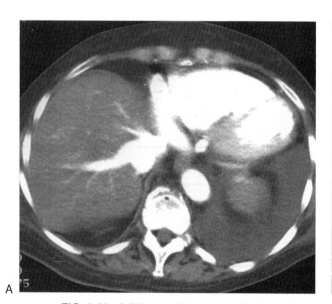

A

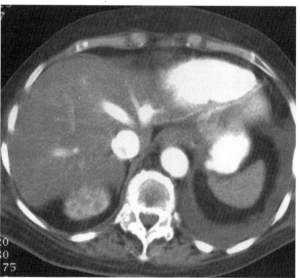

B

FIG. 8.50. A 72-year-old woman with abdominal pain. Contrast-enhanced spiral CT demonstrates cardiomegaly with marked reflux of contrast into the hepatic veins and intrahepatic inferior vena cava compatible with tricuspid regurgitation. There is also a moderate left pleural effusion.

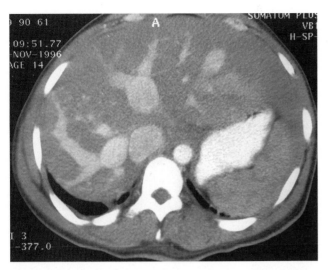

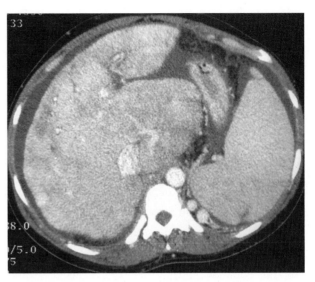

FIG. 8.51. A 55-year-old man with severe congestive heart failure. Contrast-enhanced spiral CT demonstrates marked dilation of the hepatic veins and inferior vena cava caused by right-sided heart failure.

FIG. 8.52. A 35-year-old woman with Budd-Chiari syndrome. Enhanced spiral CT demonstrates mottled enhancement of the liver and marked enlargement of the caudate lobe.

After contrast administration, there is often a "flip-flop" in liver attenuation. First, the central region of the liver will enhance, and the peripheral regions will demonstrate delayed enhancement (Fig. 8.53). On delayed images, the periphery will enhance after contrast has washed out from the central region (40,41). The CT appearance of the liver will often appear mottled, and caution is necessary not to confuse the process with an infiltrating tumor.

BILIARY DUCTS

Normal Anatomy

Intrahepatic bile ducts drain bile from the liver and empty into the right or left main hepatic ducts. They run in the portal triad adjacent to the portal vein branches and should be of water attenuation on all scans. They do not normally enhance after intravenous contrast, which allows easy differentiation from the hepatic vessels. After

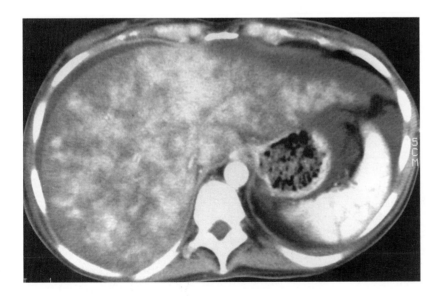

FIG. 8.53. A 45-year-old woman with Budd-Chiari syndrome. Enhanced spiral CT in the arterial phase demonstrates mottled enhancement of the liver with peripheral sparing. The inferior vena cava is compressed.

receiving drainage from the small intrahepatic ducts, the right and left hepatic ducts join to form the common hepatic duct. After the insertion of the cystic duct, the common bile duct continues inferiorly to empty into the ampulla of Vater.

In the past, visualization of intrahepatic bile ducts on CT was thought to be evidence for dilation and obstruction, as normal bile ducts were not routinely visible. However, with advancements in CT technology, it is now possible to identify normal-caliber (1- to 3-mm) intrahepatic ducts in up to 40% of patients without evidence of biliary disease (42). Recognition of this finding is important to avoid unnecessary evaluation of suspected biliary obstruction.

The extrahepatic bile ducts can be identified in most patients. In a study of 100 patients without biliary disease, the common hepatic duct was visualized in 66 patients with a mean diameter of 2.8 mm; the common bile duct was identified in 82 patients with a mean diameter of 3.6 mm (43). The normal common duct diameter is usually less than 8 mm (44), although 8 to 10 mm is typically considered indeterminate (45). Normal hepatic ducts show gradual tapering.

The wall of the extrahepatic bile ducts should measure less than 1.5 mm in thickness (43). Enhancement of the duct wall can occur in patients without biliary disease and alone is not indicative of pathology.

Normal Variants

Although normal variations in bile duct branching do exist, they are not typically visualized on CT.

Imaging Pitfalls

Pneumobilia

Following either surgical bypass or sphincterotomy or after ERCP, it is not uncommon to see air in the biliary tree (pneumobilia). The branching pattern is consistent with the anatomy of the biliary system (Fig. 8.54). Occasionally air may be present in the biliary tree as a result of the passage of a common duct stone. A potential pitfall is the misdiagnosis of pneumoperitoneum with extension of air into the porta as pneumobilia (Fig. 8.55). Another potential pitfall is the differentiation of pneumobilia from air in the portal venous system (Fig. 8.56). Portal venous air is often an ominous sign in patients with infarcted bowel. However, other causes of portal venous air have been reported, including recent surgery or tube placement (including G-tube). Portal venous air typically has a distinct branching pattern and will extend to the periphery of the liver, unlike biliary air.

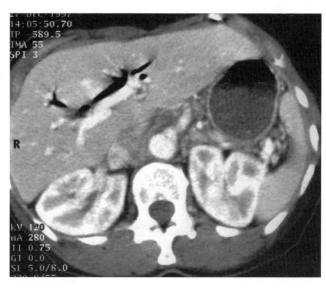

FIG. 8.54. A 45-year-old man after sphincterotomy. Enhanced spiral CT demonstrates moderate central pneumobilia.

Periportal Halo

Fluid or dilated lymphatics in the loose connective tissue of the porta triads can result in the appearance of a periportal halo. This appears as low attenuation adjacent to the portal vein branches and can be mistaken for biliary ductal dilation. However, periportal edema typically appears on both sides of the portal vein branch, whereas bile ducts run along only one side (Figs. 8.57 and 8.58) (43,46). This is an important distinctive feature. Although the CT finding of periportal edema is nonspecific, it is abnormal and commonly seen in patients with congestive

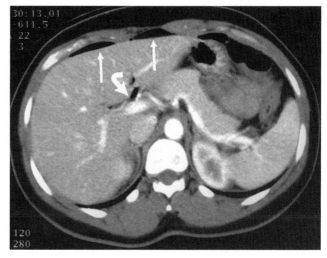

FIG. 8.55. A 29-year-old woman 2 days following laparoscopy. Contrast-enhanced spiral CT reveals pneumoperitoneum *(straight arrows)*. Free air tracks into the porta *(curved arrow)* mimicking pneumobilia.

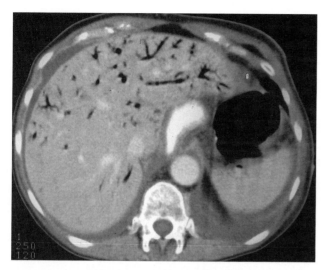

FIG. 8.56. A 59-year-old woman with ischemic bowel and portal venous air. Air in the portal venous system will be seen toward the liver periphery in contrast to pneumobilia, which is usually central.

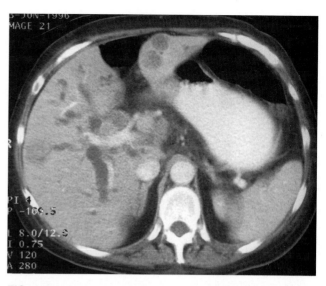

FIG. 8.58. A 55-year-old woman with cholangiocarcinoma. Enhanced spiral CT demonstrates significant intrahepatic ductal dilation. Note that in contrast to periportal edema, dilated ducts will be seen on one side of portal vein branches.

heart failure, hepatitis, liver transplant recipients, or after liver trauma. Patients with periportal adenopathy or tumors may also demonstrate a periportal halo from central obstruction of lymphatics. When a periportal halo is identified on CT, it should prompt careful evaluation for occult liver disease (47).

Periportal Fat

Periportal fat also appears as low-attenuation material adjacent to the portal vessels but should not be mistaken for dilated central bile ducts. The periportal fat will not extend into the liver parenchyma beyond the proximal portal veins.

CONCLUSION

Spiral CT has revolutionized imaging of the liver and is currently considered the imaging modality of choice for suspected liver disease. It is important for the radiologist to be familiar with the normal CT appearance of the liver and hepatic vessels and be able to recognize common anatomic variants. In addition, both conventional and spiral CT can result in various pitfalls that, if not recognized, can result in misinterpretation. This chapter discusses and illustrates a variety of these potential pitfalls and provides suggestions to avoid them.

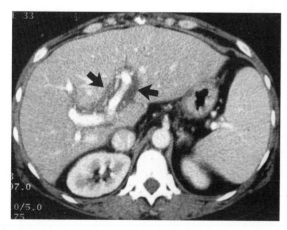

FIG. 8.57. A 38-year-old woman after liver transplant. Contrast-enhanced spiral CT reveals moderate periportal edema *(arrows)*. This should not be mistaken for biliary ductal dilation. Unlike ductal dilation, periportal edema will be present on both sides of the portal vein.

REFERENCES

1. Kasales CJ, Patel S, Hopper KD, et al. Imaging variants of the liver, pancreas and spleen. *Crit Rev Diagn Imag* 1994;35:485–543.
2. Donoso L, Martinez-Noguera A, Zidan A, Lora F. Papillary process of the caudate lobe of the liver: sonographic appearance. *Radiology* 1989; 173:631–633.
3. Auh YH, Rosen A, Rubenstein WA, et al. CT of the papillary process of the caudate lobe. *Am J Roentgenol* 1984;142:535–538.
4. Couinard C. *Le foie: Etudes anatomiques et chirurgicales.* Paris: Masson, 1957.
5. Bismuth H. Surgical anatomy and anatomic surgery of the liver. *World J Surg* 1982;:3–9.
6. Kuszyk BS, Calhoun PS, Soyer PA, Fishman EK. An interactive computer-based tool for teaching the segmental anatomy of the liver: usefulness in the education of residents and fellows. *Am J Roentgenol* 1997;169:631–634.
7. Merrill GG. Complete absence of the left lobe of the liver. *Arch Pathol* 1946;42:232–233.
8. Llorente J, Dardik H. Symptomatic accessory lobe of the liver associated with absence of the left lobe. *Arch Surg* 1971;102:221–223.
9. Yamamoto S, Kojoh K, Saito I, et al. Computer tomography of congenital absence of the left lobe of the liver. *J Comput Assist Tomogr* 1988;12:206–208.
10. Rosen A, Auh Y, Rubenstein W, et al. CT appearance of diaphragmatic pseudotumors. *J Comput Assist Tomogr* 1983;7:995–999.

11. Shirkhoda A. Diagnostic pitfalls in abdominal CT. *RadioGraphics* 1991;11:969–1002.
12. Risaliti A, De Anna D, Terrosu G, et al. Chilaiditi's syndrome as a surgical and nonsurgical problem. *Surg Gynecol Obstet* 1993;176:55–58.
13. Orangio GR, Fazio VW, Winkelman E, McGonagle BA. The Chilaiditi syndrome and associated volvulus of the transverse colon. An indication for surgical therapy. *Dis Colon Rectum* 1986;29:653–656.
14. Hashimoto M, Oomachi K, Watarai J. Accessory lobe of the liver mimicking a mass in the left adrenal gland. A case report. *Acta Radiol* 1997;38:309–310.
15. Kakitsubata Y, Kakitsubata S, Asada K, Ochiai R, Watanabe K. MR imaging of anamalous lobes of the liver. *Acta Radiol* 1993;34:417–419.
16. Sanguesa C, Esteban MJ, Gomez J, Cotina H. Liver accessory lobe torsion in the infant. *Pediatr Radiol* 1995;25:153–154.
17. Oliver JH 3d, Baron RL. Helical biphasic contrast-enhanced CT of the liver: technique, indications, interpretation, and pitfalls. *Radiology* 1996;201:1–14.
18. Hwang GJ, Kim MJ, Yoo HS, Lee JT. Nodular hepatocellular carcinomas: detection with arterial-, portal-, and delayed-phase images at spiral CT. *Radiology* 1997;202:383–388.
19. Itai Y, Moss A, Goldberg H. Transient hepatic attenuation difference of lobar or segmental distribution detected by dynamic computed tomography. *Radiology* 1982;144:835–839.
20. Ito K, Awaya H, Mitchell DG, et al. Gallbladder disease: appearance of associated transient increased attenuation in the liver at biphasic, contrast-enhanced dynamic CT. *Radiology* 1997;204:723–728.
21. Yamashita K, Jin MJ, Hirose Y, et al. CT finding of transient focal increased attenuation of the liver adjacent to the gallbladder in acute cholecystitis. *Am J Roentgenol* 1995;164:343–346.
22. Itai Y, Hachiya J, Makita K, et al. Transient hepatic attenuation differences on dynamic computed tomography. *J Comput Assist Tomogr* 1987;11:461–465.
23. Paulson EK, McDermott VG, Keogan MT, et al. Carcinoid metastases to the liver: role of triple-phase helical CT. *Radiology* 1998;206:143–150.
24. Kuszyk BS, Bluemke DA, Urban BA, et al. Portal-phase contrast enhanced helical CT for detection of malignant hepatic tumors: sensitivity based on comparison with intraoperative and pathologic findings. *Am J Roentgenol* 1996;166:91–95.
25. Keogan M, Seabourn J, Paulson E, et al. Contrast-enhanced CT of intrahepatic and hilar cholangiocarcinoma: delay time for optimal imaging. *Am J Roentgenol* 1997;169:1493–1499.
26. Yates C, Streight R. Focal fatty infiltration of the liver simulating metastatic disease. *Radiology* 1986;159:83–84.
27. Yoshikawa J, Matsui O, Takashima T, et al. Focal fatty change of the liver adjacent to the falciform ligament: CT and sonographic findings in five surgically confirmed cases. *Am J Roentgenol* 1987;149:491–494.
28. Brawer M, Austin G, Lewin K. Focal fatty change of the liver: a hitherto poorly recognized entity. *Gastroenterology* 1980;78:247–252.
29. Auh YH, Lim JH, Kim KW, et al. Loculated fluid collections in hepatic fissures and recesses: CT appearance and potential pitfalls. *RadioGraphics* 1994;14:529–540.
30. Urban BA, Fishman EK, Kuhlman JE, et al. Detection of focal hepatic lesions with spiral CT: comparison of 4- and 9-mm interspace scanning. *Am J Roentgenol* 1993;160:783–785.
31. Schultz SR, LaBerge JM, Gordon RL, Warren RS. Anatomy of the portal vein bifurcation: intra- versus extrahepatic location—implications for transjugular intrahepatic portosystemic shunts. *J Vasc Interv Radiol* 1994;5:457–459.
32. Fraser-Hill MA, Atri M, Bret PM, et al. Intrahepatic portal venous system: variations demonstrated with duplex and color Doppler US. *Radiology* 1990;177:523–526.
33. Soyer P, Bluemke DA, Choti MA, Fishman EK. Variations in the intrahepatic portions of the hepatic and portal veins: findings on helical CT scans during arterial portography. *Am J Roentgenol* 1995;164:103–108.
34. Parvey HR, Raval B, Sandler CM. Portal vein thrombosis: imaging findings. *Am J Roentgenol* 1994;162:77–81.
35. Braum S. Hepatic arteriography. In: Abrams HL, ed. *Abrams angiography: vascular and interventional radiology.* Boston: Little Brown, 1983;1479–1503.
36. Michels NA. *Blood supply and anatomy of the upper abdominal organs with a descriptive atlas.* Philadelphia: JB Lippincott, 1955.
37. Winter TC 3rd, Nghiem HV, Freeny PC, Hommeyer SC, Mack LA. Hepatic arterial anatomy: demonstration of normal supply and vascular variants with three-dimensional CT angiography. *RadioGraphics* 1995;15:771–780.
38. Lafortune M, Madore F, Patriquin H, Breton G. Segmental anatomy of the liver: a sonographic approach to the Couinaud nomenclature. *Radiology* 1991;181:443–448.
39. Holley HC, Koslin DD, Berland LV, Stanley RJ. Inhomogeneous enhancement of liver parenchyma secondary to passive congestion: contrast-enhanced CT. *Radiology* 1989;170:795–800.
40. Vogelzang RL, Anschuetz SL, Gore RM. Budd-Chiari syndrome: CT observations. *Radiology* 1987;163:329–333.
41. Murphy FB, Steinberg HV, Shires GT 3rd, Martin LG, Bernardino ME. The Budd-Chiari syndrome: a review. *Am J Roentgenol* 1986;147:9–15.
42. Liddell RM, Baron RL, Ekstrom JE, Varnell RM, Shuman WP. Normal intrahepatic bile ducts: CT depiction. *Radiology* 1990;176:633–635.
43. Marincek B, Barbier P, Becker CD, Mettler D, Rutchi C. CT appearance of impaired hepatic drainage in liver transplants. *Am J Roentgenol* 1986;147:519–523.
44. Co CS, Shea WJ Jr, Goldberg HI. Evaluation of the common bile duct diameter using high resolution computed tomography. *J Comput Assist Tomogr* 1986;10:424–427.
45. Baron RL. Computed tomography of the bile ducts. *Semin Roentgenol* 1997;32:172–187.
46. Koslin DB, Stanley RJ, Berland LL, Shin MS, Dalton SC. Hepatic perivascular lymphedema: CT appearance. *Am J Roentgenol* 1988;150:111–113.
47. Lawson TL, Thorsen MK, Erickson SJ, et al. Periportal halo: a CT sign of liver disease. *Abdom Imag* 1993;18:42–46.

Variants and Pitfalls in Body Imaging,
edited by Ali Shirkhoda.
Lippincott Williams & Wilkins, Philadelphia, © 2000.

CHAPTER 9

The Liver and Biliary System: MRI

Mark A. Brown, Tara C. Noone, and Richard C. Semelka

Current magnetic resonance imaging (MRI) techniques result in good contrast resolution and few artifacts for studies of the abdomen, but protocol developement and image interpretation remain challenging. Many of the techniques used in brain and spine imaging are unsuitable when applied to the abdomen. Respiratory motion can produce signal misregistrations of the organs on MR images. Also, the different tissue types cause signal differences that may be confused with pathologic conditions. Our goal is to describe the MR characteristics of some of the common types of normal anatomic variations as well as the artifacts that might be confused with them and with pathologic conditions.

This chapter is divided into three sections. The first section describes key aspects of the basic measurement protocols that are of importance in abdominal imaging. The reader is referred to other sources for a more complete description of the basic principles of MR imaging and characteristics of the specific pulse sequences (1–3). The second part illustrates typical examples of liver images as well as normal variations that may be encountered. The final section demonstrates images containing common artifacts that occur in imaging the abdomen and describes some options to reduce their impact.

MEASUREMENT PROTOCOLS

Pulse Sequences

A pulse sequence is the measurement technique by which an MR image is obtained. It contains the hardware

M. A. Brown: Siemens Training and Development Center, Cary, North Carolina 27511.

T. C. Noone and R. C. Semelka: Department of Radiology, University of North Carolina Hospitals, Chapel Hill, North Carolina 27599.

instructions necessary to acquire the data in the desired manner. The user-defined measurement parameters are combined with the pulse sequence to determine the actual signal intensity from a volume element. Some aspects of a pulse sequence (e.g., minimum T_R, FOV) depend on how the manufacturer has implemented the technique (e.g., gradient pulse duration) and on specific hardware characteristics of the individual scanner (e.g., maximum gradient amplitude, gradient rise time).

T_1-Weighted Techniques

T_1-weighted imaging is used in liver and biliary imaging to provide views of the underlying anatomy and to assess perfusion characteristics of various tissues. Abnormal fluid or fibrous tissue content is visualized as low-intensity signal, whereas subacute blood or proteinaceous fluid demonstrates high signal. Fat is also visualized as high-signal-intensity tissue. The predominant slice orientation is transverse. Coronal orientation is useful, as it provides good visualization of the superior and inferior margins of the lateral segment of the left lobe and the dome and inferior tip of the right lobe of the liver. Twelve to 16 slices are typically necessary for complete coverage in each plane.

Although basic spin echo has been the traditional technique of choice for neuro or orthopedic T_1-weighted imaging, it has several limitations that make it less attractive for body imaging. Relatively long T_R times are required to acquire sufficient slices for complete anatomic coverage, making the images susceptible to artifacts from respiratory or peristaltic motion. In addition, the 180-degree refocusing pulses significantly increase the amount of radiofrequency (RF) power deposited in the patient. This will limit the number of slices per scan that can be obtained without exceeding the limits of RF power deposition or specific absorption rate (SAR) of the patient. For these reasons, the preferred technique for T_1-weighted body imaging is spoiled gradient echo.

Gradient-echo sequences are a class of imaging techniques that do not use a 180-degree RF pulse for proton refocusing. The echo signal is generated only through gradient reversal. During the localization process, the imaging gradients induce proton dephasing. Application of a second gradient pulse of the same duration and magnitude but opposite polarity reverses this dephasing and produces an echo known as a gradient echo. All gradient-echo sequences have gradient reversal pulses in at least two directions, the slice selection and the readout directions, which generate the echo signal. Excitation angles less than 90 degrees are normally used.

The absence of the 180-degree RF pulse in gradient echo sequences has several important consequences for abdominal imaging. The required measurement time per slice, known as the slice loop, will be shorter than for an analogous spin-echo sequence, enabling more slices to be acquired for the same T_R. Sufficiently short T_R times can be chosen to make breath-hold scanning possible. Less total RF power is applied to the patient, so that the total RF energy deposition, as monitored by the SAR, is lower. The contrast mechanism in gradient-echo images is different from that in spin-echo images. For spin-echo images, the T_E determines the amount of T_2 weighting in the image. Static sources for proton dephasing such as the main magnetic field inhomogeneity and magnetic susceptibility differences are reversed by the 180-degree refocusing pulse. These dephasing interactions contribute to the echo signal decay in gradient-echo images, which lack this 180-degree pulse. Thus, the T_E determines the amount of T_2^* weighting in gradient echo images, where T_2^* indicates T_2 plus the additional sources of proton dephasing (1).

The simplest gradient-echo sequence is a spoiled gradient-echo sequence, also known as FLASH (fast low-angle shot) or spoiled GRASS (gradient-recalled acquisition in the steady state). This sequence uses a spoiling scheme, either gradient pulses or RF phase variation, to dephase the transverse magnetization following signal detection. As a result, only longitudinal magnetization is present at the time of the next excitation pulse (e.g., T_R). The combination of T_R and excitation angle determines the amount of T_1 weighting in the image. The spoiled gradient-echo technique is the gradient-echo counterpart of the spin-echo technique, except that T_E determines the amount of T_2^* rather than T_2 contrast.

T_2-Weighted Techniques

Conventional spin-echo T_2-weighted images are often used in abdominal imaging for tissue characterization. Fluid-filled structures such as cysts or hemangiomas have high signal intensity, whereas chronic fibrous tissue has low signal intensity, and iron-rich tissues have very low signal intensity. These images are usually acquired as part of a multiecho sequence, with proton-density-weighted images acquired at the same time as T_2-weighted images. The primary drawback to T_2-weighted imaging is artifacts caused by respiratory motion during the long measurement times. This has been alleviated in many instances by the use of fast spin-echo techniques.

Fast spin-echo (also known as turbo spin-echo) sequences are similar to standard multiecho sequences in that multiple 180-degree refocusing pulses are applied to produce multiple echoes, known as a train of echoes. However, each echo signal is acquired following a different phase-encoding gradient amplitude as well as a different T_E. A segmented gradient table is used in which each segment of the table is acquired at the same T_E within the echo train. The resultant image is produced using some or all of the echoes detected as determined by the pulse sequence design. The number of echoes used to create each image is known as the echo train length, and the time between each of the echoes is called the echo spacing. The contrast in fast spin-echo sequences is based primarily on the echoes detected following low-amplitude phase-encoding gradients and the T_Es for these echoes. The contrast is considered to be based on an effective T_E because there are echoes with different T_Es contributing to the final image. The advantage of the fast spin-echo technique is that the data collection process is more efficient and the scan time is shorter. However, because of the multiple T_Es, the T_2 content is not as pure as for a conventional spin echo. Although both hemangiomas and cysts are bright compared to normal tissue, lesion detection that is based on subtle differences of T_2 relaxation times between the tissues will be more problematic with long echo train lengths. In addition, the high signal intensity of fat in these sequences results in a different relative signal relationship between fat and other tissues/structures than that observed in conventional T_2-weighted sequences (1).

General Considerations

Although imaging of the abdomen has been a part of MRI since its earliest days, the advances in hardware performance and capabilities have produced significant improvements in image quality. The ability to implement specific techniques also depends on the particular scanner. However, the general imaging criteria have remained unchanged: T_1- and T_2-weighted images covering the entire anatomic area in one measurement whenever possible. This latter point minimizes the possibility for slice misregistration from measurement to measurement. The following discussion describes general concepts that are useful in abdominal imaging.

Breath-Hold Imaging

One of the most significant improvements in abdominal imaging has been the advent of breath-hold MRI techniques. The lengthy nature of conventional spin-echo sequences requires that these sequences be performed during patient respiration. Respiration-induced ghost images form the most problematic artifact in abdominal imaging. Signal averaging, respiratory gating of the scan, and/or reordering of the raw data collection are necessary to minimize their presence. By using spoiled gradient-echo techniques, 14 or more T_1-weighted images can be obtained with good in-plane resolution in 20 seconds or less, which is sufficiently short for complete liver coverage within a breath-hold. Spin-echo techniques are less useful because a longer slice loop reduces the number of sections that can be acquired in a measurement and, therefore, complete coverage of the liver within a single breath-hold scan may not be possible. In addition, the 180-degree refocusing pulse increases the RF power deposition, contributing to potential generation of heat within the patient.

Breath-hold T_2-weighted imaging is more problematic. As mentioned above, the use of fast spin-echo techniques enables shorter scan times. The echo train length is important in determining the scan time. Longer echo train lengths enable more echoes to be acquired per excitation pulse, reducing the number of excitation pulses necessary to collect all the raw data. For sufficiently long echo train lengths (16 or greater), the scan time can become sufficiently short to allow acquisition of T_2-weighted images within a single breath-hold yet provide a sufficient number of slices for complete coverage of the liver. For extremely long echo train lengths (100 or more), the entire raw data set for the image can be acquired following a single excitation pulse. This approach, termed half-Fourier acquisition single-shot turbo spin echo (HASTE) or single-shot fast spin echo, enables an image acquisition time of less than one second and can produce motion and artifact-free images even when the patient is unable to suspend respiration (3).

In-Phase/Out-of-Phase Gradient Echo Imaging

Magnetic resonance imaging images the mobile hydrogen nuclei (protons) within the patient. These nuclei are most frequently a part of the tissue fluid (water) or fat. The resonant frequencies for fat and water protons are slightly different because of differences in the molecular structure between the two molecules. Whereas both fat and water protons are excited by the selective RF excitation pulse, this resonant frequency difference will cause a periodic change in the phase of the fat protons relative to the water protons, a process known as phase cycling. This frequency difference (known as a chemical shift difference) and the resulting rate of phase cycling are constant with respect to time (3.5 ppm). For spin-echo techniques, the refocusing RF pulse reverses this phase cycling so that the phase of the MR signals from both the fat and water protons always contribute to the echo in the same manner; that is, the fat and water protons are described as "in phase."

The lack of a 180-degree refocusing pulse in gradient-echo imaging provides a way to affect the relative phase behavior and, thus, the relative contribution of fat and water to the image. The choice of T_E determines the phase difference between the fat and water protons at the time of the echo detection as well as the amount of T_2^* weighting. As T_E is varied, the fat protons will contribute to the signal in an oscillatory fashion relative to the water protons, causing a significantly greater change in tissue signal than that resulting from only T_2^* decay. There are two choices of T_E that are commonly used to provide known phase contributions. One is the in-phase T_E, where the two protons have the same phase. The other is the out-of-phase T_E, where the fat protons are 180 degrees out of phase from the water protons. The specific T_{ES} for the in-phase and out-of-phase times depend on the specific field strength because the absolute resonant frequency difference is field strength dependent. For 1.5-T scanners, the lowest in-phase T_E is at 4.5 milliseconds with subsequent in-phase T_{ES} occurring every 4.5 milliseconds thereafter. For 1.0-T scanners, the in-phase T_{ES} occur at 6.6 milliseconds and every 6.6 milliseconds thereafter. The out-of-phase T_{ES} occur at the midpoints between the in-phase times (1).

The change in signal contribution from fat protons in out-of-phase gradient echo imaging is particularly useful in assessing fatty infiltration of tissue. Tissues containing both fat and water protons within a voxel will have significant signal variation between the in-phase and out-of-phase images, with a lower signal intensity observed in out-of-phase images. This reduced signal can be used to demonstrate tissues that contain water and fat within the same voxel, such as fatty liver or adrenal adenomas (4).

Fat Suppression

As mentioned above, the MR signals for fat and water have intrinsically different frequencies because of the chemical shift difference. During normal imaging, both contribute to the measured signal from a tissue. Fat suppression techniques provide the ability to suppress the signal from the fat, allowing the water to be the primary source of signal. This is particularly advantageous in imaging of the pancreas, tissues that contain substantial fat, or for differentiating subacute blood from fat. Three approaches are commonly used for fat suppression: short

T_I inversion recovery (STIR), frequency-selective presaturation, and water excitation (5).

Inversion recovery (IR) sequences use a 180-degree inversion pulse applied at a user-definable inversion time (T_I) before the primary excitation pulse for the slice. The protons from both the fat and water within the tissue are excited by the pulse. Because of the differences in T_1 relaxation times between fat and water, their relative contributions to the final image can be altered by adjusting the inversion time (T_I). Excellent fat suppression can be achieved using T_I times of 150 to 170 milliseconds at 1.5 T, with the tissue water predominating in the image. The combination of IR with fast spin echo, known as fast IR or turbo IR, allows the contrast control of IR together with scan times short enough for suspension of respiration. The difficulty in using IR-based techniques is that administration of gadolinium-based contrast media shortens the water T_1 so that water protons acquire T_1 times approaching those of fat protons in a variable fashion, so that the signal intensity of gadolinium-containing water-based tissues may become unpredictable.

The other two approaches for fat suppression are based on the intrinsic difference in resonant frequency (≈ 3.5 ppm) between fat and water protons (6). One approach, known as fat saturation, uses a frequency-selective presaturation pulse centered at the fat proton frequency. This pulse is applied in the absence of a magnetic field gradient before the primary excitation pulse and saturates the fat protons so that they do not contribute signal to the echo at the time of detection. Because the gadolinium-based contrast media relax primarily the water protons in the tissue, the fat signal is still minimal following contrast agent administration. The other approach is known as water excitation. This approach uses a series or train of RF pulses that act in concert, known as a composite pulse. Between successive pulses, the fat and water protons will undergo phase cycling as described above. The timing and amplitude of each pulse in the train is such that the water protons are excited at the end of the pulse train while the fat protons remain unexcited.

One very important requirement for the frequency-dependent fat suppression techniques described above is that the magnetic field homogeneity must be very high. This ensures that the absolute frequency difference between fat and water protons is the same at all points within the magnet. Poor field homogeneity may cause incomplete fat suppression or possibly water suppression. Because the patient distorts the field homogeneity, it is often necessary to optimize the homogeneity to the individual patient or volume of tissue under observation. Automated techniques for performing this are available on many MR scanners.

NORMAL ANATOMIC VARIANTS THAT MAY MIMIC PATHOLOGY

Pitfalls in the interpretation of MR images of the liver and biliary system are not limited to artifacts arising from technical factors. Several normal variants may mimic hepatobiliary pathology. These may result from congenital anatomic variation or iatrogenic alterations of anatomy. Recognition of these normal variants precludes faulty diagnosis, which may lead to unnecessary additional imaging studies and/or intervention.

Diaphragmatic Insertions

The thoracoabdominal diaphragm is comprised of a peripheral muscular portion and a central aponeurotic portion. The muscular fibers within the periphery converge radially toward the central tendon. The muscular portion is subdivided into sternal, costal, and lumbar components, according to the origins of its muscular slips (see Chapter 5).

Occasionally, the broad muscular slips along the costal margin may produce variations in signal intensity within the liver. These are most frequently detected in the right hepatic lobe using T_1-weighted images. They may appear as longitudinal striations of decreased signal intensity along the periphery of the hepatic dome or as focal, rounded pseudolesions along the liver edge (Fig. 9.1). Diaphragmatic insertions usually are linear in appearance and demonstrate decreased signal intensity on T_2-weighted images, whereas the majority of focal hepatic masses demonstrate increased signal intensity, which provides a helpful differentiating feature.

Focal Fatty Changes and Focal Sparing

Fatty infiltration of the liver may be either homogeneous or heterogeneous and may be either diffusely or focally distributed throughout the liver parenchyma. It may have clearly demarcated margins or be ill-defined and infiltrative in appearance. Occasionally, a focus of fat within an otherwise normal liver can simulate a more ominous lesion. This entity can be differentiated from true lesions by comparing in-phase and out-of-phase T_1-weighted images (Figs. 9.2 and 9.3).

Detection of fatty infiltration using a chemical shift selective suppression technique (fat saturation) is less reliable (6). Whereas out-of-phase imaging demonstrates maximal signal loss when fat and water are present in approximately equal proportions within a voxel, as occurs in fatty infiltration, fat suppression imaging demonstrates maximal signal loss when the fat content approaches 100%. This latter finding occurs most frequently in focal fatty lesions, including lipomas and

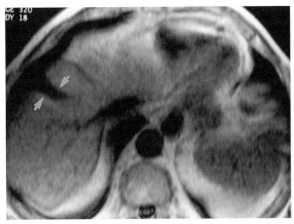 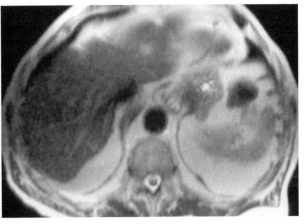

A   B

FIG. 9.1. Diaphragmatic insertions. T$_1$-weighted magnetization-prepared spoiled gradient-echo (SGE) **(A)** and T$_2$-weighted echo train spin-echo (HASTE) **(B)** transverse images. Linear striations of decreased signal intensity on T$_1$-weighted imaging represent the muscular slips of the thoracoabdominal diaphragm *(arrows)* **(A).** Scalloping along the anterolateral margin of the liver results from focal fatty invagination adjacent to the diaphragmatic slips on the HASTE image **(B).**

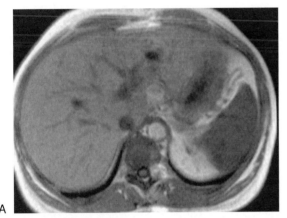 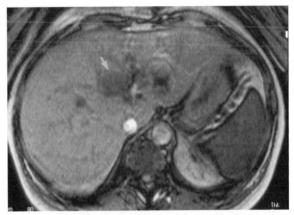

A   B

FIG. 9.2. Focal fatty infiltration. T$_1$-weighted in-phase **(A)** and out-of-phase **(B)** transverse SGE images in the same patient. Liver parenchyma within segment 4 is isointense to slightly hyperintense relative to the remainder of the liver on the in-phase image **(A).** Decrease in signal intensity of this region is apparent on out-of-phase imaging *(arrow)* **(B).** This combination of findings is consistent with the diagnosis of focal fatty infiltration.

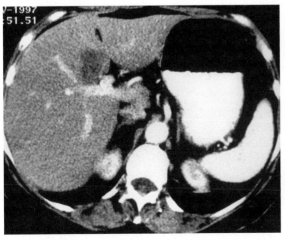 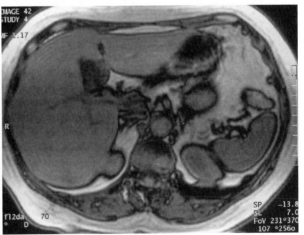

A   B

FIG. 9.3. Computed tomography scan of a patient with history of colon carcinoma shows a focal area of low density (−35 HU) in the left lobe **(A).** Because liver enzymes were normal, MRI was done to further characterize the lesion. The out-of-phase image **(B)** illustrates significant signal loss, supporting the diagnosis of focal fat. (Courtesy of A. Shirkhoda, M.D.)

angiomyolipomas. Focal fatty infiltration should be differentiated from hepatic pseudolesion, which often occurs around the falciform ligament (7).

Diffuse fatty infiltration of the liver may occur with a focus of normal, non-fat-containing liver, referred to as focal sparing. Focal fatty sparing frequently occurs adjacent to the gallbladder, the falciform ligament, or within segment 4 of the liver. Again, use of the out-of-phase imaging technique permits reliable distinction between a focus of residual normal hepatic parenchyma and focal mass lesions (Fig. 9.4).

Elongated Left Hepatic Lobe

Occasionally, the left lobe of the liver may be enlarged, extending into the left upper quadrant of the abdomen, i.e., a "wraparound liver." It may mimic normal splenic tissue or create an illusion of an exophytic mass, arising from either the spleen or the left hepatic lobe (Fig. 9.5). Enhancement features compatible with normal liver enable recognition of this anatomic variant. The liver normally demonstrates increased signal intensity relative to the spleen on T_1-weighted images and decreased signal intensity relative to the spleen on T_2-weighted images.

Riedel's Lobe

The right hepatic lobe also may be elongated relative to the remainder of the liver. Unlike an elongated left lobe, which extends transversely, a Riedel's lobe increases the craniocaudal dimension of the right lobe (Fig. 9.6). A Riedel's lobe may lead to erroneous assignment of hepatomegaly to a patient with a normal liver if only the cranio-caudal dimension of the right lobe is used to determine liver size. The contour of the elongated right lobe may aid differentiation between normal and pathologic enlargement. A Riedel's lobe frequently has a tapered inferior margin on coronal plane imaging, whereas acquired hepatomegaly often results in increases in both the transverse and craniocaudal dimensions of the liver, resulting in a rounded inferior contour. A Riedel's lobe may be distinguished from an exophytic mass, arising from the inferior aspect of the right lobe, by virtue of signal intensity identical to that of normal adjacent liver.

Aplasia/Hypoplasia

In addition to congenital anomalies resulting from excessive development of portions of the liver, anatomic variants may result from either hypoplasia or aplasia of hepatic tissue. An individual segment or an entire lobe may be involved (8). Both the lack of magnetic susceptibility artifact from clips and a past surgical history assist differentiation from iatrogenic parenchymal loss.

Situs Inversus

An extreme anatomic variant occurs when there is situs inversus. In these patients the normal relationship of the liver and spleen is reversed. They are easily differentiated by their size, shape, internal vessels and their early enhancement patterns. The normal liver enhances homogeneously, whereas early splenic enhancement is variegated. These patients will often have other congenital anomalies related to the cardiovascular, respiratory, and gastrointestinal systems.

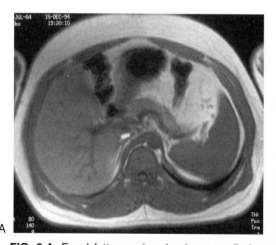 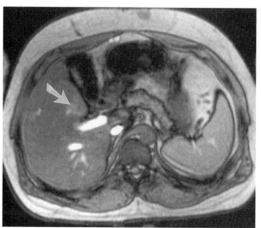

FIG. 9.4. Focal fatty sparing. In-phase spoiled gradient-echo **(A)** and out-of-phase spoiled gradient-echo **(B)**. On the in-phase image **(A)**, the liver appears homogeneous in signal intensity, reflecting the additive signal magnitude of fat and water protons on in-phase images. On the out-of-phase image **(B)**, the majority of the liver decreases in signal intensity, reflecting the diminution of signal in voxels that contain both fat and water. A small focus of liver *(arrow)* **(B)** in the medial aspect of the medial segment of the left lobe remains higher in signal than the remainder of the liver, consistent with focal sparing.

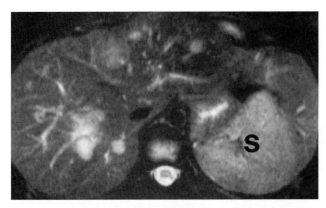

FIG. 9.5. Elongated lateral segment of the left lobe. T₂-weighted fat-suppressed echo-train spin-echo image demonstrates an elongated lateral segment of the left lobe of the liver that wraps around anterior to the spleen on T₁-weighted images or CT images because of similar signal intensity/density. On T₂-weighted images, the moderately low signal of the liver and moderately high signal of the spleen, as appreciated in this image, permit ready distinction. Note is also made of multiple moderately high signal liver lesions that represent with metastases.

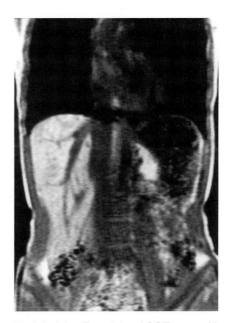

FIG. 9.6. Riedel's lobe. T₁-weighted SGE coronal image. The right portal vein extends inferiorly into the elongated right hepatic lobe in this normal variant.

Partial Hepatectomy

Hepatic anatomy may be distorted secondary to iatrogenic intervention. Lobar or segmental resections can lead to bizarre hepatic contours. Regeneration of hepatic tissue may occur between six and twelve months following resection. There may be associated variations in signal intensity and enhancement along surgical margins, simulating recurrent disease. In addition, there is frequently metallic artifact, resulting from surgical clips. This decreased signal intensity "blooming" artifact also may simulate rounded, focal hepatic lesions (Figs.

9.7–9.9). This artifact will frequently become more pronounced on spoiled gradient-echo sequences or other techniques with greater T₂ or T₂* weighting, allowing differentiation from true pathology.

Biopsy Tracts

Tracts resulting from needles, catheters, and prior cryoablation also may alter signal intensity within the

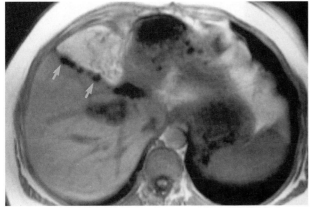
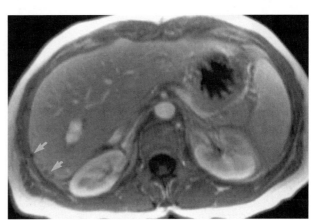

FIG. 9.7. Partial hepatectomy. T₁-weighted SGE transverse **(A)** and postgadolinium T₁-weighted SGE transverse **(B)** images. Surgical clips result in susceptibility artifact along the anterior margin of the right hepatic lobe in this patient after left hepatectomy *(arrows)* **(A).** More subtle susceptibility artifact results from clips along the posterior margin of the liver in another patient after partial right hepatectomy *(arrows)* **(B).**

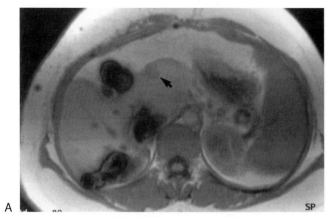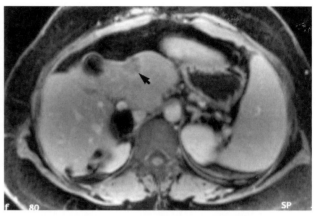

FIG. 9.8. Partial hepatectomy and magnetic susceptibility artifact simulating focal liver pathology. T_1-weighted SGE transverse **(A)** and postgadolinium T_1-weighted fat-suppressed SGE transverse **(B)** images in the same patient. Abundant magnetic susceptibility artifact results from surgical clips in this patient following partial hepatectomy **(A)**. Note a true metastasis along the anteromedial border of the remaining liver *(arrow)* **(A)**. On the postgadolinium fat-suppressed image, the susceptibility artifact is less pronounced **(B)**. In addition, continuous rim enhancement confirms the presence of a concomitant metastasis anteriorly *(arrow)* **(B)**.

involved areas of liver. Associated edema may result in focally decreased signal intensity on T1-weighted images and increased signal intensity on T2-weighted images (Fig. 9.10). Various alterations in signal intensity on both T1-weighted and T2-weighted sequences may be seen when there is associated hemorrhage. There also may be increased adjacent enhancement from reactive inflammation. Such changes frequently occur in a linear distribution, and correlation with clinical history enables exclusion of pathology.

Radiation Changes

The hepatic signal alterations resulting from radiation therapy vary according to the temporal relationship between the treatment and MR evaluation. Immediately following radiation, edematous changes within the affected liver may result. This leads to regions of decreased signal intensity on T_1-weighted images and increased signal intensity on T_2-weighted images. Over time, the affected areas may demonstrate decreased sig-

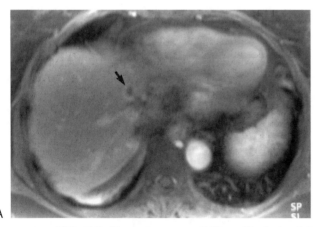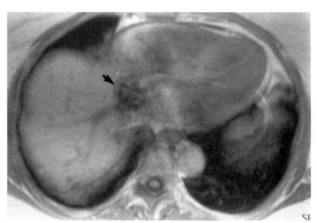

FIG. 9.9. Magnetic susceptibility artifact simulating a metastasis. T_1-weighted postgadolinium SGE transverse **(A)** and T_1-weighted pregadolinium SGE transverse **(B)** images in the same patient. **A:** An apparent continuous rim of enhancement surrounds a focus of decreased signal intensity *(arrow)* anterior to the inferior vena cava on the postgadolinium image. **B:** Correlation with the pregadolinium T_1-weighted image, which demonstrates the same finding, permits confirmation that the pseudolesion *(arrow)* resulted from a surgical clip rather than a true metastasis.

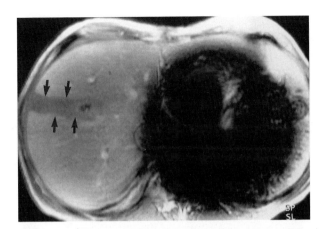

FIG. 9.10. Biopsy tract. T_1-weighted SGE postgadolinium transverse image. A linear region of decreased enhancement relative to the remainder of the liver *(arrows)* is visualized in this patient with a tract resulting from prior liver biopsy. Abundant magnetic susceptibility artifact in the left upper quadrant represents the end result of prior placement of metallic coils within the splenic artery.

nal intensity on both T_1-weighted and T_2-weighted images, reflecting the development of chronic fibrosis.

Often there is a decrease in triglyceride deposition in the hepatic parenchyma within a radiation port (9). This results in preservation of normal signal intensity relative to the remainder of a fatty liver with both fat suppression and out-of-phase imaging techniques. Increased enhancement within the confines of the port may be observed on late postgadolinium images, either from an acute radiation-induced vasculitis or from the formation of chronic granulation tissue (Fig. 9.11). Radiation changes often

have geographic margins, resulting from the well-demarcated boundaries of the treatment port, that do not correspond to hepatic segments.

Pneumobilia

Air within the biliary tree may arise in a number of settings, most commonly the result of endoscopic retrograde cholangiopancreatography (ERCP), biliary stenting, biliary–enteric anastomosis, or a patulous sphincter of Odi. Air in the biliary tree may be mistaken for a biliary calculus, as both may appear rounded with an absence of signal on all MR sequences. Differentiating features include the following: (a) air is located along the nondependent surface of the bile duct (Fig. 9.12), whereas calculi tend to be located along the dependent surface; and (b) air may create a significant magnetic susceptibility difference artifact, whereas calculi generally do not. Magnetic resonance cholangiographic sequences are less sensitive to susceptibility artifacts, so that this artifact may not be readily appreciated.

Cholecystectomy Clips

The close proximity of cholecystectomy clips to the biliary tree may at times simulate the appearance of a biliary duct calculus. Clips can be distinguished from calculi by acquisition of MR cholangiographic images in two planes, one of which is the transverse plane. In many cases, the transverse images will demonstrate the extrabiliary location of the signal void defect (Fig. 9.13) and the presence of magnetic susceptibility difference artifacts related to the clip.

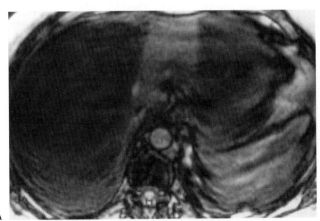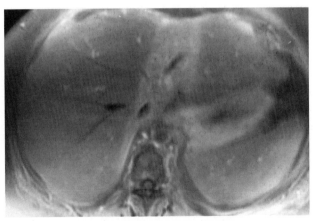

A   B

FIG. 9.11. Radiation changes. T_1-weighted out-of-phase SGE transverse **(A)** and T_1-weighted postgadolinium fat-suppressed SGE transverse images **(B)** in the same patient. An obliquely oriented band of decreased signal intensity in seen within the radiation port, anteriorly **(A)**, presumably resulting from decreased fatty infiltration within the affected area relative to the remainder of the liver. Increased signal intensity relative to the remainder of the liver is seen on the postgadolinium fat-suppressed image **(B)**. This may reflect a radiation-induced vasculitis as well as a relative lack of fatty infiltration within the affected parenchyma. (Reprinted from reference 8, with permission from the authors.)

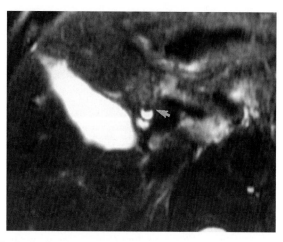

FIG. 9.12. Pneumobilia. An area of decreased signal intensity within the nondependent portion of the common bile duct resulting from magnetic susceptibility differences between tissue and air from pneumobilia *(arrow)*. (Reprinted from reference 8, with permission from the authors.)

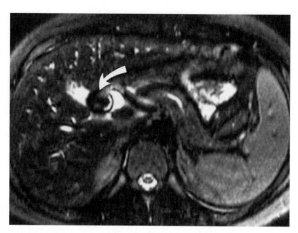

FIG. 9.13. Cholecystectomy clips. T_2-weighted fast spin-echo image showing artifact from the presence of surgical clips following cholecystectomy *(arrow)*. (Reprinted from reference 8, with permission from the authors.)

Dynamic Contrast Pitfalls

Contrast material-enhanced dynamic magnetic resonance (MR) imaging is an important technique for evaluating liver disease. However, several potential diagnostic pitfalls may be encountered, including lobar, segmental, subsegmental, and subcapsular hyperperfusion abnormalities; early-enhancing pseudolesions, particularly in the medial segment of the left hepatic lobe; heterogeneous hyperperfusion abnormalities throughout the liver; and hypointense pseudolesions due to vascular artifacts, unenhanced hepatic vessels, partial volume artifacts, magnetic susceptibility artifacts, and regenerative nodules in cirrhosis. These abnormalities sometimes have appearances similar to those of true lesions or tumor spread to the surrounding liver parenchyma on arterial-dominant phase dynamic MR images. In most cases, however, no corresponding abnormalities are seen with other pulse sequences or on delayed-phase MR images. In addition, hyperperfusion abnormalities due to readily recognizable causes are often found in characteristic locations and thus can be differentiated from true tumors (10).

COMMON MAGNETIC RESONANCE ARTIFACTS IN LIVER AND BILIARY IMAGING

Because MR artifacts are extensively discussed in Chapter 34, we briefly summarize those pertaining to the liver. In general, artifacts in MR images result from pixels that do not faithfully represent true anatomy within the patient. The appearance of the liver images is that the underlying anatomy is visualized but there are spurious signals present that do not correspond to actual tissue at that location. They may be grouped into three categories, based on their origin (1,2,7).

The first group is a consequence of motion related to the patient during the measurement. This includes both blood flow (Fig. 9.14) and gross physical motion of the liver tissue by respiration (Fig. 9.15) or peristalsis (11).

The second group of artifacts is not related to the measurement time but is generated as a result of the particular measurement technique and/or specific measurement parameters. These include chemical shift artifact (Fig. 9.16), phase cancellation artifacts (Fig. 9.17), magnetic susceptibility artifact (Fig. 9.18), aliasing artifact, and truncation artifact (Fig. 9.19).

The third group includes system-related artifacts that are produced by a malfunctioning or miscalibration of one or more of the scanner components during the data collection. They include magnetic field distortions (Fig. 9.20), system instabilities or miscalibrations (Fig. 9.21), spike (Fig. 9.22) and noise (Fig. 9.23).

In all cases, the artifacts may or may not be easily discernible from normal hepatic anatomy, particularly because they may or may not be reproducible. Our goal should be to recognize some of the more common artifacts that are encountered in liver MR imaging and take possible steps for removing or reducing their impact in the final images.

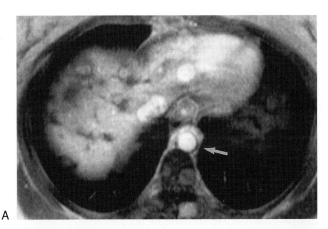

A

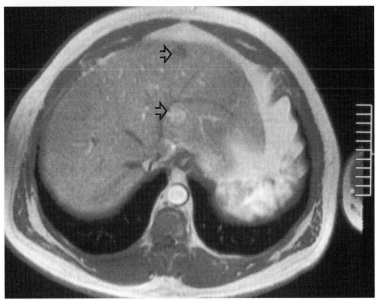

B

FIG. 9.14. Blood flow artifact. A: Flow through the slice produces multiple ghost copies of the aorta. They occur in line with the aorta *(arrow)* and are spread out in the phase-encoding direction throughout the image. B: Two ghost artifacts with different appearances *(arrows)* in the liver mimicking hepatic lesions.

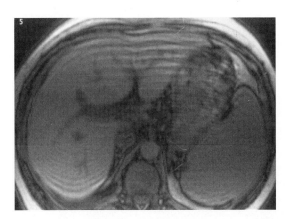

FIG. 9.15. Respiratory motion artifact. Breathing during the scan can produce multiple ghost images that superimpose on the normal anatomy. The shape of the ghosts corresponds to the moving structure.

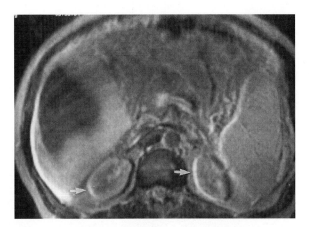

FIG. 9.16. Chemical shift artifact. Retroperitoneal fat surrounding the kidneys is incorrectly mapped (fat pixels shifted to the left) because of low receiver bandwidth on this T$_2$-weighted spin-echo image. Bright bands on left side of kidneys *(arrows)* occur from constructive addition of fat signal with water at interface, whereas black bands on the right side of the kidneys result from the misregistration.

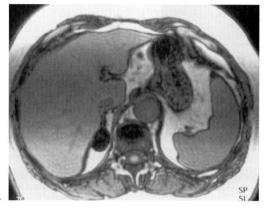
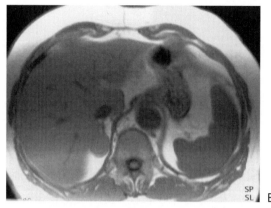

FIG. 9.17. Phase-cancellation artifact. T$_1$-weighted SGE images: **(A)** out-of-phase, T$_E$=2.2 milliseconds; and **(B)** in-phase, T$_E$=4.5 milliseconds. Note *black rings* in **A** surrounding liver and spleen caused by equal amounts of fat and water at interface, not seen in **B**. Also note reduced signal from adrenal adenoma in **A** because of significant fat content.

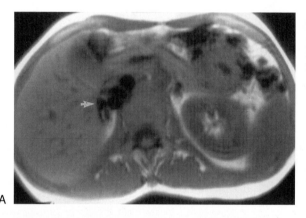
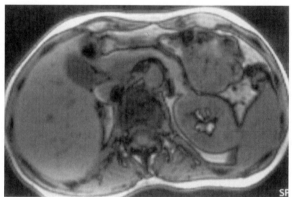

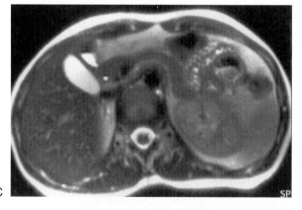

FIG. 9.18. Metal artifact from surgical clips. **A:** Transverse T$_1$-weighted SGE, T$_E$=4.5 milliseconds. **B:** Transverse T$_1$-weighted SGE, T$_E$=2.25 milliseconds. **C:** Transverse T$_2$-weighted HASTE. **D:** Coronal transverse T$_1$-weighted SGE, T$_E$=4.5 milliseconds. **E:** Coronal T$_1$-weighted SGE, T$_E$=2.25 milliseconds. Note that clip artifacts are most severe in **A** and **D** *(arrows)* and are least noticeable in **C**. Also note that pattern of distortion from clip is different in **A** than in **D**.

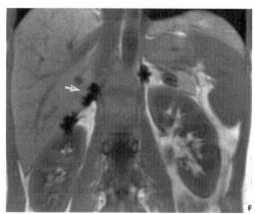
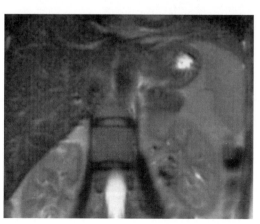

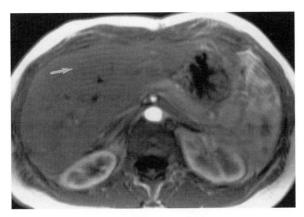

FIG. 9.19. Truncation artifact. Asymmetric echo sampling and high-amplitude signal from the abdominal wall combine to cause a ringing-like truncation artifact originating at the abdominal wall *(arrow)*.

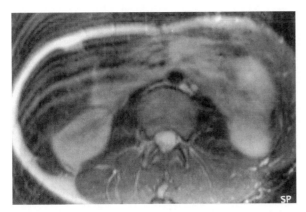

FIG. 9.20. Field inhomogeneity artifact. Poor magnetic field homogeneity causes incomplete fat saturation. Note poor suppression of subcutaneous fat on left side of figure and good suppression on the right side.

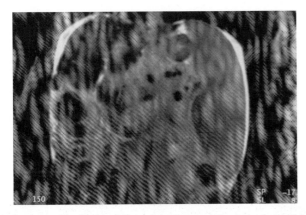

FIG. 9.21. Hardware failure. Improper detuning of receiver coil from the transmitter coil causes smearing artifacts in image.

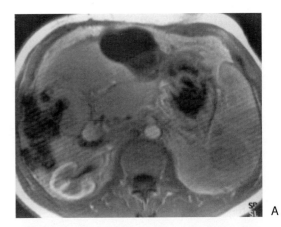

A

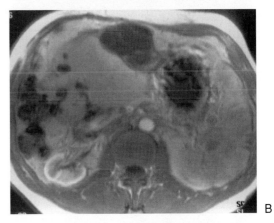

B

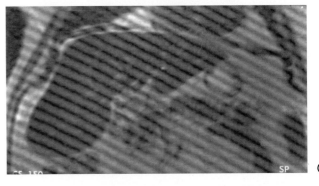

C

FIG. 9.22. Spike artifacts. **A:** T$_1$-weighted SGE showing banding from spike during data collection. **B:** Adjacent slice in scan shows no spike. **C:** T$_2$-weighted HASTE, showing different banding pattern from spike.

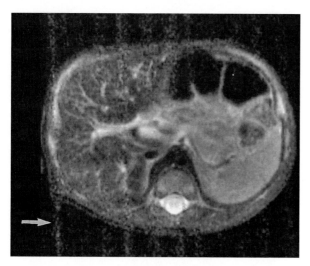

FIG. 9.23. External interference. Electrical interference caused by incomplete filtering of patient monitoring equipment. Artifacts consist of vertical stripes superimposed on image *(arrow)*.

REFERENCES

1. Brown MA, Semelka RC. *MRI: Basic principles and applications, 2nd edition,* New York: Wiley-Liss, 1999.
2. Smith RC, Lange RC. *Understanding magnetic resonance imaging.* Boca Raton, FL: CRC Press, 1998.
3. Semelka RC, Kelekis NL, Thomasson D, Brown MA, Laub GA. HASTE MR imaging: description of technique and preliminary results in the abdomen. *J Magn Reson Imag* 1994;4:759–765.
4. Mitchell DG, Grovello M, Matteucchi T, Peterson RO, Miettinen MM. Benign adenocortical masses: diagnosis with chemical shift MR imaging. *Radiology* 1992;185:345–351.
5. Soyer P, de Givry SC, Gueye C, Lenormand S, Somveille E, Scherrer A. Detection of focal hepatic lesions with MR imaging: prospective comparison of T_2-weighted fast spin-echo with and without fat suppression. T_2-weighted breath-hold fast spin-echo, and gadolinium chelate–enhanced 3-D gradient-recalled imaging. *Am J Roentgenol* 1996;166:1115–1121.
6. Outwater EK, Mitchell DG. Differentiation of adrenal masses with chemical shift MR imaging (letter to the editor). *Radiology* 1994;193:877.
7. Spelle L, Soyer P, Rondeau Y, Gouhiri M, Scherrer A, Rymer R. Nontumorous hepatic pseudolesion around the falciform ligament: prevalence on gadolinium chelate–enhanced MR examination. *Am J Roentgenol* 1997;169:795–799.
8. Semelka RC, Ascher SM, Reinhold C. *MRI of the abdomen and pelvis: a text-atlas.* New York: Wiley, 1997;26.
9. Unger EC, Lee JK, Weyman PJ. CT and MR appearances of radiation hepatitis. *J Comput Assist Tomogr* 1987;11:264–268.
10. Ito K, Mitchell DG, Honjo K, et al. Biphasic contrast-enhanced multisection dynamic MR imaging of the liver: potential pitfalls. *RadioGraphics* 1997;17:693–705.
11. Mirowitz SA. Diagnostic pitfalls and artifacts in abdominal MR imaging: a review. *Radiology* 1998;208:577–589.

Variants and Pitfalls in Body Imaging,
edited by Ali Shirkhoda.
Lippincott Williams & Wilkins, Philadelphia, © 2000.

CHAPTER 10

Hepatic Sonography

Dale B. Johnson and Mostafa Atri

Hepatic sonography is an ideal method for evaluating focal and diffuse liver abnormalities. It is noninvasive, requires no intravenous contrast or radiation, and is performed with practically no patient discomfort. The treatment options for focal liver masses such as colorectal metastasis or hepatocellular carcinoma have expanded enormously over the years. Surgeons can now resect affected liver segments safely with low morbidity and mortality. In selected patients, cryoablation and hepatic artery chemoembolization of tumors can lead to preoperative down-staging of tumors and effective palliative treatment. Therefore, knowledge of normal hepatic anatomy and its variants is important for diagnosing hepatic diseases.

Furthermore, awareness of pseudolesions and potential artifacts enable the sonographer to distinguish between real and false pathology. The dynamic nature and multiplanar aspect of sonography help identify these variants better than the other cross-sectional imaging approaches. Moreover, there is also potential for these variants to be observed more frequently with sonography, and a full knowledge of these variants and artifacts is crucial to prevent misinterpretation of these findings for pathologic entities. This chapter reviews normal and variant sonographic liver anatomy and describes many of the sonographic artifacts that may mimic true pathology.

SONOGRAPHIC TECHNIQUE

Evaluation of the liver is best performed after the patient has fasted for 8 to 12 hours before the examination. The liver is evaluated with the patient examined in the supine, right anterior oblique, and left lateral decubi-

tus positions using either a 3.5- or a 5.0-MHz curvilinear transducer. A 2.5-MHz transducer can be used in obese patients for better ultrasound beam penetration. A 7.5-MHz linear array transducer may be required to evaluate the liver surface. Subcostal views are sufficient to evaluate most of the liver, but intercostal scanning is often needed to view the more cranial aspects of the liver. Color duplex is used to assess the presence or absence as well as the direction of flow in the vascular structures.

EMBRYOLOGY AND HISTOLOGY

The liver arises as a ventral bud from the most caudal aspect of the foregut early in the fourth week (1). This ventral bud grows into the septum transversum as rapidly proliferating cell strands. The proliferating endodermal cells give rise to interlacing cords of liver cells and the intrahepatic portion of the biliary tree. These cords of hepatocytes anastomose around preexisting endothelium-lined spaces that will eventually become the hepatic sinusoids. At 3 months the liver almost fills the abdominal cavity, and its left lobe is nearly as large as its right lobe. Later, when the hematopoietic activity of the liver is assumed by the spleen and bone marrow, the relative development of the liver changes, and the left lobe actually undergoes some degeneration and becomes smaller than the right (1).

The liver is made up mainly of three cell types, including biliary epithelial cells, Kupffer cells (part of the reticuloendothelial system responsible for phagocytizing bacteria and foreign material), and hepatocytes (1). The basic functional unit of the liver is the lobule. Each lobule consists of hepatocytes that radiate out to the periphery around a central vein. These hepatocytes carry out a variety of functions including synthesis, metabolism, and excretion of a variety of compounds. The outer borders of the lobules contain the portal triad: a connective tissue septum containing branches of the hepatic artery, portal vein, and bile duct.

D. B. Johnson: Department of Diagnostic Radiology, Montreal General Hospital, Montreal, Quebec H3G 1A4, Canada.

M. Atri: Department of Medical Imaging, University of Toronto, Princess Margaret Hospital, Toronto, Ontario, M5G M9 Canada.

GROSS ANATOMY

The normal adult liver is one of the largest organs in the body and occupies most of the right upper abdomen. It weighs about 1,400 to 1,600 g. In most adults, the right lobe is as much as six times larger than the left (1). The liver is generally less than 15 cm in length when measured at the right midclavicular line in the sagittal plane from the superior to inferior liver margins (2).

Normal Segmental Anatomy

The liver consists of three lobes: the right, left, and caudate lobes. The right lobe is further subdivided into the anterior and posterior segments, whereas the left lobe is subdivided into the medial and lateral segments (3). This lobar and segmental division is based on the vascular anatomy of the liver. This knowledge has advanced the field of liver surgery to the level of being able to precisely resect only the involved segment(s) of the liver. The major hepatic veins are intersegmental and therefore course between the hepatic lobes and segments, and the major portal vein branches are intrasegmental, coursing within the hepatic segments. The only exception is the ascending or vertical portion of the left portal vein, which travels within the left intersegmental fissure.

The right lobe of the liver, the largest, is separated from the left by the major lobar fissure. This fissure is usually not visible. However, in the transverse view, the major lobar fissure is found in the imaginary plane joining the gallbladder fossa and the inferior vena cava. Part of the major lobar fissure is occasionally seen (on the transverse view) as a hyperechoic linear structure anterosuperior to the gallbladder (Fig. 10.1). In fact, this fissure is consid-

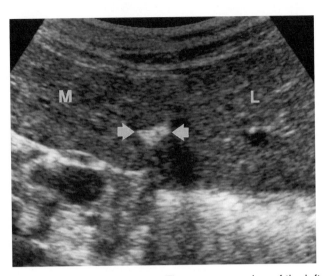

FIG. 10.2. Ligamentum teres. The transverse view of the left lobe of the liver shows an echogenic nodule *(arrows)* separating the lateral segment (L) from the medial segment (M) of the left lobe of the liver. Notice edge shadows posterior to the nodule.

ered a landmark for localization of the gallbladder when the gallbladder is contracted because of the existence of disease and difficult to identify (4). The middle hepatic vein travels through the cranial aspect of the major lobar fissure separating the anterior segment of the right lobe from the medial segment of the left lobe. The right hepatic vein travels through the right intersegmental fissure dividing the right lobe into anterior and posterior segments.

The left intersegmental fissure divides the left lobe into the medial (quadrate) and lateral segments. This intersegmental fissure can be divided into cranial, middle, and caudal thirds. The left hepatic vein, ascending portions of the left portal vein, and ligamentum teres are found in the

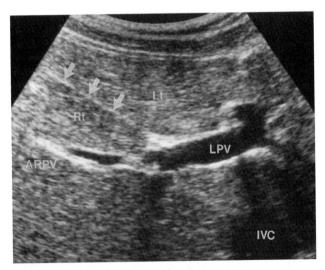

FIG. 10.1. Main interlobar fissure. The transverse view of the liver shows remaining part of the main interlobar fissure *(arrows),* which is occasionally seen cephalad to the gallbladder separating segment 4 of the left from segment 5 of the right lobe of the liver. LPV, left portal vein; IVC, inferior vena cava.

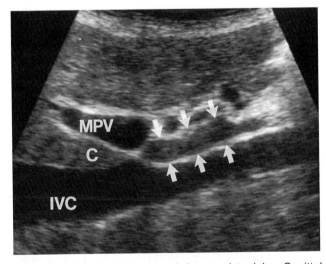

FIG. 10.3. Caudate process of the caudate lobe. Sagittal view at the level of the IVC demonstrates a nodular extension of the liver *(arrows)* caudal to the main portal vein (MPV) and the caudate lobe (C). IVC, inferior vena cava.

cranial, middle, and caudal thirds of the left intersegmental fissure, respectively. The ligamentum teres is often seen as a rounded hyperechoic structure on the transverse view and should not be confused with focal hyperechoic liver masses (Fig. 10.2). Scanning carefully through the suspected lesion in the transverse and longitudinal planes will help make this important distinction by demonstrating the elongated nature of the round ligament.

The caudate lobe of the liver is considered anatomically distinct from both right and left lobes. On the transverse view, it is located posterior to the porta hepatis, between the fissure for the ligamentum venosum and the inferior vena cava. Although it is continuous with the right lobe of the liver laterally, the caudate lobe has a distinct vascular pattern. It receives blood supply from both the right and the left portal veins and drains directly into the inferior vena cava. The proximal

horizontal portion of the left portal vein (pars transversa) travels over the anterior margin of the inferior caudate lobe, separating it from the medial segment of the left lobe of the liver. The caudate lobe is also separated from the lateral segment of the left lobe of the liver by the ligamentum venosum. The right inferior margin of the caudate lobe extends in a tongue-like projection called the caudate process between the inferior vena cava and adjacent main portal vein (Fig. 10.3). The caudate process is usually very small and therefore not seen often sonographically. When present, it should not be mistaken for a mass or adenopathy. The papillary process of the caudate lobe is a small ovoid prominence that lies above and in front of the common hepatic artery, close to the portal vein and pancreatic isthmus (Fig. 10.4) (5,6). Enlarged papillary processes are more frequently seen in patients with chronic liver disease. In

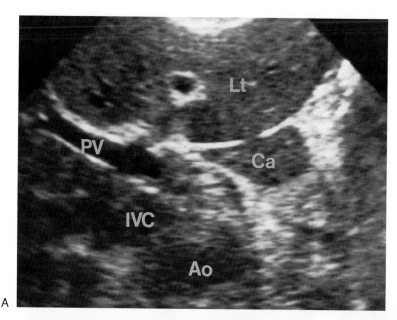

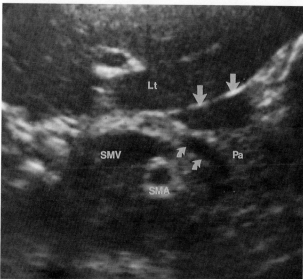

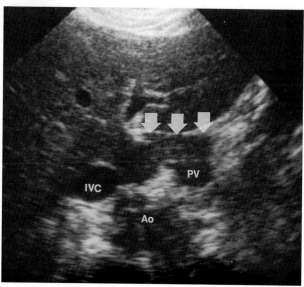

FIG. 10.4. Papillary process of the caudate lobe. Transverse views in three different patients. **A:** A separate oval-shaped papillary process (Ca) lies posterior to and separate from the lateral segment of the left lobe (Lt). **B:** A separate oval-shaped structure *(arrows)* is seen between the lateral segment of the liver (Lt) and the body of the pancreas (Pa). **C:** Medial extension *(arrows)* of the caudate lobe is seen anterior to the PV (main portal vein). Notice that all papillary processes have the same echo texture as the adjacent liver. Superior mesenteric artery and vein, SMA and SMV, splenic vein *(curved arrows)*. Ao, aorta; SMA, superior mesenteric artery; SMV, superior mesenteric vein.

one series, the papillary processes measured in transverse diameter between 8 mm and 39 mm (5). The papillary process, like the caudate process, may appear separate from the liver and thus mimic lymph nodes or a pancreatic mass. Knowledge of the anatomy, sonographic pattern, and vascular relationships of the papillary process enable its correct identification.

Functional Segmental Anatomy

The most commonly used system for mapping out the functional segmental anatomy of the liver is based on the nomenclature of Couinaud (7). According to Couinaud, a segment is the smallest functional anatomic unit of the liver. Each segment is determined by the distribution of the portal and hepatic veins with a branch of the portal vein in the center and a branch of the hepatic vein in the periphery. The liver is divided in the longitudinal plane into four sections by the right, middle, and left hepatic veins. The anterior and posterior segments of the right lobe and lateral segment of the left lobe are further divided into superior and inferior segments by an imaginary transverse plane created by a line drawn through the right and left portal veins. Eight segments are therefore recognized (Fig. 10.5), as distinguished from the five segments described in the previous section. The importance of this modified functional segmental anatomic nomenclature lies in precise localization and surgical segmental resection of liver lesions. This segmental classification and their vascular anatomy is further discussed in Chapter 11.

ANATOMIC VARIATIONS OF THE LIVER LOBES

Variant lobar and segmental anatomy has been described in the literature (8,9). In general, hypoplasia or absence of a segment or lobe of the liver is associated with hypoplasia or absence of the vascular supply. Unusual portal venous anatomy, therefore, is often the first clue to the existence of anomalies of the lobar or segmental anatomy of the liver (see the portal vein section). Absent right or left lobes of the liver are rare and constitute extreme examples of abnormal lobar anatomy. Different degrees of segmental hypoplasia are more commonly seen and often can be recognized by the variance of the size of the portal venous system or an abnormal location of the gallbladder and liver fissures. A small liver because of an absent lobe is associated with compensatory hypertrophy of the remaining liver. This may be confused with a cirrhotic liver. In the case of an absent right lobe, differentiation can be made from cirrhosis by normal architecture and contour of the remaining liver, hypertrophy of the medial segment as well as the lateral segment, and the absence of the right portal vein. In cirrhosis, the architecture and the contour of the remaining liver is abnormal, there is predominant hypertrophy of the lateral segment, and the right portal vein is present. Absent right lobe may be associated with the absence of the caudate lobe (9). Absence of liver tissue to the left of the gallbladder is diagnostic of an absent left lobe. In addition, failure to identify the falciform ligament or the ligamentum teres further supports this. In the presence of lobar or segmental hypoplasia, previous resection and

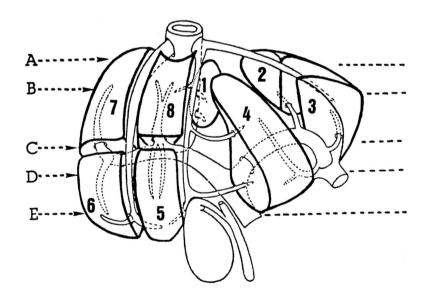

FIG. 10.5. Segmental anatomy based on the hepatic and portal venous anatomy as described by Couinaud. Clockwise lie the caudate lobe (1), superior extension of the lateral segment (2), inferior extension of the lateral segment (3), medial segment (4), inferior extension of the anterior segment of the right lobe (5), inferior extension of the posterior segment of the right lobe (6), superior extension of the posterior segment of the right lobe (7), superior extension of the anterior segment of the right lobe (8).

atrophy secondary to obstruction of the bile ducts from cholangiocarcinoma should be considered in the differential diagnosis. Rarely, accessory lobes may be seen, including a lobus vena cava along the inferior vena cava, and pons hepaticas between liver segments. Ectopic liver tissue has also been described but is also rare. Ectopic sites include the gallbladder wall, spleen, ligamentum teres, and omentum.

Accessory Fissures

Accessory fissures unrelated to the major or intersegmental fissures are well-known variants (10–13). These accessory fissures are seen as echogenic lines because of their fat content and sometimes mimic echogenic lesions. They are present mainly in the superior aspect of the liver and can sometimes extend deeply into the liver parenchyma, mimicking a major fissure. The most prominent and well-described fissure is the right inferior accessory fissure (12), which is seen within the posterior segment of the right lobe of the liver. In one series of 2,000 patients having liver sonograms, Lim et al. observed that in 15 cases, the inferior accessory fissure was present as a coronal or parasagittal fissure through the parenchyma of the posterior segment of the right hepatic lobe (12). The fissure was seen as a thin echogenic membrane

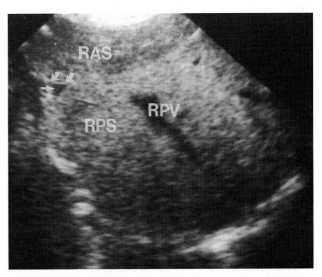

FIG. 10.7. Accessory right lobe fissure *(curved arrows)*. Transverse view of the right lobe shows a V-shaped indentation on the lateral aspect of the right lobe of the liver *(curved arrows)*, filled with ascites *(arrow)* separating the anterior segment (RAS) from the posterior segment (RPS) of the right lobe. RPV, right portal vein.

stretching downward from the right branch of the portal vein to the inferior surface of the right hepatic lobe. On cadaveric sections, the fissure was an invagination of the peritoneum directed laterally and slightly posteriorly from the medial inferior surface of the right hepatic lobe below the porta hepatis. Another relatively commonly seen fissure is the accessory fissure of the liver, located on the inferior side of the left lobe. The fissure was recognized in about 5% of 800 consecutive subjects in one series (13). This fissure separates segment 2 from segment 3 of the lateral segment of the left lobe of the liver (Fig. 10.6). The accessory right lobe fissure has not been reported. Figure 10.7 shows an indentation on the lateral aspect of the right lobe of the liver containing ascitic fluid corresponding to an imaginary line separating the anterior and posterior segments of the right lobe of the liver.

HEPATIC VASCULATURE: AN OVERVIEW

The blood supply to the liver is through the hepatic artery and the portal vein. The portal vein supplies approximately 75% of the oxygen requirement to the hepatocytes while the hepatic artery supplies the rest. Because of this dual blood supply to the liver, infarcts are rare. The importance of understanding the normal and variant vascular anatomy of the liver, however, is apparent when surgical resection or chemoembolization of a

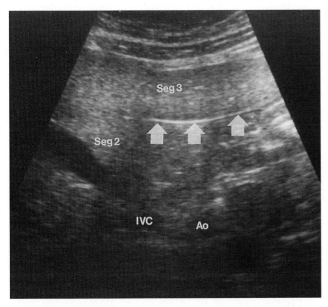

FIG. 10.6. Accessory fissure of the left lobe of the liver. Transverse view of the lateral segment of the left lobe demonstrates a horizontal line *(arrows)* separating segment 3 (Seg 3) from segment 2 (Seg 2) of the left lobe of the liver. IVC, inferior vena cava; Ao, aorta.

liver mass or masses is contemplated. In addition, preoperative knowledge of the normal and potentially variant hepatic vascular anatomy in liver transplant donors and recipients will have a significant impact on the surgical success as well. Preoperative knowledge of the precise vascular anatomy in these clinical situations is crucial to the surgical outcome.

Hepatic Veins

In approximately 70% of the population, there are right, middle, and left hepatic veins that drain into the inferior vena cava (IVC). In as much as 65% to 85% of this group, the left and middle hepatic veins have a common trunk that drains into the IVC; the remainder (15% to 35%) have separate trunks. Thirty percent of the population will have more than three hepatic veins, and absence of one or more of the hepatic veins is rare (14). Also, 30% of the population will have a right or left marginal hepatic vein(s) (Fig. 10.8). Although preoperative knowledge of this hepatic venous anatomy is not as crucial as the hepatic arterial anatomy, it is still important information.

Approximately 5% to 18% of the population have an accessory right hepatic vein. The most common of these is the inferior right hepatic vein, which is seen in 10% to 18% of the population (15,16). It drains segment 6 and enters the dorsal part of the IVC, below the level of entry of the major hepatic veins (Fig. 10.9). The middle right hepatic vein is reported in 5.5% of the population. It drains segment 5 and joins the IVC between the main right and the inferior right hepatic veins (16). Both of these veins can be larger than the main right hepatic vein (15,16).

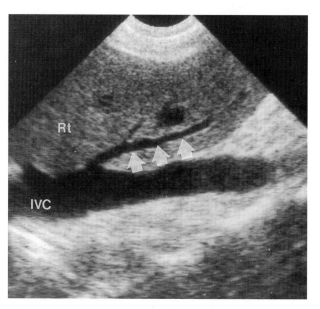

FIG. 10.9. Accessory inferior right hepatic vein. Longitudinal view of the right lobe of the liver shows an accessory inferior right hepatic vein *(arrows)* draining into the inferior vena cava (IVC). Rt, right lobe of liver.

Portal Veins

The main portal vein is formed at the confluence of the splenic and superior mesenteric veins and is approximately 8 cm in length. It travels into the liver in the porta hepatis, where it divides into left and right branches. The right portal vein further divides into anterior and posterior branches supplying the corresponding hepatic segments.

The initial horizontal portion of the left portal vein (pars transversa) gives branches to the caudate lobe and then enters the left lobe along the anterior surface of the caudate lobe before abruptly turning anteriorly. The ascending portion of the left portal vein gives branches to the medial and lateral segments of the left lobe.

Portal Vein Anomalies

Fraser-Hill et al. have described the variant portal vein anomalies using duplex and color Doppler ultrasound (17). These are divided into anomalies of the right and the left portal veins (Fig. 10.10).

Anomalies of the right portal vein includes four categories of complete absence of the main right portal vein:

1. Trifurcation of the main portal vein into the right posterior segmental, right anterior segmental, and the left portal vein (Fig. 10.11).
2. The main portal vein dividing into the right anterior segmental branch and the left portal vein. The right posterior segmental branch originates from the main portal vein (Fig. 10.12).
3. The main portal vein dividing into the right posterior segmental branch and the left portal vein. The right

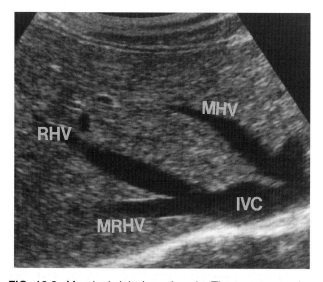

FIG. 10.8. Marginal right hepatic vein. The transverse view at the level of the hepatic veins demonstrates an accessory marginal right hepatic vein (MRHV) draining into the right hepatic vein (RHV). MHV, middle hepatic vein; IVC, inferior vena cava.

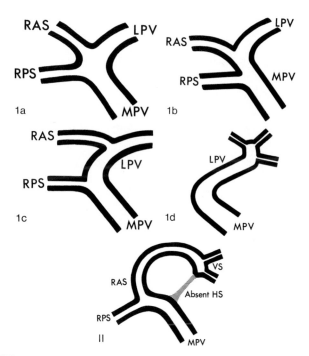

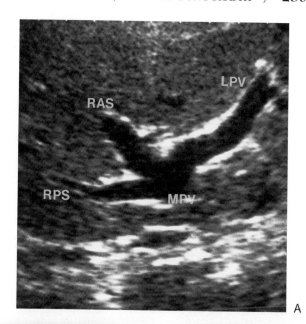

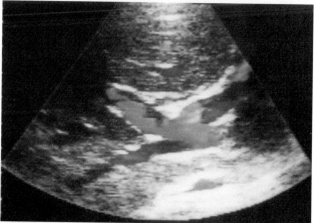

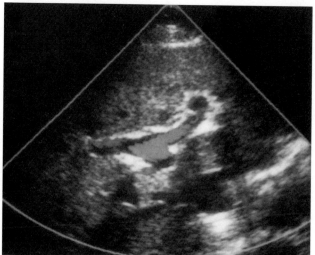

FIG. 10.10. Diagrammatic representation of portal vein anomalies. The right portal vein anomaly includes four categories (1a–1d), and the left portal vein one category (II). (Reproduced with permission from reference 18.)

FIG. 10.11. Trifurcation of the main portal vein. **A:** Transverse view shows trifurcation of the main portal vein (MPV) into the right posterior segment (RPS), the right anterior segment (RAS), and the left portal vein (LPV). Notice the right main portal vein is absent. **B:** Color representation of the same anomaly, shown in black and white. (Reproduced with permission from reference 17.)

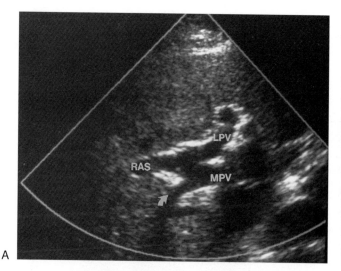

FIG. 10.12. Origin of the right posterior segment portal vein from the main portal vein. **A:** Transverse view demonstrates division of the main portal vein (MPV) into the right anterior segment (RAS) portal vein and the left portal vein (LPV). The right posterior segment vein *(curved arrow)* originates from the main portal vein (MPV). Notice that after the takeoff of the posterior segment branch, the main portal vein continues to the right. **B:** Color representation of the same anomaly, shown in black and white. (Reproduced with permission from reference 17.)

anterior segmental branch originates from the left portal vein (Fig. 10.13). Types 2 and 3 are differentiated by continuation of the portal vein to the right after the takeoff of the right posterior branch in type 2 and to the left in the type 3.

4. Complete absence of the right portal vein and its branches (Fig. 10.14). This anomaly is associated with the absence of the right lobe of the liver. Other manifestations associated with this anomaly are longer horizontal segment of the left portal vein as a result of compensatory hypertrophy of the caudate lobe and the medial segment of the left lobe. In addition, there may be indication of a subdiaphragmatic location of the gallbladder (Fig. 10.15). If the right lobe of the liver is hypoplastic, a small branch may be present originating from the portal vein (Fig. 10.16).

Anomalies of the left portal vein are generally caused by the absence of the horizontal segment of the left portal vein. Different lengths of the vertical portion of the left portal vein exist (Fig. 10.17A,B). The blood supply to the remaining left portal vein comes through an intraparenchymal connecting channel between the right anterior segmental branch of the right and the vertical portion of the left portal vein (Fig. 10.17C).

In a prospective study reported by Atri et al. (18), the prevalence of intrahepatic portal venous anomalies was reported to be as follows: trifurcation of portal vein, 10.8%; right posterior segmental branch arising from the main portal vein, 4.7%; a right anterior segmental branch

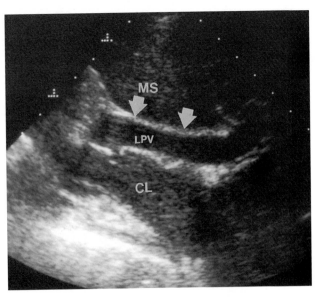

FIG. 10.14. Complete absence of the right portal vein. Transverse view shows continuation of the main portal vein (not seen on this picture) as the left portal vein (LPV). The right portal vein and the right lobe of the liver are absent. Notice the long horizontal segment of the LPV *(arrows)* corresponding to the hypertrophy of the caudate lobe (CL) and the medial segment (MS) of the left lobe.

originating from the left portal vein, 4.3%; and absence of the horizontal segment of the left portal vein, 0.2%. In this series, there was no case of absence of the right portal vein.

Congenital anomalies including atresia and stricture of the main portal vein are rare. These variants are important in two different clinical settings. One is in planning

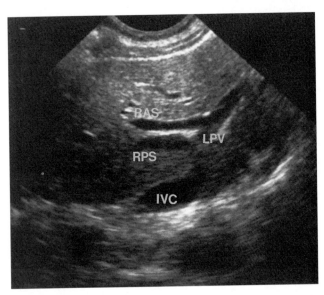

FIG. 10.13. Origin of the right anterior segment portal vein from the left portal vein. Transverse view shows the main portal vein (not seen on the picture) dividing into the right posterior segment (RPS) and the left portal vein (LPV). The right anterior segment branch originates from the left portal vein. Notice that after the takeoff of the RPS branch, the vein continues to the left. IVC, inferior vena cava. (Reproduced with permission from reference 17.)

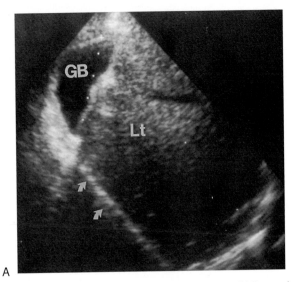

A

FIG. 10.15. Absent right lobe of the liver. **A:** Oblique ultrasound of the region of the right hemidiaphragm *(curved arrows)*. Notice that the gallbladder (GB) lies between the diaphragm and the left lobe (Lt) of the liver.

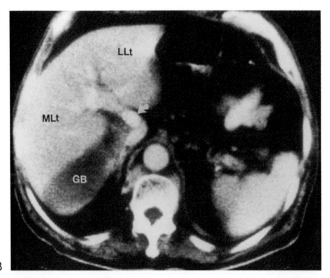

B

FIG. 10.15. *Continued.* **B:** A CT scan on the same patient also shows the GB lying between the diaphragm and the medial segment of the left lobe (MLt). The vertical portion of the left portal vein *(curved arrow)* lies between the lateral segment (LLt) and hypertrophied medial segment (Mlt) of the left lobe.

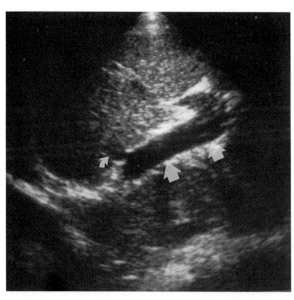

FIG. 10.16. Hypoplasia of the right lobe of the liver. A small branch of the portal vein *(curved arrow)* is seen originating from the proximal left portal vein *(arrows)* leading to the small right lobe of the liver.

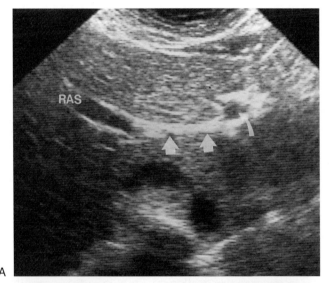

A

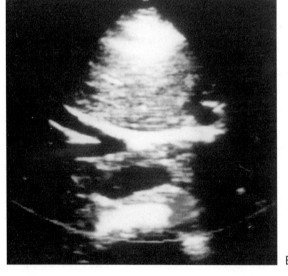

B

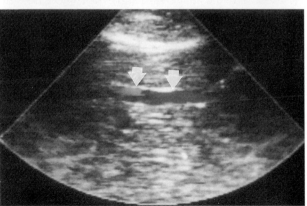

C

FIG. 10.17. Absent horizontal segment of the left portal vein. **A:** The horizontal portion of the left portal vein is absent and replaced by an echogenic band *(arrows).* A small remnant of the vertical portion remains *(curved arrow).* **B:** Color representation of the same anomaly. Notice the direction of the flow in the vertical portion of the left portal vein, which is the opposite of the normal direction. **C:** Transverse view at a level slightly above **A** and **B** shows the connecting channel *(arrows)* between the anterior segmental branch and the remaining left portal vein. Note that the direction of flow is from right to left. RAS, right anterior segment portal vein. (Reproduced with permission from reference 17.)

hepatic surgery, and the other is in the differential diagnosis of chronic portal vein thrombosis. In most cases of chronic portal vein thrombosis, the thrombosed portal vein is still evident, as opposed to those anomalies in which the involved portal vein is absent.

Hepatic Arteries

The celiac trunk, arising from the aorta, divides into the left gastric, splenic, and common hepatic arteries (19). The common hepatic artery arises from the celiac axis and travels to the right along the cephalic part of the pancreas. It then bifurcates in the region of the isthmus into the gastroduodenal artery, which travels caudally along the anterolateral surface of the pancreatic head, and the proper hepatic artery, which is a continuation of the common hepatic artery distal to the takeoff of the gastroduodenal artery. The proper hepatic artery travels cephalad toward the porta hepatis along the free margin of the gastroduodenal ligament. This artery is generally anterior to the portal vein and to the left of the common bile duct. The proper hepatic artery bifurcates (or trifurcates) into the right and relatively smaller left (and middle) hepatic arteries. Because of their smaller size, the left and middle hepatic arteries are not seen as frequently as the right one. The middle hepatic artery travels in the left intersegmental fissure and may be seen lateral to the ligamentum teres. The left hepatic artery can sometimes be seen traveling with the left portal vein in the left intersegmental fissure medial to the ligamentum teres. The intrahepatic portions of the hepatic arteries are difficult to identify sonographically because they are usually small. They, however, can be seen next to the right and left branches of the portal vein. Variations in the origin of the hepatic artery are quite common, occurring approximately 45% of the time (20). The usual (55%) arterial configuration consists of the common hepatic artery arising from the celiac axis branching into the gastroduodenal artery and proper hepatic artery. The proper hepatic artery then branches into the right and left hepatic arteries. Variations to this pattern include a replaced right hepatic artery arising from the superior mesenteric artery, replaced left hepatic artery arising from the left gastric artery, or replaced common hepatic artery arising from the superior mesenteric artery. The replaced (entire) or accessory (part) right hepatic artery arising from the superior mesenteric artery generally travels posterior to the portal vein and anterior to the IVC. In one series, 71% of the angiographically proven replaced right hepatic arteries were detected by ultrasound (21). A replaced or accessory left hepatic artery can usually be seen on the transverse view as an arterial channel within the ligamentum venosum (Fig. 10.18). This anomaly was demonstrated in 10% of normal liver ultrasound examinations in one series (22).

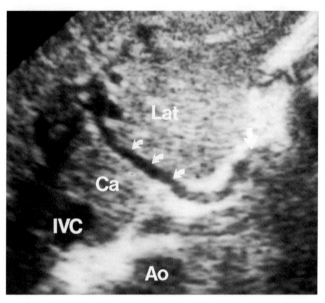

FIG. 10.18. Origin of the left hepatic artery from the left gastric artery. Transverse view shows the left hepatic artery (curved arrows) originating from the left gastric artery *(arrow)* running in the ligamentum venosum between the caudate lobe (Ca) and the lateral segment (Lat) of the left lobe. IVC, inferior vena cava; Ao, aorta.

PITFALLS AND ARTIFACTS

Shadowing Artifacts

Acoustic shadowing from the ligamentum teres or simply its increased echogenic nature can mimic a calcified mass (See Fig. 10.2). Also, attenuation of the sound beam by the echogenic fissure for ligamentum venosum can result in an apparent hypoechoic lesion in the caudate lobe (Fig. 10.19) (23). Scanning in multiple planes usually resolves this issue.

Mirror-Image Artifact

Such an artifact can be created when a hepatic lesion is located near the diaphragm, especially in a hyperechoic lesion (Fig. 10.20). This artifact results from reflection of the sound beam on the two adjacent curved surfaces, the lesion and the diaphragm (24). In some cases, during scanning, the mirror-image artifact is seen on an image different from the one that shows the true finding, and therefore, both the lesion and artifact may not be seen on the same image. In such a case, the location of the artifact that is projected over the lungs helps determine the nature of the finding.

Hyperechoic Pseudolesions

Echogenic areas in the liver include diaphragmatic slips over the superior liver surface (Fig. 10.21), involving perihepatic fat invaginating into the liver posteriorly (Figs. 10.22 and 10.23). The soft nature of the liver

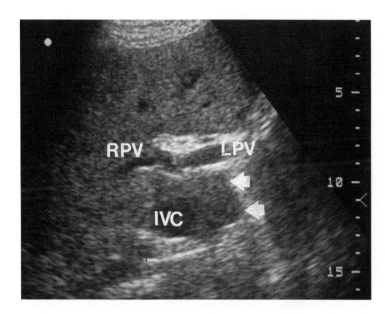

FIG. 10.19. Hypoechoic caudate lobe. Transverse view of a hypoechoic but normal caudate lobe *(arrows)* because of attenuation of sound by the portal vein or the ligamentum venosum. RPV, right portal vein; LPV, left portal vein.

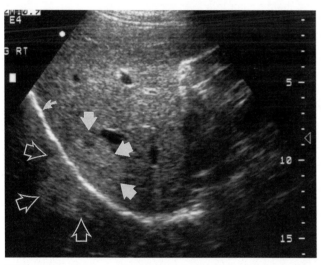

FIG. 10.20. Mirror-image artifact. Oblique view of the right lobe of the liver shows mirror-image artifact *(open arrows)* of an echogenic liver lesion *(arrows)* on the pulmonary side of the diaphragm *(curved arrow).*

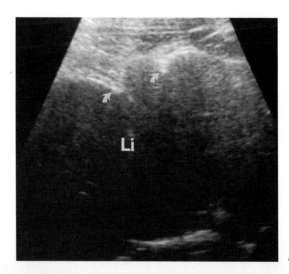

A

B

FIG. 10.21. Diaphragmatic slips. **A:** The transverse view of the right lobe of the liver shows wedge-shaped echogenic structures *(curved arrows)* protruding into the anterior aspect of the right lobe of the liver (Li). **B:** A CT scan of the same patient demonstrates the corresponding diaphragmatic slips *(arrows).*

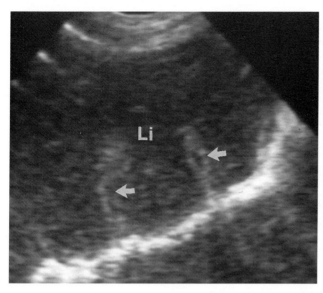
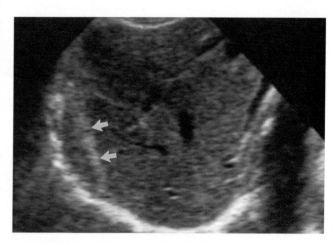

A
B

FIG. 10.22. Diaphragmatic slips. **A:** The transverse view of the right lobe of the liver shows layered triangular echogenic structures *(arrows)* protruding into the posterior aspect of the liver (Li). **B:** These structures appear elongated on the plane 90 degrees to the above plane *(arrows)*. The shape and the layered appearance of these structures help distinguished them from a true liver nodule.

allows for intraparenchymal penetration of these structures mimicking liver lesions. The shape, layered appearance of these structures representing a combination of the diaphragm, liver capsule and the intervening fat and their independent movement relative to the liver on dynamic scanning, help distinguish them from the true liver lesions. Also, careful ultrasound scanning through these lesions in the longitudinal and transverse planes will resolve the issue.

Another echogenic pseudo lesion in the liver may be present posterior to a hepatic vein as a result of through transmission of the sound beam (Fig. 10.24).

Hepatic Lobar Extension Artifact

In the left subphrenic space, the occasional extension of the left hepatic lobe between the left hemidiaphragm and the upper part of the spleen creates a crescent cephalad to the spleen which could be either hypoechoic (normal liver) (Fig. 10.25) or hyperechoic (liver with fatty infiltration) (Fig. 10.26). This can potentially mimic a subcapsular hematoma of the spleen. However, identification of portal venous branches in the liver and independent movement of the two structures help confirm the existence of this normal variant. A prominent

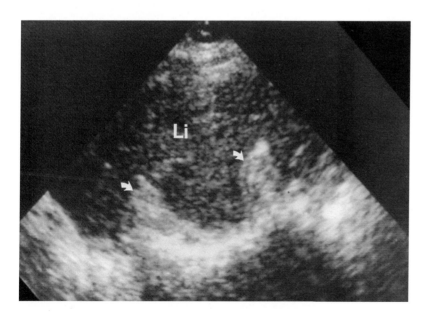

FIG. 10.23. Another example of the diaphragmatic bands.

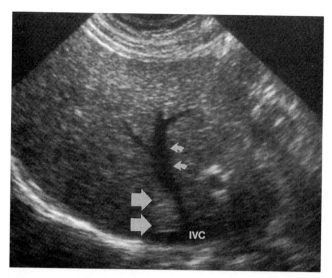

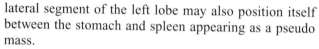

FIG. 10.24. Pseudolesion. An apparent pseudolesion *(arrows)* lying posterior to the hepatic vein *(curved arrows)*. IVC, inferior vena cava.

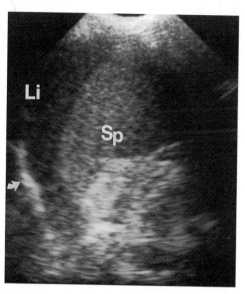

FIG. 10.25. Left subphrenic liver. Normal liver (Li) extending between the diaphragm *(curved arrow)* and the spleen (Sp).

lateral segment of the left lobe may also position itself between the stomach and spleen appearing as a pseudo mass.

The right lobe of the liver may be elongated (Reidel's lobe) and extends down as far as the right iliac crest mimicking a pelvic mass or hepatomegaly. This normal variant can be distinguished from a pelvic mass by evaluating its echopattern and its contiguity with the liver. (See also Figs. 8.10 and 9.6.)

Double-Channel Sign

A double-channel sign in the liver normally indicates the presence of bile duct dilatation. However, a visible hepatic artery following the portal vein can rarely simulate a double-channel sign. Doppler interrogation confirms the diagnosis (Fig. 10.27). This is more commonly seen in patients with cirrhosis because of hypertrophy of the hepatic arteries to compensate for the diminished portal flow.

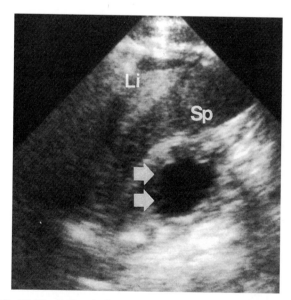

FIG. 10.26. Left subphrenic liver with fatty infiltration. The longitudinal view of the left upper quadrant demonstrates a fatty liver (Li) lying above the spleen (Sp). *Arrows* point to a pseudocyst of the pancreas.

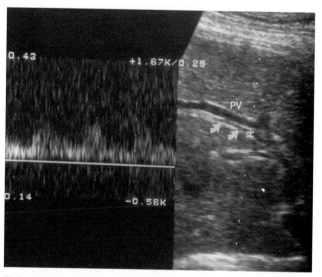

FIG. 10.27. Pseudo–double-channel sign. The transverse view of the right lobe of the liver shows double-channel *(curved arrows* and PV) sign representing hepatic artery and portal vein (PV) on pulsed Doppler examination.

In summary, hepatic sonography is an excellent way to evaluate the liver for focal and diffuse diseases. It is also a crucial part of the pretherapeutic evaluation. Recognition of normal anatomic variations aids the sonographer in readily distinguishing between normal and pathologic processes.

REFERENCES

1. Elias H, Sherrick JC. Development of the human liver. In: *Morphology of the liver*. New York: Academic Press 1969;265–293.
2. Gosink BB, Leymaster CE. Ultrasonic determination of hepatomegaly. *J Clin Ultrasound* 1981;9:37–44.
3. Lafortune M, Madore F, Patriguin H, et al. Segmental anatomy of the liver: A sonographic approach to Couinaud nomenclature. *Radiology* 1991;181:443–448.
4. Callen PW, Filly RA. Ultrasonographic localization of the gallbladder. *Radiology* 1979;133:687–691.
5. Donoso L, Martinez-Noguera A, Zidan A, et al. Papillary process of the caudate lobe of the liver: sonographic appearance. *Radiology* 1989;173:631–633.
6. Brown BM, Filly RA, Callen PW. Ultrasonic anatomy of the caudate lobe. *J Ultrasound Med* 1982;1:189–192.
7. Dodd GD III. An American guide to Couinaud's numbering system. *Am J Roentgenol* 1993;161:574–575.
8. Belton RI, VanZandt TF. Congenital absence of the left lobe of the liver: A radiologic diagnosis. *Radiology* 1983;147:184.
9. Radin DR, Colletti PM, Ralls PW, et al. Agenesis of the right lobe of the liver. *Radiology* 1987;164:639–642.
10. Parulekar SG. Ligaments and fissures of the liver: Sonographic anatomy. *Radiology* 1979;130:409–411.
11. Auh YH, Rubenstein WA, Zirinsky K, et al. Accessory fissures of the liver: CT and sonographic appearance. *Am J Roentgenol* 1984;143:565–572.
12. Lim JH, Ko YT, Hau MC, et al. The inferior accessory hepatic fissure: sonographic appearance. *Am J Roentgenol* 1987;149:495–497.
13. Martinoli C, Cittadini G, Conzi R, et al. Sonographic characterization of an accessory fissure of the left hepatic lobe determined by omental infolding. *J Ultrasound Med* 1992;11:103–107.
14. Cosgrove DO, Arger PH, Coleman BG. Ultrasonic anatomy of the hepatic veins. *J Clin Ultrasound* 1987;15:231–235.
15. Makuuchi M, Hasegawa H, Yamazaki S, et al. The inferior right hepatic vein: Ultrasonic demonstration. *Radiology* 1983;148:213–217.
16. Cheng YF, Huang TL, Chen CL, et al. Variations of the middle and inferior right hepatic vein: application in hepatectomy. *J Clin Ultrasound* 1997;25:175–182.
17. Fraser-Hill M, Atri M, Bret PM, et al. Intrahepatic portal venous system: Variations demonstrated with duplex and color Doppler ultrasound. *Radiology* 1990;177:523–526.
18. Atri M, Bret PM, Fraser-Hill M. Intrahepatic portal venous variations: Prevalence with ultrasound. *Radiology* 1992;184:157–158.
19. Abams HL, ed. *Abrams angiography: Vascular and interventional radiology, 3rd ed.* Boston: Little, Brown, 1983.
20. Kadir S. *Atlas of normal and variant angiographic anatomy.* Philadelphia: WB Saunders, 1991.
21. Bret PM, Reinhold C, Herba M, et al. Replaced or accessory right hepatic artery: Can ultrasound replace angiography. *J Clin Ultrasound* 1988;16:245–249.
22. Nichols DM, Cooperberg PL. Sonographic demonstration of the aberrant left hepatic artery. *J Ultrasound Med* 1984;3:219–221.
23. Mitchell SE, Gross BH, Spitz HB. The hypoechoic caudate lobe: an ultrasonic pseudolesion. *Radiology* 1982;144:569–572.
24. Robinson DE, Wilson LS, Kossoff G. Shadowing and enhancement in ultrasonic echograms by reflection and refraction. *J Clin Ultrasound* 1981;9:181–188.
25. Laing FC. Commonly encountered artifacts in clinical ultrasound. *Semin Ultrasonogr* 1983;4:27.

Variants and Pitfalls in Body Imaging,
edited by Ali Shirkhoda.
Lippincott Williams & Wilkins, Philadelphia, © 2000.

CHAPTER 11

The Liver: CT Arterial Portography

Lilliam M. Diaz-Sola, Hoon Ji, and Pablo R. Ros

In liver tumor imaging, computed tomography arterial portography (CTAP) has been found to be the most sensitive preoperative imaging study for focal liver lesions, although it lacks specificity (Fig. 11.1). The reported sensitivity of CTAP is 81% to 91% in series correlated with surgical findings (1,2). This is even more significant for lesions larger than 1.5 to 2.0 cm (Fig. 11.2) (3–6).

Unfortunately, CTAP is plagued with many pitfalls and normal variations in addition to its invasive nature. The revolution in imaging techniques over the past several years has created a wide array of choices for clinicians investigating patients with suspected hepatic disease. Nevertheless, to date, CTAP has a prominent function in patient selection and surgical planning in cases of hepatic metastases from colorectal carcinoma and primary malignant hepatic tumors (7). A well-performed and interpreted CTAP study can precisely describe the size, number, and segmental location of existing hepatic focal lesions and demonstrate their relationship to the inferior vena cava, hepatic veins, portal vein branches, and porta hepatis.

HEPATIC SEGMENTAL ANATOMY AND USEFULNESS OF COMPUTED TOMOGRAPHY ARTERIAL PORTOGRAPHY FOR SURGICAL PLANNING

In 1982, Bismuth (8) created a hepatic segmental nomenclature system that combined two prior systems. Bismuth's system is surgically relevant because all hepatic segments, with the exception of the caudate lobe, are defined by three oblique vertical scissurae, corresponding to the planes described by the course of the right, left, and middle hepatic veins, and by an oblique horizontal scissura, which is defined by the course of the right and left portal veins (Fig. 11.3).

Bismuth's system is currently the one most frequently used because of the need for a precise terminology secondary to advances in hepatic surgical imaging and tumor ablative techniques. Surgeons can now obtain precise preoperative information that allows performance of wedge resection, subsegmentectomy, segmentectomy, lobectomy, or trisegmentectomy, either alone or in combination with ablative techniques (either surgical or percutaneous) such as cryotherapy or intratumoral injections of ethanol (8,9).

Helical (spiral) CTAP also can be used to estimate liver volume preoperatively and, therefore, to determine precisely the percentage of liver that will remain after resection of all metastases (10). This is another reason why helical CTAP has become an important preoperative diagnostic tool in surgical planning: patient survival following hepatic resection decreases sharply if less than 35% of the liver volume remains after surgery. Furthermore, it has been suggested that preoperative emboliza-

L. M. Diaz-Sola: Division of Body Imaging and Magnetic Resonance Imaging, Department of Radiology, University of Florida College of Medicine, Gainesville, Florida 32610.

H. Ji: Department of Radiology, Ajou University, Suwon, Korea; and Brigham and Women's Hospital, Harvard Medical School, Boston, Massachusetts 02115.

P. R. Ros: Department of Radiology, Brigham and Women's Hospital, Harvard Medical School, Boston, Massachusetts 02115.

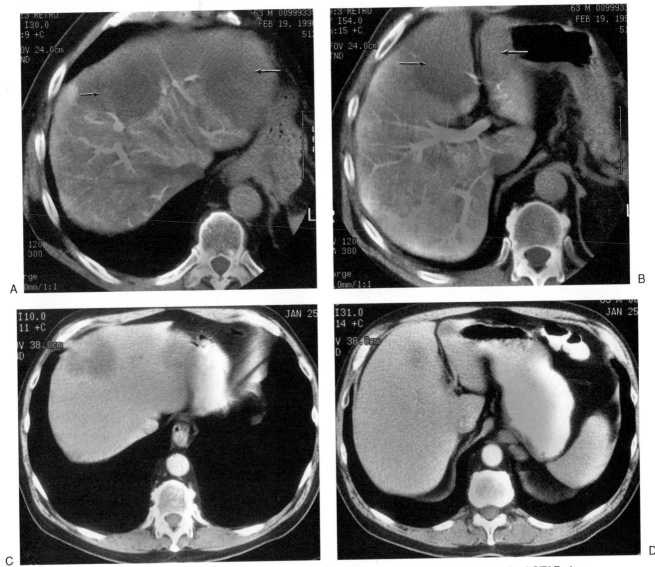

FIG. 11.1. Metastatic liver disease: CTAP compared to intravenous helical CT. **A,B:** Helical CTAP showing well-defined hypodense lesions in segments 8, 2 *(arrows),* 4a, 4b, and 3 **(B)** *(arrows).* **C,D:** Intravenous helical CT (portal phase) showing above-described lesions. Note that on CTAP, lesions are better defined and show greater extension than on triphasic helical CT examination.

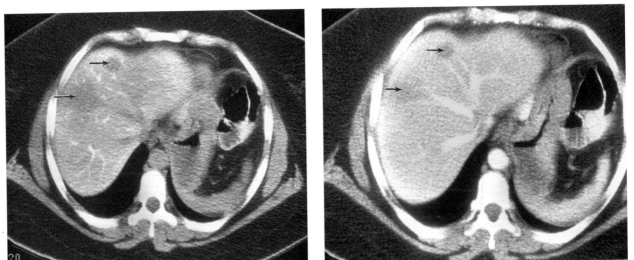

FIG. 11.2. Metastatic liver disease. **A,B:** Helical CTAP early **(A)** and late **(B)** phases clearly showing *(arrows)* focal hypodense metastatic lesions at segments 8 and 4a.

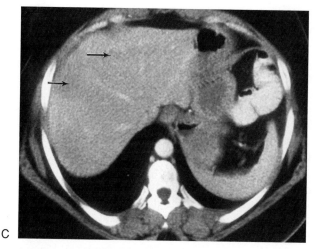

FIG. 11.2. *Continued.* **C:** A 4a metastatic lesion, which measures less than 2 cm in diameter, was virtually not seen on intravenous helical CT examination.

TECHNIQUE OF HELICAL COMPUTED TOMOGRAPHY ARTERIAL PORTOGRAPHY

In helical or spiral CT, x-ray output and table translation can be continuous without interscan delays, which permits the radiographic images to be obtained from a volume data set acquired during a single 20-second breath-hold. Motion artifact and misregistration are practically eliminated (11–13). Selective delivery of contrast material to the intrahepatic portal system is achieved through injection of contrast through the splenic or superior mesenteric artery. Hepatic images are then obtained before systemic circulation of the contrast material occurs in order to achieve a significant difference in attenuation values between nonenhancing hepatic parenchymal lesions and enhancing disease-free liver (11,14). These differences in attenuation values relate to the fact that the normal liver parenchyma receives 75% of its blood supply from the portal vein, as opposed to metastases and primary liver neoplasms, which are supplied by the hepatic artery (11,14) and have no significant portal enhancement.

Conventional angiographic examination of the celiac and superior mesenteric arteries is initially performed to demonstrate the hepatic arterial supply and to determine normal anatomy versus variants (i.e., displaced hepatic artery). During this examination, patency of the superior

tion of the right portal vein in surgical candidates for right lobectomy secondary to metastases may lead to increased percentages of postoperative liver volume through hypertrophy of the left lobe after induction of atrophy in the right lobe (10).

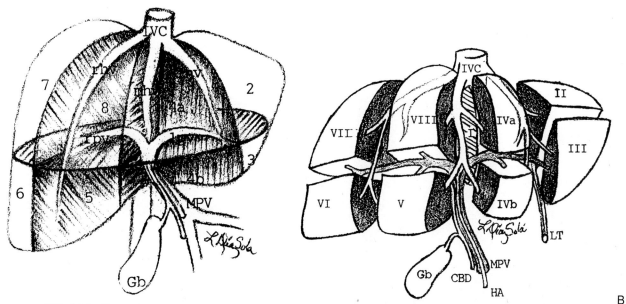

FIG. 11.3. Bismuth hepatic segmental nomenclature system. **A:** Planes are defined by vertical and horizontal planes formed by hepatic and portal veins, respectively. The caudate lobe itself is considered as segment 1 in this nomenclature system. IVC, inferior vena cava; rhv, right hepatic vein; mhv, middle hepatic vein; lhv, left hepatic vein; rpv, right portal vein; mpv, main portal vein; lpv, left portal vein; gb, gallbladder; CBD, common bile duct; LT, ligamentum teres; HA, hepatic artery. **B:** Exploded view of Bismuth hepatic segmental nomenclature system.

mesenteric and splenic arteries and splenic, superior mesenteric, and portal veins is evaluated (1,2). A minimal amount of contrast material should be used in order to avoid tumoral enhancement through arterial perfusion and a subsequent decrease in liver-to-lesion attenuation value differences on CTAP (1,2).

Some authors propose catheter placement in the splenic artery rather than in the superior mesenteric artery, arguing a greater and more homogeneous enhancement of the hepatic parenchyma as well as fewer nontumorous perfusion defects (15). However, this approach may not always be possible, particularly in patients with prior splenectomy or thrombosis of the splenic vein.

A displaced right hepatic artery may be encountered in approximately 25% of patients. This is the cause of one of the major technical pitfalls in spiral CTAP. A displaced right hepatic artery arises from the proximal portion of the superior mesenteric artery instead of the celiac trunk and directly supplies a portion of the right hepatic lobe (14,16,17). Contrast material injection into the superior mesenteric artery will cause preferential arterial enhancement of a displaced hepatic artery, with subsequent obliteration of any focal parenchymal lesions present in the right hepatic lobe segment supplied by the displaced hepatic artery (Fig. 11.4) (14,16,17). Furthermore, the amount of contrast material available for CTAP will be reduced and diluted, causing a suboptimal portographic effect (14,16,17).

After the conventional angiographic examination has been performed, the catheter is placed in the proximal portion of the superior mesenteric artery. The catheter is then connected to a heparin-saline drip infusion and securely stabilized and protected for the patient's transport to the CT suite.

The following CTAP protocol is an example currently being used in our institution.

With a GE 9800 helical CT scanner (General Electric, Milwaukee, WI), we use a table speed of 5 mm/sec and 5-mm collimation (1:1 pitch). Volume data are acquired at 120 kVp and 200 to 250 mA during a 20-second breath-hold. A volume of 150 ml of iodinated contrast medium is injected at a rate of 3 ml/sec. When the catheter is placed in the hepatic artery, the contrast material is diluted to a 30% concentration. With a power injector (Med Rad CT power injector, Med Rad, Pittsburgh, PA), a delay of up to 70 seconds may be used, beginning scanning from the dome of the diaphragm through the liver. Some authors advocate the use of a shorter scanning delay (30 and 20 seconds) (15, 18). However, we believe that when scanning in a cranial to caudal fashion a 40 second delay provides a more consistent enhancement of the hepatic veins and still permits all sections to be obtained within the period of peak hepatic enhancement, which lasts approximately 70 seconds after initiation of the contrast injection.

NORMAL FINDINGS

In helical CTAP, normal liver parenchyma undergoes a homogeneous attenuation increase of approximately 150 to 175 Hounsfield units (HU) (Fig. 11.5) (13). When scanning is done in a caudal fashion from the diaphragm, a slight progressive increase in hepatic parenchymal attenuation value will occur on inferior scans because of buildup of contrast medium in the extravascular compartment (Fig. 11.6) (13). Anatomic structures not supplied by the portal vein, including gallbladder, biliary

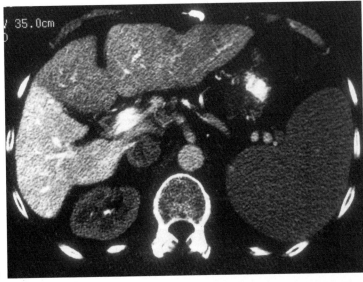
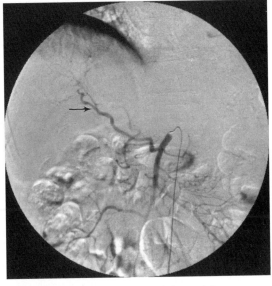

FIG. 11.4. Replaced right hepatic artery. **A:** Helical CTAP arterial phase showing preferential arterial enhancement of right hepatic lobe. Note the relative hyperattenuation of the entire left lobe. **B:** Digital subtraction arteriogram of the superior mesenteric artery showing a displaced right hepatic artery.

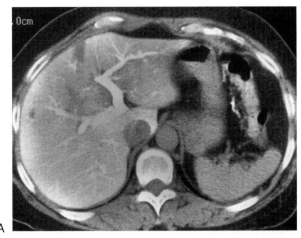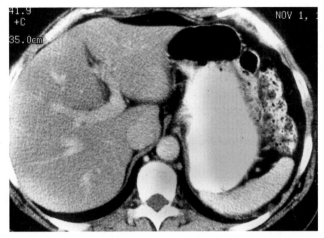

FIG. 11.5. Attenuation differences between helical CTAP and helical intravenous CT. Attenuation values for both liver parenchyma and portal vein are much higher in helical CTAP **(A)** than in intravenous CT **(B)**. Also note small perfusion defect seen at the periphery of segments 4b and 5 seen only in CTAP.

tree, hepatic arteries, hepatic fissures, and capsule, and diaphragm and other perihepatic structures, do not enhance (13).

The portal and hepatic veins undergo a homogeneous attenuation increase of approximately 250 to 300 HU (see Fig. 11.6) (13). The inferior vena cava may show no, mixed, or high attenuation (13). Some CTAP studies may show some enhancement in the aorta, which may be on the basis of systemic recirculation of contrast material or secondary to the initial interventional angiographic examination (13). Portions of the pancreas or bowel wall may show prominent enhancement with superior mesentery artery injections, and the spleen will significantly enhance if the splenic artery is injected (15).

PITFALLS IN COMPUTED TOMOGRAPHY ARTERIAL PORTOGRAPHY

CTAP has been found to be the most sensitive preoperative imaging method in the detection of malignant hepatic lesions. However, when compared with other diagnostic techniques such as intravenous CT, transabdominal sonography, or magnetic resonance (MR) imaging, CTAP has a false-negative rate of 9% to 19% (1–6,19), particularly if focal masses are smaller than 1.0 cm (1,20). False-negative CTAP have also been described in focal fatty liver (21), diffuse hepatocellular disease with portal hypertension (22), capsular and subcapsular metastases (1,19), peritoneal carcinomatosis (1,19), and

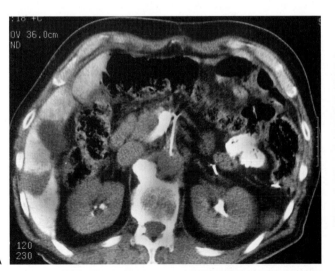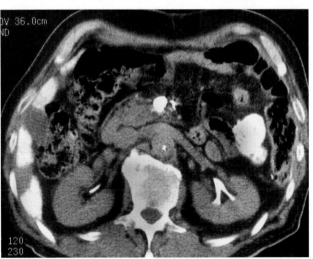

FIG. 11.6. Lesion versus normal structure (gallbladder). **A:** Helical CTAP examination showing a metastatic hypodense lesion at segment 6. Gallbladder is seen more anteromedially. **B:** Note slight progressive increase in parenchymal attenuation value seen when scanning in a craniocaudal fashion in a lower CT section compared to **A.**

in advanced metastatic disease of the liver, where centrally located lesions may cause compression or occlusion of the portal vein (1,14). In addition, in patients with severe cirrhosis, it may be very difficult to differentiate between nodular regeneration and dysplastic nodules from hepatocellular carcinoma (Fig. 11.7).

Another important CTAP pitfall relates to that of false-positive diagnoses. This may occur in cases with focal benign hepatic lesions, extrahepatic cholangiocarcinoma, or nonenhancing normal intrahepatic or perihepatic anatomic structures (1,15,19). Pseudolesions are also caused by vascular variations of the portovenous system, parenchymal perfusion defects caused by portal vein compression or occlusion by centrally located tumors, and so-called round central perfusion defects that are rare and of unknown etiology (14,22,23).

CTAP perfusion defects may be classified as neoplastic and nonneoplastic (15). Both of these perfusion defects are of important clinical significance because they may alter management.

Neoplastic Perfusion Defects

Neoplastic perfusion defects may be secondary to metastases, hepatocellular carcinoma, or benign neoplasms.

Metastases are supplied by the hepatic artery; therefore, when CTAP is performed, they present as focal, well-circumscribed round low-attenuation lesions that contrast sharply with adjacent enhancing normal hepatic parenchyma (Fig. 11.8) (1,15). Metastases may be difficult to differentiate from other focal hepatic parenchymal lesions (14,20).

Similar findings may be seen in patients with hepatocellular carcinoma. However, this type of neoplasm may present in association with segmental or lobar perfusion defects caused by portal vein tumoral thrombus (15,22). CTAP has been found to have a sensitivity of 72% in hepatocellular carcinoma, lower than that for metastatic lesions (1,15,22). This may be related to the fact that hepatocellular carcinoma is multicentric, with approximately 25% of cases having multiple satellite lesions

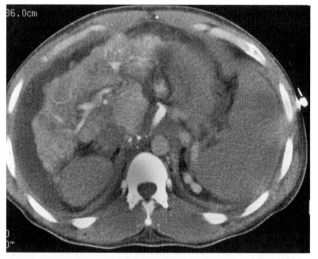

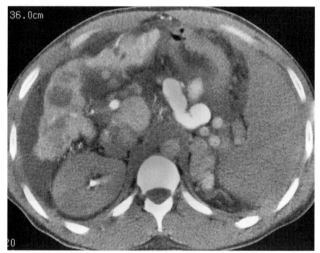

FIG. 11.7. CTAP in cirrhosis. **A:** Helical CTAP portovenous phase showing ascites, splenomegaly, and changes of the liver consistent with diffuse hepatic cirrhosis and portal hypertension. **B:** Multiple nodular hypodense areas are seen throughout the liver parenchyma, particularly at segments 5 and 6. These may represent areas of dysplastic nodules versus hepatocellular carcinoma. Delay imaging may be of help in some cases, showing areas of focal nodular regeneration with some degree of enhancement on delay images. **C:** Extensive splenic venous collaterals showing marked enhancement with contrast material, which is also seen at the superior mesenteric vein. This extensive vascular collateralization contributes to poor hepatic parenchymal enhancement as seen in **A** and **B**.

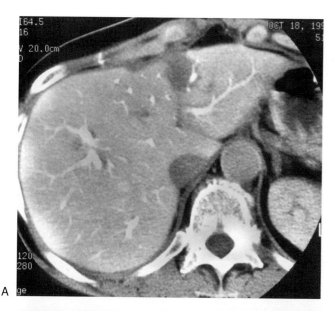

A

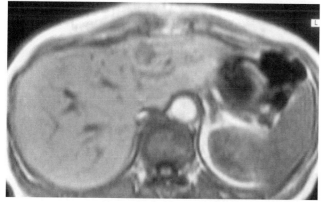

B

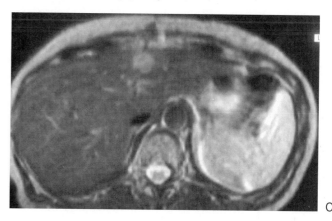

C

FIG. 11.8. Neoplastic perfusion defect. **A:** Helical CTAP showing a neoplastic perfusion defect secondary to a metastatic lesion identified in segment 4a. **B,C:** MRI examination, as seen on T_1W **(B)** and T_2W **(C)** image confirms metastases.

smaller than 2.0 cm. Also, even though hepatocellular carcinoma is usually supplied by the hepatic artery, in approximately 6% of cases, these neoplasms may have some concomitant portal supply because of arterioportal shunting at the tumor periphery. Furthermore, if there is a large central hepatocellular carcinoma, many peripheral lesions will not be detected because of peripheral perfusion defects secondary to portal vein tumoral thrombus and/or compression of portal vein branches.

False-negative diagnoses are usually found in technically inadequate CTAPs in which regions of hyperattenuating or diminished parenchymal enhancement and areas of diffuse nontumoral mottling are seen (1,22). False-positive results may be seen in patients with hepatocellular disease such as cirrhosis with dysplastic nodules and areas of confluent hepatic fibrosis (see Fig. 11.7). Nevertheless, dysplastic nodules will show some degree of enhancement, as most of them are primarily supplied by the portal system (1,22).

Benign hepatic neoplasms and other benign focal lesions may also cause focal perfusion defects in CTAP. These include hemangioma, focal nodular hyperplasia,

hepatocellular adenoma, focal fatty change, focal fibrosis, metastases (without neoplastic cells) previously treated with ablative techniques, subcapsular and parenchymal hematomas, and abscesses and cysts (1,15). Benign focal lesions almost never cause perfusion defects secondary to vascular occlusion (1,15).

Nonneoplastic Perfusion Defects

In CTAP, it is not uncommon to encounter multiple or single perfusion defects that are not caused by normal anatomic structures or benign and malignant neoplasms (1,14,23). These perfusion defects have been classified as (a) pseudolesions (small, triangular or square, peripheral or central perfusion defects); (b) large, round central defects; and (c) flow defects (larger subsegmental, segmental, or lobar perfusion defects) (1,14,15,23).

Pseudolesions most commonly occur in the medial segment of the left hepatic lobe (Fig. 11.9). They occur in approximately 15% of CTAP studies and present with a round, oval, or square configuration (1,14,23). Perihepatic venous anomalies are thought to be the cause of this

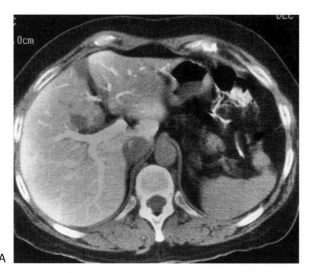
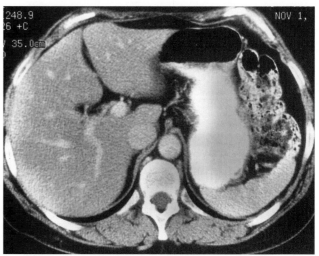

FIG. 11.9. Nonneoplastic perfusion defect. **A:** Helical CTAP showing nonneoplastic perfusion defect or pseudolesion seen in medial segment of left hepatic lobe. Another perfusion defect is seen at periportal region. **B:** Helical CT portovenous phase showing homogeneous parenchymal enhancement with no focal lesions identified, confirming their pseudolesion nature.

type of perfusion defect (24). It has been found that in approximately 6% to 14% of the population, the right gastric vein drains directly into segment 4 instead of the main portal vein as seen in most people (24). Furthermore, pseudolesions occurring in the central portion of the liver, adjacent to the falciform fissure, are thought to be caused by parabiliary venous system aberrant vessels (Fig. 11.10) (24,25). In addition, anatomic variations in the portal perfusion of the peripheral subcapsular hepatic parenchymal microvasculature are thought to be the cause of peripheral subcapsular pseudolesions (see Fig. 11.9) (23).

Large, round central perfusion defects that may simulate those caused by neoplasm are seen with CTAP. However, these rare perfusion defects are not caused by focal parenchymal lesions, nor do they follow the characteristics of a pseudolesion or flow defect. These large, round perfusion defects are of unknown etiology, although abnormal venous vasculature or variations in the portal venous system are the most likely cause (see Fig. 11.10).

Flow defects usually cause larger perfusion defects than those seen with pseudolesions. These may be secondary to obstructive or nonobstructive condition (15). In obstructive flow defects, a centrally located metastasis or hepatocellular carcinoma causes obstruction by either extrinsic compression, invasion or tumoral thrombosis of an adjacent portal vein branch (Fig. 11.11) (2,14,26). Larger flow defects have a segmental or lobar distribution with well-defined borders surrounded by normal enhancing hepatic parenchyma. This finding has been named the "straight line" sign (1,14,26).

Nonobstructive flow defects are seen in heterogeneous hepatic parenchymal enhancement secondary to portal blood flow asymmetries.

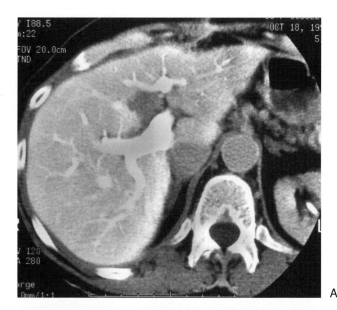

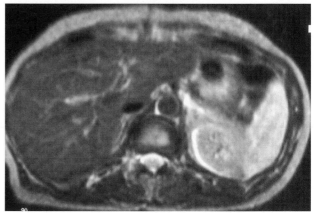

FIG. 11.10. Central pseudolesion. **A:** Helical CTAP showing pseudolesion in the central part of the liver. **B:** MRI examination on T$_2$W image demonstrates normal liver without focal lesion.

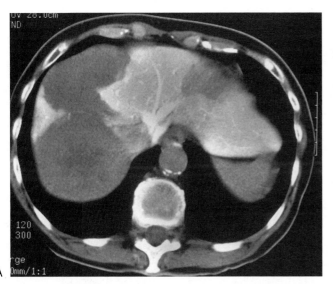
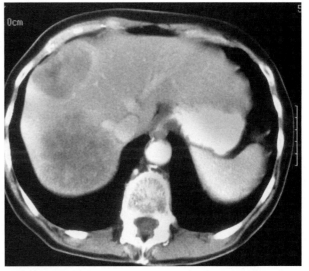

FIG. 11.11. Perfusion defect. **A:** Helical CTAP showing two well-defined hepatic lesions in a patient with metastatic liver disease. However, other defects are also seen. An obstructive flow defect is seen between two large metastases. Another perfusion defect is seen in left hepatic lobe. **B:** Comparison is done to helical CT examination, which does not show the above-described perfusion defects.

COMPLEMENTARY TECHNIQUES AND IMAGING

In order to increase the accuracy and sensitivity of CTAP, CT hepatic arteriography may be performed simultaneously. This technique permits arterial perfusion characterization of metastases and hepatomas (27,28). A higher accuracy for detecting hypervascular hepatic masses has been reported. However, this technique is more time-consuming and complicated because it requires placement of a second indwelling

catheter in the hepatic artery. Furthermore, limited results are obtained in patients with a displaced right hepatic artery.

Delayed CTAP done at approximately 4 to 5 hours after contrast administration has been proposed by some authors for further characterization of neoplastic versus nonneoplastic perfusion defects (Fig. 11.12) (1,15,29). On delayed CTAP images, nonneoplastic perfusion defects show some degree of enhancement similar to that of normal hepatic parenchyma (1,15,29). Furthermore, delayed CTAP may demonstrate perfusion defects not visualized

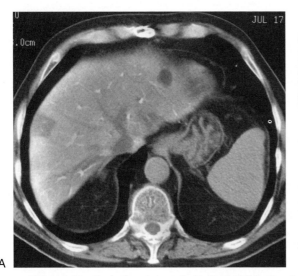
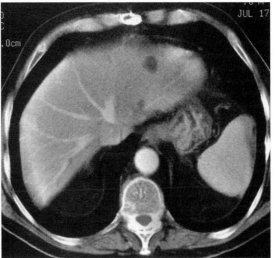

FIG. 11.12. Perfusion defect. **A:** Helical CTAP showing peripheral lesion at right hepatic lobe. **B:** Delayed image demonstrates normal enhancement. Two small cysts are seen in the left lobe.

on early CTAP (1,15,29). Delayed CTAP images may be obtained as early as in 10 minutes.

Another drawback of CTAP is its lack of specificity, requiring further diagnostic work-up such as ultrasound or CT-guided percutaneous biopsy for a definite diagnosis in most cases. Delayed imaging may occasionally increase the specificity.

CTAP is gradually falling into disfavor because of its pitfalls, invasive nature, and recent developments in helical CT and MR. Recent advances in CT and MR imaging have greatly improved the assessment of liver neoplasms. Multiphasic helical CT can image the liver in a single breath-hold during the optimal contrast enhancement. Magnetic resonance imaging with specific contrast agents for liver, which significantly increase the tumor-to-liver contrast, can be also used. Multiphasic CT and MR are considered to be comparable to CTAP for detection of liver lesions with higher specificity. Some authors have proposed the use of ferumoxide-enhanced MR imaging instead of CTAP for the detection of hepatic lesions, particularly metastases (30). Ferumoxide-enhanced MR imaging has been found to be as sensitive as CTAP, noninvasive, more cost-effective, and to have greater specificity.

In conclusion, CTAP is described as the most sensitive diagnostic imaging technique for the detection of focal hepatic lesions such as hepatocellular carcinoma and metastases. Unfortunately, it is associated with many pitfalls. But most of these come from normal or deviated vascular supply, and usually found at the constant location in the liver. Thorough knowledge of CTAP's potential pitfalls and normal variations is therefore very important for an optimal diagnostic yield.

REFERENCES

1. Soyer P, Bluemke DA, Fishman EK. CT during arterial portography for the preoperative evaluation of hepatic tumors: how, when, why? *Am J Roentgenol* 1994;163:1325–1331.
2. Merine D, Takayasu K, Wakas E. Detection of hepatocellular carcinoma: comparison of CT during arterial portography with CT after intra-arterial injection of iodized oil. *Radiology* 1990;175:707–710.
3. Soyer P, Levesque M, Elias D, Zertoun G, Roche A. Preoperative assessment of resectability of hepatic metastases from colonic carcinoma: CT portography vs. sonography and dynamic CT. *Am J Roentgenol* 1992;159:741–744.
4. Soyer P, Laissy JP, Sibert A, et al. Focal hepatic masses: comparison of detection during arterial portography with MR imaging and CT. *Radiology* 1994;190:737–740.
5. Soyer P, Levesque M, Caudron C, Elias D, Zertoun G, Roche A. MRI of liver metastases from colorectal cancer vs. CT during arterial portography. *J Comput Assist Tomogr* 1993;17:67–74.
6. Soyer P, Levesque M, Elias D, Zeitoun G, Roche A. Detection of liver metastases from colorectal cancer: comparison of intraoperative US and CT during arterial portography. *Radiology* 1992;183:541–544.
7. Nelson RC, Chzman JL, Sugarbaker PH, Munay DR, Bernardino ME. Preoperative localization of focal liver lesions to specific liver segments: utility of CT during arterial portography. *Radiology* 1990; 176:89–94.
8. Bismuth H. Surgical anatomy and anatomical surgery of the liver. *World J Surg* 1982;6:3–9.
9. Soyer P, Bluemke DA, Bliss DF, Woodhouse CE, Fishman EK. Surgical segmental anatomy of the liver: demonstration with spiral CT during arterial portography and multiplanar reconstruction. *Am J Roentgenol* 1994;163:99–103.
10. Soyer P, Roche A, Elias D, Levesque M. Hepatic metastases from colorectal cancer: influence of hepatic volumetric analysis on surgical decision-making. *Radiology* 1992;184:695–697.
11. Bluemke DA, Fishman EK. Spiral CT arterial portography of the liver. *Radiology* 1993;186:576–579.
12. Zeman RK, Fox SM, Silverman PM, et al. Helical (spiral) CT of the abdomen. *Am J Roentgenol* 1993;160:719–725.
13. Bluemke DA, Fishman EK. Spiral CT of the liver. *Am J Roentgenol* 1993;160:787–792.
14. Nelson RC, Thompson GH, Chezman JL, Harred RK II, del Pilar Fernandez M. CT during arterial portography: diagnostic pitfalls. *RadioGraphics* 1992;12:705–718.
15. Lupetin AR, Cammisa BA, Beckman I, et al. Spiral CT during arterial portography. *RadioGraphics* 1996;16:723–743.
16. Little AF, Baron RL, Peterson MS, et al. Optimizing CT portography: prospective comparison of injection into the splenic versus superior mesenteric artery. *Radiology* 1994;193:651–655.
17. Paulson EK, Baker ME, Hilleren DJ. CT arterial portography: causes of technical failure and variable liver enhancements. *Am J Roentgenol* 1992;159:745–749.
18. Graf O, Dock WI, Lammer J, et al. Determination of optimal time window for liver scanning with CT during arterial portography. *Radiology* 1994;190:43–47.
19. Soyer P, Lacheheb D, Levesque M. False-positive CT portography: correlation with pathologic findings. *Am J Roentgenol* 1993;160:285–289.
20. Sexton CC, Zeman RK. Correlation of computed tomography, sonography, and gross anatomy of the liver. *Am J Roentgenol* 1983;141: 711–718.
21. Hanger J, Prez C, Coscojuela P, Sanchis E, Traid C. Hepatic metastases: false-negative CT portography in cases of fatty infiltration. *J Comput Assist Tomogr* 1991;15:320–322.
22. Oliver JM III, Baron RI, Dodd GD III, Peterson MS, Can BL. Does advanced cirrhosis with portosystemic shunting affect the value of CT arterial portography in the evaluation of the liver? *Am J Roentgenol* 1995;164:333–337.
23. Peterson MS, Baron RL, Dodd GD III, et al. Hepatic parenchymal perfusion defects detected with CTAP: imaging–pathologic correlation. *Radiology* 1992;185:149–155.
24. Matsui O, Takahashi S, Kadoya M, et al. Pseudolesion in segment IV of the liver at CT during arterial portography: correlation with aberrant gastric venous drainage. *Radiology* 1994;193:31–35.
25. Couinaud C. The parabiliary venous system. *Surg Radiol Anat* 1988; 10:311–316.
26. Tyrrel RT, Kaufman SL, Bernandino ME. Straight-line sign: appearance and significance during CT portography. *Radiology* 1989;173: 635–637.
27. Freeny PC, Marks WM. Hepatic perfusion abnormalities during CT angiography: detection and interpretation. *Radiology* 1986;159: 685–691.
28. Chezman JL, Bernardino ME, Kaufman SH, Nelson RC. Combined CT arterial portography and CT hepatic angiography for evaluation of the hepatic resection candidate: work in progress. *Radiology* 1993;189: 407–410.
29. Perkerson RB Jr, Erwin BC, Baumgartner BR, et al. CT densities in delayed iodine hepatic scanning. *Radiology* 1985;155:445–446.
30. Senterre E, Taourel P, Bouvier Y, et al. Detection of hepatic metastases: ferumoxides-enhanced MR imaging versus unenhanced MR imaging and CT during arterial portography. *Radiology* 1996;200:785–792.

Variants and Pitfalls in Body Imaging,
edited by Ali Shirkhoda.
Lippincott Williams & Wilkins, Philadelphia, © 2000.

CHAPTER 12

The Gallbladder and the Biliary Tract

Gary G. Ghahremani and Andrea Laghi

COMPUTED TOMOGRAPHY AND ULTRASOUND

Anatomic variants and developmental anomalies involving the gallbladder or bile ducts are common. The majority are detected incidentally at surgery or autopsy, but they are also being recognized with an increasing frequency during radiologic imaging for evaluation of suspected biliary symptoms or unrelated abdominal disorders (1–4). An unusual topography or configuration of the gallbladder and biliary tract may present as a diagnostic challenge to practicing radiologists. It can also predispose these structures to intraoperative mishaps and iatrogenic injuries, particularly when the field of view is limited during laparoscopic cholecystectomy (5–8).

The purpose of this chapter is to review the spectrum of biliary tract variants and anomalies, with emphasis on their imaging features and the potential pitfalls that may hamper their correct diagnosis.

Embryologic Considerations

Development of the hepatobiliary system begins in the third week of fetal life, when a bifid bud sprouts from the ventral aspect of the primitive foregut. The larger cephalic portion of this endodermal diverticulum is called pars hepatica, representing the anlage for liver parenchyma and intrahepatic bile ducts. The smaller caudal segment, pars cystica, leads to the formation of the gallbladder and extrahepatic ducts. When the embryo is 5 to 7 weeks old,

G. G. Ghahremani: Department of Radiology, Evanston Hospital, Northwestern University Healthcare, Evanston, Illinois 60201.

A. Laghi: Department of Radiology, University of Rome "La Sapienza," Policlinico Umberto I, 00161 Rome, Italy.

the proliferating endodermal cells undergo vacuolization to establish a patent lumen for these structures. With progressive maturation of the liver, the intrahepatic ducts grow along the portal vein branches and discharge the excreted bile by the 12th week (1–3). Therefore, it is during the first trimester of pregnancy that the normal development of the hepatobiliary system can be affected by genetic or environmental factors as well as local or systemic conditions.

The Gallbladder

The gallbladder is invisible on abdominal radiographs unless its lumen contains contrast material or gas, radiopaque calculi or milk of calcium bile, or its walls are calcified as a porcelain gallbladder. However, the gallbladder is usually well demonstrated routinely by sectional imaging modalities, particularly in the fasting state when it becomes distended with bile (9–12). It often appears as a pear-shaped structure attached to the inferior surface of the right and quadrate lobes of the liver, often protruding into the interlobar fissure.

Gallstones and cholecystitis are prevalent among the American adult population and account for almost 600,000 operations per year and over $5 billion of annual health care expenditure in the United States (13–15). Various radiologic techniques are being utilized for evaluation of patients with suspected biliary tract disorders, but sonography is currently the method of choice (9,10). This examination is best performed with a real-time ultrasound and a 5.0-MHz transducer. The patients are usually instructed to fast for 12 hours because a bile-filled gallbladder would improve the visibility of intraluminal calculi and masses as well as the assessment of gallbladder wall thickness and mucosal septations. Because each sonographic image covers only a thin sagittal or transverse section of limited depth, however, the entire gallbladder cannot be viewed at the same time. This represents a potential source of diagnostic error, particularly if small calculi are hidden in the gallbladder neck or cystic duct, obscured by gas in the duodenum or colon, or if the gallbladder is shrunken or malpositioned (9,10,16).

Technical limitations that are inherent to sectional imaging by CT or MRI may also interfere with the demonstration of gallbladder diseases (9–12,17,18). Therefore, each examination must be tailored and carefully reviewed to assure a complete visualization of the gallbladder and bile ducts for accurate diagnosis of calculi or pathologic processes.

Anatomic variations and congenital anomalies involving the gallbladder position, shape, and number are frequently encountered on routine abdominal imagings (2–4). However, most have no clinical significance, but their recognition is important because they may predispose to gallbladder diseases, serve as a potential source of confusion and diagnostic pitfalls for radiologists, and increase the risk of inadvertent injury during biliary tract surgery or intervention (5–10).

Positional Anomalies of the Gallbladder

Floating Gallbladder

A common cause of gallbladder malposition is its excessive mobility because of a loose mesenteric attachment (1–4,19). Normally the gallbladder is fixed in a subhepatic location by the peritoneum covering its surface. In about 4% to 5% of individuals, however, the gallbladder and part of the cystic duct are suspended beneath the liver by a mesentery of variable length, a condition known as "floating, wandering, or pendulous gallbladder." Such a mobile gallbladder may migrate to the middle or left side of the abdomen for a considerable distance from the liver (Fig. 12.1), or it may gradually elongate as a tubular structure protruding into the pelvis (Fig. 12.2). It can also herniate through the foramen of Winslow and undergo spontaneous torsion and ischemic necrosis (20–23). Furthermore, a floating gallbladder in an unusual position can simulate a soft tissue mass or cystic lesion on CT or sonograms (2–4). However, a careful evaluation often shows its connection to the hilus of the liver and the absence of gallbladder in its usual subhepatic fossa.

Intrahepatic Gallbladder

In approximately 9% of the population, the gallbladder is partially or completely embedded within the liver parenchyma, thus referred to as an "intrahepatic gallbladder." It can resemble a liver cyst, abscess, or necrotic metastasis on ultrasound or CT sections (Fig. 12.3A), though its relationships to the interlobar fissure and the cystic duct can provide clues to the correct diagnosis (2–4,10).

An intrahepatic gallbladder is prone to develop calculi because the surrounding liver will interfere with its emptying and function. Furthermore, its involvement by an acute cholecystitis may have a confusing clinical presentation because of its deep location and paucity of peritoneal signs on physical examination (24,25). Its resection by either open cholecystectomy or laparoscopic approach can also be difficult because of the inherent risk of inducing liver injury and hemorrhage (5–7). The accumulation of bile or blood in the vacated region of intrahepatic gallbladder will frequently mimic its original appearance or that of a liver cyst or abscess on postoperative CT exams (Fig. 12.3B).

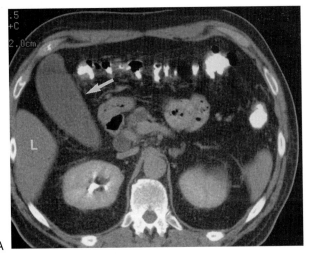
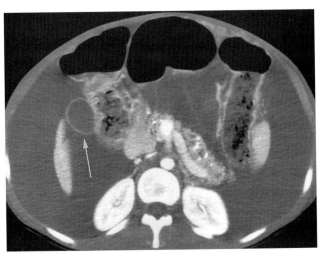

FIG. 12.1. Computed tomographic appearance of the floating gallbladder in two cases. **A:** The excessively mobile gallbladder in this patient presents as a large intraperitoneal mass *(arrow)* that extends posteromedially with distinct separation from the right lobe of the liver (L). **B:** The mobile gallbladder *(arrow)* of this man with chronic calcific pancreatitis is floating within the pool of ascites.

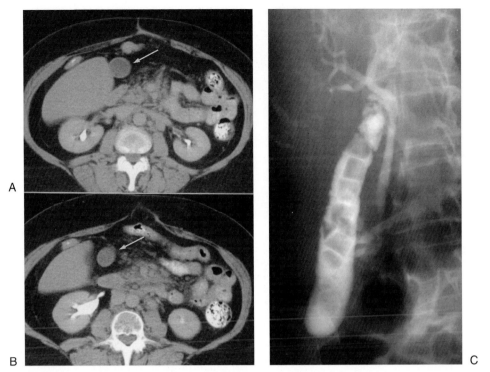

FIG. 12.2. Radiologic features of a pendulous gallbladder. **A,B:** Contrast-enhanced CT sections of the midabdominal region show the gallbladder seen as a tubular structure medial to the liver *(arrows).* **C:** Radiograph obtained following ERCP demonstrates a markedly elongated gallbladder with multiple radiolucent stones that were invisible on CT.

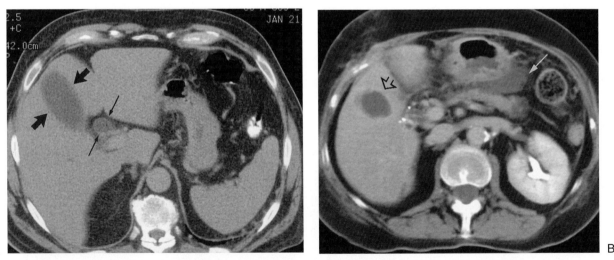

FIG. 12.3. Computed tomographic findings in two patients with intrahepatic gallbladder. **A:** The gallbladder is embedded deep within the liver parenchyma *(large arrows),* but its neck extends into the interlobar fissure *(small arrows).* **B:** Computed tomographic scan 10 days after cholecystectomy reveals a bile collection in the fossa of resected intrahepatic gallbladder *(open arrow)* and within the lesser sac *(white arrow).* The cause of bile leakage was insecure ligation of the cystic duct stump.

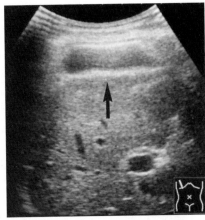
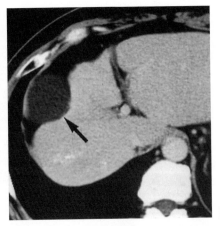

FIG. 12.4. Imaging of a suprahepatic gallbladder. **A:** Sonogram of the liver in an oblique sagittal projection shows a well-defined fluid collection anterior to the right lobe *(arrow)*, mimicking a perihepatic abscess, hematoma, biloma, or ascites. **B:** Computed tomogram reveals a malpositioned gallbladder *(arrow)* between the right hemidiaphragm and atrophic right lobe. (Courtesy of Dr. S. Naganuma, Akita University Hospital, Akita, Japan.)

Suprahepatic Gallbladder

This rare congenital anomaly is associated with hypoplasia of the anterior segment of the right lobe of the liver and upward migration of the hepatic flexure of the colon (26–28). Similar findings are observed when the right hepatic lobe is atrophic from cirrhosis. The ectopic gallbladder will be visible in the right subdiaphragmatic space on CT or sonography but may closely simulate a perihepatic fluid collection or an abscess (Figs. 12.4, and 12.5).

Retrohepatic and Retrorenal Gallbladder

These represent two unusual types of gallbladder malposition posterior to the liver or right kidney, respectively (3,19,29,30). In such instances the ectopic gallbladder, if

not specified with cholangiographic contrast media, can be mistaken for a renal, adrenal, or hepatic cyst on sectional imaging studies (Fig. 12.6). Radiopaque calculi in the malpositioned gallbladder can mimic calcified cysts or tumors of the neighboring organs. Furthermore, the anomalous location of the gallbladder may lead to difficulties in surgical or interventional management and increase the risk of iatrogenic injuries (7,31).

Left-Sided Gallbladder

Transposition of the gallbladder to the left upper abdomen is typically seen in patients with total situs inversus (2–4,19,29). The anatomic relationships among the liver, gallbladder, and other viscera remain normal

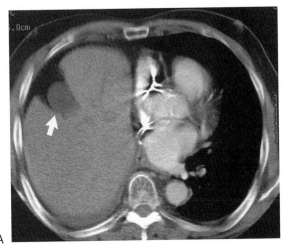
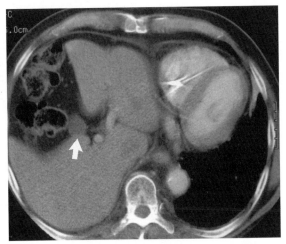

FIG. 12.5. Computed tomographic diagnosis of a suprahepatic gallbladder. **A:** The upper section shows the gallbladder fundus protruding anteriorly toward the dome of the liver *(arrow)*. **B:** Another section 7 cm caudad demonstrates the gallbladder neck *(arrow)* and hepatic flexure of the colon occupying the space of the hypoplastic right lobe. Note that the right hemidiaphragm is elevated, thus accounting for a much higher position of the liver and gallbladder as compared to the heart and left lung.

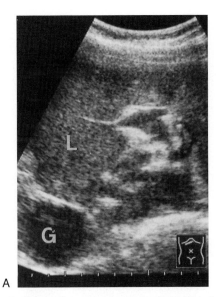 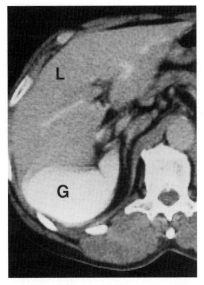

FIG. 12.6. Imaging of a retrohepatic gallbladder. **A:** Sonogram of the liver through the right subcostal region demonstrates the malpositioned gallbladder (G) as a cystic structure behind the right lobe of the liver (L). **B:** Computed tomogram following opacification of the gallbladder with contrast material confirms its retrohepatic location. (Courtesy of Dr. S. Naganuma, Akita University Hospital, Akita, Japan.)

except for their mirror-image topography (Fig. 12.7A). A left-sided gallbladder may also occur in patients with a floating gallbladder and midgut malrotation caused by defective mesenteric attachment (Fig. 12.7B), or as an isolated anomaly (32–34).

In the majority of about 50 reported cases, the gallbladder was located beneath the left hepatic lobe and to the left of the falciform ligament, with its cystic duct crossing the midline to join either the common bile duct or the left hepatic duct. Therefore, if the gallbladder is invisible in its normal location on CT or sonograms, one should consider the possibility of a left-sided gallbladder and carefully search the area under the left hepatic lobe.

Possible coexistence of other congenital anomalies (e.g., polysplenia, interruption of the inferior vena cava with hemiazygos continuation) should also be sought in such patients. Two recent articles provide detailed description of sonographic and CT findings of various anomalies associated with gallbladder malposition (29,35).

Acquired Gallbladder Malposition

In patients with liver atrophy caused by cirrhosis, the gallbladder tends to migrate anteriorly into the peritoneal compartment between the liver and abdominal wall (36,37). The radiologic findings in this condition can

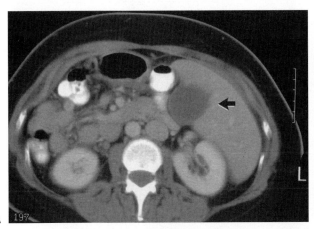 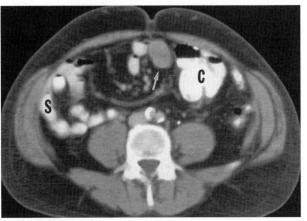

FIG. 12.7. Computed tomographic appearance of left-sided gallbladder in two different cases. **A:** In this patient with total situs inversus, the liver and gallbladder *(arrow)* occupy the left upper quadrant *(arrow),* and their relationships to other abdominal viscera are maintained in a mirror image of normal anatomy. Notice that the superior mesenteric artery (SMA) is to the right of its venous counterpart. **B:** Left-sided gallbladder presenting as a left subumbilical cyst or mass *(arrow).* The coexistent midgut malrotation accounted for anomalous position of the cecum (C) and small bowel loops (S).

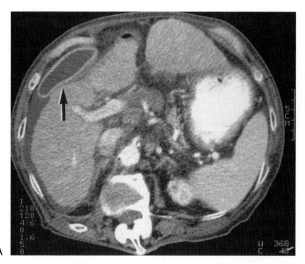
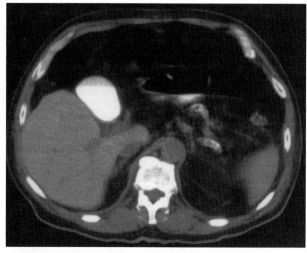

FIG. 12.8. Two examples of acquired gallbladder malposition depicted by CT. **A:** In this patient with liver cirrhosis and ascites, the gallbladder had immigrated anteriorly into the right perihepatic space *(arrow);* it could be mistaken for a cyst or abscess. **B:** In this patient with a markedly atrophic liver, the antehepatic gallbladder was opacified as a result of vicarious excretion of contrast material after carotid angiography. (Courtesy of Dr. Ali Shirkhoda, William Beaumont Hospital, Royal Oak, Michigan.)

resemble a suprahepatic gallbladder of congenital nature (Fig. 12.8). An acquired malposition of the gallbladder may also occur following segmental hepatectomy or right nephrectomy, particularly when a mobile gallbladder prolapses into the surgically vacated space.

Developmental Anomalies of the Gallbladder

Gallbladder Agenesis

The gallbladder is congenitally absent in certain animal species, such as in rats and horses. In humans, however, agenesis of the gallbladder and cystic duct is encountered with an incidence of about one per 6,000 live births, with a preponderance of 3:1 for women and some evidence for familial occurrence (1–3). Coexistent anomalies are found in up to 50% of the cases; these include congenital heart defects, imperforate anus, rectovaginal or tracheoesophageal fistulas, asplenia, horseshoe kidneys, and various other malformations.

In the majority of over 200 reported cases, the gallbladder agenesis was an unexpected finding at surgery or autopsy (38–42). About half of these patients had experienced postprandial pain or biliary colic, fatty food intol-

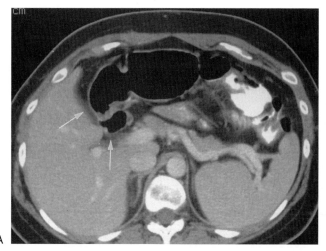
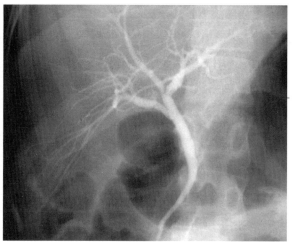

FIG. 12.9. Imaging features of gallbladder agenesis. **A:** Computed tomogram of the upper abdomen shows prolapse of the gastric antrum and duodenal bulb into the gallbladder fossa *(arrows),* but no gallbladder could be visualized by this exam or prior sonography. **B:** Endoscopic retrograde cholangiogram confirms the congenital absence of gallbladder and cystic duct, but the biliary tract is otherwise normal. Again, note that the gas-filled antrum and bulb occupy the vacant subhepatic fossa.

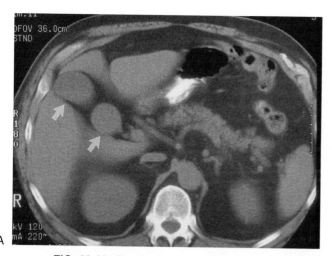
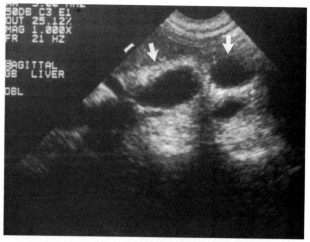

FIG. 12.10. Duplication of gallbladder. **A:** Computed tomogram of the abdomen incidentally disclosed the presence of two round structures *(arrows)* within a wide interlobar fissure. **B:** Sonogram of the same region in sagittal oblique projection shows clear separation of the two gallbladders *(arrows)* and their cystic ducts.

erance, and other symptoms that were actually caused by an associated biliary tract dyskinesia or choledocholithiasis (40). The nonvisualization of the gallbladder on preoperative imaging studies was usually attributed to its shrinkage from chronic cholecystitis, hence subjecting some patients to unnecessary surgery for cholecystectomy and an unpleasant surprise about the absent gallbladder (39–42). Therefore, it is important to consider this anomaly when the gallbladder and cystic duct are invisible by sonography, CT, or cholangiography (Fig. 12.9).

A hypoplastic or rudimentary gallbladder is often present in patients with cholestasis since early childhood. The underlying cause for arrested growth of the gallbladder in such cases can be biliary atresia, neonatal hepatitis or cholangitis, and cystic fibrosis (3,43).

Gallbladder Duplication

Duplication of the gallbladder is reported to occur in approximately one per 5,000 individuals, but it is common among the domesticated mammals (1–3,44). A true duplication (vesica duplex) consists of two separate gallbladders and cystic ducts. The latter may join before entering the common duct (Y-type), or both may connect to it at different sites (H-type). Usually the two gallbladders are located adjacent to each other within the gallbladder fossa (Fig. 12.10). The accessory one may also be intrahepatic or malpositioned elsewhere and drain into the left or right hepatic ducts. Not infrequently one or both gallbladders are involved by pathologic processes or harbor calculi (44–46). Therefore, the correct identification of this anomaly would be important to avoid intraoperative mishaps or future need for a second surgery.

A bilobed gallbladder (vesica divisa) has two adjoining chambers divided by a cleft, but in contrast to true duplication, there is a single neck and cystic duct. A somewhat

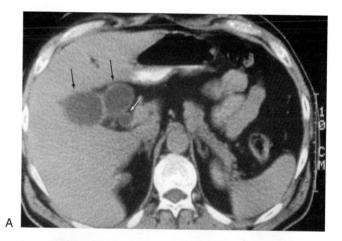

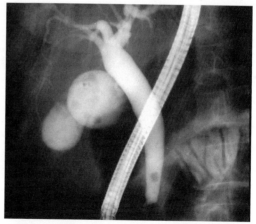

FIG. 12.11. Bilobed gallbladder with cholelithiasis. **A:** Computed tomogram of the abdomen in this patient presenting with postprandial pain demonstrated three cystic structures in the subhepatic region, caused by two adjoining gallbladders *(black arrows)* and their shared cystic duct *(white arrow)*. **B:** Endoscopic retrograde cholangiogram confirms this anomaly and reveals multiple radiolucent stones in both gallbladders and in the common bile duct, although these calculi were not detectable on CT.

similar configuration may be seen when a large congenital diverticulum of the gallbladder is present (1,44).

The correct diagnosis of a duplicated or bilobed gallbladder can be made if its lumen is well opacified by oral cholecystography, direct cholangiography, or endoscopic retrograde cholangiopancreatography ERCP. However, these anomalies may also be recognized on sonograms or CT (Fig. 12.11). The differential diagnosis of two cystic structures within the gallbladder fossa should include a choledochal cyst, gallbladder diverticulum, compartmentalized gallbladder resulting from folding or phrygian cap, focal adenomyomatosis, and periocholecystic fluid or abscess (3,44–46).

Variations of Gallbladder Configuration

Considerable variations in size and shape of the gallbladder are observed on imaging studies, depending on its anatomy and degree of luminal distension with bile, involvement by pathologic processes, and extrinsic compression by the adjacent structures (3,10).

Gallbladder Septations

The most common variation of gallbladder shape is the so-called phrygian cap deformity, which occurs in about 5% of the population. Named after a headgear worn by liberated Greek slaves in the ancient country of Phrygia, it is characterized by a mucosal septum or fold in the fundus of gallbladder (1–4). On cross-sectional CT or sonographic views, the phrygian cap may simulate a duplicated or bicameral gallbladder. Furthermore, its presence can lead to stasis and stone formation within the septated fundus.

Spiral folds of Heister are normally present in the cystic duct. Their function is to regulate filling and emptying of the gallbladder according to intraluminal pressure within the biliary tract. In some patients the spiral folds or mucosal septa may extend into the gallbladder neck and mimic a gallstone on CT image (Fig. 12.12). They can also obscure the sonographic visualization of small calculi that are hidden between the spiral folds (3,10).

Multiseptated Gallbladder

This is a rare congenital anomaly wherein a network of mucosal septa divide the gallbladder into interconnecting chambers (2,47–49). This condition is attributed to incomplete vacuolization of developing gallbladder or excessive infolding of its epithelial lining. Although a multiseptated gallbladder can have a normal shape and function, it is prone to develop calculi. Its unique appearance as a honeycomb or multicystic gallbladder is usually well depicted on oral cholecystogram, CT, or sonography (2–4,47–49). Nevertheless, it should be differentiated from somewhat similar findings caused by desquamated gallbladder epithelium and polypoid cholesterolosis (3,50,51).

Gallbladder Deformities

An unusual gallbladder configuration caused by congenital or acquired processes can be a source of confusion on imaging studies (4,9,10). For example, the gall-

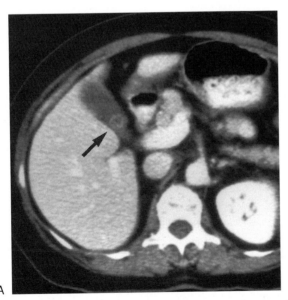 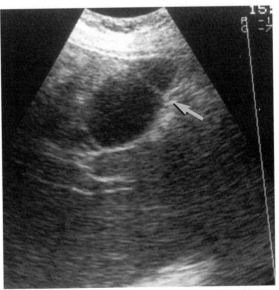

FIG. 12.12. Gallbladder septation simulating a gallstone. **A:** Contrast-enhanced CT of the abdomen shows a ring-like density in the gallbladder neck, suggesting an intraluminal stone with peripheral calcification *(arrow).* **B:** Ultrasound exam reveals a thin mucosal fold as the source of pseudocalculus effect. (Courtesy of Dr. Ali Shirkhoda, William Beaumont Hospital, Royal Oak, Michigan.)

bladder on longitudinal section may appear bilobular or compartmentalized because of an hour-glass configuration produced by localized circumferential narrowing of the lumen. An axial CT section of the same constricted area can also simulate a gallstone because of volume averaging.

Gallbladder Diverticula

A distorted polycystic structure may be seen instead of the round or pear-shaped gallbladder on CT or sonograms. This unusual configuration can result from either congenital gallbladder diverticula or acquired pseudodiverticula caused by adenomyomatosis (1–3,10,52). The latter condition is characterized by mucosal proliferation and outpouching into the hypertrophied muscular layers of the gallbladder wall, forming Rokitansky-Aschoff sinuses. They can develop in a focal, segmental, or diffuse manner. On sonograms these intramural pseudodiverticula appear as multiple anechoic areas within the thickened gallbladder wall and may contain echogenic foci caused by calculi (52,53). The CT features of adenomyomatosis are particularly striking when there is diffuse involvement. In such cases the deformed and lobulated gallbladder is surrounded by clusters of cystic elements, which may protrude into the adjacent liver parenchyma (Fig. 12.13).

The Bile Ducts

The complexity of hepatobiliary development results in enormous architectural variations of the intrahepatic and extrahepatic ducts. These are best demonstrable by direct cholangiography. Sonography and CT are primarily used for evaluation of the gallbladder and pathologic processes causing bile duct dilation (9,10). The applica-

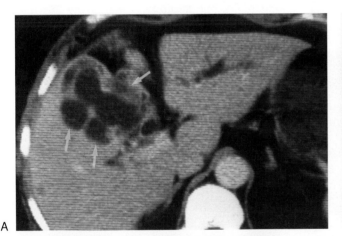
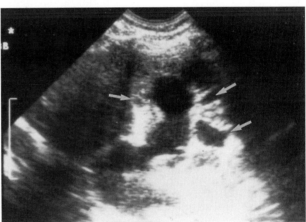
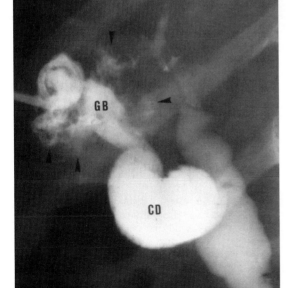

FIG. 12.13. Distorted gallbladder caused by pseudodiverticula formed by adenomyomatosis. **A:** Computed tomogram of the liver shows multicystic appearance of the gallbladder with numerous intramural outpouchings that extend into the liver parenchyma *(arrows).* **B:** Sonogram demonstrates the markedly thickened walls and deformed lumen of the gallbladder *(arrows).* **C:** Injected contrast material through percutaneous cholecystostomy has opacified the distorted gallbladder (GB) and its intramural pseudodiverticula *(arrowheads)* as well as the dilated cystic duct (CD) because of an impacted stone in the distal dilated common bile duct. (Courtesy of Dr. J.I. Hwang, Veterans General Hospital, Taiwan, Republic of China.)

tions of MR cholangiography are evolving at this time, though recent studies have shown its value in preoperative assessment of some biliary tract anomalies (11, 12,54,55).

Pitfalls in Imaging the Intrahepatic Ducts

The intrahepatic ducts are normally located anterior to their corresponding portal vein branches. Both of them converge on the porta hepatis, where their larger central parts can be distinguished by sonography or contrast-enhanced CT (9,10). However, peripheral intrahepatic ducts of normal caliber are barely visible on CT and particularly difficult to depict in the presence of fatty liver (56,57). These technical limitations also hamper the visualization of obliterated intrahepatic ducts in infants with biliary atresia. Nevertheless, sonography is being used in such patients to evaluate the liver parenchyma and its increased periportal echoes caused by associated fibrosis, to exclude other potential sources of obstructive jaundice, and to search for often coexisting anomalies

such as choledochal cyst and an atretic or hypoplastic gallbladder (58).

Anatomic variation and anomalies of the intrahepatic ducts are obviously better appreciated on cross-sectional imaging if there is biliary tract dilation. For instance, an aberrant duct that drains either the posterior or anterior segment of the right lobe in up to 20% of individuals (59,60) usually joins the main hepatic or common hepatic duct in the porta hepatis. It may be ligated inadvertently during cholecystectomy and result in a segmental biliary obstruction that is detected by postoperative imaging exams (Fig. 12.14). The radiologic diagnosis of this ductal anomaly and management of its iatrogenic injuries are described by several authors (7,61,62). There are also other small accessory ducts, which emerge from the liver and course along the gallbladder fossa to join the extrahepatic ducts in the triangle of Calot. They can be transected at cholecystectomy and present with bile leakage and peritonitis (5–7,63).

These complications are usually well demonstrated by CT or sonography, but detection of underlying bile duct

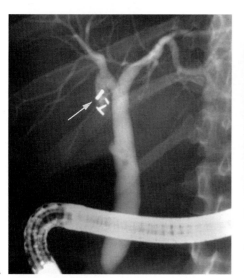

A

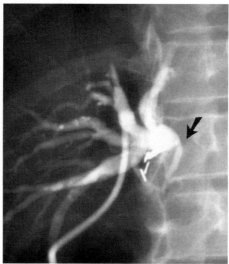

B

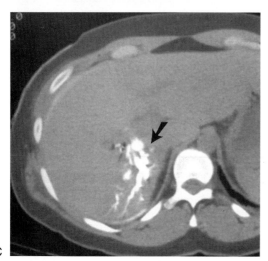

C

FIG. 12.14. Inadvertent ligation of an aberrant right hepatic duct causing segmental cholestasis. **A:** Endoscopic retrograde cholangiogram done 4 weeks after cholecystectomy shows a normal biliary tract except for a nonopacified branch of the right hepatic duct *(arrow)*. **B:** Cholangiogram through a percutaneous biliary catheter demonstrates the dilated ducts in the posterior segment of the right lobe. It drained through an aberrant connection with the cystic duct *(arrow)*, which had been ligated at surgery. **C:** Subsequent CT scan shows retained contrast material in the dilated bile ducts of the posterior segment of right hepatic lobe *(arrow)*.

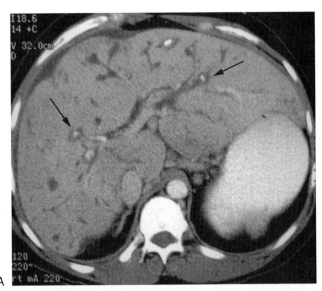

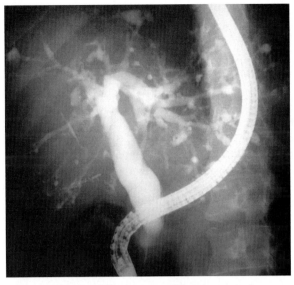

FIG. 12.15. Imaging features of Caroli disease. A: Contrast-enhanced CT shows multifocal areas of intrahepatic ductal dilation, some encircling of the opacified portal vein branches *(arrows),* accounting for the so-called "central dot sign." B: Endoscopic retrograde cholangiogram demonstrates numerous areas of saccular ectasia in the intrahepatic ducts. (Courtesy of Dr. Richard M. Gore, Evanston Hospital—Northwestern University, Evanston, Illinois.)

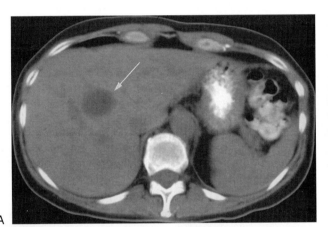

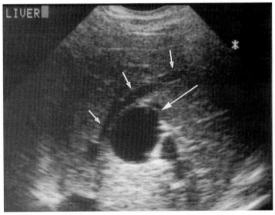

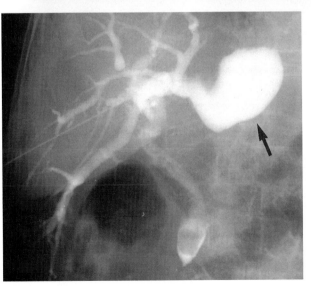

FIG. 12.16. Intrahepatic bile duct aneurysm. A: Computed tomogram of the upper abdomen shows a 4-cm low-attenuation round lesion in the right hepatic lobe *(arrow);* it could represent a possible cyst, abscess, metastasis, or an intrahepatic gallbladder. B: Sagittal sonogram of the same area shows this cystic structure *(arrow)* to be anterior to the portal vein branches *(short arrows);* it also lacked their Doppler flow characteristics. C: Transhepatic cholangiogram of another patient with a similar finding demonstrates the aneurysmal dilation of an intrahepatic duct.

abnormality would require direct cholangiography by T-tube, percutaneous, or endoscopic approach (6,59–63). An alternative noninvasive method is MR cholangiography, using fast spin-echo sequence (FSE) or the half-Fourier rapid acquisition with relaxation enhancement (RARE). Recent studies have documented the value of MR cholangiography for diagnosis of various biliary tract anomalies, such as aberrant right hepatic duct and low-inserting cystic duct (54,55).

Dilation of the biliary tract in adults is usually caused by an acquired obstruction from an impacted stone, stricture, or tumor. However, some congenital anomalies are manifested by nonobstructive dilation of the intrahepatic ducts. Hence, these entities must be differentiated from obstructing biliary lesions despite some similarities of their radiologic findings. A typical example is Caroli disease, which is characterized by segmental or diffuse cavernous ectasia of the intrahepatic ducts (64,65). This entity is often associated with recurrent cholangitis and stone formation but may also include hepatic fibrosis and renal tubular ectasia. The key feature for CT and sonographic diagnosis of Caroli disease is the presence of dilated saccular intrahepatic ducts, which surround the portal vein branches and make them appear as intraluminal protrusions and bridges (Fig. 12.15).

On rare instances a localized aneurysmal dilation of an intrahepatic duct may occur as an isolated anomaly related to congenital weakness of the wall, the presence of a partially obstructing epithelial diaphragm, or subsequent to focal pathologic processes (67). Its CT appearance as a well-circumscribed area of low attenuation within the liver can simulate an intrahepatic gallbladder, a liver cyst or lipoma, or a cavitating metastasis. However, cholangiography and other imaging studies would assist in clarifying the precise nature of ductal aneurysm and its differential diagnosis (Fig. 12.16).

Pitfalls in Imaging the Extrahepatic Ducts

The extrahepatic ducts in the porta hepatis are often visible on sonograms because the liver provides an acoustic window, but the common bile duct may be obscured by duodenal or colonic gas (10). However, the extrahepatic bile ducts are usually well demonstrated by high-resolution or spiral CT, particularly when they are dilated. During arterial and portal phases of a contrast-enhanced CT, the walls of the gallbladder and extrahepatic ducts show a moderate degree of transient opacification, whereas their bile-filled lumen will have a much lower attenuation than the liver and pancreas. On axial images, therefore, the ring-like appearance of these ducts may resemble radiolucent gallstones with a thin layer of peripheral calcification (Fig. 12.17). A similar pitfall in CT diagnosis of biliary calculi is the occasional occurrence of a "pseudocalculus defect" caused by spiral folds or septae in the gallbladder neck (see Fig. 12.12) or by thickening of inflamed gallbladder wall. In this situation, the low attenuation of the edematous submucosal layer can be misinterpreted as intraluminal fluid surrounding a pseudostone image created by the contrast-enhanced mucosa (9,68).

The right and left main hepatic ducts unite in the hilus of the liver to form the common hepatic duct. It is usually 2 to 4 cm long and lies anterior to the portal vein, which serves as the reference structure for its CT or sonographic identification (10,69). The cystic duct inserts into the right side of the common hepatic duct in about 90% of cases. In the remaining 10% of individuals, however, the cystic duct coils around it to join its anterior, posterior, or medial aspect.

A frequent variation seen in up to half of the patients is a more proximal or distal union of hepatic and cystic ducts (10,60,70). When they join low at a distance from

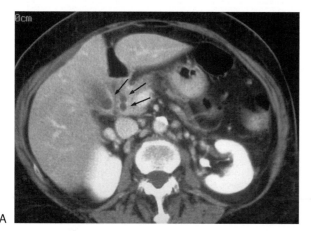
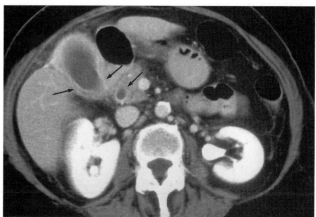

FIG. 12.17. Contrast-enhanced walls of the extrahepatic biliary tract during spiral CT examination. **A:** This image shows three low-attenuating circular structures in the porta hepatis, representing the gallbladder neck and cystic and common hepatic ducts *(arrows)*. Their contrast-enhanced walls and the low density of intraluminal bile would simulate calculi with peripheral calcification. **B:** Another CT section 3 cm caudad demonstrates the contrast-enhanced walls of the gallbladder and common bile duct *(arrows)*.

the porta hepatis, both ducts will be elongated and have a parallel course for several centimeters before merging to form a short common bile duct. On imaging studies, therefore, the adjoining segments of common hepatic and cystic ducts appear like a double-barrel structure (see Fig. 12.17A). It is often difficult to correctly identify and separate them even at surgery because both are enclosed within a shared sheath of connective tissues. This can lead to mishaps such as inadvertent ligation of the common hepatic duct with resultant biliary obstruction, ductal transection causing postoperative bile leakage, and misplacement of a T-tube into the cystic duct (5–7). To prevent such iatrogenic complications, it is a common practice to leave a long cystic duct stump behind at cholecystectomy. This may become a site of bile stasis, inflammation, and calculi.

Patients with an elongated and low-inserting cystic duct have an increased incidence of gallstones (71). They are also predisposed to develop the Mirizzi syndrome in which an impacted stone in the gallbladder neck or cystic duct would result in obstructive jaundice secondary to extrinsic compression and blockage of the adjacent common hepatic duct. The correct diagnosis of Mirizzi syndrome is usually made by cholangiography, but CT and ultrasound features of it include the demonstration of a large calculus in the cystic duct junction with the common hepatic duct, local inflammatory reaction in the

hepatoduodenal ligament, and dilated gallbladder and intrahepatic ducts (72).

The common bile duct is usually 4 to 8 cm long and about 6 to 9 mm in diameter. It is divided into suprapancreatic, intrapancreatic, and ampullary segments. In 80% to 90% of individuals, the common bile duct and pancreatic duct have a shared orifice as they empty into papilla of Vater, but they have two separate openings in the remaining 10% to 20% of cases. Occasionally, the common bile duct inserts into the pancreatic duct about 2 to 3 cm from the ampulla. This anomalous junction allows reflux of the pancreatic juice, thereby damaging the common duct wall and causing its luminal dilation to form a choledochal cyst (73).

Choledochal cyst is usually manifested during the first year of life, but delayed presentation in children or adults will occur in 20% to 30% of cases. The classic triad of right upper abdominal pain, palpable mass, and jaundice is noted in approximately a third of patients, though nearly all have at least one of these findings (10,58).

The correct diagnosis of a choledochal cyst can be made by several imaging techniques, including direct cholangiography, hepatobiliary scintigraphy, sonography, CT, and MR cholangiography (73,74). The most common appearance is a large saccular or fusiform dilation of the common duct (type 1), seen in about 75% of patients (Fig. 12.18). Another 2% of the cases present as a large diver-

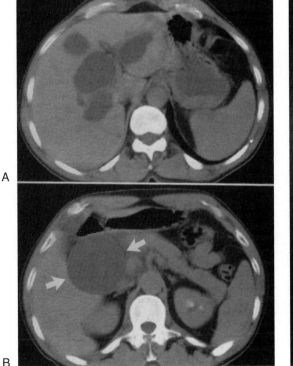

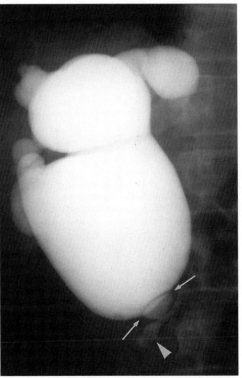

FIG. 12.18. Choledochal cyst in an adult. **A,B:** Two CT sections of the upper abdomen demonstrate the massively dilated intrahepatic ducts proximal to a large choledochal cyst *(arrows)*. **C:** Percutaneous transhepatic cholangiogram reveals a mucosal diaphragm *(white arrows)* and aberrant insertion of the common duct into the pancreatic duct, which harbors one small stone *(arrowhead)*.

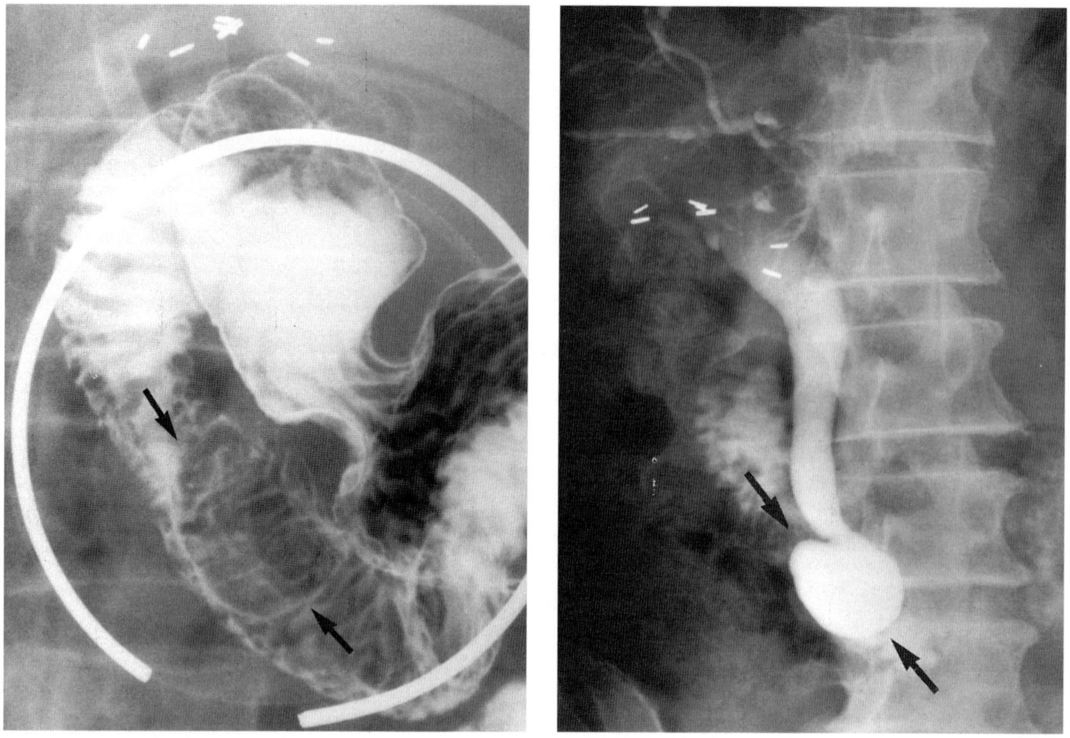

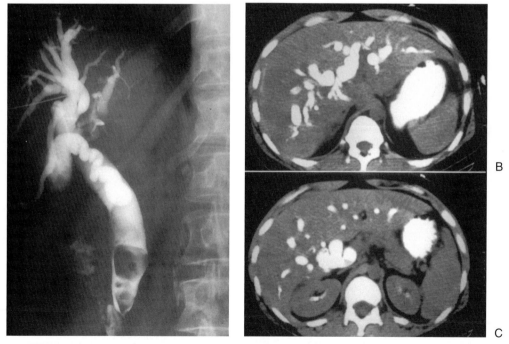

FIG. 12.19. Radiologic appearance of a choledochocele. **A:** Upper gastrointestinal series of this postcholecystectomy patient with recurrent biliary tract symptoms revealed a well-defined intramural mass in the duodenum *(arrows)*. **B:** Endoscopic retrograde cholangiogram showed a large choledochocele *(arrows)*, which caused intermittent biliary tract obstruction.

FIG. 12.20. Imaging similarities of acquired and congenital biliary tract obstruction. **A:** Transhepatic cholangiogram of this patient shows dilated intra- and extrahepatic ducts caused by multiple calculi in the common duct. **B,C:** Subsequent CT exam demonstrates the retained contrast material in dilated intrahepatic ducts; their saccular appearance resembles the congenital bile duct ectasia associated with Caroli disease.

ticulum protruding from the common duct (type 2). In both instances the rest of biliary tract may appears otherwise normal, although the thin-walled cyst may simulate a double gallbladder or pancreatic pseudocyst on imaging examinations. About 18% to 20% of patients will have multiple areas of aneurysmal dilation involving both the intra- and extrahepatic ducts (type 4). The least frequent presentation in 1% to 2% of cases is a choledochocele (type 3), a localized ballooning of the intraduodenal segment of the common bile duct (10,73). It appears as a cystic lesion in the head of the pancreas or duodenal wall on radiologic studies, but its precise nature is best demonstrated by various cholangiographic methods (Fig. 12.19).

As a general rule the presence of segmental or diffuse biliary tract dilation is readily appreciated on sonograms, CT, or MRI of the abdomen. However, it is important to carefully assess the most distal extent of ductal involvement on consecutive imaging sections. Every attempt should be made to distinguish congenital anomalies causing ectasia of bile ducts (e.g., Caroli disease and choledochal cysts) from dilation proximal to an impacted stone, tumor, or other pathologic processes (Fig. 12.20). The practicing radiologist should also keep it in mind that the appearance of a gallstone can be simulated by normal anatomic structures, as seen with pseudocalculus effect of gallbladder septae, contrast-enhanced mucosa, or ductal walls (see Figs. 12.12 and 12.17). On the other hand, the majority of gallstones that are not radiopaque will be invisible on CT because their attenuation is similar to that of the intraluminal bile itself (see Figs. 12.2 and 12.11). They may even escape sonographic detection if obscured by spiral folds and septations or by the gas and echoreflective material in the adjacent duodenum or colon (9,10).

In summary, frequent topographic variations and anomalies involving the gallbladder and bile ducts are major sources of diagnostic pitfalls in the CT and ultrasound hepatobiliary system that are described or illustrated in the first section of this chapter. These selected examples and the quoted references reflect a much broader range of potential problems that may be encountered in the clinical practice of biliary tract radiology.

MAGNETIC RESONANCE CHOLANGIOPANCREATOGRAPHY

Magnetic resonance cholangiopancreatography (MRCP) can now be reasonably considered as part of the routine imaging modalities for the evaluation of the biliary tree (12,54,75). Although MRCP images resemble those obtained with conventional cholangiographic techniques (i.e., intravenous, percutaneous, or endoscopic retrograde cholangiography), peculiar diagnostic criteria should be adopted in selected cases because of typical pitfalls occurring in MRCP images. The knowledge of certain anatomic variants and pitfalls is mandatory in order to improve the

overall diagnostic accuracy, limiting the number of false-positive and false-negative examinations.

Anatomic Variants

Anatomic variants of biliary ducts are mostly related to developmental anomalies occurring during the embryonic life. They are represented by dilation of both extra- and intrahepatic ducts and by the anomalies of the common bile duct (CBD) and cystic duct. The former have been classified by Todani (76) into different subtypes and include diverticula of the CBD and cystic dilation of intrahepatic bile ducts (Caroli's disease). In Caroli's disease, MRCP may provide the clue for the diagnosis, represented by the demonstration of communication among the multiple intrahepatic cystic dilations, obtained on both source and maximum intensity projection (MIP)-reconstructed images. The demonstration of the biliary origin of the cysts permits a differential diagnosis with other entities such as multiple simple cysts and intrahepatic abscesses (77).

Other anatomic variants of great clinical interest, especially with the advent of laparoscopic procedures, are the accessory ducts and the anomalous insertion of the cystic duct. Anomalous ducts are present in up to 18% of patients and are more frequent on the right biliary system (78). Anomalous ducts draining segments VII or VIII and joining either the CBD or the cystic duct are those of critical surgical importance because they can be inadvertently transected during a laparoscopic procedure (Fig. 12.21).

Insertion of the cystic duct in the CBD is extremely variable, although it is most commonly found on the lateral aspect of the middle third of CBD. Both low and high insertions exist. Low insertion with a long cystic duct running medially and parallel to the CBD may be a cause of a pitfall because it may look like a dilated CBD. To overcome this pitfall, either the source images should be

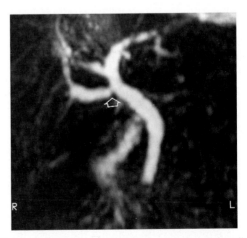

FIG. 12.21. This MIP-reconstructed image reveals mild stricture at the level of anomalous insertion of the posterior right hepatic duct into the common bile duct *(arrow)*. Normal appearance of the common bile duct and binary bifurcation is noted.

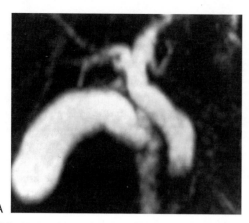 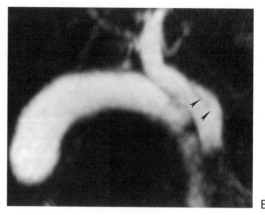

FIG. 12.22. Low insertion of the cystic duct. **A:** On coronal MIP image, a dilated common bile duct is depicted. **B:** Oblique projection reveals the low insertion of the cystic duct *(arrowheads),* simulating dilated common bile duct.

evaluated or the MIP images should be examined in oblique projections (79) (Fig. 12.22).

Pitfalls

Common pitfalls in MRCP may be divided into three groups, according to the different clinical indications: (a) pitfalls in diagnosing choledocholithiasis; (b) pitfalls in the evaluation of biliary strictures; and (c) pitfalls in the ampullary region.

Pitfalls in Diagnosing Choledocholithiasis

Diagnosis of choledocholithiasis with MRCP is relatively easy, and it is based on the same criteria used for conventional cholangiography; a stone, in fact, is depicted as an oval-shaped low-signal-intensity structure surrounded by hyperintense bile. The accuracy of MRCP in diagnosing stones is strictly dependent on the knowledge of common pitfalls, which may lead to erroneous interpretation. Most common pitfalls are (a) lack of stones on MIP-reconstructed images, (b) diffuse low signal intensity of CBD secondary to multiple stones, mimicking biliary stricture, (c) susceptibility artifacts caused by pneumobilia, and (d) air bubbles mimicking small stones.

Small Stone

As far as MIP-related artifacts are concerned, usually no difficulties occur in detecting large stones (more than 10 mm in diameter), even on MIP-reconstructed images, where a filling defect surrounded by hyperintense bile can be easily recognized. But for identification of small stones, it is necessary to evaluate the source images. In fact, on MIP projectional images, small stones are canceled out by the hyperintense signal from the bile surrounding the stone. This pitfall is similar to what happens at endoscopic retrograde cholangiography, where over-

filling of the CBD with contrast medium may lead to missing small stones. In our series of 51 patients with choledocholithiasis, stones were visible on MIP images in 56.8% of the cases, with visualization strictly dependent on size. But even relatively large stones (ranging between 5 and 10 mm) could be missed on MIP reconstructions (54.2% in our series). As a consequence, the analysis of both MIP and source images should be considered mandatory in all cases (80) (Fig. 12.23).

Multiple Stones

Another pitfall may occur when multiple stones completely fill the CBD; the result is a completely inhomogeneous low signal of the CBD because of the very small amount of bile among the multiple impacted stones, with marked dilation of proximal biliary ducts. The MRCP image may look like proximal binary stricture. Also in this case, source images may give the clue for a correct interpretation of the images (Fig. 12.24).

Pneumobilia

Air can frequently be present in the bile ducts (pneumobilia), in particular in patients with previous operation on the biliary system (biliary-enteric anastomoses, sphincterotomy). Pneumobilia may cause susceptibility artifacts, which are usually limited to a minimum by the use of a sequence, such as turbo spin echo, which is very stable with regard to this kind of artifact. In very rare situations, the excessive amount of air may create a complete inhomogeneity in the signal of the CBD, limiting the diagnostic value of the examination.

Air Bubbles

In patients who underwent sphincterotomy, air bubbles represent a common finding and may sometimes create

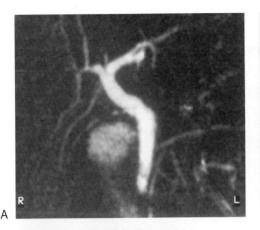

A

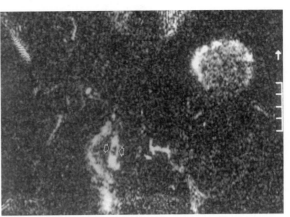

B

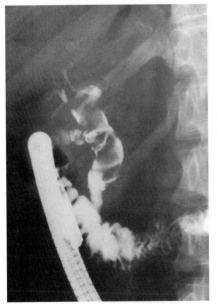

C

FIG. 12.23. Missing small stone on MIP image. **A:** Coronal MIP-reconstructed image shows normal appearance of the common bile duct in a patient who previously had a cholecystectomy. **B:** On the source image, an 8-mm stone is depicted as a low-signal-intensity round filling defect *(arrows)*. **C:** Stone extraction is performed at endoscopic retrograde cholangiography.

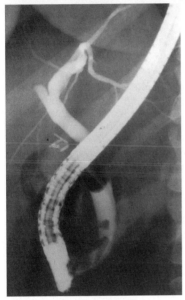

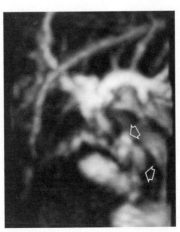

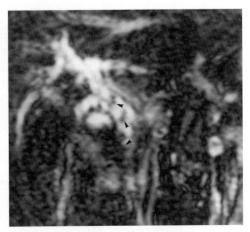

A,B

C

FIG. 12.24. Multiple stones pitfall. **A:** Endoscopic retrograde cholangiography reveals multiple stones filling the common bile duct. **B:** On MIP-reconstructed image, marked dilation of intrahepatic ducts is observed; the common bile duct is hardly visible *(arrows)* because of inhomogeneous signal; MRCP findings may simulate a stricture at the level of the biliary bifurcation. **C:** Source image reveals multiple stones *(arrowheads)* filling the common bile duct with small amount of bile.

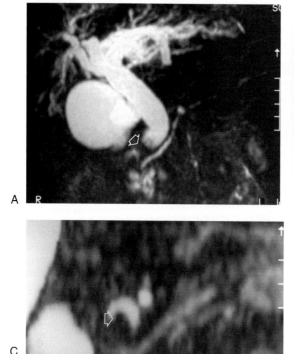

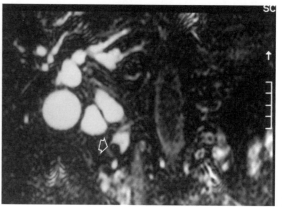

FIG. 12.25. Common bile duct stone. **A:** The MIP-reconstructed image shows obstructing stones in the distal portion of the common bile duct *(arrow)*. **B:** Stones are better evaluated on source image *(arrow)*. **C:** Typically, on axial image (multiplanar reformation of 3-D data sets), stone is in dependent portion of the common bile duct, and this is how it can be differentiated from air bubbles.

problems in the differential diagnosis with small stones. This is because bubbles and stones have the same appearance on MRCP images, as is the case on conventional cholangiography. A useful trick to differentiate between small stones and air bubbles is represented by the generation of MRCP images on a plane orthogonal to the long axis of the CBD (usually an axial oblique plane). These additional images may be obtained either by reformatting the volumetric data on the axial plane (if a 3-D sequence has been acquired) or, if working with 2-D images, by acquiring a second set of images. The evaluation of CBD on the axial plane demonstrates stone to be in the dependent part of the CBD, whereas air bubbles lie in the nondependent part (Figs. 12.25 and 12.26).

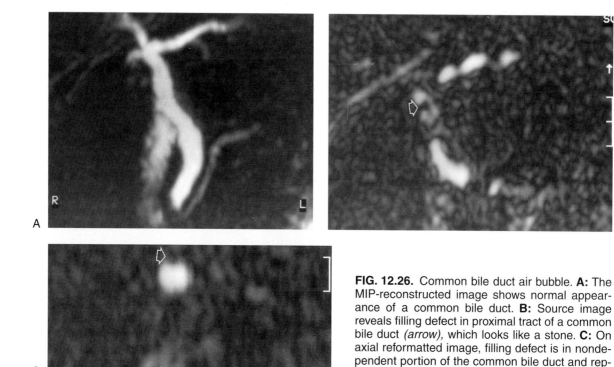

FIG. 12.26. Common bile duct air bubble. **A:** The MIP-reconstructed image shows normal appearance of a common bile duct. **B:** Source image reveals filling defect in proximal tract of a common bile duct *(arrow)*, which looks like a stone. **C:** On axial reformatted image, filling defect is in nondependent portion of the common bile duct and represents an air bubble, not a stone.

Pitfalls in the Evaluation of Biliary Strictures

When a biliary stricture is diagnosed, pitfalls may occur in characterizing the nature and also in evaluating the degree of the stricture. Causes of artifacts have to be found in the reduced matrix size of MR images compared with conventional films and in artifacts related to MIP reconstructions.

As far as the characterization of the stricture is concerned, the evaluation of MRCP images alone is not sufficient to obtain a correct diagnosis. In fact, the reduced matrix size limits the evaluation of fine details (i.e., mucosal irregularities); lack of injection of contrast medium on one side provides a physiologic image of the stricture but, on the other side, limits the evaluation of additional features (distensibility, etc.). But MRCP has the further advantage of being part of a complete abdominal evaluation; as a consequence, the contemporary evaluation of both MRCP and conventional images may help in stricture characterization.

Another pitfall may occur in the evaluation of the degree of the stricture, usually overestimated on MIP-reconstructed images. In fact, the small amount of bile in a tight stricture is completely canceled out on MIP images, producing a false image of complete obstruction. This pitfall may be limited either by the analysis of source images, where even a very small amount of bile can be detected, or by the evaluation of secondary signs, represented by the degree of dilation of bile ducts above the stricture.

The other possible diagnostic problem in biliary stricture is the lack of visualization of distal collapsed common bile duct, preventing a correct evaluation of the length of the stricture.

There are also situations in which a stricture may be mimicked. This is the case of the right hepatic artery crossing the CBD. In normal anatomy, the right hepatic artery runs posterior to the proximal tract of the CBD and can produce an extrinsic impression on the CBD. In some cases, the extrinsic impression may mimic a mild stricture (Fig. 12.27). The typical location as well as the evaluation of both source images and axial T$_2$-weighted images may help in distinguishing between these two entities. Finally, a small intrahepatic stone, wedged in a segmentary duct, surrounded by a very low amount of bile and causing dilation of intrahepatic ducts may produce a false image of intrahepatic stricture (Fig. 12.28).

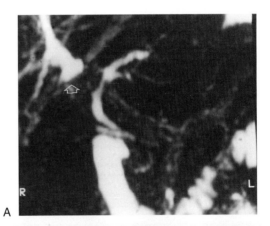

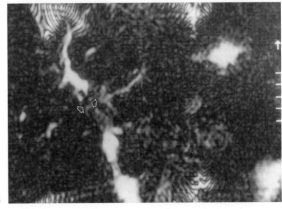

FIG. 12.27. Pseudostricture caused by right hepatic artery. **A:** The MRCP image shows normal appearance of a common bile duct. **B:** On source image, extrinsic impression *(arrow)* on the posterior aspect of the proximal common bile is noted as a result of the right hepatic artery crossing the common bile duct.

FIG. 12.28. Pseudostricture caused by stone. **A:** Marked dilation of segmentary intrahepatic duct resembling an intrahepatic stricture *(arrow)*. **B:** On source image, a small stone *(arrows)* surrounded by a very small amount of bile is shown.

Pitfalls in the Ampullary Region

The evaluation of the ampullary region is particularly difficult on MRCP because of the small size of the distal tract of the CBD containing little bile and producing poor signal. A useful trick to improve the visualization of the region is represented by the administration of tap water before the examination in order to fill and distend the duodenum. In this way, small protrusions caused by papillary inflammations can be more easily detected. Additionally, the evaluation of conventional T_1-weighted MR images can be helpful in ruling out the presence of mass lesions in ampullary and periampullary regions (Fig. 12.29). However, a differential diagnosis between small ampullary tumor (Fig. 12.30) and papillary stricture secondary to inflammation cannot be obtained in all cases.

Other pitfalls are related to the diagnosis of small stones wedged in the papilla (if no fluid surrounds the stones, the detection could be very difficult) and to the atypical appearance of the morphology of the distal tract of the CBD mimicking wedged stones; in both cases the evaluation of source images is mandatory to improve the diagnostic accuracy.

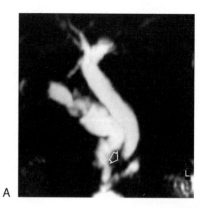
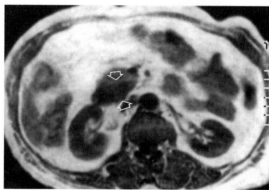

FIG. 12.30. Periampullary tumor. **A:** Same morphology of the stricture as in Fig. 12.29 is evident in another patient. **B:** On spin-echo T_1-weighted image, a solid periampullary lesion is shown. The MRCP findings indicate a periampullary tumor.

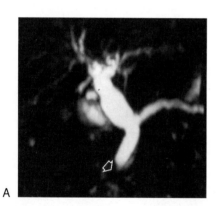
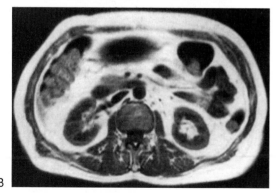

FIG. 12.29. Periampullary stricture. **A:** The MRCP images show distal common bile duct stricture. **B:** The evaluation of axial spin-echo T_1-weighted image reveals no mass lesion. The MRCP findings are suggestive of an inflammatory stricture.

REFERENCES

1. Hatfield PM, Wise RE. Anatomic variation in the gallbladder and bile ducts. *Semin Roentgenol* 1976;11:157–169.
2. Schulte SJ. Embryology, normal variation, and congenital anomalies of the gallbladder and biliary tract. In: Freeny PC, Stevenson GW, eds. *Margulis and Burhenne's alimentary tract radiology, 5th ed.* St Louis: Mosby-Year Book, 1994;1251–1274.
3. Gore RM, Ghahremani GG, Fernbach SK. Gallbladder and biliary tract: Anomalies and anatomic variations. In: Gore RM, Levine MS, Laufer I, eds. *Textbook of gastrointestinal radiology.* Philadelphia: WB Saunders, 1994;1620–1635.
4. Meilstrup JW, Hopper KD, Thieme GA. Imaging of gallbladder variants. *Am J Roentgenol* 1991;157:1205–1208.
5. Ghahremani GG. Postsurgical and traumatic lesions of the biliary tract. In: Gore RM, Levine MS, Igor I, eds. *Textbook of gastrointestinal radiology.* Philadelphia: WB Saunders, 1994;1762–1778.
6. Ghahremani GG, Crampton AR, Bernstein JR, Caprini JA. Iatrogenic biliary tract complications: Radiologic features and clinical significance. *RadioGraphics* 1991;11:441–456.
7. Ghahremani GG. Postsurgical biliary tract complications. *Gastroenterologist* 1997;5:46–57.
8. Ward EM, LeRoy AJ, Bender CE, Donohue JH, Hughes RW. Imaging of complications of laparoscopic cholecystectomy. *Abdom Imag* 1993;18:150–155.
9. Turner MA. Diagnostic methods and pitfalls in the gallbladder. *Semin Roentgenol* 1991;26:197–208.
10. Zeman RK, Burrell MI. *Gallbladder and bile duct imaging: a clinical radiological approach.* New York: Churchill Livingstone, 1987;47–104.
11. Reinhold C, Bret PM, Guibaud L, Barkun AN. MR cholangiopancreatography: potential clinical applications. *RadioGraphics* 1996;16:309–320.
12. Guibaud L, Bret PM, Reinhold C, Atri M, Barkun AN. Bile duct

obstruction and choledocholithiasis: diagnosis with MR cholangiography. *Radiology* 1995;197:109–115.

13. Diehl AK. Epidemiology and natural history of gallstone disease. *Gastroenterol Clin North Am* 1991;20:1–19.

14. Johnston DE, Kaplan MM. Pathogenesis and treatment of gallstones. *N Engl J Med* 1993;328:412–421.

15. NIH Consensus Conference. Gallstones and laparoscopic cholecystectomy. *JAMA* 1993;269:1018–1024.

16. Rosenthal SJ, Cox GG, Wetzel LH, et al. Pitfalls and differential diagnosis in biliary sonography. *RadioGraphics* 1990;10:285–311.

17. Anderson CM, Saloner D, Tsuruda JS, et al. Artifacts in maximum-intensity projection display of MR cholangiograms. *Am J Roentgenol* 1990;154:623–629.

18. Reuther G, Kiefer B, Tuchmann A, Pesendorfer FX. Imaging findings of pancreaticobiliary duct diseases with single-shot MR cholangiopancreatography. *Am J Roentgenol* 1997;168:453–459.

19. Blanton DE, Bream CA, Mandel SR. Gallbladder ectopia: a review of anomalies of position. *Am J Roentgenol* 1974;121:296–300.

20. Bach DB, Satin R, Palayew M, et al. Herniation and strangulation of the gallbladder through the foramen of Winslow. *Am J Roentgenol* 1984;142:541–542.

21. Merine D, Meziane M, Fishman EK. CT diagnosis of gallbladder torsion. *J Comput Assist Tomogr* 1987;11:712–713.

22. Yeh HC, Weiss MF, Gerson CD. Torsion of the gallbladder: the ultrasonographic features. *J Clin Ultrasound* 1989;17:123–125.

23. Levard G, Weil D, Barret D, Barbier J. Torsion of the gallbladder in children. *J Pediatr Surg* 1994;29:569–570.

24. Lusink C, Sali A. Intrahepatic gallbladder and obstructive jaundice. *Med J Aust* 1985;142:53–54.

25. Wysong CB, Gorten RJ. Intrahepatic gallbladder. *South Med J* 1980;6:825–826.

26. Faintuch J, Machado MC, Raia AA. Suprahepatic gallbladder with hypoplasia of the right lobe of the liver. *Arch Surg* 1980;115:658–659.

27. Youngwirth LD, Peters JC, Perry MC. The suprahepatic gallbladder: an unusual anatomical variant. *Radiology* 1983;149:57–58.

28. Van Gansbeke D, DeToeuf J, Cremer M, Engelholm L, Struyven J. Suprahepatic gallbladder: a rare congenital anomaly. *Gastrointest Radiol* 1984;9:341–343.

29. Naganuma S, Ishida H, Konno K, et al. Sonographic findings of anomalous position of the gallbladder. *Abdom Imag* 1998;23:67–72.

30. Nardi PM, Yaghoobian J, Ruchman RB. CT demonstration of retrohepatic gallbladder in severe cirrhosis. *J Comput Assist Tomogr* 1988;12:969–970.

31. Feldman L, Venta L. Percutaneous cholecystostomy of an ectopic gallbladder. *Gastrointest Radiol* 1988;13:256–258.

32. Banzo I, Carril JM, Arnal C, et al. Left-sided gallbladder: an incidental finding on hepatobiliary scintigraphy. *Clin Nucl Med* 1990;15:358–359.

33. Newcombe JF, Henley FA. Left-sided gallbladder: a review of the literature and report of a case associated with hepatic duct carcinoma. *Arch Surg* 1964;88:494–497.

34. Pradeep VM, Ramachandran K, Sasidharan K. Anomalous position of the gallbladder: ultrasonographic and scintigraphic demonstration in four cases. *J Clin Ultrasound* 1992;20:593–597.

35. Maetani Y, Itoh K, Kojima N, et al. Portal vein anomaly associated with deviation of the ligamentum teres to the right and malposition of the gallbladder. *Radiology* 1998;207:723–728.

36. Gore RM, Ghahremani GG, Joseph AE, et al. Acquired malposition of the colon and gallbladder in patients with cirrhosis: CT findings and clinical implications. *Radiology* 1989;171:739–742.

37. Brown BD, Gerscovich EO, Lais BR. Migrating gallbladder in alcoholic liver cirrhosis mimicking true ectopia: CT findings. *Eur J Radiol* 1994;19:34–36.

38. Bennion RS, Thompson JE, Tompkins RK. Agenesis of the gallbladder without extrahepatic biliary atresia. *Arch Surg* 1988;123:1257–1260.

39. Vanek VW, Lyras L. Agenesis of the gallbladder. *Contemp Surg* 1988;32:39–34.

40. Richards RJ, Taubin H, Wasson D. Agenesis of the gallbladder in symptomatic adults. A case and review of the literature. *J Clin Gastroenterol* 1993;16:231–233.

41. Azmat N, Francis KR, Mandava N, Pizzi WF. Agenesis of the gallbladder revisited laparoscopically. *Am J Gastroenterol* 1993;88:1269–1270.

42. Watemberg S, Rahmani H, Avrahami R, et al. Agenesis of the gallbladder found at laparoscopy for cholecystectomy: an unpleasant surprise. *Am J Gastroenterol* 1995;90:1020–1021.

43. McHugo JM, McKeown C, Brown MT, et al. Ultrasound findings in children with cystic fibrosis. *Br J Radiol* 1987;60:137–141.

44. Diaz MJ, Fowler W, Hnatow BJ. Congenital gallbladder duplication: preoperative diagnosis by ultrasonography. *Gastrointest Radiol* 1991;16:198–200.

45. Garfield HD, Lyons EA, Levi CS. Sonographic findings in double gallbladder with cholelithiasis of both lobes. *J Ultrasound Med* 1988;7:589–591.

46. Chouhan AL, Chouhan S, Chouhan MK. Duplication of gallbladder associated with cholelithiasis: sonographic detection. *J Clin Ultrasound* 1995;23:556–557.

47. Adear H, Burki Y. Multiseptate gallbladder in a child: incidental diagnosis on sonography. *Pediatr Radiol* 1990;20:192–194.

48. Lev-Toaff AS, Friedman AC, Rindsberg SN, et al. Multiseptate gallbladder: incidental diagnosis on sonography. *Am J Roentgenol* 1987;148:1119–1120.

49. Saimura M, Ichimiya H, Naritomi G, et al. Multiseptate gallbladder: biliary manometry and scintigraphy. *J Gastroenterol* 1996;31:133–136.

50. Wales LR. Desquamated gallbladder mucosa: unusual sign of cholecystitis. *Am J Roentgenol* 1982;139:810–812.

51. Price RJ, Stewart ET, Foley WD, et al. Sonography of polypoid cholesterolosis. *Am J Roentgenol* 1982;139:1197–1200.

52. Hwang JI, Chou YH, Tsay SH, et al. Radiologic and pathologic correlation of adenomyomatosis of the gallbladder. *Abdom Imag* 1998;23:73–77.

53. Fowler RC, Reid WA. Ultrasound diagnosis of adenomyomatosis of the gallbladder. *Clin Radiol* 1988;39:402–406.

54. Taourel P, Bret PM, Reinhold C, Barkun AN, Atri M. Anatomic variants of the biliary tree: diagnosis with MR cholangiopancreatography. *Radiology* 1996;199:521–527.

55. Fulcher AS, Turner MA, Capps GW, Zfass AM, Baker KM. Half-Fourier RARE MR cholangiopancreatography: experience in 300 subjects. *Radiology* 1998;207:21–32.

56. Liddell RM, Baron RL, Ekstrom JE, Varnell RM, Shuman WP. Normal intrahepatic bile ducts: CT depiction. *Radiology* 1990;176:633–635.

57. Quint LE, Glazer GM. CT evaluation of bile ducts in patients with fatty liver. *Radiology* 1984;153:755–756.

58. Stringer DA. *Pediatric gastrointestinal imaging.* Toronto: BC Decker, 1989;471–506.

59. Puente SG, Bannura GC. Radiological anatomy of the biliary tract: variations and congenital abnormalities. *World J Surg* 1983;7:271–276.

60. Hamlin JA. Radiological anatomy and anomalies of the extrahepatic biliary ducts. In: Berci G, Buschieri A, eds. *Bile ducts and bile duct stones.* Philadelphia: WB Saunders, 1997;9–19.

61. Christensen RA, Van Sonnenberg E, Nemcek AA Jr, D'Agostino HB. Inadvertent ligation of the aberrant right hepatic duct at cholecystectomy: radiologic diagnosis and therapy. *Radiology* 1992;183:549–553.

62. Seely JM, Cooperberg PL, Mathieson JR, et al. Inadvertent ligation of the right hepatic duct at cholecystectomy: long-term imaging findings. *Am J Roentgenol* 1994;162:1109–1111.

63. Rappoport AS, Diamond AB. Cholangiographic demonstration of postoperative bile leakage from aberrant biliary ducts. *Gastrointest Radiol* 1981;6:273–276.

64. Choi BI, Yeon KM, Kim SH, Han MC. Caroli disease: central dot sign in CT. *Radiology* 1990;174:161–163.

65. Marchal GJ, Desmet VJ, Proesmans WC, et al. Caroli disease: high-frequency US and pathologic findings. *Radiology* 1986;158:507–511.

66. Boyle MJ, Doyle GD, McNulty JG. Monolobar Caroli disease. *Am J Gastroenterol* 1989;84:1437–1441.

67. Terada T, Nakanuma Y. Solitary cystic dilation of the intrahepatic bile duct: morphology of two autopsy cases and a review of the literature. *Am J Gastroenterol* 1987;82:1301–1305.

68. Middleton WD, Thorsen MK, Lawson TL, et al. False positive diagnosis of gallstones due to thickening of the gallbladder wall. *Am J Roentgenol* 1987;149:941–944.

69. Rosenthal SJ, Cox GG, Wetzel LH, et al. Pitfalls and differential diagnosis in biliary sonography. *RadioGraphics* 1990;10:285–311.

70. Shaw MJ, Dorsher PJ, Vennes JA. Cystic duct anatomy: an endoscopic perspective. *Am J Gastroenterol* 1993;88:2102–2106.

71. Kubota Y, Yamaguchi T, Tani K, et al. Anatomical variation of pancreaticobiliary ducts in biliary stone diseases. *Abdom Imag* 1993;18:145–149.

72. Cruz FO, Barriga P, Tocornal J, Burhenne HJ. Radiology of the Mirizzi

syndrome: diagnostic importance of the transhepatic cholangiogram. *Gastrointest Radiol* 1983;8:249–253.

73. Savader SJ, Benenati JF, Venbrux AC, et al. Choledochal cysts: classification and cholangiographic appearance. *Am J Roentgenol* 1991;156: 327–331.

74. Akhan O, Demirkazik FB, Ozmen MN, Ariyurek M. Choledochal cysts: ultrasonographic findings and correlation with other imaging modalities. *Abdom Imag* 1994;19:243–247.

75. Barish MA, Yucel EK, Soto JA, Chuttani R, Ferrucci JT. MR cholangiopancreatography: efficacy of three-dimensional turbo spin-echo technique. *Am J Roentgenol* 1995;165:295–300.

76. Todani T, Watanabe Y, Narusue M. Congenital bile ducts cyst. *Am J Surg* 1977;134:263–269.

77. Pavone P, Laugh A, Catalano C, Materia A, Basso N, Passariello R. Caroli's disease: evaluation with N/IR cholangiopancreatography (MRCP). *Abdom Imag* 1996;21:117–119.

78. Hayes MA, Goldenberg IS, Courtney CB. The developmental basis for bile duct anomalies. *Surg Obstet* 1985;107:447.

79. David V, Reinhold C, Hochman M, et al. Pitfalls in the interpretation of NM cholangiopancreatography. *Am J Roentgenol* 1998;170: 1055–1059.

80. Laugh A, Pavone P, Catalano C, et al. *Pitfalls in the evaluation of common bile duct stones at NM cholangiography.* Paper presented at the 8th Annual ESGAR Meeting and Postgraduate Course "Clinical Gastrointestinal Radiology; Update for the New Millennium," Amsterdam, The Netherlands, June 25–28, 1997;65.

Variants and Pitfalls in Body Imaging,
edited by Ali Shirkhoda.
Lippincott Williams & Wilkins, Philadelphia, © 2000.

CHAPTER 13

The Spleen

Dixon Gilbert and Abraham H. Dachman

The spleen is a soft, reddish purple, highly vascular organ located in the posterior portion of the left upper quadrant. It measures an average 12 cm long by 7 cm wide by 4 cm thick and weighs approximately 150 g (normal range of 100 to 250 g) (1). It has unique structural and functional features and is the largest of the lymphatic organs, which include the lymph nodes, tonsils, and thymus (2). The spleen receives 4% of the cardiac output with 350 L of blood perfusing this organ each day with a transit time of approximately 25 seconds (3).

The immune response of the spleen is not completely understood, though the spleen is important in initiation of humoral and cellular immune response. The lymphatic tissue of the spleen is unique in that whole blood perfuses the Malpighian corpuscle rather than only the lymphatic elements as in other lymphatic organs. Therefore, this organ is able to respond quickly to blood-borne antigens; it removes aged erythrocytes, abnormal cells, and foreign particles from the circulation. Though the spleen is the major site of blood filtration and is therefore potentially exposed to a variety of pathogenic organisms and metastases, splenic abscesses and metastasis are uncommon. This may be because of the extensive phagocytic activity of the macrophages in the spleen. The spleen also sequesters red blood cells and platelets for release in times of need. The average spleen sequesters 30% of all platelets. In addition, the spleen is a hematopoietic organ during gestation, and multipotential cells within the spleen can hypertrophy and function as hematopoietic cells postnatally in times of need.

EMBRYOLOGY

Multiple aggregations of mesenchymal cells develop in the dorsal mesogastrium during the sixth week of gestation in order to form the embryonic spleen (4). These mesenchymal cells will proliferate and coalesce to eventually form the spleen. At this stage of development, the greater curvature of the stomach is directed posteriorly, and the dorsal mesogastrium extends from the greater curvature to the posterior abdominal wall. With further development, the greater curvature rotates to the left, and the dorsal mesogastrium balloons to the left, also carrying the spleen. Further proliferation of these mesenchymal cells causes the spleen to bulge to the left of the dorsal mesogastrium; this action places the spleen almost completely intraperitoneal just below the left hemidiaphragm. When the dorsal mesogastrium balloons, it also carries the splenic vessels and the dorsal pancreas. Much of the left side of the dorsal mesogastrium posterior to the spleen fuses with the parietal peritoneum overlying the left hemidiaphragm, the left adrenal gland, and the left kidney. With this process, most of the pancreas and splenic vessels become located in the anterior pararenal compartment of the retroperitoneum.

This ballooning of the dorsal mesogastrium also forms the splenorenal ligament, the gastrosplenic ligament, the anterior layer of the renal (Gerota's) fascia, and the omental bursa (lesser sac). The splenorenal ligament is the portion of the dorsal mesogastrium that extends from the spleen to the left kidney; this ligament contains the tip of the pancreatic tail and the splenic vessels and directs them toward the splenic hilum. The gastrosplenic ligament is formed by the anterior portion of the dorsal mesogastrium, which extends from the greater curvature to the spleen. The anterior layer of the renal fascia is formed as the visceral peritoneum on the left side of the dorsal

D. Gilbert and A. H. Dachman: Department of Radiology, University of Chicago Hospital, Chicago, Illinois 60637.

mesogastrium fuses with the parietal peritoneum of the posterior abdominal wall. The splenic hilar structures, the splenorenal ligament, and the gastrosplenic ligament form the left wall of the omental bursa.

The spleen achieves its characteristic form, position, and organ relationships by the third month of fetal life. The original mesenchymal cells differentiate to form all of the elements of the spleen, including the functioning parenchymal cells and the supporting stromal tissue, such as the capsule, trabeculae, and venous sinuses. The white pulp, red pulp, and lymphatic nodules become distinguishable by the sixth month. The hematopoietic cells produce both white and red blood cells until late in fetal life. The lymphatic nodules continue to produce lymphocytes and monocytes after birth.

MICROSCOPIC ANATOMY

The spleen is comprised of a dense connective tissue stroma and functional parenchymal cells (3). The supporting stroma forms a connective tissue framework; this includes the capsule externally and the trabeculae internally. The dense capsule is less than 1 mm thick and covers the entire spleen except at the hilum where the splenic artery, vein, lymphatics, and nerves enter and leave. The trabeculae extend deep into the internal substance of the spleen. A thin visceral peritoneum that covers the capsule and a tiny volume of lubricating peritoneal fluid allow for physiologic movement of the spleen during respiration, changes in body position, and trunk movements.

The functional parenchyma of the spleen is comprised of red and white pulp. The white pulp is typically composed of round or elliptical areas of densely aggregated lymphocytes, plasma cells, macrophages, and other free cells. These cells are arranged as periarterial lymphatic sheaths or nodules, which are also known as Malpighian or splenic corpuscles. The gross color of the white pulp results from these closely packed lymphocytes.

The white pulp is surrounded by a larger area of red pulp, which is comprised of terminal branches of the central arteries, splenic sinuses, and splenic cords (of Billroth), which are filled with systemic blood. The high content of erythrocytes produces the gross color of the red pulp. The splenic sinuses are composed of long, anastomosing dilated, capillary-like channels. These channels are periodically joined together by longitudinal slit-like spaces; all types of blood cells can easily pass through these spaces into the splenic cords. The splenic sinuses ultimately coalesce to form pulp veins, which in turn drain into the trabecular and then splenic veins. The splenic cords occupy all of the red pulp between the pulp arteries, sinuses, and veins. The cords contain red blood cells, macrophages, lymphocytes, granulocytes, and platelets and are supported by a sparse network of reticular cells and fibers that lack an endothelial lining. Some of the macrophages in the splenic cords are arranged as sheaths around the branches of the central arteries and can monitor the passage of cells between the sinuses and cords. These macrophages also phagocytize damaged erythrocytes and foreign antigens.

The blood traveling through the red pulp can enter either the open or closed circulation of the spleen. Blood cells that enter the splenic cords form the open circulation of the spleen; these cells migrate freely back and forth between the sinuses and cords with no predefined pathway. However, a portion of blood traverses directly from the splenic cords into endothelium-lined venous sinuses; this pathway is deemed the closed circulation.

GROSS ANATOMY

The spleen is often a complete intraperitoneal structure in location and underlies the posterior ninth through 11th ribs. It is classically described as having two poles, anterior and posterior, but is obliquely oriented with its long axis following the posterior course of the tenth rib. The superior portion is relatively superior, posterior, and medial with the lower pole directed inferiorly, anteriorly, and laterally. The superior portion is located in the upper left paravertebral gutter under the left hemidiaphragm. The left adrenal and kidney lie posterior to the inferior portion of the spleen. The spleen lies lateral to the greater curvature of the stomach. The pancreatic tail approaches the splenic hilum in the region of the splenorenal ligament.

The spleen is a pliable organ with three major surfaces that are molded by the surrounding organs. The diaphragmatic surface is convex and faces posteriorly, superiorly, and laterally. The gastric surface is concave and faces anteromedially and slightly superiorly. The renal surface is also concave and faces posteromedially and slightly inferiorly. The spleen typically has two hila, or depressions, in the surface where the major vessels enter or leave the spleen; these are most often on the gastric surface. The pancreatic tail enters the splenorenal ligament as it exits the retroperitoneum. The splenic flexure of the colon is typically described as contacting the inferior pole of the spleen and may leave an impression; it may also be located anteriorly between the spleen and the stomach. The splenic capsule is clearly delineated from these organs by the surrounding mesenteric fat.

The splenic artery is a branch of the celiac trunk that originates just above the neck of the pancreas. This artery is large for the size of the spleen and gives off branches to the stomach (short gastric and sometimes the left gastroepiploic) as well as the pancreas (including the dorsal pancreatic artery). The branches to the pancreas affix this artery to the pancreas. The splenic artery is notable for its tortuosity, which is unique among normal arteries. It takes a winding course along the upper border of the pancreas traversing posterolaterally toward the splenic hilum. Approximately 4 cm before the hilum, the splenic artery branches into two or three terminal branches. These terminal branches again branch several times just before entering the spleen to form six to 36 vessels, which separately enter the spleen at a single hilum or, more commonly, two hila.

The splenic vein most commonly begins as a confluence of three major trunks and runs inferiorly and anteriorly along the pancreas near the splenic artery. As the splenic vein parallels the pancreas, the peripancreatic fat may be mistaken for a dilated pancreatic duct (5). This vein also receives branches from the left gastroepiploic, short gastric, and pancreatic veins, and at the neck of the pancreas, it joins the superior mesenteric vein to form the portal vein. Unlike the splenic artery, the splenic vein is not tortuous.

Lymphatic drainage of the spleen exits the splenic hila and drains into the celiac lymphatic trunk. Innervation of the spleen is primarily sympathetic from levels T5 through T9; this innervation arrives at the spleen via the celiac ganglion and allows for contraction of smooth muscle in the capsule for vasoconstriction.

COMPUTED TOMOGRAPHY: TECHNIQUE

Helical scanning permits acquisition of the entire spleen in a single breath-hold, thus eliminating artifacts from respiratory motion and misregistration of lesion location. As with liver scanning, the ability to perform rapid scanning permits not only arterial and redistribution phase scanning but also calculation of splenic perfusion and sequential delayed images to help characterize vascular lesions. For general abdominal scanning, an infused study is sufficient, but pre- and postcontrast infused studies may be useful for optimally showing calcifications and quantifying change in enhancement.

On nonenhanced scans, the spleen is homogeneous and slightly less dense than the normal liver with an attenuation value of approximately 40 to 60 Hounsfield units (HU) (6). The omental and mesenteric fat that surrounds the spleen provides sharp demarcation of the splenic capsule and its vessels. The splenic artery is tortuous and may appear curvilinear, round, or elliptical on any section of the scan as its wandering course leads the artery into and out of the plane of scanning.

Contrast-enhanced scanning is indicated to evaluate parenchymal lesions or to better delineate splenic from pancreatic or adrenal abnormalities. Bolus infusion will provide dense enhancement of the hilar vessels and the spleen. Routine abdominal CT protocols are usually optimized for detection of liver lesions and are therefore usually performed with a 2- to 3-cc/sec injection, a scan delay of 60 to 70 seconds, a collimation of 5 to 10 mm, and a pitch of 1:1. Initial heterogeneous enhancement should become homogeneous with time, and eventually the enhanced splenic parenchyma should be 5 to 10 HU less dense than the liver.

PITFALLS

Heterogeneous Enhancement

During the arterial phase of contrast enhancement, splenic heterogeneity is expected and should not be mistaken for disease. The more rapid the injection rate, the more pronounced the pattern (7). Other conditions that may exaggerate heterogeneous enhancement include decreased cardiac output and delayed transit time as a result of splenic vein thrombosis, portal vein thrombosis, or portal hypertension (7,8). The proposed etiology for this heterogeneity is that the flow rate of blood varies through the different histologic components of the spleen. As the terminal arteries transport blood into the splenic parenchyma, it is first carried into the white pulp before being discharged into the relatively larger-volume red pulp. The red pulp is comprised of splenic sinuses and cords. A portion of the blood is transferred from the splenic sinuses and perfuses slowly through the splenic cords before entering the venous sinuses; this is known as the open circulation. However, some of the blood bypasses the splenic cords and travels from the splenic sinuses directly into the endothelium-lined venous sinuses; this more direct, faster pathway is known as the closed circulation. The relatively faster perfusion through the closed circulation may explain why the normal spleen

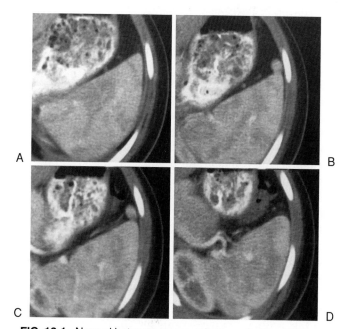

FIG. 13.1. Normal heterogeneous splenic perfusion, CT scan. **A–D:** Helical CT done with intravenous contrast administered at 2 cc/sec with a 70-second scan delay. This mottled or striated appearance is commonly seen during arterial weighted phase or early redistribution phase of splenic enhancement.

(continued on next page)

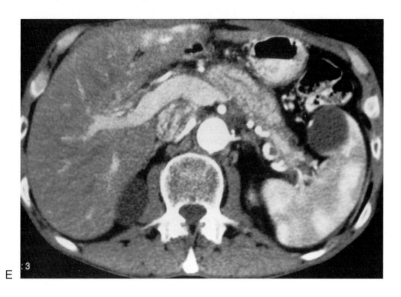

E

FIG. 13.1. *Continued.* E: Heterogeneous peripheral enhancement of the spleen during early arterial phase of CT scanning. Incidentally noted is the low-attenuation splenic cyst seen anteriorly. (Courtesy A. Shirkhoda, M.D., William Beaumont Hospital.)

appears heterogeneous when imaged during the early phase of perfusion; the central portion of the spleen may enhance homogeneously while the more peripheral red pulp may appear heterogeneous or mottled with apparent focal areas of decreased enhancement (9). Patterns of heterogeneous enhancement have been described as "serpentine," "cord-like," "mottled," or "striped." The term "zebra spleen" has been applied (10). By 2 minutes postinjection, the normal spleen should demonstrate a homogeneous enhancement pattern (Fig. 13.1).

Variation in Position

Position of the spleen is related to the length of the splenorenal ligament, which is typically several centimeters long. The splenorenal ligament is formed by the fusion of the dorsal mesogastrium and the parietal peritoneum of the posterior parietal wall. There is often some mobility to the spleen even with a normal length, so that its position may differ slightly between the supine and prone positions (11). This may have implications in radiation therapy planning, for example. If the fusion of the dorsal mesogastrium with the parietal peritoneum of the posterior abdominal wall proceeds too far, this ligament is obliterated, creating a "bare area" on the spleen (12) so that a surface of the spleen is not intraperitoneal in location (Fig. 13.2). This can place the spleen in direct contact with the kidney. The spleen may also be positioned partly dorsal to the kidney (13).

If incomplete fusion occurs, the splenorenal ligament can be elongated and create a wandering spleen (14,15). In this setting, the position of the spleen can vary over time; the spleen may be located in its normal position in the left upper quadrant or may descend lower into the abdomen or pelvis (Fig. 13.3). Wandering spleen may become symptomatic as a result of torsion, which may be

intermittent or may result in splenic infarction. Occasionally, a wandering spleen remains asymptomatic and is not detected until adulthood.

Differentiation from Adjacent Organs

An elongated left hepatic lobe can extend to and hug the spleen, creating the appearance of splenomegaly,

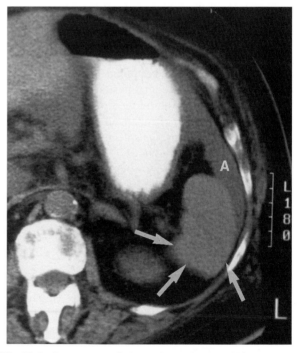

FIG. 13.2. Bare area of the spleen. Ascites (A) is demonstrated lateral and ventral to the spleen. In this case, the bare area of the spleen *(arrows)* along the renal margin as well as the dorsal and hilar margins are anatomically separated from the peritoneal cavity and do not interface with the ascitic fluid.

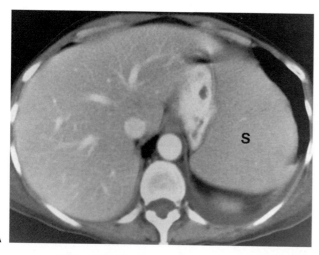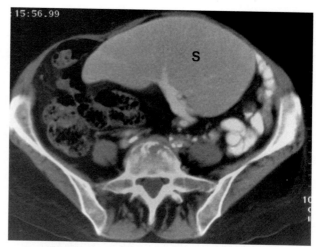

FIG. 13.3. Wandering spleen. **A:** The spleen (S) is located in the left upper quadrant. **B:** Computed tomogram obtained 1 year later for evaluation of lower abdominal mass. The spleen (S) has now rotated and descended into the anterior portion of the upper pelvis. There is no evidence of splenic infarct or torsion. No abnormal mass was seen. (Courtesy A. Shirkhoda, M.D., William Beaumont Hospital.)

splenic mass, or fracture (16) (Fig. 13.4). This is more likely to be a pitfall in thin patients or children who have little peritoneal fat and may present a problem in sonography as well as CT (17).

The inferior portion of the spleen can approach the left kidney and create the appearance of a renal mass. Coronal reconstruction images can be helpful to delineate the two organs (Fig. 13.5).

Accessory Spleen

The mesenchymal cells that form the spleen may fail to coalesce completely. If most of the mesenchymal masses fuse to form a spleen of normal size and shape but one or a few of these masses fail to fuse, an accessory spleen, or spleniculus, is formed (Fig. 13.6). Accessory spleens are found in approximately 10% of the population (18,19) and are most commonly located in the splenic hilum (75%). Spleniculi can also be embedded in the pancreatic tail (20%), in the gastrosplenic ligament, or along the splenic artery in the retroperitoneum and can cause mass effect on the gastric fundus (18,19). Multiple accessory spleens, or polysplenia, occurs when more than one of the mesenchymal masses fails to fuse with the true spleen. Polysplenia can occur in association with cardiovascular anomalies such as levoisomerism or partial situs inversus

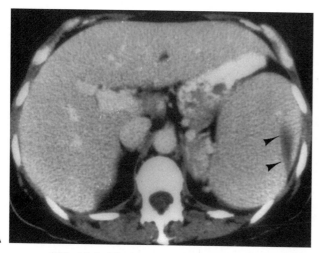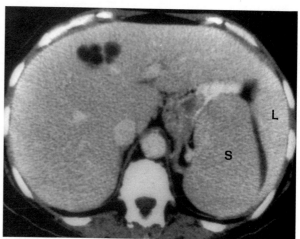

FIG. 13.4. Elongated left lobe of the liver hugging the spleen. **A:** On a single image, a hypodense line *(arrowheads)* is seen at the lateral aspect of the spleen and could be mistaken for splenic laceration. **B:** A more cephalad image clearly shows the elongated left lobe of the liver (L) separated from the spleen (S).

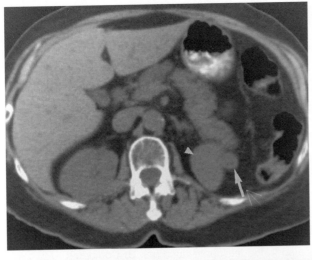

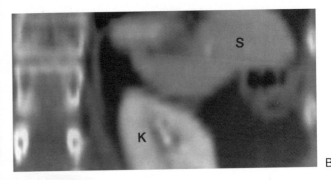

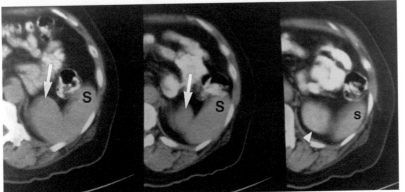

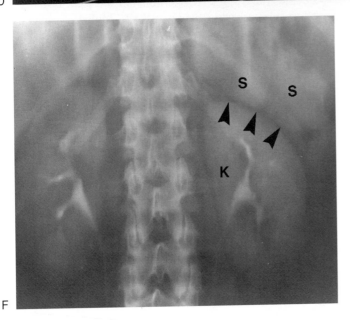

FIG. 13.5. Splenic tissue suggestive of left renal mass. **A:** Unenhanced CT image demonstrates a soft tissue density suggestive of mass *(arrow)* on the left kidney *(arrowhead)*. **B:** Coronal reconstruction images convincingly demonstrate contiguity with the spleen (S) of unusual shape (K, kidney). **C–E:** On a different patient, three axial sections from enhanced CT imaging demonstrate soft tissue density *(arrow)*, which could represent normal splenic (S) configuration or possible renal mass (kidney, *arrowhead*). **F:** Plane film tomography from intravenous pyelogram demonstrates normal kidney with normal variant splenic lobulations (S). Note the radiolucent fat plane *(arrowheads)*, which clearly separates the kidney and spleen.

(20,21). Accessory spleens should demonstrate a synchronous pattern of enhancement with the spleen during all phases of scanning but may resemble mass or adenopathy.

In addition, an accessory spleen can increase in size over time, particularly in a patient who has undergone splenectomy (Fig 13.7).

An accessory spleen or a medial extension of the spleen can also extend into the adrenal fossa and mimic an adrenal nodule. On careful evaluation of the enhancement pattern, the tissue characteristics will follow the splenic parenchyma during all phases of enhancement. Nuclear medicine SPECT scanning can also aid in discrimination (Fig. 13.8).

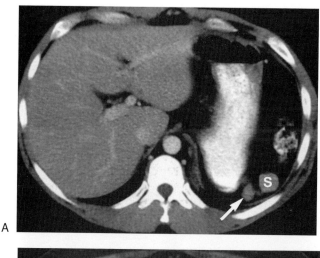

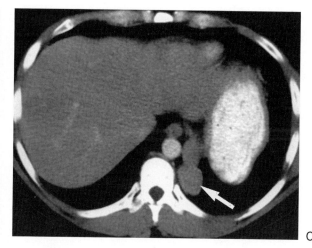

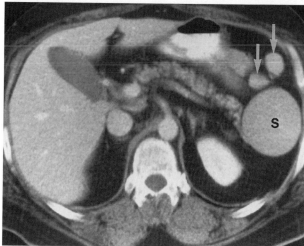

FIG. 13.6. Accessory spleen in three patients. **A:** Accessory spleen *(arrow)* medial to the inferior pole of the normal spleen (S). **B:** Two small accessory spleens *(arrows)* ventral to the main splenic body (S). **C:** Accessory spleen *(arrow)* in an unusual location abutting the diaphragm in the left paraspinal region. (Courtesy A. Shirkhoda, M.D., William Beaumont Hospital.)

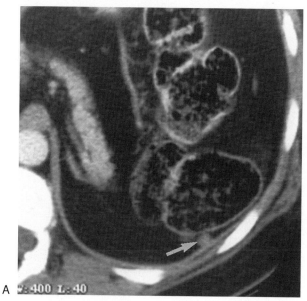

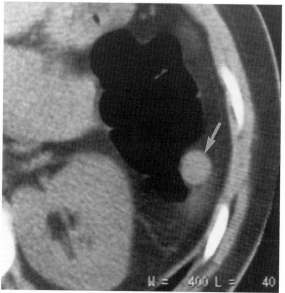

FIG. 13.7. Growth of accessory spleen. **A:** Small accessory spleen *(arrow)* adjacent to the splenic flexure in a patient who had a splenectomy. **B:** A later CT demonstrates hypertrophy of this accessory spleen *(arrow).*

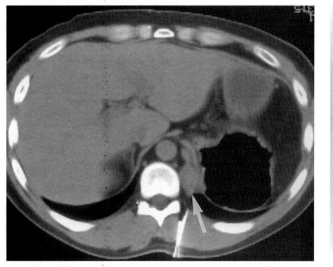
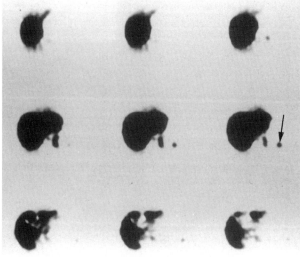

FIG. 13.8. Accessory spleen mimicking adrenal nodule. **A:** Unenhanced CT demonstrates soft tissue density *(arrow)* in the left suprarenal region in this postsplenectomy patient. A needle biopsy was initiated to rule out adrenal mets, but the procedure was aborted. **B:** Technetium-99m sulfur colloid SPECT in axial plane proves this tissue to represent accessory spleen *(arrow)*. (Courtesy A. Shirkhoda, M.D.)

Variation in Splenic Contour

The mesenchymal masses may all coalesce to form a single spleen, but portions of these masses may only partially fuse. This can create splenic lobulations, notches, or clefts. The lobulations are most commonly located on the inferior or anteromedial aspect of the spleen, may be supplied by a separate splenic artery, and may produce extrinsic impression on the stomach. Splenic clefts can have a sharp appearance and may extend 2- 3 cm into the splenic parenchyma (Fig. 13.9). The portions of the spleen which are divided by the cleft may only be joined

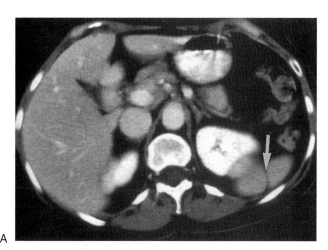
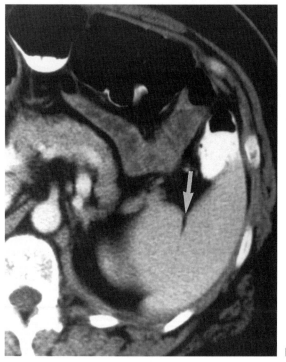

FIG. 13.9. Splenic cleft. **A:** Hypodense line *(arrow)* in the inferior pole of the spleen could be confused with a splenic laceration. Note the homogeneous parenchymal enhancement, the clearly defined splenic margins, and the normal appearance of the surrounding fat, convincing evidence that this is a normal variant. (Courtesy A. Shirkhoda, M.D., William Beaumont Hospital.) **B:** Normal variant splenic cleft *(arrow)* in a different patient.

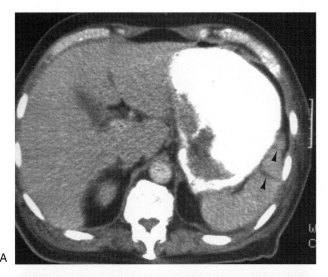

A

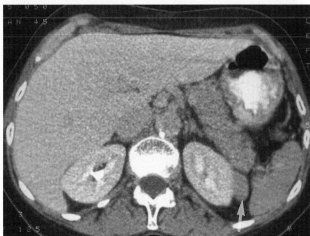

B

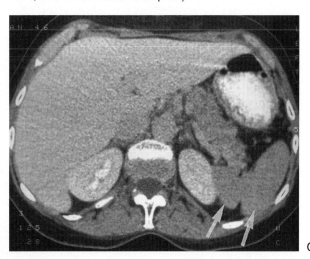

C

FIG. 13.10. Splenic lobulations. **A:** Two well-defined lobulations *(arrowheads)* in the superior pole of the spleen. **B:** In a second patient, there appears to be either an accessory spleen or a renal mass *(arrow)* on a single CT section. **C:** A second more caudal image demonstrates that this tissue is contiguous with the spleen *(arrows)* and represents splenic lobulations. (Courtesy A. Shirkhoda, M.D., William Beaumont Hospital.)

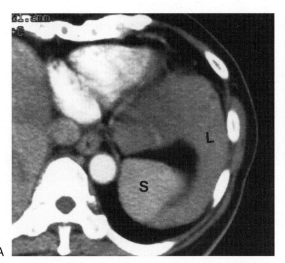

A

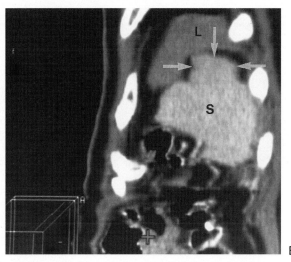

B

FIG. 13.11. Splenic lobulation. **A:** Elongated left lobe of the liver (L) hugs the spleen (S), but splenic lobulation is not apparent on the axial images. **B:** Sagittal reconstruction images clearly separate the liver (L) from the spleen (S). Of note is splenic lobulation *(arrows),* which is not apparent on the axial images.

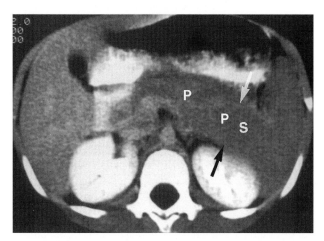

FIG. 13.12. Splenic tongue mimicking pancreatic mass. Hypodense splenic tongue (S) abuts the pancreas (P) in this patient with minimal intraperitoneal fat. *Arrows* identify the interface between these organs. (Courtesy A. Shirkhoda, M.D., William Beaumont Hospital.)

The mesenchymal masses may also fuse and form a remnant of normal tissue in the splenic hilum, known as a splenic tongue. The splenic tongue can be difficult to distinguish from the tail of the pancreas (Fig. 13.12). A splenic tongue can also extend toward the stomach and create a worrisome extrinsic mass effect (Fig. 13.13).

Congenital Cysts

Splenic cysts may be congenital, posttraumatic, or parasitic in origin. A true splenic cyst, also known as epidermoid, epithelial, or congenital cyst, should have an epithelial lining. It has been hypothesized that a true cyst is created by an infolding of the peritoneal epithelium or by collections of mesothelial cells that become trapped in the splenic sulci (Fig. 13.14A) (10,11). Further, a splenic cyst can be accompanied by other normal splenic variations, as shown in this case of wandering spleen with large splenic cyst (Fig. 13.14B).

Computed Tomography Arterial Portography Defects

Splenic perfusion defects have been observed on CT portography that are similar to those previously described for early arterial-phase enhancement during peripherally infused CT scanning. In a study that correlated CTAP to either 4- to 6-hour delayed CT, follow-up

together by a narrow bridge of tissue; this should not be confused with splenic laceration. Splenic lobulation is a more subtle variation of splenic cleft with shorter extension of the cleft into the parenchyma; this may also be multiple (Fig 13.10). Splenic lobulations may also be more apparent with multiplanar imaging (Fig. 13.11).

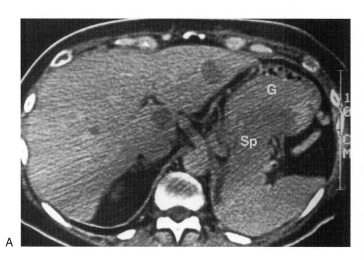

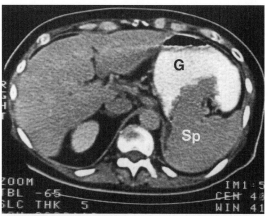

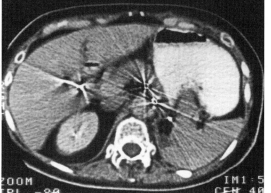

FIG. 13.13. Splenic tongue creating extrinsic mass effect on the stomach. **A:** Without contrast in the gastric lumen (G), the medial extension of the spleen (Sp) cannot be differentiated from the stomach. **B:** However, additional imaging performed immediately following administration of oral contrast demonstrates the gastric lumen (G) and the splenic tongue (Sp) more clearly. (Courtesy A. Shirkhoda, M.D., William Beaumont Hospital.)

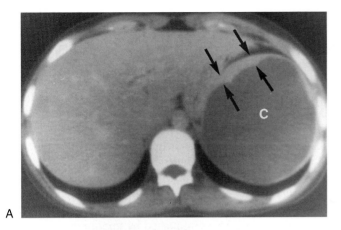

A

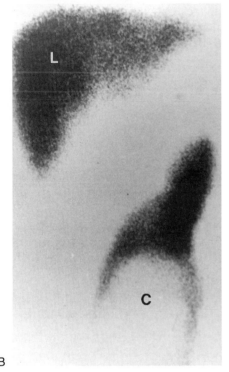

B

FIG. 13.14. Congenital splenic cyst. **A:** Single section from axial CT demonstrates large, well-defined hypodense region within the spleen, which represents a congenital splenic cyst (C). Thin rim of normally enhancing spleen is also seen *(arrow)*. **B:** In a second patient, anterior view of a Tc-99m sulfur colloid nuclear medicine imaging demonstrates the spleen, which has descended into the pelvis with a rounded, well-defined region of absent radiopharmaceutical activity representative of splenic cyst (C) in this wandering spleen.

CT, or MRI, splenic perfusion defects were demonstrated in 14 of 46 (30%) patients. These defects were usually wedge-shaped and peripheral, but a few were round. Only one patient had an infarct based on a correlative study, and all had normal spleens by inspection at laparotomy (22). These were assumed to be perfusion-related defects. Thus, it is important not to assume that splenic defects at CTAP represent space-occupying lesions (Fig. 13.15).

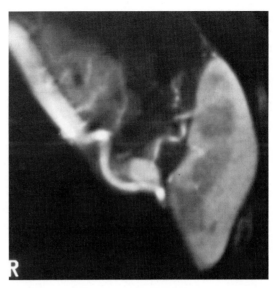

FIG. 13.15. Axial image during CT portography demonstrates heterogeneous enhancement pattern in this normal spleen.

MAGNETIC RESONANCE

Single breath-hold MRI techniques and intravenous administration of gadolinium chelate have improved evaluation of the spleen. The T_1 and T_2 relaxation times of spleen are similar to those of the kidney and longer than those of the liver. The proton density of the spleen is similar to that of the liver.

Technique

Magnetic resonance imaging of the spleen should include at least T_1-weighted and T_2-weighted sequences. Spin-echo (SE), spoiled gradient-echo (SGE), and inversion recovery sequences are most often used to generate T_1-weighted images. Spin-echo or echo train spin-echo (e.g., fast spin-echo or turbo spin-echo) sequences are most frequently used to generate T_2-weighted images. Short tau inversion recovery (STIR) may also be used as a T_2-weighted sequence. Chemically selective fat suppression may be added to improve the dynamic range of tissue signal intensities, to remove chemical shift artifact, and to reduce phase artifact.

Contrast enhancement is becoming routine in MR imaging of the spleen. The most common approach is to administer a nonspecific extracellular gadolinium-based contrast agent (e.g., gadolinium-DTPA) as a rapid intravenous bolus with serial imaging using a spoiled gradient echo sequence [e.g., fast multiplanar spoiled gradient echo (FMPSPGR) or fast low angle shot (FLASH)]. Ideally, the entire spleen should be imaged in a single breath-hold, and the first contrast-enhanced series of images should be obtained within 30 seconds after the bolus injection. Fat suppression is often added to at least one contrast-enhanced SGE image series.

Normal Appearance and Pitfalls

The spleen has a homogeneous appearance on conventional spin-echo MR images. The spleen may also demonstrate homogeneous appearance on gadolinium-infused images; however, on breath-hold contrast-enhanced studies, the normal spleen often demonstrates unique enhancement patterns such as arciform, mottled, peripheral heterogeneous appearance as with CT (Fig. 13.16). This appearance may be related to variations in flow rates through the open and closed circulation of the red pulp as previously described. A second possible reason is that the red pulp enhances rapidly, and the white pulp enhances slowly. Delayed imaging of the normal spleen will show a homogeneous pattern within 2 minutes.

Flow artifacts are also common and are most conspicuous in the phase-encoding direction (23). Therefore, when imaging is performed in the transverse plane with horizontal phase-encoding direction, flow artifacts that can simulate splenic lesion are seen just lateral to the aorta or the inferior vena cava. These artifacts can be diminished by swapping the phase- and frequency-encoding directions, although artifacts may remain just anterior and posterior to the aorta or the inferior vena cava (16).

Magnetic susceptibility artifacts also occur during MR imaging of the spleen. The fast gradient-echo techniques, which are commonly employed for evaluation of the spleen, are particularly sensitive to magnetic susceptibility artifacts. This can result in large areas of signal void around surgical clips or other metallic foreign bodies. These artifacts can be diminished by minimizing T_E and maximizing receiver bandwidth (16).

In addition, filming techniques used in MRI scanning are often optimized to evaluate the liver; the spleen may

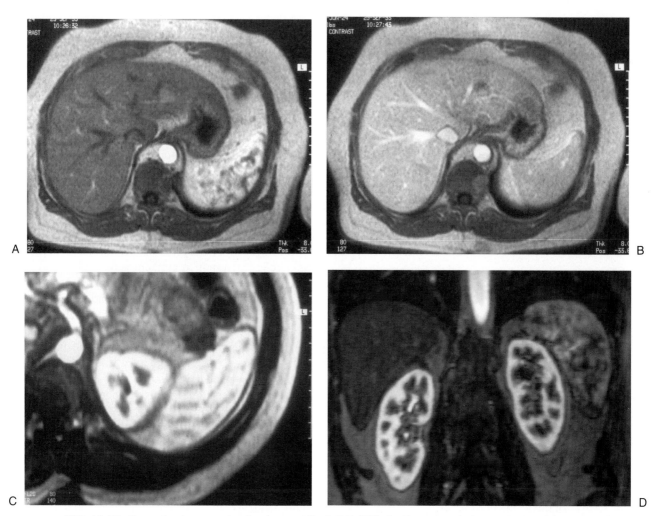

FIG. 13.16. Normal spleen, contrast-enhanced flash 2-D MRI. **A:** Scanning during early arterial phase of gadolinium demonstrates heterogeneous enhancement. **B:** Delayed images in same patient demonstrate homogeneous signal intensity and enhancement pattern. **C:** In a different patient, early arterial weighted scanning demonstrates a striated enhancement pattern, a normal variant. **D:** Coronal image during early arterial phase demonstrates mottled enhancement of the spleen. (Courtesy A. Shirkhoda, M.D., William Beaumont Hospital.)

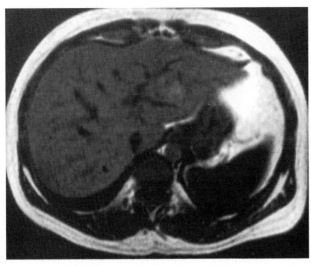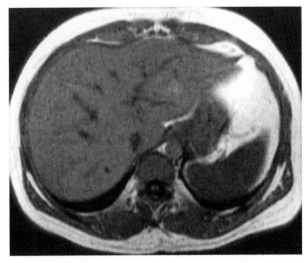

A   B

FIG. 13.17. Normal spleen, gadolinium-enhanced flash 2-D MRI. **A:** On original images filmed to opti-mize hepatic assessment, the spleen demonstrates diffusely black signal and cannot be adequately evaluated. **B:** Following refilming with new window and level settings, this normal spleen can be ade-quately evaluated.

show diffusely high or low signal intensity, depending on the sequence used, when filmed for hepatic contrast, which severely limits evaluation of the spleen. If splenic assessment is indicated, image window settings should be closely monitored to insure that evaluation of the spleen is satisfactory (Fig 13.17).

ACKNOWLEDGMENT

The authors thank David Casalino for contributing to the MR portions of this chapter.

REFERENCES

1. Anson BJ, McVay CB. *Surgical anatomy, 5th ed.* Philadelphia: WB Saunders, 1971;633–639.
2. Defiore MSH. *Atlas of human histology, 2nd ed.* Philadelphia: Lea & Febiger, 1963.
3. MacPherson AIS, Richmond J, Stuart AE. *The spleen.* Springfield, IL: Charles C Thomas, 1973.
4. Moore KL. *The developing human.* Philadelphia: WB Saunders, 1973.
5. Seidelmann FE, Cohen WN, Bryan PJ, et al. CT demonstration of the splenic vein–pancreatic duct relationship: the pseudodilated pancreatic duct. *Am J Roentgenol* 1977;129:17–21.
6. Mategrano VC, Petasnick J, Clark J, et al. Attenuation values in computed tomography of the abdomen. *Radiology* 1977;125:135–140.
7. Urban BA, Fishman EK. Helical CT of the spleen. *Am J Roentgenol* 1998;170:997–1003.
8. Miles KA, McPherson SJ, Hayball MP. Transient splenic inhomogene-ity with contrast-enhanced CT: mechanism and effect of liver disease. *Radiology* 1995;194:91–95.
9. Rabushka LS, Kawashima A, Fishman EF. Imaging of the spleen: DT with supplemental MR examination. *RadioGraphics* 1994;14:307–332.
10. Glazer GM, Axel L, Goldberg HI, et al. Dynamic CT of the normal spleen. *Am J Roentgenol* 1981;137:343–346.
11. Ball WS, Wicks JD, Medttle FA Jr. Prone–supine change in organ posi-tion: CT demonstration. *Am J Roentgenol* 1980;136:815–820.
12. Vibhakar SD, Bellon EM. The bare area of the spleen: a constant CT feature of the ascitic abdomen. *Am J Roentgenol* 1984;141:953–955.
13. Hopper KD, Chantelois AE. The retrorenal spleen. *Radiology* 1987;165:85.
14. Gordon DH, Burrell MI, Levin DC, et al. Wandering spleen: the radio-logical and clinical spectrum. *Radiology* 1977;125:39–46.
15. Herman TE, Siegel MJ. CT of acute splenic torsion in children with wandering spleen. *Am J Roentgenol* 1991;156:151–153.
16. Katsuyoshi I, Mitchell DG, et al. Gadolinium-enhanced MR imaging of the spleen: Artifacts and potential pitfalls. *Am J Roentgenol* 1996;167:1147–1151.
17. Li DKB, Cooperberg PL, Graham MF, Callen P. Pseudoperisplenic fluid collection: a clue to normal liver and spleen echogenic texture. *J Ultrasound Med* 1986;5:397.
18. Miller EJ, Nowak E, Hair L, et al. Retroperitoneal accessory spleen. *Am Surg* 1990;56:293–294.
19. Hargrove MD Jr, Kilpatrick ZM. Pseudotumor of the gastric fundus caused by an accessory spleen. *J LA State Med Soc* 1969;121:386–387.
20. Peoples WM, Moller JH, Edwards JE. Polysplenia: a review of 146 cases. *Pediatr Cardiol* 1983;4:129–137.
21. Winer-Muram HT, Tonkin IL, Gold RE. Polysplenia syndrome in the asymptomatic adult: computed tomography evaluation. *J Thorac Imag* 1991;6:69–71.
22. Nazarian LN, Wechsler RJ, Grady CK, et al. The frequency, appear-ance, and significance of splenic perfusion defects on CT arterial por-tography. *Abdom Imag* 1996;21:53–57.
23. Arena L, Morehouse HT, Satir J. MR Imaging artifacts that simulate disease: how to recognize and eliminate them. *RadioGraphics* 1995;15:1373–1394.

SUGGESTED READINGS

Glazer GM, Axel L, Goldberg HI, et al. Dynamic CT of the normal spleen. *Am J Roentgenol* 1981;137:343–346.
Koehler RE. Spleen. In: Lee JKT, Sagel SS, Stanley RJ, eds. *Computed body tomography.* New York: Raven Press, 1983;243–256.
Kormano M, Partanen K, Soimakallio S, et al. Dynamic contrast enhance-ment of upper abdomen: effects of contrast medium and body weight. *Invest Radiol* 1983;18:364–367.

Partanen K, Soimakallio S, Kivimaki T, et al. Dynamic topography of the contrast enhancement of the spleen. *Eur J Radiol* 1984;4:101–106.

Piekarski J, Federle MP, Moss AA, et al. Computed tomography of the spleen. *Radiology* 1980;135:683–689.

Stephens DH, Sheedy PF, Hattery RR, et al. Computed tomography of the liver. *Am J Roentgenol* 1977;128:579–590.

Vermess M, Doppman JL, Sugarbaker P, et al. Clinical trials with a new intravenous liposoluble contrast material for computed tomography of the liver and spleen. *Radiology* 1980;137:217–222.

Vermess M, Doppman JL, Sugarbaker PH, et al. Computed tomography of the liver and spleen with intravenous lipoid contrast material: review of 60 examinations. *Am J Roentgenol* 1982;138:1063–1071.

Variants and Pitfalls in Body Imaging,
edited by Ali Shirkhoda.
Lippincott Williams & Wilkins, Philadelphia, © 2000.

CHAPTER 14

The Pancreas

Ali Shirkhoda and Richard M. Gore

Familiarity with the normal anatomy and anatomic variants of the pancreas on cross-sectional imaging studies is important in order to diagnose subtle and complex pancreatic pathology. Knowledge of the embryology and development of this gland is also needed to recognize the various pancreatic anomalies and to differentiate them from neoplasms. Errors and variations at several critical periods in the development of the pancreas are responsible for the majority of anomalies (1–4). The clinical manifestations of these anomalies and anatomic variations are wide ranging, varying from asymptomatic to being inconsistent with life (5).

EMBRYOLOGIC CONSIDERATIONS

The pancreas develops from two buds originating from the endodermal lining of the duodenum (Fig. 14.1A). One is the dorsal pancreatic bud, which is in the dorsal mesentery and is seen as a diverticulum of the foregut before 28 days of gestation (6). It grows into the dorsal mesentery. The other is the ventral pancreatic bud located close to the bile duct, and it appears as an invagination at the biliary–duodenal angle between 30 and 35 days of fetal life. These two buds soon grow into a pair of branching ductal systems, each with its own central duct (Fig. 14.1B). The ventral pancreas rotates posterior to the duodenum and abuts the dorsal pancreas, where they eventually fuse (Fig. 14.1C). In the mature pancreas, the ventral part becomes the inferior portion of the head and uncinate process, while the dorsal part becomes the body and tail of the pancreas. After the fusion, a new duct connects the distal portion of the dorsal pancreatic duct with the shorter duct of the ventral pancreas to form the main pancreatic duct or the duct of Wirsung. In approximately 91% of adults, this duct enters the duodenum at the major papilla or ampulla of Vater (Fig. 14.2A). The proximal portion of the dorsal pancreatic duct usually atrophies, but it may persist as a small accessory duct of Santorini entering into the duodenum at the minor papilla (Fig. 14.2B). The ductal system may fail to fuse, and the original double system persists in up to 10% of adults (7) (Fig. 14.2C).

In the third month of fetal life, the islets of Langerhans develop as clusters of cells derived from the terminal ductules. They finally become separate from the ductules when the endocrine portion of the pancreas develops, and insulin secretion begins at approximately the fifth month. The acini develop from the terminal ductal cells and collectively along with the ductal system become the exocrine portion of the pancreas. The weight of the pancreas, which is 5 to 5½ g at birth, will increase to 15 g at 1 year of age (8).

During the process of pancreatic fusion, a wide spectrum of anomalies and anatomic variants may develop. These include agenesis, aplasia, hypoplasia, pancreatic divisum, and annular pancreas (9).

IMAGING PROTOCOL

When the pancreas is evaluated with CT, helical scanning is preferred, and two protocols are applicable. One is routine scanning of the pancreas in patients with known or suspected pancreatitis, and the other is tailored to diagnose and stage for a possible neoplasm. In pancreatitis, routine abdominal scanning with a 5- to 8-mm slice thickness and a 7- to 8-mm reconstruction interval is generally adequate. However, when pancreatic tumor is suspected, slice thickness should be 3 to 4 mm with a reconstruction interval of 4 to 5 mm. In both cases, intravenous and oral contrast should be used, and in suspected neoplasm, dual-phase scanning is recommended (10).

A. Shirkhoda: Department of Diagnostic Radiology, William Beaumont Hospital, Royal Oak, Michigan 48073.

R.M. Gore: Department of Radiology, Evanston Hospital, Northwestern University Healthcare, Evanston, Illinois 60201.

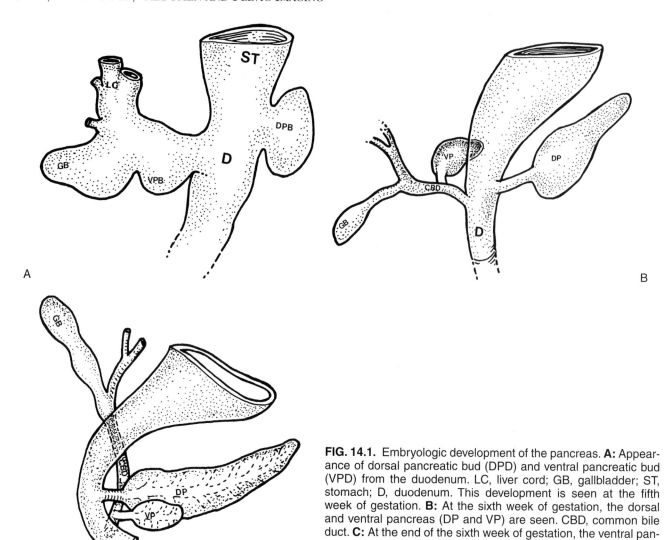

FIG. 14.1. Embryologic development of the pancreas. **A:** Appearance of dorsal pancreatic bud (DPD) and ventral pancreatic bud (VPD) from the duodenum. LC, liver cord; GB, gallbladder; ST, stomach; D, duodenum. This development is seen at the fifth week of gestation. **B:** At the sixth week of gestation, the dorsal and ventral pancreas (DP and VP) are seen. CBD, common bile duct. **C:** At the end of the sixth week of gestation, the ventral pancreas rotates posterior to the duodenum and makes contact with the dorsal pancreas, where they will fuse with each other.

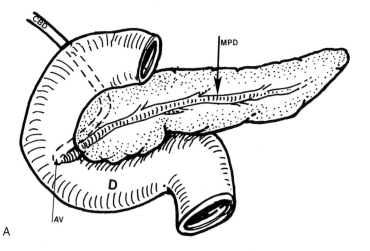

FIG. 14.2. Major types of ductal anatomy. **A:** In the mature pancreas, the distal portion of the dorsal pancreatic duct is connected with the short duct of the ventral pancreas to form the main pancreatic duct (MPD) or the duct of Wirsung, which enters the duodenum (D) at the ampulla of Vater (AV). **B:** The accessory pancreatic duct (APD) or the duct of Santorini may remain patent and empty into the minor papilla (MiP). This duct does communicate with the main pancreatic duct (MPD), which in turn empties into the ampulla of Vater (AV). **C:** If the ductal system fails to fuse, then pancreas divisum will develop, in which the dorsal pancreatic duct (DPD) and ventral pancreatic duct (VPD) are isolated. The ventral duct and common bile duct (CBD) drain into the ampulla of Vater (AV), while the dorsal duct will drain into the minor papilla (MiP). (Modified from reference 5 with permission.)

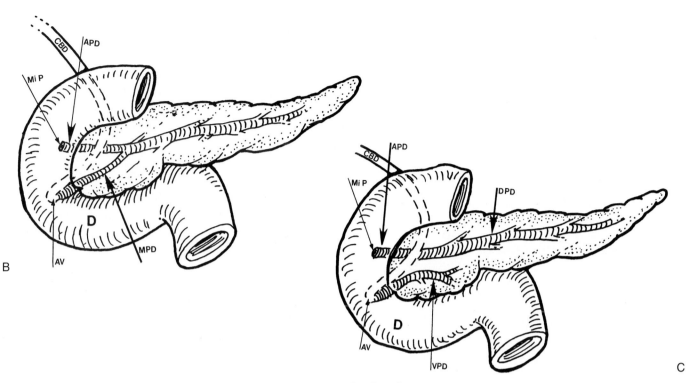

FIG. 14.2. *Continued.*

For MR imaging, breath-hold fat-suppressed sequences are preferred. Also, thin slices should be obtained in a search for a tumor.

ANATOMIC VARIATIONS

Positional Variants

The pancreas is deeply seated in the anterior aspect of the retroperitoneal space behind the posterior parietal peritoneum. It is located in the anterior pararenal space and is normally surrounded by fat. Traditionally, it is divided into five parts: the uncinate process, head, neck, body, and tail. The head, neck, and body are retroperitoneal while the tail extends into the peritoneum ensheathed in the splenorenal ligament. It is connected to the splenic flexure by the splenorenal and phrenicocolic ligaments. The transverse mesocolon attaches to the anterior surface of the head and the inferior aspect of the body and tail of the gland (11). The position and configuration of the pancreas are often variable. For example, the head, which is not fixed in position, almost invariably maintains a constant relationship lateral to the second portion of the duodenum and medial to the superior mesenteric vessels. Occasionally, the pancreas lies entirely to the left of the aorta, where the head and uncinate process maintain their normal relationship, encircling the displaced superior mesenteric vessels, while

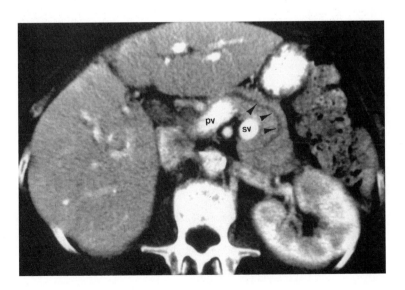

FIG. 14.3. Folding of the pancreatic tail, a positional variant in which the tail of the pancreas circles the splenic vein (SV), where it gets near the superior mesenteric artery, which is seen just medial to the portal vein (PV). The pancreatic duct *(arrowheads)* is identified.

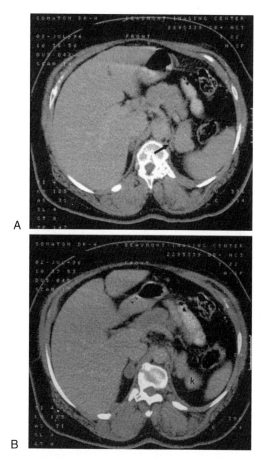

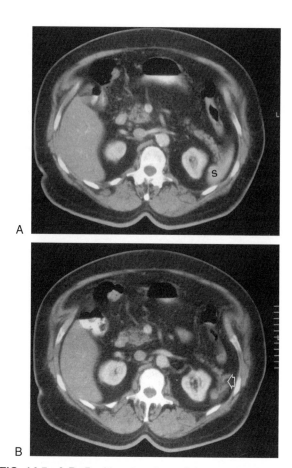

FIG. 14.4. Proximity of the tail and left adrenal, a normal variant. **A:** The pancreatic tail is anterolateral to the left kidney near the left adrenal *(arrow)*. In the lower image **(B)**, there is a right adrenal adenoma. The tail of the pancreas is seen medial to the left kidney (K) and the left crus of the diaphragm.

FIG. 14.5. A,B: Positional variant of the pancreatic tail. The tail of the pancreas is anterolateral to the left kidney *(open arrow)* and inferior to the tip of the spleen (S).

the pancreatic body remains in intimate contact with the splenic vein. This normal variant has been attributed to increased laxity in the retroperitoneal connective tissue that accompanies the aging process (12).

The splenic vein is an important anatomic landmark of the pancreas, outlining the dorsal margin of the body and tail. However, the tail may curve dorsal and medial to the splenic vein (Fig. 14.3), occasionally extending near the left adrenal gland, simulating an adrenal mass (Fig. 14.4). Occasionally, the pancreatic tail may lie anterolateral to the kidney, where it may appear as a pseudomass on images below the level of spleen (Fig. 14.5). When the left kidney is absent, the tail of the pancreas may be displaced into the renal fossa lateral to the spine (Fig. 14.6), where it should not be confused with a mass lesion (13). Although a deep cleft separating the two distinct pancreatic moieties may be identified on CT in pancreatic divisum. Many contour abnormalities may represent a spectrum of fusion anomalies.

Variants of Size and Configuration

The normal anteroposterior diameter of the head of the pancreas is approximately 3 cm, that of the neck and body

is up to 2.5 cm, and that of the tail is about 2 cm (14). Normally, there is gradual tapering from the head to the tail without abrupt alteration in size or contour. However, it is well known that the size and shape of the pancreas are variable, and occasionally, this tapering may not be seen. In these individuals, the body and tail may have almost the same thickness (Fig. 14.7), or occasionally, the tail may actually be thicker than the body of the pancreas (Fig. 14.8).

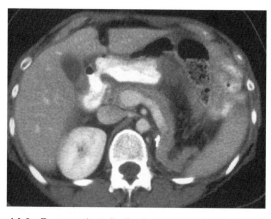

FIG. 14.6. Pancreatic tail displacement after left nephrectomy. The tail of the pancreas is displaced medially and posteriorly. Because of the medial displacement of the spleen, the pancreatic tail has bent.

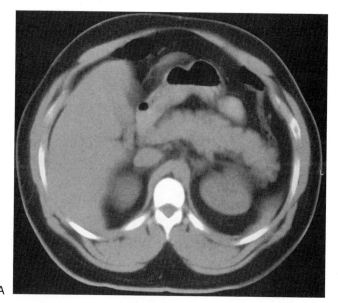

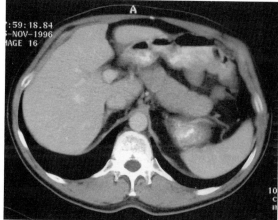

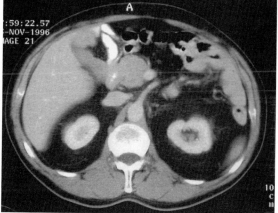

FIG. 14.7. Variants of pancreatic size. **A:** The body and tail of the pancreas have almost similar thickness. This 37-year-old man had no illness related to the pancreas, and the CT remained unchanged in 18 months of follow-up. **B,C:** In this 51-year-old man, the thickness of the body and tail are the same, being about 3.5 cm. The pancreatic head is proportionately prominent and measures about 4 cm in AP diameter.

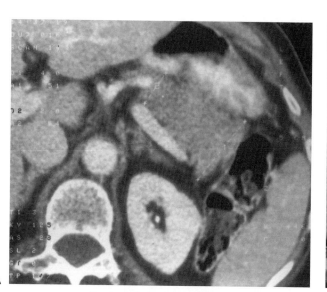

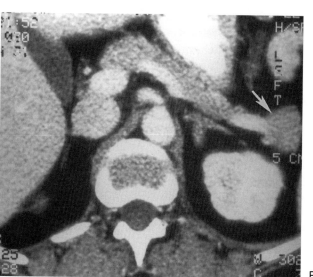

FIG. 14.8. Normal prominence of the pancreatic tail. **A:** The AP diameter of the tail of the pancreas is 4 cm, which is twice as thick as the body, which is only 2 cm. This was an incidental finding and remained unchanged at 2-year follow-up. **B:** The prominence of the tail of the pancreas *(arrow)* was stable in two different CT scans done within an interval of about 20 months. Its enhancement pattern is similar to that of the normal pancreas, and it was considered to be a normal variation.

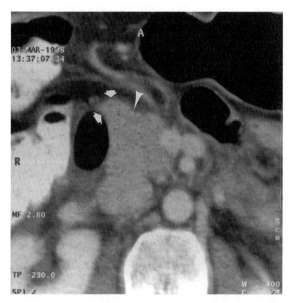

FIG. 14.9. Normal variation of lateral contour of the pancreatic head. Lobulation of the pancreatic head with anterior orientation of the pancreatic lobules *(arrows)*. Note that the lobulation is lateral to the anterior-superior pancreatoduodenal artery *(arrowhead)*.

The size of the pancreas is generally related to age, and there is a gradual decrease in size with advancing age. As a result, overall proportions of the gland (including symmetry, density and contour) are considered more important than absolute measurements in assessing the presence of a subtle mass.

In some individuals, the pancreas can be diffusely prominent in the absence of pathology. The normal lobular architecture, attenuation, tissue texture, and signal intensity of the parenchyma are maintained; there are no alterations in the peripancreatic fat; and the pancreatic duct is not dilated. These features distinguish a normal prominent pancreas from one affected by pancreatitis (15).

The contour abnormalities of the head and neck have been well described in pancreatic divisum (3), but there is actually a spectrum of fusion patterns of the dorsal and ventral anlagen (15,16). This results in discrete lobules of normal tissue in the pancreatic head, which is usually seen lateral to the gastroduodenal or the anterior-superior pancreaticoduodenal artery (Fig. 14.9).

Fatty Infiltration

In cases of complete fatty replacement, the pancreas may not be seen on CT, as it has the same density of retroperitoneal fat (10) (Fig. 14.10). This phenomenon occasionally is seen in a segment of the gland (Fig. 14.11). Sonographically, it results in increased echogenicity of the gland (Fig. 14.12). Fatty infiltration is more frequently seen in elderly and obese patients and is associated with

overall decreased volume of the pancreas (17). When associated with obesity, fatty infiltration is likely reversible. It can also be associated with diabetes mellitus, alcoholism, cystic fibrosis, chronic pancreatitis, chronic steroid ingestion, and the Schwachman syndrome in children. Focal sparing of the normal pancreas from fatty infiltration can give the appearance of a slightly hyperdense mass on CT (Fig. 14.13) that is difficult to distinguish from a tumor (18). This process usually occurs within the head, and endoscopic retrograde cholangiopancreatography (ERCP)

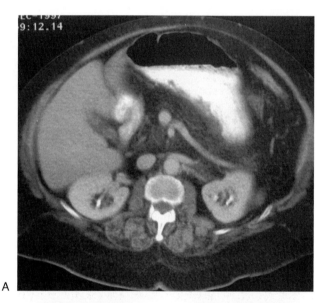

A

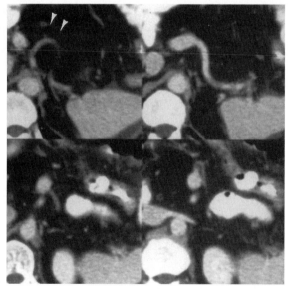

B

FIG. 14.10. Total fatty infiltration of the pancreas. **A:** There is indication of total fatty infiltration of the pancreas. The normal vascular anatomic landmarks of the pancreas are seen on this image. **B:** Four continuous images of the pancreas at 4-mm intervals reveal complete fatty replacement of the head, body, and tail of the pancreas. Note the normal orientation of the splenic vein with the body and tail. The *arrowheads* point to the pancreatic duct.

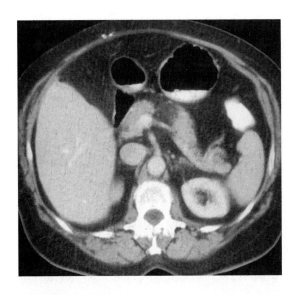

FIG. 14.11. Partial fatty infiltration. There is focal fatty infiltration involving the pancreas near the neck region. This was a 64-year-old woman who had a work-up for diverticulitis.

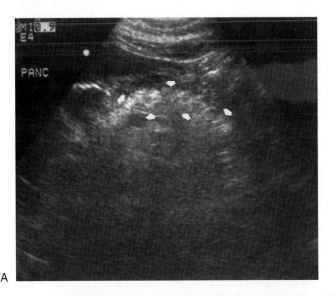

FIG. 14.12. Echogenic pancreas as a result of diffuse fat infiltration. **A:** Axial sonogram reveals significant increased echogenicity of the pancreas *(arrowheads)* in comparison to the normal left lobe of the liver. **B:** Corresponding CT reveals pancreatic fatty infiltration. **C:** An axial sonogram of a normal pancreas from a different patient is shown to demonstrate the relatively higher echogenicity of the pancreas *(open arrows)* compared to the adjacent liver.

A

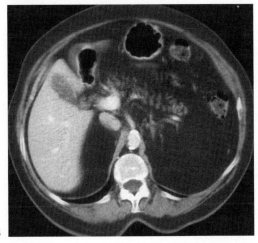

B

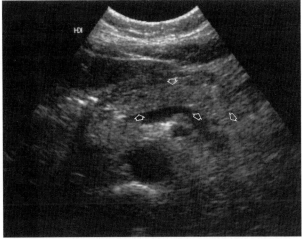

C

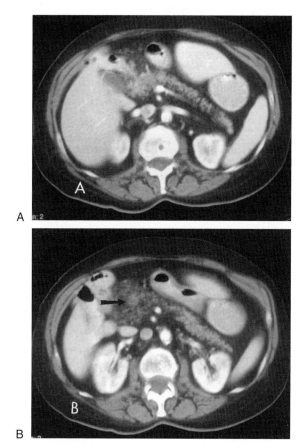

FIG. 14.13. (A) Focal sparing of the normal pancreas. Fatty infiltration is predominantly confined to the head of the pancreas. However, focal sparing of pancreatic tissue in the region of the head *(arrow)* (B) can give the appearance of a small hyperdense lesion.

or MRI may be needed to exclude a neoplasm. Fatty infiltration can also alter the normal configuration of the pancreas (Fig. 14.14).

Fatty Cleft and Pseudofracture

Peripancreatic fat can invaginate into the pancreas and produce an appearance similar to that of a cleft (Fig. 14.15). Such a pattern on CT in a traumatized patient can be confused with a fracture of the pancreas. However, serum pancreatic enzymes are usually normal, and the peripancreatic fat remains clear, in patients with the fatty cleft.

Sonographic Pitfalls

On sonograms, the pancreas is usually isoechoic or slightly hyperechoic with respect to the liver (see Fig. 14.12C). Although the head and body are visualized in the majority of patients, visualization of the tail may require filling the stomach with water to avoid artifacts from the overlying gas. The normal pancreatic duct may be seen in about 80% of normal subjects as a thin hypoechoic line outlined by echogenic walls (Fig. 14.16) and measures up to 2 mm in width (15).

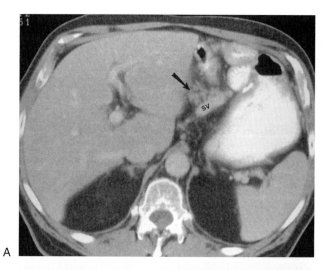

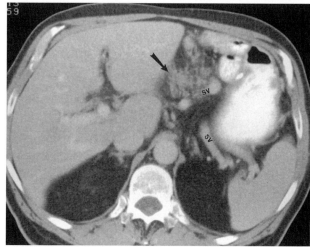

FIG. 14.14. Fatty infiltration and high position of the pancreas. A portion of the body of the pancreas is near the gastrohepatic ligament. Note that the relationship of the splenic vein (SV) and pancreas is maintained. There has not been any prior surgery in this patient.

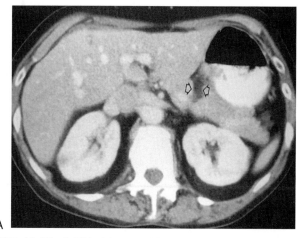

FIG. 14.15. A: This 61-year-old woman had abdominal CT to rule out visceral injury from a car accident. Peripancreatic fat invagination into the pancreas *(open arrows)* represents a pseudofracture. This should not be confused with pancreatic fracture in a traumatized patient.

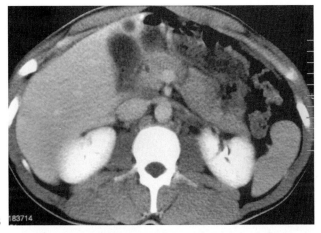

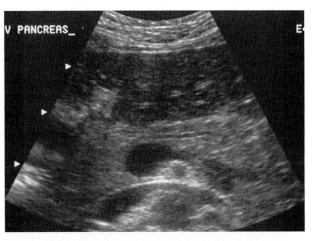

B

FIG. 14.15. *Continued.* **B:** Similar finding in a 38-year-old woman after a fall from a bicycle. In both patients, the serum pancreatic enzymes remained normal. In the second case, a six month follow-up CT showed no change.

FIG. 14.16. Normal pancreatic duct. The normal duct is seen as a thin hypoechoic stripe outlined by echogenic walls.

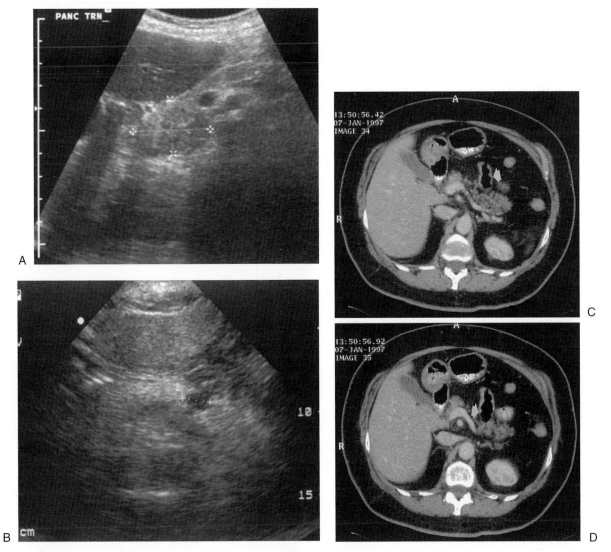

A

B

C

D

FIG. 14.17. A: Pancreatic pseudomass on sonogram. On this axial image, a mass was suspected to originate from the head of the pancreas as outlined by the *cursor.* However, the CT scan (not shown) revealed no mass in the region. It is presumed that this is a duodenum filled with food material. **B:** In this 68-year-old woman, a hypoechoic mass was suspected in the region of the body of the pancreas as outlined by the *cursor.* **C,D:** Two adjacent CT images obtained at 4-mm slice thickness and at 4-mm intervals reveals that there is a loop of bowel adjacent to the body of the pancreas *(arrows).* There was no indication of any pancreatic mass lesion.

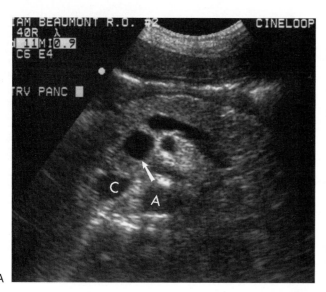 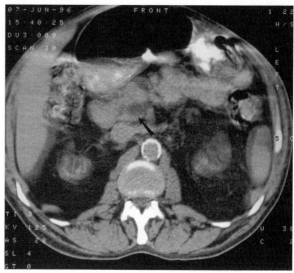

FIG. 14.18. A: Distal CBD mimicking hypoechoic mass. The hypoechoic mass *(arrow)* was thought to be present in the region of the head of the pancreas. Because of overlying gas, communication with the dilated common bowel duct could not be established. A, aorta, C, IVC. **B:** A CT scan was done with a great deal of difficulty because of the patient's inability to hold breath. The dilated common bile duct *(arrow)* is seen.

Adjacent bowel near the head (Fig. 14.17A) or the body of the pancreas (Fig. 14.17B) can mimic a hypoechoic pancreatic mass, and CT may be needed to rule out a tumor (Fig. 14.17C,D). In addition, a dilated distal common bile duct may suggest an anechoic mass in the pancreatic head (Fig. 14.18A). Again, CT may be necessary to avoid this pitfall (Fig. 14.18B).

Other structures that can simulate the pancreas or pancreatic pathology on ultrasound include the posterior part (segment 2) of the lateral segment of the left lobe of the liver, which is less echogenic than the anterior part (segment 3) because of the sound attenuation caused by the perivascular fat. The papillary process of the caudate lobe and an enlarged portocaval lymph node can also be mistaken for the pancreas. A horseshoe kidney (see Fig. 17.1) and retroperitoneal fibrosis, when seen as a midline band, can also simulate a pancreatic mass (17).

Sonographically, there are three normal structures that can potentially simulate a dilated pancreatic duct. First, the fat plane separating the posterior margin of the pancreas from the splenic vein can simulate the duct. Second, the splenic artery or vein can also simulate a dilated duct, particularly when the vessels are tortuous and undergo volume averaging with the pancreas.

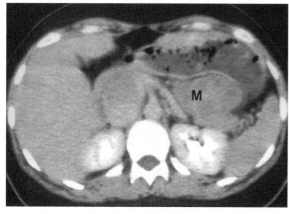 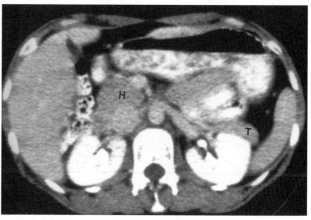

FIG. 14.19. Bowel loops mimicking pancreatic mass. **A:** On this axial image, there appears to be a retrogastric mass (M) with apparent mass effect on the gastric wall. **B:** Repeat CT scan with additional oral contrast proved the nature of the mass to be unopacified bowel loops. The pancreatic head (H) and tail (T) are better seen in this image.

Finally, the collapsed gastric antrum sandwiched between the left lobe of the liver anteriorly and pancreas posteriorly can be mistaken for a dilated pancreatic duct (17).

Computed Tomography Density Pitfalls

On routine abdominal CT, the attenuation value of the pancreas is similar to muscle and fluid-filled bowel. For this reason, oral contrast is important in differentiating a pancreatic mass from unopacified bowel loops

(11) (Figs. 14.19 and 14.20). A calcified and tortuous splenic artery may occasionally mimic pancreatic calcification on routine abdominal CT (Fig. 14.21). However, thin slices will generally reveal the tubular nature of the calcified vessel. In addition, a tortuous enhanced splenic artery should not be mistaken for a small vascular pancreatic tumor (Fig. 14.22). A perivaterian duodenal diverticulum can fill with contrast, simulating a distal common bile duct stone or pancreatic calcification. Debris within a duodenal diverticulum can also simulate a mass or pancreatic abscess.

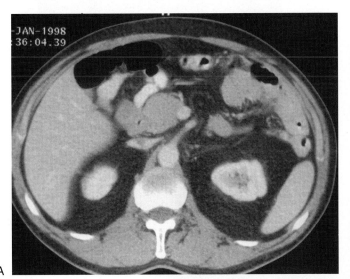

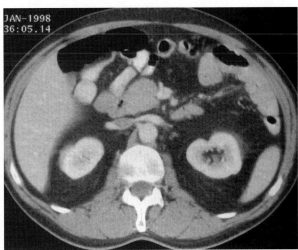

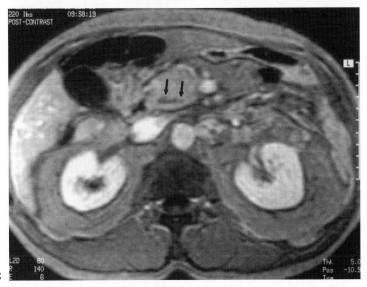

FIG. 14.20. Pancreatic pseudomass. A,B: A CT scan in this 51-year-old man was interpreted as showing a prominent head of the pancreas measuring 4.2 cm in AP diameter. An ERCP was normal. **C:** Post-contrast flash 2-D MR image reveals the proximity of the duodenum with the posterior aspect of the head of the pancreas *(arrows)*. Retrospectively, one can appreciate in **A** the subtle density difference of the duodenum and the head of the pancreas. The duodenum has added approximately 12 mm in thickness to the normal 3-cm pancreatic head.

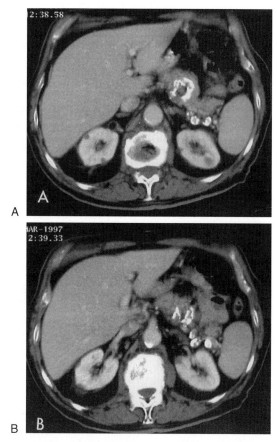

FIG. 14.21. Calcified splenic artery mimicking pancreatic calcification. **A,B:** On these two sequential axial CT images, the tortuous and calcified splenic artery mimics pancreatic calcification. Thin-slice axial images are often capable of illustrating the communication of the calcification and its tubular nature (as seen in A).

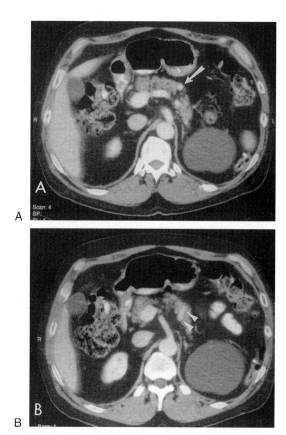

FIG. 14.22. Pancreatic pseudonodule. **A,B:** The tortuous noncalcified and enhanced splenic artery can occasionally mimic a small vascular pancreatic tumor *(arrow)* **(A).** Again, thin slices can establish communication of the enhanced nodule with the splenic artery as seen in **B** *(arrowheads).*

PANCREAS DIVISUM

Pancreas divisum is a common congenital anomaly of pancreatic development in which the dorsal and ventral pancreatic anlagen fail to fuse (see Fig. 14.2C). As a result, there are two separate drainages into the duodenum: the pancreatic head and uncinate process are drained by the duct of Wirsung through the major papilla, while the body and tail are drained by the duct of Santorini through the minor papilla (6). This anomaly is seen in 4% to 11% of autopsy series and 3% to 4% of ERCP examinations (16).

On CT, contour abnormalities of the pancreatic head and neck have been identified in some patients with pancreatic divisum. In 12 patients studied by Zeman et al., five patients had enlargement of the pancreatic head (5). The CT can occasionally suggest the diagnosis of pancreas divisum when two distinct pancreatic moieties or an unfused ductal system is identified on thin collimation scans (5,21) (Fig. 14.23). The two moieties may cause pancreatic head enlargement or may be separated by a fat

cleft (Fig. 14.24). Sometimes fatty replacement of the dorsal pancreas may delineate it from the ventral moiety. This can manifest sonographically as a difference in echo texture between the components of the pancreatic head. The portion formed from the ventral bud may be less echogenic than the dorsal aspect, presumably because of a difference in the relative fat content. This process may be more readily evident in older patients because of increasing fatty deposition with age. It should not be confused with a pathologic condition.

When spared from atrophy and pancreatitis affecting the body and tail, the pancreatic head may suggest a pseudotumor on CT and ultrasound studies. In alcoholics, isolated ventral pancreatitis may occasionally be observed, which suggests a synergism between the effects of alcohol and bile reflux into the ventral pancreas. The dorsal pancreas is spared this reflux because of the pancreas divisum. Although ERCP has been the traditional means for confirming the diagnosis of pancreas divisum (21) (see Fig. 14.23), magnetic resonance cholangiopancreatography (MRCP) has the potential to replace ERCP in this regard (21–24).

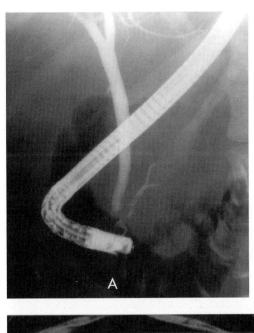

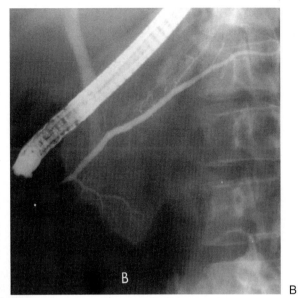

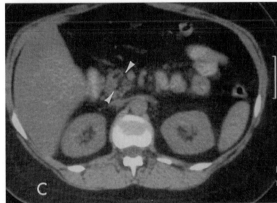

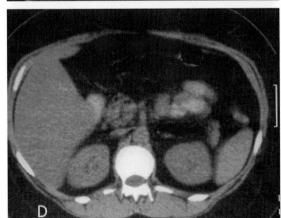

FIG. 14.23. Pancreas divisum: **A:** ERCP in this 54-year-old woman with prior history of pancreatitis reveals opacification of the common bile duct and only small branches of the pancreatic ducts in the region of the head. With probable diagnosis of pancreas divisum and the fact that only the ventral pancreatic duct is opacified, a search for the cannulation of minor papilla was made. **B:** Injection through the minor papilla resulted in opacification of the dorsal pancreatic duct. **C,D:** On the noncontrast CT images, in the region of the head, there appears to be a small fatty cleft *(arrow)* **(C)** presumably separating the ventral from the dorsal pancreatic moiety. **C** and **D** images are 4 mm apart.

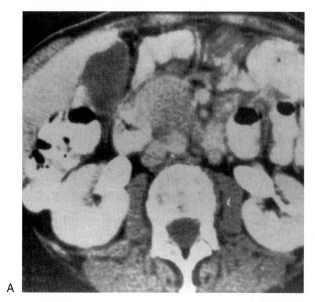
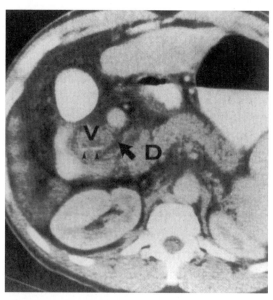

A

B

FIG. 14.24. A: Pancreatic head enlargement secondary to pancreas divisum. Contrast-enhanced CT section at the level of the pancreatic head illustrates that divisum can mimic a focal pancreatic mass. B: Separation of the dorsal and ventral pancreas by a fat cleft. Contrast-enhanced CT section at the level of the pancreatic head reveals an oblique fat cleft *(arrow)* separating the ventral (V) from dorsal (D) pancreas. Note how the two moieties are present at the same craniocaudal level. Residual iodinated contrast material is present in the ventral pancreatic duct *(arrowheads)* after ERCP. (Reproduced with permission from reference 5.)

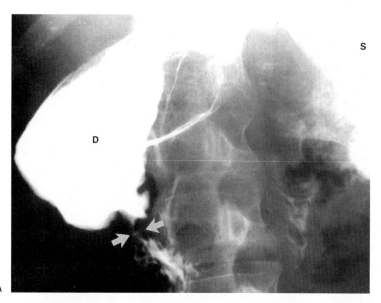

A

FIG. 14.25. Annual pancreas. This 38-year-old man presented with recurrent epigastric fullness for several years. A: Film from an upper gastrointestinal series shows a dilated, fluid-filled stomach (S) and duodenum (D) proximal to narrowing *(arrows)* of the second portion of the duodenum. B: This CT scan confirms the gastric (S) and duodenal dilation. C: This scan shows the obstructing band of pancreatic tissue *(arrows)* that can simulate a tumor. D, fluid-filled duodenum; P, pancreatic head. (From Gore RM, Fernbach SK, Ghahremani GG. Pancreas anomalies and anatomic variants. In: Gore RM, Levine MS, Laufer I, eds. *Textbook of gastrointestinal radiology.* Philadelphia: WB Saunders, 1994;2122–2132, with permission.)

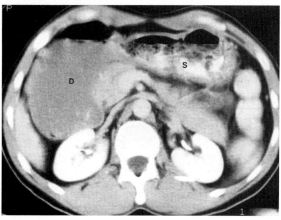

B

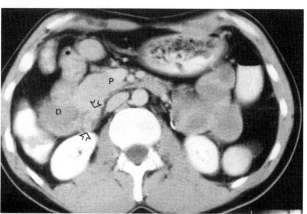

C

ANNULAR AND SEMIANNULAR PANCREAS

In this anomaly, the annulus is often a flat band of pancreatic tissue completely encircling the second portion of the duodenum. In nearly half of the patients, this congenital anomaly may manifest clinically in the neonate, and in the other half, it remains asymptomatic until adulthood (25,26). The findings on computed tomography are often nonspecific and may show enlargement of the pancreatic head that has a central region of low density representing fluid within the narrowed duodenal segment (Fig. 14.25). If oral contrast is used, then the central region will have high attenuation because of the contrast material (27,28). If the duodenum is not sufficiently opacified with fluid or barium, then only pancreatic head enlargement may be seen. Annular pancreas can thus be confused with a neoplasm, particularly in adults with obstructive symptoms.

ECTOPIC PANCREATIC TISSUE

Organs that derive from entoderm, including the pancreas, are potential sites of pancreatic ectopia. Presence of ectopic pancreas in such organs is the result of heteroplastic differentiation of parts of embryonic entoderm that do not normally produce pancreas (7). In about 25%, these nests lie in the gastric antrum, and 28% in proximal portion of the duodenum (Fig. 14.26). Less frequent sites

of involvement include the jejunum, ileum, Meckel's diverticulum, colon, appendix, mesentery, omentum, liver, gallbladder, spleen, bile ducts, esophagus, mediastinal cysts, fallopian tubes, and bronchoesophageal fistula (29–32). When located in the walls of the duodenum and stomach, the lesion is usually composed of normal pancreatic tissue including islet cells and a small duct, whereas the islet cells are usually absent at other sites.

The diagnosis of ectopic and heterotopic pancreas usually established by conventional barium studies (Fig. 14.26). Rarely, CT may show large intramural cystic collections in the stomach and duodenum. Their typical submucosal location gives a classic radiographic appearance of a small collection of barium with a central niche or umbilication. Differential diagnosis includes peptic ulcer disease, gastric polyp, Brunner's gland adenoma, leiomyoma, leiomyosarcoma, lymphoma, and metastasis to the stomach from malignant melanoma or Kaposi's sarcoma (33,34).

PANCREATIC AGENESIS

Total agenesis of the pancreas is incompatible with life. However, several partial variants of pancreatic agenesis have been reported, most commonly agenesis of the dorsal anlage (32,33). The cause is uncertain, but primary

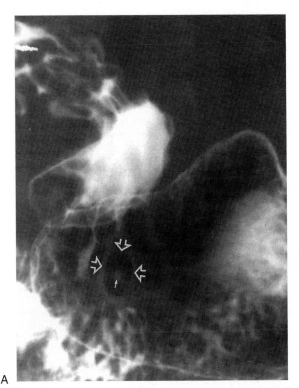
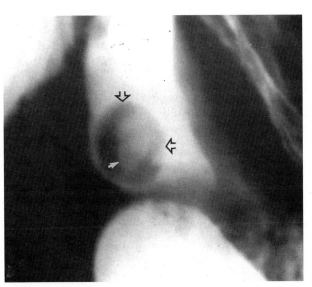

FIG. 14.26. Ectopic pancreas. Ectopic nests of pancreatic tissue are present in the gastric antrum **(A)** and duodenal bulb **(B)**. The mound of pancreatic tissue is signified by the *open arrows*. The *solid arrows* show the draining duct. (From Gore RM, Fernbach SK, Ghahremani GG. Pancreas anomalies and anatomic variants. In: Gore RM, Levine MS, Laufer I, eds. *Textbook of gastrointestinal radiology.* Philadelphia: WB Saunders, 1994;2122–2132, with permission.)

dysgenesis of the dorsal bud and ischemic insult to the developing pancreas are possible explanations (34). Agenesis of the dorsal pancreas may be partial or complete. In complete agenesis, the pancreatic neck, body, and tail and duct of Santorini are absent. When partial agenesis is present, a remnant of the duct of Santorini and the minor papilla are present, and a variable amount of pancreatic body develops. Agenesis of the dorsal pancreas has also been reported as part of the polysplenia syndrome (39).

In the differential diagnosis of pancreatic agenesis on CT, other etiologies such as idiopathic fatty replacement and atrophy after severe pancreatitis should be considered. On CT scan, the absence of pancreatic tissue ventral to the splenic vein with a normal pancreatic head is characteristic of agenesis of the dorsal pancreas (36).

REFERENCES

1. Durie PR. Inherited and congenital disorders of the exocrine pancreas. *Gastroenterologist* 1996;4(3):169–187.
2. Grendell JH, Ermak TH. Anatomy, histology, embryology, and developmental anomalies of the pancreas. In: Feldman M, Scharschmidt BF, Sleisenger MH, eds. *Gastrointestinal and liver disease, 6th ed.* Philadelphia: WB Saunders, 1998:761–770.
3. Rizzo RJ, Szucs RA, Turner MA. Congenital abnormalities of the pancreas and biliary tree in adults. *RadioGraphics* 1995;15:49–67.
4. Torra R, Alos L, Ramos J, Estivill X. Renal-hepatic-pancreatic dysplasia: an autosomal recessive malformation. *J Med Genet* 1996;33(5):409–412.
5. Zeman RK, McVay LV, Silverman PM, et al. Pancreas divisum: thin-section CT. *Radiology* 1988;169:395–398.
6. Gray SW, Skandalakis JE, Skandalakis LJ. Embryology and congenital anomalies of the pancreas. In: Howard JM, Jordan GL, Reber HA, eds. *Surgical diseases of the pancreas.* Philadelphia: Lea & Febiger, 1987:37–45.
7. Schneck CD, Dabezies MA, Friedman AC. The pancreas—embryology, histology, gross anatomy, and normal imaging of the pancreas. In: Friedman AC, Dachman AH, eds. *Radiology of the liver, biliary tract, and pancreas.* St Louis: CV Mosby, 1994:715–742.
8. Kloppel G, Heitz PU. Pancreatic pathology. In: Kloppel G, Heitz PU, eds. *Pancreatic diseases.* Edinburgh: Churchill Livingstone, 1984; 225–232.
9. Kozu T, Suda K, Toki F. Pancreatic development and anatomical variation. *Gastrointest Endosc Clin North Am* 1995;5(1):1–30.
10. Hollett MD, Jorgensen MJ, Jeffrey RB. Quantitative evaluation of pancreatic enhancement during dual-phase helical CT. *Radiology* 1995; 195:359–361.
11. Kasales CJ, Patel S, Hopper KD, et al. Imaging variants of the liver, pancreas, and spleen. *Crit Rev Diagn Imag* 1994;35(6):485–543.
12. Faeber EN, Friedman AC, Dabezies MA. The pancreas: anomalies and congenital disorders. In: Friedman AC, Dachman AH, eds. *Radiology of the liver, biliary tract, and pancreas.* St Louis: CV Mosby, 1994; 743–762.
13. Shirkhoda A. Diagnostic pitfalls in abdominal CT. *RadioGraphics* 1991;11:969–1002.
14. Kreel L, Haertel M, Katy D. Computed tomography of the normal pancreas. *J Comput Assist Tomogr* 1977;1:290.
15. Mirowitz SA. *Pitfalls, variants, and artifacts in body MR imaging.* St Louis: CV Mosby, 1996.
16. Ross BA, Jeffrey RR, Mindelzun RE. Normal variation in the lateral contour of the head and neck of the pancreas mimicking neoplasm: evaluation with dual phase helical CT. *Am J Roentgenol* 1996;166:799–801.
17. Atri M, Finnegan PN. The pancreas. In: Rumack CM, Wilson SR, Charboneau JW, eds. *Diagnostic ultrasound, 2nd ed.* Philadelphia: Lippincott-Raven, 1998;225–278.
18. Jacobs JE, Coleman BG, Arger PH, et al. Pancreatic sparing of focal fatty infiltration. *Radiology* 1994;190:437.
19. Hadidi A. Pancreatic duct diameter: Sonographic measurement in normal subjects. *J Clin Ultrasound* 1983;11:17.
20. Agha FP, Williams KD. Pancreas divisum: incidence, detection, and clinical significance. *Am J Gastroenterol* 1987;82:315–320.
21. Silverman PM, McVay L, Zeman RK, et al. Pancreatic pseudotumor in pancreas divisum: CT characteristics. *J Comput Assist Tomogr* 1989;13:140–141.
22. Laghi A, Catalano C, Panebianco V, Messina A, DiGirolamo M, Pavone P. Pancreas divisum: demonstration of a case with cholangiopancreatography with magnetic resonance. *Radiol Med (Torino)* 1997;93(5):648–650.
23. Bret PM, Reinhold C, Taourel P, Guibaud L, Atri M, Barkun AN. Pancreas divisum: evaluation with MR cholangiopancreatography. *Radiology* 1996;199(1):99–103.
24. Brinberg DE, Carr MF, Premkumar A, et al. Isolated ventral pancreatitis in an alcoholic with pancreas divisum. *Gastrointest Radiol* 1988;13:323–326.
25. Johnston DWB. Annular pancreas: a new classification and clinical observations. *Can J Surg* 1978;21:241–244.
26. Kiernan PD, ReMine SG, Kiernan PC, et al. Annular pancreas. Mayo Clinic experience from 1957 to 1976 with review of the literature. *Arch Surg* 1980;115:46–50.
27. Urayama S, Kozarek R, Ball T, et al. Presentation and treatment of annular pancreas in an adult population. *Am J Gastroenterol* 1995;90(6):995–999.
28. Inamoto K, Ishikawa Y, Itoh N. CT demonstration of annular pancreas: case report. *Gastrointest Radiol* 1983;8:143–145.
29. Ben-Baruch D, Sandbank Y, Wolloch Y. Heterotopic pancreatic tissue in the gallbladder. *Acta Chir Scand* 1986;152:557–558.
30. Carr MJT, Deiranya AK, Judd PA. Mediastinal cyst containing mural pancreatic tissue. *Thorax* 1977;32:512–516.
31. Eklof O. Accessory pancreas in the stomach and duodenum: clinical features, diagnosis, and therapy. *Acta Chir Scand* 1961;121:19–20.
32. Mito T, Nakazawa S, Yoshino J, et al. A case of adult intussusception due to the inverted Meckel's diverticulum with ectopic pancreas which showed characteristic findings of MRI. *Nippon Shokakibyo Gakkai Zasshi* 1998;95(4):326–332.
33. Burke GW, Binder SC, Barron AM, et al. Heterotopic pancreas: gastric outlet obstruction secondary to pancreatitis and pancreatic pseudocyst. *Am J Gastroenterol* 1989;84:52–55.
34. Claudon M, Verain AL, Bigard MA, et al. Cyst formation in gastric heterotopic pancreas: report of two cases. *Radiology* 1988;169:659–660.
35. Schnedl WJ, Reisinger EC, Schreiber F, et al. Complete and partial agenesis of the dorsal pancreas in one family. *Gastrointest Endosc* 1995;42:485–487.
36. Macari M, Giovanniello G, Blair L, Krinsky G. Case report: diagnosis of agenesis of the dorsal pancreas with MR pancreatography. *Am J Roentgenol* 1998;170:144–146.
37. Deignan RW, Nizzero A, Malone DE. Agenesis of the dorsal pancreas: cause of diagnostic error on abdominal sonography. *Clin Radiol* 1996;51:145–146.
38. Gold RP. Agenesis and pseudo-agenesis of the dorsal pancreas. *Abdom Imag* 1993;18:141–144.
39. Sener RN, Alper H. Polysplenia syndrome: a case associated with transhepatic portal vein, short pancreas, and left inferior vena cava with hemiazygos continuation. *Abdom Imag* 1994;19:64–66.

Variants and Pitfalls in Body Imaging,
edited by Ali Shirkhoda.
Lippincott Williams & Wilkins, Philadelphia, © 2000.

CHAPTER 15

The Gastrointestinal Tract: CT

Michael Macari and Emil J. Balthazar

During the last decade, computed tomography (CT) has become either the primary imaging modality or an essential secondary examination used to evaluate patients with a variety of abdominal complaints. When CT is performed, incidental irrelevant findings and normal variants are often encountered. Recognition of these variants and pitfalls is essential to avoid misdiagnosing these conditions as disease. In most instances, if optimal CT techniques are performed, these pitfalls can be avoided. In this chapter, optimal CT techniques, normal CT anatomy, and clues to the appropriate diagnosis of the variants and pitfalls related to the gastrointestinal tract are discussed.

COMPUTED TOMOGRAPHY TECHNIQUES FOR IMAGING THE GASTROINTESTINAL TRACT

Computed tomography of the gastrointestinal tract is performed: (a) to diagnose suspected primary gastrointestinal disease, (b) to assess the nature and extent of involvement in patients with known gastrointestinal disease, and (c) to detect associated complications of primary gastrointestinal disorders (1). In this section, the CT techniques used to achieve optimal evaluation of the gastrointestinal tract are discussed.

Routine CT examinations of the abdomen generally result in inadequate evaluation of the gastrointestinal tract. To obtain a clinically useful CT study of the gastrointestinal tract, several general principles need to be followed, including: (a) optimizing the technical parameters of the CT scanner for the clinical indication of the study, (b) achieving optimal enhancement of the bowel wall and surrounding structures, and (c) achieving adequate visualization and distention of the gastrointestinal lumen.

Optimizing technical parameters for CT evaluation of the gastrointestinal tract is facilitated by the use of helical (spiral) scanning. With helical CT, the entire gastrointestinal tract can be evaluated in two or three breath-holds in most patients. Helical CT, coupled with the use of 1 mg of IV glucagon, can essentially eliminate motion artifacts related to intestinal peristalsis. For most indications, 7-mm collimation, pitch 1 to 1.5, and reconstruction intervals every 6 to 7 mm allow adequate CT evaluation. If there is known or suspected pathology in a certain area of the gastrointestinal tract, narrow collimation (3 to 5 mm) can be used to evaluate that region. If only axial incremental CT scanning is available, the examination is optimized by the liberal use of 5-mm sections over the area of interest. This can be performed during the initial phase of scanning if the site of abnormality is known or during repeated scanning at the end of the initial examination.

The evaluation of the gastrointestinal wall is facilitated by performing CT during the late arterial or early portal phase of IV iodinated contrast enhancement. This can be easily achieved with helical CT scanning. To obtain adequate visualization of a gastrointestinal lesion, iodinated contrast material may be injected in a single phase via an 18- to 20-gauge IV catheter inserted into an arm vein and connected via tubing to an automatic power injector. A total of 150 ml of 60% diatrizoate is injected at a steady rate of 2 to 2.5 ml/sec. Scanning is initiated 60 seconds after the beginning of contrast injection. A dual-phase technique may be used in a helical CT by scanning during the arterial and venous circulation of contrast material. If helical CT is not available, adequate enhancement is obtained by injecting 50 ml of 60% diatrizoate at a rate of 1.5 ml/sec followed by 100 ml at a rate of 0.8 ml/sec. When the location of the lesion is known, the rate of contrast administration and timing of scanning are appropriately tailored. The presence, degree, and pattern of enhancement of the bowel wall and intestinal lesion are some of the most important parameters used in the differential diagnosis of gastrointestinal disorders (1).

M. Macari and E. J. Balthazar: Department of Radiology, Abdominal Imaging, New York University, Tisch–Bellevue Medical Center, New York, New York 10016.

Visualization of the intestinal lumen, its mucosal surface, and the true thickness of the intestinal wall are essential for evaluating diseases related to the gastrointestinal tract. This requires that the intestinal tract be cleaned and its lumen well distended with contrast material. Patients should routinely fast before elective CT examinations, and adequate preparation of the colon, if not contraindicated, should be carried out when colonic pathology is suspected or known to be present.

Although endoscopy and barium esophagram remain the primary modalities used to evaluate the esophagus, these techniques allow accurate evaluation mainly of the mucosa. Evaluation of the wall of the esophagus and periesophageal tissues is facilitated by the use of CT (2). In cases of suspected esophageal disease, the use of an esophageal paste immediately before scanning aids in optimal evaluation (Esopho-CAT; E-Z-Em, Westbury, NY). A barium paste mixture developed specifically for CT of the esophagus has demonstrated consistent ability to opacify the esophageal lumen and allows a better assessment of wall thickness (3).

Distention of the stomach is essential for evaluating both primary gastric pathology and pathology related to the pancreas and perigastric structures. Positive (dilute barium or iodine) or negative (gas or water) contrast may be used for gastric distension. We have been routinely using EZ gas (E-Z-Em, Westbury, NY) because gastric distension can be achieved easily and rapidly, and it is well tolerated by patients. Recently the use of water (two cups given right before CT scanning with 1 mg of IV

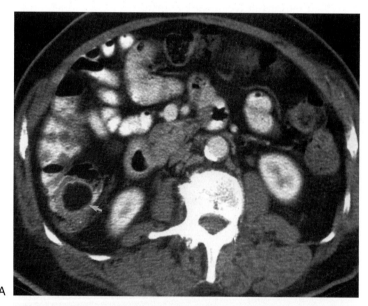

A

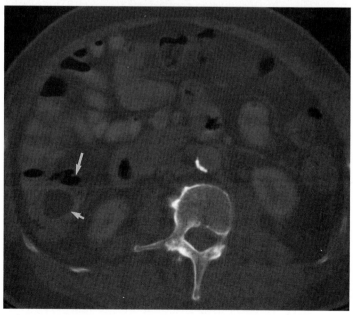

B

FIG. 15.1. Colonic lipoma in a patient with intermittent abdominal pain. **A:** Axial CT of the abdomen using standard abdominal CT settings (window 440, level 15). In the ascending colon, lipoma can be mistaken for intraluminal air *(arrow).* **B:** Same axial CT section using wider window settings (window 1,400, level −250). Colonic lipoma *(short arrow)* is now easily recognizable adjacent to gas *(long arrow)* in the colon.

glucagon) has gained acceptance in our practice as a negative oral contrast agent. This technique has been demonstrated to be well tolerated and efficacious for evaluating the stomach and proximal bowel (4). It can achieve accurate evaluation of the wall of the stomach and duodenum in approximately 90% of patients, and adequate distention of the stomach and duodenum is obtained in 80% of these patients (4). Whether gas or water is used, the key to avoiding false-positive and false-negative diagnosis is to adequately distend the stomach (5).

Evaluation of the duodenum is helped by obtaining adequate luminal distention with oral contrast. As with the stomach, either positive or negative contrast may be used. A recent evaluation of water as an oral contrast agent demonstrated it to be very effective in evaluating the wall of the duodenum (4).

Optimal visualization of the small intestine requires adequate opacification and distention of its lumen. Distention is difficult to achieve, but luminal opacification is obtained by the administration of positive contrast material. Oral administration of 800 cc of barium sulfate suspension 2.1% (Readi-CAT 2; E-Z-EM, Westbury, NY) or dilute (2%) water-soluble contrast ingested in small increments beginning approximately 1 hour before scanning is usually adequate to opacify the small bowel (6). In cases of suspected lower abdominal or pelvic pathology, more time may be required to ensure adequate opacification of the terminal ileum and cecum. For suspected distal ileal, appendiceal, or cecal pathology, obtaining a single CT slice at the beginning of the examination at the level of cecum to determine if oral contrast is present will avoid repeated CT scanning. Alternatively, for cases of suspected appendicitis, positive contrast material may be administered per rectum (7).

When CT is performed to evaluate the colon, meticulous cleansing and preparation are essential. Preparation of the colon similar to that obtained for a barium enema examination (24-hour Fleet prep) is usually sufficient for CT scanning of the colon. As with all segments of the gastrointestinal tract, differentiation of collapsed or contaminated colonic loops from pathologic processes may be difficult and confusing unless the colonic lumen is seen well. Visualization of the colonic lumen can be achieved by the oral administration of diluted (2%) Gastrografin 10 to 12 hours before the CT examination is performed. To secure adequate colonic distention, however, insufflation of rectal air or a dilute contrast enema is distinctly superior. We prefer the use of air insufflation because it can be rapidly and easily performed, it is well tolerated by patients and allows exquisite visualization of the colonic lumen and wall. Routine use of rectal air (15 pumps through a red rubber catheter) and 1 mg glucagon IV in evaluating cases of suspected colonic pathology is preferred by us and others. In addition, routine use of rectal air when evaluating patients with gynecologic or colorectal malignancies will aid in better defining pelvic pathology and in detecting tumor involvement of the rectosigmoid wall.

Finally when reading CT scans of the abdomen, appropriate window and level settings are essential to avoid missing pathology. Standard settings for evaluating the abdomen are 400 HU window and 10 to 40 HU level. However, subtle pathology may be overlooked when these window and level settings are used (Figs. 15.1 and 15.2). In cases of suspected intraperitoneal air or subtle

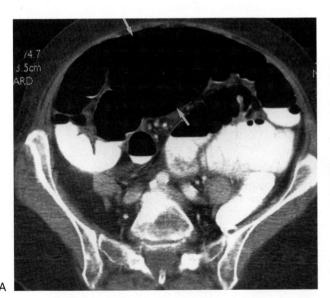
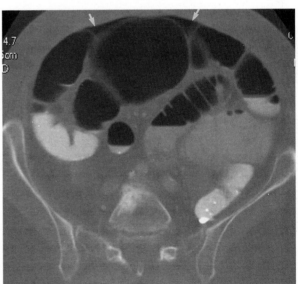

A   B

FIG. 15.2. Perforated colonic carcinoma with subtle extraluminal gas. **A:** Axial CT of the abdomen using standard abdominal CT settings. Distended loops of bowel *(arrows)* are identified, but intraperitoneal free air is not visualized. **B:** Axial CT with wider window settings (window 1,400, level -250). The extraluminal gas is now easily identified *(arrow).* The use of wider window settings enhances visualization of small amounts of intraperitoneal free air.

changes in the omental or mesenteric fat, wider window and lower level settings (1,000 HU window and -100 HU level) should be surveyed for optimal evaluation. This can be done by monitoring CT images at the CT console. A quick interaction with the data set, using several window and level settings at the CT console before standard photography is performed, will increase the accuracy of detection and evaluation of a gastrointestinal lesion. In cases of suspected trauma or bony metastases, skeletal evaluation is facilitated by interaction with data obtained using bone windows at the CT console. If the case is interpreted via a PACS (Picture-Archiving and Communication Systems) monitor, then several appropriate preset or manual windows should be applied before a final report is rendered.

ESOPHAGUS

Normal Anatomy and Anatomic Variants

There is variation in the apparent thickness of the wall of the normal esophagus at CT (2,3,8). This is primarily related to the degree of distention during the CT examination. Because the lumen of the esophagus is often collapsed, the thickness of the wall may be difficult to determine. The true thickness of the esophageal wall can be appreciated when a small amount of air is present in the lumen. When the esophagus is distended, the normal thickness of the esophageal wall is 1 to 2 mm (Fig. 15.3).

The esophagus is located in the posterior mediastinum in the midline anterior to the dorsal spine. In the upper and midthorax it is positioned posterior to the trachea

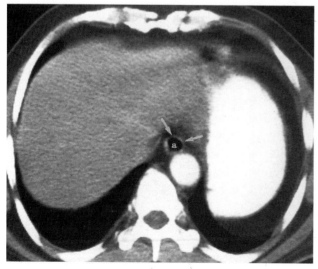

FIG. 15.3. Normal thickness of the esophageal wall. Axial CT at the level of the distal esophagus demonstrates the esophageal wall as a thin structure, measuring 1 to 2 mm *(arrows).* A small amount of air (a) is present in the lumen of the esophagus. This is a normal finding.

and heart, adjacent to and to the right of the descending aorta. In the lower thorax, the esophagus follows the aorta and enters the esophageal hiatus located anterior to and to the right of the aorta. Aneurysms of the aorta and cardiac enlargement may displace the esophagus from its normal position. When collapsed, the esophagus may be difficult to identify, particularly in patients with little mediastinal fat.

Aberrant Right Subclavian Artery

Between the esophagus and the spine, a small amount of adipose tissue is often identified, but soft tissue masses should not be present. An anatomic variant occasionally seen posterior to the upper esophagus is the aberrant right subclavian artery (Fig. 15.4). This represents the most common anomaly of the aortic arch and great vessels and occurs in approximately one in 200 individuals (9–11). The artery originates as the last branch of the aortic arch and passes obliquely to the right, posterior to the esophagus. The aberrant right subclavian artery forms a vascular ring around the esophagus, but it is seldom clinically significant. On contrast-enhanced CT, the aberrant subclavian artery is seen as a tubular enhancing structure crossing behind the esophagus. On an unenhanced CT, it should not be confused with a soft tissue mass in the posterior mediastinum.

Diagnostic Pitfalls

The indications for esophageal CT include staging of esophageal carcinoma, evaluation of primary diseases involving the esophageal wall such as duplication cysts and stromal tumors, and detection of mediastinal conditions that secondarily affect the esophagus (2,3,8). The following are some common pitfalls that should be avoided.

Esophageal Air

The presence of air in the esophageal lumen is a normal finding. It is frequently identified, and it is related to swallowed air or regurgitation of gas from the stomach (see Fig. 15.3). Small amounts of intraluminal gas should be expected to be present, and it helps in identifying the esophagus and demonstrating the true thickness of the wall of the esophagus. When the esophagus is distended and air/fluid levels are present within it, an obstructing lesion such as carcinoma or achalasia should be considered and ruled out (Fig. 15.5) (2).

Esophageal Thickening

Mild circumferential thickening of the esophageal wall is a normal finding without significance and is frequently related to incomplete distention. However, true esophageal wall thickening may be diagnosed when the

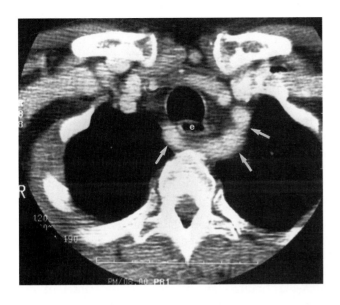

FIG. 15.4. Aberrant right subclavian artery. Axial CT in the upper thorax demonstrates the enhancing aberrant right subclavian artery *(arrows)* posterior to the esophagus (e). Normally only mediastinal fat is present posterior to the esophagus.

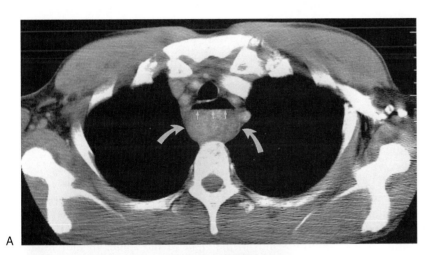

A

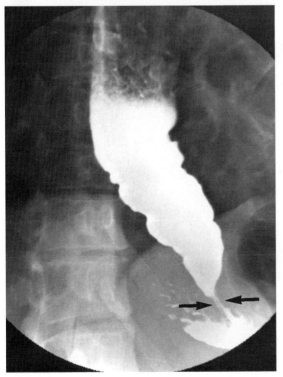

B

FIG. 15.5. Achalasia presenting with distended esophagus containing air and residual food. **A:** On the axial CT in the upper thorax, a markedly dilated esophagus is identified in the mediastinum *(curved arrows)*. Note air–fluid level *(small arrows)*. An obstructing lesion should be suspected. **B:** Conventional esophagram. Classic appearance of achalasia with distention, retained secretions, and distal beaking *(arrow)*.

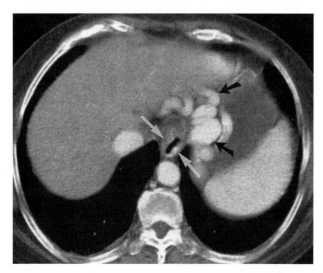

FIG. 15.6. Circumferential thickening of the distal esophageal wall caused by sclerotherapy treatment of varices. Axial CT at the level of the distal esophagus. Thickened appearance of the wall of the esophagus is consistent with endoscopic sclerotherapy treatment for varices *(white arrows)*. Extensive gastroesophageal and mediastinal varices are still present *(black arrows)*.

lumen is distended with gas and is often related to a neoplasm or inflammation. In addition, it could be related to endoscopic sclerotherapy, which has become a widely practiced form of treatment for bleeding esophageal varices (12). Sclerotherapy has been reported to produce a homogeneous circumferential thickening or a laminated appearance of the distal esophageal wall (Fig. 15.6) (12,13). This laminated

appearance, consisting of concentric layers of high and low attenuation, may be seen when CT is performed after sclerotherapy (12). The inner low-attenuation layer probably represents edema and or necrosis. It appears to represent an acute reaction to the injection of a sclerosing agent because it is not seen in patients who had sclerotherapy treatment in the past (12).

Hiatal Hernia

Apparent thickening of the distal esophagus is often caused by the presence of a sliding hiatal hernia (2). This should not be confused with esophageal neoplasm. At CT, a sliding hiatal hernia can be recognized when the following findings are present: (a) separation of the diaphragmatic crura can be seen in most patients with sliding hiatal hernia; (b) identification of rugal folds within the thickened area of apparent distal esophagus; and (c) continuity with the infradiaphragmatic cardia of the stomach on sequential axial images (Fig. 15.7). If the etiology of esophageal thickening is still unclear, repeat CT with effervescent granules and prone positioning may aid in differentiating collapsed hiatal hernia from neoplasm.

STOMACH

Normal Anatomy and Anatomic Variants

The stomach is located in the upper abdomen with the fundus below the left diaphragm and the body extending inferiorly and to the right of the spine. In individuals

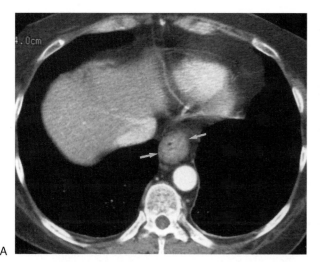
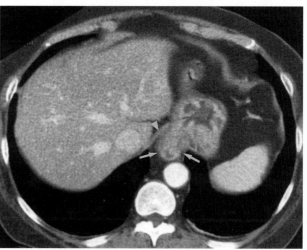

A   B

FIG. 15.7. Hiatal hernia mimicking distal esophageal neoplasm. **A:** Axial CT at the level of the distal esophagus. Diffuse apparent thickening of the region of the distal esophagus is present *(arrows)*. A small amount of oral contrast is trapped within folds. **B:** Axial CT image 2 cm caudal to **A**. Hiatal hernia *(arrows)* is demonstrated in continuity with the more proximal portion depicted in **A** *(arrows)*. Also note separation of the right diaphragmatic crus *(arrowhead)*. If etiology of distal esophageal thickening is in doubt, an oral effervescent agent and scanning with the patient prone may be helpful.

who have a high transverse stomach, the body and fundus are visualized at the same level with the fundus located posteriorly and the body anteriorly. The pyloric channel is located posterior to the distal antrum, connecting with the triangular-shaped duodenal bulb (Fig. 15.8).

The thickness of the gastric wall on a CT examination varies from 1 to 3 mm when well distended but may be up to 2 cm when collapsed (14). If the stomach is not adequately distended, it may appear thickened and thus may simulate inflammatory or neoplastic processes that cause gastric wall thickening (Fig. 15.8). If the wall thickening is concentric and symmetric, and if it involves mainly the proximal stomach, the process is usually benign. Normal rugal folds situated mainly in the gastric fundus extend evenly along the greater curvature of the stomach toward the gastric antrum. On CT these rugal folds tend to thicken preferentially in the greater curvature of the stomach. They can often be identified on CT as traversing the entire width of an apparently thickened stomach.

The appearance is often seen as a normal variant and is related to either rugal hypertrophy or frequently to incomplete gastric distention.

If the etiology of the gastric wall thickening is in doubt, repeat CT after the stomach is distended with water or effervescent granules or the patient is repositioned in a prone or lateral decubitus position is helpful in ruling out gastric pathology (Fig. 15.9) (5). If thickened rugal folds are detected as a focal abnormality in a well-distended stomach, a pathologic condition related to gastritis or possibly neoplasm should be ruled out (Fig. 15.10). In these cases, correlation with upper gastrointestinal series or endoscopy will be required for further evaluation.

Diagnostic Pitfalls

The following examples are some of the more common pitfalls that should be avoided in evaluating CT examinations of the stomach.

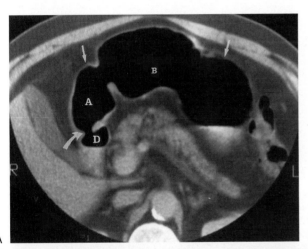

A

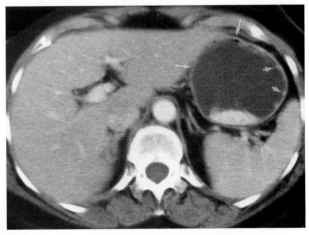

B

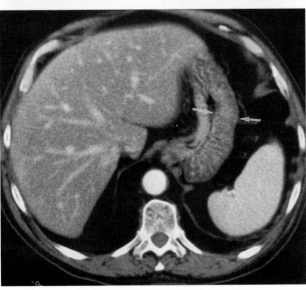

C

FIG. 15.8. Normal appearance of the stomach at CT. A: Axial view of air-distended distal stomach. The wall of the stomach is barely perceptible, measuring between 1 and 2 mm *(arrows)*. Note duodenal bulb (D), gastric antrum (A), gastric body (B), and pylorus *(curved arrow)*. B: Water-filled distended proximal stomach with residual barium. The gastric wall is uniformly thin, measuring between 1 and 2 mm *(arrows)*. Note normal effaced rugal folds *(small arrows)*. C: Collapsed stomach. In this case, the empty stomach is completely collapsed, and its wall measures more than 2 cm in thickness *(arrows)*. However, the normal-appearing rugal folds traversing the wall of the stomach, predominantly along the greater curvature, allow a confident diagnosis of collapsed stomach to be made and a pathologic condition ruled out.

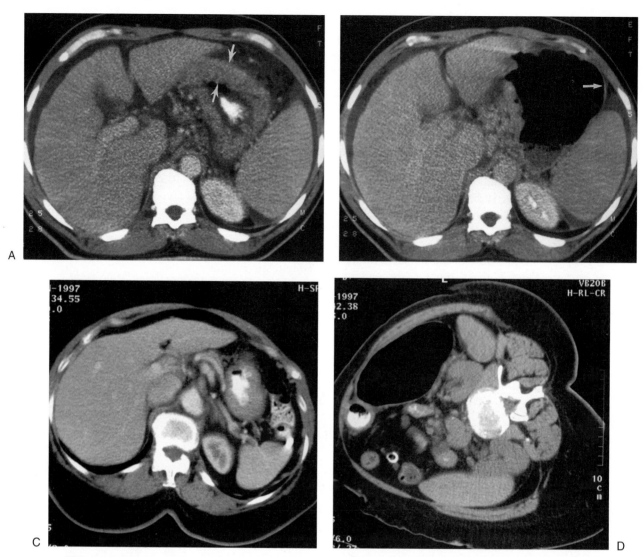

FIG. 15.9. Incomplete gastric distention mimicking neoplasm. **A,B:** Axial CT at the level of the stomach **(A)**. The stomach demonstrates circumferential and symmetric wall thickening *(arrows)*. Axial CT after the administration of effervescent granules **(B).** The stomach is now well distended, and the normally thin wall is barely perceptible *(arrow)*. This case illustrates the importance of distending the stomach for adequate evaluation. (Reproduced with permission from reference 14.) **C,D:** Axial CT of the stomach in a different patient **(C)**. Again, circumferential thickening of the stomach is present. Same patient after effervescent granules and decubitus positioning **(D).** The thin gastric wall is now clearly identified after these maneuvers. Occasionally prone or decubitus imaging will help distend a hollow viscus, thus eliminating an erroneous diagnosis of pathologic bowel thickening. (Figures courtesy of Ali Shirkhoda, M.D.)

Gastric Pseudotumor

Axial CT imaging of the region of the cardia and gastroesophageal (GE) junction often demonstrates a transitional segment of wall thickening that can be mistaken for a soft tissue tumor (Fig. 15.11). This finding is present at the GE junction in up to one-third of patients on CT imaging and is seen at the level of the fissure for the ligamentum venosum (14). The finding on axial CT scanning is related to incomplete distention as well as to the oblique course of the GE junction entering the gastric cardia (see Fig. 15.11) (14). Visual-

ization of a focal area of wall thickening in a well-distended stomach that is not located at the level of the GE junction should be considered abnormal until proven otherwise.

Gastric Fundus and Gastric Diverticula

The gastric fundus is the most dependent portion of the stomach in the supine position. On CT, it extends posteriorly to the level of the left adrenal gland and top of the left kidney. The presence of intraluminal air and or con-

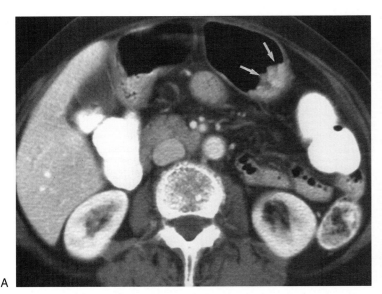
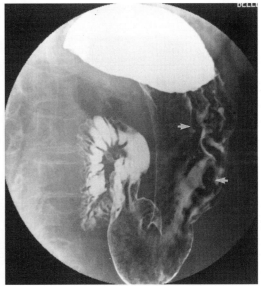

FIG. 15.10. Hypertrophic gastritis mimicking neoplasm. A: Axial CT at the level of the gastric body. Focal thickening along the greater curvature is suspicious for gastric neoplasm (arrows). B: Upper GI series. Thickened folds along the greater curvature (small arrows) are identified. Biopsy confirmed hypertrophic gastritis.

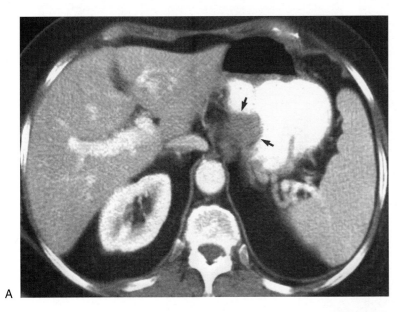

FIG. 15.11. Gastric pseudotumor. A: Axial CT scan at the level of the gastroesophageal (GE) junction. Focal thickening (arrows) is present at the level of the GE junction representing pseudotumor. B: Schematic diagram of pseudotumor. This finding is often observed at the level of the fissure for the ligamentum venosum and is due to oblique course of gastroesophageal junction, incomplete distention, and axial scanning. (Reproduced with permission from reference 14). C: Occasionally, the gastric pseudotumor is present even if the stomach is well distended. In this case, an infiltrative process was thought to be present in the posterior wall of the stomach. The patient had an endoscopy and a thick mucous material was seen covering the normal dependent gastric wall.

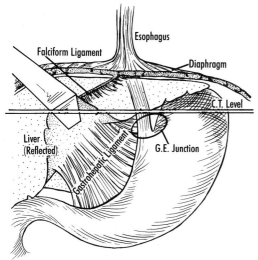
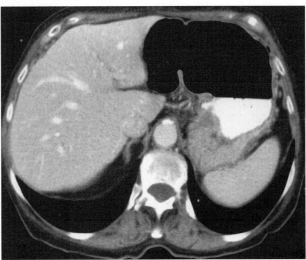

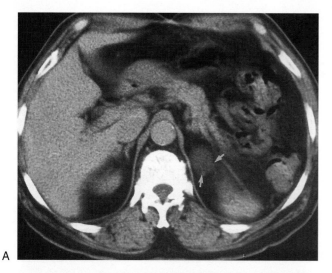

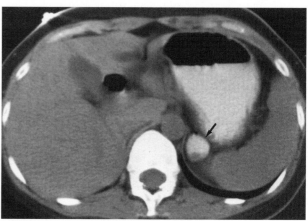

FIG. 15.12. Gastric diverticulum mimicking adrenal neoplasm. **A:** Axial CT demonstrates low-left retroperitoneum *(arrow).* It is in the region of the adrenal gland. **B:** Axial CT slightly cephalad to **A** in the same patient. The low density mass *(arrows)* is again noted posterior to the pancreas (p). Small gas bubble *(curved arrow)* and continuity with the body of the stomach help identify this structure as a gastric diverticulum. **C:** Axial CT in a different patient. In this patient the gastric diverticulum is filled with positive contrast material *(arrow).* These diverticula should not be confused with adrenal masses.

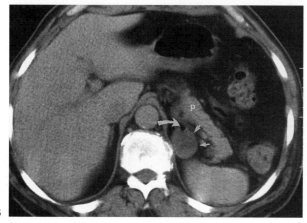

trast material in the stomach facilitates its recognition on CT examinations.

Most gastric diverticula arise from the gastric fundus posterior to the esophagogastric junction. There is still controversy regarding whether they are congenital or acquired in origin (15). During embryologic development, the diverticulum may be entrapped and located in the retroperitoneum (15). Because of its posterior location, diverticula are often situated adjacent to or overlapping the left adrenal gland. When filled with fluid, they may simulate an adrenal mass on CT study (Fig. 15.12A). Careful evaluation of CT images performed with narrow collimation will usually demonstrate a separate adrenal gland. Furthermore, the true nature of a gastric diverticulum is often apparent by the visualization of air or oral contrast within the diverticulum (Fig. 15.12B,C).

DUODENUM AND SMALL BOWEL

Normal Anatomy and Anatomic Variants

Except for the duodenal bulb and a short postbulbar segment, the duodenum is located in the retroperitoneum.

The third portion of the duodenum is positioned behind the superior mesenteric artery (SMA) and superior mesenteric vein (SMV) and anterior to the aorta and inferior vena cava (IVC) (Fig. 15.13). In the absence of previous surgery, if this portion of the duodenum is missing, the presence of small bowel malrotation should be strongly considered. The remainder of the small bowel (jejunum and ileum) is located within the peritoneal cavity.

When the small bowel lumen is well opacified with water, the normal valvulae conniventes are often identified (Fig. 15.14). On CT scans, when the small bowel is filled with positive contrast material, its wall is barely perceptible, measuring not more than 1 to 2 mm (16). Thickness of the wall greater than 3 mm in a distended loop of small bowel should be considered suspicious (17). With inadequate distention, however, the normal intestinal wall may appear circumferentially thickened (Figs. 15.15 and 15.16) and mimic intrinsic intestinal pathology.

If the small bowel wall appears thickened to more than 3 mm in maximum width despite adequate distention, a neoplastic or inflammatory condition should be suspected. Some secondary findings can help in differentiating normal collapsed small bowel loops from pathologic

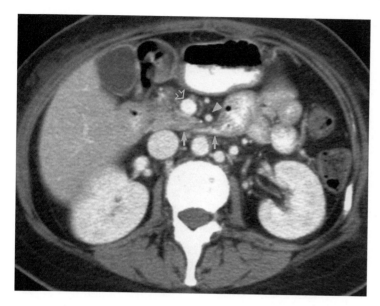

FIG. 15.13. Normal anatomy of a transverse portion of the duodenum. Axial CT at the level of the superior mesenteric artery and vein (SMA/SMV). The transverse duodenum *(arrows)* is identified posterior to the SMA and SMV and anterior to the aorta and inferior vena cava. Normally the SMA *(arrowhead)* is posterior, to the left, and slightly smaller in diameter than the SMV *(open arrow)*.

conditions; they include visualization of peri-intestinal fat stranding, mesenteric adenopathy, extraluminal air or fluid collections, and a "target" or "halo" configuration to the small bowel wall (17). The multilayered target appearance (two or three concentric circumferential rings of varying attenuation) is not a specific finding but, when visualized, implies the presence of an abnormal intestinal wall and generally excludes malignancy (17). The "target" configuration is explained by the enhancing mucosa and muscularis during the IV contrast bolus study with the lower intermediate circumferential layer of density representing the edematous submucosa (17). On contrast-enhanced CT scans, the target appearance is seen in the following conditions: Crohn's disease, ulcerative colitis, infectious enteritis, ischemic enteritis, radiation enteritis, bowel edema, and fat deposition associated with burned-out inflammatory conditions.

A common problem when evaluating CT scans of the abdomen and pelvis is differentiating partially filled and collapsed loops of small bowel from pathologically thickened loops and soft tissue masses in the peritoneal cavity (14). If adequate opacification of the small intestine with positive contrast is not achieved, these loops of small bowel may be mistaken for pathologic processes such as mesenteric and peritoneal tumor deposits. In these cases, the collapsed loops of bowel can often be followed sequentially on serial CT scans. When this is possible, the collapsed small bowel loops can be confidently differentiated from peritoneal tumor. Whenever possible, CT scans should be prospectively monitored, and additional oral contrast should be given with delayed imaging to help differentiate unopacified small bowel from tumors (Fig. 15.17). If the small bowel is fluid filled and contains gas, it may mimic an abscess. Differentiating abscesses

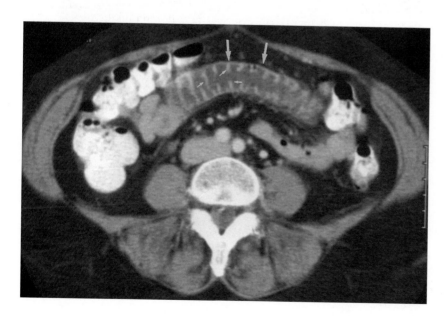

FIG. 15.14. Normal fluid-filled loop of small bowel. Axial CT of the lower abdomen. Fluid-filled and distended loop of small bowel demonstrates thin jejunal wall *(arrows)* and multiple thin valvulae conniventes *(small arrows)* within the loop of small bowel. The normal small bowel wall and the folds measure 1 to 2 mm.

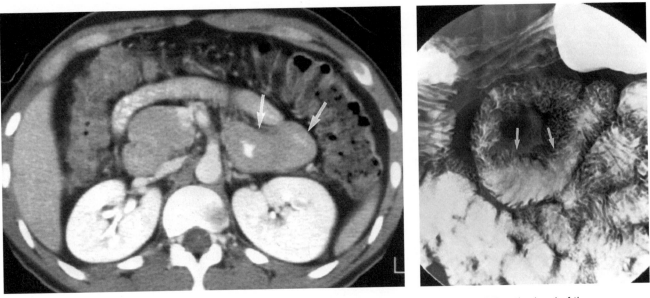

FIG. 15.15. Unopacified and nondistended small bowel mimicking tumor. **A:** Axial CT at the level of the SMA. Several loops of proximal jejunum are identified and appear markedly thickened. They are suspicious for neoplasm *(arrows)*. **B:** Spot film from small bowel series in the same patient. Proximal small bowel *(arrows)* is normal without evidence for neoplasm or thickened folds. This case demonstrates the pitfalls of fluid-filled small bowel mimicking neoplasm.

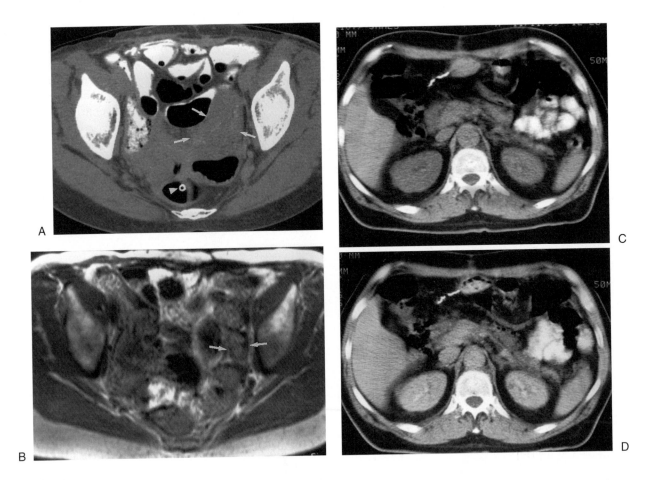

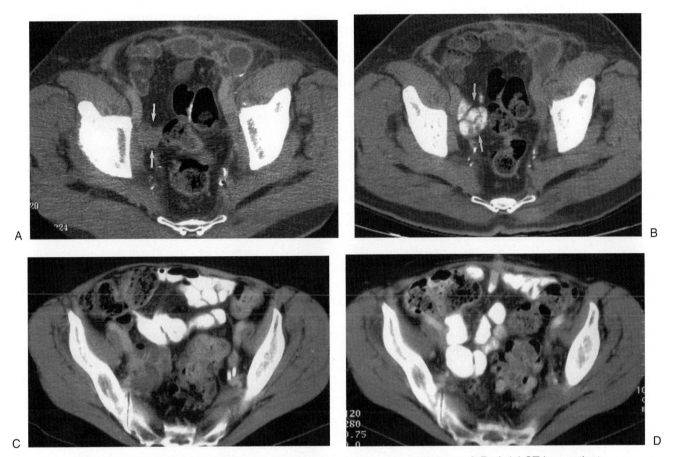

FIG. 15.17. Unopacified small bowel mimicking recurrent tumor or abscess. **A,B:** Axial CT in a patient who has undergone cystectomy for bladder cancer. **A:** Irregular soft tissue mass near the right obturator internus muscle is suspicious for recurrent neoplasm *(arrows)*. **B:** A 30-minute delayed CT scan in the same patient. The soft tissue mass is now opacified with positive oral contrast material *(arrows)*, confirming previous finding as unopacified small bowel. This case demonstrates the importance of delayed CT, sometimes with additional positive oral contrast to help differentiate small bowel from neoplasm. **C,D:** In a different patient suspected for pelvic inflammatory disease, CT shows an abnormal collection **(C)** in the right side of the pelvis that, on delayed scan **(D)**, proved to be unopacified bowel loops. **(C** and **D** courtesy of Ali Shirkhoda, M.D.)

FIG. 15.16. Unopacified and nondistended small bowel mimicking tumor. **A,B:** Axial CT of the pelvis in a patient who has undergone hysterectomy for cervical cancer **(A)**. Apparent soft tissue mass in the left pelvis is present and is suspicious for recurrent neoplasm *(arrows)*. Patient was given colonic air via a rectal tube *(arrowhead)*. Axial MR image in the same patient **(B)**. Multiple folds are identified in the small bowel loops *(arrows)*, confirming that the soft tissue mass depicted on CT is unopacified small bowel. Delayed CT images would have solved the problem on CT, and MRI would not be necessary (see Fig. 15.17). **C,D:** Axial CT in a different patient who had a prior gastrectomy. Soft tissue structure in the omentum is suspicious for omental neoplasm **(C)**. Delayed CT, gas, and oral contrast are now present within this structure **(D)**, allowing a confident diagnosis of bowel to be made. **(C** and **D** courtesy of Ali Shirkhoda, M.D.)

from fluid-filled small bowel is facilitated by recognizing stranding of the mesenteric fat and mass effects, which are present with abscess but not with fluid-filled bowel (Fig. 15.18). Occasionally it may be difficult to distinguish abscess from bowel. Again, in these cases, delayed CT imaging with additional oral contrast material will aid in differentiating water- and gas-filled small bowel from tumors or abscesses.

Diagnostic Pitfalls

Duodenal Diverticulum

Duodenal diverticula consisting of mucosal and submucosal herniations through defects in the muscular wall are identified in 2% to 5% of patients during the upper GI series (18,19). After the colon, the duodenum is the second most common location for gastrointestinal diverticula (18). There continues to be controversy whether they are congenital or acquired. These diverticula most frequently occur along the medial aspect of the second portion of the duodenum adjacent to the ampulla of Vater and are often seen as incidental findings (18) (Fig. 15.19). At CT examination, duodenal diverticula are seen as sharply contoured small fluid- and or air/fluid-filled structures located adjacent to the medial aspect of the duodenum in the region of the head of the pancreas. Rarely diverticula may become complicated and may be seen in symptomatic individuals. Complications are related to duodenal obstruction, bleeding, or perforation (18).

At CT, duodenal diverticula may mimic an abscess or perforated ulcer. A sealed-off duodenal ulcer occurring along the medial wall of the duodenum can be mistaken for a duodenal diverticulum. The associated inflammatory response, the irregular contour, and the acute clinical presentation seen with ulcers and abscesses help to differentiate these entities. If there is doubt, an upper gas-

trointestinal series will be required to differentiate these conditions.

In some instances a duodenal diverticulum, when fluid filled, may be mistaken for a low-attenuation pancreatic neoplasm. Decubitus positioning is helpful in differentiating it from a pancreatic neoplasm by allowing gas to enter the diverticulum (see Fig. 15.19).

Malrotation

The primitive gut, which develops during the first 4 weeks of gestation, is divided into three parts: the foregut, the midgut, and the hindgut (9). The portions of the gastrointestinal tract derived from the foregut are the pharynx, esophagus, stomach, and proximal duodenum to the level of the ampulla of Vater. The midgut gives rise to the remainder of the duodenum, small intestine, appendix, and the ascending and proximal transverse colon. The remainder of the colon, rectum, and superior portion of the anal canal are derived from the hindgut (9).

Midgut malrotation occurs when the small bowel and its attached mesentery fails to complete the normal counterclockwise rotation around the axis of the superior mesenteric artery during embryologic development (20). In adults, the condition has no clinical significance unless recurrent crampy abdominal pain occurs secondary to intermittent partial intestinal torsion (21,22). Midgut volvulus associated with malrotation and caused by inappropriate fixation of the midgut mesentery to the posterior abdominal wall represents an abdominal emergency (21).

At CT, in the normal individual, the SMA and SMV have a constant relationship. The SMV is positioned ventral and to the right of the SMA (see Fig. 15.13). Reversal of this normal relationship is suggestive of intestinal malrotation (Fig. 15.20) unless an abdominal tumor is present causing mass effect on these vessels (23). In a

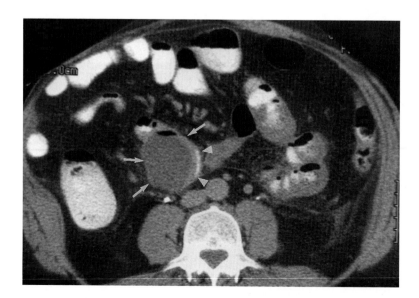

FIG. 15.18. Abscess mimicking small bowel. Axial CT scan in the midabdomen. Fluid- and gas-filled structure with sharp border and clear surrounding fat is present near the mesentery *(arrows)*. Recognizing mass effect on adjacent contrast-filled loop of small bowel *(arrowheads)* helps to differentiate this structure as an abscess as opposed to fluid-filled small bowel loop. At surgery, appendicitis with interloop abscess was confirmed.

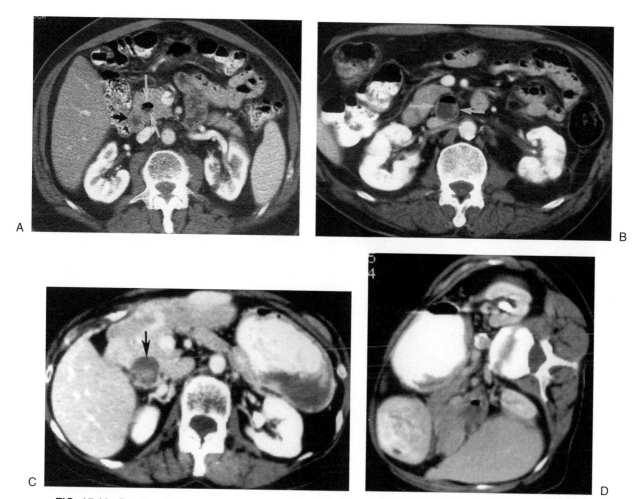

FIG. 15.19. Duodenal diverticulum. **A:** Axial CT at the level of the pancreatic head. Air-filled structure *(arrows)* medial to the second portion of the duodenum *(black arrow)* is identified as a common finding for duodenal diverticulum. **B:** Axial CT in a different patient. Similar presentation with air–fluid level in a duodenal diverticulum located in a typical location at the junction of second and third portions of the duodenum (arrows). Lack of surrounding inflammatory response helps to exclude abscess or perforated ulcer. **C,D:** In a different patient, there appears to be a low-density mass *(arrow)* behind the head and uncinate process of the pancreas **(C)**. In the lateral decubitus position **(D)**, presence of an air bubble within the mass proves its identity as a duodenal diverticulum. **(C** and **D** reproduced with permission from reference 14.)

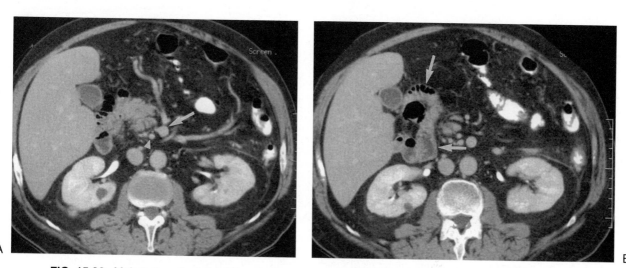

FIG. 15.20. Malrotation. **A:** Axial CT at the level of the SMA and SMV. There is reversal of the normal position of the SMA *(arrowhead)* and SMV *(arrow)*. In this patient the SMA is to the right of the SMV. **B:** A CT scan 2 cm caudal to **A.** The duodenum is in the right abdomen *(arrows)* and not in its normal location in the retroperitoneum between the SMA and SMV (see Fig. 15.13).

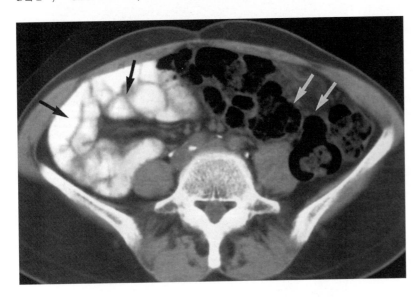

FIG. 15.21. Complete nonrotation. Axial CT of the upper pelvis. The entire small bowel *(black arrows)* is in the right side of the abdomen, and the colon is in the left abdomen *(white arrows)*. Findings are typical of nonrotation of the midgut. This is often an incidental finding on CT.

review of 182 CT scans in pediatric patients, a reversal of the normal position (SMV to the left of the SMA) was demonstrated in 16 cases (8.2%). In only three of these 16 patients was malrotation confirmed with upper gastrointestinal series. In the adult patient, if reversal of the normal position of the SMA and SMV is demonstrated in an otherwise normal abdomen, the possibility of malrotation should be suggested. The diagnosis is confirmed by the absence of the horizontal retroperitoneal segment of the duodenum, by the location of the jejunal loops in the right upper quadrant, and by the location of the colon in the left hemiabdomen (Fig. 15.21). If reversal of the position of the SMA and SMV is the only finding at CT, an upper gastrointestinal series is recommended to confirm the diagnosis of a partial intestinal malrotation.

Transient Intussusception of the Small Bowel

Intestinal intussusception occurs when one segment of the gastrointestinal tract (intussusceptum) invaginates into an adjacent segment (intussuscipiens) (24). Although common in children, intussusception is less common in adults, with only 5% of all cases occurring later in life (24). At CT, enteroenteric intussusceptions present as a complex mass (25). The CT appearance of intestinal intussusceptions is variable but generally consists of a segment of collapsed intestine (the intussusceptum), often with attached mesentery and blood vessels, located within a more dilated adjacent segment of bowel (intussuscipiens). The appearance on cross section consists of a peripheral ring of intestine (intussuscipiens) containing a

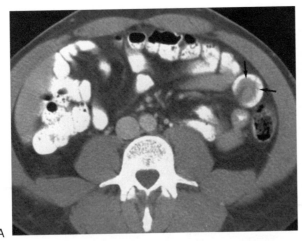
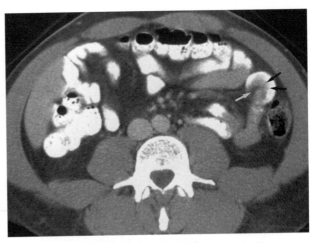

FIG. 15.22. Transient intussusception without identifiable lead point. **A:** Axial CT scan of the lower abdomen. A filling defect is present within a loop of small bowel *(arrows)*. **B:** Axial CT 1 cm caudal to **A**. The adjacent low-attenuation intraluminal mesenteric fat *(white arrow)* is better seen on this image and identifies the abnormality as intussuscepting bowel *(black arrow)*. Small bowel series (not shown) demonstrated no identifiable cause. In this patient, the small bowel intussusception was transient, without a lead point, and the patient did not require surgery.

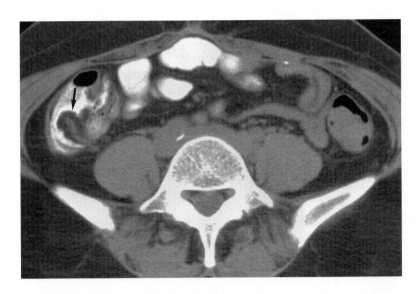

FIG. 15.23. Lipomatous hypertrophy of the ileocecal valve. Axial CT scan at the level of the cecum. Lipomatous hypertrophy of the ileocecal valve is detected *(arrow)*. Note the marked low-attenuation tissue of the ileocecal valve, a common normal variant.

collapsed loop of bowel (intussusceptum) and adjacent mesenteric fat. In adults, up to 90% of intussusceptions are caused by a leading mass (24). The exact cause of an intussusception is often not identified at CT, and in these cases the etiology of the intussusception can not be established (25). Cases of mild intermittent intussusceptions presenting without associated bowel obstruction or intraluminal mesenteric fat are sometimes seen on CT and may have no clinical significance. They can occur in patients with enteritis, pancreatitis, sprue, edematous bowel, or be idiopathic. The CT findings in these patients should be interpreted with caution, in the correct clinical setting, and should be correlated with a small bowel examination before surgery is contemplated (Fig. 15.22). Documenting a lead point is important in that most patients with transient intussusception not caused by a leading mass do not require surgery.

Lipomatous Hypertrophy of the Ileocecal Valve Versus Neoplasm

The ileocecal valve is often visualized during abdominal CT. It is located on the medial aspect of cecum approximately 3 to 4 cm from the cecal caput (26). Occasionally, a slightly thickened (2 to 3 cm) ileocecal valve is identified during CT examination. Demonstration of fat attenuation within a thickened ileocecal valve is diagnostic of benign lipomatous infiltration and has no clinical significance (Fig. 15.23). It excludes the presence of an inflammatory or neoplastic condition. This is an incidental finding when present and requires no further evaluation.

APPENDIX

Normal Anatomy and Anatomic Variants

The appendix is a small-caliber blind-ending tube ranging from 2 cm to 20 cm and averaging 9 cm in length (26). Two-thirds of appendices are retrocecal (26). McBurney's point (located at the junction of the lateral and middle thirds of a line connecting the umbilicus and anterior superior iliac crest) is recognized as the surface landmark for locating the appendix at surgery (27). Although most appendices can be found in the right lower quadrant, other locations such as lower pelvis, midabdomen, and subhepatic are not unusual. Its usual location is posterior or inferior to the cecal caput and anterior to the right psoas muscle. A survey of 275 double contrast barium enemas demonstrated that only 35% of appendices were located within 5 cm of McBurney's point (27). Computed tomography is able to visualize a normal appendix in over 50% of individuals and an abnormal appendix in virtually all cases. If the appendix is not visualized in the right lower quadrant, a careful search for the right colon and cecum will usually detect it in a different location (Fig. 15.24). The detection of an inflamed appendix or appendiceal abscess in an aberrant location can explain the confusing clinical presentation that these patients often present with.

Diagnostic Pitfalls

Fluid-Filled Distal Ileum Mimicking Acute Appendicitis

When patients are evaluated for suspected acute appendicitis, it is imperative that the terminal ileum and small bowel be well opacified with positive oral contrast material. This aids in identifying the abnormal appendix and differentiates it from fluid-filled small bowel (Fig. 15.25). It is necessary to wait 1 to 2 hours after the patient ingests oral contrast material before the CT exam is performed for suspected appendicitis. We routinely obtain a single CT slice at the level of the iliac crest to document the presence of oral contrast material in the cecum. If oral contrast material is identified in the cecum, then CT with IV contrast is initiated to evaluate for possible appendicitis.

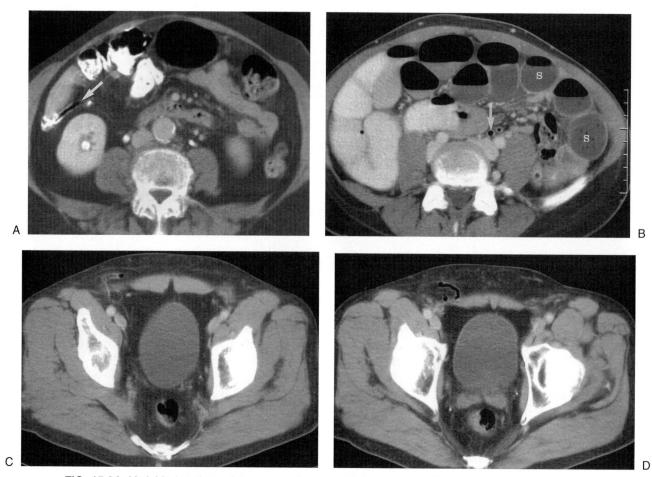

FIG. 15.24. Variable locations of the appendix. **A:** Axial CT at the inferior edge of the liver. Air-filled appendix is identified in the subhepatic region *(arrow)*. In this patient, if appendicitis developed, symptoms may mimic acute cholecystitis. **B:** Axial CT in a patient with nonrotation and small bowel obstruction. In this patient the normal air-filled appendix is identified in the left side of the abdomen *(arrow)*. Note distended small bowel loops (S), some of which are present in the right side of abdomen. **C,D:** Pelvic CT images show presence of appendix in right groin within inguinal canal. (**C** and **D** courtesy of Ali Shirkhoda, M.D.)

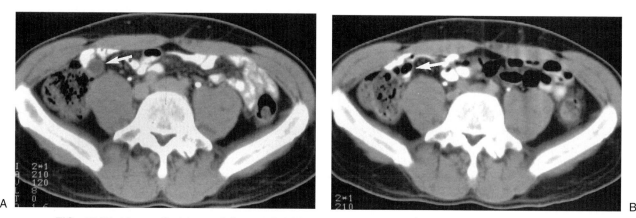

FIG. 15.25. Unopacified loop of ileum mimicking appendicitis. **A:** Axial CT of the lower abdomen demonstrates a fluid-filled tubular structure ventral to the psoas muscle *(arrow)*. **B:** Delayed CT scan in same patient. Oral contrast opacification of the distal ileum *(arrow)* is now present. In cases of suspected appendicitis, opacification of the distal ileum and cecum with positive contrast material is essential. (Case courtesy of Ali Shirkhoda, M.D.)

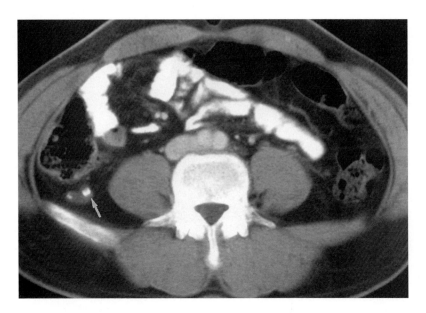

FIG. 15.26. Incidental identification of appendicolith. Axial CT scan of the upper pelvis in a trauma patient. Calcified appendicolith is present within the appendix *(arrow)*. In this patient there was no CT evidence for appendicitis, and the patient was asymptomatic.

Appendicolith

Appendicitis is caused by an obstructive process (fecalith or tumor) of the appendiceal lumen causing stasis and secondary infection. At CT, a calcified appendicolith may be present in the appendix or within the abscess cavity following appendiceal perforation. The incidence of appendicoliths in patients with appendicitis has been reported to be 25% to 40% (28). Occasionally, however, an appendicolith may be detected at CT without evidence of appendicitis (28) (Fig. 15.26). If the wall of the appendix is not thickened, its lumen not distended, and periappendiceal inflammatory changes not identified at CT, the presence of an appendicolith should be considered an incidental finding of limited clinical significance. Patients with appendicoliths have a high incidence of

developing appendicitis later. The mere detection of an appendicolith, however, is not diagnostic of appendicitis.

COLON

Normal Anatomy and Anatomic Variants

On CT scans, the thickness of the normal colonic wall does not exceed 2 to 3 mm (20). This measurement should be made when the colon is at least partially distended and imaged transaxially. In any distended segment of colon, if the wall thickness measures over 4 mm, it should be considered abnormal (20). When the colon is evaluated, careful attention should be given to the degree of distention because nondistended segments of colon will appear thickened at different levels and may mimic disease (Figs. 15.27 and 15.28). The correct interpreta-

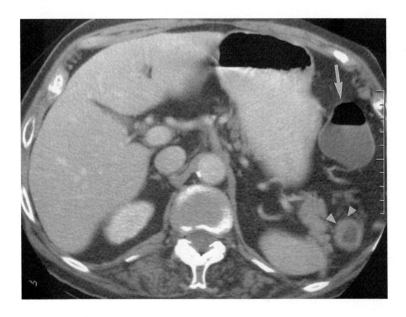

FIG. 15.27. Normal colonic wall: effect of degree of luminal distention. Axial CT at the level of the splenic flexure. The well-distended proximal portion of the splenic flexure *(arrow)* demonstrates a thin colonic wall measuring 1 to 2 mm. In the posterior and distal portion of the splenic flexure, the colon is not well distended and appears thickened *(arrowheads)*. This case demonstrates the variable thickness of the normal colonic wall depending on the degree of distention.

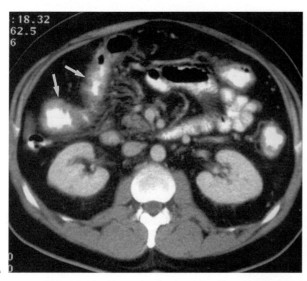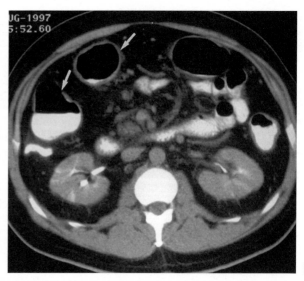

FIG. 15.28. Normal colonic wall: effect of degree of luminal distention. **A:** Axial CT demonstrates apparent thickening of the hepatic flexure *(arrows).* **B:** After insufflation of rectal air, the normal colonic wall is identified *(arrows).* (Case courtesy of Ali Shirkhoda, M.D.)

tion of the true thickness of the colonic wall should, therefore, be correlated to the degree of distention before any clinical implications can be inferred. Furthermore, when fluid and oral contrast are present as a mixture within the colon, a CT appearance mimicking wall thickening may be encountered (Fig. 15.29). The presence of minute amounts of gas in these segments of colon allows for accurate interpretation of this finding. Additional findings, when present, help in establishing the presence and nature of a suspected colonic wall abnormality. Loss of haustration, edema, shagginess, target sign, and peri-

colic inflammation are findings that, when present, help in confirming colonic wall pathology.

Positional Anomalies

Axial CT images visualize the colon on transverse sections in its ascending and descending retroperitoneal segments and on longitudinal sections in its transverse and sigmoid sections. The position of the colon, its larger size, haustral pattern, and fecal contents allow its relatively easy detection and evaluation by CT imaging. The

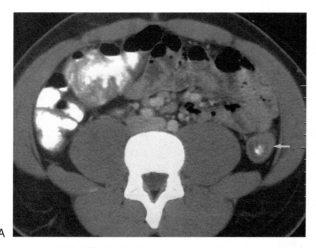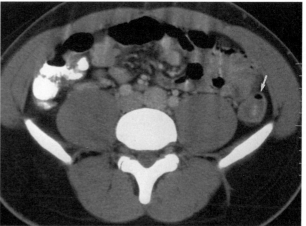

FIG. 15.29. Fluid in the descending colon mimicking thickening of the wall. **A:** Axial CT of the descending colon. Positive oral contrast material is noted within the nondistended descending colon. The wall appears circumferentially thickened and multilayered, suggesting inflammation *(arrow).* **B:** Axial CT slightly caudal to **A**. An air–fluid level is present, allowing apparent thickening to be identified as residual fluid within the colon. The wall of the colon measures only 1 to 2 mm *(arrow).* If any doubt, insufflation of air through the rectum and repeat scanning would be helpful.

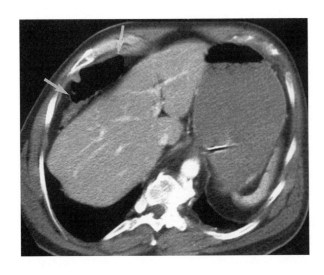

FIG. 15.30. Subdiaphragmatic hepatic flexure (Chilaiditi syndrome). Axial CT at the level of the liver. The hepatic flexure *(arrows)* is interposed between the liver and the diaphragm. This condition is usually asymptomatic. It may become important when one is attempting percutaneous liver biopsy.

ascending and descending colon are retroperitoneal, whereas the transverse and sigmoid colon are located within the peritoneal cavity, have a mesentery, and may be quite redundant.

Positional anomalies of the colon result from embryologic abnormalities in bowel rotation and fixation (29). The most common positional anomaly is the mobile cecum and ascending colon. In these cases, the cecum and ascending colon have a long mesentery, which attaches these segments of the colon to the retroperitoneum. Although most of these patients are asymptomatic, the condition does predispose the patient to cecal volvulus.

Hepatodiaphragmatic interposition may cause abdominal symptoms in a small percentage of patients (32). It is a potential pitfall in that occasionally it can be mistaken for subdiaphragmatic abscess or free air on abdominal and chest radiographs. The occurrence of hepatodiaphragmatic interposition is more common when the patient is supine than erect (2.4% vs. 0.3%) (32). This condition needs to be recognized when one is carrying out interventional liver procedures because most percutaneous procedures are performed with the patient supine. On CT examinations the true nature of subdiaphragmatic interposition is easily recognized by detecting haustrations and continuity with the right and transverse colon (Fig. 15.30).

Other less common positional anomalies include retrogastric and retrosplenic colon (Fig. 15.31), interposition of the colon between the kidney and psoas, and retropancreatic colon (29–32). The most dramatic is nonrotation, when the entire colon is situated in the left abdomen and the small bowel is on the right (see Fig. 15.21).

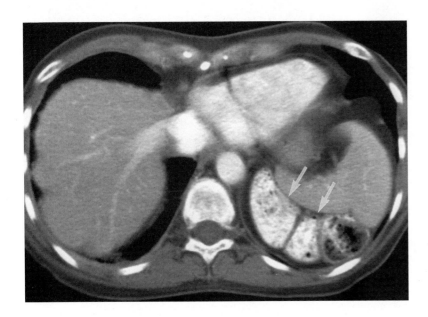

FIG. 15.31. Retrosplenic colon. Axial CT at the level of the spleen. Contrast-filled colon *(arrow)* is located entirely posterior to the spleen and stomach. This is a normal variant in this asymptomatic patient.

Diagnostic Pitfalls

Submucosal Fat Deposition

On contrast-enhanced CT, the "target" or "halo" appearance within the colon usually implies the presence of an inflammatory or ischemic process within that segment of bowel (17). This is secondary to edema in the submucosa causing low attenuation interposed between the enhancing mucosa and muscularis layers. Rarely, the target appearance has been identified in patients with scirrhous carcinomas of the colon (33). A target appearance within the bowel wall may also be caused by the presence of submucosal fat deposition (Fig. 15.32) (34). This is occasionally seen in patients with long-standing inflammatory bowel disease and does not imply active inflammation (34). The etiology is not entirely clear and may be in part related to chronic steroid use that these patients often receive. It has also been reported in patients without a history of inflammatory bowel disease who have been treated with high doses of chemotherapy (35).

Giant Sigmoid Diverticulum

Giant colonic diverticula usually occur in the elderly and almost always occur within the sigmoid colon (36). Patients may be asymptomatic or have signs and symptoms related to a mass or sudden onset of abdominal pain (36). The development is related to a ball-valve mechanism allowing gas to enter the diverticulum but not to exit (36,37). These are pseudodiverticula in that they do not contain a true muscular layer similar to the other sigmoid diverticula (37). On plain abdominal radiographs they usually appear as a sharply marginated large gas density located in the left pelvis. At CT a cystic well-defined gas-containing structure with thin walls is seen adjacent to the sigmoid colon (Fig. 15.33). An air–fluid level may be identified within the diverticulum. The finding should not be confused with abscess. Elective surgery is usually indicated for all confirmed cases of giant sigmoid diverticula.

Colonic Edema

Colonic edema is usually seen in patients with severe colitis of different etiologies and colonic ischemia. In addition, in patients with cirrhosis, intestinal edema develops often and can be identified on barium studies and CT examinations of the gastrointestinal tract. The edema most often occurs in the small bowel and less frequently in the stomach and colon (38). Factors leading to the development of gastrointestinal edema in these patients include low oncotic pressure (hypoalbuminemia) and portal hypertension (increased hydrostatic pressure),

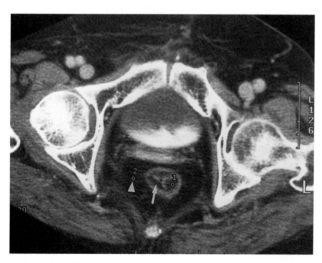

FIG. 15.32. Submucosal fat deposition. Axial CT at the level of the rectum. The submucosa of the rectum demonstrates diffuse low attenuation *(arrow),* similar to the perirectal fat *(arrowhead).* Region-of-interest cursors in the submucosa of the rectum and in the perirectal fat measured -53 HU consistent with fat. This finding has been described in patients with chronic ulcerative colitis and in patients on high-dose cytoreductive chemotherapy. It should not be confused with the "target" or halo appearance consistent with an acute inflammatory condition. In these cases, the low attenuation in the submucosa represents edema, not fat.

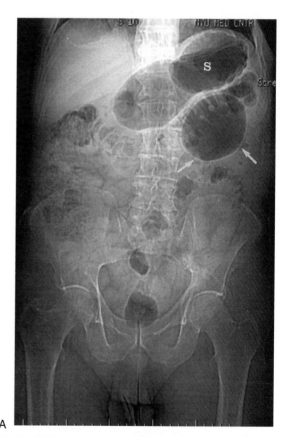

FIG. 15.33. Giant sigmoid diverticulum mimicking loculated free air or abscess. **A:** Anteroposterior CT scout view. Abnormal gas collection is present in the left upper abdomen *(arrows).* S, stomach.

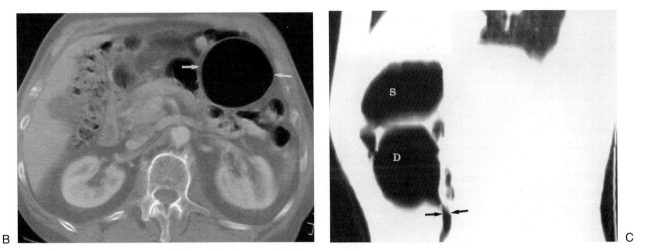

B

C

FIG. 15.33. *Continued.* **B:** Computed tomography scan at the level of the gas collection. Thin-walled sharply contained gas collection is identified in the left upper quadrant *(arrows).* **C:** Sagittal 2-D reformatted CT image using lung window settings (window 1,200, level –700). **D:** The gas collection is communicating with a loop of redundant sigmoid colon *(arrows),* suggesting diagnosis of a giant sigmoid diverticulum. S, stomach. Surgical resection confirmed diagnosis of giant sigmoid diverticulum.

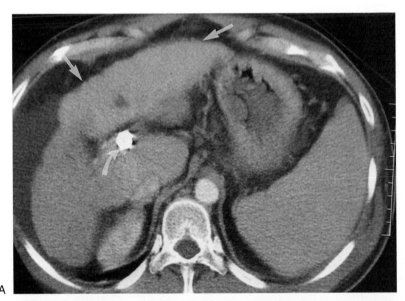

A

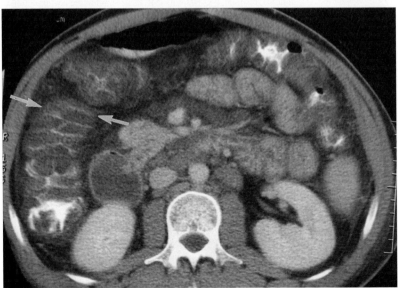

B

FIG. 15.34. Colonic edema in a cirrhotic patient mimicking acute inflammation. **A:** Axial CT of the liver. Nodular surface contour *(arrow)* and intrahepatic shunt *(curved arrow)* consistent with known diagnosis of cirrhosis in patient following transjugular intrahepatic portosystemic shunt (TIPS) procedure. Notice the undistended stomach with apparent thickened wall. **B:** Axial CT of the lower abdomen. Diffuse circumferential wall thickening and distorted haustral pattern are present in the right colon *(arrows).* Patient was being treated with lactulose for hepatic encephalopathy and was otherwise asymptomatic. At colonoscopy the colonic mucosa was shown to be normal. Edema, predominately in the right colon, is often identified in patients with cirrhosis. In asymptomatic patients this reflects a combination of low oncotic pressure and portal hypertension.

which probably plays the dominant role because it correlates best with its unusual distribution in patients with cirrhosis (38). In the colon, confusing radiographic changes may be detected mimicking acute colitis. Colonic edema in patients with cirrhosis appears similar to edema within the colon caused by any other etiology (Fig. 15.34). The wall of the colon is thickened, haustrations are altered, and a target appearance may be present as a result of low-density edema within the submucosa. At endoscopy the mucosa will appear normal. Colonic edema related to cirrhosis has a tendency to commonly involve the right side of the colon, although the entire colon may be involved. Differential diagnosis is based on the presence of other CT findings (cirrhosis, varices) and the clinical presentation.

REFERENCES

1. Balthazar EJ. CT of the gastrointestinal tract: principles and interpretation. *Am J Roentgenol* 1991;156:23–32.
2. Noh HM, Fishman EK, Forastiere AA, Bliss DF, Calhoun PS. CT of the esophagus: spectrum of disease with emphasis on esophageal carcinoma. *RadioGraphics* 1995;15:1113–1134.
3. Noda Y, Yasuhiro O, Akihito N, et al. Technical note: New barium paste mixture for helical (slip ring) CT evaluation of the esophagus. *J Comput Assist Tomogr* 1996;20:773–776.
4. Winter TC, Ager JD, Nghiem HV, Hill RS, Harrison SD, Freeny PC. Upper gastrointestinal tract and abdomen: water as an orally administered contrast agent for helical CT. *Radiology* 1996;201:365–370.
5. Fishman EK, Urban BA, Hruban RH. CT of the stomach: spectrum of disease. *RadioGraphics* 1996;16:1035–1054.
6. Gore RM, Balthazar EJ, Ghahremani GG, Miller FH. CT features of ulcerative colitis and Crohn disease. *Am J Roentgenol* 1996;167:3–15.
7. Rao PM, Rhea JT, Novelline RA, et al. Helical CT technique for the diagnosis of appendicitis: prospective evaluation of a focused appendix examination. *Radiology* 1997;202:139–145.
8. Picus D, Balfe DM, Koehler RE, et al. Computed tomography in the staging of esophageal carcinoma. *Radiology* 1983;146:433–438.
9. Moore KL. The digestive system. In: Moore KL, ed. *The developing human, clinically oriented anatomy, 3rd ed.* Philadelphia: WB Saunders, 1982;227–254,329–332.
10. McLoughlin MJ, Weisbrod G, Wise DJ, et al. Computed tomography in congenital anomalies of the aortic arch and great vessels. *Radiology* 1981;138:399–403.
11. Gamsu G. The mediastinum. In: Moss AA, Gamsu G, Genant HK, eds. *Computed tomography of the body with magnetic resonance imaging, 2nd ed.* Philadelphia: WB Saunders, 1992;63–64.
12. Mauro MA, Jaques PF, Swantkowski TM, Staab EV, Bozymski EM. CT after uncomplicated esophageal sclerotherapy. *Am J Roentgenol* 1986; 147:57–60.
13. Halden WJ, Harnsberger HR, Mancuso AA. Computed tomography of esophageal varices after sclerotherapy. *Am J Roentgenol* 1983;140: 1195–1196.
14. Shirkhoda A. Diagnostic pitfalls in abdominal CT. *RadioGraphics* 1991;11:969–1002.
15. Hulnick DH, Balthazar EJ. Gastric duplication cyst: gastrointestinal series and CT correlation. *Gastrointest Radiol* 1987;12:106.
16. Balthazar EJ. CT of the gastrointestinal tract: principles and interpretation. *Am J Roentgenol* 1991;156:23–32.
17. Gore RM, Balthazar EJ, Ghahremani GG, Miller FH. CT features of ulcerative colitis and Crohn disease. *Am J Roentgenol* 1996;167:3–15.
18. Scudamore CH, Harrison RC, White TT. Management of duodenal diverticula. *Can J Surg* 1982;25:311–314.
19. Pugash RA, O'Brien EO, Stevenson GW. Perforating duodenal diverticulitis. *Gastrointest Radiol* 1990;15:156–158.
20. Shatzkes D, Gordon DH, Haller JO, Kantor A, De Silva R. Malrotation of the bowel: malalignment of the superior mesenteric artery–vein complex shown by CT and MR. *J Comput Assist Tomogr* 1990;14: 93–95.
21. Berdon WE. The diagnosis of malrotation and volvulus in the older child and adult: a trap for radiologists. *Pediatr Radiol* 1995;25: 101–103.
22. Zerin MJ, DiPietro MA. Mesenteric vascular anatomy at CT: normal and abnormal appearances. *Radiology* 1991;179:739–742.
23. Nichols DM, Li DK. Superior mesenteric vein rotation: a CT sign of midgut malrotation. *Am J Roentgenol* 1983;141:707–708.
24. Agha FP. Intussusception in adults. *Am J Roentgenol* 1986;146: 527–531.
25. Merine D, Fishman EK, Jones B, Siegelman SS. Enteroenteric intussusception: CT findings in nine patients. *Am J Roentgenol* 1987;148: 1129–1132.
26. Curtin KR, Fitzgerald SW, Nemcek AA Jr, Hoff FL, Vogelzang RL. CT diagnosis of acute appendicitis: Imaging findings. *Am J Roentgenol* 1995;164:905–909.
27. Ramsden WH, Mannion RAJ, Simpkins KC, deDombal FT. Is the appendix where you think it is—and if not does it matter? *Clin Radiol* 1993;47:100–103.
28. Malone AJ Jr, Wolf CR, Malmed AS, Melliere BF. Diagnosis of acute appendicitis: value of unenhanced CT. *Am J Roentgenol* 1993;160: 763–766.
29. Holemans JA, Rankin SC. Retropancreatic colon interposed between the spleen and left diaphragmatic crus: CT appearance. *J Comput Assist Tomogr* 1997;21:389–390.
30. Oldfield AL, Wilbur AC. Retrogastric colon: CT demonstration of anatomic variations. *Radiology* 1993;186:557–561.
31. Prassopoulous P, Gourtsoyiannis N, Cavouras D, Pantelidis N. Interposition of the colon between the kidney and psoas muscle: A normal anatomic variation studied by CT. *Abdom Imag* 1994;19:446–448.
32. Prassopoulous PK, Raissaki MT, Gourtsoyiannis N. Hepatodiaphragmatic interposition of the colon in the upright and supine position. *J Comput Assist Tomogr* 1996;20:151–153.
33. Balthazar EJ, Siegel SE, Megibow AJ, Scholes J, Gordon R. CT in patients with scirrhous carcinoma of the GI tract: Imaging findings and value for tumor detection and staging. *Am J Roentgenol* 1995;165: 839–845.
34. Jones B, Fishman EK, Hamilton SR, et al. Submucosal accumulation of fat in inflammatory bowel disease: CT/pathologic correlation. *J Comput Assist Tomogr* 1986;10:759–763.
35. Muldowney SM, Balfe DM, Hammerman A, Wick MR. "Acute" fat deposition in bowel wall submucosa: CT appearance. *J Comput Assist Tomogr* 1995;19:390–393.
36. Kricun R, Stasik JJ, Reither RD, Dex WJ. Giant colonic diverticulum. *Am J Roentgenol* 1980;135:507–512.
37. Gallagher JJ, Welch JP. Giant diverticula of the sigmoid colon. *Arch Surg* 1979;114:1079–1083.
38. Balthazar EJ, Gade MF. Gastrointestinal edema in cirrhotics. *Gastrointest Radiol* 1976;1:215–223.

Variants and Pitfalls in Body Imaging,
edited by Ali Shirkhoda.
Lippincott Williams & Wilkins, Philadelphia, © 2000.

CHAPTER 16

The Peritoneum, Retroperitoneum, and the Fascial Planes

Robert E. Mindelzun and Hossein Jadvar

The peritoneal and extraperitoneal spaces and their fascial planes create complex three-dimensional structures with unique radiologic characteristics. Anatomic variations and pathologic conditions create appearances that are often difficult to interpret and subsequently lead to serious misinterpretation (1). Before embarking on an evaluation of the images, the radiologist should avail himself or herself of an appropriate history, especially of prior radiation or surgery (Fig. 16.1), which may alter or even result in new structures and anatomic relationships (Figs. 16.2 and 16.3). In addition, it is important to realize that although cross-sectional imaging, particularly computed tomography (CT), has given us a unique understanding of normal anatomic planes and boundaries, there are a subset of patients who will have anatomic variations or incompletely developed fascial planes (Fig. 16.4).

COMPUTED TOMOGRAPHY

Numerous techniques are available for performing CT of the abdomen. These include protocols that opacify the bowel (with positive or negative oral contrast agents), the vessels (with varying volumes and injection rates), and specialized injections to solve specific clinical problems (2–5). A typical protocol would include contrast-enhanced 5- to 7-mm axial images from the dome of the

diaphragm to the symphysis pubis. Intravenous 60% iodinated contrast injection by a mechanical injector with a volume of 150 ml is injected using a variety of protocols. For example, it may be infused at 2.5 ml/sec for 20 seconds followed by 1 ml/sec for 100 seconds and scanning for 40 seconds after the start of infusion provides reliable contrast enhancement. Oral contrast is used to delineate the stomach and the bowel and to improve conspicuity of the mesenteries and of structures adjacent to the bowel wall. Each radiologist needs to be familiar with a variety of protocols, as no one technique is appropriate for every clinical question. For example, in a patient with a presumptive diagnosis of lymphoma, one will usually need to administer large volumes of positive oral contrast in order to differentiate bowel loops from enlarged lymph nodes. On the other hand, administration of positive contrast agents may mask coproliths (as in appendicitis) or calcified lesions such as ovarian malignancies (Fig. 16.5) (5). High injection rates and rapid image acquisition, especially with helical scanners, will produce unusual flow patterns. A typical example is the marbled appearance of the spleen or the corticomedullary differentiation of the kidneys.

Helically acquired data may be reconstructed and reformatted for detailed analysis of a specific finding. Determination of the CT number in Hounsfield units (HU) is valuable in characterizing lesions or fluid collections. This is especially important when one is trying to differentiate processes that have similar patterns of spread but slightly different tissue characteristics (Fig. 16.6). Window settings (level and width) can also be manipulated as necessary when the images are reviewed in order to enhance the detectability of some lesions. These settings include liver (level 70 to 80 HU, width 150 HU), lung

R. E. Mindelzun: Department of Radiology, Stanford University School of Medicine, Stanford, California 94305.

H. Jadvar: Joint Program in Nuclear Medicine, Harvard Medical School, and Division of Nuclear Medicine, Department of Radiology, Brigham and Women's Hospital, and Massachusetts General Hospital, Boston, Massachusetts 02164.

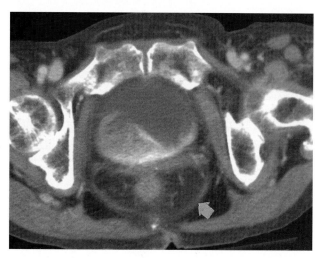

FIG. 16.1. Thickening of the perirectal fascia *(arrow)* secondary to prior radiation therapy.

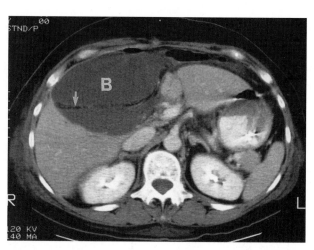

FIG. 16.2. Postoperative visualization of an omental patch *(arrow)* in a patient who underwent a left hepatic lobe resection for malignancy. Postoperatively the patient developed a large biloma (B) that has lifted the omentum off the liver surface.

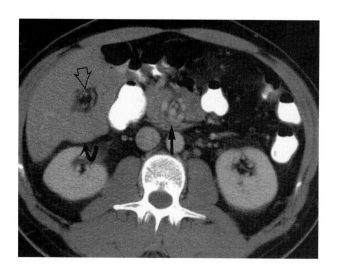

FIG. 16.3. Malrotation of the bowel creates a pseudomass lesion in the right abdomen. Note the swirl sign created by central mesenteric vessels *(straight arrow)* and the right-sided mass near the liver caused by loops of small intestine *(curved black arrow)*. Identifying the swirl sign as well as the fat-laden mesentery within this soft tissue mass *(open arrow)* helps to establish the correct diagnosis.

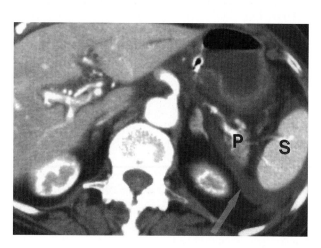

FIG. 16.4. Variation in the formation of the retroperitoneal and intraperitoneal fascial planes. In this patient with pancreatitis there is extravasation of fluid *(arrow)* behind the pancreas (P) with extension of the fluid around the spleen (S) along the so-called bare area of the spleen.

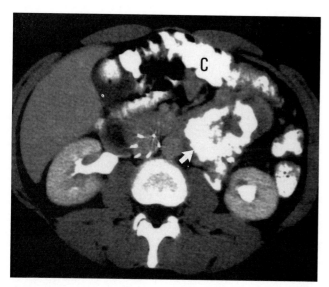

FIG. 16.5. Densely calcified *(arrow)* ovarian carcinoma that could be readily mistaken for contrast material. C, transverse colon.

(level −500 HU, width 2,000 HU), soft tissue (level 30 to 50 HU, width 400 HU), and bone (level 600 HU, width 2,000 HU). A pixel matrix of 512×512 is commonly used. Three-dimensional reconstruction is effective in conceptualizing the various spaces and the relationship of the lesions to the surrounding organs and fascial planes. Rapid technologic changes and physician variability necessitate individual familiarity with local equipment. A flexible approach usually best serves the patient.

ANATOMY OF THE PERITONEUM

The peritoneum forms a closed sac invaginated by the digestive system (6). The portion that contacts the body wall is the parietal peritoneum. This is separated from the transversalis fascia by a layer of extraperitoneal connective tissue and fat. The visceral peritoneum is closely applied to the surface of the digestive tract. The peritoneal cavity and its multiple compartments lie between these two layers and normally contain only a small amount of fluid (7). Fluid dynamics, respiratory motion, gravity, and anatomic barriers dictate the spread of disease processes within the peritoneal cavity and their appearance on cross-sectional imaging studies (8). On current scanners, the peritoneum is faintly visible as a thin line, which is smooth, nonenhancing, without nodularity or calcification. When a calcification is seen, especially in an area of fluid stasis such as an anatomic recess, a tumor should be suspected even when the calcification has a rather benign appearance (Fig. 16.7). Common sites of tumor deposition are the *cul-de-sac,* the hepatorenal fossa, the paracolic gutters, the omenta, the roots of the mesenteries, the subphrenic spaces, the peritoneal ligaments, and the lesser sac.

The Mesenteries

The mesenteries are comprised of two peritoneal folds that connect the bowel (jejunum, ileum, transverse and sigmoid colons) to the retroperitoneum (9,10). A mesentery carries the neurovascular and lymphatic bundles to

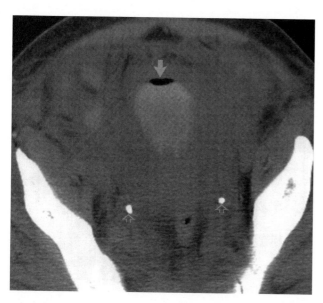

FIG. 16.6. Loss of normal retroperitoneal fascial and fat planes secondary to generalized permeation of the subperitoneal tissues by extensive extraperitoneal lymphomatosis (non-Hodgkin). The urinary bladder *(white arrow)* and the ureters *(open arrow)* are identified after contrast administration.

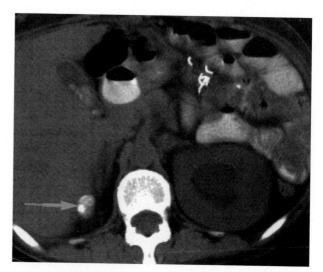

FIG. 16.7. Focal calcification in Morison's pouch. This benign-appearing calcification *(arrow)* is caused by a metastatic serous adenocarcinoma of the ovary with spread throughout the peritoneum. Any peritoneal calcification in a woman should be regarded with suspicion, as malignant tumors may have a very innocent appearance. This patient, in addition, demonstrates gallstones and hydronephrosis of the left kidney secondary to the ovarian tumor.

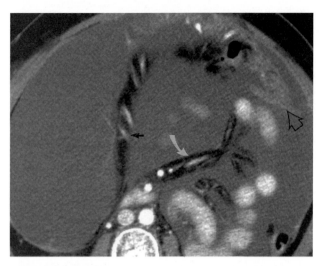

FIG. 16.8. Malignant ascites demonstrating the tree-like configuration of the floating small bowel mesentery *(curved white arrow)*. The right colonic mesentery *(black arrow)* is also visualized. Note in addition the enhancing peritoneum as well as the thickened omentum *(open arrow),* which are characteristic of peritoneal carcinomatosis.

the intestines. The root of small bowel mesentery measures about 15 cm. It extends in an oblique direction from the middle of the pancreas in the left upper quadrant to the ileocecal valve in the right lower quadrant. The small bowel mesentery is fan-shaped, and its connection to the jejunum and ileum can usually be recognized because of its capacious fat content (Fig. 16.8). The transverse mesocolon begins to the right side at the infra-ampullary portion of the descending duodenum, crosses the pancreatic head, runs along the inferior aspect of the body and tail of the pancreas, and extends to the spleen on the left. It merges with the root of the small bowel mesentery at the uncinate process of the pancreas. It serves as an impor-

tant pathway for the extension of pancreatitis. A diffuse increase in the density of the mesentery (misty mesentery) associated with engorgement of the vessels and enhancement of slightly enlarged lymph nodes can be seen in sclerosing retractile mesenteritis (Fig. 16.9). The sigmoid mesocolon forms an inverted V with the apex located at the left common iliac artery division, the left segment descending along the medial to the left psoas major muscle, and the right segment descending into the pelvis to the level of the third sacral vertebra. The sigmoid mesocolon usually contains a large amount of fat that surrounds the sigmoid vessels. Branches of the left colic artery bifurcate early and are seen as two parallel vessels extending as vasa recti to the sigmoid colon wall. On occasion this mesentery will contain massive amounts of fat (lipomatosis), which can be mistaken for an extrinsic tumor on colonoscopy and barium enema (see Fig. 16.10). Abscesses in the sigmoid mesocolon may sometimes be mistaken for the colon itself (Fig. 16.11). The ascending and descending colon are normally retroperitoneal in their location, although on occasion the right colon will be on a long mesentery that allows it to move freely in the peritoneal cavity (Fig. 16.12). A persistent unilateral (rarely bilateral) mesocolon may result if the embryonic mesenteries of the ascending colon do not fuse with the parietal peritoneum. The appendix is normally intraperitoneal even when retrocecal in location. On occasion, however, a retrocecal appendix will be extraperitoneal, leading to retroperitoneal inflammation in appendicitis that may have confusing clinical and radiographic presentations (Fig. 16.13).

The Peritoneal Ligaments

An abdominal ligament consists of two folds of peritoneum that support a structure (6). The primitive dorsal

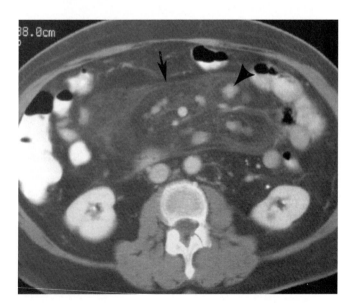

FIG. 16.9. Sclerosing retractile mesenteritis. There is diffuse infiltration *(arrow)* of the mesentery (misty mesentery) with enhancement of the mesenteric lymph nodes *(arrowhead).* The adjacent bowel is normal, and there is no evidence of lymphadenopathy.

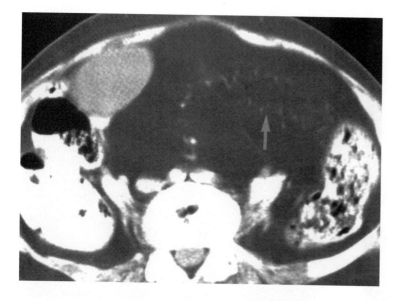

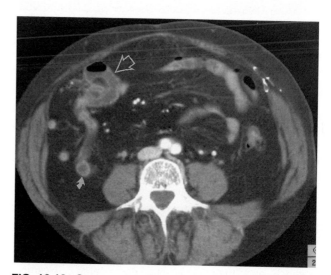

FIG. 16.10. The subperitoneal continuum is evident in this patient with pelvic lipomatosis with fat extending from the extraperitoneal pelvis into the sigmoid mesentery. Differentiation from a lipomatous tumor is established by the presence of well-organized parallel vessels *(arrow)*, which represent sigmoid arteries to the colon.

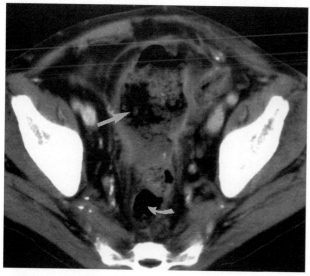

FIG. 16.11. Massive pelvic abscess *(straight arrow)* containing large amounts of air and debris, mistaken for a dilated sigmoid colon. The rectum *(curved arrow)* is noted posterior to the mass which resulted from a perforated sigmoid diverticulum.

FIG. 16.12. Cecum on a long mesentery. The cecum *(open arrow)* is noted anteriorly and is defined by fat within the ileocecal valve. Note the terminal ileum *(curved arrow)*, which extends to the cecum laterally, and the numerous loops of small intestine with their corresponding mesenteries.

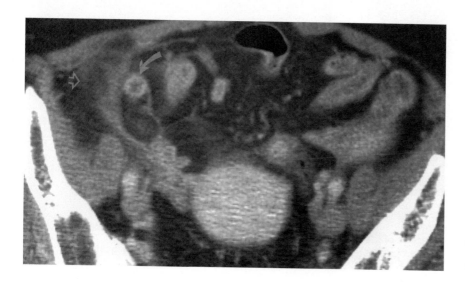

FIG. 16.13. Inflammation of the pelvic extraperitoneal space–lateral pathway *(open arrow)* secondary to rupture of a retroperitoneal appendix *(arrow)*.

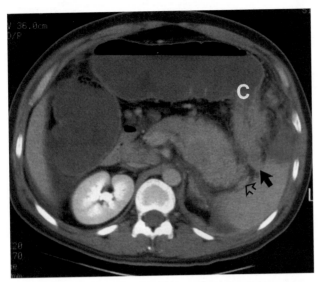

FIG. 16.14. Lymphoma extending from the gastrosplenic *(black arrow)* into the phrenicocolic ligament with invasion of the colon (C). The short splenorenal ligament *(open arrow)*, which extends to the pancreas, is also involved.

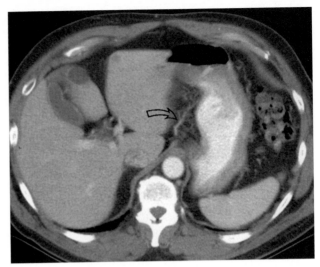

FIG. 16.16. Gastrohepatic ligament identified by the presence of the left gastric artery *(arrow)*.

mesentery gives rise to the gastrophrenic, gastropancreatic, gastrosplenic, splenorenal, phrenicocolic, and gastrocolic ligaments in the upper abdomen. The primitive ventral mesentery forms the falciform, gastrohepatic, and hepatoduodenal ligaments (8). These ligaments can serve as conduits (Fig. 16.14) or as barriers to the spread of disease (9). The gastrohepatic ligament is recognized by the presence of fat as well as the left gastric artery, coronary vein, and gastrohepatic lymph nodes (Figs. 16.15–16.18). It represents an important conduit of disease between the stomach and liver (11). The gastrosplenic ligament

extends between the splenic hilum and the greater curve of the stomach (Figs. 16.19–16.22). It is very variable in size and contains the left gastroepiploic and short gastric vessels. With the splenorenal ligament and the gastrocolic ligament, it provides an important conduit among the stomach, the spleen, and the anterior pararenal space (see Fig. 16.14). The five primary pathways for the extension of intraperitoneal and retroperitoneal diseases are the gastrohepatic/hepatoduodenal ligaments, the splenorenal/ gastrosplenic ligaments, the transverse mesocolon/gastrocolic ligaments, the small bowel mesentery, and the sigmoid mesocolon (8). Incomplete formation of the abdominal ligaments may lead to incomplete fixation of

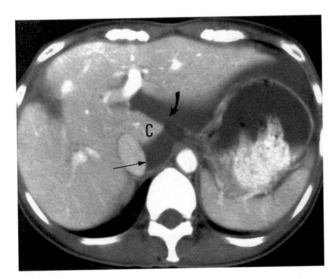

FIG. 16.15. Visualization of the gastrohepatic ligament *(curved arrow)* in the presence of large amounts of ascitic fluid. Fluid has also extended into the superior recess of the lesser sac *(straight arrow)* with compression of the caudate lobe of the liver (C).

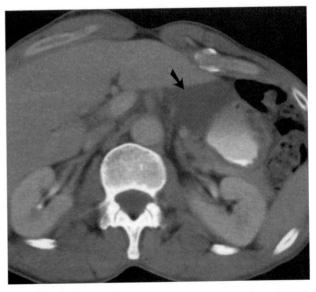

FIG. 16.17. Fluid *(arrow)* trapped by the gastrohepatic ligament (lesser omentum).

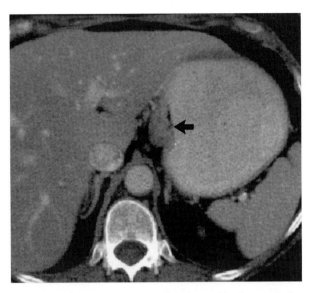

FIG. 16.18. Enlarged lymph nodes *(arrow)* in the gastrohepatic ligament (lesser omentum) secondary to lymphoma.

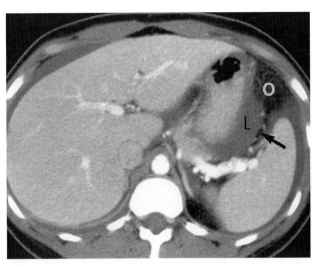

FIG. 16.19. Gastrosplenic ligament *(arrow)* extending to the greater omentum (O). Fat and vessels are noted within both the ligament and the omentum. Medial to the gastrosplenic ligament is the lesser sac (L), which contains fluid in this patient with ascites.

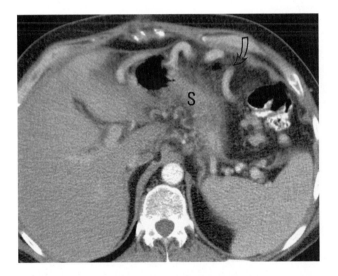

FIG. 16.20. Gastroepiploic varices traverse the gastrosplenic ligament in this patient with portal hypertension. S, stomach.

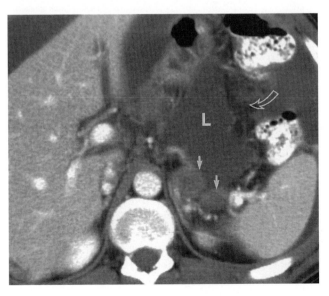

FIG. 16.21. Metastatic adenocarcinoma with tumor nodules lying on the splenorenal ligament *(straight arrow)*. A large amount of fluid is noted within the lesser sac (L), identified medial to the gastrosplenic ligament *(open arrow)*.

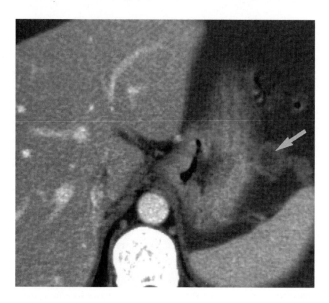

FIG. 16.22. Tumor nodule *(arrow)* on the surface of the spleno-renal ligament.

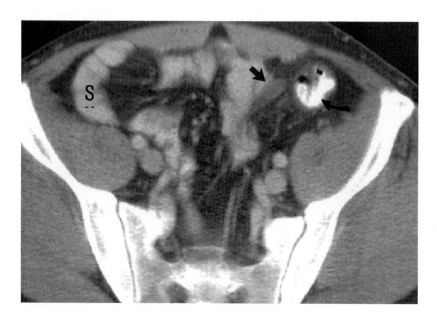

FIG. 16.23. Left-sided appendicitis. Nonrotation of the bowel characterized by the presence of the cecum *(curved arrow)* in the left pelvic fossa and the small intestine (S) in the right lower quadrant. Clinically the patient was thought to have diverticulitis, but identification of the dilated appendix *(straight arrow)* aids in establishing the correct diagnosis of left-sided appendicitis.

solid and hollow abdominal organs resulting in torsion, obstruction, or unusual clinical presentation (Fig. 16.23).

The Omenta

The omenta are specialized ligaments. The lesser omentum (gastrohepatic ligament) is a double-layer membrane that connects the lesser curvature of the stomach to the liver. The greater omentum (gastrocolic ligament) is composed of four layers resembling an apron that connects the greater curvature of the stomach to the transverse colon (12). The greater omentum is usually readily identified because of its fat content and the many vessels that permeate through it (Figs. 16.24 and 16.25). The greater omentum can be quite variable in size and sometimes takes on a mass-like configuration (Fig.

16.26). In some patients, the anterior and posterior layers of the greater omentum do not fuse, allowing fluid from the lesser sac to dissect inferiorly mimicking an omental mass (Fig. 16.27). On occasion, infarction of the omentum will take on the appearance of a peritoneal mass (Fig. 16.28). A similar confusing appearance may occur when the omentum (the abdominal policeman) is recruited in the isolation of an intra-abdominal infection, giving the omentum a mass-like appearance reminiscent of a tumor (Fig. 16.29). Any calcification in the omentum should be suspected of being malignant in origin (Fig. 16.30). The peritoneum communicates with the lesser sac (anteriorly bounded by stomach and posteriorly by peritoneum over the pancreas) through the foramen of Winslow (epiploic foramen) (13). Fluid collection in the lesser sac may be mistaken for tumors (Fig. 16.31). The caudate lobe of the

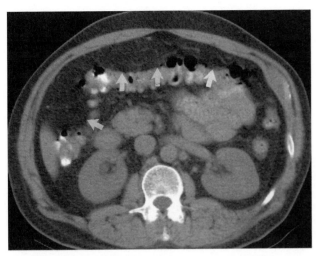

FIG. 16.24. Normal omentum. The omentum *(white arrows)* is identified as a fat-laden structure located anterior to the transverse colon and permeated by numerous blood vessels. In most patients there is enough fat within the omentum to cause separation of the colon from the anterior abdominal wall. The omentum should be carefully scrutinized in all patients, as it is a common site for metastases as well as for infection.

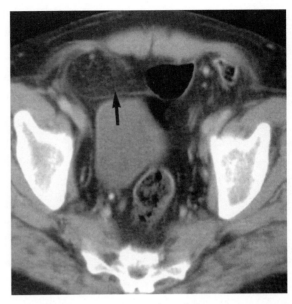

FIG. 16.26. Ball-like configuration of the greater omentum *(black arrow),* which extended into a large right inguinal hernia. This mass could be differentiated from a lipomatous tumor by evaluating the progression of the omentum into the inguinal sac. (Courtesy Dr. Ali Shirkhoda.)

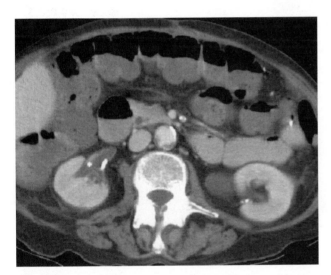

FIG. 16.25. Patient with ovarian cancer who has undergone an omentectomy. The absence of the omentum can be surmised by the close apposition of the transverse colon to the anterior abdominal wall.

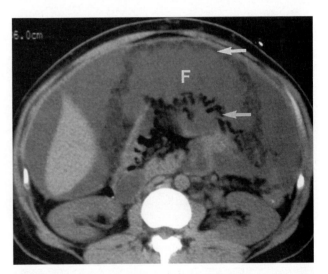

FIG. 16.27. Congenital separation of the anterior and posterior *(arrows)* leaves of the greater omentum. Fluid (F) between these leaves extends inferiorly as a continuation of the lesser peritoneal sac. In this young man with diffuse carcinomatosis, this fluid was misinterpreted as an intra-abdominal mass. The key to the diagnosis is the recognition of the fat contained within the omental apron.

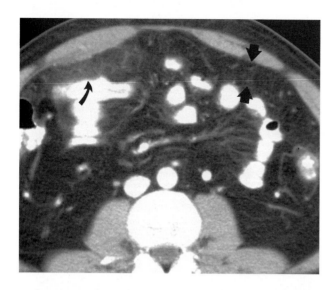

FIG. 16.28. Infarction of the omentum. This patient was admitted with the presumptive diagnosis of appendicitis characterized by right lower quadrant pain and fever. Note the characteristic focal region of omental infiltration *(curved arrow)*. The normal omentum is seen between the *straight black arrows*. There is also spasm of the adjacent right rectus muscle, resulting in asymmetry of the muscles.

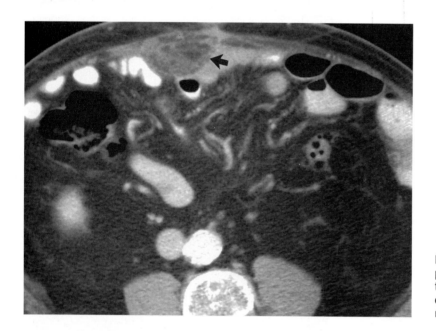

FIG. 16.29. Inflammation of the omentum (in a patient with jejunal perforation) simulates a tumor of the omentum *(arrow)*. The omentum commonly isolates an area of inflammation resulting, in a tumor-like region.

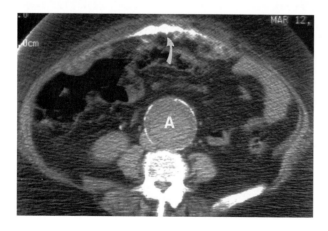

FIG. 16.30. Calcified metastases in the greater omentum mistaken for a calcified abdominal mesh. The patient was being evaluated for an aortic aneurysm (A) and was noted to have calcifications in the region of the anterior peritoneum. At surgery she had diffuse peritoneal carcinomatosis secondary to a serous adenocarcinoma of the ovary.

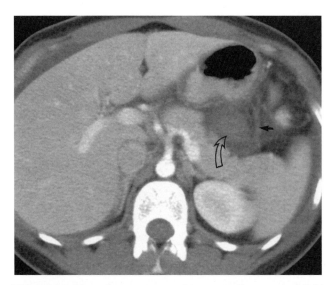

FIG. 16.31. Pseudomass created by a small amount of fluid *(curved arrow)* in the lateral compartment of the lesser sac. Note the gastroepiploic vessels within the gastrosplenic ligament identifying the lateral border of the lesser sac.

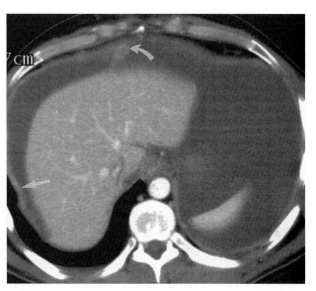

FIG. 16.32. Metastatic adenocarcinoma with seeding of the peritoneal surfaces. There is thickening and irregularity of the peritoneal surface covering the diaphragm *(straight arrow).* In addition, a tumor nodule *(curved arrow)* has lodged on the surface of the falciform ligament.

liver invaginates the superior recess of the lesser sac (14). Fluid collections or masses (see Fig. 16.15) within this recess may mimic intrahepatic masses on sectional images (15).

The Peritoneal Spaces

Peritoneal reflections and mesenteric attachments subdivide the peritoneal cavity into compartments that are well described by Meyers (8). The transverse mesocolon represents a major barrier that divides the abdominal cavity into a supramesocolic and an inframesocolic compartment. The supramesocolic compartment is divided into perihepatic and perisplenic spaces. In the supine patient, the posterior extension of the perihepatic space (Morison's pouch–hepatorenal fossa) is the most dependent recess in the upper abdomen (16). The left coronary and triangular ligaments of the liver separate the left suprahepatic space into anterior and posterior sections (17,18). The posterior left suprahepatic space is located anterosuperior to the lesser sac, separated from it by the lesser omentum and the stomach, and is continuous with the gastrohepatic space inferiorly and the lesser sac (19). The falciform ligament represents a triangular fold of parietal peritoneum raised by the obliterated umbilical vein that ascends from the umbilicus to the anterior surface of the liver. As it divides the prehepatic space, it may serve as a barrier to fluid and free air and as a site of deposition of metastatic disease (20) (Figs. 16.32 and 16.33).

The inframesocolic compartment is further divided into the smaller right infracolic space and the larger left infracolic space by the obliquely oriented root of the small bowel mesentery (8,13,16,17). The right infracolic

space is bounded inferiorly by the cecum and terminal ileum junction. The left infracolic space is open toward the pelvis. The right paracolic gutter is continuous superiorly with the right perihepatic space and the right subphrenic space. In contrast, the left paracolic gutter is separated from the left subphrenic space by the presence of the phrenicocolic ligament. The superior and inferior

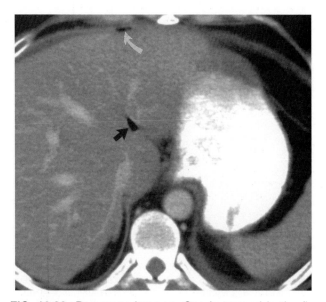

FIG. 16.33. Pneumoperitoneum. Gas is trapped in the fissure for the ligamentum venosum *(black arrow).* A small gas collection is also trapped to the left of the falciform ligament *(white arrow),* where there is fluid to its right. (Courtesy Dr. Ali Shirkhoda.)

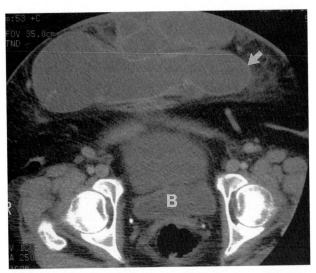

FIG. 16.34. Massive intraperitoneal fluid within a large pannus mimicking dilated fluid-filled loops of small intestine. A pendulous abdomen can lead to abnormal configurations, which may be especially troublesome, when the fluid is loculated by extensive septa, as was seen in this case. Free fluid is seen anterior to the bladder (B).

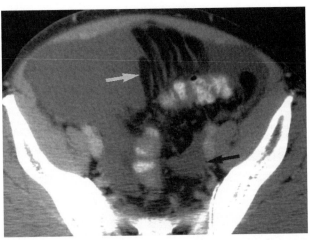

FIG. 16.36. Fat-laden appendices epiploicae *(white arrow)* floating within extensive ascites. Fluid is noted to extend between the individual appendices. The intersigmoid fossa is filled with fluid *(black arrow)*.

ileocecal recesses are located above and below the terminal ileum, respectively. The intersigmoid recess is situated along the undersurface of sigmoid mesocolon. Intraperitoneal compartments extend posteriorly to the posterior subhepatic or hepatorenal space, the retropancreatic recess, the paracolic gutters, and the pararectal fossae. Fluid collections in these locations may mimic

retroperitoneal masses. In addition, when large amounts of fluid are present in the peritoneal cavity, structures that are usually not visible may sometimes become prominent (Figs. 16.34 and 16.35). This is exemplified by appendices epiploicae, which are seen to float within ascites (Fig. 16.36). On the other hand, it is important to be certain when identifying generalized density as fluid that one is not dealing with a diffuse permeation of cellular elements such as malignant lymphomatosis (peritoneal or

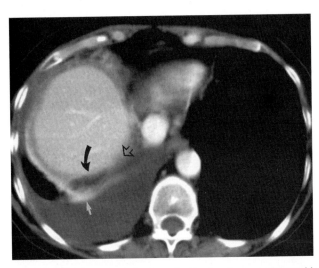

FIG. 16.35. Ascites and pleural effusion in a patient with ovarian carcinomatosis. Fat within the bare area of the liver *(curved arrow)* is visualized as intraperitoneal fluid defines its right lateral border. A pleural effusion defines the right diaphragm *(open arrow)*. Fluid is prevented from reaching the bare area of the liver because of the presence of the right and left coronary ligaments. Right lower lobe compressive atelectasis is also present *(small white arrow)*.

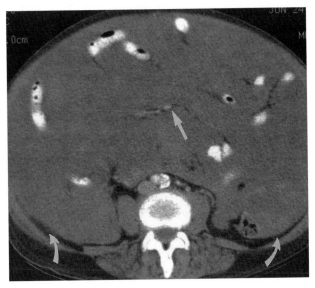

FIG. 16.37. Intraperitoneal lymphomatosis mimicking ascites. In this patient with generalized primary intraperitoneal lymphomatosis, there is compression of multiple loops of small intestine and their respective mesenteries *(straight arrow)*. The high density of the cellular infiltrate as well as its mass effect, which compresses the posterior pararenal spaces *(curved arrows)* differentiates this from free fluid within the peritoneal cavity.

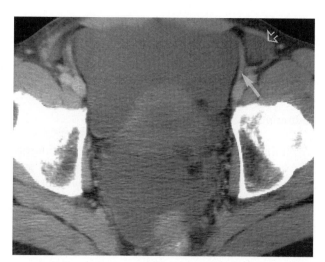

FIG. 16.38. Inguinal fossa fluid mimicking a mass *(open arrow)*. Fluid in the medial or in the lateral compartment of the inguinal fossa can often mimic a mass or an extraperitoneal process. The correct diagnosis is established by identifying the inferior epigastric artery *(arrow),* surrounded by fat, which defines the medial border of the fluid collection.

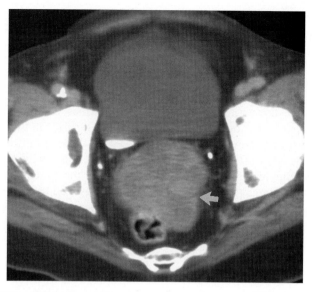

FIG. 16.40. Dropped metastases *(arrow)* in the pouch of Douglas.

retroperitoneal) (Fig. 16.37). In such circumstances, intravenous contrast administration as well as measurements of Hounsfield units may be helpful.

The pelvis, which is anatomically continuous with the paracolic gutters, forms the most dependent portion of the peritoneal cavity. The pelvic peritoneal cavity is subdivided into the midline pouch of Douglas (rectovaginal pouch in women, rectovesical pouch in men), the lateral paravesical recesses, and the medial and lateral inguinal fossae (Fig. 16.38).

Ascitic fluid and, by inference, other pathologic fluids follow predictable patterns of flow that direct physicians in their evaluation of abnormal processes (8,13). Because of the deep and dependent nature of the pelvic peritoneal cavity, many infections (Fig. 16.39) and half of all seeded metastases will involve the pouch of Douglas (Fig. 16.40). Fluid then flows preferentially to the right lower quadrant to the inferior portion of the small bowel mesentery and right paracolic gutter. Fluid may also extend on the left side to involve the superior sigmoid mesocolon. On the right side, fluid will then pass to the posterior subhepatic space and subsequently to a subdiaphragmatic location. It is important to recognize these preferred sites

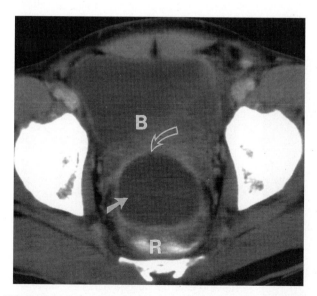

FIG. 16.39. Large abscess *(solid arrow)* in the pouch of Douglas. Note the tiny gas collection *(open arrow)* that characterizes this fluid collection as an abscess. There is marked compression of the rectum (R). B, urinary bladder.

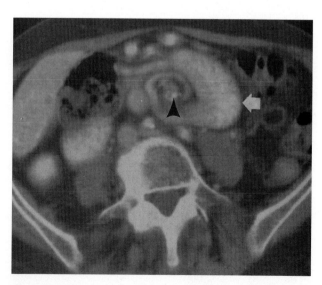

FIG. 16.41. Malrotation of the small intestine *(white arrow),* which is noted to swirl around the superior mesenteric artery *(arrowhead).*

of malignant deposits, infection, and fluid accumulation in order not to overlook their pathologic significance. Optimal opacification of the bowel lumen will help in isolating lesions and in differentiating them from normal unopacified structures.

Embryonic development and rotation of the gut determine the peritoneal relationship to various abdominal organs. An abnormal alignment of the superior mesenteric artery and vein as well as a swirl of the small intestine (Fig. 16.41) can suggest rotation abnormalities. Incomplete fusion of the mesentery of the ascending colon to the posterior abdominal wall may lead to bowel obstruction or volvulus. Abnormal peritoneal bands (Ladd bands), which are associated with abnormal gut rotation, may cause proximal bowel obstruction. A failure in the development of mesenteric lymphatic tissue may result in lymphangiectasia and possibly lymphangioma.

Abdominal Hernias

Abnormal congenital or acquired openings in structures surrounding the peritoneum can result in the development of a wide variety of abdominal hernias. These are typically classified as internal or external hernias (21–24). External hernias, which protrude through a defect of the abdominal wall, are more common. They

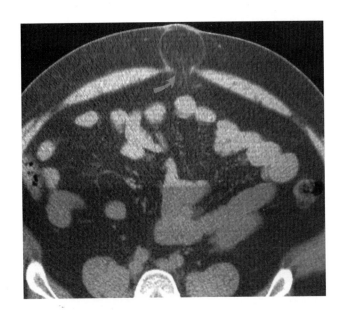

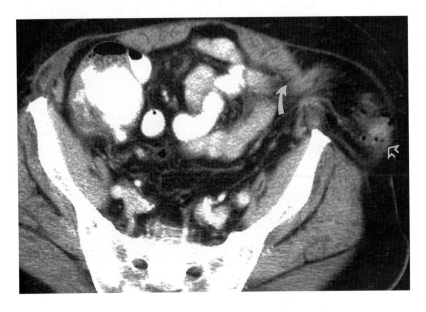

FIG. 16.42. Herniation of the omentum *(arrow)* into a small umbilical hernia. Small omental vessels are noted to pass into the hernial sac. It is important not to overlook such small hernias, as they may cause cryptic abdominal pain and omental infarction.

FIG. 16.43. Spigelian hernia. Herniation of the colon *(open arrow)* along the linea semilunaris *(curved arrow)* at the aponeurotic union of the transverse abdominal and internal and external oblique muscles. This hernia is caused by a congenital weakness of the posterior layer of the transversalis fascia and is usually located at the level of the iliac crest.

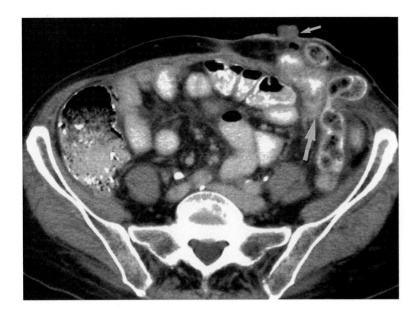

FIG. 16.44. Incisional hernia adjacent to a colostomy *(small white arrow)*. Loops of small intestine *(large arrow)* are noted to herniate adjacent to the colon. These types of hernias can be difficult to identify clinically and are ideally visualized by CT.

contain a wide variety of abdominal tissues such as properitoneal fat, the greater omentum, loops of bowel, and visceral organs surrounded by peritoneum. When the herniated elements are composed primarily of fat, they may mimic a fatty tumor (Fig. 16.42) or lead to a clinically occult infarction. Small hernias are important to recognize, as they are difficult to diagnose clinically and may result in obstruction, ischemia, or perforation. Abdominal wall hernias include umbilical (see Fig. 16.42), Spigelian (Fig. 16.43), incisional (Fig. 16.44), inguinal (indirect and direct) (Fig. 16.45), femoral (Fig. 16.46), perineal (Fig. 16.47), obturator, sciatic, Petit's (Fig. 16.48), and Grynfeltt's hernias (25–27). Richter hernias represent hernias in which one wall of the bowel pro-

trudes through the opening. They are usually not associated with obstruction but may cause abdominal pain, vascular compromise and perforation. Hernias need to be differentiated from other anatomic structures that have a similar appearance. Knowing the anatomic location of these abnormalities can help in establishing the proper diagnosis (29) and avoiding pitfalls (Fig. 16.49).

Internal hernias involve protrusion of the bowel through the peritoneum or mesentery into an abdominal cavity. Fifty percent of internal hernias are paraduodenal

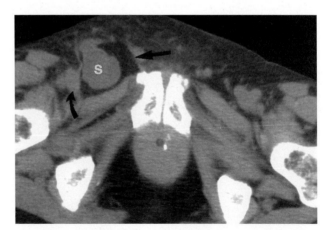

FIG. 16.46. Surgically proven femoral hernia in a patient with small bowel obstruction. The hernial sac *(arrow)* contains properitoneal fat and a loop of small bowel (S). The femoral vein *(curved arrow)* is displaced laterally. A femoral hernia can be distinguished from an inguinal hernia by recognition that the neck of the femoral hernia is below the inguinal ligament and lateral to the pubic tubercle. Femoral hernias are important to identify because they are difficult to diagnose clinically and are more likely to incarcerate and strangulate.

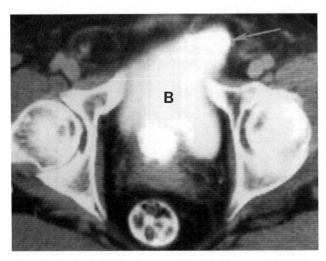

FIG. 16.45. Herniation of the urinary bladder (B) into the left inguinal canal *(arrow)*.

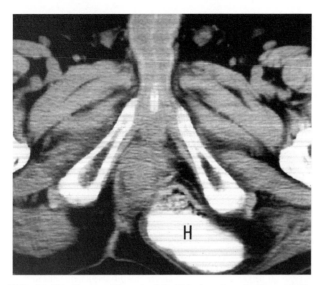

FIG. 16.47. Perineal hernia (H). This is a hernia through the urogenital diaphragm. It is associated with defects in the levator ani or coccygeus muscles. The large hernia in the left ischiorectal fossa is displacing the rectum to the right.

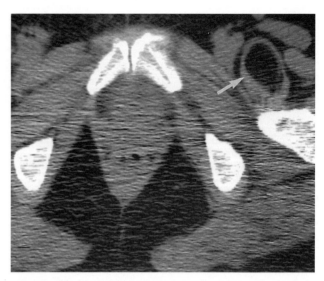

FIG. 16.49. Fat in the iliopsoas bursa. This was originally misdiagnosed as a femoral hernia.

in location (Figs. 16.50 and 16.51). These hernias can be very difficult to diagnose clinically, and patients often have symptoms for years before the correct diagnosis is made. Other internal hernias are classified as pericecal, transmesenteric, supravesical, sigmoid, and retropancre-

atic colonic (Fig. 16.52), depending on the anatomic location of the herniation (28). Fluid commonly collects in the sigmoid fossa and may take on the appearance of a mass or hernia (Fig. 16.53). The diaphragm as it separates the abdomen from the chest is pierced by the aorta, the

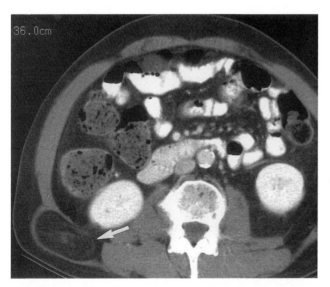

FIG. 16.48. Petit's hernia *(arrow)*. This inferior lumbar hernia is bordered inferiorly by the iliac crest, posteriorly by the latissimus dorsi muscle, and anteriorly by the external oblique muscle. A Grynfeltt's (superior) lumbar hernia is found inferior to the 12th rib.

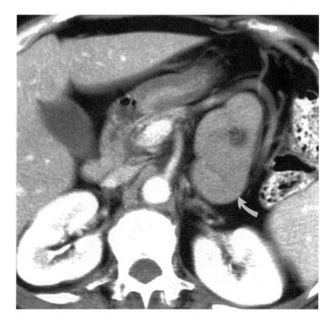

FIG. 16.50. Left paraduodenal hernia into the fossa of Landzert. The herniated loops of jejunum *(curved arrow)* lie behind the inferior mesenteric vein. The herniated bowel is noted to lie medial to the descending colon, explaining why these hernias are referred to as mesocolic hernias by surgeons.

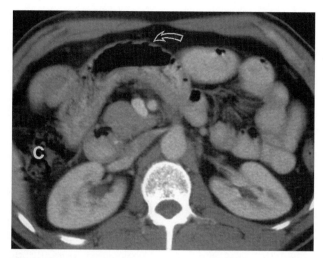

FIG. 16.51. Right paraduodenal hernia. Herniated loops of jejunum *(curved arrow)* extend within the right mesocolon to the ascending colon (C).

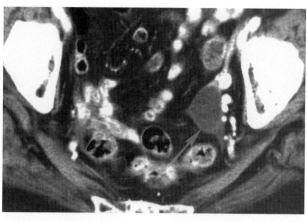

FIG. 16.53. Collection of fluid *(white arrow)* in the intersigmoid fossa simulates a cystic mass lesion in the pelvis. The correct interpretation rests on the triangular configuration of the mass, which is typical of fluid trapped by the sigmoid mesentery. On occasion a laterally placed normal ovary will have a similar appearance.

vena cava, and the esophagus. Herniation of retroperitoneal and abdominal contents through the diaphragm into the chest is not uncommon.

In addition herniation through the foramen of Bochdalek (Fig. 16.54) are seen posteriorly, and herniation through the foramen of Morgagni (Fig. 16.55) may

be seen anteriorly. These can sometimes be mistaken for mesenchymal tumors.

Abnormal body configurations and alignments such as seen in scoliosis may create unusual appearances, which may be especially difficult to interpret on cross-sectional imaging (Fig. 16.56). Reformatting these images may be helpful in establishing a proper diagnosis.

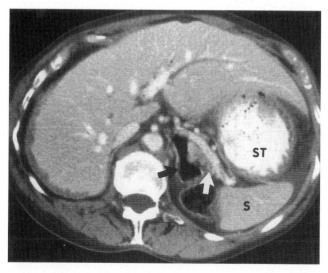

FIG. 16.52. Retropancreatic herniation of the colon. The colon *(black arrow)* is noted posterior to the pancreas *(white arrow)*. This was caused by a congenital internal herniation. Note also the irregular notching of the liver surface secondary to ovarian carcinomatosis. S, spleen; ST, stomach.

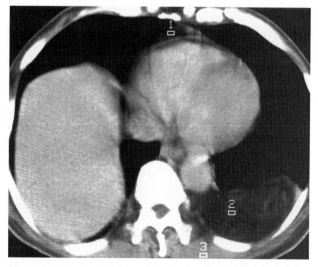

FIG. 16.54. Bochdalek hernia. A large amount of retroperitoneal fat (2) is noted to pass through the foramen of Bochdalek. Vessels throughout the fat as well as the irregular outer border indicate that this represents a hernia rather than a lipomatous tumor.

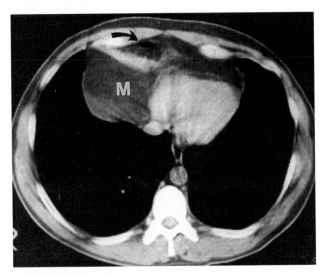

FIG. 16.55. Morgagni hernia. The omentum (M) and the colon *(arrow)* have herniated into the chest.

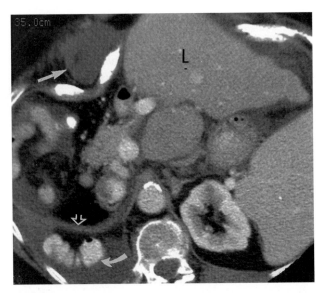

FIG. 16.56. Marked thoracolumbar scoliosis creating a pseudoherniation of the right lateral abdominal wall. A collection of ascitic fluid *(straight arrow)* is noted lateral to the ribs. The liver (L) is displaced medially. The deformity is so severe that it has also caused the colon *(curved arrow)* to protrude behind the diaphragm *(open arrow)*.

ANATOMY OF THE RETROPERITONEUM

The retroperitoneum is bounded anteriorly by the peritoneum, posteriorly by the spine and psoas and quadratus lumborum muscles, superiorly by the 12th ribs and diaphragm attachments, and inferiorly by the pelvic rim. Important structures within the retroperitoneum include the kidneys, ureters, adrenals, pancreas, duodenum, ascending and descending colon, abdominal aorta, inferior vena cava, lymphatics, and nerves. In interpreting abnormalities of the retroperitoneum, it is important to

remember that slowly developing processes tend to remain within the space of origin, whereas rapidly accumulating collections, as seen in acute hemorrhage, can extend into expandable potential compartments that are not normally evident (30).

The retroperitoneum is traditionally divided into three compartments (Fig. 16.57). The anterior pararenal space contains the ascending and descending portions of the colon, the duodenum, and the pancreas. It extends between the posterior parietal peritoneum and the anterior renal fascia and is bounded laterally by the lateroconal fascia. The perirenal space contains a large amount of fat that permits good visualization of the kidneys and adrenal glands (31,32). It is discontinuous across the midline because of fusion of the renal fascial layers with connective tissues around the aorta and inferior vena cava. Inferiorly, the perirenal space is open and forms an inverted cone. The ureter, surrounded by fat, passes through its apex (33). The posterior pararenal space is continuous with the properitoneal fat and contains no organs. It is a potential space filled with fat that is outlined anteriorly by the posterior renal fascia, posteriorly by the transversalis fascia, and

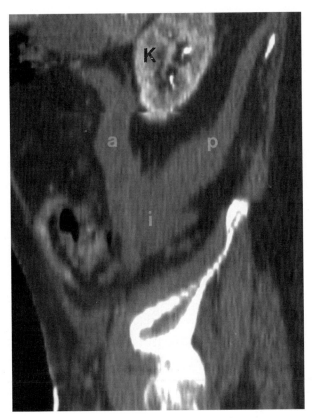

FIG. 16.57. The fluid-filled infraconal space (I) is noted to represent a continuation of the anterior pararenal space (a) and the posterior pararenal space (p). The perirenal space is clearly identified by fat that extends anterior and posterior to the kidney (k). Abnormal processes that begin in one of the usual retroperitoneal compartments can migrate inferiorly and at the inferior cone of renal fascia converge to create a mass.

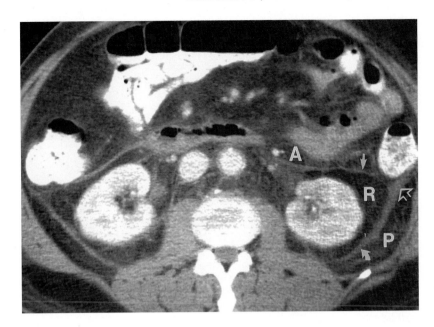

FIG. 16.58. Thickening of Gerota's *(straight arrow)* and Zuckerkandl's *(curved arrow)* fascias secondary to prior pancreatitis. The lateroconal fascia *(open arrow)* is also thickened. At the time of the study the patient did not have any symptoms referable to the prior inflammation. R, perirenal space; P, posterior pararenal space; A, anterior pararenal space.

medially is bounded by the psoas and quadratus lumborum muscles. The infraconal compartment is the caudal continuation of the anterior and posterior pararenal spaces (33). On computed tomography, retroperitoneal fascial planes are visible in virtually all patients, becoming more evident with advancing age. Thickening of these tissues usually indicates evidence of a prior pathologic process but should not be misinterpreted as a sign of active disease (Fig. 16.58).

Retromesenteric planes have also been described (30). These lie anterior to the anterior pararenal space, extending superiorly to the diaphragm near the esophageal hiatus, inferiorly to the pelvis along the anterolateral surface of the psoas muscle, and laterally, running along the posterior surface of the descending colon (30). The anterior interfascial space (most commonly involved in pancreatitis) is the space between the anterior pararenal space and

the anterior renal fascia (30). The posterior interfascial space (most commonly involved in renal hemorrhage, urinoma, or ruptured aortic aneurysm) is between the posterior pararenal space and the perirenal space. Fluid, when it dissects these interfascial planes, may be mistaken for inflammation (Fig. 16.59) or even a tumor. The three primary retroperitoneal spaces merge superiorly under the diaphragm. The anterior pararenal space is contiguous with the bare area of the liver as defined by the coronary ligaments. Large amounts of fat can sometimes be seen in this region displacing the liver anteriorly (Fig. 16.60), thus mimicking a fatty tumor.

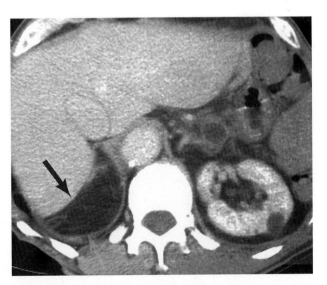

FIG. 16.60. Extensive retroperitoneal fat *(white arrow)* extending behind the liver. The bare area *(black arrow)* of the liver is in continuity with the retroperitoneal compartments and can serve as a two-way conduit for the spread of diseases between the liver and the retroperitoneal compartments.

FIG. 16.59. Interfascial compartment fluid *(curved arrow)* secondary to an adrenal hemorrhage. Blood is also noted adjacent to the psoas muscle *(black arrow).*

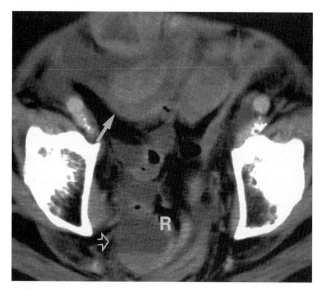

FIG. 16.61. Extraperitoneal hemorrhage after femoral artery catheterization. A large collection of blood is noted in the prevesical space *(arrow),* with dissection along the paravesical space posteriorly *(open arrow)* displacing the rectum (R) to the left.

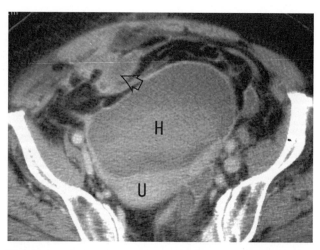

FIG. 16.62. Subperitoneal perivesical hematoma secondary to surgery for an ovarian tumor. The high-density fluid collection (H) is noted to be compressing the uterus (U) posteriorly and splaying the broad ligaments bilaterally. Extraperitoneal fluid collections can readily mimic intraperitoneal masses but can usually be identified by their spread to other extraperitoneal fluid compartments. In this case blood is noted to dissect anterior to the prevesical space *(arrow).*

The pelvic extraperitoneal compartments, although not as well known as the retroperitoneal spaces, are critically important for understanding the appearance of diseases in the pelvis. The prevesical space (space of Retzius) is an extraperitoneal compartment bounded posteriorly by the umbilicovesical fascia that contains the obliterated umbilical arteries (33–35) (Figs. 16.61 and 16.62). This space may hold up to 3,000 ml of fluid. Posterior to this fascia is the perivesical space that contains the bladder and the urachus. The intraperitoneal *cul-de-sac* separates the posterior perivesical space from the rectum. The paravesical space (lateral pathway) lies between the pelvic wall and the visceral pelvic fascia. Fluid col-

lections are common in this space, especially after femoral catheterization, and are usually oblong in shape (Fig. 16.63). They need to be carefully differentiated from regional adenopathy. The extraperitoneal tissues are currently felt to represent a subperitoneal continuum with pathways between tissues such as the retroperitoneal spaces, the mesenteries, the extraperitoneal pelvis, the bare area of the liver, and others. Disease processes such as hemorrhage, inflammation, or tumor spread along these conduits to remote sites (35) (see Figs. 16.10 and 16.64). For example, an extraperitoneal bladder rupture may dissect from the perivesical tissues into the lateral pelvic pathway, then via the anterior pararenal space to

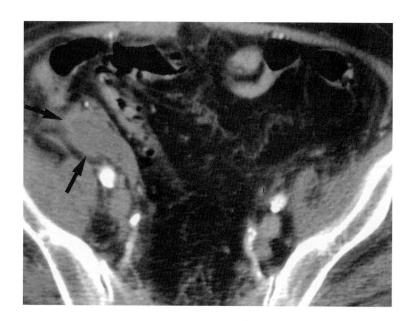

FIG. 16.63. Mass in the right paravesical space *(black arrows)* caused by hemorrhage secondary to a recent femoral artery catheterization. This type of mass can sometimes be difficult to differentiate from adenopathy, although the latter would usually be more nodular and localized.

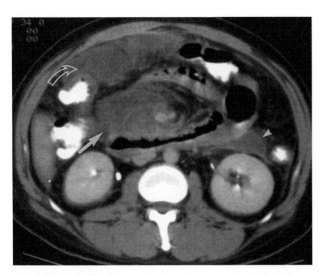

FIG. 16.64. Spread of pancreatitis through the subperitoneal compartments. In addition to inflammation of the anterior pararenal space *(arrowhead),* there is extension of the pancreatic exudate into the small bowel mesentery *(straight arrow)* and into the transverse mesocolon-omentum *(curved arrow).*

the retropancreatic paraduodenal space. Alternatively, using the same pathway, a tumor such as a neuroblastoma or lymphangioma (originating above the kidneys) may spread to the extraperitoneal inguinal region. For a complete understanding of these pathways, the reader is referred to the works of Oliphant, Berne, and Meyers (36,37).

REFERENCES

1. Shirkhoda A. Diagnostic pitfalls in abdominal CT. *RadioGraphics* 1991;11:969–1002.
2. Malone AJ Jr, Wolf CR, Malmed AS, Melliere BF. Diagnosis of acute appendicitis: value of unenhanced CT. *Am J Roentgenol* 1993;160(4): 763–766.
3. Rao PM, Rhea JT, Noveline RA, et al. Helical CT technique for the diagnosis of appendicitis: prospective evaluation of a focused appendix CT examination. *Radiology* 1997;202(1):139–144.
4. Balthazar EJ, Birnbaum BA, Yee J, Megibow AJ, Roshkow J, Gray C. Acute appendicitis: CT and US correlation in 100 patients. *Radiology* 1994;190(1):31–35.
5. Lane MJ, Katz DS, Ross BA, Clautice-Engle TL, Mindelzun RE, Jeffrey RB Jr. Unenhanced helical CT for suspected acute appendicitis. *Am J Roentgenol* 1997;168(2):405–409.
6. Putz R, Pabst R, eds. *Sobotta atlas of human anatomy, 12th ed, vol 2.* Baltimore: Williams & Wilkins, 1996;130–259.
7. DeMeo JH, Fulcher AS, Austin RF Jr. Anatomic CT demonstration of the peritoneal spaces, ligaments, and mesenteries: normal and pathologic processes. *RadioGraphics* 1995;15(4):755–770.
8. Meyers MA. *Dynamic radiology of the abdomen: normal and pathologic anatomy, 4th ed.* New York: Springer-Verlag, 1994;55–57,170–171.
9. Mindelzun RE. Diseases of the mesenteries. In: Ferrucci J, ed. *Radiology: diagnosis, imaging, intervention, vol 48.* Philadelphia: JB Lippincott, 1997;1–11.
10. Sivit CJ. CT of mesentery-omentum peritoneum. *Radiol Clin North Am* 1996;34(4):863–884.
11. Balfe DM, Mauro MA, Koehler RE. Gastrohepatic ligament: normal and pathologic CT anatomy. *Radiology* 1984;150:485–490.
12. Sompayrac SW, Mindelzun RE, Silverman PM, Sze R. The greater omentum. *Am J Roentgenol* 1997;168:683–687.
13. Meyers MA. Peritoneography. Normal and pathologic anatomy. *Am J Roentgenol Radiol Ther Nucl Med* 1973;117(2):353–365.
14. Jeffrey RB, Federle MP, Goodman PC. Computed tomography of the lesser peritoneal sac. *Radiology* 1981;141(1):117–122.
15. Dodds WJ, Foley WD, Lawson TL, Stewart ET, Taylor A. Anatomy and imaging of the lesser peritoneal sac. *Am J Roentgenol* 1985;144(3): 567–575.
16. Rubenstein WA, Auh YH, Zirinsky K, Kneeland JB, Whalen JP, Kazam E. Posterior peritoneal recesses: assessment using CT. *Radiology* 1985; 156(2):461–468.
17. Chiu LC, Yiu VS, Schapiro RL. A primer in computed tomographic anatomy. VII. Peritoneal and extraperitoneal compartments, spaces, and fasciae. *J Comput Assist Tomogr* 1979;3(1):57–74.
18. Chou CK, Liu GC, Chen LT, Jaw TS. MRI demonstration of peritoneal ligaments and mesenteries. *Abdom Imag* 1993;18(2):126–130.
19. Min PQ, Yang ZG, Lei QF, et al. Peritoneal reflections of left perihepatic region: Radiologic–anatomic study. *Radiology* 1992;182(2):553–557.
20. Rubenstein WA, Auh YH, Whalen JP, Kazam E. The perihepatic spaces: computed tomographic and ultrasound imaging. *Radiology* 1983; 149(1):231–239.
21. Nyhus LM, Condon RE, eds. *Hernia, 3rd ed.* Philadelphia: JB Lippincott, 1989.
22. Miller PA, Mezwa DG, Feczko PJ, Jafri ZH, Madrazo BL. Imaging of abdominal hernias. *RadioGraphics* 1995;15(2):333–347.
23. Stamm ER, Pretorius DH, Olson LK. Abdominal wall CT: a pictorial essay. *Comput Radiol* 1985;9(5):271–278.
24. Zarvan NP, Lee FT Jr, Yandow DR, Unger JS. Abdominal hernias: CT findings. *Am J Roentgenol* 1995;164(6):1391–1395.
25. Ghahremani GG, Jimenez MA, Rosenfeld M, Rochester D. CT diagnosis of occult incisional hernias. *Am J Roentgenol* 1987;148:139–142.
26. Lubat E, Gordon RB, Birnbaum BA, et al. CT diagnosis of posterior perineal hernia. *Am J Roentgenol* 1990;154:761–762.
27. Chenoweth J, Vas W. Computed tomography demonstration of inferior lumbar (Petit's) hernia. *Clin Imag* 1989;13:164–166.
28. Estrada RL, Mindelzun RE. The retropancreatic colon: a congenital anomaly. *Abdom Imag* 1997;22(4):426–428.
29. Steinbach LS, Schneider R, Golman AB, Kazam E, Ranawat CS, Ghelman B. Bursae and abscess cavities communicating with the hip. Diagnosis using arthrography and CT. *Radiology* 1985:156(2):303–307.
30. Molmenti EP, Balfe DM, Kanterman RY, Bennett HF. Anatomy of the retroperitoneum: observations of the distribution of pathologic fluid collections. *Radiology* 1996;200(1):95–103.
31. Beaulieu CF, Mindelzun RE, Dolf J, Jeffrey RB. The infraconal compartment: a multidirectional pathway for spread of disease between the extraperitoneal abdomen and pelvis. *J Comput Assist Tomogr* 1997; 21(2):223–228.
32. Auh YH, Rubenstein WA, Markisz JA, Zirinsky K, Whalen JP, Kazam E. Intraperitoneal paravesical spaces: CT delineation with US correlation. *Radiology* 1986;159(2):311–328.
33. Bechtold RE, Dyer RB, Zagoria RJ, Chen MYM. The perirenal space: relationship of pathologic processes to normal retroperitoneal anatomy. *RadioGraphics* 1996;16:841–854.
34. Raptopoulos V, Touliopoulos P, Lei QF, Vrachliotis TG, Marks SC Jr. Medial border of the perirenal space: CT and anatomic correlation. *Radiology* 1997;205:777–784.
35. Roy C. The extraperitoneal paravesical pelvic spaces. In Meyers MA, ed. *Dynamic radiology of the abdomen, 4th ed.* Springer Verlag, New York 1994;332–335.
36. Oliphant M, Berne M, Meyers MA. The subperitoneal spaces of the abdomen and pelvis: planes of continuity. *Am J Roentgenol* 1996: 167(6):1433–1439.
37. Oliphant M, Berne AS, Meyers MA. Bi-directional spread of disease via the subperitoneal space: the lower abdomen and left pelvic. *Abdom Imag* 1993;18(2):117–125.

Variants and Pitfalls in Body Imaging,
edited by Ali Shirkhoda.
Lippincott Williams & Wilkins, Philadelphia, © 2000.

CHAPTER 17

The Kidneys

Marco A. Amendola

Variations of renal anatomy and development as well as technical artifacts inherent to the different imaging techniques used to evaluate the kidneys may present diagnostic problems and potential pitfalls. In many situations a complementary study with a different imaging modality will clarify the issue (Fig. 17.1). In other instances recognition of an artifact may prompt a change or modification of the technique in the same examination that may resolve the problem. In this chapter, the discussion is limited to ultrasound (US), computed tomography (CT), and magnetic resonance imaging (MRI), with mention of other complementary studies only where appropriate.

EMBRYOLOGIC CONSIDERATIONS

The permanent kidney develops from repeated branching of the ureteric bud and differentiation of its surrounding metanephric blastema. In the human embryo, the kidney is made of the summation of multiple separate small kidneys or renunculi, each of which has its own cortex and medulla and drains into a separate calyx (1). This fetal renunculus is the future renal lobe. Hodson described the renal lobe as a central mass of medullary tissue enveloped by a cortical layer on all sides except where the papilla emerges (1). In the human fetus, these lobes are well demarcated by sulci, first visible with the naked eye at 10 weeks of gestational age. Fusion of these lobes occurs during the late second trimester, with the apposing portions of the cortex of two adjacent renunculi forming the cloisons, septa, or columns of Bertin (2). As fusion of the lobes progresses in infancy, the renal surface becomes smoother, and the interlobar grooves are less prominent.

M. A. Amendola: Department of Radiology, University of Miami School of Medicine, Miami, Florida 33101.

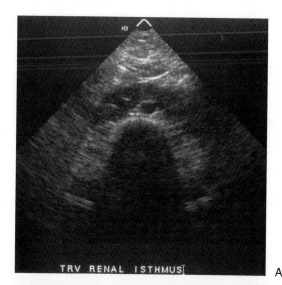

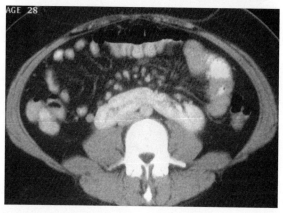

FIG. 17.1. Horseshoe kidney. **A:** Transverse ultrasound of horseshoe kidney simulating a midline retroperitoneal mass or adenopathy surrounding the aorta. **B:** Contrast-enhanced CT scan readily clarifies the anatomy. (Case courtesy of Dr. A. Shirkhoda, William Beaumont Hospital.)

ANATOMIC VARIANTS

Persistent Fetal Lobation

In some individuals, one or more renal interlobar grooves persist throughout childhood and into adult age. These remnants of the fusion of fetal renunculi can be mistaken for renal scars or tumors at renal imaging. However, interlobar grooves are sharply defined markings, linear on sagittal and triangular on cross-sectional views of the kidneys. They are located in the center of a column of Bertin and surrounded on either side by cortex that is of normal thickness when studied with US, CT, or MRI and of normal echogenicity when studied with sonography. In contrast, renal scars are thicker, less sharply defined, and always accompanied by loss of cortex (2). Radionuclide studies using cortical agents and possibly power Doppler ultrasound may show poor perfusion beneath scars (3). In addition, the indentations in the surface of the kidney produced by fetal lobation lie between the renal pyramids or calyces, unlike scars that lie directly over the calyces.

Junctional Parenchymal Defects

Anatomic variants closely related to persistent fetal lobation include the so-called parenchymal junctional defect and the interrenicular junction (4,5). In this situation, a prominent indentation of the renal surface incorporates perirenal fat and invaginates the anterior surface of the upper third of the kidney toward the hilum, representing the most visible remnant of fetal lobation. On CT scans, as one follows the direction of the renal sinus on axial sections from upper to lower pole, the renal sinus turns from an oblique anteroposterior axis to a horizontal one (Fig. 17.2). At the site of fusion of these two masses of metanephric blastema, a roughly triangular echogenic

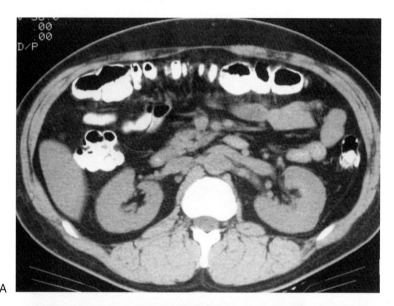

A

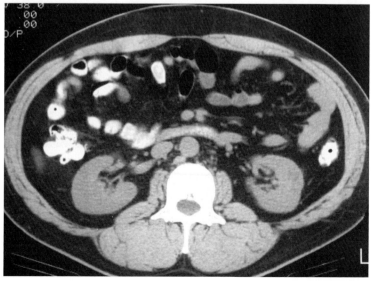

B

FIG. 17.2. Junctional parenchymal defect on CT. Depiction of junctional parenchymal defect in consecutive axial CT scans. Note the change of orientation of the renal sinus turning from an oblique AP axis **(A)** to a more horizontal one from superior to inferior **(B).**

focus or mass can be seen on sagittal ultrasound scans, most commonly in the anterosuperior or posteroinferior margins of the kidney (4). These echogenic foci may simulate cortical renal scars with loss of parenchyma or, when round, may mimic a solid echogenic mass such as a small angiomyolipoma. They have been aptly termed by Carter et al. junctional parenchymal defects (4). In order to differentiate it from pathologic conditions one must rely on its characteristic anterior and superior location and trace it medially and slightly inferiorly into the renal sinus. An interrenicular septum appears as an echogenic line connecting the junctional defect to the renal hilum. The echogenic line that extends from the renal sinus to the perinephric fat has been also called the anterior junction line (6). Because it is oriented more horizontally than vertically, it is best appreciated on sagittal scans (Fig. 17.3). These

findings are three times more frequent in the right side but can be seen in the left kidney, especially in patients with splenomegaly, and they can also be seen in the inferior half of either kidney (4–6). Similar findings can be seen with CT scanning on the left side and in a posteromedial location (Fig. 17.4). A somewhat related pitfall is the one found secondary to surgical filling of renal cortical wedge resections of renal tumors with vascularized retroperitoneal fat. Postoperative appearances at CT simulate angiomyolipomas and at ultrasonography usually hyperechoic or less commonly isoechoic masses (7,8). On sonography the

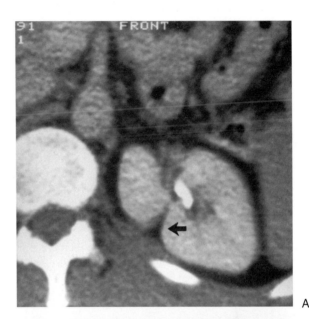

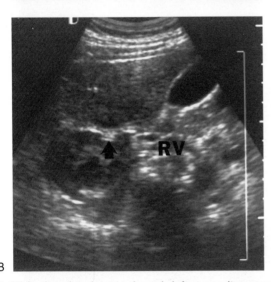

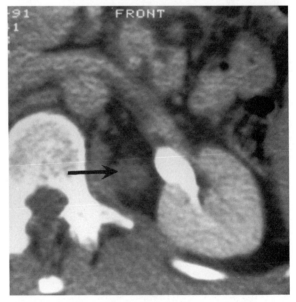

FIG. 17.3. Junctional parenchymal defect on ultrasound. **A:** The sagittal sonogram shows a triangular echogenic focus in the anterior renal parenchyma. **B:** A transverse image at the level of the renal vein (RV) demonstrates the echogenic defect *(arrow)* to be continuous with the anteriorly directed renal sinus.

FIG. 17.4. Junctional defect and hilar lip. **A:** Junctional defect seen in the left kidney posteromedially just inferior to the renal hilus *(arrow)* on a contrast-enhanced CT scan. **B:** On an adjacent axial image, the impression of a small mass medial to the renal pelvis *(arrow)* is created. *Continued on next page.*

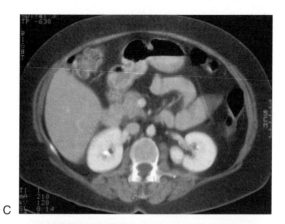

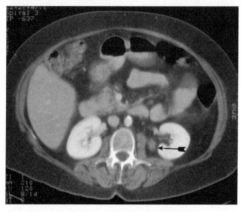

FIG. 17.4. *Continued.* **C:** A CT scan of a different patient demonstrating a left renal hilar lip. **D:** On a slightly inferior CT image, the presence of a lymph node posterior to the renal hilus is simulated *(arrow)*. (Cases courtesy of Dr. A. Shirkhoda, William Beaumont Hospital.)

echogenic lesions are not associated with the renal sinus and therefore can be separated from the normal variants. Knowledge of the prior renal surgery may obviate an unnecessary further work-up.

Renal Hilar Lip

Another example of normal junctional parenchyma creating a potential pitfall is the so-called hilar lip (9). Although this is usually not a problem when found on IVU or angiography, it may present a problem on CT scans because of the usual limitation of this technique to the axial plane. Coronal and sagittal reconstructions could be useful, although they are not usually necessary when one realizes the presence of this normal variant (see Fig. 17.4).

Column of Bertin

The hypertrophic column of Bertin (Fig. 17.5) is a normal variant that has also been termed congenitally large septum of Bertin, cloison, and also lobar dysmorphism (10–16). The column of Bertin consists of normal functioning cortical tissue, extending from the cortex to the renal sinus, that separates the medulla into segments. They were first described in 1744 by the French anatomist Bertin as "cloisons," meaning septa, to indicate internal partitions, although Bertin's word has been mistranslated for many years as "columns." Thanks to Hodson, the original meaning has been restored (1,14). When the cortices of immediately adjacent lobes fuse, they form the septum of Bertin. The most prominent septa occur in the midzone of the kidney, at the junction of the upper pole and the midkidney, where excessive infolding of cortical tissue is most likely to occur. This is the most frequent location of a congenitally

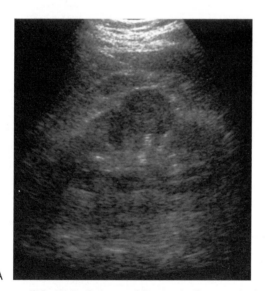

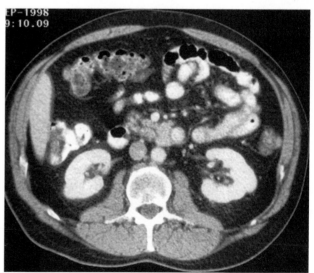

FIG. 17.5. Column of Bertin. **A:** On a sagittal sonogram of the left kidney, it was initially thought to represent a tumor in the midrenal region. **B:** Computed tomography scans through the area show no evidence of tumor, and findings are consistent with a so-called hypertrophic column of Bertin. (Case courtesy of Dr. A. Shirkhoda, William Beaumont Hospital.)

large septum of Bertin and of partial division of a duplex kidney. Partial duplication of the kidney including presence of a bifid pelvis is very common in kidneys with a congenitally large septum of Bertin. This variant is bilateral in 60% of cases. When a mass-like lesion is suspected at sonography, the diagnosis of a column of Bertin can be made with a high degree of certainty when all or most (at least three) of the following criteria are met: (a) the mass is associated with two renal sinus systems, (b) it is located between the overlapping parts of the two renal sinus systems, usually at the junction between the upper one-third and lower two-thirds of the kidney, (c) it contains renal cortex and pyramids of normal size and echo pattern, (d) the renal cortex within junctional parenchyma is demarcated by a junctional parenchymal line and defect, and (e) the renal cortex within junctional parenchyma is continuous with the adjacent renal cortex of the same subkidney (11). Further imaging to demonstrate that the suspected mass really corresponds to normal functioning renal tissue can be obtained using radionuclide scanning, contrast-enhanced CT, or MRI. Power Doppler and contrast Doppler studies may accomplish similar objectives, although this has not yet been fully substantiated in the literature.

Peripelvic Cysts Simulating Hydronephrosis

Peripelvic cysts, also known as renal sinus cysts and thought to be of congenital or lymphatic origin, are usually small and multiple, and although they insinuate in between calyces, they do not cause hydronephrosis. These water-containing structures often mimic hydronephrosis on ultrasound studies because they often parallel the normal calyces and renal pelvis (17). Scanning in a plane that shows the infundibula connecting at the renal hilum may solve the problem. At excretory urography or contrast-enhanced CT, the extraluminal position of these cysts is clearly outlined, and instead of hydronephrosis, an attenuated spidery collection is demonstrated.

Prominent Extrarenal Pelvis Simulating Hydronephrosis

Occasionally a large extrarenal pelvis may be quite prominent and on sonography or CT simulates hydronephrosis and an ureteropelvic junction obstruction. Absence of calyceal dilation on ultrasound and opacification on delayed CT represent a helpful clue.

Hypoechoic Perirenal Fat

The perirenal fat can be variable in amount and in echogenicity from highly echogenic (most often) to relatively hypoechoic (18,19). This is likely related to the number of bridging septa within the perirenal fat (20). Another potential explanation for the occasional hypo- or anechoic sonographic appearance of fat is the presence of pure sebum, known to be liquid at body temperature, with

lack of significant tissue interfaces within it (21). Correlative CT scans have shown that the hypoechoic fat is less dense on CT than the rest of the perirenal fat (18). This has also been documented in certain ovarian cystic teratomas (22). The hypoechoic perinephric fat may be confused with fluid collections. Indicators of hypoechoic fat include the presence of linear, regular internal echoes, lack of posterior wall enhancement, compressibility in real time, lack of mass effect, and common bilaterality around the kidneys (19). When clinically indicated, CT scans may be necessary to differentiate this normal variant from a true pathologic condition.

CONGENITAL ANOMALIES

Congenital renal anomalies represent another category of potential pitfalls in renal imaging. Familiarity with the different congenital anomalies and their diverse presentations is usually sufficient to avoid misinterpretation. Examples illustrated include horseshoe kidney (see Fig. 17.1), cross-fused ectopia (Fig. 17.6), pelvic kidney (Fig. 17.7), and duplication anomalies (Fig. 17.8).

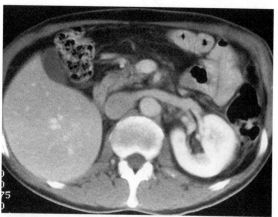

A

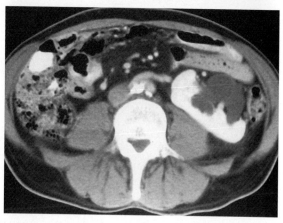

B

FIG. 17.6. Cross-fused ectopia. **A:** The right kidney is not present in the right renal fossa at the level of the left renal vein. Note medial position of the right lobe of the liver occupying the right renal fossa. **B:** At a lower level, the inferior portion of the crossed right kidney, which is fused to the left kidney, is apparent with its anteriorly malrotated renal pelvis. *Continued on next page.*

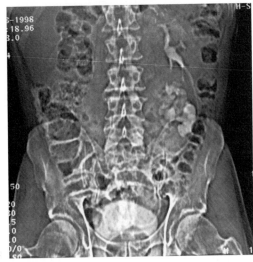

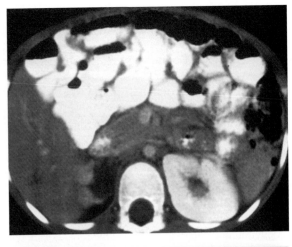

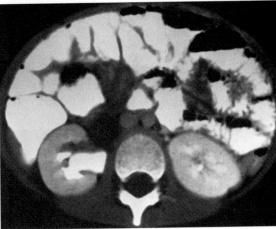

FIG. 17.6. *Continued.* **C:** Digital radiograph from CT scans clarifies the abnormal anatomy. (Case courtesy of Dr. A. Shirkhoda, William Beaumont Hospital.)

FIG. 17.8. Duplication with obstruction. **A:** Duplication anomaly with obstructed upper pole moiety simulating a complex right upper pole cystic mass. **B:** Dilated nonopacified obstructed ureter from the upper pole moiety is seen ventral to opacified pelvicalyceal system of the lower moiety. Figure continues on next page.

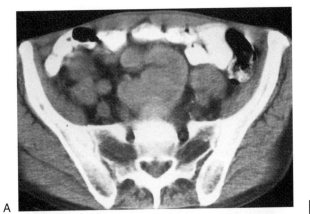

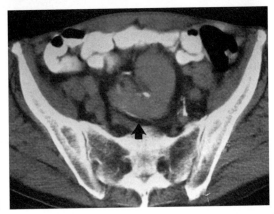

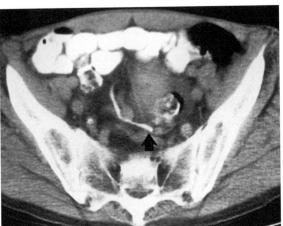

FIG. 17.7. Pelvic kidney. **A:** Centrally placed pelvic kidney simulates a solid pelvic mass on this unenhanced CT image. Faint corticomedullary differentiation is the clue that it represents a pelvic kidney. **B:** Contrast excretion into collecting system and ureter *(arrow)* is present in a delayed scan. **C:** Opacification of the ureter *(arrow)* at the lower level clarifies the real etiology of the mass as a pelvic kidney.

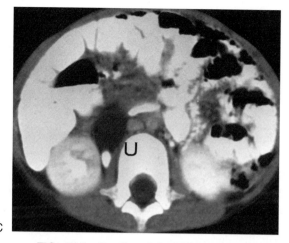

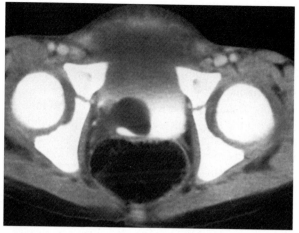

C

D

FIG. 17.8. *Continued.* **C:** Dilated upper ureter (u) anterior to the opacified ureter draining the lower renal moiety. **D:** Filling defect in the right side of the bladder confirming the presence of an ectopic ureterocele from a duplicated ureter draining the obstructed upper pole moiety. (Case courtesy of A. R. Sedaghat, M.D., Teheran, Iran.)

TECHNICAL ARTIFACTS

Sonographic Artifactual Duplication

When the kidney is studied with ultrasound, a common artifact is caused by refraction of the sound beam between the spleen and perisplenic fat, resulting in apparent duplication of upper pole of the kidney. Less often it simulates a suprarenal mass rather than a renal abnormality. The mechanism of production of this artifact and its substantiation using *in vitro* models have been well described by Middleton and Melson (23) and are depicted in Fig. 17.9. A sound beam that enters and exits

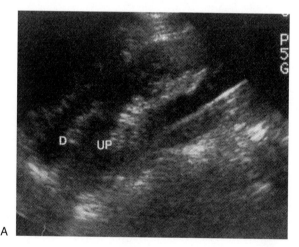

A

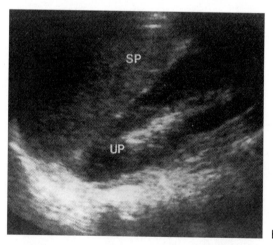

B

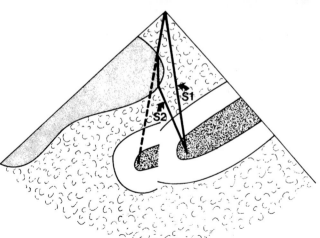

C

FIG. 17.9. Pseudoduplication. **A:** Longitudinal sonogram of the left kidney shows apparent duplication (D) of the upper pole. The spleen is barely seen. **B:** At deep inspiration, and with the transducer positioned so that the spleen covers the entire kidney, the upper pole is displayed correctly without artifactual duplication. UP, upper pole of kidney; SP, spleen. **C:** Drawing showing production of the renal duplication artifact. Sound traveling entirely in fat below the spleen (S$_1$) is not refracted, and therefore, the infrasplenic portion of the left kidney is accurately displayed on the image. Sound traveling through the tip of the spleen (S$_2$) is refracted inferiorly as it enters and exits the spleen, allowing it to reflect off the upper pole of the kidney in a location similar to S$_1$. Because localization of reflecting interfaces assumes a straight path for the sound *(dotted line)*, the upper pole is duplicated in a more superior location. (Reprinted with permission from Middleton WD, Melson GL. Renal duplication artifact in US imaging. *Radiology* 1989;773:427–429.)

the lower pole of the spleen is refracted inferiorly. If the upper pole of the kidney is positioned appropriately, this inferiorly refracted sound may reflect from it. Because the sound is assumed to have traveled in a straight line, the upper pole of the kidney is localized incorrectly in the image, creating the false appearance of upper pole duplication. To overcome this problem during real-time examination, one needs to move the transducer superiorly so that the sound beam travels completely through the spleen and does not encounter an interface between spleen and fat. With the patient taking a deep inspiration, and with the transducer repositioned so that the spleen covers the entire kidney, the upper pole is depicted accurately without artifactual duplication. There is increased incidence of this artifact in obese patients, presumably because of their greater amount of perisplenic fat. It is

much less commonly seen in the right side, most likely because most longitudinal images of the right kidney show the liver covering the majority or all of the kidney (23).

Computed Tomography Technical Artifacts

Conventional axial CT of the kidney is a well-established and highly effective diagnostic modality; however, there are several artifacts in renal CT that are technical in nature. They include different types of partial volume effects (Figs. 17.10 and 17.11) and motion-related artifacts like the pseudosubcapsular hematoma (Fig. 17.12). With conventional axial CT, partial volume averaging of renal masses with surrounding normal parenchyma or with perirenal fat may result in spurious attenuation mea-

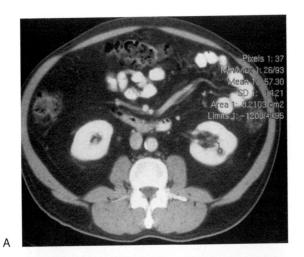

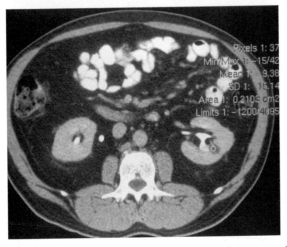

FIG. 17.10. Volume averaging. A: Computed tomography scan of a patient during nephrographic phase shows a small left renal lesion; with a 7-mm slice thickness, it was measured to have an attenuation value of 57.30 HU and therefore mimicked a solid lesion. B: During pyelogram, with a 2-mm slice thickness, the attenuation value was 9.38 HU, consistent with a simple cyst. (Case courtesy of Dr. A. Shirkhoda, William Beaumont Hospital.)

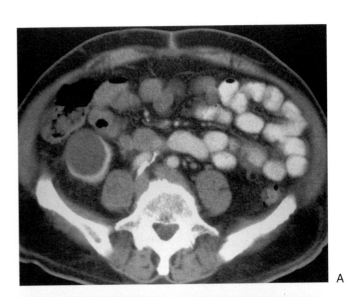

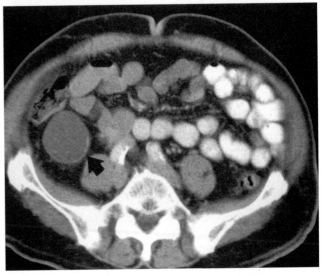

FIG. 17.11. Partial volume effect. A,B: A cyst hanging from the lower pole of the right kidney with a thin rim of the renal parenchyma *(arrow)* **(B)**, as seen on the image above it **(A)**. It can mimic a cyst with a thick wall.

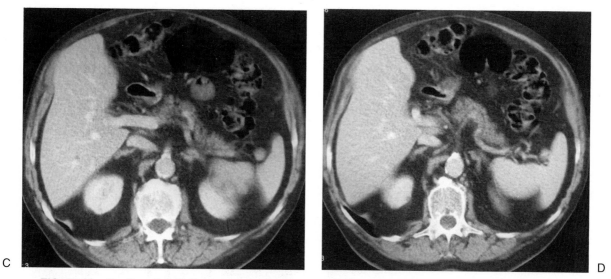

FIG. 17.11. *Continued.* **C,D:** Partial volume averaging between the spleen and the upper pole of the left kidney mimicking a renal mass **(C)**, but the spleen and kidney are clearly seen in the image below **(D).** (Cases courtesy of Dr. A. Shirkhoda, William Beaumont Hospital.)

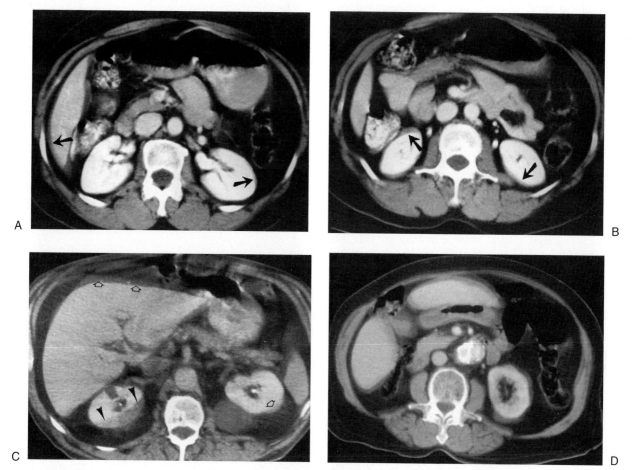

FIG. 17.12. Pseudosubcapsular hematoma. **A,B:** An apparent left subcapsular or perirenal fluid collection is seen on CT scans secondary to respiratory motion. Clues to the diagnosis are the bilaterality in two different levels, presence of artifact near the liver *(arrows)* **(B),** and the double line of the anterior abdominal musculature indicating the inappropriate movement during scanning. Although this artifact was more prevalent in older and slower scanning CT units, it is still possible in new faster machines. **C,D:** Similar findings of pseudosubcapsular hematomas of the kidneys and liver *(arrows)* **(C)** in two different patients. Note also a renal cyst arising from the posterior aspect of the left kidney in **C.** (Case courtesy of Dr. A. Shirkhoda, William Beaumont Hospital.)

surements both before and after intravenous contrast enhancement (24). This is the case with a small lesion less than twice the image collimation that is not centered perfectly within the image. If a small cyst does not occupy the entire thickness of the CT slice, partial volume averaging with the normal adjacent renal parenchyma will spuriously increase the attenuation value of the renal cyst (see Fig. 17.10A). This can be reduced or eliminated by using CT sections with the slice thickness thinner than the size of the renal cyst (see Fig. 17.10B). The volumetric image acquisition of helical CT and its ability to reconstruct an image at the precise level of the center of a renal mass will obviate this type of partial volume artifacts. Another pitfall of partial volume averaging is the occurrence of a pseudo-thick-walled renal cyst located at either renal pole (25). This artifact is generated by obtaining axial cuts including the renal parenchyma surrounding the base of the cyst (see Fig. 17.11A,B). Familiarity with this appearance is usually enough to resolve the issue, but if doubt persists, finer slices or reformatting in sagittal or coronal planes will be diagnostic. In the measurement of attenuation values of renal cysts, it must be remembered that the presence of any streak artifact within the cyst will result in spuriously elevated values, and measurements should be obtained from the portion of the cyst free of artifact (26).

ARTIFACT CAUSED BY THE SPLENORENAL RELATIONSHIP

Organs adjacent to the kidney, particularly the spleen, can lead to artifacts created by partial volume averaging. This may occur with normal and abnormal spleen (26). For example, in some patients with a prominent median aspect of the spleen, partial volume averaging with the upper pole of the left kidney may incorrectly suggest the presence of an upper pole left renal mass (see Fig. 17.11C,D). In most instances this can be ascertained from the axial CT images using thinner slices, but in some cases, if CT reformatting is not diagnostic or available, complementary imaging techniques with direct multiplanar capabilities such as US or MRI may be helpful.

MOTION ARTIFACTS ON COMPUTED TOMOGRAPHY

Patient motion during CT imaging of the kidneys can cause artifacts that simulate the appearance of a subcapsular fluid collection (see Fig. 17.12). This may also be confused with other pathology in the perirenal space, for example, perirenal lymphoma. Clues to the presence of an artifact include the presence of similar findings in the liver or contralateral kidney, evidence of motion of the anterior abdominal wall musculature, and its normal visualization in adjacent CT images (26).

ARTIFACTS AND PITFALLS CAUSED BY CONTRAST EXCRETION

With the advent of helical (spiral) CT scanning, it is now possible to image the kidneys very rapidly after administration of intravenous contrast material, and a new variety of artifacts inherent to this particular technique have become encountered. Some of these artifacts are related to the three phases of intravenous contrast enhancement of the kidney.

The cortical or corticomedullary phase (CMP) normally occurs between 25 and 80 seconds after the start of the injection of the IV bolus of contrast material. In this phase, there is rapid and intense enhancement of the renal cortex going from its unenhanced attenuation of 30 to 40 HU to densities of 145 to 185 HU at 40 to 50 seconds. However, there is minimal enhancement of the renal medulla to a mean of 50 to 60 HU at 40 seconds (27–29). The difference in enhancement between the cortex and medulla is marked and can approach 100 HU (Fig. 17.13).

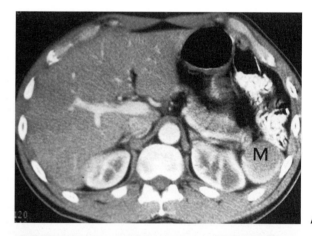

A

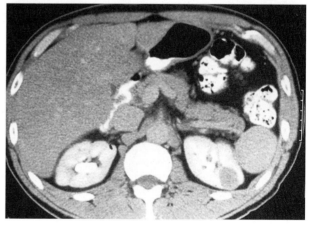

B

FIG. 17.13. False-negative cortical lesion at CMP of spiral CT. **A:** No renal masses were prospectively identified on this CMP image. A low-attenuation splenic mass (M) is noted. **B:** A solid hypodense renal mass can be easily detected in the posterolateral aspect of the middle of the left kidney on an EP image obtained at a similar level. (Reprinted with permission from Cohan RH, et al. Renal masses: assessment of corticomedullary-phase and nephrographic-phase CT scans. *Radiology* 1995;196:445–451.)

The nephrographic phase (NP) begins about 85 to 120 seconds after the start of IV injection of contrast. In this phase there is homogeneous dense enhancement of the renal cortex and medulla without any contrast material being excreted into the collecting system. The attenuation of both the cortex and medulla ranges between 120 and 170 HU depending on the rates of injection and volume of contrast employed.

The excretory phase (EP) begins when contrast material is first excreted into the renal calyces. It usually starts about 3 minutes after the beginning of the bolus injection of contrast. There is no corticomedullary differentiation with homogeneous nephrograms that have slightly lower density and attenuation value compared to the nephrographic phase.

Clinically significant errors can be made when images are obtained only during CMP. For example, a hypovascular solid renal tumor mass may be initially interpreted as normal renal medulla when only unenhanced images and images during CMP are reviewed (see Fig. 17.13). There are reports of hypervascular cortical renal carcinomas enhancing to the same degree as normal renal cortical tissue during CMP and thus not being easily identified (27,30).

If images are obtained only during nephrographic phase, a poorly enhanced renal medulla may be mistaken for a real lesion and result in a false-positive diagnosis (29–33). Delayed scans through the area in the excretory phase are essential to avoid this pitfall (Figs. 17.14 and 17.15). On the other hand, a mass that appears to represent a simple cyst on CMP imaging may demonstrate a thin, enhancing wall indicating a complex cystic lesion when imaged in the NP (Fig. 17.16). This is probably secondary to delayed enhancement of the wall of the

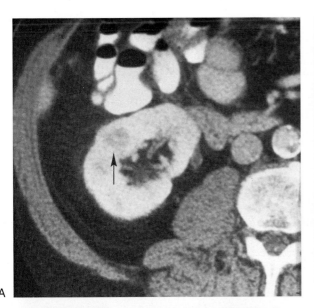

A

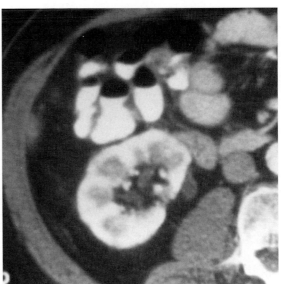

B

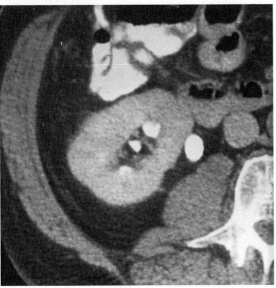

C

FIG. 17.14. False-positive cortical lesion at NP of spiral CT. **A:** Nephrographic-phase image shows a rounded area of decreased attenuation in the anterior aspect of the middle of the right kidney *(arrow)*. This was suspected to be a solid, heterogeneously enhancing mass. **B,C:** Both CMP **(B)** and delayed **(C)** images fail to demonstrate any abnormality in the region. In retrospect, the low-attenuation area was believed to represent normal renal medulla that had not yet enhanced homogeneously and to the same extent as the renal cortex. (Reprinted with permission from Cohan RH, et al. Renal masses: assessment of corticomedullary-phase and nephrographic-phase CT scans. *Radiology* 1995;196:445–451.)

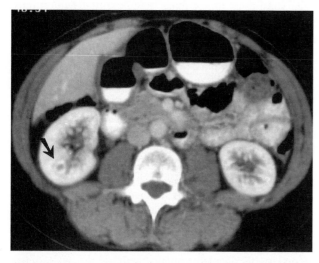

A

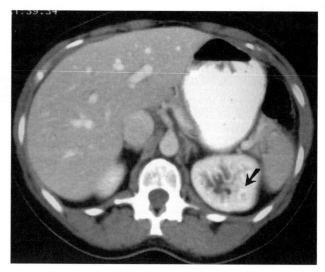

B

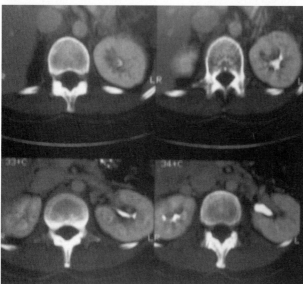

C

FIG. 17.15. Pseudocortical lesions. **A,B:** Areas of rim enhancement in the kidney seen during helical scanning simulating small abscesses or tumors *(arrows)*. These are probably secondary to axial images obtained through the renal pyramids as seen in the nephrographic phase. **C:** Occasionally, this pitfall is seen during the pyelographic phase. (Case courtesy of Dr. A. Shirkhoda, William Beaumont Hospital.)

necrotic cystic renal carcinoma not apparent on the CMP images. In doubtful cases, an ultrasound examination can be very helpful.

Imaging the kidneys only during CMP may result in difficulty differentiating a small simple renal cyst from unopacified medulla (Fig. 17.17). The presence of the cyst usually becomes obvious during NP or EP imaging. The lack of contrast excretion into the pelvicalyceal system during the CMP and NP makes it difficult to differentiate a focally dilated calyx from a hypodense mass unless delayed scans through the area are obtained (Fig. 17.18). Even relatively large pelvicalyceal filling defects may be missed if excretory-phase films are not available for review (Fig. 17.19).

Multiple peripelvic cysts can be confused with hydronephrosis during the CMP or nephrographic phase (Fig. 17.20A) because it is not possible to realize (as in a similar situation in US) that they are not connecting

together. Excretory-phase CT images (Fig. 17.20B) or a digital film or CT topogram (Fig. 17.20C) at the end of the study will avoid this pitfall. Occasionally CMP images may be helpful in diagnosing vascular abnormalities such as AVM or renal artery aneurysms and differentiate them from a calcified renal tumor (Fig. 17.21).

A problem that may be encountered with excretory-phase images is the production of streak artifacts emanating from the dense contrast in the collecting system (see Fig. 17.18). This is more common when the study is obtained with nonionic contrast material that achieves a higher concentration than ionic media because of its lesser diuretic effect secondary to its lower osmolarity (34).

Another contrast-material-related artifact on CT scanning is related to the occurrence of urinary excretion of orally ingested Gastrografin intended for bowel opacification. This unusual situation is significantly more likely to

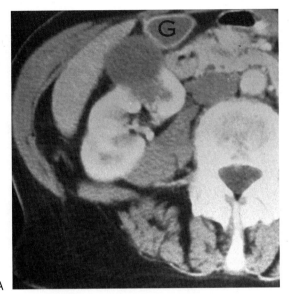
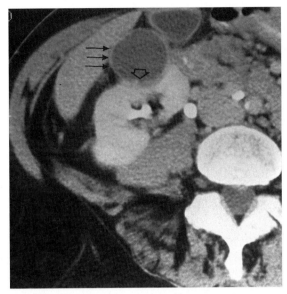

A   B

FIG. 17.16. Problems with characterization of renal masses on spiral CT. **A:** Corticomedullary-phase scan shows a homogeneous mass in the anterior aspect of the right kidney. The mass had an attenuation value similar to that of water and adjacent gallbladder (G) and, therefore, makes one believe that it represents a simple cyst. **B:** Nephrographic-phase image obtained at the same level shows a thin enhancing wall *(solid arrows)* that was not previously apparent. Note that the slightly irregular interface of the mass with the renal parenchyma *(open arrow)* is also more apparent on the NP image. The mass was characterized as a complex cyst. The lesion was found to be necrotic renal cancer at surgery. (Reprinted with permission from Cohan RH, et al. Renal masses: assessment of corticomedullary-phase and nephrographic-phase CT scans. *Radiology* 1995;196:445–451.)

occur in patients with diseases involving the intestinal wall such as inflammatory bowel disease, radiation enteritis, ischemia, and bowel perforation, in which there is increased absorption of the contrast and subsequent renal excretion (35). The differential diagnosis of a radiopaque density in the pelvicalyceal system on CT includes stone disease, bleeding, pus, and a fungus ball. These processes are usually unilateral, unlike the occurrence of bilateral contrast excretion, but in questionable cases ultrasound or plain film correlation may be useful (35).

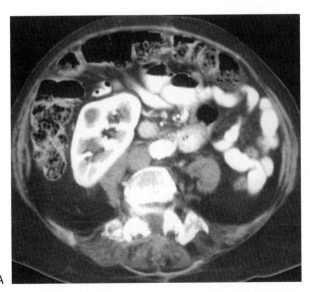
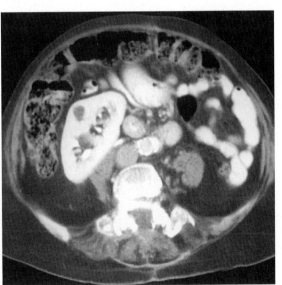

A   B

FIG. 17.17. Missing cortical lesion at CMP of spiral CT. **A:** Small cyst in the anterior aspect of the right kidney is difficult to be seen at CMP since it simulates unopacified medullary tissue. **B:** The lesion becomes obvious in the EP images. (Courtesy of A. Shirkhoda, M.D.)

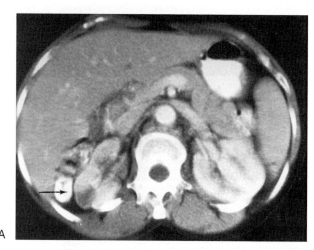
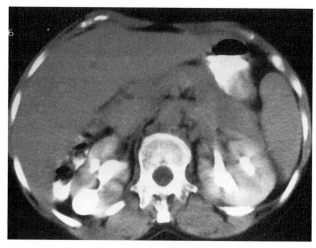

FIG. 17.18. Chronic atrophic pyelonephritis simulating a mass in CMP of spiral CT. **A:** In the CMP, a hypodense mass is suggested in the posterior and inferior aspect of the right kidney *(arrow).* **B:** Delayed scan through the same area in the EP reveals the presence of a hydrocalyx with marked cortical thinning overlying it, consistent with changes of chronic pyelonephritis and not a real mass. Note also the streak artifacts emanating from the dense contrast in the collecting system, more marked in the left kidney.

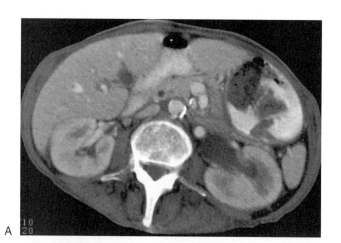

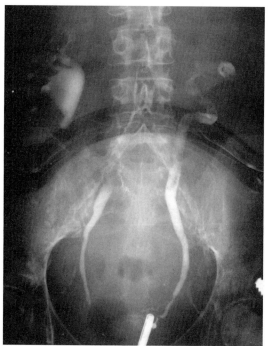

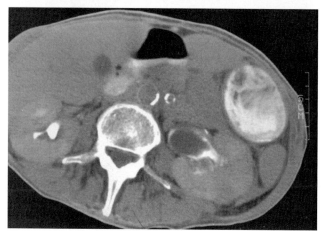

FIG. 17.19. Missing renal pelvic mass at CMP of spiral CT. **A:** A transitional cell carcinoma in the left pelvic region that is easily missed on CMP. **B:** It is clearly seen on the delayed image. **C:** Retrograde pyelography confirms the presence of a large polypoid tumor in the left renal pelvis and proximal left ureter. (Case courtesy of Dr. A. Shirkhoda, William Beaumont Hospital.)

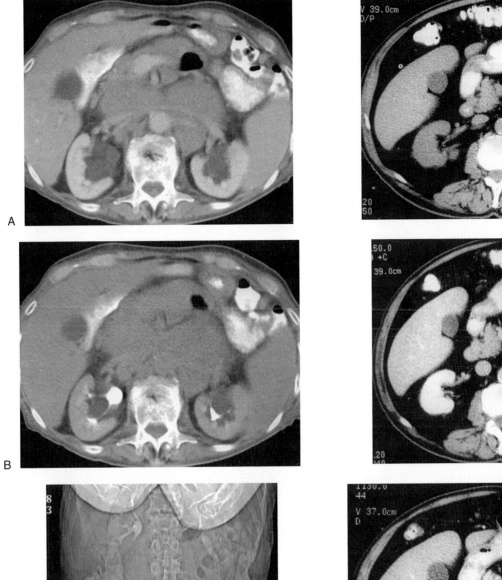

A

B

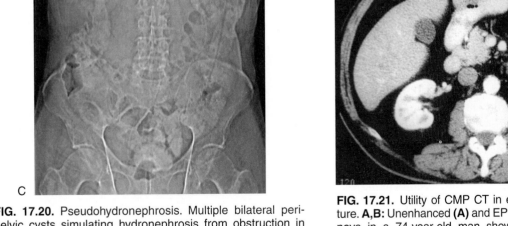

C

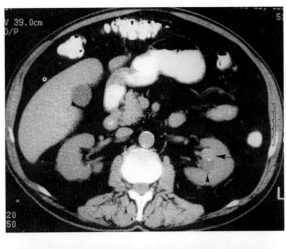

A

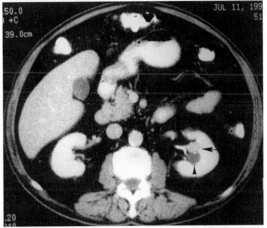

B

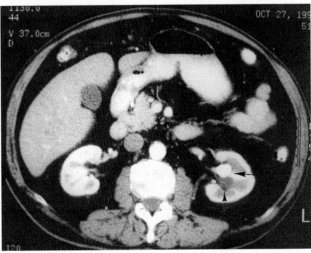

C

FIG. 17.20. Pseudohydronephrosis. Multiple bilateral peripelvic cysts simulating hydronephrosis from obstruction in this patient with lymphoma and retroperitoneal adenopathy. **A:** Early-phase postcontrast CT was thought to represent hydronephrosis. **B:** Delayed excretion phase illustrating the cysts in the central sinus of the kidney. **C:** Digital CT scans at the end of the spiral study show the spidery appearance of collecting system of the right kidney without any evidence of hydronephrosis. The left kidney is partially obscured by the patient's arm. The ureters are deviated by retroperitoneal nodes. (Case courtesy of Dr. A. Shirkhoda, William Beaumont Hospital.)

FIG. 17.21. Utility of CMP CT in evaluation of renal vasculature. **A,B:** Unenhanced **(A)** and EP images **(B)** through the kidneys in a 74-year-old man show an abnormal soft tissue *(arrows)* in the left renal sinus, immediately anterior to a parapelvic cyst *(arrowheads)*. This mass was initially suspected to represent a renal neoplasm; however, the presence of a thin rim of peripheral calcification visible only on the precontrast images **(A)** and enhancement identical to that of the aorta suggested a vascular etiology such as a renal artery aneurysm. **C:** The CMP image shows that the mass enhances intensely to the same extent as the abdominal aorta. This confirms its vascular nature, which represents a renal artery aneurysm. (Reprinted with permission from reference 24.)

ARTIFACTS AND PITFALLS ON MAGNETIC RESONANCE IMAGING

Magnetic resonance imaging, in addition to anatomic variants and congenital anomalies similar to those discussed in CT scanning and artifacts such as partial volume averaging and motion-related ones, has also demonstrated a wide variety of novel imaging artifacts. A detailed technical discussion of these is beyond the scope of this chapter, and the reader is directed to the related chapter in this book or other authoritative sources (37–43). Also we specifically exclude the wide spectrum of artifacts caused by defective components or malfunctions of the imaging system and limit our discussion to some artifacts that may cause diagnostic pitfalls in imaging the kidneys with MRI.

Chemical Shift Artifacts

An MRI artifact is defined as presence or absence of any signal intensity that does not have an anatomic basis in the image (37). One of the magnetic field perturbation artifacts with relevance to imaging of the kidneys is the chemical shift caused by the change in resonant frequency experienced by protons in different chemical environments, typically fat and water in proton MR imaging (38). The protons of fatty triglycerides are chemically shielded by their electron clouds and therefore resonate at slightly lower frequencies than water protons in the same tissue. This shift in resonance frequency has been measured to be 3.5 parts per million (ppm) or a difference of about 225 Hz at 1.5 T (39). In MRI, spatial position is assigned along the frequency-encoding direction on the basis of resonant frequency. If both H_2O and fat protons coexist in a voxel, the signal emitted by the lipid protons has a lower frequency than that of water protons. So when the system frequency is set to H_2O, the signal from the fat protons appears to have arisen from water protons in another voxel in a lower part of the field. When image intensities are assigned in the final image, the location of fat protons is spatially mismapped toward the lower part of the readout gradient field. This pixel misregistration artifact appears as a dark border along one interface and a bright border on the opposite interface and consistently appears as a line perpendicular to the direction of the read or frequency-encoding gradient. The appearance of the artifact depends on the direction of the read gradient (i.e., increasing or decreasing) and the order of substances in the field (i.e., water to fat or fat to water). In the instance of a fat-to-water interface in an increasing field, a dark space appears at the boundary corresponding to a separation of data between the water and fat signals. Conversely, a water-to-fat boundary in an increasing field may appear bright, corresponding to an overlap of data from the fat and water signals (44,45). Thus, for the MR imager used for collection of these data (this may vary with the direc-

tion of the frequency encoding in different machines) in the particular case of the normal kidneys viewed on axial images of the abdomen, the artifact appears as a low-intensity line seen on the right side of the kidney, i.e., on the lateral aspect of the right kidney and on a medial aspect of the left kidney (Fig. 17.22). On the left side of the kidney (medial aspect of the right kidney and lateral aspect of the left kidney), there is a similar but high-intensity line that in some cases may be more difficult to appreciate because it merges with the adjacent high-intensity fat (44,45). Similar artifacts can be seen on coronal images. Identification and recognition of this chemical shift misregistration artifact is important so as not to confuse it with real anatomic structures, such as calcification, fluid collections, or a tumor pseudocapsule (44,45). It must be noted that the chemical shift artifact

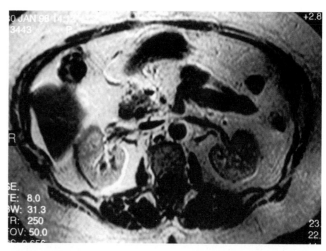

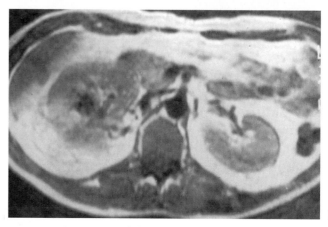

FIG. 17.22. Chemical shift artifact. **A:** Axial MRI showing a low-intensity line on the lateral aspect of right kidney and medial aspect of left kidney and bright bands on medial aspect of right kidney and lateral surface of left kidney. **B:** Magnetic resonance image of exophytic renal angiolipoma. Note relative lack of chemical shift artifact in the area where the fatty mass abuts the perirenal fat, indicating its lipid content.

varies as a function of field strength among other factors (46,47), and therefore, the finding may vary in studies obtained with different units. The lack of the artifact may be of diagnostic help in some situations. For example, in our experience with renal angiomyolipomas with a prominent fatty component, arising as an exophytic mass from the kidney, we have observed a relative lack of chemical shift artifact (48). As a result, in some areas the contour of the mass is difficult to discern, and it appears to blend with a perinephric fat, which has some similar magnetic resonance properties (see Fig. 17.22).

The chemical shift artifact can be reduced by using the widest receive bandwidth in keeping with good signal-to-noise ratio (SNR) and the smallest field of view (FOV) possible. If the bandwidth is reduced to increase the SNR, chemical saturation can be used to saturate out the signal from either fat or water (49).

Phase Cancellation Artifact

There is a second artifact induced by the chemical shift phenomenon, which is the phase cancellation artifact, also called "chemical shift artifact of the second kind," observed especially in out-of-phase gradient-echo (GRE) images (Fig. 17.23). In a GRE sequence, fat and water protons go in and out of phase with one another as a function of echo time (T_E). At 1.5 T, the period of alternation is about 4.4 milliseconds. Therefore, at T_E = 2.2, 6.6, 11.0, and 15.4 milliseconds, fat and water fall out of phase with one another in GRE images at 1.5 T (39). Then GRE images acquired with T_Es near these values will demonstrate this artifact. In boundary voxels that contain equal amounts of fat and water, such as at the interface between

kidney and perirenal fat, their signals cancel each other, resulting in a signal void with a black halo along the entire fat–water interface. Because this is a phase cancellation effect, it is not limited to the frequency-encoding direction as the chemical shift artifact of the first kind. It must be emphasized that the T_E values that generate this phase cancellation artifact are dependent on the field strength of the magnet because the difference in precessional frequency between fat and water is proportional to the main magnetic field strength. At 1.5 T, fat precesses 220 Hz less than water, whereas at 1.0 T the difference is 147 Hz. At 1.0 T, the in-phase images occur at T_E times of 6.7, 13.5, and 20 milliseconds, whereas at 1.5 T, in-phase images occur at T_Es of 4.5, 9, 13.5, and 18 milliseconds (42).

The out-of-phase T_E times are midway between the in-phase times. To reduce this artifact when using a gradient-echo pulse sequence, one must select a T_E that generates an echo when fat and water are in phase, as noted above, so that their signals add constructively (49). For example, at 1.5 T, selecting a T_E that is a multiple of 4.2 milliseconds such as 8.4 milliseconds reduces this artifact, whereas at a T_E of 10.4 milliseconds, a chemical shift artifact of the second kind will be produced.

Wrap-Around Artifacts

Wrap-around artifacts, or aliasing, occur if the specified field of view (FOV) is smaller than the actual extent of the anatomy (50). An object or organ can be wrapped around to the opposite side, and in some cases a renal mass can be simulated (Fig. 17.24). One of the several ways to eliminate the phase wrap-around artifact is to increase the FOV to encompass the entire anatomic area

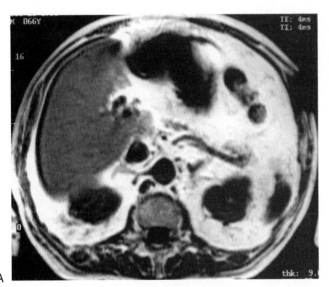
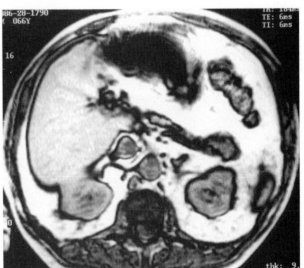

FIG. 17.23. Phase cancellation artifact. **A:** In-phase gradient-echo image. **B:** Corresponding out-of-phase image. Fat and water protons have opposite phases. For voxels with equal amounts of fat and water, such as the boundary between kidney and perirenal fat, there is cancellation of signal, creating a dark ring around the kidney.

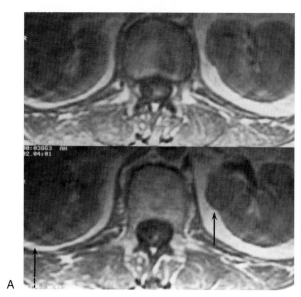

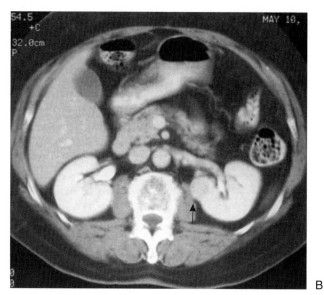

FIG. 17.24. Wrap-around artifact simulating a renal mass. **A:** On MRI of the spine, there is a suggestion of bilateral renal masses *(arrows)*. **B:** On follow-up contrast-enhanced CT scan a small left renal mass, later proven to be a renal cell carcinoma, is well depicted, corresponding to the MRI exam. However, no mass is present in the right kidney, confirming that the pseudomass on the MRI was secondary to a wrap-around artifact.

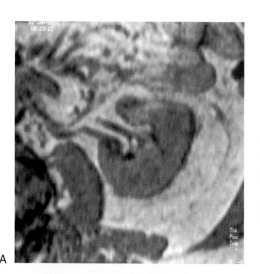

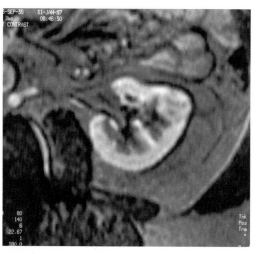

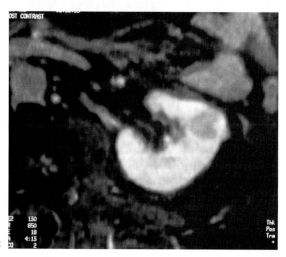

FIG. 17.25. Small renal cell carcinoma missed on breath-hold gradient sequence. **A:** The tumor is not seen on the precontrast 2-D FLASH. **B:** It is possible to overlook its presence on the dynamic perfusion sequence. **C:** It is best illustrated on the delayed T_1 fat-saturation image. (Case courtesy of Dr. A. Shirkhoda, William Beaumont Hospital.)

in that direction. Antialiasing, no-phase-wrap software is also available in the most recent commercial MR units.

Gadolinium-Enhanced Pitfalls

The normal renal enhancement patterns with gadolinium contrast have been well described for different MRI sequences including fat saturation (51–55). In contrast-enhanced MRI of the kidneys using dynamic scanning with gadolinium-based compounds, some artifacts may occur quite similar to the ones observed with contrast-enhanced CT. Small renal carcinomas may not be visible with noncontrast scans and also become virtually isointense with normal kidney in dynamic perfusion images. In these patients delayed scans and fat saturation techniques may provide useful additional information (Fig. 17.25).

REFERENCES

1. Hodson CJ. The lobar structure of the kidney. *Br J Urol* 1972;44:246–261.
2. Patriquin H, Lefaivre JF, Lafortune M, Russo P, Boisvert J. Fetal lobation—an anatomo-ultrasonographic correlation. *J Ultrasound Med* 1990;9:191–197.
3. McGahan JP, Goldberg BB. Urinary tract. In: *Diagnostic ultrasound. A logical approach.* Philadelphia: Lippincott-Raven, 1998;801–858.
4. Carter AR, Horgan JG, Jennings TA, Rosenfield AT. The junctional parenchymal defect: A sonographic variant of renal anatomy. *Radiology* 1985;154:499–502.
5. Hoffer FA, Hanabergh AM, Teele RL. The interrenicular junction: A mimic of renal scarring on normal pediatric sonograms. *Am J Roentgenol* 1985;145:1075–1078.
6. Kenney IJ, Wild SR. The renal parenchymal junctional line in children: Ultrasonic frequency and appearances. *Br J Radiol* 1987;60:865–868.
7. Papanicolau N, Harbury OL, Pfister RC. Fat-filled postoperative renal cortical defects: Sonographic and CT appearance. *Am J Roentgenol* 1988;151:503–505.
8. Millward SF, Lanctin HP, Lewandowski BJ, et al. Fat-filled post-operative renal pseudotumor: Variable appearance in ultrasonography images. *Can Assoc Radiol J* 1992;43:116–119.
9. Kolbenstvedt A, Lien HH. Isolated renal hilar lip on computed tomography. *Radiology* 1982;143:150.
10. Leekam RN, Matzinger MA, Brunelle M, et al. The sonography of renal columnar hypertrophy. *J Clin Ultrasound* 1983;11:491–494.
11. Yeh HC, Halton KP, Shapiro RS, et al. Junctional parenchyma: Revised definition of hypertrophied column of Bertin. *Radiology* 1992;185:725–732.
12. Lafortune M, Constantin A, Breton G, Vallee C. Sonography of the hypertrophied column of Bertin. *Am J Roentgenol* 1986;146:53–59.
13. Dalla Palma L, Rossi M. Advances in radiological anatomy of the kidney. *Br J Radiol* 1982;55:404–412.
14. Hodson CJ, Mariani S. Large cloisons. *Am J Roentgenol* 1982;139:327–332.
15. Mahony BS, Jeffrey RB, Laing F. Septa of Bertin: A sonographic pseudotumor. *J Clin Ultrasound* 1983;11:317–319.
16. DallaPalma L, Bazzocchi M, Cressa C, Tomasini G. Radiological anatomy of the kidney revisited. *Br J Radiol* 1990;3:680–690.
17. Zagoria RJ, Tung GA. The renal sinus, pelvocalyceal system, and ureter. In: *Genitourinary radiology. The requisites.* St Louis: CV Mosby, 1997;152–191.
18. Brammer HM, Smith WS, Lubbers PR. Septated hypoechoic perirenal fat on sonograms: A pitfall in renal sonography. *J Ultrasound Med* 1992;11:361–363.
19. Spencer GM, Rubens DJ, Roach DJ. Hypoechoic fat: A sonographic pitfall. *Am J Roentgenol* 1995;164:1277–1286.
20. Kunin M. Bridging septa of the perinephric space: Anatomic, pathologic and diagnostic considerations. *Radiology* 1986;158:3631–3635.
21. Behan M, Kazam E. The echographic characteristics of fatty tissues and tumors. *Radiology* 1978;129:143–151.
22. Sheth S, Fishman EK, Buck JL, et al. The variable sonographic appearance of ovarian teratomas: Correlation with CT. *Am J Roentgenol* 1988;151:331–334.
23. Middleton WD, Melson GL. Renal duplication artifact in ultrasound imaging. *Radiology* 1989;173:427–429.
24. Yuh BI, Cohan RH. Helical CT for detection and characterization of renal masses. *Semin US CT MR* 1997;18:82–90.
25. Segal AG, Spitzer RM. Pseudo thick-walled renal cyst by CT. *Am J Roentgenol* 1979;132:827.
26. Shirkhoda A. Diagnostic pitfalls in abdominal CT. *RadioGraphics* 1991;11:969–1002.
27. Cohan RH, Sherman LS, Korobkin M, Bass JC, Francis IR. Renal masses: Assessment of corticomedullary-phase and nephrographic-phase CT scans. *Radiology* 1995;196:441–445.
28. Birnbaum BA, Jacobs JE, Ramchandani P. Multiphasic renal CT: Comparison of renal enhancement during the corticomedullary and nephrographic phases. *Radiology* 1996;200:753–758.
29. Szolar DH, Kammerhuber F, Altziebler S, et al. Multiphasic helical CT of the kidney- increased conspicuity for detection and characterization of small (<3 cm) renal masses. *Radiology* 1997;202:211–217.
30. Herts BR, Epstein DM, Paushter DM. Spiral CT of the abdomen: Artifacts and potential pitfalls. *Am J Roentgenol* 1993;161:1185–1190.
31. Zeman RK, Zeiber G, Hayes WS, et al. Helical CT of renal masses: The value of delayed scans. *Am J Roentgenol* 1996;167:771–776.
32. Kopka L, Fischer U, Zoeller G, et al. Dual-phase helical CT of the kidney: Value of the corticomedullary and nephrographic phase for evaluation of renal lesions and preoperative staging of renal cell carcinoma. *Am J Roentgenol* 1997;169:1573–1578.
33. Silverman SG, Pearson GDN, Seltzer SE. Small (<3 cm) hyperechoic renal masses: Comparison of helical and conventional CT for diagnosing angiomyolipoma. *Am J Roentgenol* 1996;167:877–881.
34. Sussman SK, Illescas PF, Opalacz JP, Yirga P, Foley LC. Renal streak artifact during contrast enhanced CT: Comparison of high versus low osmolality contrast media. *Abdom Imag* 1993;18:180–185.
35. Apter S, Gayer G, Amitai M, Hertz M. Urinary excretion of orally ingested Gastrografin on CT. *Abdom Imag* 1998;23:297–300.
36. Silverman PM, Cooper C, Zeman RK. Lateral arcuate ligaments of the diaphragm: anatomic variations at abdominal CT. *Radiology* 1992;185:105–108.
37. Wesbey G, Adamis MK, Edelman RR. Artifacts in MRI: description, causes and solutions. In: Edelman RR, Hesselink JR, Zlatkin MB, eds. *Clinical magnetic resonance imaging.* Philadelphia: WB Saunders, 1996;88–144.
38. Henkelman RM, Bronskill MJ. Artifacts in magnetic resonance imaging. *Rev Magn Reson* 1987;2:1–126.
39. Elster AD. MR Artifacts. In: Elster AD, ed. *Questions and answers in magnetic resonance imaging.* St Louis: CV Mosby, 1994;134–161.
40. Porter BA, Hastrup W, Richardson ML, et al. Classification and investigation of artifacts in magnetic resonance imaging. *RadioGraphics* 1987;7:271–287.
41. Mirowitz SA. Adrenals, kidneys and retroperitoneum. In: Mirowitz SA, ed. *Pitfalls, variants and artifacts in body MR imaging.* St Louis: CV Mosby, 1996;181–209.
42. Brown MA, Semelka RC. Artifacts. In: Brown MA, Semelka RC, eds. *MRI, basic principles and applications.* New York: Wiley-Liss, 1995;87–101.
43. Semelka RC, Kelekis NL. Kidneys. In: Semelka RC, Ascher SM, Reinhold C, eds. *MRI of the abdomen and pelvis, a test-atlas.* New York: Wiley-Liss, 1997;379–469.
44. Soila KP, Viamonte M Jr, Starenwicz PM. Chemical shift misregistration effect in magnetic resonance imaging. *Radiology* 1984;153:819–821.
45. Weinreb JC, Brateman L, Babcock EE, et al. Chemical shift artifact in clinical magnetic resonance imaging at 0.35 T. *Am J Roentgenol* 1985;145:183–185.
46. Apicella PL, Mirowitz SA, Borello J. Chemical shift misregistration artifacts: Increased conspicuity following intravenous administration of Gadopentetate Dimeglumine. *Magn Reson Imag* 1994;12:675–678.
47. Wachsberg RH, Mitchell PG, Rifkin MD, et al. Chemical shift artifact along the section-select axis. *J Magn Reson Imag* 1992;2:1589–1591.
48. Amendola MA. Comparison of MR imaging and CT in the evaluation of renal masses. *Crit Rev Diagn Imag* 1989;29:117–150.
49. Westbrook C, Kaut C. Artifacts and their compensation. In: *MRI in practice, 2nd ed.* London: Blackwell Science, 1998;158–182.
50. Wood ML. Artifact identification and elimination. In: Riederer ST,

Wood ML, eds. *Categorical course in physics: the basic physics of MR imaging.* Chicago: RSNA Publications, 1997;59–69.

51. Semelka RC, Chen W, Hricak H, et al. Fat-saturation MR imaging of the upper abdomen. *Am J Roentgenol* 1990;155:1111–1116.

52. Eilenberg SS, Lee JKT, Brown JJ, et al. Renal masses: Evaluation with gradient-echo Gd-DTPA-enhanced dynamic MR imaging. *Radiology* 1990;176:333–338.

53. Semelka RC, Hricak H, Stevens SK, et al. Combined gadolinium-enhanced and fat-saturation MR imaging of renal masses. *Radiology* 1991;178:803–809.

54. Mirowitz SA, Gutierrez E, Lee JKT, et al. Normal abdominal enhancement patterns with dynamic gadolinium-enhanced MR imaging. *Radiology* 1991;180:637–640.

55. Semelka RC, Hricak H, Tomei E, et al. Obstructive nephropathy: Evaluation with dynamic Gd-DTPA-enhanced MR imaging. *Radiology* 1990;575:797–803.

Variants and Pitfalls in Body Imaging,
edited by Ali Shirkhoda.
Lippincott Williams & Wilkins, Philadelphia, © 2000.

CHAPTER 18

The Adrenals

Patrick O'Kane and Eric K. Outwater

Because the adrenal glands are small, clinically inaccessible, and prone to develop significant pathology, sectional body imaging plays a critical role in their assessment. This chapter first reviews the anatomy and normal appearance of the adrenals as seen on various imaging modalities. Then the diagnostic challenges posed by intrinsic and adjacent normal and abnormal structures are discussed, and the imaging strategies for evaluating them is presented.

ADRENAL ANATOMY

Each adrenal gland is composed of two embryologically, anatomically, and functionally distinct endocrine organs, the cortex and the medulla (Fig. 18.1). The cortex derives from a combination of mesoderm and coelomic epithelium that arises near the urogenital ridge. Early in embryonic life, chromaffin neural crest cells of the sympathetic system invade these mesenchymal cells to form the medulla. The adrenal cortex arises from the same region that supplies ovarian thecal and testicular interstitial cells, which explains the occasional finding of adrenal rests within the gonads. The neuroectodermal origin of the medulla explains why ectopic medullary tumors such as pheochromocytomas and neuroblastomas can occur anywhere along the sympathetic chain. The cortex is divided microscopically into three layers, the zona glomerulosa, the zona fasciculata, and the zona reticularis. These produce aldosterone (zona glomerulosa), glucocorticoids, and dehydroepiandrosterone. The zona fasciculata cells, in particular, are lipid-laden. The medulla produces epinephrine and norepinephrine as well as a number of noncatecholamine hormones (1,2).

P. O'Kane: Department of Radiology, Temple University Medical Center, Philadelphia, Pennsylvania 19140.

E. K. Outwater: Department of Radiology, Arizona Health Sciences Center, Tucson, Arizona 85724-5067.

The adrenals lie within the perinephric space, which is enclosed by Gerota's fascia. The anterior and posterior leaves of the fascia fuse above the kidneys to enclose the adrenals. Typically, the adrenals are made up of a body, a lateral limb, and a medial limb (Fig. 18.2). The shape is variable, however, and trefoil, quadrifolate, and globular configurations, among others, have been reported.

The right adrenal lies anteromedial to and just above the right kidney between the right crus of the diaphragm and the liver, directly posterior to the inferior vena cava. It usually resembles an elongated and inverted Y (3). The left adrenal is more variable in appearance and location. It is located anteromedial to the left kidney, lying between the left crus of the diaphragm and the splenic vein. It tends to be less elongated than the right adrenal, with a shape that has been likened to Napoleon's hat (3).

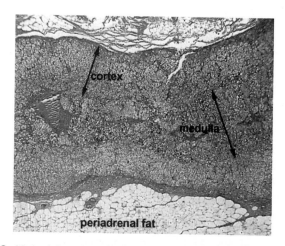

FIG. 18.1. Adrenal structure. Histologic slide shows the clear lipid-laden cells of the adrenal cortex surrounding the basophilic cells of the adrenal medulla. The adrenal is surrounded by periadrenal fat.

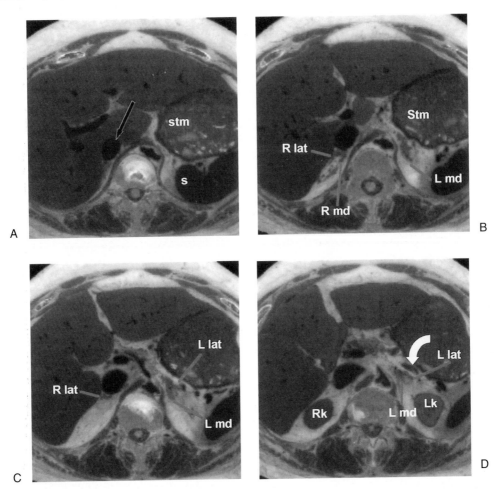

FIG. 18.2. Cadaver section showing normal adrenal anatomy from its superior **(A)** to its inferior **(D)** part. Note the relationship between the adrenal glands and the adjacent diaphragmatic crura. The right adrenal gland is located directly behind the inferior vena cava *(arrow)* **(A)**. The left adrenal is behind the splenic vein *(curved arrow)* **(D)**. Both are anteromedial to the upper pole of the kidneys. Stm, stomach; S, spleen; Rk, right kidney; Lk, left kidney; Rlat, lateral limb of the right adrenal; Lmd, medial limb of the left adrenal.

In the adult, the adrenals normally measure 4 to 6 cm in greatest dimension and weigh about 4 g each. The limbs normally range between 3 mm and 6 mm in width. Each is no wider than the adjacent crus of the diaphragm. The body contains both cortical and medullary tissue, while the limbs are composed almost exclusively of cortical tissue. In adults, the medulla comprises about 10% of the gland.

Blood supply to the adrenals arises from three main sources. The superior pole is supplied by branches from the inferior phrenic artery, the midpole is supplied by a branch from the aorta, and the lower pole is supplied by branches from the renal artery (2). The adrenal gland is unique in that its venous drainage is less subject to variation than its arterial supply. Drainage is usually via a single central vein (4). The right adrenal drains into the inferior vena cava via a very short connection, and the left adrenal drains into the left renal vein. The draining vein originates at the hilum of the adrenal gland, along its lateral aspect. Frequently there is a corresponding bulge on the medial aspect of the gland, which can give the gland a globular appearance. Lymphatic drainage is into lateral aortic nodes (5).

NORMAL APPEARANCE ON CROSS-SECTIONAL IMAGING

The ultrasound appearance of the adrenals varies greatly with age. The glands appear relatively large in fetal life and can be identified after the 26th week of gestation (6). In the second trimester, the adrenal glands appear larger than the kidneys and can be mistaken for them (Fig. 18.3). At this stage they contain a central echogenic component, believed to correspond to the medulla, surrounded by a thick hypoechoic layer representing the cortex. At term, the adrenals weigh about the same as they do in the adult. In infants, the adrenals appear relatively prominent (7) (Fig. 18.4). They

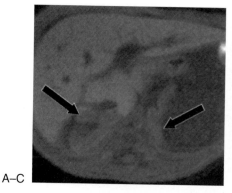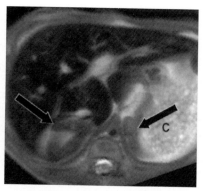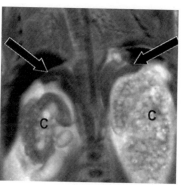

A–C

FIG. 18.3. Postmortem MRI of a 22-week fetus showing normal adrenal glands *(arrows)*. Note relatively large size compared with the adult gland. **A:** On a T1-weighted axial image there is faint cortico-medullary differentiation. The signal intensity of the adrenals *(arrows)* is less than that of liver (TR/TE = 400/13). **B:** Adrenal glands *(arrows)* are isointense to muscle on a T2-weighted axial image (TR/TEeff = 4,000/120). The adrenal limbs are thicker than the adjacent crus. **C:** T2-weighted coronal image shows a trilaminar appearance similar to that seen on ultrasound (TR/TEeff = 3,000/168). Bilateral cystic renal dysplasia (C) was from bladder outlet obstruction.

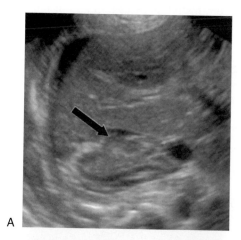

A

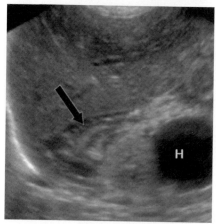

B

FIG. 18.4. Normal ultrasound appearance of a neonatal right adrenal gland *(arrow)*. Transverse **(A)** and sagittal **(B)** images show a central echogenic layer and a hypoechoic cortical layer. Note incidental right hydronephrosis (H).

decrease markedly in size in the first few weeks of extrauterine life and then gradually grow until puberty. In adults, they have a uniform intermediate echo texture on ultrasound and attenuation value on CT (Fig. 18.5), with no differentiation between cortex and medulla. The average width for the right adrenal gland is 6 mm, and that of the left adrenal gland is 8 mm (8). Larger measurements are nonspecific and could represent hyperplasia or tumors (Fig. 18.6).

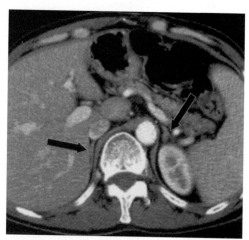

FIG. 18.5. Normal CT appearance of adrenal glands *(arrows)*. The right adrenal gland is located directly behind the inferior vena cava. The left adrenal is behind the splenic vein and artery. They are either thinner than or have the same thickness as the adjacent smooth diaphragmatic crura and display homogeneous density.

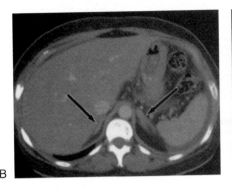
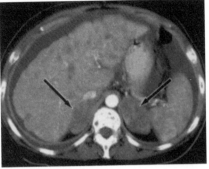

A,B

FIG. 18.6. Adrenal enlargement. A: Initial CT study shows slightly thickened adrenal glands *(arrows)* in a patient with a primary carcinoma of the breast. The appearance is indistinguishable from hyperplasia. B: Same patient 11 months later with marked growth of bilateral adrenal metastases.

On CT, normal adrenal tissue is similar in attenuation to unenhanced renal parenchyma. Usually, though not always, the glands are well defined by a surrounding fat plane separating them from adjacent organs (see Fig. 18.5). The margins of the glands should be sharp, and infiltrating margins may suggest hemorrhage or metastases (see Fig. 18.6).

On MRI, the signal intensity of the adrenal glands is close to that of normal liver on all non-fat-suppressed spin-echo sequences (Fig. 18.7). When fat-saturation techniques are used, the adrenals appear isointense to liver on T_1-weighted sequences and hyperintense on T_2-weighted sequences. They show moderate enhancement following administration of gadolinium or mangafodir, a

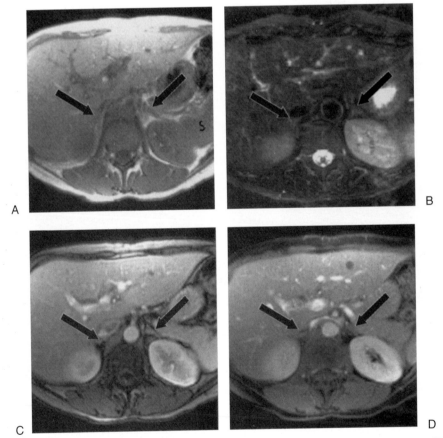

FIG. 18.7. Normal MR appearance of adrenal glands. A: T1-weighted gradient-echo image (TR/TE = 150/4.2) shows the adrenals *(arrows)* as thin structures with signal intensity similar to that of spleen (S). B: T2-weighted fat-suppressed fast spin-echo image (TR/TEeff = 7,500/104) shows intermediate-signal-intensity adrenal glands *(arrows)*. C: Postgadolinium image (TR/TE = 170/2.2) taken during the venous phase shows enhancement of the adrenals *(arrows)* similar to the liver. D: Delayed postgadolinium image (TR/TE = 150/2.3) shows enhancement *(arrows)* less than the liver, indicating greater washout of contrast.

manganese-containing liver contrast agent (9). Following administration of gadolinium, the gland enhances and shows homogeneous enhancement by 2 to 4 minutes, and the contrast washes out by 5 minutes (see Fig. 18.7) (10).

ADVANTAGES AND LIMITATIONS OF IMAGING MODALITIES

Sonography

The advantages of ultrasound are its lack of ionizing radiation, its instant and real-time multiplanar imaging capability, its ability to evaluate flow characteristics, its comparative insensitivity to motion, and its relatively low cost. Its limitations include dependence on operator skill and patient body habitus, high false-negative rate, and poor visualization of the normal adrenal (Fig. 18.8). In children, the adrenal glands are relatively large and are comparatively well visualized on ultrasound. Therefore, it is the initial study of choice for evaluating pediatric adrenals. In adults, however, ultrasound is not very useful for assessing the adrenal glands and, at best, has a limited role in serial follow-up studies. However, adrenal pathology occasion-

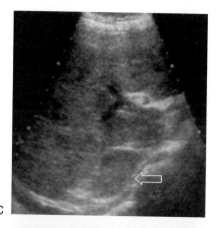
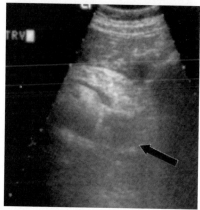

FIG. 18.8. C: Transverse view shows that the mass is separate from the liver. **D:** Left adrenal metastasis *(arrow)* is difficult to visualize as a discrete mass.

ally can be identified or suspected on ultrasound studies done for other indications (Fig. 18.9). In patients with large retroperitoneal tumors, where the organ of origin is difficult to determine on CT, the multiplanar capabilities of ultrasound may enable detection of a tissue plane between

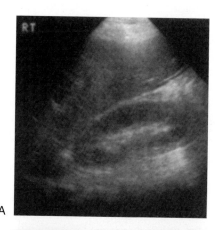
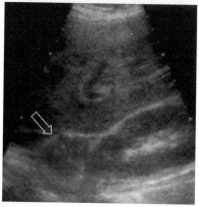

FIG. 18.8. Bilateral adrenal metastases, showing ultrasound's technical limitations and dependence on operator skill. **A:** Sagittal view shows no abnormality. **B:** Parasagittal view angulated medially shows a right suprarenal mass *(arrow).*

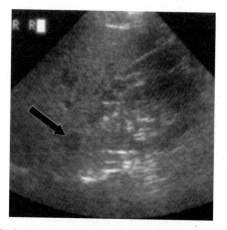

FIG. 18.9. Adrenal adenoma found incidentally on abdominal ultrasound examination. Sagittal view shows the hypoechoic small adenoma *(arrow)* above the kidney, demonstrating a tissue plane between the mass and the renal parenchyma.

tumor and adjacent organs. The limit of detectability is on the order of 2 cm. When a low-density lesion is located on an unenhanced CT scan, ultrasound may be helpful for determining whether the lesion is solid or cystic.

Computed Tomography

Computed tomography is the study of choice for the initial evaluation of adrenal glands. It is a mature modality that is widely available, and high-quality images are obtained easily in a wide variety of patients and clinical situations. Usually, even suboptimal CT images are often adequate for interpretation. However, CT, although sensitive, is nonspecific except for lipomas and adrenal adenomas that contain enough lipid to be low in attenuation. The main disadvantages of CT are exposure to ionizing radiation and the risks associated with use of iodinated contrast.

Magnetic Resonance Imaging

Although not yet as sensitive in detecting small masses as CT, MRI is more specific; currently it is the best noninvasive means available for distinguishing benign from malignant lesions. Several pathologic processes have distinctive signal characteristics, and the multiplanar capability of MRI can be helpful in elucidating structural features and in staging tumor spread. At present MRI is most frequently used to characterize lesions detected on CT. This modality continues to evolve, and continued improvements in imaging techniques, along with ever-shorter imaging times, suggest that MRI may shortly become the dominant modality for evaluating the adrenals, at least in patients in whom the *a priori* suspicion of an adrenal lesion is moderate or high. The main disadvantage of MRI is cost. In addition, it is more prone to artifacts than CT, and it requires more patient compliance.

Magnetic resonance imaging is the modality of choice for evaluating a suspected neuroblastoma because of its superior sensitivity for detecting vascular encasement and spinal involvement. Computed tomography, however, is more sensitive for detecting internal calcification within the tumor, which can be helpful in establishing the diagnosis. As a general rule, CT is probably the best modality for evaluating hyperfunctioning tumors and hyperplasia; MRI is probably best for distinguishing pheochromocytomas or neuroblastomas; and the two modalities are about equally effective (18,22) in evaluating for metastases versus adrenal adenoma (11–15).

IMAGING CONSIDERATIONS AND PROPER PROTOCOLS

Dedicated searches for adrenal pathology may require tailoring the search to the specific problem. For example,

pheochromocytomas and neuroblastomas frequently occur in extra-adrenal locations, and imaging must take this into account. Functional adenomas, especially aldosteronomas, can be small and require dedicated thin-collimation CT. Cortisol-secreting tumors tend to be more conspicuous because they tend to be larger and because they induce abundant retroperitoneal fat, which outlines the adrenals.

Computed Tomography Imaging

Thin-section helical CT provides excellent visualization of the adrenals, easily demonstrating 8-mm lesions. Thin sections also serve to prevent artifactually low Hounsfield unit (HU) readings caused by partial volume effects. Three-millimeter slices usually suffice. When a known adrenal lesion is being studied, unenhanced images should be obtained so that the attenuation of the lesion can be determined. In many instances, however, an adrenal mass is discovered incidentally in the course of a study done for other reasons, and no unenhanced images are available. In these instances, delayed images to assess the rate and degree of contrast washout may be helpful. Care must be taken when selecting the region of interest for density measurement to avoid spurious density readings caused by volume averaging with adjacent fat.

Incidental adrenal adenomas are common. The adrenal glands also are a common site for metastatic lesions, and differentiating between the two is a perennial challenge (16,17). Computed tomography is the initial study in these patients. Most adenomas are homogeneous, sharply marginated, and less than 3 cm in size, but metastases can appear morphologically identical. Because of their lipid content, adenomas tend to be low in attenuation on unenhanced CT, and a HU number of less than 15 in a homogeneous nonnecrotic lesion measuring less than 3 cm is highly suggestive of adenoma (18–22). However, there are pitfalls. Volume averaging between a solid lesion and periadrenal fat can give a falsely low attenuation number. Simple cysts or necrotic metastases can also be low in attenuation. Furthermore, adenomas larger than 3 cm are relatively common and have been reported in almost 3% of autopsy series (23). Hence, both false-positive and false-negative diagnoses are possible, and up to 30% of scans are inconclusive. Nevertheless, lesions found incidentally in patients with normal endocrine profile and without a known primary tumor and that meet size and density criteria are treated empirically as nonfunctioning adenomas in standard practice.

One frequent problem is that adrenal masses are often discovered incidentally on contrast-enhanced scans, where no determination can be made about intrinsic lesion density. To address this problem, attempts have been made to differentiate the enhancement patterns of adenomas and nonadenomas. On dynamic enhancement, adenomas show only moderate enhancement, whereas malignant lesions show relatively strong and prolonged enhancement. One study found that density of less than 30 HU within an adrenal lesion on a 1-hour delayed post-contrast study strongly suggests that the lesion is an adenoma (24). Other studies comparing ratios of immediate to delayed attenuation have found relatively rapid washout from adenomas (25).

Magnetic Resonance Imaging

Because the adrenals are small and thin, they are prone to motion and chemical shift artifacts. Careful attention to both spatial resolution and signal-to-noise ratio is needed to produce readable images. A multicoil designed for imaging the abdomen gives a better signal-to-noise ratio than a body coil. Motion- and flow-related artifact can be limited by using respiratory compensation and by applying superior and inferior saturation pulses. Fat-saturated sequences both reduce motion artifacts and increase the visibility of small differences in tissue contrast.

As with CT, MR protocols vary depending on whether the examination is focused exclusively on the adrenals or encompasses a larger portion of the abdomen. An adrenal examination requires axial T1- and T2-weighted sequences. T1-weighted images are needed for specific identification of lipid, fat, and hemorrhage. T2-weighted images are needed to evaluate for cysts and tumors. In most patients, contrast-enhanced sequences using a dynamic technique can be helpful. Additional sagittal or coronal sequences can be added as needed to evaluate lesion origin or extension. T1-weighted images are acquired using gradient-echo techniques, which enable both in- and out-of-phase sequences and rapidly acquired dynamic contrast-enhanced images. T2-weighted images are acquired using fast spin-echo (FSE) sequences, typically with a TR of about 4,000 and TE of at least 90. Matrix size is usually 256×256 or 192×256, and one or two excitations or signal averages (NEX) are used. The field of view should be small, usually 25 to 35 cm. Slice thickness generally varies from 4 mm to 8 mm. The choice of slice thickness depends in part on the extent of coverage desired and in part on the gradient-switching abilities of the system. Thinner slices require stronger gradients, which in turn affect the minimum TE that the system can achieve. If the system must increase TE to achieve these gradients, then lipid and water protons may not be truly in opposite phase on out-of-phase images.

Chemical shift techniques are currently the most sensitive MR imaging method to distinguish adenomas from nonadenomas (26–31). This technique takes advantage of the fact that protons in water resonate at a slightly different frequency from protons in lipid. Hence, the overall signal strength from any voxel containing both water and lipid varies cyclically with echo time, depending on whether the individual signals from the components are in phase or out of phase at the chosen echo time. (Note

that voxels containing pure water or pure fat will not be affected in this way.) Because adenomas contain lipid whereas most metastases do not, the technique is a powerful way to distinguish between the two. As with other techniques, however, volume-averaging with adjacent tissue limits the ability to characterize masses smaller than about 1 cm.

In- and out-of-phase signal intensities can be assessed visually or quantitatively as, for example, (SI of adrenal mass)/(SI of spleen) on opposed-phase images versus (SI of mass)/(SI of spleen) on in-phase images. In- and out-of-phase techniques, unlike conventional SE sequences, are highly sensitive to small amounts of lipid. Lipid-containing lesions show a drop in signal intensity on out-of-phase sequences with these techniques (18,27,31–34). On MRI, an adrenal lesion that does not lose at least 10% of its signal intensity on opposed-phase images is not considered to be an adenoma (35). Because adenomas contain lipid and most metastases do not, the presence of lipid in an adrenal lesion is frequently interpreted as indicating that the lesion is an adenoma (see Fig. 18.18C,D). However, metastases from renal cell carcinoma and hepatocellular carcinoma, as well as primary adrenocortical carcinoma, also can contain lipid (36–38). Although a drop in intensity on out-of-phase sequences strongly indicates presence of an adenoma, it is not pathognomonic, and in a patient with renal cell carcinoma, for example, biopsy may be required to make the diagnosis. It is considered atypical for an adenoma to appear lipid-free. In at least one of these patients, the tumor recurred after resection (39).

In addition to the true exceptions to the rule that lipid-containing lesions are benign, artifactual drops in signal intensity on opposed-phase images can also cause confusion. Edge effects on out-of-phase images can cause an apparent drop in signal intensity in small masses, which can falsely suggest that they contain lipid.

Because both adenomas and metastases to the adrenal are common, an adrenal gland occasionally may contain both. In patients with a primary malignant tumor, it is essential to evaluate any preexisting adrenal lesions for change, and any growth in a previously identified adenoma should be scrutinized closely. Again, opposed-phase MRI can be helpful in differentiating between an adenoma and a coexisting metastatic focus. Obviously, the distinction is crucial when a site for biopsy is being chosen (40).

The liver is often used as a standard for judging adrenal intensity on MRI. However, the liver is prone to conditions that alter its signal characteristics, such as fatty infiltration or iron overload. Therefore, before using it as a reference, one must first ensure that the liver itself is normal. For example, a classic rule of thumb is that adrenal adenomas tend to be lower in signal than liver on T_2-weighted images, and malignancies tend to be higher. This rule is not reliable, however, not only because both benign and malignant lesions can be atypical but also because the signal characteristics of the liver itself are variable. For example, a liver with increased iron deposits will be abnormally low in signal on T2-weighted images. In such instances, adrenal adenomas will appear relatively high in signal, suggesting malignancy. On the other hand, a fatty or edematous liver will be abnormally bright on T2-weighted images, which could make a malignant adrenal lesion appear benign. Other structures less prone to signal abnormalities can be substituted as reference standards, such as renal parenchyma, spleen, or paraspinous muscles or, for T2-weighted images, cerebrospinal fluid or bile.

The signal intensity of adrenal adenomas tends to resemble that of a normal adrenal gland on all conventional spin-echo sequences, and metastases tend to be hyperintense to a normal adrenal gland on T2-weighted images. Both can be atypical, however. Subacute hemorrhage can be hyperintense on both T1- and T2-weighted images. In about two-thirds of patients, necrotic tumors tend to be heterogeneously low in signal on T1-weighted images and high on T2-weighted images. Pheochromocytomas are isointense to normal liver on T1-weighted images and markedly hyperintense on T2-weighted images in about two-thirds of patients.

ADJACENT NORMAL STRUCTURES THAT CAN MIMIC ADRENAL MASSES

There are several classic pitfalls in adrenal imaging. Among these are encroaching normal structures or variants, such as stomach or a gastric diverticulum, splenules, renal cysts or focal prominences, or a lobulated diaphragmatic crus. In many instances, confusion can be avoided by carefully following normal structures on adjacent images or, in case of CT, by repositioning the patient or giving a glass of water and reimaging. In some patients, however, adjacent structures can closely mimic adrenal pathology, and additional imaging using a different modality may be needed. The left adrenal is more prone to these difficulties than the right because there are more structures adjacent to it. Obviously, every precaution should be taken to avoid biopsying a pseudomass.

Left Adrenal

Vessels

Vascular structures such as normal and tortuous splenic vessels or splenic artery aneurysms can mimic an adrenal mass (Figs. 18.10 and 18.11). Varices from the left inferior phrenic vein, in particular, can closely mimic a left adrenal mass (41–44). The presence of vessels can be confirmed either by pre- and postcontrast CT (see Fig. 18.11) or MRI showing flow voids (Fig. 18.12) or by Doppler ultrasound.

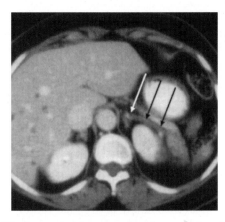

FIG. 18.10. Computed tomography of a splenic artery mimicking an enlarged left lateral adrenal limb in a patient with hyperaldosteronism. The adrenal glands are slightly thickened and nodular. What is apparently the lateral limb of the left adrenal is actually part of the splenic artery *(arrows)*. Renal and hepatic cysts are seen incidentally.

Spleen

Variations in splenic shape or contour are common. The tip of the spleen may be oriented in such a way as to simulate a left adrenal mass (Fig. 18.13) The spleen or, more frequently, an accessory splenule can abut the left adrenal gland and mimic an adrenal mass (Fig. 18.14A) (44–48). It may become necessary to obtain multiplanar reconstruction to establish the anatomic relations (47). On CT, the enhancement pattern matches the spleen rather than the adrenal, and on MRI, signal characteristics match the rest of the splenic tissue. Ultrasound is less helpful than CT or MRI in making the distinction between splenule and adrenal gland, although splenules will be isoechoic to the spleen.

Pancreas

The tail of the pancreas can abut the left adrenal gland and cause a pseudomass on CT (Fig. 18.14B) (49,50). Either ultrasound or MRI can be helpful in making the distinction in difficult cases. On MRI, on fat-suppressed T1-weighted images, the normal pancreas is higher in signal than adrenal tissue and can readily be distinguished from it.

Stomach

A gastric diverticulum, the gastric antrum itself, or a gastric mass such as a leiomyoma can mimic a left adrenal mass (Fig. 18.15) on CT or MRI (44,50–52). Gastric diverticula can be distinguished from adrenal pathology by reimaging after changing patient position, by giving more oral contrast, or by giving fizzies. Leiomyomas may require imaging by other modalities to make a definitive diagnosis.

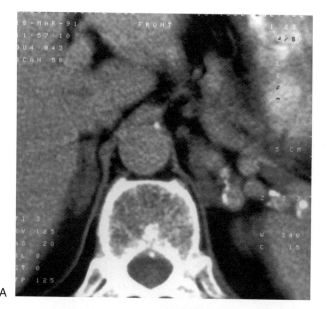

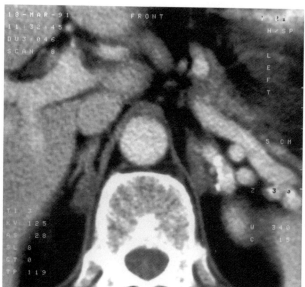

A

B

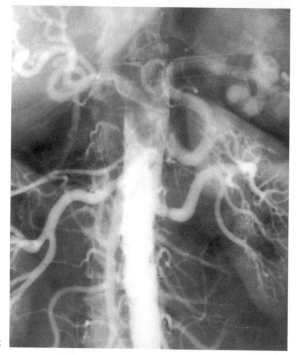

C

FIG. 18.11. Tortuous splenic artery mimicking calcified left adrenal nodule. **A,B:** Pre- and postcontrast CT scans show a tortuous and calcified splenic artery adjacent to the left adrenal mimicking an adrenal nodule. **C:** Aortic arteriogram shows the tortuous splenic artery curving above the left renal artery into the adrenal fossa, leading to a lobulated small splenic artery aneurysm. (Courtesy of A. Shirkhoda, M.D.)

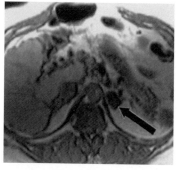

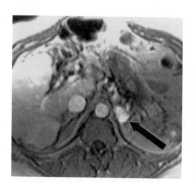

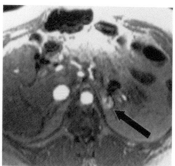

A–C

FIG. 18.12. Spontaneous splenorenal shunt *(arrow)* mimicking an adrenal mass in a patient with cirrhosis. **A:** T1-weighted precontrast image shows a periadrenal mass isointense to the IVC (TR/TE = 150/1.5). **B:** Postgadolinium image shows intense enhancement, matching that of the IVC (TR/TE = 150/1.5). **C:** Image from a magnetic resonance angiographic sequence shows flow-related enhancement, proving that the lesion is vascular in nature (TR/TE = 32/4.9).

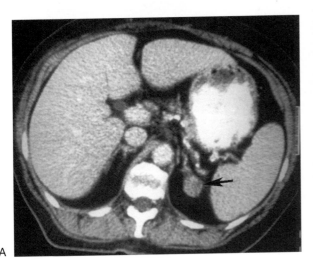

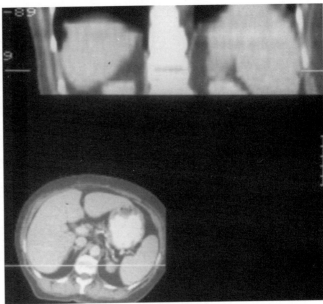

A

B

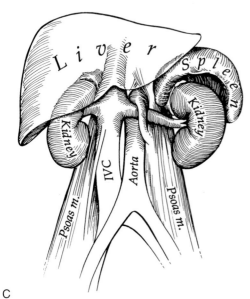

FIG. 18.13. Splenic tip simulating an adrenal mass on CT. **A:** Computed tomography scan shows an apparent left adrenal nodule *(arrow)* adjacent to the lateral limb of the left adrenal. **B:** Coronal reconstruction reveals the splenic tip in the adrenal fossa. **C:** Corresponding drawing shows horizontally oriented spleen with tip projecting over and medial to the upper pole of the kidney in the left adrenal fossa. (Reproduced with permission from reference 47.)

C

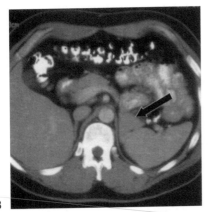

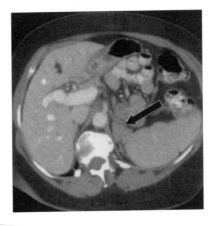

A,B

FIG. 18.14. Pancreatic and splenic lobulations simulating an adrenal mass on CT. **A:** Computed tomography image shows splenic lobulation *(arrow)* simulating a left adrenal mass. During surgery, the left adrenal gland was normal. **B:** Computed tomography image in a patient with scoliosis shows a triangular structure representing the pancreatic tail *(arrow)* simulating an adrenal mass. Contiguous images showed connection to the pancreas. If a pseudotumor is suspected, thin sections should be obtained, and the left adrenal gland specifically identified. (**B** courtesy of A. Shirkhoda, M.D.)

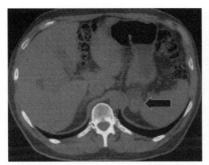 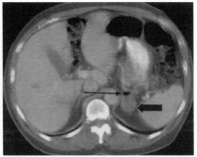

FIG. 18.15. Gastric diverticulum mimicking an adrenal mass on CT. **A:** Noncontrast image shows mass-like structure *(arrow)*. **B:** Contrast-enhanced image at a later date with oral and intravenous contrast shows the mass *(thick arrow)* to be a gastric diverticulum that now contains air *(thin arrow)*.

Diaphragmatic crura may be lobular and protrude into the left adrenal fossa, mimicking an adrenal gland or a nodule.

Right Adrenal

Right Kidney

Dynamic contrast enhancement on either CT or MRI is particularly useful in instances of focal lobation of the kidney because the lobation will enhance like the rest of the renal cortex.

Gallbladder

The gallbladder neck can mimic a right adrenal cyst (Fig. 18.16) if it lies more posterior than normal (53). For the same reason, a gallstone in the gallbladder neck can mimic a calcified adrenal nodule (Fig. 18.17).

Bowel

Fluid-filled loops of small bowel or colon can be confused with a right adrenal gland mass on CT (44,52). If careful review of adjacent images does not clarify matters, repeat imaging with better oral contrast, MRI, or ultrasound can be used to make the distinction (51).

Other Causes

Other causes of right adrenal pseudotumors are right inferior phrenic vein varices, tortuous or dilated renal vessels, or a dilated IVC.

A–C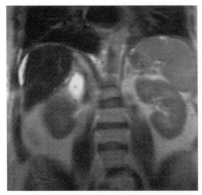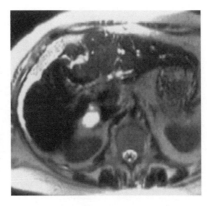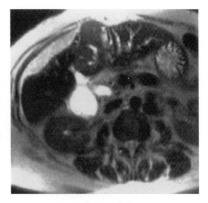

FIG. 18.16. Gallbladder mimicking a right adrenal cyst. **A:** Coronal FSE T2-weighted image shows a high-intensity mass in the expected location of the right adrenal gland (TR/TEeff = 19,960/99). **B:** Axial FSE T2-weighted image shows that the apparent mass represents the neck of the gallbladder. The adrenal gland is seen medial to the mass. **C:** Axial FSE T2-weighted image at a lower level shows stones within the dependent part of the gallbladder.

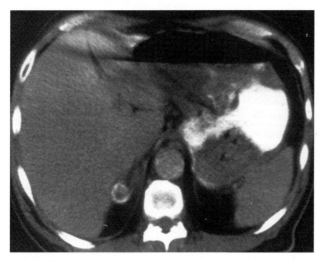

FIG. 18.17. Gallstone simulating calcified adrenal mass on CT. Ring-shaped calcification in the right adrenal fossa represents a gallstone in the right adrenal fossa. Cephalad adjacent thin slices showed connection with the gallbladder. (Figure courtesy of A. Shirkhoda, M.D.)

Adjacent Pathology That Can Mimic Adrenal Masses

Hepatic, renal, and pancreatic pathologic processes such as tumors, cysts, pseudocysts, and phegmons can invade or encroach on the adrenals, giving the appearance of an adrenal abnormality. The multiplanar capabilities of MRI as well as application of different pulse sequences (Fig 18.18) can help in making the distinction. Coronal images tend to be especially useful in distinguishing renal from adrenal processes (Fig. 18.19).

Large masses in the region of the adrenal glands are often difficult to ascribe to adrenal, renal, hepatic, pancreatic, or nonspecific retroperitoneal origin (54–56). Large masses either obliterate or displace the adrenal glands, making them difficult to identify. Several clues can help to suggest an adrenal origin for a large mass. On the right side, the adrenal gland lies posterior to the inferior vena cava (IVC), so that large masses of the right adrenal displace the IVC anteriorly (see Fig. 18.19), not leftward or posteriorly, as hepatic masses will, or leftward as renal masses will. On the left side, large masses origi-

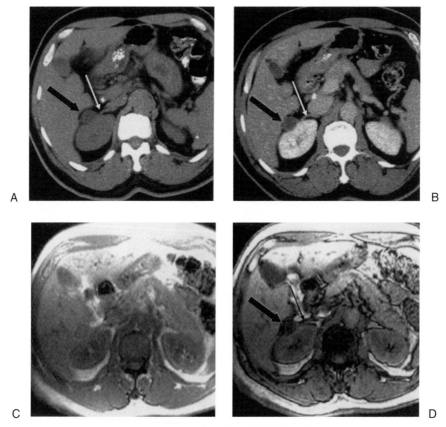

FIG. 18.18. Adrenal adenoma mimicking renal mass. Precontrast **(A)** and contrast-enhanced **(B)** CT images show relatively hypovascular right mass *(thick arrow),* which raised concern for a renal cell carcinoma. Note normal-appearing limb of adrenal gland *(thin arrow).* The precontrast attenuation is -6.2 HU; the postcontrast attenuation is 21.4 HU. **C:** In-phase gradient-echo image (TR/TE = 110/4.2) shows mass isointense to kidney. D: Opposed-phase gradient-echo image (TR/TE = 120/3.5) shows loss of signal consistent with adrenal adenoma *(thick arrow).* The ratio of the signal intensity of the adenoma relative to spleen is 0.83 on the in-phase image and 0.35 on the opposed-phase image, indicating the presence of lipid.

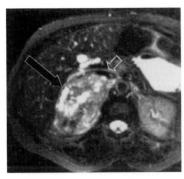
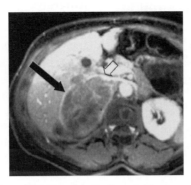
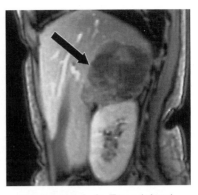

A–C

FIG. 18.19. Large mass of indeterminate origin in the right upper quadrant *(arrow)*. **A:** T2-weighted axial MR image (TR/TEeff = 8,571.4/144) shows a mass that displaces the inferior vena cava anteriorly *(open arrow)*. **B:** Gadolinium-enhanced axial T1-weighted gradient-echo image (TR/TE = 100/2.3) shows the displaced and compressed inferior vena cava. **C:** Sagittal T1-weighted gradient-echo image (TR/TE = 130/2.3) shows the mass superior to the right kidney *(arrow)*, displacing it inferiorly. The mass was found to be an adrenal schwannoma at surgery.

nating from the adrenal gland displace the pancreas and splenic vein anteriorly and the kidney inferiorly (Fig. 18.20). Imaging in the sagittal or coronal planes with ultrasound or MRI may help confirm or exclude involvement of these adjacent organs. Although the origin of many large masses may be difficult to determine, attention to the vector of displacement of adjacent organs is often helpful (56).

Extralobar sequestrations and bronchopulmonary foregut malformations can mimic a neuroblastoma in prenatal and pediatric studies (Fig. 18.21) (57–61). Rarely, bronchopulmonary foregut malformations and esophageal duplication cysts have been reported as incidental retroperitoneal masses in adults. Ultrasound generally shows these as hyperechoic, well-defined masses. On CT they tend to be low in attenuation and show little or no enhancement on postcontrast images. On MRI they appear intermediate in signal intensity on T1-weighted images and high on T2-weighted images (62).

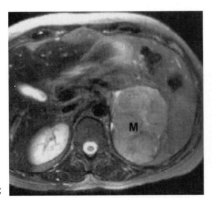
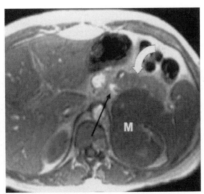
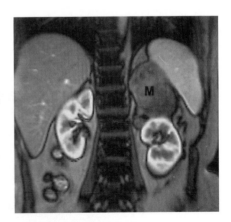

A–C

FIG. 18.20. Localizing a large left suprarenal mass to the adrenal in a patient with adrenocortical carcinoma. **A:** T2-weighted axial MR image (TR/TEeff = 4,767/104) shows a large suprarenal mass (M) that is hyperintense to liver and paraspinous muscle, displacing pancreas anteriorly and spleen laterally. **B:** On in-phase T1-weighted gradient-echo axial image (TR/TE = 120/4.2), mass (M) is hypointense to liver and paraspinous muscle. The anterior displacement of the splenic vein *(straight arrow)* and pancreas *(curved arrow)* are well demonstrated. **C:** Postgadolinium coronal T1-weighted gradient-echo image (TR/TE = 120/2.3) shows a poorly enhancing mass (M) displacing the kidney inferiorly.

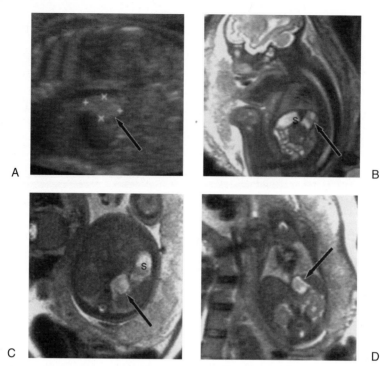

FIG. 18.21. Left suprarenal mass mimicking neuroblastoma. Fetal ultrasound **(A)** shows hyperechoic left suprarenal mass *(arrow)*. Sagittal **(B)**, axial **(C)**, and coronal **(D)** T2-weighted single-shot FSE images from fetal MRI show left suprarenal mass *(arrow)* with signal approaching that of fluid. S, stomach. Although the mass was found to be compatible with an extralobar sequestration, the newborn underwent exploratory surgery to exclude neuroblastoma. Adrenal gland was normal at surgery.

ADRENAL ANOMALIES

Adrenal anomalies are relatively rare. Variations in appearance often accompany renal anomalies, such as renal agenesis or ectopia (2,7). In such instances, the gland often assumes a flattened or pancake appearance (Fig. 18.22). Usually it maintains its normal position in the abdomen however, regardless of renal location or agenesis. Other relatively common adrenal anomalies include agenesis, hypoplasia, and congenital hyperplasia. Congenital hyperplasia results from various defects in cortisol synthesis and leads to a variety of virilizing and salt-wasting syndromes. In heterotopia, islands of adrenal tissue are found along the route of embryologic develop-

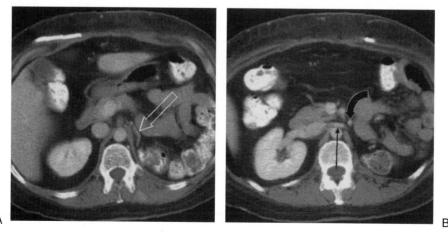

FIG.18.22. Adrenal morphology in a patient with left renal agenesis. **A:** Computed tomography scan shows a flattened vertical left adrenal gland *(arrow)* slightly more inferior than its usual location. **B:** Computed tomography scan inferior to **A** shows the left adrenal vein *(curved arrow)* emptying into the remnant left renal vein *(thin arrow)*.

ment (2). Adrenal gland tissue has been detected under the capsule of the liver and in the kidneys. Fused or horseshoe adrenal glands occur in conjunction with a wide range of other anomalies, including genitourinary, central nervous system, and situs abnormalities (6). In these instances, the fused portion can pass either between the inferior vena cava and the aorta or posterior to the aorta (63).

SUMMARY

Because they are small, surrounded by complex structures, and prone both to primary tumors and to metastases, the adrenal glands pose a challenge to imagers, requiring careful attention to choice of modality and imaging technique as well as to interpretation. Potential pitfalls include artifacts, encroaching adjacent normal or abnormal structures, and atypical appearances of intrinsic pathologic processes.

REFERENCES

1. Rubin E, Farber JL. *Pathology, 2nd ed.* Philadelphia: JB Lippincott, 1994;1128–1143.
2. Page DL, DeLellis RA, Hough AJ. Tumors of the adrenal. In: Hartmann WH, Sobin LH, eds. *Atlas of tumor pathology, vol 23.* Washington, DC: Armed Forces Institute of Pathology, 1986;9–10.
3. Brownlie K, Kreel L. Computer assisted tomography of normal suprarenal glands. *J Comput Assist Tomogr* 1978;2:1–10.
4. Schneck CD. Sectional anatomy of the genitourinary system. In: Resnik MI, Rifkin MD, eds. *Ultrasonography of the urinary tract.* Baltimore: Williams & Wilkins, 1991.
5. Novick AC, Pontes ES, Streem SB. *Stewart's operative urology.* Baltimore: Williams & Wilkins, 1989.
6. Burton EM, Strange ME, Edmonds DB. Sonography of the circumrenal and horseshoe adrenal gland in the newborn. *Pediatr Radiol* 1993; 23:362–364.
7. Mitty HA. Embryology, anatomy, and anomalies of the adrenal gland. *Semin Roentgenol* 1988;23:271–279.
8. Vincent JM, Morrison ID, Armstrong P, Reznek RH. The size of normal adrenal glands on computed tomography. *Clin Radiol* 1994;49: 453–455.
9. Mitchell DG, Outwater EK, Matteucci T, Rubin DL, Chezmar JL, Saini S. Adrenal gland enhancement at MR imaging with Mn-DPDP. *Radiology* 1995;194:783–787.
10. Krestin GP, Steinbrich W, Friedmann G. Adrenal masses: evaluation with fast gradient-echo MR imaging and Gd-DTPA-enhanced dynamic studies. *Radiology* 1989;171:675–680.
11. Neumann HP, Berger DP, Sigmund G, et al. Pheochromocytomas, multiple endocrine neoplasia type 2, and von Hippel-Lindau disease *N Engl J Med* 1993;329:1531–1538. [Published erratum appears in *N Engl J Med* 1994;331(22):1535.]
12. Velchik MG, Alavi A, Kressel HY, Engelman K. Localization of pheochromocytoma: MIGB, CT, and MRI correlation. *J Nucl Med* 1989;30:328–336.
13. Dietrich RB, Kangarloo H, Lenarsky C, Feig SA. Neuroblastoma: The role of MR imaging. *Am J Roentgenol* 1987;148:937–942.
14. Fletcher BD, Kopiwoda SY, Strandjord SE, Nelson AD, Pickering SP. Abdominal neuroblastoma: Magnetic resonance imaging and tissue characterization. *Radiology* 1985;155:699–703.
15. Freitas JE. Adrenal cortical and medullary imaging. *Semin Nucl Med* 1995;25:235–230.
16. Korobkin M, Francis IR, Kloos RT, Dunnick NR. The incidental adrenal mass. *Radiol Clin North Am* 1996;34:1037–1054.
17. Kloos RT, Gross MD, Francis IR, Korobkin M, Shapiro B. Incidentally discovered adrenal masses. *Endocr Rev* 1995;16:460–484.
18. Outwater EK, Siegelman ES, Huang AB, Birnbaum BA. Adrenal

masses: correlation between CT attenuation value and chemical shift ratio at MR imaging with in-phase and opposed-phase sequences. *Radiology* 1996;200:749–752. [Published erratum appears in *Radiology* 1996;201(3):880.]
19. Miyake H, Takaki H, Matsumoto S, Yoshida S, Maeda T, Mori H. Adrenal nonhyperfunctioning adenoma and nonadenoma: CT attenuation value as discriminative index. *Abdom Imag* 1995;20:559–562.
20. Korobkin M, Brodeur FJ, Yutzy GG, et al. Differentiation of adrenal adenomas from nonadenomas using CT attenuation values. *Am J Roentgenol* 1996;166:531–536.
21. Korobkin M, Francis IR. Imaging of adrenal masses. *Urol Clin North Am* 1997;24:603–622.
22. Korobkin M, Giordano TJ, Brodeur FJ, et al. Adrenal adenomas: relationship between histologic lipid and CT and MR findings. *Radiology* 1996;200:743–747.
23. Commons RR, Callaway CP. Adenomas of the adrenal cortex. *Arch Intern Med* 1948;81:47.
24. Korobkin M, Brodeur FJ, Francis IR, Quint LE, Dunnick NR, Goodsitt M. Delayed enhanced CT for differentiation of benign from malignant adrenal masses. *Radiology* 1996;200:737–742.
25. Cirillo RL Jr, Bennett WF, Vitellas KM, Poulos AG, Bova JG. Pathology of the adrenal gland: imaging features. *Am J Roentgenol* 1998;170: 429–435.
26. Schwartz LH, Panicek DM, Koutcher JA, et al. Adrenal masses in patients with malignancy: prospective comparison of echo-planar, fast spin-echo, and chemical shift MR imaging. *Radiology* 1995;197: 421–425.
27. Korobkin M, Lombardi TJ, Aisen AM, et al. Characterization of adrenal masses with chemical shift and gadolinium-enhanced MR imaging. *Radiology* 1995;197:411–418.
28. Tsushima Y, Ishizaka H, Matsumoto M. Adrenal masses: differentiation with chemical shift, fast low-angle shot MR imaging. *Radiology* 1993; 186:705–709.
29. Slapa RZ, Jakubowski W, Dabrowska E, et al. Magnetic resonance imaging differentiation of adrenal masses at 1.5 T: T2-weighted images, chemical shift imaging, and Gd-DTPA dynamic studies. *Magma* 1996; 4:163–179.
30. Mayo-Smith WW, Lee MJ, McNicholas MM, Hahn PF, Boland GW, Saini S. Characterization of adrenal masses (<5 cm) by use of chemical shift MR imaging: observer performance versus quantitative measures. *Am J Roentgenol* 1995;165:91–95.
31. Bilbey JH, McLoughlin RF, Kurkjian PS, et al. MR imaging of adrenal masses: value of chemical-shift imaging for distinguishing adenomas from other tumors [see comments]. *Am J Roentgenol* 1995;164: 637–642.
32. McNicholas MM, Lee MJ, Mayo-Smith WW, Hahn PF, Boland GW, Mueller PR. An imaging algorithm for the differential diagnosis of adrenal adenomas and metastases. *Am J Roentgenol* 1995;165: 1453–1459.
33. Martin J, Sentis M, Puig J, et al. Comparison of in-phase and opposed-phase GRE and conventional SE MR pulse sequences in T1-weighted imaging of liver lesions. *J Comput Assist Tomogr* 1996;20:890–897.
34. Outwater EK, Siegelman ES, Radecki PD, Piccoli CW, Mitchell DG. Distinction between benign and malignant adrenal masses: value of T1-weighted chemical-shift MR imaging. *Am J Roentgenol* 1995;165: 579–583.
35. Gilfeather M, Woodward PJ. MR imaging of the adrenal glands and kidneys. *Semin Ultrasound CT MR* 1998;19:53–66.
36. Outwater EK, Bhatia M, Siegelman ES, Burke MA, Mitchell DG. Detection of lipid in renal clear cell adenocarcinomas on opposed-phase gradient echo MR images. *Radiology* 1997;205:103–107.
37. Schlund JF, Kenney PJ, Brown ED, Ascher SM, Brown JJ, Semelka RC. Adrenocortical carcinoma: MR imaging appearance with current techniques. *J Magn Reson Imag* 1995;5:171–174.
38. Leroy-Willig A, Bittoun J, Luton JP, et al. *In vivo* MR spectroscopic imaging of the adrenal glands: distinction between adenomas and carcinomas larger than 15 mm based on lipid content. *Am J Roentgenol* 1989;153:771–773.
39. Outwater EK, Mitchell DG, Rubenfeld IG. Correction to a previously published case: recurrence of invasive adrenocortical tumor after excision of atypical adenoma. *Radiology* 1997;202:531–532.
40. Schwartz LH, Macari M, Huvos AG, Panicek DM. Collision tumors of the adrenal gland: demonstration and characterization at MR imaging. *Radiology* 1996;201:757–760.

41. Brady TM, Gross BH, Glazer GM, Williams DM. Adrenal pseudo-masses due to varices: angiographic-CT-MRI-pathologic correlations. *Am J Roentgenol* 1985;145:301–304.

42. Vogler JB, Helms CA, Callen PW. *Normal variations and pitfalls in imaging.* Philadelphia: WB Saunders, 1986.

43. Mitty HA, Cohen BA, Sprayregen S, Schwartz K. Adrenal pseudotumors on CT due to dilated portosystemic veins. *Am J Roentgenol* 1983;141:727–730.

44. Berliner L, Bosniak MA, Megibow A. Adrenal pseudotumors on computed tomography. *J Comput Assist Tomogr* 1982;6:281–285.

45. Beahrs JR, Stephens DH. Enlarged accessory spleens: CT appearance in postsplenectomy patients. *Am J Roentgenol* 1980;135:483–486.

46. Gooding GA. The ultrasonic and computed tomographic appearance of splenic lobulations: a consideration in the ultrasonic differential of masses adjacent to the left kidney. *Radiology* 1978;126:719–720.

47. Shirkhoda A. Diagnostic pitfalls in abdominal CT. *RadioGraphics* 1991;11:969–1002.

48. Stiris MG. Accessory spleen versus left adrenal tumor: computed tomographic and abdominal angiographic evaluation. *J Comput Assist Tomogr* 1980;4:543–544.

49. Churchill RJ, Reynes CJ, Love L. Pancreatic pseudotumors: computed tomography. *Gastrointest Radiol* 1978;3:251–256.

50. Mirowitz SA. *Pitfalls, variants, and artifacts in body MR imaging.* St Louis: CV Mosby, 1996.

51. Marks WM, Goldberg HI, Moss AA, Koehler FR, Federle MP. Intestinal pseudotumors: a problem in abdominal computed tomography solved by directed techniques. *Gastrointest Radiol* 1980;5:155–160.

52. Schwartz JM, Bosniak MA, Megibow AJ, Hulnick DH. Right adrenal pseudotumor caused by colon: CT demonstration. *J Comput Assist Tomogr* 1988;12:153–154.

53. Papanicolaou N, Pfister RC. Adrenal pseudotumor: gallbladder simulating a right adrenal mass. *J Comput Tomogr* 1985;9:171–172.

54. Jow W, Satchidanand S, Spinazze E, Lillie D. Malignant juxtadrenal schwannoma. *Urology* 1991;38:383–386.

55. Maekawa S, Mizutani Y, Terachi T, Okada Y, Yoshida O. A case of exophytic hepatic hemangioma mimicking adrenal tumor. *Hinyokika Kiyo—Acta Urol Jpn* 1997;43:123–126.

56. Harris RD, Heaney JA, Sueoka BL, Burke PR. Retroperitoneal leiomyosarcoma: a rare cause of adrenal pseudotumor on CT and MRI. *Urol Radiol* 1988;10:186–188.

57. Fenton LZ, Williams JL. Bronchopulmonary foregut malformation mimicking neuroblastoma. *Pediatr Radiol* 1996;26:729–730.

58. Goldstein I, Gomez K, Copel JA. The real-time and color Doppler appearance of adrenal neuroblastoma in a third-trimester fetus. *Obstet Gynecol* 1994;83:854–856.

59. McVicar M, Margouleff D, Chandra M. Diagnosis and imaging of the fetal and neonatal abdominal mass: an integrated approach. *Adv Pediatr* 1991;38:135–149.

60. Matzinger MA, Matzinger FR, Matzinger KE, Black MD. Antenatal and postnatal findings in intra-abdominal pulmonary sequestration. *Can Assoc Radiol J* 1992;43:212–214.

61. Swanson SJ, Skoog SJ, Garcia V, Wahl RC. Pseudoadrenal mass: unusual presentation of bronchogenic cyst. *J Pediatr Surg* 1991;26:1401–1403.

62. Daneman A, Baunin C, Lobo E, et al. Disappearing suprarenal masses in fetuses and infants. *Pediatr Radiol* 1997;27:675–681.

63. Shafaie FF, Katz ME, Hannaway CD. A horseshoe adrenal gland in an infant with asplenia. *Pediatr Radiol* 1997;27:591–593.

Variants and Pitfalls in Body Imaging,
edited by Ali Shirkhoda.
Lippincott Williams & Wilkins, Philadelphia, © 2000.

CHAPTER 19

The Bladder, Prostate, and the Testis

Zafar H. Jafri and Leopold Fregoli

This chapter briefly discusses the common anatomic variants and diagnostic pitfalls encountered with the imaging of the urinary bladder and the adjacent spaces, prostate, scrotum, and testicles. Correct recognition of anatomic landmarks and their variants are essential to avoid misinterpretation, which results in errors in diagnosis and management of the patient. Therefore, familiarity with the normal anatomy and embryology is essential to avoid such mistakes.

URINARY BLADDER AND THE ADJACENT SPACES

Bladder Embryology

The male pronephros, mesonephros, and mesonephric duct are three embryologic systems whose complex interactions result in the eventual formation of the urogenital system. The cloaca and portions of the mesonephric ducts form the urinary bladder. The cloaca is divided by the urorectal septum into a dorsal rectum and ventral urogenital sinus. The urogenital sinus, in turn, is comprised of three parts: a posteriorly positioned phallic segment, a pelvic portion, and a vesicourethral portion. The mesonephric ducts are absorbed by the vesicourethral portion and become the area of the trigone of the bladder and portions of the prostatic urethra. The remaining vesicourethral portions develop into the body of the bladder and the remainder of the prostatic urethra. An elongated extension from the allantois is then noted to extend to the umbilicus. This is known as the urachus. The male mesonephric or Wolffian duct continues to

develop into the epididymis, the vas deferens, and the ejaculatory ducts (1,2).

Normal Anatomy

The bladder is located centrally within the extraperitoneal fat, anterior and inferior to the peritoneum. Anatomically it consists of an apex, a superior surface, two inferolateral surfaces, a base, and a neck. The bladder apex ends as the medial umbilical ligament. The only portion of the urinary bladder that is covered by peritoneum is its superior surface. Recognition of extraperitoneal and intraperitoneal paravesical spaces is essential to correctly interpret the etiology of fluid collections surrounding the urinary bladder. The bladder trigone resides at the base, and the bladder neck is pierced by the internal urethral orifice.

The bladder wall is made up of several layers, which include the transitional epithelium or urothelium, the submucosa, the muscular layer, and the serosa. The muscular layers of the bladder wall are referred to as the detrusor muscle. The serosal layer is limited to the superior surface of the bladder and is separated from the peritoneal reflection by perivesical fat. Located immediately above and behind the internal urethral orifice is the bladder trigone. Three angles make up this trigone: two posterolateral angles formed by the ureteral orifices and an anteroinferior angle formed by the internal urethral orifice.

The superior, middle, and inferior vesical arteries provide arterial branches to the urinary bladder. These arteries arise from the anterior division of the internal iliac artery. Small arteries from the obturator, inferior gluteal, uterine, and vaginal arteries also feed this richly vascular structure. The vesical veins are short and unite into rich

---

Z. H. Jafri and L. Fregoli: Department of Diagnostic Radiology, Division of Uroradiology, William Beaumont Hospital, Royal Oak, Michigan 48073.

pudendal plexus that ultimately terminate into the internal iliac vein (3).

When appropriately distended, the bladder wall has a thickness of less than 5 mm on CT, and on enhanced studies, it enhances uniformly. The layers of the bladder wall, which include the mucosa, lamina propria, superficial and deep muscles, and serosa, cannot be distinguished. Approximately 1 to 2 minutes following intravenous injection of contrast medium, enhancement of the bladder wall becomes apparent. Opacification of the bladder lumen is seen after approximately 5 to 10 minutes (4).

Bladder anatomy is well delineated with magnetic resonance imaging (MRI). The aforementioned layers of the bladder wall can, at times, be distinguished. On proton density-weighted images, the mucosa and the lamina propria can be discerned from the muscle layer, given their higher signal intensity. The muscle layer consists of bundles of smooth muscle, which demonstrate an intermediate signal intensity similar to that of skeletal muscle on T_1-weighted images and a low signal intensity on T_2-weighted images. Although indicated as such, the serosa is not a true layer of the bladder wall. It is in contact with the bladder only at its dome and actually represents the peritoneal covering. This layer is too thin to be recognized on MR images (5).

Intraperitoneal Paravesical Space

The intraperitoneal paravesical spaces can be subdivided into anterior and posterior paravesical spaces. The anterior paravesical space can be further subdivided into supravesical space and medial inguinal fossae.

The supravesical space extends above the bladder between the medial umbilical folds and may contain small bowel loops and the dome of the urinary bladder. The medial umbilical folds can occasionally be visualized on computed tomography, especially in patients with abundant surrounding perivesical and intraperitoneal fat (Fig. 19.1).

The medial inguinal fossae lie between the medial and lateral umbilical folds. These fossae are occupied by cecum or ilium on the right and sigmoid colon on the left. The lateral inguinal fossae lie between the lateral umbilical folds and the lateral parietal peritoneum and are the smallest of the anterior paravesical fossae (Fig. 19.2).

The posterior intraperitoneal paravesical space is a potential space formed by the reflections of the peritoneum from the posterior wall of the urinary bladder on the rectum. In women this is subdivided by the uterus and ovaries into vesicouterine space, rectouterine pouch or *cul-de-sac*, ovarian fossae, and pararectal fossae.

With cross-sectional imaging in patients with presence of intraperitoneal fat, the extraperitoneal and intraperi-

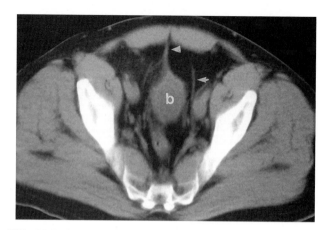

FIG. 19.1. Medial umbilical folds. Axial CT scan at the level of the dome of the urinary bladder demonstrates the medial umbilical folds *(arrow)* near the lateral aspect of the bladder. The obliterated urachus is seen in midline as medial umbilical ligament *(arrowhead)*.

toneal spaces can be delineated. The prevesical collection, which can typically have a molar tooth appearance, can be differentiated from intraperitoneal fluid such as ascites, which displaces the urinary bladder inferiorly but not posteriorly (6).

Extraperitoneal Paravesical Spaces

The umbilicovesical fascia surrounds the urachus, obliterated umbilical arteries, and urinary bladder. This

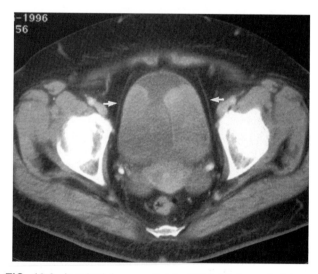

FIG. 19.2. Inguinal fossae. Pelvic CT following administration of contrast medium in a 60-year-old woman with carcinoma of the uterus demonstrates a mosaic pattern of the urinary bladder caused by admixing of contrast and urine. The medial umbilical folds are well seen separating the medial and lateral inguinal fossae *(arrows)*.

fascia is triangular with its apex at the umbilicus and, coursing around the urinary bladder, it blends with the visceral layer of the pelvic fascia along the lateral aspect of the lower uterus or seminal vesicles and rectum.

The umbilicovesical fascia divides the anterior extraperitoneal fat into perivesical and prevesical spaces. The bladder, umbilical artery, and urachus lie within the perivesical space, whereas the prevesical space is located predominantly anterior and lateral to the umbilicovesical fascia. This is a large compartment that extends up to the umbilicus and communicates with the preperitoneal space in the anterior abdominal wall and flanks.

The pubovesical ligament forms the anteroinferior boundaries of both the peri- and prevesical spaces. Clinically the prevesical space is more significant than the perivesical space (Fig. 19.3). The prevesical space behind the pubic symphysis is also known as the space of Retzius. The space between the posterior aspect of the bladder and lower uterine segment in women and seminal vesicle in men is in continuity with the perivesical space (7).

The prevesical fascia represents fused peritoneal layers that line the medial recesses of the medial inguinal fossae. This is not commonly seen on CT scans. Fluid collections in the prevesical spaces can assume a molar tooth

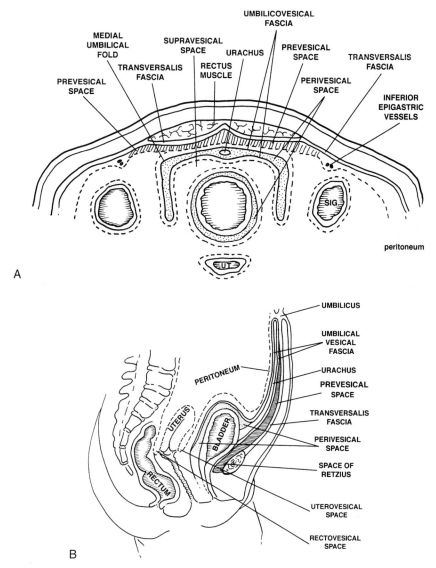

FIG. 19.3. Paravesical spaces. **A:** Schematic drawing at the level of the midpelvis in the axial plane demonstrates the relationship of the urinary bladder to the paravesical spaces. **B:** Schematic drawing in midsagittal plane illustrates the relationship of bladder and uterus to the intra- and extraperitoneal paravesical spaces. (**A,B:** Courtesy Alexander Cacciarelli, M.D., William Beaumont Hospital.)

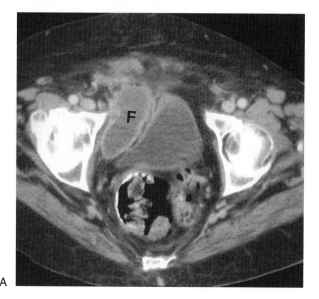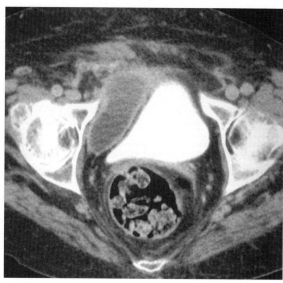

FIG. 19.4. Extraperitoneal perivesical fluid. **A:** Computed tomography scan through the pelvis obtained several months following a spontaneous rectus sheath and retroperitoneal hematoma demonstrates a fluid collection (F) along the right anterolateral aspect of the urinary bladder. **B:** Delayed images obtained 15 minutes later confirm the nature of the collection to extraperitoneal space as a chronic perivesical seroma.

appearance as fluid collects between the umbilicovesical fascia and transverse fascia. The fluid in the prevesical space can extend into the rectus sheath, along the round ligament, vas deferens, spermatic cord, and femoral sheath. This consists of downward prolongation of transversalis fascia anteriorly and iliac fascia posteriorly. The fluid can also extend laterally and posteriorly and come in contact with the iliopsoas muscle and retroperitoneum (7,8) (Fig. 19.4).

Bladder Diverticula

Diverticulum of the urinary bladder may present as a cystic pelvic mass that, in female patients, may occasionally appear as a complex cystic ovarian mass not obviously connected with urinary bladder. If it gets infected, it may simulate a deep pelvic abscess. The size of these bladder diverticula may vary from a small pea size to large, giant diverticulum that may lead to urinary retention secondary to ureteral compression and renal failure (9).

Urinary bladder diverticula are usually acquired most commonly as a result of bladder outlet obstruction and are most common in men. Before diverticular formation, a spectrum of changes is evident ranging from simple bladder wall thickening to trabeculation. The end result is mucosal herniation through the detrusor muscle fibers, which is usually solitary but can be multiple (Figs. 19.5–19.7). There is also the rare congenital variant that can be seen in normal healthy children or patients with Menkes', Williams', and Ehlers-Danlos syndromes (10,11).

The numerous complications that may be associated with diverticula or that may complicate the course of patients with this entity place a great deal of emphasis on the correct diagnosis. Possible complications include infection, rupture, calculus formation, and neoplasm (12,13). The prognosis of diverticula that contain neoplasm is not favorable, as there is usually early invasion, given their lack of a muscular barrier. An additional complication is that of vesicoureteral reflux as a result of a strategically placed diverticulum, which alters the normal antireflux mechanism of the distal ureter. This is known as the Hutch diverticulum.

Vesical diverticula can usually be well delineated on CT, ultrasound, and MR imaging as well as by cystography (14). The diagnosis can be easy if the diverticulum is filled with contrast material; however, when these entities are devoid of contrast material, it can sometimes be difficult to differentiate a bladder diverticulum from other perivesical fluid collections or masses such as ovarian cysts, seminal vesicle cysts, or loculated ascites. The degree of bladder filling thus strongly influences the establishment of the correct diagnosis. In the age of fast dynamic CT scanners, an examination simply outruns the renal excretion of contrast material and filling of the bladder (Figs. 19.8–19.10). Color Doppler US can sometimes demonstrate a jet phenomenon within the diverticulum; however, the sonographic diagnosis depends on the demonstration of a communication between the bladder and the perivesical pseudocollection (Fig. 19.11) (15).

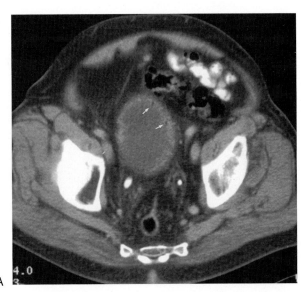
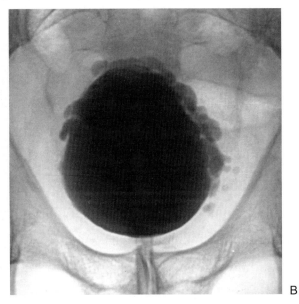

FIG. 19.5. Bladder wall thickening. **A:** Helical CT scan obtained in an 81-year-old man demonstrates diffuse thickening of the wall of the urinary bladder with subtle hypodense crypts involving the inner wall (arrows). **B:** Contrast cystogram demonstrates markedly trabeculated bladder with multiple small outpouchings consistent with multiple diverticuli. These findings are commonly seen with chronic bladder outlet obstruction.

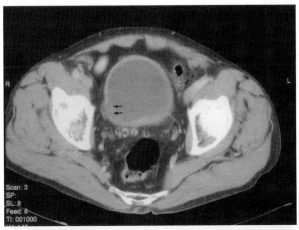
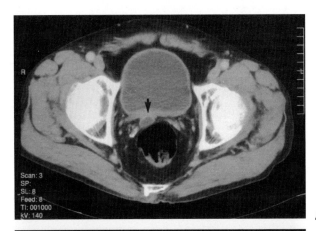

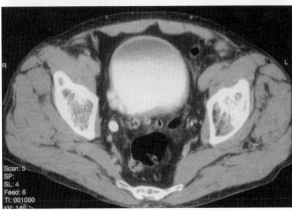
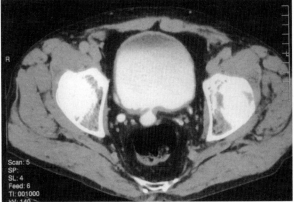

FIG. 19.6. Small bladder diverticuli. **A:** Helical CT of the pelvis in the arterial phase demonstrates lobulated right lateral wall of the urinary bladder *(arrows)*. The wall of the bladder is also thickened. **B:** Delayed image confirms this to represent multiple bladder diverticuli secondary to chronic bladder outlet obstruction by BPH.

FIG. 19.7. Small posterior bladder diverticulum. Two images of the pelvis obtained during helical scans. In the early arterial phase **(A)**, a focal low-density mass is seen posterior to the urinary bladder *(arrow)* that, on delayed images, fills with contrast medium, confirming a bladder diverticulum. On the initial scan the findings may be confused as a perivesical lymph node.

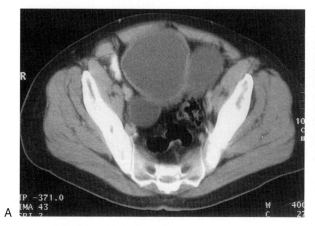
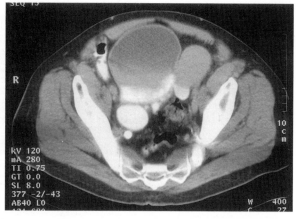

FIG. 19.8. Multiple bladder diverticuli. Early **(A)** and delayed **(B)** helical CT scans at the midpelvis level demonstrate two fluid-filled structures adjacent to the urinary bladder that, on delayed image, fills with contrast medium, confirming multiple bladder diverticuli. On the initial scan the findings may be confused with adnexal cysts.

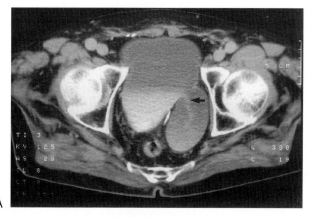
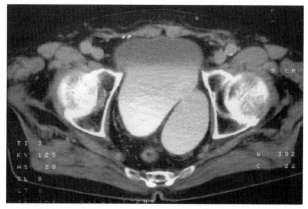

FIG. 19.9. Large bladder diverticulum. Early **(A)** and delayed **(B)** images at the level of the midpelvis demonstrate a fluid-filled structure communicating with the bladder. On the initial image **(A)**, spillage of contrast is faintly seen *(arrow);* this was confirmed on delayed scan **(B)** as a large bladder diverticulum.

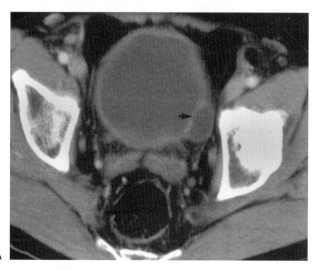
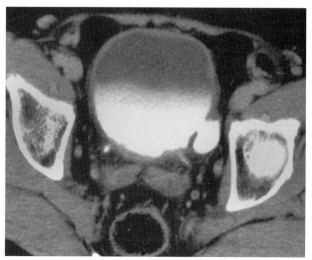

FIG. 19.10. Bladder wall thickening and diverticulum. **A:** Contrast-enhanced helical CT of the pelvis in a 58-year-old man with carcinoma of the prostate demonstrates a fluid structure adjacent to the left lateral wall of the bladder *(arrow).* **B:** Six-minute delayed images obtained at the same level show filling of the diverticulum with contrast. In addition, there is diffuse thickening of the bladder wall caused by chronic obstruction by an enlarged prostate.

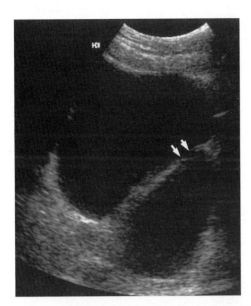

FIG. 19.11. Large bladder diverticulum. Sagittal sonogram of the pelvis demonstrates a fluid-filled mass posterior to the urinary bladder with a defect in the posterior wall *(arrows)* indicating the neck of a large bladder diverticulum. Flow of urine through the neck may be detectable by Doppler ultrasound.

Ureterovesical Jet Phenomenon

The ureterovesical jet occurs when densely opacified urine from the ureter enters the more dilute urine in the bladder and appears as a stream exiting the ureteral orifice. This jet of urine can also be seen on gray-scale sonography as a stream of echogenic bubbles entering the urine-filled bladder from the ureter. This represents a nor-

mal finding seen in patients with normal excretion and can also aid in the diagnosis of obstructive uropathy (16). The frequency and size of ureteral jets are variable and range from 1 per minute to a continuous stream, depending on diuresis and nervous system stimulation. Doppler techniques are more sensitive to moving low-level reflectors than is gray-scale sonography. Therefore, one may evaluate this phenomenon with Doppler techniques rather than with gray-scale sonography alone (Fig. 19.12) (17).

Under normal conditions two to six ureteral contraction waves form per minute. The ureteral jet is usually directed anteromedially under normal circumstances. Although real-time ultrasound can depict ureteral jets, color Doppler ultrasound demonstrates ureteric jets more reliably provided the bladder is not overfilled and the patient is well hydrated (Figs. 19.13 and 19.14). Laterally placed ureteral orifice as seen by ureteral jets has also been correlated with the presence of vesicoureteral reflux in children (18,19).

With the introduction of the contrast-enhanced spiral or helical CT, the phenomenon of ureterovesical jet is being observed almost daily. The findings are variable, depending on the timing of the scan through the bladder. Bilateral jets may be observed as the contrast enters the bladder, or the bladder may demonstrate confusing and deceptive variable densities, which may be mistaken for intravesical masses (Figs. 19.15–19.17). Recognition of these artifacts is important and can be easily obviated by obtaining delayed images through the bladder. Similarly, such findings may also be observed during HASTE sequence (Fig. 19.18) or gadolinium-enhanced MR imaging when the ureteral jet creates swirling artifacts with the urinary bladder (Figs. 19.19).

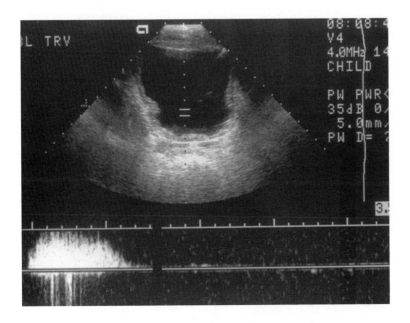

FIG. 19.12. Turbulent ureterovesical jet. Turbulence at the site of the right ureteral jet seen on Doppler not visible at gray scale in an 8-year-old child with recurrent urinary tract infection.

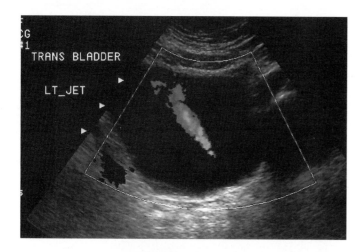

FIG. 19.13. Left ureterovesical jet. Transverse sonogram of the urinary bladder demonstrates a left ureteric jet. After entering the bladder it propagates to the opposite anterior urinary bladder wall.

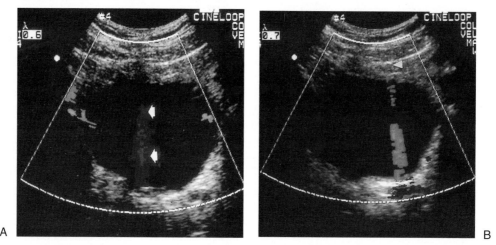

A   B

FIG. 19.14. Bilateral ureterovesical jet. **A:** Transverse sonogram of the urinary bladder demonstrates a right ureteric jet. Ureteric jets propagate from the UV junction and splash along the opposite anterior bladder wall. Note that this is a true ureteric jet. **B:** Transverse sonogram of the urinary bladder suggests the presence of a left ureteric jet.

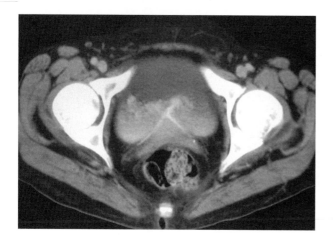

FIG. 19.15. Bilateral ureterovesical jet on CT. Contrast scan at the level of the UVJ demonstrates bilateral ureteral jets with layering of contrast in the dependant portion.

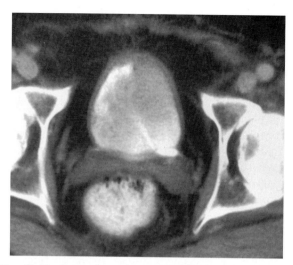

FIG. 19.16. Prominent left ureterovesical jet. Contrast-enhanced helical CT at the level of the seminal vesicles demonstrates a large left ureteral jet resulting in admixing of contrast and urine.

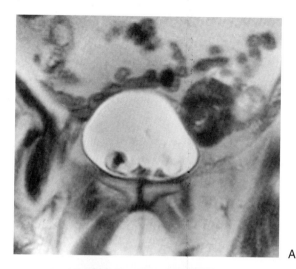

A

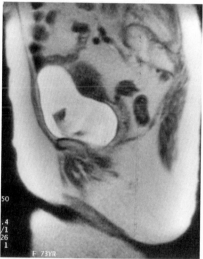

B

FIG. 19.18. Ureterovesical jet on MRI. Coronal **(A)** and sagittal **(B)** T_2-weighted HASTE (half-Fourier single-shot turbo spin echo) images of the bladder reveal curvilinear areas of low signal within the bladder lumen caused by bladder jets. Typically, bladder jets are seen on postcontrast T_1-weighted imaging sequences. The jets are seen here because of spin dephasing by slush in the bladder.

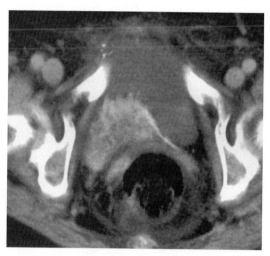

FIG. 19.17. Bladder pseudotumor from UV jet on CT. Helical CT at the level of the ureterovesical junction demonstrates a left ureteral jet with inhomogeneous mixing of contrast and urine. Such findings should not be mistaken for a mass at the base of the bladder.

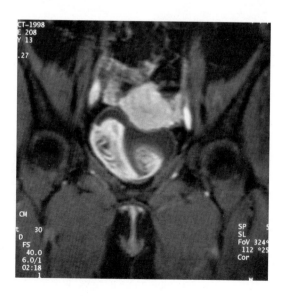

FIG. 19.19. Bladder pseudotumor from UV jet on MRI. Coronal fat saturation T_1-weighted contrast-enhanced gradient-echo image shows nonuniform mixing of excreted MR contrast in the urinary bladder, which should not be mistaken for an enhancing bladder neoplasm.

Bladder Herniation

Bladder herniation accounts for 1% to 4% of inguinal hernias; they are usually direct hernias and commonly right sided. Bladder hernias in women are more commonly associated with femoral hernias; however, most patients are men over 50 years of age with either direct or indirect hernia. In addition to obesity, contributing factors include bladder outlet obstruction and loss of bladder tone (20).

The majority of bladder hernias are asymptomatic, being discovered incidentally at surgery. Failure to recognize may result in inadvertent bladder perforation during herniorrhaphy. In the past, intravenous urography and cystographic examinations were performed to diagnose and assess these hernias. The findings included transient herniation (bladder ears) to marked prolapse of the bladder through the femoral or inguinal canals. At times erect and prone films may be required to better demonstrate the findings.

Recently, however, the bladder hernias are discovered as incidental findings during pelvic CT examinations performed for some unrelated conditions. The diagnosis is obvious in most of the situations and may require delayed scans if contrast has not reached the bladder (Fig. 19.20). At times, coronal or sagittal reconstruction may help to further delineate and confirm the findings (Fig. 19.21). Computed tomographic evaluation before surgery would also clarify the anatomy and any associated complications of this condition including hydronephrosis, calculi, and strangulation. Rarely the intraperitoneal fat may herniate, resembling lipoma of the spermatic cord (Fig. 19.22). One must also remember to scan through the scrotum when this entity is suspected, as it may otherwise go undetected (21).

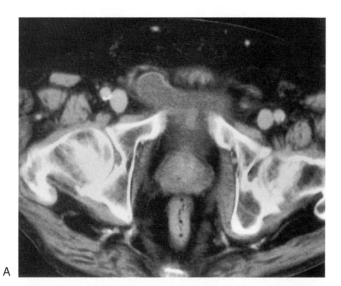

A

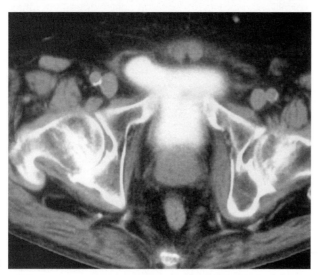

B

FIG. 19.20. Bladder herniation. **A:** Computed tomography scan obtained during staging of colon carcinoma of this 64-year-old man demonstrates abnormal protrusion of the urinary bladder into the right external inguinal ring. **B:** Delayed images obtained at the same level confirm the contrast-filled bladder herniation through the right external inguinal ring, suggesting a direct inguinal hernia.

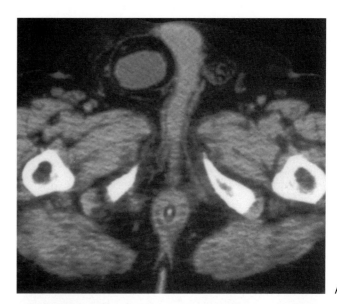

A

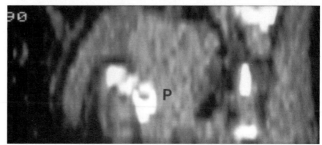

B

FIG. 19.21. Bladder herniation. **A:** Pelvic CT at the level of inferior pubic ramus demonstrates a round fluid-filled mass in the right spermatic canal. **B:** Reconstructed sagittal image confirms this to be herniated urinary bladder over the os pubis secondary to an enlarged prostate (P).

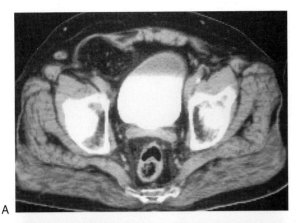

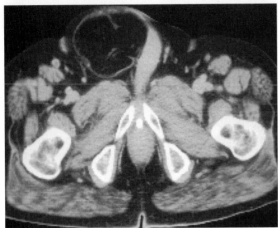

FIG. 19.22. Peritoneal fat herniation. **A:** Computed tomography scan of the pelvis in a 68-year-old man with a history of chronic cough demonstrates herniation of intraperitoneal fat with bulging of the transverse oblique muscle. **B:** Scan obtained several centimeters below **A** demonstrates a round fat density in the spermatic canal. Such herniation may resemble a lipoma of the spermatic cord, which commonly presents as a focal fatty mass in the paratesticular region.

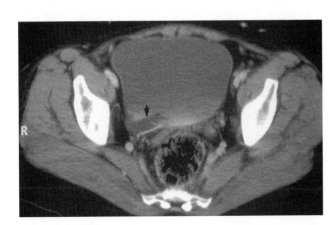

FIG. 19.23. Pseudolesion from contrast–urine mixture. This CT scan through the lower pelvis in a 44-year-old woman with lower extremity edema demonstrates an artifact created with excreted contrast medium and urine in the bladder simulating an irregular filling defect *(arrow)*. Subsequent delayed scan and ultrasound confirmed the normal appearance of the urinary bladder.

Pseudomasses

One of the main advantages of helical CT is being consistently able to obtain scans in the arterial phase of the injection, which results in excellent opacification and enhancement of the intraabdominal organs. Because a majority of the scans are routinely obtained only as a single helical scan, the time interval between the abdominal and pelvic images is markedly minimized, which results in imaging of the pelvis in the late arterial and early venous phases of injection. The urinary bladder is mostly imaged when the excreted contrast has not yet reached it or is in the early phase of entry. Such timing of the scan results in bizarre contrast/urine admixing patterns not previously seen (see Figs. 19.15–19.17). Recognition of these admixing artifacts will obviate mistakes in interpretation of these findings as pathologic processes (Fig. 19.23). In a majority of such cases recognition and, if necessary, delayed images will clarify the nature of the artifacts and pseudolesions (Figs. 19.24 and 19.25).

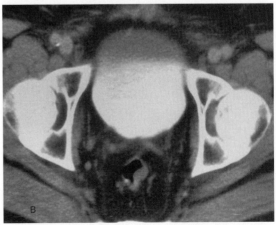

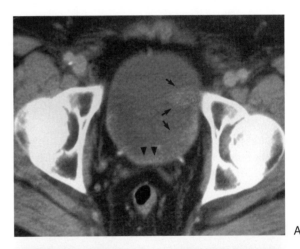

FIG. 19.24. Pseudotumors of the bladder. **A:** Pelvic CT in the early phase of a helical CT scan demonstrates a patchy area of increased density along the left lateral aspect of the urinary bladder *(arrows)*. There is also apparent thickening of the posterior bladder wall *(arrowheads)*. **B:** Delayed scan obtained several minutes later demonstrates a normal lumen of the bladder. The initial pitfall was secondary to poor admixing of urine and contrast in the early phase of the scanning.

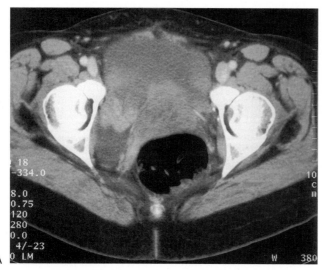
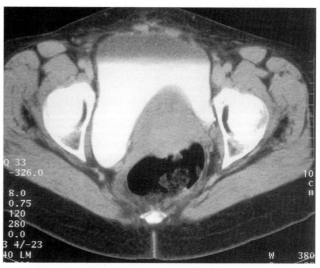

FIG. 19.25. Lobulated bladder pseudotumor. **A:** Contrast scan in the early phase of a helical CT scan demonstrates a lobular enhancing mass on the right side of the pelvis. A right adnexal mass was questioned. **B:** Delayed images clearly confirm this to represent extension of the urinary bladder posteriorly. The finding on the initial scan was caused by poor mixing of contrast with urine.

The distended urinary bladder has long been used as a sonographic window to identify the pelvic structures during transabdominal sonography of the female pelvis. Identification of a normal filled urinary bladder does not present a problem in the majority of situations. It has a characteristic anterior midline location posterior and cephalad to symphysis pubis (22). Proper gain settings will avoid mismatch artifacts at the interface of the anterior abdominal wall and the anterior wall of the bladder (Fig. 19.26). Large distended urinary bladder diverticu-

lum or urine refluxed into the vagina can sometimes be mistaken for a pathologic cystic pelvic mass, and rarely an ovarian neoplasm with a mural nodule or clots has been erroneously confused for a urinary bladder containing a Foley catheter (Figs. 19.27 and 19.28). It is always prudent to identify the urinary bladder, and, if necessary, a scan can be repeated following bladder voiding to con-

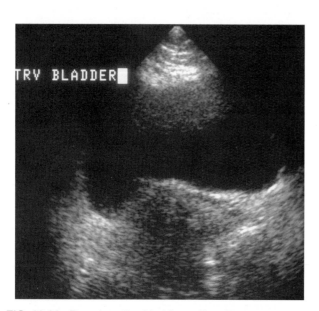

FIG. 19.26. Reverberation bladder artifact. Transverse sonogram of the pelvis with a distended urinary bladder demonstrates low-level echoes obscuring detail of the anterior bladder wall. A strong mismatch of sound at the soft tissue–fluid interface is responsible for these artifactual echoes.

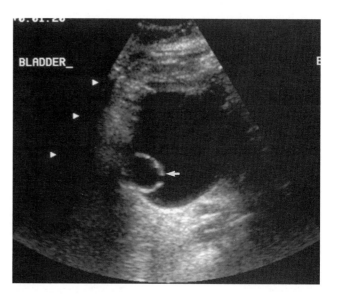

FIG. 19.27. Ovarian mass mimicking bladder. Eighty-six-year-old woman with a history of carcinoma of the breast demonstrates a cystic mass with a mural nodule in the right adnexal region (arrow). This initially was mistaken for a urinary bladder containing a Foley balloon. The bladder was empty and collapsed. Follow-up CT scan of the pelvis (not shown) obtained a week later confirms this mass to be arising from the right ovary. Surgery was deferred because of the patient's severe debilitation.

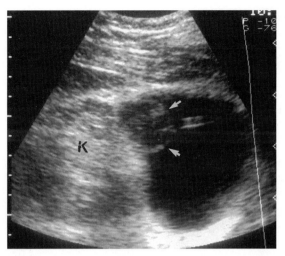

FIG. 19.28. Intravesical hematoma. Sagittal sonogram of the transplant kidney (k) in the left lower quadrant demonstrates a stent with a surrounding hematoma mimicking a Foley balloon *(arrows)*.

firm the findings observed in an extravesical mass. Likewise, in patients who undergo transvaginal sonogram with Foley catheter in the urinary bladder, a novice sonographer can mistake a Foley balloon for an ectopic pregnancy (Fig. 19.29). The majority of these errors can be avoided if definitive identification of a urinary bladder is made. The most common cystic mass that has been shown to simulate urinary bladder include ovarian cystadenomas, lymphoceles, ovarian and parovarian cysts, urinoma, hematoma, fluid-filled bowel loop, or even a pancreatic pseudocyst. A chronic rectus sheath hematoma or loculated ascites may also simulate a urinary bladder. In situations where the diagnosis is in doubt, a postvoid or postcatheterization repeat ultrasound will document a change in size and volume of the bladder and will result in correct identification of the structure in question.

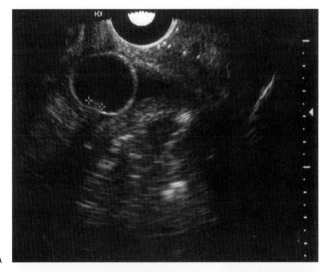

A

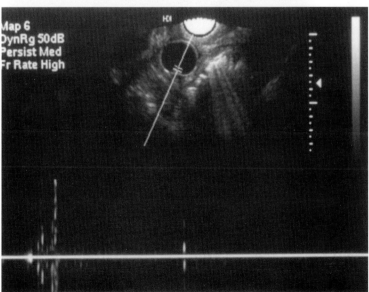

B

FIG. 19.29. Pseudogestational sac. **A:** Transvaginal sonogram of a female pelvis demonstrates a sharply marginated round structure with a small intraluminal echogenic area. This Foley balloon in a collapsed urinary bladder was erroneously mistaken for a gestational sac containing a fetus *(cursors)*. **B:** Obtaining a Doppler signal was also attempted. Recognition of normal anatomy will obviate such pitfalls.

Intravaginal Pessary

Genital prolapse in women is quite common, and some degree of prolapse occurs in nearly 50% of parous women. It is considered one of the most common indications for hysterectomy in noncancerous patients (23).

Uterine prolapse occurs when there is disruption or injury to the endopelvic fascia and levator ani muscles. Major risk factors include women with congenital anomalies such as exstrophy of the urinary bladder, trauma to the pelvic musculature secondary to vaginal delivery, and aging probably related to estrogen depletion. Other factors include obesity, chronic lung disease, and constipation. Uterine prolapse is often associated with concomitant rectocele, cystocele, and/or an enterocele.

Nonsurgical conservative management approaches include pelvic floor exercises (Kegel) and use of vaginal pessaries to mechanically support prolapsed tissues. There are wide varieties of pessaries that are available in the market, and recognition of these various types will make it possible to identify them correctly during various imaging studies, as no imaging studies are required in the routine management of these pessaries (Figs. 19.30 and 19.31) (24).

Urachal Remnant

Urachus is a remnant located between the umbilicus and urinary bladder. It lies in the space of Retzius behind the transversalis fascia and anterior to the peritoneum. During fetal life the lumen gets obliterated and forms the median umbilical ligament. In children a normal urachal

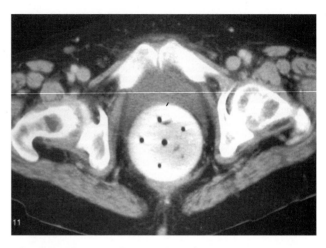

FIG. 19.31. Pessary. Contrast CT of the lower pelvis demonstrates a large radiopaque Gellhorn (silicone flexible, multiple drain) pessary in the vagina.

remnant can be seen as a hypoechoic area at the dome of the bladder in nearly 60% of pelvic sonograms (Fig. 19.32). In adults it is difficult to image on sonography but is observed frequently on routine computed tomography (25).

Rectus Sheath and Subfascial Hematoma

The rectus abdominis muscle extends from the fifth rib to the pubic bone. It is enclosed within the rectus sheath. Above the arcuate (semilunar) line of Douglas the anterior rectus sheath is composed of aponeurosis of the internal and external oblique muscles, and the posterior rectus sheath consists of aponeurosis of the transversus abdominis and the internal oblique muscle. Below the arcuate line, which is about half way between the umbilicus and

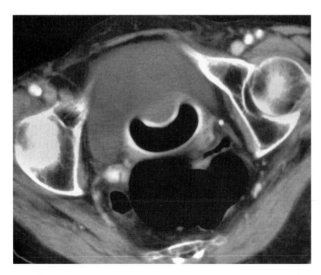

FIG. 19.30. Pessary. Contrast-enhanced CT of the lower pelvis demonstrates a semicircular foreign body in the vagina consistent with a pessary. (There are several different shapes and sizes of pessaries available on the market.)

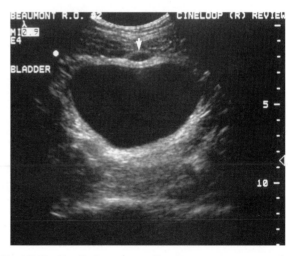

FIG. 19.32. Urachal remnant. Transverse sonogram of the bladder shows the urachal remnant as a small midline anechoic structure anterior to the urinary bladder *(arrow)*.

pubic symphysis, the aponeurosis of the posterior rectus sheath passes anterior to the muscle, leaving only the transversalis fascia separating the rectus muscle from the peritoneum. The blood supply to the rectus abdominis muscle is via the superior and inferior epigastric arteries. The inferior epigastric artery enters the rectus sheath at the level of the arcuate line (26).

Hemorrhage into the rectus sheath is a well-known complication of anticoagulation, and such therapy is considered the most common predisposing factor. Other etiologies include postoperative hematoma secondary to vigorous retraction, inadequate hemostasis, and a sawing effect of the abdominal wall sutures (27). The correct diagnosis of a rectus sheath hematoma is made on initial presentation in fewer than 50% of cases and can be mistaken for a hernia, tumor, appendicitis, and so on. With the patient supine, the head is elevated, and the mass is palpated. In such position, if the mass becomes fixed and more constricted, it indicates a rectus sheath mass (Fothergill's sign), whereas an intraabdominal mass becomes less prominent. Hematomas above the arcuate line are usually small and confined to one side of the midline. However, fluid collections below the arcuate line can enlarge, cross the midline, and dissect down into the pelvis. This prevesical space can accommodate fluid up to 2,500 cc, sometimes without evidence of a palpable mass (28).

Ultrasound and CT can correctly localize these hematomas and fluid collection in nearly 100% of cases. The density and echo pattern of hematomas are variable depending on their age (Fig. 19.33). Fresh hematomas are

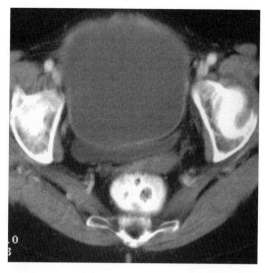

FIG. 19.34. Hematoma mimicking bladder. Axial helical CT scan of the lower pelvis with oral and intravenous contrast medium demonstrates a large low-density mass anterior to the urinary bladder secondary to a liquefied hematoma in the anterior prevesical space. Although it initially mimics the bladder, note should be made that the bladder is compressed and displaced posteriorly by this fluid collection.

hyperdense on CT, whereas subacute and chronic hematomas may have a fluid density. Because of its extraperitoneal location, rectus sheath hematomas displace the urinary bladder posteriorly in contrast to intraperitoneal fluid such as ascites, which displaces the urinary bladder inferiorly (Fig. 19.34).

Penile Prosthesis Reservoir

Several forms of treatment are currently available for patients with erectile dysfunction. The form of therapy primarily depends on the cause of impotence. These can be broadly classified into psychogenic, neurogenic, endocrinologic, pharmacologic, and vasogenic causes. Of all the treatments available, penile prosthesis plays a major role in management of such patients when other less aggressive options fail.

In many instances these protheses are seen as incidental findings on abdominal radiographs, CT scans, and MRI studies. There are four basic types of penile prosthesis: (a) semirigid nonmalleable rods; (b) semirigid malleable rods; (c) mechanical devices; and (d) inflatable penile protheses. Inflatable prostheses are of different types and can exist in erect (inflated) or flaccid (deflated) states. The implants create an artificial erection by transferring fluid from a reservoir into the penile cylinders. These reservoirs are usually implanted just deep to the rectus abdominis muscle (Fig. 19.35), and their appearance and recognition help in correctly iden-

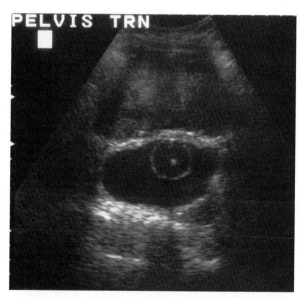

FIG. 19.33. Rectus sheath hematoma. Transabdominal sonogram of the pelvis in an axial plane reveals a complex cystic nature of rectus sheath hematoma. Compressed urinary bladder with Foley balloon posteriorly. Patient was on coumadin, a common predisposing factor.

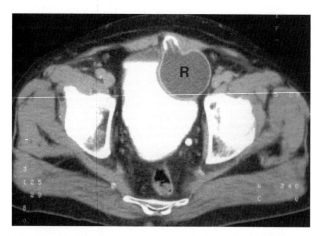

FIG. 19.35. Penile implant reservoir. This CT of the lower pelvis demonstrates an inflated reservoir (R) in the anterior pelvis deep to the left rectus abdominis muscle and compressing the anterolateral wall of the urinary bladder.

tifying them on routine examinations. Common complications include fluid leaks, erosions, pump malfunction and migration, cylinder dilatation and buckling, and separation of connecting tubing. The reservoir most frequently erodes into the bladder, and CT may demonstrate and localize the eroded reservoir but not identify the cause until exploratory surgery is performed (29,30). Because of the proximity of the reservoir with the urinary bladder, it can be mistaken for bladder diverticulum on CT (Fig. 19.36).

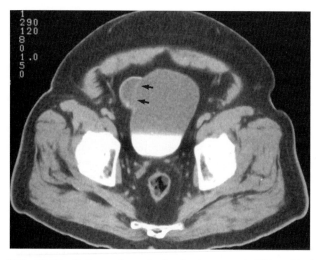

FIG. 19.36. Collapsed penile implant reservoir. This CT of the lower pelvis in a 65-year-old diabetic patient demonstrates a semicircular fluid density abutting the right anterior wall of the bladder (arrows). This represents a collapsed reservoir of a penile implant. The finding may be confused with a broad-based bladder diverticulum.

PROSTATE

Prostate Embryology

The prostate is the major accessory sex gland in men and is often evaluated by digital exam and transrectal ultrasound.

Embryologically it has its roots in and around the pelvic portion of the urogenital sinus, where, on about the 78th day of gestation, the endodermal precursors of its tubuloalveolar glands grow into the mesenchymal forebears of its fibromuscular components. The Wolffian ducts open into the area that eventually becomes the verumontanum. Two laterally positioned depressions that become the eventual prostate are seen on either side of the verumontanum and are known as Muller's hillock. The appearance of the gland is noted by the development of five areas of solid epithelial tissue at approximately 12 weeks. All these events occur under the influence of fetal gonadal secretion of testosterone and its conversion to dehydrotestosterone by 5α-reductase. The prostate grows from the size of a pea in a newborn infant to a large chestnut in a young adult (1,2,32).

Prostate Ultrasound Technique

Optimal scanning technique is important when transrectal prostate ultrasound is performed to avoid pitfalls in the diagnosis of the diseases of the prostate and seminal vesicles. The prostate can be demonstrated by several approaches including transabdominal, transperineal, endourethral, and transrectal scanning. The transrectal approach by far is best in demonstrating normal zonal anatomy of the prostate. The end-viewing transducer is typically utilized, which allows for both axial and sagittal multiplanar imaging. The transrectal probe should be at least 5 MHz, with the vast majority up to 7 to 8 MHz.

Before the examination, an enema may be administered in order to clean the rectum. It is important for the radiologist to review any previous studies in addition to important data such as PSA trends, history of prostatitis, and family history. The examination is then explained to the patient in order to ease anxiety and apprehension.

With the patient in the left lateral decubitus position, a digital rectal exam is performed to evaluate for possible rectal anomalies/abnormalities, suspected nodules, and to assess for overall gland size and position. Appropriate lubrication precedes gentle insertion of the probe into the rectum.

It is imperative that the prostate gland be examined in a systematic manner. One can begin in the transverse or sagittal plane. Many consider beginning the examination at the level of the seminal vesicles, which lie just cephalad to the prostatic base. If one begins in the transverse plane, a slow and thorough sweeping motion is utilized, with images obtained at approximately 5-mm intervals. The examination includes assessment of glandular size, symmetry, overall echo appearance, focal areas of nodularity, capsular integrity, and an assessment of the neurovascular bundles.

Once adequate examination in the transverse plane is established, the prostate is then interrogated in the sagittal plane simply by turning the probe counterclockwise from the 9-o'clock to the 6-o'clock position. When the tip of the probe is pointed to the patient's left, the left side of the gland is being examined. Again, a slow thorough sweeping motion is utilized with images being obtained from left to right or vice-versa. Routine use of color Doppler is encouraged, particularly when a suspicious area is being interrogated as well as when biopsy is contemplated. Technical factors including color sensitivity and gain are set so that normal vessels are not seen. An abnormality is suspected when increased vascularity is identified. Appropriate measurement of the gland dimensions is obtained in three planes to assess gland volume to correlate with the patient's PSA levels (32).

Prostate Anatomy

The zonal anatomy of the normal prostate has been described in detail by McNeal in 1968. Four glandular zones anatomically divide the prostate gland as they surround the prostatic urethra. These zones are named as to their position in relation to the prostatic urethra and include the peripheral zone (PZ), transitional zone (TZ), central zone (CZ), and the periurethral glandular zone. The fibromuscular stroma represents a nonglandular area that is located on the anterior surface of the gland (Fig. 19.37).

The largest zone is the PZ, which accounts for 70% of the glandular tissue. The posterior, lateral, and apical regions of the prostate are made up of the PZ, which surrounds the central zone posteriorly. The distal urethral segment is also surrounded by the PZ.

The base of the prostate is predominently the central zone (CZ), which contains 25% of the glandular prostatic tissue. The central zone surrounds the ejaculatory ducts as they course from the seminal vesicles to the verumontanum (Fig. 19.38). An anatomic barrier does not exist between the PZ and the CZ. This is an important factor for progression of tumor.

Adjacent to the proximal urethral segment is the TZ. In the normal situation this zone makes up approximately 5% of the glandular tissue. The transitional zone consists of two small paraurethral lobes at the midprostate level. Interestingly, as the site of origin of benign prostatic hypertrophy, this glandular zone can comprise a much larger portion of the gland.

The longitudinal smooth muscle of the proximal urethra contains the periurethral glands, which form approximately 1% of the glandular volume. As noted previously, the anterior fibromuscular stroma comprises the anterior third of the prostate gland. The prostate capsule averages about 5 mm thick at the cephalad, posterior, and lateral aspect and becomes thicker anteriorly to form the anterior fibromuscular stroma.

The average dimensions of the seminal vesicles are 27 × 15 mm, and they are angled at 20 to 30 degrees lateral to the prostate base (see Figs. 19.32–19.34).

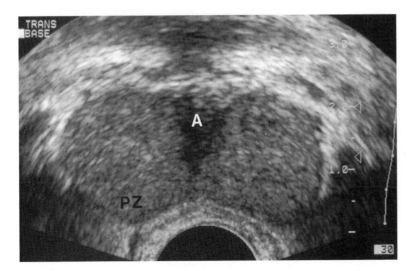

FIG. 19.37. Normal prostate sonogram. Axial scan at the level of the base of the prostate demonstrates a homogeneous echo pattern of the outer gland peripheral zone (PZ) and a hypoechoic anterior fibromuscular stroma (A).

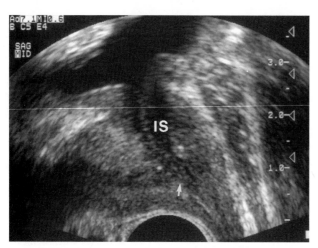

FIG. 19.38. Normal prostate sonogram. Sagittal scan at the midgland level demonstrates the urethra as a tubular structure. The ejaculatory duct is also seen entering the urethra at the level of the verumontanum *(arrow)*. Note: the area of the internal sphincter (IS) is quite hypoechoic.

Pitfalls and Variants

The most common errors in imaging of the prostate with endorectal ultrasound are improper gain setting and keeping the high-risk peripheral zone outside the optimal focal zone. This usually results in false-positive abnormal echoes (usually hypoechoic), which can be mistaken for pathology (Fig. 19.39).

The seminal vesicles are seen as paired tubular, cigar-shaped structures. Their echo pattern may be variable and can demonstrate solid or a more fluid-filled appearance depending on the degree of their distension (Figs. 19.40 and 19.41). Unusual angulation of the endorectal probe

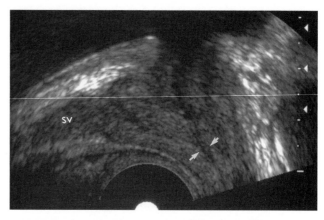

FIG. 19.40. Echogenic seminal vesicles. Sagittal sonogram of a normal prostate toward midline demonstrates the more echogenic seminal vesicles (sv) with the ejaculatory duct *(arrows)* entering the intraprostatic urethra.

may demonstrate a portion of the base of the prostate and the seminal vesicles on the same image (Fig. 19.42). The seminal vesicles are normally symmetric, and any variation must be considered an abnormal finding (32). In longitudinal images, the fat is seen surrounding the seminal vesicle and base of the prostate (Fig. 19.43); however, the seminal vesicles and vas deferens may extend into the central zone and may appear as bilateral basilar hypoechoic areas. In such instances the fat between the rectum, seminal vesicle, and base of the prostate may not be present.

The ejaculatory duct muscle bundles, which are normally no more than 2 mm, may be abnormally large and hypertrophied and appear as hypoechoic areas on sonographic images (Fig. 19.44). Normally, the ejaculatory ducts may also be mildly dilated. Rarely in 2% of patients

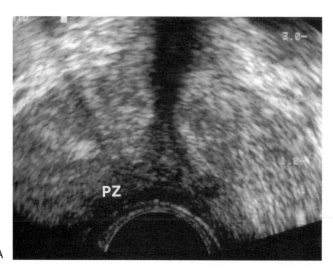

A

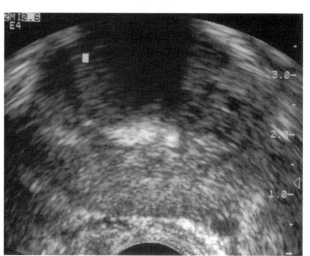

B

FIG. 19.39. Prostate sonogram: pseudolesion. **A:** Axial scans of the prostate at the midgland level demonstrate a hypoechoic anterior fibromuscular stroma. The peripheral zone (PZ) demonstrates a diffuse hypoechoic band because the PZ is out of the focal zone. **B:** Same patient when the scans were obtained by withdrawing the transducer results in demonstration of a normal homogeneous echo pattern of the peripheral zone.

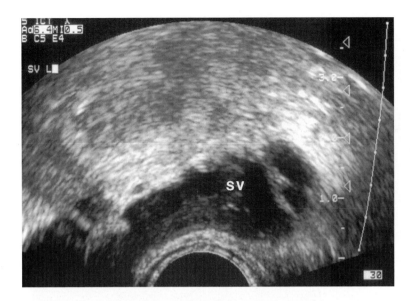

FIG. 19.41. Cystic seminal vesicles. Transverse sonogram demonstrates the left seminal vesicle (sv) as a tubular fluid-filled structure.

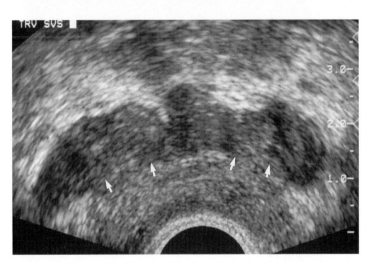

FIG. 19.42. Hypoechoic seminal vesicles. Transverse scan at the level of the base of the prostate demonstrates a portion of the seminal vesicle *(arrows)* because of the unusual angle of the endorectal probe.

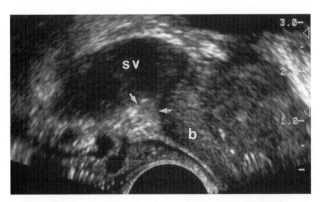

FIG. 19.43. Normal fat near the prostate base. Sagittal scan of the prostate demonstrates normal fat plane *(arrow)* between the seminal vesicle (sv) and base (b) of the prostate.

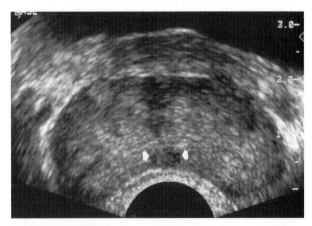

FIG. 19.44. Periejaculatory duct muscle. Axial scan demonstrates a hypoechoic region *(arrows)* in the midperipheral zone representing the smooth muscle surrounding the ejaculatory duct.

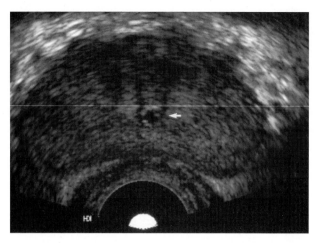

FIG. 19.45. Utricle cyst. Axial scan of the prostate near the base demonstrates a small cyst of the utricle as a hypoechoic area in the midline near the urethra *(arrow)*.

a central cystic utricle may be observed as a midline hypoechoic structure (Fig. 19.45) (33).

Benign Prostate Hypertrophy

Benign prostatic hyperplasia (BPH) is a common disorder affecting men over the age of 50. Such conditions will affect the neighboring organs, as the growth can extend posteriorly toward the rectum without any adverse physiologic effect. However, growth toward the urethra can result in pressure on the trigone, thereby producing irritative symptoms (35).

Clinically, the diagnosis of BPH is made using the American Urologic Symptoms Index (incomplete emptying, frequency, intermittency, urgency, weak stream, hesitancy and nocturia). The most important urologic change associated with BPH is the change in shape of the prostate as it grows more round (35,36).

Diagnosis of BPH using ultrasound is relatively reliable and quick. However, at times enlargement of the median lobe will protrude into the urinary bladder, especially on CT scan, and can be mistaken for an intravesical mass (Figs. 19.46 and 19.47). Correct recognition of

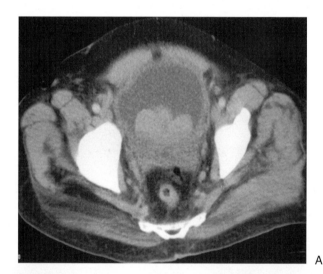

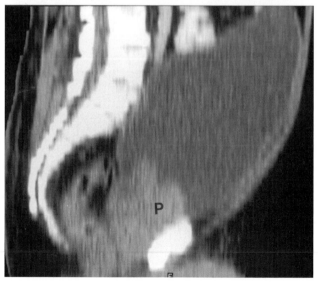

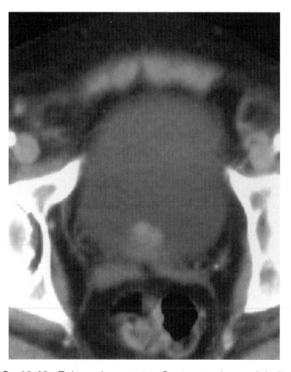

FIG. 19.46. Enlarged prostate. Contrast-enhanced helical CT scan at the level of the seminal vesicles demonstrates a mass-like density protruding into the base of the bladder secondary to an enlarged median lobe of the prostate.

FIG. 19.47. Enlarged prostate BPH. A: Axial helical CT of the lower pelvis demonstrates a lobulated mass protruding from the base of the bladder. There is also thickening of the bladder wall. **B:** Sagittal reconstruction clearly demonstrates this mass to represent an enlarged prostate (p) and bladder outlet obstruction secondary to BPH.

median lobe enlargement will avoid other unnecessary invasive work-up in such patients.

Prostate Calcification

Prostatic calcification is a common finding on transrectal ultrasound. This is often seen in patients with BPH and is situated in the periurethral location in the area between the enlarged central gland and the outer peripheral zone. These calcifications are easy to recognize and are considered a benign process (Fig. 19.48). However, calcifications may also be seen in the peripheral zone, mostly related to prior infection or infarction. This may clinically present as hard nodules on digital rectal examination. In addition, the diffuse calcification involving PZ also results in acoustic shadowing and will limit the evaluation of prostate (Fig. 19.49) (37,38).

TESTICLE

Testicular Embryology

The testes develop from the genital ridge as a central mass of cells. Arising from the surface epithelium of this central cellular mass are a series of epithelial cords. The embryologic testis is made up of a surface epithelium overlying the epithelial cords, which are separated by the tunica albuginea. The rete testis is formed by the convergence of the epithelial cords toward the hilum. The epithelial cords also form the seminiferous tubules. Development of the efferent ductal system is from the residual mesonephros. The subsequent connection of the efferent ducts with the seminiferous tubules results in formation of the functional testis. At this time the testes are attached to the posterior abdominal cavity by peritoneum. Descent of the testes and supporting structures through

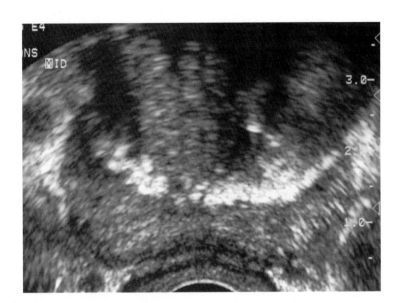

FIG. 19.48. Diffuse prostatic calcification. Transrectal axial ultrasound of the prostate demonstrates diffuse calcification between the enlarged inner gland and the peripheral zone along the surgical capsule. These are typical calcifications seen as concretions of corpora amylacea.

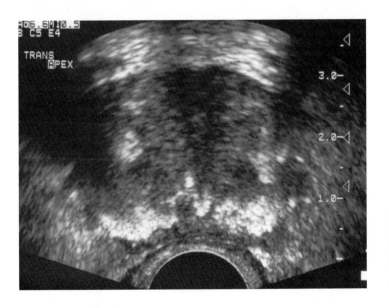

FIG. 19.49. Peripheral zone calcification. Transrectal ultrasound of the prostate near the apex of the gland demonstrates diffuse bright echoes with acoustic shadowing involving the peripheral zone (PZ). Such findings are commonly seen in patients with prior inflammation.

the inguinal canal and into the scrotum is guided by the eventual formation of the gubernaculum testis (1,2,39, 40).

Normal Anatomy

The normal testis is a firm, elliptical gland measuring approximately 3 to 5 cm in length, 2 to 3 cm in anterior/posterior diameter, and 2 to 3 cm in width. In adults, the volume of the testes (length × width × thickness/2) ranges from 16 to 20 cc. It is enclosed within the dense fibrous capsule of the tunica albuginea. Along the superior and posterior aspect of the testis, the tunica albuginea projects into the testis as the mediastinum testis (Fig. 19.50).

The epididymis is located posterolateral to the testis. The head of the epididymis overlies the superior pole of the testis and consists of 10 to 20 efferent ductules, which become highly convoluted on leaving the testis. These ductules join, forming a single duct (the duct of the epididymis), which courses along the posterolateral aspect of the testis as the body and tail of the epididymis. Beyond the tail, this duct becomes the ductus deferens, straightening and ascending behind the testis into the spermatic cord.

With the advent of color Doppler scrotal imaging, familiarity with the vascular anatomy of the testis has become a necessity. The testicular arteries arise anteriorly from the aorta just below the renal arteries and course through the spermatic cord along with the artery of the vas deferens and cremasteric artery. At the posterosuperior aspect of the testis, the testicular artery divides into multiple branches that pierce and course within the deep layers of the tunica albuginea, forming the tunica vasculosa at the periphery of the testis. The tunica vasculosa supplies centripetal branches, which supply the testicular parenchyma and run toward the mediastinum testis in a distribution parallel to the lobular anatomy of the testis. At or just before the mediastinum testis, these centripetal arteries give off recurrent rami, which run in the opposite direction back toward the periphery of the testis. The transtesticular or transmediastinal artery that passes through the mediastinum may appear as a hypoechoic band (Fig. 19.51) (40,41). Testicular venous drainage is directed posteriorly where multiple (10-12) veins anastomose forming the pampiniform plexus. They are usually single and unilateral (50%) but may be multiple and bilateral. The testicular vein drains into the inferior vena cava on the right and into the renal vein on the left side.

Sonographic Anatomy

Sonographically, the testis is of uniform, homogeneous, medium-level echo texture. The mediastinum testis may be seen as a sagittally oriented, echogenic linear structure in the medial or superoposterior portion of the testis parallel to the epididymis.

The rounded or triangular shaped epididymal head is seen along the superior and posterior aspect of the testis, demonstrating a coarser echo pattern than that of the testis (Fig. 19.52). The body and tail of the epididymis are less echogenic than the head and may be identified on the dorsal aspect of the testis.

Normal vascular structures are readily identified with color Doppler. The main testicular artery and capsular and centripetal branches demonstrate a low-impedance flow pattern with high levels of antegrade flow. The centripetal branches flow toward the mediastinum testis and then arborize into recurrent rami that branch back and flow in the opposite direction.

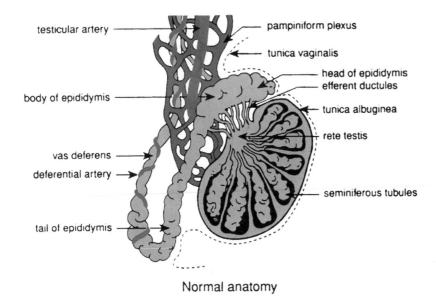

testicular artery — pampiniform plexus

tunica vaginalis

head of epididymis
efferent ductules

body of epididymis — tunica albuginea

rete testis

vas deferens

deferential artery

seminiferous tubules

tail of epididymis

Normal anatomy

FIG. 19.50. Normal testicular anatomy. A longitudinal drawing of a testicle showing different anatomic parts. (Reproduced with permission from Sheth, S. Inflammatory conditions of the epididymis and testis. In: Jafri, SZH, Diokno AC, Amendola MA (eds.). *Lower genitourinary radiology: Imaging and Intervention.* New York: Springer Verlag, 1998.

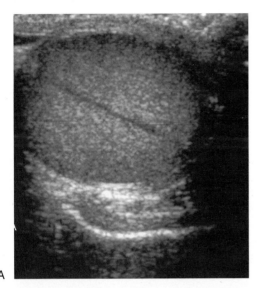

A

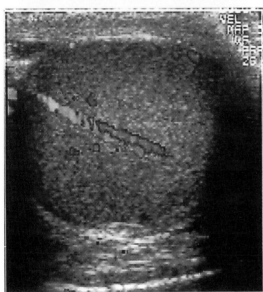

B

FIG. 19.51. Transtesticular vessels. **A:** Sagittal and color Doppler sonogram of the right testicle demonstrates a transtesticular hypoechoic band coursing obliquely through the testicle. **B:** Color Doppler (shown in black and white) image on the same testicle shows transtesticular artery and vein, which corresponds to the hypoechoic band.

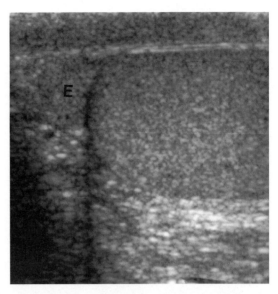

E

FIG. 19.52. Normal epididymis. Sagittal sonogram of the right hemiscrotum demonstrates epididymal head as a triangular structure (E) and homogeneous low-level echoes of normal testicular parenchyma.

Sonographic Technique and Related Artifacts

Before sonographic evaluation of the scrotum, one must obtain adequate historical information. This will aid in guiding the examination. Scrotal ultrasound is best performed with the patient in the supine position. A towel is placed over the abducted thighs with the scrotum resting on this towel. The penis is placed onto the abdomen and is covered with a towel. Certain pathologic entities may warrant deviation of the examination technique from the accepted standard. For example, with additional evaluation of varicoceles and inguinal hernias, scanning with the patient upright is helpful. A generous amount of coupling gel is added as a means of eliminating image degrading air inclusions (Fig. 19.53) (42).

Sonographic evaluation of the scrotum should be performed with high-resolution, real-time scanners with frequencies in the range of 5 to 10 MHz. The linear array transducer is preferred, given superior spatial resolution in the near field. The unaffected testis is used for adjustment of technical parameters, which include gain and time gain compensation. Once ideal parameters are selected, the scrotum is imaged in a continuous manner in both the longitudinal and transverse planes. Direct comparison of both testicles is of utmost importance, and is accomplished in the transverse plane.

Color Doppler sonography has become a standard in scrotal evaluation. It provides useful information regarding blood flow. Color gain and, therefore, sensitivity should be adjusted and maximized without compromising background noise. Many advocate sensitivity settings of 7 cm or less. Given inherent variability between ultrasound equipment with respect to their sensitivity for detecting blood flow, the asymptomatic testicle is used as the control. An additional means of resolving this dilemma is to scan the testicles side by side. It is imperative that one verifies blood flow or the lack thereof with pulsed-Doppler waveform analysis, as flash artifact has comforted many into believing that flow exists when none does. This error of interpretation can be of grave consequence to the patient (Figs. 19.54 and 19.55) (43).

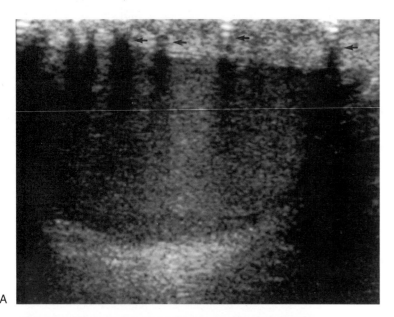

A

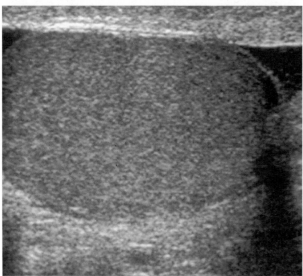

B

FIG. 19.53. Contact artifacts. **A:** Sagittal sonogram of the right testicle demonstrates multiple reverberating artifact with ring down shadow caused by poor contact of the scrotal skin with the transducer *(arrows).* **B:** Same patient: rescanning with adequate amount of ultrasonic gel eliminates such artifacts.

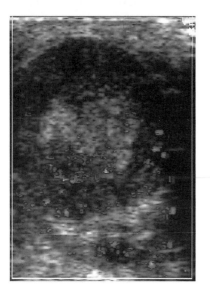

FIG. 19.54. Infarcted testis with flow artifacts. Sagittal sonogram of the left testicle demonstrates color-encoded pixels with deep hues of red and blue (shown in black and white). These areas do not have a linear configuration of vascular structures. The testicle is also diffusely enlarged with central areas of increased echogenicity. Patient underwent orchiectomy, which confirmed an infarcted testicle. The color hues (shown in black and white) demonstrate findings secondary to artifacts from motion and flash. At low flow sensitivity settings (low pulse repetition frequency), the color write priority will prevail and assign color to nonflow areas. This should not be confused with flow.

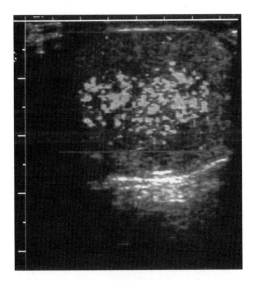

FIG. 19.55. Flow artifacts. Sagittal sonogram of the right testicle demonstrates an apparent central area of arterial flow. These power-encoded pixels correspond to the focal zone of the transducer (shown in black and white). This greater intensity of the beam at the focal zone results from a nonuniform transition between the focal zone and other positions of the beam. This artifact has also been referred to as banding.

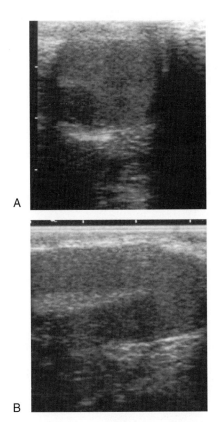

FIG. 19.56. Testicular pseudolesion. Transverse **(A)** and sagittal **(B)** scans of the testicle obtained in a 12-year-old child demonstrate a focal hypoechoic area immediately posterior to the mediastinum testis. A focal mass was initially suspected; however, a follow-up scan (not shown) failed to reproduce this artifact. This probably represents refractory shadow from mediastinum testis.

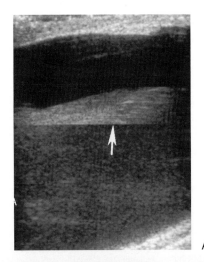

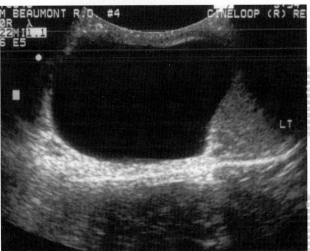

FIG. 19.57. Focal-zone-related artifact. **A:** Sagittal sonogram of the scrotum demonstrates a focal band of increased echogenicity at 2 cm depth *(arrow)*. This results from the transition between focal zones of this transducer (L10, 5 MHz). **B:** Sagittal sonogram with another transducer (C4, 2 MHz) on the same patient demonstrates a completely anechoic epididymal cyst.

The horizontal hyperechoic line artifact is a result of reverberating echoes from the transducer/gel interface. Refractory shadows produced by the mediastinum testis can be problematic to the unweary eye. Misinterpretation of these shadows as hypoechoic intratesticular lesions can be avoided by utilizing transducer directed compression and/or by altering the scan plane (Fig. 19.56). Refractory shadows can also result from obliquely oriented testicular septae.

There are few artifacts that are quite inherent to the design of the transducer. This is especially true of the multiple focused transducers, which can create a linear band of artifacts both on scanning the testicle as well as in imaging of hydroceles and fluid collection. Recognition of such artifacts will avoid errors in misinterpretation. Such artifacts can be corrected by rescanning the scrotum with a curved linear transducer (Fig. 19.57).

In summary, this chapter briefly discussed the normal anatomy and illustrated several pitfalls and variants that can be seen during routine daily imaging of the bladder, prostate, and scrotum. Perhaps there are many more that one may encounter in this rapidly changing technology. Recognition of such variables and pitfalls will result in proper interpretations of the images and avoid errors that may result in unnecessary additional work-up of such findings in the patients.

REFERENCES

1. Moore KL, Persaud TVN. The urogenital system. In: *The developing human, clinically oriented embryology, 6th ed.* Philadelphia: WB Saunders, 1998;315–318.
2. Rana MW. Genital system. Chapter 18. In: *Key facts in embryology.* New York: Churchill Livingston, 1984;173–189.
3. Hollinshead WH, Rosse C. Abdomen. In: *Textbook of anatomy, 4th ed.* New York: Harper & Row, 1985;735–813.
4. Husband JES. Computed tomography of the bladder. In: Jafri SZH, Diokno AC, Amendola MA, eds. *Lower genitourinary radiology. Imaging and intervention.* New York: Springer Verlag, 1998.
5. Maynor CH, Kliewer MA, Hertzberg BS, Paulson EK, Keogan MT, Carroll BA. Urinary bladder diverticula: sonographic diagnosis and interpretive pitfalls. *J Ultrasound Med* 1996;16:189–194.
6. Auh YH, Rubenstein WA, Markisz JA, Zirinsky K, Whalen JP, Kazam E. Intraperitoneal paravesical spaces: CT delineation with US correlation. *Radiology* 1986;159:311–317.
7. Auh YH, Rubenstein WA, Schneider, M, Reckler JM, Whalen JP, Kazam E. Extraperitoneal paravesical spaces: CT delineation with US correlation. *Radiology* 1986;159:319–328.
8. Mastromatteo JF, Mindell HJ, Mastromatteo MF, Magnant MB, Sturtevant NV, Shuman WP. Communications of the pelvic extraperitoneal spaces and their relation to the abdominal extraperitoneal spaces: helical CT cadaver study with pelvic extraperitoneal injections. *Radiology* 1997;202:523–530.
9. Farhi J, Dicker D, Goldman JA. Giant diverticulum of the bladder simulating ovarian cyst. *Int J Gynecol Obstet* 1991;36:55–57.
10. Blane CE, Zerin JM, Bloom DA. Bladder diverticula in children. *Radiology* 1994;190:695–697.
11. Babbitt DP, Dobbs J, Boedecker, RA. Multiple bladder diverticula. In: Williams elfin facies syndrome. *Pediatr Radiol* 1979;8:29–31.
12. Itoh N, Kounami T. Spontaneous rupture of a bladder diverticulum: ultrasonographic diagnosis. *J Urol* 1994;152:1206–1207.
13. Patel U, Furie DM, Lee WJ. CT of infected bladder diverticulum. *J Comput Assist Tomogr* 1991;15:498–499.
14. Thickman D, Mintz M, Arger P, Coleman B. CT Imaging of the unusually shaped bladder. *J Comput Assist Tomogr* 1984;8:801–803.
15. Weingardt JP, Nemcek AA Jr, Miljkovic SC. The diverticular jet effect: Color Doppler differentiation of bladder diverticula from other pelvic fluid collections. *J Clin Ultrasound* 1994;22:397–400.
16. Burge HJ, Middleton WD, McClennan BL, Hildebolt CF. Ureteral jets in healthy subjects and in patients with unilateral ureteral calculi: comparison with color Doppler US. *Radiology* 1991;180:437–442.
17. Price CI, Adler RS, Rubin JM. Ultrasound detection of differences in density: explanation of the ureteric jet phenomenon and implications for new ultrasound applications. *Invest Radiol* 1989;24:876–883.
18. Jequier S, Paltiel H, Lafortune M. Ureterovesical jets in infants and children: duplex and color Doppler US studies. *Radiology* 1990;175:349–353.
19. Levine D, Filly RA. Using color Doppler jets to differentiate a pelvic cyst from a bladder diverticulum. *J Ultrasound Med* 1994;13:575–577.
20. Bell ED, Witherington R. Bladder hernias. *Urology* 1980;15:127–130.
21. Izes BA, Larsen CR, Izes JK, Malone MJ. Computerized tomographic appearance of hernias of the bladder. *J Urol* 1993;149:1002–1005.
22. Vick CW, Viscomi GN, Mannes E, Taylor KJW. Pitfalls related to the urinary bladder in pelvic sonography: a review. *Urol Radiol* 1983;5:253–259.
23. Thompson JD. Surgical correction of defects in pelvic support. In: *Operative gynecology, 8th ed.* Philadelphia: Lippincott-Raven, 1998;951–968.
24. Sarto GE. Genital prolapse. In: Wallis LA, ed. *Textbook of women's health.* Philadelphia: Lippincott-Raven, 1998;747–753.
25. Cacciarelli AA, Kass EJ, Yang SS. Urachal remnants: sonographic demonstration in children. *Radiology* 1990;174:473–475.
26. Fukuda T, Sakamoto I, Kohzaki S, et al. Spontaneous rectus sheath hematomas: clinical and radiological features. *Abdom Imag* 1996;21:58–61.
27. Ray CE Jr, Wilbur AC. CT diagnosis of concurrent hematomas of the psoas muscle and rectus sheath: case report and review of anatomy, pathogenesis, and imaging. *Clin Imag* 1993;17:22–26.
28. Wiener MD, Bowie JD, Baker ME, Kay HH. Sonography of subfascial hematoma after cesarean delivery. *Am J Roentgenol* 1987;148:907–910.
29. Cohan RH, Ohl DA. Radiology of penile prosthesis. In: Jafri SZH, Diokno AC, Amendola MA, eds. *Lower genitourinary radiology: imaging and intervention.* Berlin: Springer Verlag, 1998;390–400.
30. Shandera KC, Thompson IM. Urologic prosthesis. *Emerg Med Clin North Am* 1994;12:729–748.
31. Nguyen HT, Etzell J, Jurek PJ. Normal human ejaculatory duct anatomy: a study of cadaveric and surgical specimens. *J Urol* 1996;155:1639–1642.
32. Rifkin MD. Embryology, anatomy and pathogenesis of diseases of the prostate, seminal vesicles and surrounding structures. In: *Ultrasound of the prostate, 2nd ed.* Philadelphia: Lippincott-Raven, 1997;3–14.
33. Villers A, Terris MK, McNeal JE, Stamey TA. Ultrasound anatomy of the prostate: the normal gland and anatomical variations. *J Urol* 1989;143:732–738.
34. Strasser H, Janetschek G, Reissigl A, Bartsch G. Prostate zones in three-dimensional transrectal ultrasound. *Urology* 1996;47:485–490.
35. Mauroy B. Bladder consequences of prostatic obstruction. *Eur Urol* 1997;32(suppl 1):3–8.
36. Kojima M, Naya Y, Inoue W, et al. The American Urological Association symptom index for benign prostatic hyperplasia as a function of age, volume and ultrasonic appearance of the prostate. *J Urol* 1997;157(6):2160–2165.
37. Casillas J. Imaging of the benign conditions of the prostate and seminal vesicles. In: Jafri SZH, Diokno AC, Amendola MA, eds. *Lower genitourinary radiology: imaging and intervention.* New York: Springer Verlag, 1998;177–194.
38. Mahoney JE, Rivkin MD. Benign prostatic hyperplasia: an overview of clinical and imaging characteristics and treatment options. In: *Ultrasound of the prostate, 2nd ed.* Philadelphia: Lippincott-Raven, 1997.
39. Hricak H, Hamm B, Kim B. Anatomy and embryology. In: *Imaging of the scrotum.* New York: Raven Press, 1995;1–5.
40. Shirkhoda AS, Vrachliotis T, Bis KG. Undescended testis. In: Jafri SZH, Diokno AC, Amendola MA, eds. *Lower genitourinary radiology: imaging and intervention.* New York: Springer Verlag, 1998;238–249.
41. Fakhry J, Khoury A, Barakat K. The hypoechoic band: a normal finding on testicular sonography. *Am J Roentgenol* 1989;153:321–323.
42. Middleton WD, Bell MW. Analysis of intratesticular arterial anatomy with emphasis on transmediastinal arteries. *Radiology* 1993;189:157–160.
43. Hricak H, Hamm B, Keri B. Imaging techniques, anatomy, artifacts and bioeffects. In: *Imaging of the scrotum.* New York: Raven Press, 1995;11–36.

Variants and Pitfalls in Body Imaging,
edited by Ali Shirkhoda.
Lippincott Williams & Wilkins, Philadelphia, © 2000.

CHAPTER 20

The Female Pelvis

Catherine A. D'Agostino, Robin J. Warshawsky,
Gwen N. Harris, and John S. Pellerito

From birth to menopause, numerous pathologic conditions can affect the female genitourinary tract, which may present diagnostic challenges. Ultrasound has become established as the procedure of choice in the initial investigation of pelvic disease, followed by computed tomography (CT) and magnetic resonance imaging (MRI). An understanding of normal anatomic variants and potential diagnostic pitfalls is essential for the proper work-up and management of pelvic disorders.

ANATOMY

The female pelvis contains the uterus, fallopian tubes, ovaries, urinary bladder, and bowel. The uterus is located between the two layers of the broad ligament laterally, the bladder anteriorly, and the rectosigmoid colon posteriorly. It is divided into two major portions—the body and cervix. The superior area of the body is called the fundus and the areas of the body where the fallopian tubes enter the uterus are called the cornua. The vagina lies in the midline and extends from the cervix to the vestibule of the external genitalia.

The endometrium is the inner lining of the myometrium, and immediately lateral to the junction of the cervix and lower uterine segment are the parametrial uterine vessels. The normal postpubertal uterus varies considerably in size, and the maximum dimensions of the nulliparous uterus are approximately 8 cm in length by 5 cm in width by 4 cm in anteroposterior (AP) diameter. Multiparity can increase the size of the uterus. The postmenopausal uterus is usually smaller in size (1). The fallopian tubes run laterally from the uterus in the upper free margin of the broad ligament. Each tube is divided into intramural, isthmic, ampullary, and infundibular portions (2). The ovaries are located anterior to the ureter and the anterior branch of the internal iliac artery. They are elliptical in shape, with the long axis usually oriented vertically. Normally there are multiple small cystic structures within the periphery of each ovary during the years of active menstrual cycles, representing follicles at various stages of development. The best method for determining ovarian size is by obtaining a volume measurement. This is made with measurements in two planes and based on the formula for a prolate ellipse (length × width × height × 0.523). The mean normal ovarian volume in a woman of menstruating age is approximately 10 cc (3). The normal range about this mean is wide (3). Following menopause the ovaries decrease in size.

IMAGING TECHNIQUES

Ultrasound

The standard transabdominal sonogram is performed with a distended urinary bladder, which provides an acoustic window to view the pelvic organs. The urinary bladder is considered filled when it allows visualization of the fundus of the uterus. A 3.5-MHz transducer is usually adequate for evaluating the entire pelvis. Imaging of the uterus and adnexa is performed in both the sagittal and transverse planes. The adnexae may be optimally imaged by scanning obliquely from the contralateral side through the distended bladder.

Transvaginal transducers range in frequency from 4 to 9 MHz. With the urinary bladder empty, the transducer is inserted into the vagina with the patient in a supine or

R. J. Warshawsky: Department of Radiology, North Shore University Hospital, Manhasset, New York 11030.

C. A. D'Agostino, G. N. Harris, and J. S. Pellerito: Department of Radiology, New York University School of Medicine, New York, New York; and Department of Radiology, North Shore University Hospital, Manhasset, New York 11030.

Trendelenburg position. The probe can be rotated from 0 degrees to 90 degrees about its long axis to obtain any plane of section from sagittal to coronal. The probe can be manipulated to position the structure of interest within the focal zone of the transducer.

Transvaginal images provide a more limited field of view but with higher resolution than transabdominal images. Depending on the reason for evaluation, a survey by transabdominal scan is almost always necessary prior to transvaginal scanning. This survey reduces the possibility of overlooking pathology such as a pelvic mass lying outside the field of view of the transvaginal probe (4).

Saline infusion sonohysterography enhances transvaginal ultrasound examination of the uterine cavity. The sonohysterography catheter is inserted into the uterus through the cervical os. Sterile saline is then slowly instilled into the uterine cavity while imaging is performed with the transvaginal probe. Diffuse and focal endometrial and subendometrial abnormalities are better evaluated with this technique (5).

Computed Tomography

Optimal pelvic CT requires adequate opacification of bowel with oral contrast. This is essential to avoid mistaking unopacified bowel for masses, adenopathy, or an abscess (6). Typically, 750 to 1,000 cc of oral contrast is administered 45 to 60 minutes prior to scanning. Rectal air or contrast may also be helpful in select cases to evaluate the rectosigmoid colon, and distinguish it from gynecologic neoplasms (6,7). In addition, intravenous contrast should be administered with a power injector unless it is medically contraindicated. Vascular enhancement is important to distinguish vessels from lymph nodes, to enhance the myometrium, to delineate the endometrium, and to distinguish avascular or hypodense tumors from enhancing myometrium and cervix. In some cases, delayed scans of the pelvis may be required to clarify important findings or to completely opacify the bladder (7). Thin collimation (5 mm or smaller) should be used to avoid volume averaging (6). Some authors also advocate scanning the pelvis from the inferior aspect to the superior part to optimize the vascular enhancement (7,8).

Magnetic Resonance Imaging

Pelvic MRI is ideally performed with the use of a dedicated multicoil (phased array). This provides a better signal-to-noise ratio than the body coil and produces high-resolution images. The routine field of view is 20.0 cm, and the routine slice thickness is 5.0 mm. Glucagon can be administered to minimize bowel peristalsis.

Axial T1-weighted images provide excellent anatomic delineation of pelvic fat planes, easily outline any lymph nodes, and allow tissue characterization of fatty and hemorrhagic masses. Fat suppressed T1-weighted images will confirm the fatty versus hemorrhagic nature of pelvic

masses and increase the conspicuity of hemorrhagic deposits of endometriosis. T2-weighted images are used to evaluate uterine zonal anatomy, facilitate identification of the ovaries, and highlight pathology. Sagittal images are best for uterine anatomy and pathology, and axial and coronal images are often best for the adnexa. Coronal oblique images can be used to evaluate uterine anomalies. The role of gadolinium in pelvic imaging is limited and may be useful for tumor staging.

EMBRYOLOGY AND CONGENITAL ANOMALIES

The female genital tract develops from paired embryologic structures called the müllerian ducts, which give rise to the fallopian tubes, uterus, and the upper two-thirds of the vagina. Congenital anomalies of the uterus and vagina are caused by arrested development or failure of fusion of the müllerian ducts (9). Uterine malformations may also be due to failure of resorption of the median septum. The American Fertility Society has classified these anomalies as hypoplasia or agenesis (class I), unicornuate (class II), didelphic (class III), bicornuate (class IV), septate (class V), or arcuate (class VI). These anomalies are well evaluated with both transvaginal ultrasound and MRI. Transvaginal ultrasound examination of uterine hypoplasia will demonstrate a small uterine size. However, a very small uterine corpus may be missed on transabdominal ultrasound, which may mimic uterine agenesis (10). A unicornuate uterus, or class II anomaly, results from varying degrees of developmental arrest of one müllerian duct. On ultrasound, there is loss of the normal pear shape of the uterus, with the fundus appearing asymmetric and one cornual area being smaller than usual (11). On MRI, there is an asymmetric configuration of the uterus, and an atretic, rudimentary horn may be identified (12).

Uterus didelphys, or a class III anomaly, results from complete lack of fusion of the müllerian ducts. These patients are generally asymptomatic. In a nonpregnant patient, ultrasound shows two symmetric uterine horns, each of which has an endometrial cavity and a cervix. MRI shows complete separation of the uterine horns, two cervices, and a vaginal septum (Fig. 20.1) (12). The diagnosis is generally made on physical exam by the finding of two cervices. In pregnancy, there is enlargement of both horns, with decidual reaction of the endometrium seen in the nongravid horn (11).

A bicornuate uterus, or class IV anomaly, has a single cervix and results from varying degrees of lack of fusion of the corpus. On ultrasound, a bilobed external uterine contour is demonstrated (Fig. 20.2). Ultrasound and MRI depict a large fundal cleft (>1 cm), divergent uterine horns, and a single cervix (Fig. 20.3) (12). CT may also demonstrate two horns in a bicornuate uterus, which should not be mistaken for a tumor (Fig. 20.4). An obstructed horn may simulate an adnexal mass (Fig. 20.5).

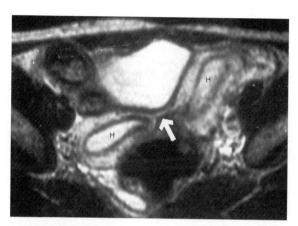

FIG. 20.1. Uterus didelphys. Axial T2-weighted magnetic resonance imaging (MRI) showing widely separated *(arrow)* uterine horns (H).

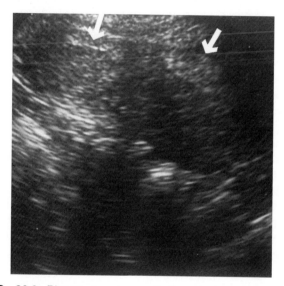

FIG. 20.2. Bicornuate uterus. Endovaginal scan demonstrates diverging uterine horns *(arrows).* There is a large cleft at the uterine fundus.

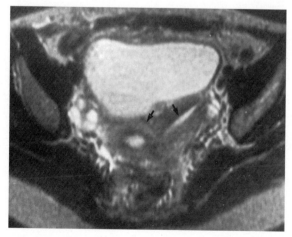

FIG. 20.3. Bicornuate uterus. Axial T2-weighted MRI demonstrates separated uterine horns *(arrow).* Note presence of multiple ovarian follicles.

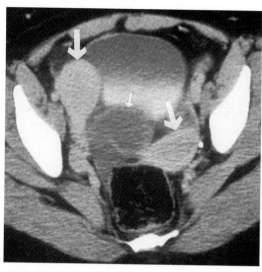

FIG. 20.4. Bicornuate uterus and right hydrosalpinx *(small arrow).* Axial contrast-enhanced computed tomography (CT) shows separated uterine horns *(large arrows).*

A septate uterus, or class V anomaly, occurs when there are varying degrees of failure of absorption of the midline septum. The septum may be partial (involving the endometrial cavity) or complete (extending into the endocervical canal), but the external uterine contour is normal. The septate uterus is the most common anomaly, and is associated with a 90% abortion rate, which is felt to be related to poor vascularity of the septum. On ultrasound, an echogenic area, with echogenicity similar to myometrium, may be seen dividing the endometrial canals (Fig. 20.6). MRI is useful in diagnosing a septate uterus, in which case the fundus is convex, flat, or has a small notch (<1 cm) (Fig. 20.7). Both partial and complete septa have signal intensity similar to myometrium (12).

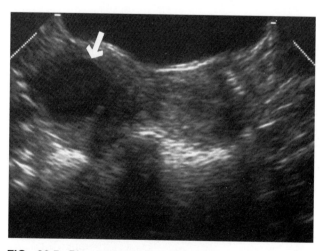

FIG. 20.5. Bicornuate uterus. Transverse transabdominal ultrasound image of the pelvis showing an obstructed right horn *(arrow)* simulating an adnexal mass.

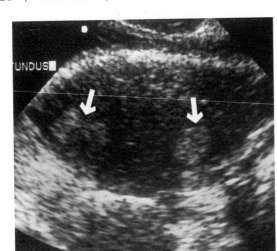

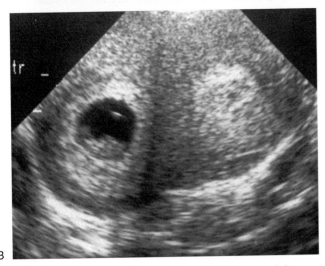

FIG. 20.6. Septate uterus. **A:** Endovaginal ultrasound demonstrating two endometrial canals *(arrows)*, with a rounded fundus. **B:** Septate uterus with a pregnancy. Endovaginal ultrasound shows a pregnancy in the right horn and thickened endometrium in the left horn.

Additional uterine anomalies may result from *in utero* exposure to diethylstilbestrol (DES), a synthetic estrogen used between 1940 and 1970 to prevent miscarriage in pregnant women with bleeding; 35 to 69 percent of women who were exposed to DES while *in utero* can be shown to have uterine anomalies such as hypoplasia, T shape, constrictions, and small marginal irregularities (13).

Congenital vaginal obstruction may present in the neonatal period or at the time of menarche. In infancy, vaginal obstruction may be secondary to vaginal atresia, high-grade stenosis, transverse septum, or an imperforate membrane. A transverse vaginal septum is caused by a lack of canalization of the vaginal plate, which generally occurs at the junction of the middle and upper thirds of the vagina (14). Transverse vaginal septum is associated with renal anomalies. Vaginal obstruction that presents in

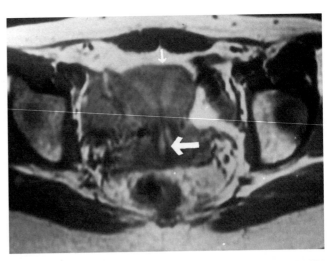

FIG. 20.7. Complete septate uterus. Axial T2-weighted MRI showing septum extending to the cervix *(arrow)*. Note mildly convex fundal contour *(small arrow)*.

pubertal girls is usually secondary to an imperforate hymen, which is caused by failure of perforation of the hymen formed at the junction of the urogenital sinus and the paired müllerian ducts. Patients present with recurrent lower abdominal pain or an abdominal mass. There is no increased incidence of other congenital anomalies in patients with imperforate hymen. MRI, CT, and sonographic findings of hydrometrocolpos include a tubular, predominantly cystic, midline mass, representing the dilated uterus and vagina, between the rectum and bladder (Fig. 20.8). The vagina is usually filled with blood, and may be five to nine times larger than the uterus (Fig. 20.9). Fluid may be present within the uterus or vagina (Fig. 20.10).

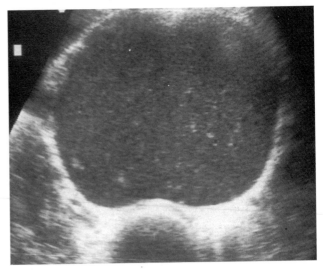

FIG. 20.8. Hematometrocolpos. Transverse transabdominal ultrasound demonstrating distended vagina filled with hemorrhage.

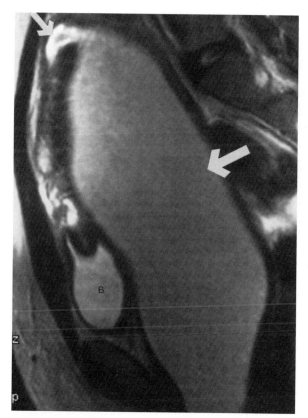

FIG. 20.9. Hematometrocolpos. Sagittal T2-weighted MRI revealing a markedly distended vagina *(arrow)* and mildly distended uterus *(small arrow)* filled with hemorrhage. Urinary bladder (B).

Another vaginal congenital anomaly is the Gartner's duct cyst, which lies within the roof of the vagina and develops from the remnants of the wolffian duct. Additional vestigial structures include the Bartholin glands, which open on the labia majora just within the vaginal vestibule and may become infected (15).

The most common developmental anomaly of the ovary is bilateral ovarian agenesis, as seen in Turner's syndrome. Other anomalies are rare and include absence of one ovary, ectopic ovary, third ovary, accessory ovaries, and congenital displacements. The para-ovarian cyst is a congenital cyst located within the broad ligament that develops from vestigial structures of the mesonephron (15).

NORMAL ANATOMIC VARIANTS

Wandering Spleen

The wandering spleen is a congenital variant in which there is marked laxity of the suspensory splenic ligaments (Fig. 20.11). This allows the spleen to move in the

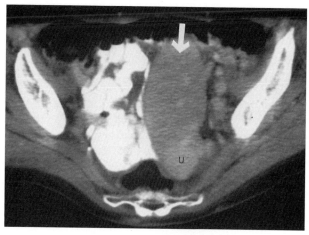

A

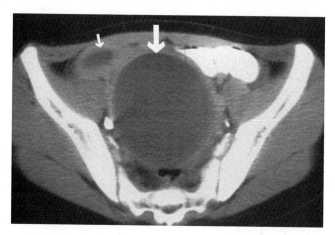

FIG. 20.10. Hematometrocolpos. Axial contrast-enhanced CT showing distended fluid-filled vagina *(arrow)* and fluid-filled uterus *(small arrow)*.

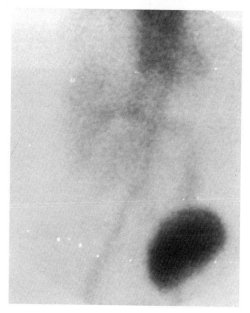

B

FIG. 20.11. Wandering spleen. **A:** Axial contrast-enhanced CT through the pelvis demonstrates an ectopic location of the spleen *(arrow)*. U, uterus. **B:** Technetium (Tc) 99m sulfur colloid scan confirms the pelvic location of the spleen.

abdomen, often mimicking a mass in the abdomen or in the pelvis. This is a rare entity, which is more common in women (16). On CT, there is absence of the spleen in its normal anatomic location, and a mass with the shape and enhancement characteristics of the spleen is present in an ectopic location. An ectopic spleen may be difficult to visualize on ultrasound due to overlying bowel gas. If there is uncertainty about the diagnosis, technetium (Tc) 99m–sulfur colloid imaging may resolve the issue. Although a wandering spleen is generally clinically insignificant, it may undergo torsion (16).

Pelvic Kidney

A pelvic kidney lies in the true pelvis and may be unilateral, bilateral, crossed, or solitary (Fig. 20.12). The left kidney is most commonly involved, occurring in about 70% of patients (17). On CT, a pelvic kidney may be mistaken for a pathologic mass, particularly if intravenous contrast is not utilized.

Renal Transplant

In adults, most renal transplants are placed in an extraperitoneal location in the iliac fossa (18). Although it generally has a reniform appearance, a transplant kidney may sometimes be confused with a pelvic mass on CT, particularly if intravenous contrast has not been administered, or if the transplant is nonfunctional and atrophic or calcified (Fig. 20.13).

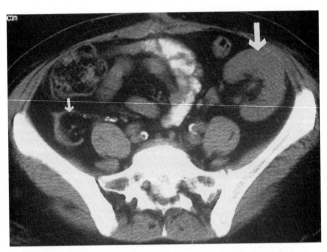

FIG. 20.13. Renal transplant. Noncontrast CT demonstrates a left iliac fossa renal transplant *(arrow)* and an older, atrophic right iliac fossa transplanted kidney *(small arrow)*.

DIFFERENTIAL DIAGNOSIS AND PITFALLS

Uterus

Uterine Leiomyomas

Uterine leiomyomas are frequently encountered benign neoplasms that contain collagen and smooth muscle. On ultrasound, leiomyomas are most often solid, with echogenicity similar to that of the uterus (Fig. 20.14). However, with degeneration, the appearance may become more cystic or complex (19).

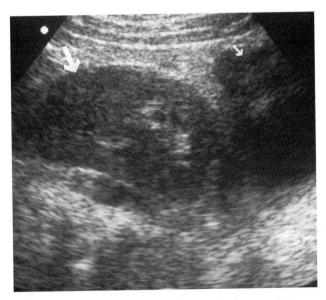

FIG. 20.12. Pelvic kidney. Longitudinal ultrasound image showing a pelvic kidney *(large arrow)* superior to the bladder *(small arrow).*

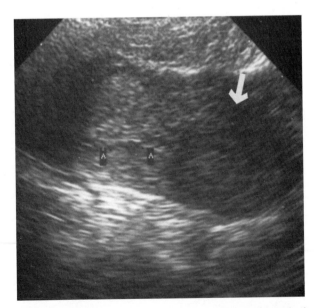

FIG. 20.14. Uterine myoma. Transverse image through the fundus with a left lateral myoma *(arrow)*. *Arrowheads* indicate the endometrial canal with increased through transmission.

The most common CT appearance of uterine leiomyomas is an enlarged uterus with a lobulated contour. Additional findings may include a deformed endometrial cavity and focal uterine masses, with or without calcifications (7). Approximately 10% of uterine leiomyomas contain calcifications, which is the most specific sign of a leiomyoma. Noncalcified leiomyomas, particularly the pedunculated ones, may be mistaken for other pelvic masses, including ovarian and other extra-uterine masses (20). A degenerating leiomyoma may appear as a low attenuation mass, which may mimic a neoplasm of the endometrium, cervix, or ovary. In these cases, ultrasound may help to distinguish leiomyomas from other adnexal masses (Fig. 20.15). A mass extending from and contiguous with the uterus is consistent with a fibroid. The pedicle attachment to the uterus may not always be clearly shown with ultrasound. Performing a transvaginal ultrasound may be helpful in some cases. In addition, Doppler imaging of a fibroid mass may demonstrate an arterial waveform with the characteristic uterine notch, which indicates a uterine rather than an adnexal origin (21). In more difficult cases, MRI may help to characterize uterine myomas (Fig. 20.16) (20).

Endometrial Polyp

Endometrial polyps may cause uterine bleeding, although most are asymptomatic. Malignant degeneration is uncommon. The size of polyps ranges from microscopic to more than 5 cm. They typically appear as diffuse or focal thickening of the endometrium (22).

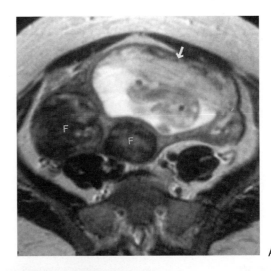
A

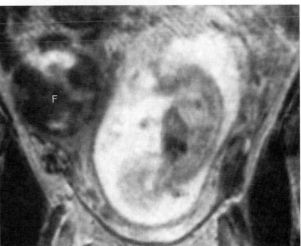
B

FIG. 20.16. Uterine myoma. **A:** Axial T2-weighted MRI demonstrates a right lateral exophytic degenerating fibroid (F). An ultrasound exam questioned whether this lesion represented an adnexal mass or a myoma. Note gravid uterus *(small arrow)*. **B:** Coronal T2-weighted MRI confirms a mixed signal intensity myoma (F) projecting from a gravid uterus.

Cystic spaces within an abnormally thickened endometrium on transvaginal sonograms are noted with polyps (23). Individual polyps are better visualized when they are outlined by intracavitary fluid, as with sonohysterography (Fig. 20.17). Submucosal fibroids may simulate an endometrial polyp, which can be distinguished by a sonohysterogram.

Endometrial Carcinoma

Eighty-five percent of patients with endometrial carcinoma are postmenopausal. The role of unopposed estrogens as a contributory factor to endometrial hyperplasia and carcinoma has been well established (24). The threshold for an abnormally thickened endometrium has been

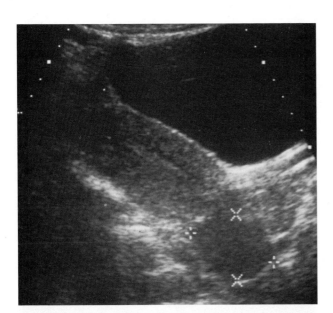

FIG. 20.15. Uterine myoma. Sagittal view of the pelvis showing an exophytic posteriorly located leiomyoma simulating an adnexal mass.

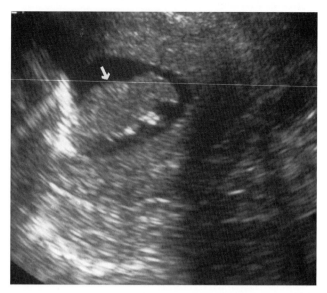

FIG. 20.17. Endometrial polyp. Sonohysterogram revealing a polypoid mass *(arrow)* projecting into a fluid-filled endometrial cavity.

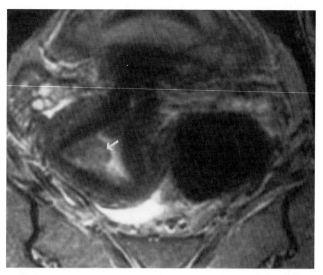

FIG. 20.19. Endometrial carcinoma. A coronal T2-weighted MRI demonstrates a polypoid lesion *(arrow)* with intermediate signal intensity in the endometrial cavity.

set by several groups as a double-layer thickness greater than 5 or 6 mm in a postmenopausal patient who is not on hormones (Fig. 20.18) (25). In general, the risk of endometrial carcinoma increases with the degree of endometrial thickening (26). In addition to endometrial thickening, sonographic findings of more advanced, invasive endometrial carcinoma include mixed echogenicity of the myometrium and a lobular contour of the uterus (27).

Magnetic resonance imaging can identify abnormalities within the endometrial cavity in 81% to 84% of cases (Fig. 20.19), but cannot reliably distinguish endometrial carcinoma from adenomatous hyperplasia. Blood clots

are one of the major pitfalls in differential diagnosis. MRI can assess the depth of myometrial invasion in stage I tumors. For overall staging of endometrial carcinoma, the accuracy of MRI has been reported to range from 85% to 92% (28).

Postpartum Uterus

Computed tomography findings in the normal postpartum uterus include uterine enlargement as well as fluid in the endometrial canal (Fig. 20.20). In addition, intrauterine gas has been reported to occur in 21% of asymptomatic patients and should not be mistaken for infection

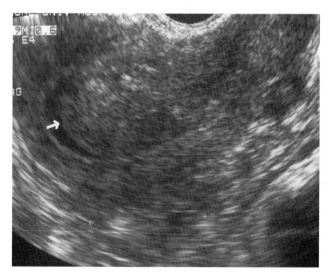

FIG. 20.18. Endometrial carcinoma. Endovaginal sagittal image revealing a large mass *(arrow)* occupying most of the endometrial cavity, outlined by a small amount of fluid.

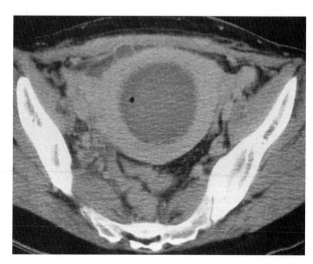

FIG. 20.20. Postpartum uterus. Transaxial contrast-enhanced CT shows fluid and a small amount of air in a very large endometrial cavity.

(29). An air-fluid level within the endometrial cavity may be seen with endometritis, and thus it is important to be aware of the clinical scenario (30). Other findings that have been reported in the postpartum pelvis include widening of the sacroiliac joints occasionally containing gas (29). The appearance of the uterus following cesarean section may be confusing and can mimic abscess, phlegmon, and dehiscence. It is common to see uterine discontinuity without incisional necrosis or dehiscence following cesarean section (31). After cesarean section, droplets of air are often seen in the subcutaneous fat, rectus sheath, parametrium, and paravesical spaces (6). Low-density parametrial fluid collections and air are also commonly seen and are felt to be clinically insignificant (31).

Molar Pregnancy

Molar pregnancy occurs in 1:200 to 1:1,500 pregnancies in the United States. About 20% of these patients develop persistent gestational trophoblastic disease, invasive mole, and choriocarcinoma. In the first trimester, moles may be difficult to diagnose sonographically.

Molar pregnancies from 8 to 12 weeks may show only thickened echogenic endometrium. From 18 to 20 weeks, cystic spaces grow to nearly 1 cm and are readily apparent (Fig. 20.21A,B). These vesicular spaces account for the typical snowstorm appearance (Fig. 20.21C) (32). Duplex and color-flow Doppler can demonstrate abnormal vascularity within areas of endometrium (33). A pattern of arteriovenous shunting and high diastolic flow is demonstrated. MRI of gestational trophoblastic disease shows an enlarged uterus containing an endometrial mass of heterogeneous signal intensity. Patients with myometrial invasion show myometrial disruption with distortion of the normal zonal anatomy of the uterus (34).

Nabothian Cyst

Retention (nabothian) cysts of the cervix are commonly seen during routine sonography (Fig. 20.22). They may vary in size from a few millimeters to 4 cm, and may be single or multiple (Fig. 20.23). They represent obstructed glands of the cervical canal and may be associated with healing chronic cervicitis (35).

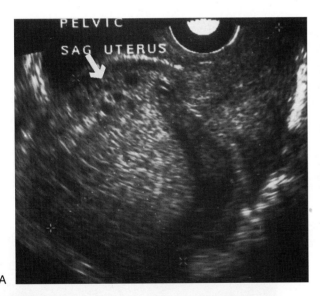

A

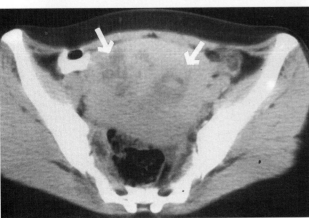

B

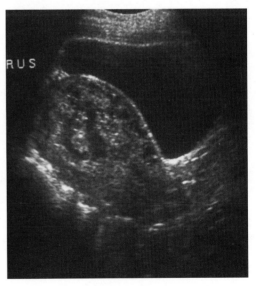

C

FIG. 20.21 Molar pregnancy. **A:** Sagittal endovaginal ultrasound image showing an echogenic mass with cystic areas in the endometrial cavity *(arrow)*. **B:** Axial CT in the same patient shows irregular hypodense areas centrally in the uterus *(arrows)*. **C:** In another patient, sagittal ultrasound shows numerous hypoechoic areas in the endometrial canal.

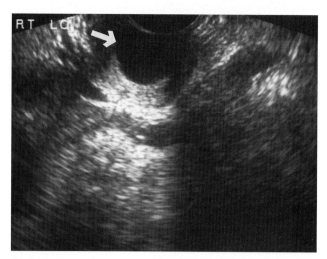

FIG. 20.22. Nabothian cyst. Endovaginal image reveals a cystic structure *(arrow)* initially thought to be adnexal. MRI confirmed this to be a nabothian cyst in the cervix.

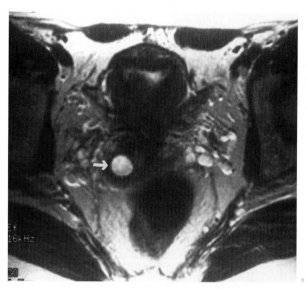

FIG. 20.23. Nabothian cyst. Axial T2-weighted MRI demonstrating a sharply marginated T2 hyperintense structure in the cervix *(arrow)*. On ultrasound, this was mistaken for an adnexal cyst.

Cervical Lymphoma

Malignant lymphoma arising from the uterine cervix is a very rare entity (Fig. 20.24). Approximately 1% of extranodal primary lymphoma has been reported in the female reproductive tract, and 0.12% to 0.6% are confined to the uterine cervix. Abnormal vaginal bleeding is the most common presentation (36). The differential diagnosis for a cervical mass includes cervical carcinoma or cervical fibroid. Cervical fibroids account for fewer than 3% of fibroids. Cervical carcinoma is usually diagnosed clinically but may present as a solid retrovesical mass on ultrasound associated with hydrometra or hematometra. MRI is

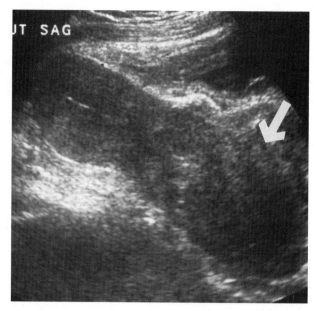

FIG. 20.24. Cervical lymphoma. Sagittal transabdominal image of the uterus reveals a large cervical mass *(arrow)*.

the modality of choice for staging cervical carcinoma, with overall accuracy rates of 76% to 83% (37).

Adnexa

Dermoid

Cystic teratomas make up approximately 10% to 15% of ovarian neoplasms, and 10% to 15% of them are bilateral. Since ectodermal elements generally predominate, they are virtually always benign and are also called dermoid cysts. Their sonographic appearance is extremely variable. A cystic mass with an echogenic mural nodule may be seen (Fig. 20.25). The dermoid plug usually con-

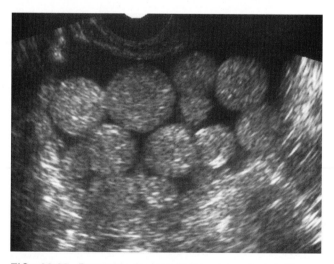

FIG. 20.25. Dermoid. Endovaginal sonogram reveals an adnexal mass containing multiple rounded echogenic areas representing fat within a dermoid.

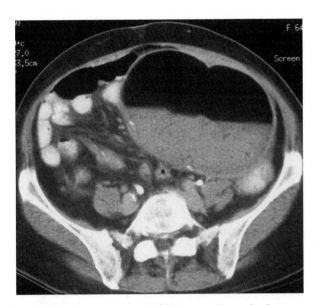

FIG. 20.26. Dermoid. Axial CT image through the upper pelvis shows a large fat containing mass.

tains hair, teeth, or fat (38). Low attenuation is demonstrated on CT scans (Fig. 20.26) (39). On MRI, the fat or sebaceous material within the cyst is similar to the intensity of subcutaneous fat on all pulse sequences. The use of fat suppression improves characterization and distinguishes cystic teratomas from hemorrhagic masses (40). It is important to keep in mind that an echogenic dermoid may demonstrate acoustic shadowing similar to bowel gas and may therefore be difficult to detect on ultrasound (Fig. 20.27).

Endometriosis

Endometriosis occurs when endometrial tissue is found in an ectopic location, outside the uterus. Approximately 25% of infertile women age 20 to 55 years are found to have endometriosis at laparoscopy, and 30% to 40% of women with endometriosis experience infertility (41). Patients may present with pain, dysmenorrhea, dyspareunia, or infertility. There is no correlation between symptoms and extent of disease (19). The most common sites of implantation are the ovaries, cul-de-sac posterior uterine wall, uterosacral ligaments, anterior uterine wall, and dome of the bladder (42). Laparoscopy is the standard of reference for the diagnosis of endometriosis. Although MRI cannot replace laparoscopy in the staging of endometriosis, it can assess extraperitoneal sites of involvement or lesions hidden by dense adhesions. MRI can also be used to characterize adnexal masses as well as to evaluate response to treatment for patients in whom a diagnosis of endometriosis has already been made (41). The MRI appearance of a large (>1 cm) endometrioma is a homogeneous hyperintense mass on T1-weighted images (Fig. 20.28). Small endometriomas may appear hyperintense on T1-weighted images regardless of the appearance on T2-weighted images (41). Fat saturated T1-weighted images may also be used to increase the conspicuity of small peritoneal implants (42). Pelvic ultrasound may be normal because the endometrial deposits are often very small and dispersed throughout the peritoneal cavity. An endometrioma or chocolate cyst is a focal collection of blood that may be anechoic or complex with low-level echoes or fluid debris levels seen on ultrasound (19). However, the sonographic appearance is nonspecific.

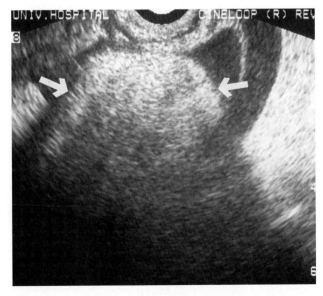

FIG. 20.27. Dermoid. Endovaginal ultrasound shows an echogenic mass *(arrows)* with attenuation of the sound beam, which could be confused with bowel.

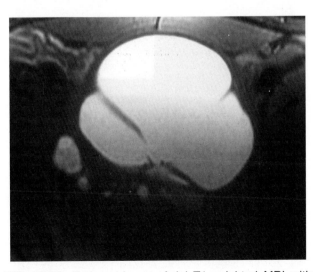

FIG. 20.28. Endometriomas. Axial T1-weighted MRI with fat suppression demonstrating several T1 hyperintense lesions.

Ovarian Torsion

Torsion of the ovary is caused by complete or partial rotation of the ovary on its axis, with resulting compromise in lymphatic and venous drainage. Ultimately, there may be loss of arterial perfusion and infarction. Torsion usually occurs in association with an adnexal mass. There is an increased risk of ovarian torsion during pregnancy. Patients present with severe lower abdominal pain, nausea, and vomiting (43). The sonographic appearance is of an enlarged ovary or adnexal mass, often with peripheral follicles (Fig. 20.29A). Free fluid is found in one-third to two-thirds of patients. Color Doppler has been used to assist in the diagnosis of ovarian torsion; however, the Doppler findings may be variable depending on the chronicity and degree of torsion. Arterial waveforms have been reported in cases of proven torsion during color and pulsed Doppler examination. This finding may be related to the dual blood flow to the ovary, from both the ovarian artery and ovarian branches of the uterine artery, or to incomplete or chronic torsion (44). On occasion, there may also be torsion of the fallopian tube, which may mimic an ovarian mass (Fig. 20.30).

CT and MRI are generally not needed for the diagnosis of ovarian torsion, but several findings have been reported in ovarian torsion with infarction. These findings include a lack of enhancement and engorged blood vessels on the affected side (Fig. 20.29B) (45).

Tubo-Ovarian Abscess

Pelvic inflammatory disease is one of the most common gynecologic diseases affecting young women

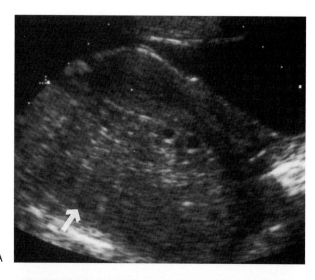

A

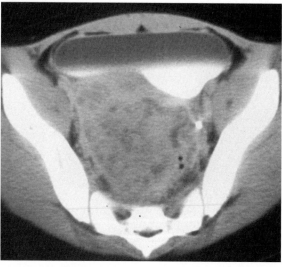

B

FIG. 20.29. Ovarian torsion. **A:** Sagittal view of the pelvis demonstrates a complex mass *(arrow)* posterior to the uterus. **B:** Axial CT scan thorough the pelvis shows a large complex mass in the cul-de-sac.

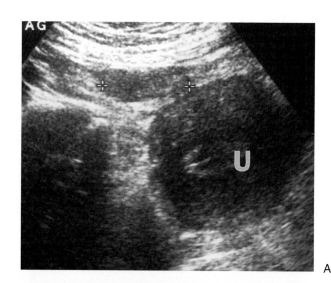

A

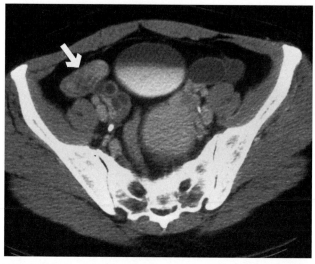

B

FIG. 20.30. Torsion of a right hydrosalpinx. **A:** Sagittal ultrasound image shows a solid tubular mass *(cursors)* superior to the uterus (U). **B:** Axial CT image shows an ovoid heterogeneous soft tissue *(arrow)* in the right pelvis initially thought to represent a solid mass.

between 15 and 24 years of age. Patients may present with fever, lower abdominal pain, and an elevated white blood cell count. The most common pathogens are *Chlamydia trachomatis* and *Neisseria gonorrhoeae* (19). The infection begins in the cervix and, if untreated, may spread to the endometrium and fallopian tubes.

Ultrasound may show hydrosalpinx and adnexal masses. Tubo-ovarian abscesses may appear as unilocular or multilocular complex masses with thickened walls (Fig. 20.31). CT may be useful in severe cases of pelvic inflammatory disease or if the ultrasound findings are equivocal. CT findings include unilateral or bilateral adnexal masses, hydrosalpinx, and ascites (Fig. 20.32). Air seen within an adnexal mass is strongly suggestive of a tubo-ovarian abscess (7).

Hydrosalpinx may be demonstrated on MRI where interdigitating mucosa within a hydrosalpinx appears as longitudinal thin ridges within the dilated tube (42). A

tubo-ovarian abscess may have variable signal intensity on MR, depending on the hemorrhagic content of the fluid. Simple fluid will be high signal intensity on T2-weighted images. The walls of a tubo-ovarian abscess will enhance following gadolinium administration (42). Hydro- or pyosalpinx may also be depicted with ultrasound and CT (Fig. 20.33).

Ectopic Pregnancy

Ectopic pregnancy represents approximately 1.4% of all reported pregnancies. Tubal pregnancies, most commonly within the ampullary portion, account for approximately 98% of all ectopic pregnancies (46). Transvaginal

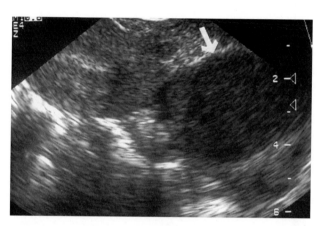

FIG. 20.31. Tubo-ovarian abscess. Endovaginal sonogram reveals a complex mass *(arrow)* with low-level echoes, which can mimic a hemorrhagic cyst, endometrioma, or neoplasm.

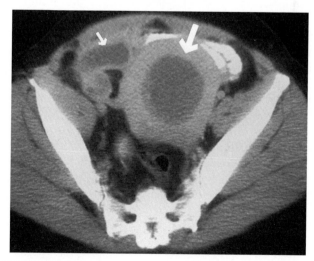

FIG. 20.32. Pyometria and right pyosalpinx. Axial CT image shows fluid-filled endometrial cavity *(large arrow)* and tubular hydrosalpinx *(small arrow)*.

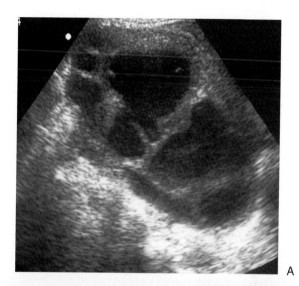

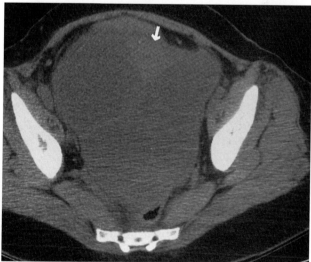

FIG. 20.33. Pyosalpinx. **A:** Transabdominal sonogram shows a complex mass with hypoechoic areas with low-level echoes and septations/folds. A tubular nature was demonstrated on real-time scanning. **B:** Axial CT without contrast showing a complex cystic pelvic mass posterior to the uterus *(arrow)*.

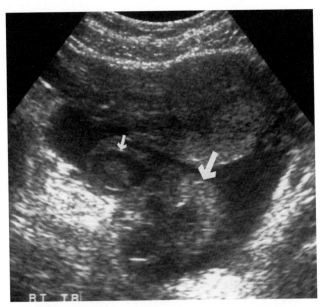

FIG. 20.34. Ruptured ectopic. Transverse transabdominal sonogram shows a heterogeneous mass in the cul-de-sac representing hemorrhage in the fallopian tube *(large arrow)*. Note adjacent corpus luteal cyst *(small arrow)* and surrounding free fluid.

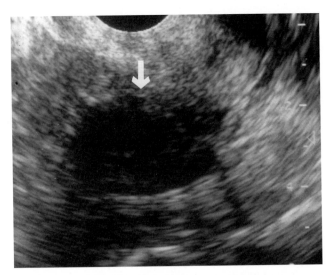

FIG. 20.35. Thecoma. Endovaginal sonogram shows a hypoechoic adnexal mass *(arrow)* with posterior attenuation of the sound beam consistent with a fibrous tissue tumor.

sonography is the imaging procedure of choice. Ectopic pregnancy presents as an adnexal ring or extrauterine embryo in 54% of cases. A pseudogestational sac is recognized as an irregular intrauterine sac or endometrial thickening, representing a decidual reaction related to elevated human chorionic gonadotropin (HCG) titers (47). Pseudogestational sacs do not demonstrate a double decidual sac sign, yolk sac, fetal pole, or placental flow on Doppler imaging (48). The presence of echogenic free fluid (hemoperitoneum) or blood clots in the posterior cul-de-sac in pregnant patients without sonographic evidence of an intrauterine pregnancy should strongly suggest the presence of a ruptured ectopic pregnancy (Fig. 20.34) (49).

A corpus luteum cyst, hemorrhagic cyst, tubo-ovarian abscess, and endometrioma can mimic the appearance of an adnexal ring, and therefore ectopic pregnancy should not be suggested without correlating clinical and laboratory data.

Thecoma

Thecomas account for less than 1% of all ovarian tumors arising from ovarian stroma, as do fibromas. Thecomas and fibromas may be difficult to distinguish; 70% of thecomas occur in postmenopausal women. They are unilateral, almost always benign, and frequently show clinical signs of estrogen production. Tumors with an abundance of thecal cells are classified as thecomas, whereas those with fewer thecal cells and abundant fibrous tissue are classified as fibrothecomas and fibromas.

The sonographic appearance is characteristic. Thecomas and fibromas present as a hypoechoic mass with marked posterior attenuation of the sound beam (Fig. 20.35). This is a result of the homogeneous fibrous tissue in these tumors (50). The main differential diagnosis is that of a Brenner tumor or pedunculated uterine fibroid. Not all thecomas and fibromas show this characteristic appearance. A variety of sonographic appearances have been reported, including a mass of mixed echogenicity or an anechoic mass (51). This is explained by the known tendency for edema and cystic degeneration to occur within these tumors.

Cystadenocarcinoma

Ovarian serous cystadenocarcinoma is the most common malignant tumor of epithelial origin (52). It may be quite large and usually presents as a multilocular cystic mass containing multiple papillary projections, arising from the cyst wall, and septa. The septa and walls may be thickened, measuring greater than 2 mm (Fig. 20.36A,C). Echogenic solid material may be seen within the loculations. Ascites is frequent. The use of Doppler ultrasound may be useful, as it has been shown that malignant ovarian masses are associated with arteriovenous shunting and increased diastolic flow (RI <0.4) (Fig. 20.36B) (53). The resistive index (RI) is calculated by subtracting the end-diastolic velocity from the peak systolic velocity and then dividing by the peak systolic velocity.

Oophoropexy

Surgical transposition of the ovaries, or oophoropexy, refers to repositioning of the ovaries in premenopausal patients who are to undergo pelvic radiation therapy and wish to preserve ovarian function. Most often, lateral

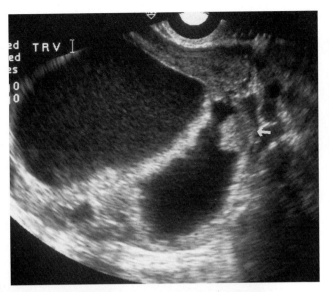

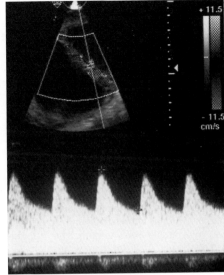

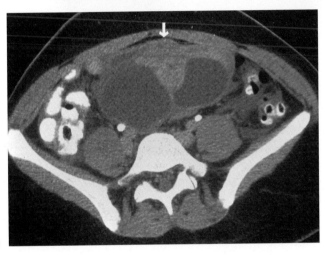

FIG. 20.36. Cystadenocarcinoma. A: Endovaginal sonogram showing a complex adnexal mass with nodularity *(arrow)* and thick septations. B: Doppler interrogation of the septation demonstrates low-resistance (RI = 0.4) flow. C: Axial CT shows a complex mass with large mural nodule *(arrow)*.

transposition is performed, in which the ovary is tacked lateral to the cecum, usually in association with a surgical clip (6). On CT, the transposed ovaries can be seen in the paracolic gutters near the iliac crests. Transposed ovaries are usually of soft tissue attenuation and are important to recognize in order to avoid misinterpretation as a mural mass or peritoneal implant. Cysts commonly occur within transposed ovaries and may then be mistaken for pathologic entities such as an abscess, hematoma, lymphocele, or cystic neoplasm (54).

Pelvic Arteriovenous Malformation

Pelvic arteriovenous malformations (AVMs) are uncommon lesions, but more common in women than in men. This diagnosis is rarely suspected until the lesion is demonstrated on an imaging study, such as CT or MRI, performed to evaluate pelvic symptoms (Fig. 20.37). Intravenous contrast plays a very important role in differentiating AVMs from nodes or other masses on CT. When performing ultrasound with Doppler imaging, color flow

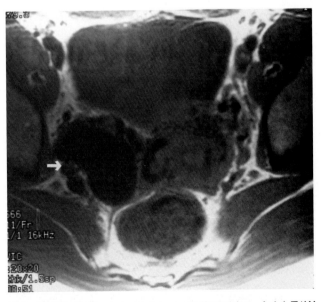

FIG. 20.37. Pelvic arteriovenous malformation. Axial T1W MRI revealing multiple tubular regions of signal void *(arrow)* representing vessels.

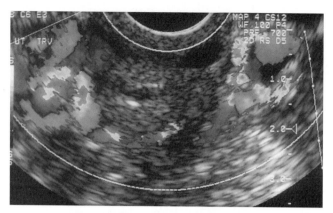

FIG. 20.38. Enlarged parametrial vessels. Endovaginal ultrasound with color Doppler shows prominent parametrial vessels (varices) in a multiparous female. This should not be confused with a pelvic AVM, and may be associated with pelvic congestion syndrome.

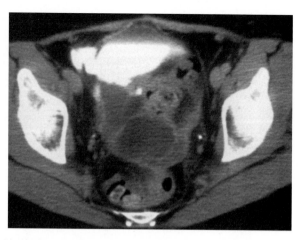

FIG. 20.39. Cystic mesothelioma. Contrast-enhanced CT of the pelvis demonstrates a cystic mesothelioma mimicking a cystic adnexal mass or pelvic inflammatory disease.

can demonstrate the communication between the artery and vein. This guides placement of the Doppler gate precisely over the fistulous communication. The feeding artery has a low-resistance flow profile and the distended recipient vein contains high-velocity flow signals resembling those of an artery (55). Angiography provides the most specific information regarding patterns of arterial supply and venous drainage. While deriving blood supply from multiple sources, the major nidus of the lesion is generally on one side of the pelvis. Surgery should be reserved for lesions that are judged to be completely resectable. For other lesions, staged selective embolization using deeply penetrating permanent embolic materials provides the best results (56).

Pelvic Congestion Syndrome

Enlarged, tortuous para-uterine vessels are seen in association with the pelvic congestion syndrome. These varicosities may involve the external and internal genitalia (57). Patients with this syndrome may present with complaints of nonspecific pelvic pain. Endovaginal sonography using color-flow Doppler demonstrates vascular flow within these enlarged veins (Fig. 20.38).

Miscellaneous

Cystic Mesothelioma of the Peritoneum

Cystic mesothelioma of the peritoneum is a rare neoplasm that tends to occur along the surfaces of the pelvic viscera. It is unrelated to prior asbestos exposure. Although it does not metastasize, it does tend to recur locally (58). Radiographically, cystic mesothelioma appears as a multicystic diffuse lesion, and it involves the peritoneum, omentum, and pelvic and abdominal viscera. On ultrasound, the lesion may appear as multilocular cystic masses. On CT, the appearance is of a thin-walled multilocular cystic lesion of fluid attenuation (Fig.

20.39). The differential diagnosis includes ovarian neoplasms such as cystadenoma and cystadenocarcinoma, as well as teratoma, endometriosis, lymphangioma, pseudomyxoma peritonei, and mesenteric and omental cysts (58).

Mucocele of the Appendix

Mucocele of the appendix refers to a cystic mass of the appendix resulting from an abnormal accumulation of mucus. The ultrasound appearance is that of a complex, predominantly cystic mass. The echogenicity within the mass depends on the mucus within it; however, there is usually good through-transmission (59). On CT, the mass is usually of low attenuation, with thin, well-defined walls, in the right lower quadrant (Fig. 20.40). There may be thin calcification within the wall. No adjacent inflammatory changes are present, in contradistinction to

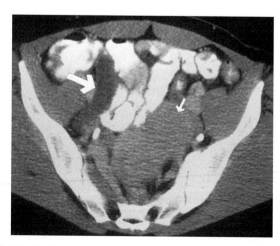

FIG. 20.40. Mucocele. Axial CT image reveals a tubular fluid density structure in the right pelvis, initially felt to represent a hydrosalpinx *(large arrow)*. Note fibroid uterus *(small arrow)*.

appendicitis (59). Adequate bowel opacification is important to distinguish a mucocele from unopacified bowel. Based on its tubular cystic appearance, a mucocele may be mistaken for a hydrosalpinx. However, tracing the origin of the mass to the base of the cecum should aid in making this differentiation.

Pelvic Neurofibromatosis

Neurofibromatosis is an autosomal dominant disorder with manifestations in the skin, nervous system, and bone. Retroperitoneal plexiform neurofibromas have a characteristic appearance, consisting of bilateral, symmetric, low-attenuation masses in a parapsoas or presacral location (60). Within the pelvis, neurofibromas may be unilateral. CT demonstrates nodular soft tissue masses anterior to the sacrum and extending to the pelvic sidewalls. The masses are often of slightly lower attenuation than enhanced muscle (Fig. 20.41). This type of soft tissue pelvic mass may be mistaken for adenopathy. It is therefore important to obtain a pertinent clinical history and to search for ancillary findings such as enlargement of the sacral foramina, which would suggest a neurogenic origin for the mass (61).

Urachal Cyst

The urachus may remain partially or completely patent. If it is completely patent, a fistulous urinary tract exists between the bladder and the umbilicus. If the urachus closes at the umbilical and bladder ends, but remains patent in the central portion, a urachal cyst may develop, lined by either transitional or metaplastic epithelium. Carcinomas, particularly adenocarcinomas, have been reported to arise in such cysts (62). On ultrasound or CT, a urachal cyst appears as a cyst seen superior to the bladder near the midline (63). These cysts may sometimes calcify (Fig. 20.42).

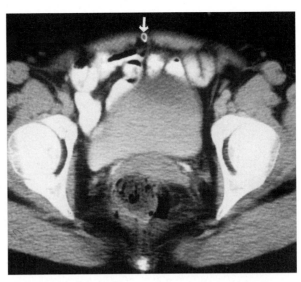

FIG. 20.42. Urachal remnant. Axial contrast-enhanced CT shows a calcified urachal remnant in the midline *(arrow)*.

Ovarian Vein Thrombosis

Ovarian vein thrombosis may be a complication of postpartum endometritis (64), obstetric and gynecologic surgery, and pelvic inflammatory disease. Symptoms at presentation include lower abdominal pain, flank pain, fever, and tachycardia.

The sonographic appearance is of a tubular anechoic or hypoechoic structure extending cranially from the adnexa. Doppler interrogation demonstrates absent flow. Overlying bowel may sometimes obscure a thrombosed ovarian vein. However, CT with contrast readily demonstrates characteristic findings of a dilated ovarian vein with a low-attenuation center and peripheral enhancement of the wall (Fig 20.43A) (65). The right ovarian vein is involved in 80% to 90% of cases, and there may be extension of thrombus into the inferior vena cava (Fig 20.43B) (64). MRI utilizing flow-sensitive pulse sequences may also confirm the diagnosis.

Gelfoam and Surgicel

Absorbable surgical hemostatic agents such as gelatin sponge (Gelfoam) and oxidized regenerated cellulose (Surgicel) may mimic an abscess on CT or ultrasound, and have been reported to mimic a mass on MRI (66,67). On ultrasound, Surgicel or gelatin sponge may be seen as a complex mass with both hypoechoic and hyperechoic components. The echogenic component is felt to represent air trapped within the folds of the material (66). Similarly, on CT, these materials appear as collections of air surrounded by postoperative hematoma in the operative bed (Fig. 20.44). The gas collections are often focal and linear, which is an atypical appearance for air in a gas-forming abscess (68). In a postoperative patient in whom an echogenic mass or collection of air is seen in the post-

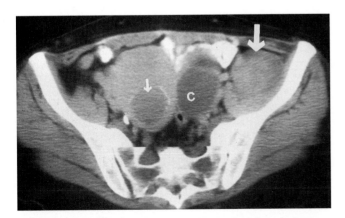

FIG. 20.41. Neurofibroma. Axial CT of the pelvis showing a soft tissue density mass in the left iliac fossa *(large arrow)* in a patient with known neurofibromatosis. Note the calcified uterine myoma *(small arrow)* and left adnexal cyst (c).

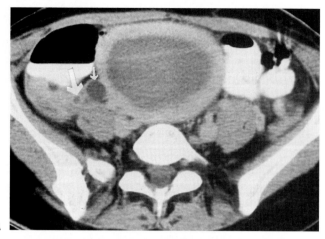
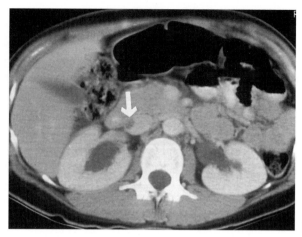

FIG. 20.43. Ovarian vein thrombosis. **A:** Contrast-enhanced CT in a postpartum patient demonstrates low density within the right ovarian vein *(large arrow)*, with an enhanced wall. Note right hydroureter *(small arrow)* and an enlarged, postpartum uterus. **B:** There is extension of the ovarian vein clot into the inferior vena cava *(arrow)*.

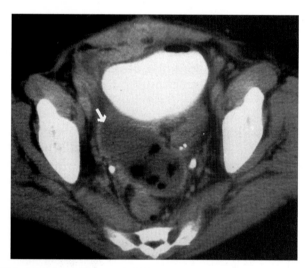

FIG. 20.44. Gelfoam mimicking an abscess. Axial contrast-enhanced CT shows a collection of air and fluid with peripheral enhancement *(arrow)* mimicking abscess.

operative bed, the differential diagnosis should include abscess. Direct communication with the surgeons is important to ascertain whether Surgicel or Gelfoam was used. In patients with clinical signs of infection, it sometimes may be necessary to aspirate these collections to exclude a concomitant abscess (66,68).

REFERENCES

1. Platt JF, Bree RL, Davidson D. Ultrasound of the normal nongravid uterus: correlation with gross and histopathology. *J Clin Ultrasound* 1990;18:15.
2. Jones HW III, Wentz AC, Burnett LS. *Novak's textbook of gynecology,* 11th ed. Baltimore: Williams & Wilkins, 1987.
3. Cohen H, Tice H, Mandel F. Ovarian volumes measured by ultrasound: bigger than we think. *Radiology* 1990;177:189.
4. Leibman AJ, Kruse B, McSweeney MB. Transvaginal sonography:

comparison with transabdominal sonography in the diagnosis of pelvic masses. *AJR* 1988;151:89.
5. Goldstein SR. Saline infusion sonohysterography for the patient with abnormal bleeding. *Appl Radiol* 1997;26:33.
6. Langer JE, Jacobs JE. High-resolution computed tomography of the female pelvis: spectrum of normal appearances. *Semin Roentgenol* 1996;31:267.
7. Urban BA, Fishman EK. Helical (spiral) CT of the female pelvis. *Radiol Clin North Am* 1995;33:933.
8. Walsh JW. Computed tomography of gynecologic neoplasms. *Radiol Clin North Am* 1992;30:817.
9. Carrington BM, Hricak H, Nuruddin RN. Müllerian duct anomalies: MR imaging evaluation. *Radiology* 1990;176:715.
10. Mintz MC, Grumbach K. Imaging of congenital uterine anomalies. *Semin Ultrasound CT MR* 1988;9:167.
11. Malini S, Valdes C, Malinak LR. Sonographic diagnosis and classification of anomalies of the female genital tract. *J Ultrasound Med* 1984; 3:397.
12. Pellerito JS, McCarthy SM, Doyle MB, Glickman MG, DeCherney AH. Diagnosis of uterine anomalies: relative accuracy of MR imaging, endovaginal sonography, and hysterosalpingography. *Radiology* 1992; 183:795.
13. Van Gils APG, Tjon A, Than RTO, Falke THM, Peters AAW. Abnormalities of the uterus and cervix after diethylstilbestrol exposure: correlation of findings on MR and hysterosalpingography. *AJR* 1989; 153:1235.
14. States LJ, Bellah RD. Imaging of the pediatric female pelvis. *Semin Roentgenol* 1996;31:312.
15. Netter F. *The Ciba collection of medical illustrations, reproductive system, part II,* 5th ed. West Caldwell, NJ: Ciba Pharmaceutical, 1974.
16. Lee JKT, Sagel SS, Stanley RJ, Heiken JP. *Computed body tomography with MRI correlation,* 3rd ed. Philadelphia: Lippincott-Raven, 1998.
17. Pollack HM. *Clinical urography.* Philadelphia: WB Saunders, 1990.
18. Oliver JH III. Clinical indications, recipient evaluation, surgical considerations, and the role of CT and MR in renal transplantation. *Radiol Clin North Am* 1995;33:435.
19. Coleman BG. Transvaginal sonography of adnexal masses. *Radiol Clin North Am* 1992;30:677.
20. Casillas J, Joseph RC, Guerra JJ. CT appearance of uterine leiomyomas. *Radiographics* 1990;10:999.
21. Pellerito JS, Troiano RN, Quedens-Case C. Common pitfalls of endovaginal color flow imaging. *Radiographics* 1995;15:37.
22. Johnson MA, Graham MF, Cooperberg PL. Abnormal endometrial echoes: sonographic spectrum of endometrial pathology. *J Ultrasound Med* 1982;1:161.
23. Hulka CA, Hall DA, McCarthy K, Simeone JF. Endometrial polyps, hyperplasia and carcinoma in postmenopausal women: differentiation with endovaginal sonography. *Radiology* 1994;191:755.

24. Ettinger B. Optimal use of postmenopausal hormone replacement. *Obstet Gynecol* 1988;72:315.

25. Granberg S, Wikland M, Karlsson B, Norstrom A, Friberg LG. Endometrial thickness as measured by endovaginal ultrasonography for identifying endometrial abnormality. *Am J Obstet Gynecol* 1991;164:47.

26. Varner ED, Sparks JM, Cameron CD, Roberts LL, Soong SJ. Transvaginal sonography of the endometrium in postmenopausal women. *Obstet Gynecol* 1991;78:195.

27. Requard CK, Wicks JD, Mettler FA. Ultrasonography in staging of the endometrial adenocarcinoma. *Radiology* 1981;140:781.

28. Hricak H, Stern JL, Fisher MR, et al. Endometrial carcinoma staging by MR imaging. *Radiology* 1987;162:297.

29. Garagiola DM, Tarver RD, Gibson L, Rogers RE, Wass JL. Anatomic changes in the pelvis after uncomplicated vaginal delivery: a CT study on 14 women. *AJR* 1989;153:1239.

30. Rooholamini SA, Au AH, Hansen GC, et al. Imaging of pregnancy-related complications. *Radiographics* 1993;13:753.

31. Twickler DM, Setiawan AT, Harrell RS, Brown CEL. CT appearance of the pelvis after cesarean section. *AJR* 1991;156:523.

32. Javniax E, Campbell S. Ultrasonographic assessment of placental abnormalities. *Am J Obstet Gynecol* 1990;163:1650.

33. Desai RK, Desberg AL. Diagnosis of gestational trophoblastic disease: value of endovaginal color flow Doppler sonography. *AJR* 1991;157:787.

34. Barton JW, McCarthy SM, Kohorn EI, Scoutt LM, Lange RC. Pelvic MR imaging findings in gestational trophoblastic disease, incomplete abortion, and ectopic pregnancy; are they specific? *Radiology* 1993;186:163.

35. Fogel SR, Slasky BS. Sonography of nabothian cysts. *AJR* 1982;138:927.

36. Abbas MA, Birdwell R, Katz DS, Chang H, Ostrow K. Primary lymphoma of the cervix in a heart transplant patient. *AJR* 1996;167:1136.

37. Kim SH, Choi BI, Han JK. Preoperative staging of uterine carcinoma: comparison of CT and MRI in 99 patients. *J Comput Assist Tomogr* 1993;17:633.

38. Quinn SF, Erichson S, Black WC. Cystic ovarian teratomas: the sonographic appearance of the dermoid plug. *Radiology* 1985;155:477.

39. Sheth S, Fishman EK, Buck JL, et al. The variable sonographic appearances of ovarian teratomas: correlation with CT. *AJR* 1988;151:331.

40. Stevens SK, Hricak H, Campos Z. Teratomas versus cystic hemorrhagic adnexal lesions: differentiation with proton-selective fat-saturation MR imaging. *Radiology* 1993;186:481.

41. Bis KG, Vrachliotis TG, Agrawal R, Shetty AN, Maximovich A, Hricak H. Pelvic endometriosis: MR imaging spectrum with laparoscopic correlation and diagnostic pitfalls. *Radiographics* 1997;17:639.

42. Outwater EK, Schiebler ML. Magnetic resonance imaging of the ovary. *MRI Clin North Am* 1994;2:245.

43. Rumack CM, Wilson SR, Charboneau JW. *Diagnostic ultrasound.* New York: Mosby, 1998.

44. Rosado WM, Trambert MA, Gosink BB, Pretorius DH. Adnexal torsion: diagnosis by using Doppler sonography. *AJR* 1992;159:1251.

45. Kimura I, Togashi K, Kawakami S, et al. Ovarian torsion: CT and MR imaging appearances. *Radiology* 1994;190:337.

46. Cartwright PS. Ectopic pregnancy. In: Jones HW III, Wentz AC, Burnett LC, eds. *Novak's textbook of gynecology,* 11th ed. Baltimore: Williams & Wilkins, 1988:479.

47. Fleischer AC, Pennell RG, McKee MS, et al. Ectopic pregnancy: features at transvaginal sonography. *Radiology* 1990;174:375.

48. Dillon EH, Quedens-Case, C, Ramos IM, Holland CK, Taylor KJ. Endovaginal pulsed and color flow Doppler in first trimester pregnancy. *Ultrasound Med Biol* 1993;19:517.

49. Nyberg DA, Hughes MP, Mack LA, Wang KY. Extrauterine findings of ectopic pregnancy at transvaginal US: importance of echogenic fluid. *Radiology* 1991;178:823.

50. Athey PA, Malone RS. Sonography of ovarian fibromas/thecomas. *J Ultrasound Med* 1987;6:431.

51. Stephenson WM, Laing FC. Sonography of ovarian fibromas. *AJR* 1985;144:1239.

52. Kurman RJ. *Blaustein's pathology of the female genital tract,* 3rd ed. New York: Springer-Verlag, 1987.

53. Fleischer AC, McKee MS, Gordon AN, et al. Transvaginal sonography of postmenopausal ovaries with pathologic correlation. *J Ultrasound Med* 1990;9:637.

54. Bashist B, Friedman WN, Killackey MA. Surgical transposition of the ovary: radiologic appearance. *Radiology* 1989;173:857.

55. Taylor KJW, Burns PN, Wells PNT. *Clinical applications of Doppler ultrasound,* 2nd ed. New York: Raven Press, 1995.

56. Berenstein A, Kricheff I. Catheter and material selection for transarterial embolization II. materials. *Radiology* 1979;132:631.

57. Craig O, Hobbs JT. Vulval phlebography in the pelvic congestion syndrome. *Clin Radiol* 1974;25:517.

58. O'Neil JD, Ros PR, Storm BL, Buck JL, Wilkinson EJ. Cystic mesothelioma of the peritoneum. *Radiology* 1989;170:333.

59. Madwed D, Mindelzun R, Jeffrey RB. Mucocele of the appendix: imaging findings. *AJR* 1992;159:69.

60. Bass JC, Korobkin M, Francis IR, Ellis JH, Cohan RH. Retroperitoneal plexiform neurofibromas: CT findings. *AJR* 1994;163:617.

61. Paling MR. Plexiform neurofibroma of the pelvis in neurofibromatosis: CT findings. *J Comput Assist Tomogr* 1984;8:476.

62. Cotran RS, Kumar V, Robbins SL. *Robbins' pathologic basis of disease.* Philadelphia: WB Saunders, 1989.

63. Di Santis DJ, Siegel MJ, Katz ME. Simplified approach to umbilical remnant abnormalities. *Radiographics* 1991;11:59.

64. Langer JE, Dinsmore BJ. Computed tomographic evaluation of benign and inflammatory disorders of the female pelvis. *Radiol Clin North Am* 1992;30:831.

65. Quane LK, Kidney DD, Cohen AJ. Unusual causes of ovarian vein thrombosis as revealed by CT and sonography. *AJR* 1998;171:487.

66. Melamed JW, Paulson EK, Kliewer MA. Sonographic appearance of oxidized cellulose (Surgicel): pitfall in the diagnosis of postoperative abscess. *J Ultrasound Med* 1995;14:27.

67. Hoefner EG, Soulen RL, Christensen CW. Gelatin sponge mimicking a pelvic neoplasm on MR imaging. *AJR* 1991;157:1227.

68. Young ST, Paulson EK, McCann RL, Baker ME. Appearance of oxidized cellulose (Surgicel) on postoperative CT scans: similarity to postoperative abscess. *AJR* 1993;160:275.

Variants and Pitfalls in Body Imaging,
edited by Ali Shirkhoda.
Lippincott Williams & Wilkins, Philadelphia, © 2000.

CHAPTER 21

Abdominal and Pelvic Vasculature: CT

John L. Roberts

Spiral computed tomography (CT) scanning represents a significant step forward in the interpretation of CT images. The ability to supply contrast to the various organ structures in a timely and reproducible manner has resulted in greater conspicuity of pathology. It also has allowed CT scans to be less likely to be affected by respiratory motion and has virtually eliminated respiratory misregistration. However, some limitations in interpretation have become evident, mainly as a result of the timing of the IV bolus and the fact that different organ systems require different scanning parameters for optimal display. Vascular flow artifacts have also been observed, resulting in potential pitfalls in diagnosis.

FLOW-RELATED ARTIFACTS

The degree of enhancement of a vessel is determined by the size of the blood pool and cardiac output relative to the timing of the scan. If venous structures, for example, are scanned too early following an injection of contrast, poor mixing of enhanced and nonenhanced blood can result in "apparent" venous thrombosis (1,2). This is most commonly seen in the inferior vena cava (IVC) near its junction with the renal veins (Figs. 21.1 and 21.2). At this level, opacified blood from the kidneys, which has a relatively short circulation time, meets with unopacified blood draining the lower extremities (longer circulation time), with the resulting appearance of a central low-density "filling defect." More cephalad, these two types of venous blood have a chance to mix and become more homogeneous. This phenomenon can also be seen at the confluence of the common iliac veins (3). To complicate matters further, an unusual flow phenomenon occurs

J.L. Roberts: Department of Diagnostic Radiology, William Beaumont Hospital, Royal Oak, Michigan 48073.

when foot veins are utilized for injections and there is mixing of opacified and nonopacified blood at the proximal aspect of the IVC (Fig. 21.3). Delayed scanning or repeat scanning both before and after IV contrast can help determine if this is artifact or represents thrombosis. Also, enlargement of the involved vein (with thrombosis) as well as the presence of collaterals can help in this differentiation.

Layering of contrast can occur in venous structures when flow is especially sluggish. This will be accentuated when long breath-holds are performed with a Valsalva maneuver, which is often required for spiral scanning. In this case, the denser contrast-enhanced blood will layer along the posterior wall of the vein (Fig. 21.4). Retrograde flow within the vena cava can occur in the setting of caval valvular incompetence. Contrast can actually bypass the systemic circulation when the right atrium is enlarged as a result of tricuspid insufficiency. Contrast will be seen within the IVC before it appears in the aorta because of reflux from the right atrium (Fig. 21.5). This should not be mistaken with the foot injection of contrast material.

Another cause of flow-related artifact, particularly when spiral technique is used, is IVC cut-off (4). Most supine patients, while in deep inspiration, will demonstrate this effect with the result of local collapse of the IVC near the hemidiaphragm and reduction or cessation of venous return to the heart. This would result in the delay of the mixing of opacified and nonopacified blood within the IVC and accentuate any pre-existing flow artifact, causing pseudothrombosis. Inferior vena cava cut-off does not usually occur during normal quiet respiration.

Flow artifacts, although more commonly seen in large-caliber vessels, can also be present in small vessels such as in the portal vein and superior mesenteric vein (5).

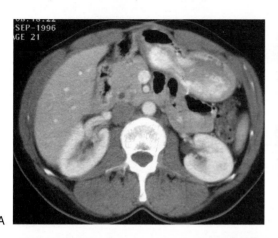

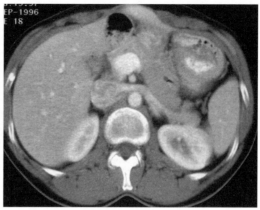

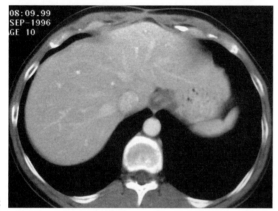

FIG. 21.1. Mixing of contrast-enhanced blood simulating a thrombus. **A:** Contrast-enhanced CT scan at a level below the renal veins shows nonopacified blood within the IVC. The blood in the IVC derives from the lower extremities and has not received contrast from the IV injection at this time. **B:** Computed tomography scan at the level of the left renal vein. Contrast-enhanced blood from the renal veins mixes with the unenhanced blood from the IVC, resulting in a bizarre density pattern caused by turbulence and can simulate thrombus formation. **C:** Computed tomography scan at a much higher level shows a vena cava that is of intermediate but relatively homogeneous density because of more complete mixing of enhanced and nonenhanced blood than is present in **B.**

Flow artifacts in these vessels are rare on conventional scanning but are common on spiral scanning because of improved vascular enhancement and rapid scanning technique. These artifacts can simulate venous thrombosis. To sort out this dilemma, a set of delayed scans can be performed at the level of the questioned vessel.

A pseudothrombosis may also be seen relating to partial volume effects. This can be seen in the portal vein or the IVC, which is enveloped by low-density fat. Spiral scanning may actually be of benefit in this scenario, as the volumetrically obtained raw data can be reconstructed with variable slice thickness and overlap.

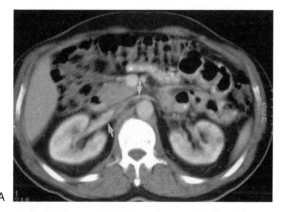

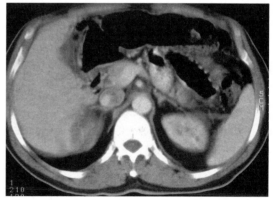

FIG. 21.2. Laminar flow within the inferior vena cava. **A:** Computed tomography scan at the level of the renal veins. Both renal veins *(arrows)* contain contrast-enhanced blood. The IVC receiving non-contrast-enhanced blood from the lower extremities is of lower attenuation. **B:** At a slightly higher level, because of a laminar flow pattern within the IVC, a bizarre central luminal enhancement pattern is seen suggesting the presence of eccentric thrombus.

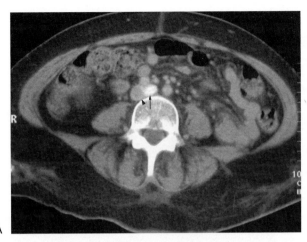
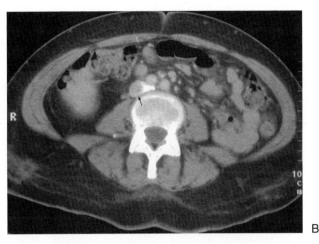

FIG. 21.3. Left foot injection resulting in pseudothrombus. **A:** Contrast-enhanced CT scan at the level of the common iliac vessels after a left foot venous injection. The left common iliac vein (LCIV) demonstrates marked enhancement *(arrow)*, while the right common iliac vein (RCIV) shows no enhancement *(arrowhead)*. **B:** Computed tomography scan at the level of the caval bifurcation. There is incomplete mixing of opacified (LCIV) and nonopacified (RCIV) blood, creating a pseudothrombus effect within the IVC *(arrow)*.

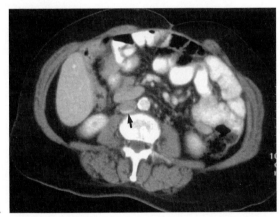
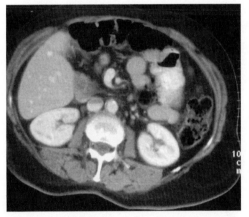

FIG. 21.4. Layering of contrast within the IVC from sluggish flow. A contrast/noncontrast fluid level can be seen when there is sluggish flow within the IVC. **A:** Contrast-enhanced spiral CT scan at the level of the lower pole of the kidneys. A small amount of contrast is seen within the IVC along its posterior wall (arrow). **B:** A contrast/noncontrast fluid level is seen within the IVC on a scan just below the renal hila. The contrast within the IVC at this level is caused by reflux of contrast-enhanced blood from the renal veins.

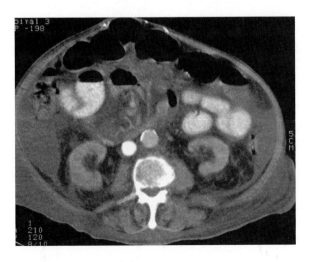

FIG. 21.5. Regurgitant flow into the IVC from tricuspid insufficiency. Contrast-enhanced CT scan in an 85-year-old patient with a history of leg swelling and tricuspid insufficiency. During the early phase, the IVC is seen as greatly enhancing, even more so than the aorta. The bolus of intravenous contrast delivered via an arm vein refluxed into the IVC from a large right atrium because of tricuspid insufficiency.

Pseudothrombosis of the right ovarian vein can be seen, usually in multiparous women, secondary to valve incompetency and retrograde flow into the left ovarian vein (6). On CT, one can appreciate asymmetry in the enhancement of the ovarian veins when scanning is performed during the early phase of spiral scanning (Figs. 21.6 and 21.7). The IVC and right gonadal vein contain

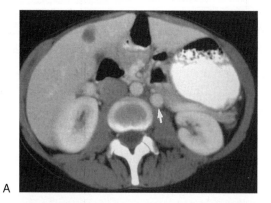

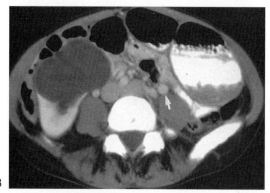

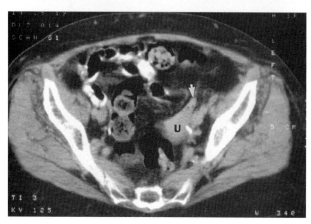

FIG. 21.6. Prominent left ovarian vein simulating adenopathy. **A:** Contrast-enhanced CT scan below the level of the renal hila. An enhancing structure *(arrow)* is seen just anterior to the left ureter. This corresponds to a very prominent left ovarian vein, which drains into the left renal vein at a higher level. Differential considerations include adenopathy or a duplication of the IVC. **B:** At a slightly lower level, the left ovarian vein has a position just lateral to the ureter. **C:** Within the pelvis, the left ovarian vein *(arrow)* lies anterolateral to the uterus (U) and separate from the left external iliac artery and vein.

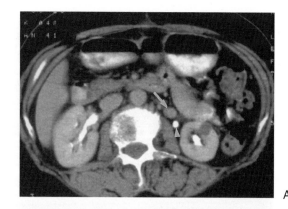

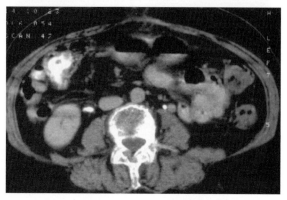

FIG. 21.7. Prominent left ovarian vein mimicking adenopathy. **A:** Contrast-enhanced CT scan near the renal hilum shows an enhancing mass *(arrow)* to the left of the aorta and anterior to the ureter *(arrowhead),* which corresponds to a very prominent left ovarian vein. Note a very prominent enhanced IVC to the right of the aorta. On an unenhanced scan, the left ovarian vein could be mistaken for hydronephrosis or lymphadenopathy. **B:** Computed tomography scan just above the aortic bifurcation shows continued presence of the left ovarian vein lateral to the left ureter. This excludes the possibility of caval duplication.

little or no IV contrast with early scanning, but the renal veins opacify early, and retrograde flow into the left ovarian vein can occur because of incompetent or absent valves in the cephalic portion of the left ovarian vein. This situation occurs because of the normal venous drainage of the ovarian veins: the right ovarian vein drains directly into the IVC, whereas the left ovarian vein empties into the left renal vein. The result is that the left ovarian vein will enhance while the right ovarian vein does not, which suggests the presence of thrombus within the right ovarian vein. Misdiagnosis can be avoided by recognizing the lack of opacification of the IVC. The diagnosis of pseudothrombus can be confirmed by obtaining a delayed CT when the IVC is opacified.

Although there are problems regarding the timing of IV contrast and flow artifacts, the benefits of IV contrast are far greater with the ability to differentiate normal vasculature (Figs. 21.8 and 21.9), and normal variations in vascular anatomy from pathology.

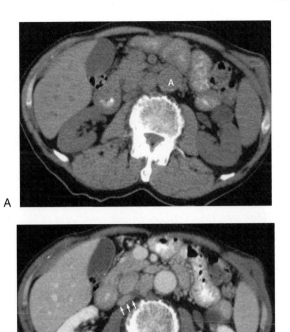

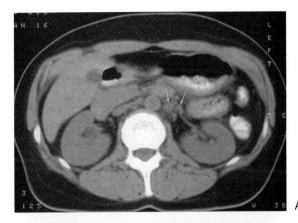

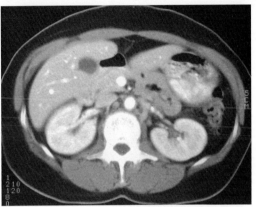

FIG. 21.8. Benefit of IV contrast in a patient with lymphadenopathy. **A:** Noncontrast CT scan at the level of the renal hila. The aorta (A) can be identified by the calcification within its wall. However, numerous rounded soft tissue densities are seen to its right, and identification of the IVC is difficult. **B:** Contrast-enhanced CT scan at the same level as A shows enhancement of the IVC *(arrows)* with the other two rounded densities representing lymph nodes.

FIG. 21.9. Paraaortic vascular structures simulating lymphadenopathy. **A:** Initial noncontrast CT scan at the level of the renal hila demonstrates several soft tissue masses in a left paraaortic location *(arrows)*. These were considered suspicious for lymphadenopathy at this location. **B:** Postcontrast CT scan at the same level shows that these soft tissue densities enhance significantly and to an equal degree at the inferior vena cava. These represent tortuous venous collaterals.

FAT IMPINGEMENT ON THE INFERIOR VENA CAVA

Focal fat collections associated with the subdiaphragmatic portion of the IVC have been described (7–9). Focal round or oval fat-containing collections will be seen adjacent to the medial border of the hepatic portion of the IVC but can appear intraluminal as well (Fig. 21.10). The density measurement should clearly indicate fat density but can be variable because of volume averaging relating to the small size of the collections or thick slices. Such a fat collection can measure up to 2.2 cm, and coronal reformatted images will confirm their extraluminal origin (Fig. 21.10C). This phenomenon always occurs above the confluence of the hepatic veins and the IVC and relates to subdiaphragmatic paraesophageal fat extending laterally and superiorly to impinge on the IVC.

Fat impingement on the IVC is seen in approximately 0.5% of patients, and no symptomatology has been attributed to this process. These have been followed with repeat scans and have never demonstrated any progression of the apparent defect. Although there has been some

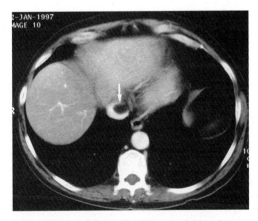

FIG. 21.10. Pericaval fat collection mimicking intracaval fat or thrombosis. **A:** Postcontrast CT scan at the level of the caval hiatus of the diaphragm shows an apparent intraluminal fat collection *(arrow)* associated with the anteromedial margin of the IVC. An acute angle is seen within the IVC posterior to the low attenuating mass, suggesting an intraluminal position. The mass has an attenuation value of –35 Hounsfield units. *Continued on next page.*

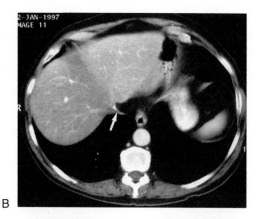

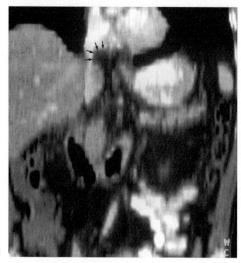

FIG. 21.10. *Continued.* **B:** Computed tomography scan at a slightly more caudal level demonstrates a more severe narrowing of the IVC with only an apparent small amount of contrast-enhanced blood *(arrow)* being seen laterally within the cava. **C:** Coronal reconstruction demonstrates that this fatty mass *(arrows)* is continuous with the subdiaphragmatic, paraesophageal fat. Note the significant narrowing of the diameter of the IVC at this level.

conjecture that this entity possibly relates to a shrunken right hepatic lobe (cirrhosis) or mediastinal lipomatosis, this is generally not considered to be the case.

Differential considerations for focal fat collections associated with the IVC would include: (a) bland thrombus, (b) primary tumors (leiomyosarcoma), and (c) secondary tumor extention (hepatic, renal, or adrenal in origin). Fat density measurements should exclude other possibilities, although extention of renal angiomyolipoma into the IVC could measure fat density. This is extremely rare and would be associated with an obvious renal mass.

CONGENITAL ANOMALIES OF VENOUS RETURN

Congenital anomalies of the inferior vena cava and renal veins are not uncommon and occur with a preva-

lence of up to 17%. Knowledge of these anomalies is essential for correct interpretations of CT scans. Only then can false-positive diagnoses of adenopathy or mass be avoided. Fundamental familiarity with these variations on CT can obviate the need for more invasive procedures such as angiography or FNA. Anomalies of the IVC can be categorized as malformations of the renal, the suprarenal, and the infrarenal segments (10).

Renal Venous Anomalies

Congenital anomalies involving the left renal vein can be divided into (a) a retroaortic left renal vein (1% to 3%) or (b) the more common circumaortic venous ring (1% to 9%).

The embryologic development of the IVC and renal veins is quite complex. Paired supracardinal veins are present, being positioned dorsal to the developing aorta. A series of midline anastomotic communications develop between the supracardinal veins. Normally, the right-sided IVC is formed from the persistence of the right supracardinal vein and simultaneous regression of the left supracardinal vein and the posterior anastomotic communications. The persistence of the left supracardinal vein or the midline anastomatosis produces the various IVC and left renal vein variants.

The normal course of the left renal vein is anterior to the aorta and results from the persistence of the intersubcarinal anastomosis, which passes anterior to the abdominal aorta. In the case of a retroaortic left renal vein, the preaortic anastomosis completely regresses, while the retroaortic anastomosis persists along with a short segment of the left supracardinal vein. The result is a left renal vein that passes entirely posterior to the aorta. The left retroaortic renal vein typically is below that of the right renal vein (34.8 ± 23 mm) (11). It is common to have the left retroaortic renal vein course posterior to the aorta and then ascend some distance in a left paraaortic location, simulating adenopathy or mass (Fig. 21.11).

A circumaortic left renal vein can be considered a true vascular ring, although only rarely will any symptom result from this variant. This variant will result from the persistence of the left supracardinal vein and the midline dorsal anastomosis. Computed tomography scanning will demonstrate two left renal veins with the preaortic left renal vein almost always being the larger of the two and emptying into the IVC at a higher level relative to the retroaortic counterpart (39 ± 17.4 mm) (Fig. 21.12). The preaortic left renal vein merges the IVC at a similar level to the corresponding right renal vein (2 ± 9 mm).

The renal veins do not always take a direct horizontal course to enter the hilum of their corresponding kidney. The kidneys may be displaced by an adjacent soft tissue mass, by organomegaly, or by emphysema such that the renal hila may not be opposite the origin of its renal vein. In this situation, the renal vein may have to ascend or

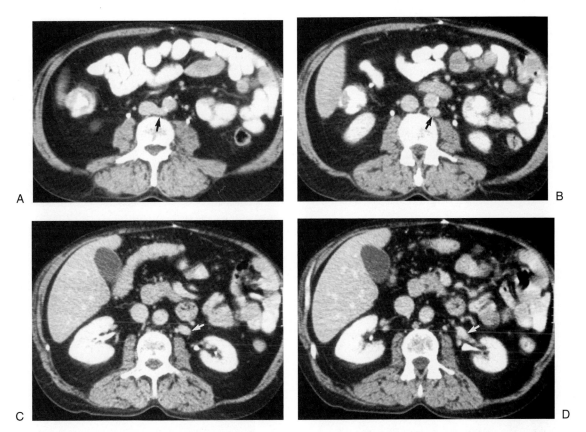

FIG. 21.11. Retroaortic left renal vein. **A:** Contrast-enhanced CT scan at the level of the origin of the left renal vein *(arrow)*, typically at a level below the renal hilum in the case of a retroaortic left renal vein. **B,C:** The left renal vein *(arrow)* at a slightly higher level than **A,** coursing posterior to the aorta and then ascending in a left paraaortic location, **C** *(arrow)*. **D:** Finally, the left renal vein *(arrow)* enters the left renal hilar area anterior to the left kidney's collecting system.

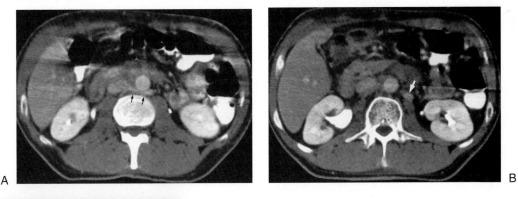

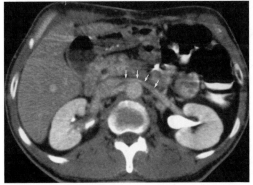

FIG. 21.12. Circumaortic left renal vein. **A:** Contrast-enhanced CT scan below the level of the renal hila. Note the rather diminutive retroaortic left renal vein *(arrows)*. **B:** At a slightly more cephalic level, the retroaortic left renal vein is seen ascending toward the left renal hilum and appears on CT scan as an enhancing nodular density *(arrow)*. **C:** At a still higher level, a second left renal vein drains into the IVC traveling anterior to the aorta *(arrows)*.

descend a distance in order to reach its final entry into its kidney. Because CT scans are limited to the axial plane, the vertically oriented vein may appear as a round or ovoid structure, in which case, adenopathy may be suspected when no intravenous contrast is given (Figs. 21.13 and 21.14). Enhancement with intravenous contrast would help to characterize these pitfalls. Coronal reconstructions in the plane of the renal vein may be of value in this regard, although the veins usually also course in an anterior-posterior plane as well making evaluation difficult. Cine-mode display should make it easier to trace the appropriate renal vein from its origin to insertion in most cases.

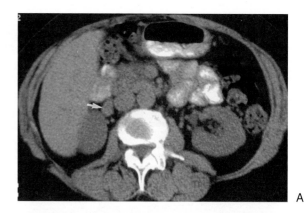

A

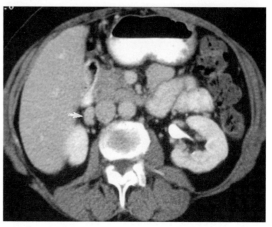

B

FIG. 21.14. Prominent, tortuous renal vein simulating adenopathy. **A:** Noncontrast CT above the level of the right renal hilum shows a soft-tissue mass *(arrow)* just to the right of the inferior vena cava. This was considered suspicious for adenopathy in this cancer patient. **B:** Postcontrast CT scan at the same level as **A.** The soft tissue mass *(arrow)* enhances 30 Hounsfield units and to a level equal to that of the inferior vena cava. This corresponds to a tortuous and somewhat prominent right renal vein.

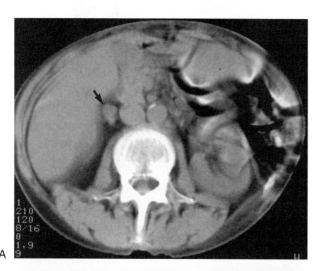

A

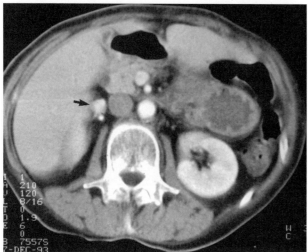

B

FIG. 21.13. Right renal vein simulating paracaval lymphadenopathy. **A:** Noncontrast CT scan at the level of the upper pole of the right kidney shows a 1.6-cm soft tissue density *(arrow)* to the right of the inferior vena cava. This was felt to represent adenopathy, and the patient was scheduled for biopsy. **B:** Two weeks later, a postcontrast prebiopsy scan at the same level demonstrates that this mass *(arrow)* is clearly vascular in origin and corresponded was related to the right renal vein. Biopsy was deferred.

Infrarenal IVC Anomalies

Infrarenal anomalies of the IVC can be subgrouped into: (a) left-sided IVC (transposition), (b) duplication of the IVC, and (c) retrocaval ureter. Each of these anomalies has a characteristic appearance that can be reliably recognized so as not to be confused for pathology. Each also has a characteristic embryologic basis for its appearance (12).

Transposition or anomalous left-sided inferior vena cava (Fig. 21.15) results from the persistence of the left supracardinal vein in conjunction with the regression of the right supracardinal vein. It is present in about 0.2% to 0.5% of the population. The left-sided IVC almost always crosses the midline at the level of the renal veins in order to eventually empty into the right-sided vena cava above the level of the kidneys. The left-sided IVC will not generally appear above the level of the renal hila. The left IVC will typically cross over the midline via the left renal

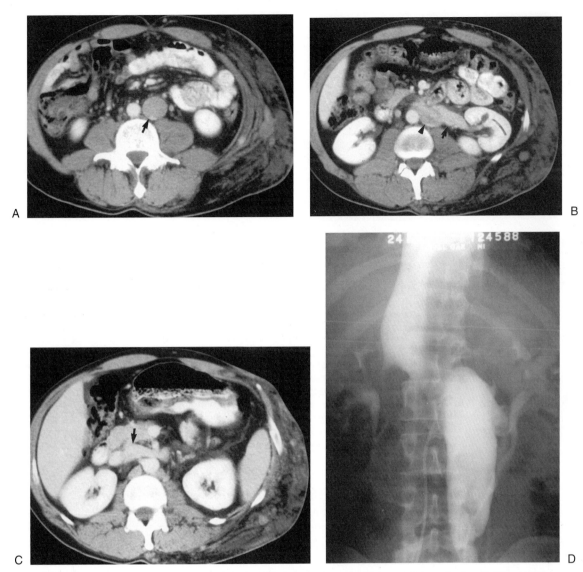

FIG. 21.15. Left-sided inferior vena cava. **A:** Contrast-enhanced CT scan below the level of the kidneys demonstrates a large-caliber left-sided vena cava *(arrow)* to the left of the aorta. Note some layering of contrast in the dependent portion of the IVC. **B:** Computed tomography scan at the level of the left renal vein *(arrow)*. The poorly opacified IVC *(arrowhead)* empties into the enhanced left renal vein (notice mixture of densities) before crossing over anterior to the aorta. **C:** Computed tomography scan at a level just above the renal hila. The IVC *(arrow)* is now situated in its normal position (to the right of the aorta). A preaortic left renal vein crosses between the SMA and aorta. (Note is made of a large cavernous hemangioma in the patient's left abdominal wall.) **D:** Venogram demonstrates a large left-sided vena cava that crosses midline at the level of the left renal vein to lie on the right side of the spine above the renal veins.

vein itself and may cross anterior (more common) or posterior to the aorta and rarely cross over caudal to the left renal vein.

Duplication of the IVC (Fig. 21.16) occurs in up to 3% of individuals (13) and results from the persistence of both the right and left supracardinal veins. In the vast majority of cases, the left-sided IVC drains into the left renal vein, which then crosses anterior to the aorta to empty into the right-sided IVC. The anastomosis between the right and left IVC is variable, and the left IVC can cross over at a more caudal level and may cross posterior to the aorta. Most commonly, the left-sided IVC is formed by direct drainage from the left common iliac vein. In this scenario, both IVCs will be of similar caliber. However, it is not uncommon for the left common iliac vein to bifurcate, resulting in a variable amount of blood crossing over the midline to join the right common iliac vein to form a normal or right-sided IVC. In this case, the left IVC will be smaller than its right counterpart, the extent of which is determined by differential distribution

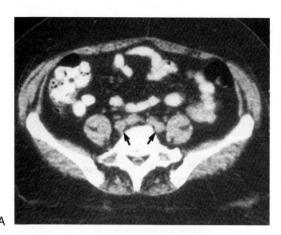
A

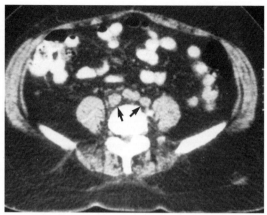
B

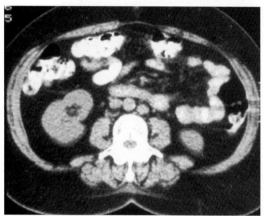
C

FIG. 21.16. Duplication of the inferior vena cava. **A:** Contrast-enhanced CT scan at a level just below the aortic bifurcation. Note the common iliac veins *(arrows)* in their normal location, posterior to their corresponding common iliac arteries. **B:** At a slightly higher level, the aorta is just beginning to bifurcate (the aorta almost always bifurcates at a level higher than the IVC). Here, the common iliac veins remain widely separated *(arrows)*. **C:** At the level of the lower poles of the kidneys, venous structures persist on both sides of the aorta, representing both the right- and left-sided IVC *(arrows)*. The left-sided IVC will drain at a higher level into the left renal vein, which will cross over anterior to the aorta to empty into the right-sided IVC such that above the level of the renal hilum there is only one inferior vena cava (right-sided only).

of flow from the left common iliac vein. When the left IVC is small, it can be mistaken for a large gonadal vein. This situation can be clarified as the left IVC continues caudally as the left common iliac vein, whereas a prominent gonadal vein will course toward the left inguinal canal (male) or the left ovary (female).

The retrocaval ureter is very rare (less than 0.1%) (14) and results from the persistence of the right posterior cardinal vein rather than the right supracardinal vein. This results in a right-sided IVC, which will displace the descending right ureter both medially and posteriorly relative to the IVC (Fig. 21.17). This anomaly can result in

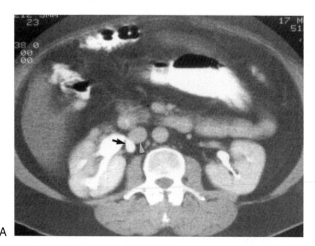
A

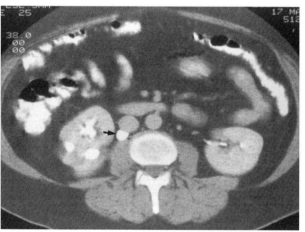
B

FIG. 21.17. Retrocaval ureter. A: Contrast-enhanced CT at a level just below the right renal hilum. Note that the opacified ureter *(arrow)* is initially posterior and medial to the IVC *(arrowhead)*. **B:** At a level just caudal to **A**, the ureter *(arrow)* begins to course medially and is situated behind the IVC.

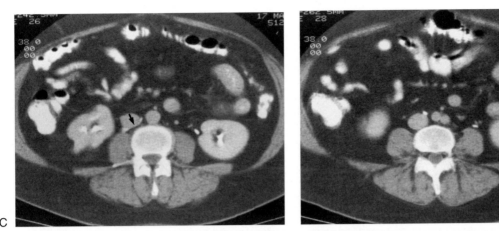

C   D

FIG. 21.17. *Continued.* **C,D:** Still more caudally, the ureter *(arrow)* takes a horizontal course posterior to the IVC and ends up medial to the IVC as demonstrated in **D.**

hydronephrosis because of potential mass effect by the IVC on the ureter. Relative obstruction can then result in an increased risk of infection and nephrolithiasis.

Suprarenal IVC Anomalies

Interruption of the IVC with azygous (Fig. 21.18) or hemiazygous (Fig. 21.19) continuation occurs with a prevalence of less than 1% (11). This condition results from failure in the development of the hepatic and right subcardinal venous anastomatosis. The hepatic segment of the IVC fails to develop. Venous return from below the diaphragm is achieved via the azygous/hemiazygous system (from the supracardinal system). Either azygous or hemiazygous continuation may occur, although azygous continuation is far more common. The hepatic

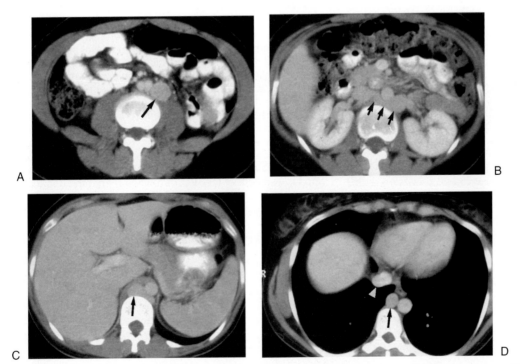

FIG. 21.18. Interruption of the inferior vena cava with azygous continuation. **A:** Contrast-enhanced CT scan at the level of the aortic bifurcation. The IVC is poorly opacified and exists as a left-sided IVC *(arrow).* **B:** At the level of the renal hila, the left-sided IVC joins the left renal vein and crosses midline as a retroaortic left renal vein *(arrows).* **C:** At a higher level, the venous drainage continues as a large azygous vein in its retrocrural location *(arrow).* Note the absence of the intrahepatic vena cava at this level. **D:** Within the chest, the suprahepatic components of the IVC reconstitute *(arrowhead)* from the hepatic veins while the azygous vein *(arrow)* courses in its normal location.

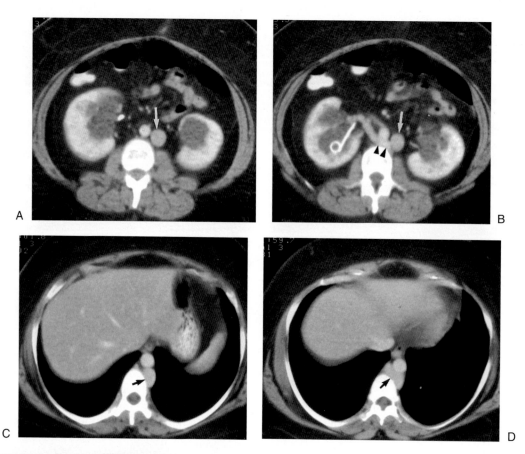

FIG. 21.19. Interruption of the inferior vena cava with hemiazygous continuation. **A:** Contrast-enhanced CT scan at a level below the renal hila showing a left-sided IVC *(arrow)* and bilateral hydronephrosis. **B:** The vena cava *(arrow)* continues on the left side of the aorta but receives a retroaortic right renal vein *(arrowheads)*. The patient has a right stent. **C:** Above the level of the kidneys, the cava ascends as a dilated hemiazygous vein *(arrow)*. Note a normal-sized azygous vein at this level and the absence of an intrahepatic vena cava. **D:** At T9, the hemiazygous vein communicates *(arrow)* and empties into the azygous vein as it does in the normal situation. **E:** At T8, venous drainage continues as a dilated azygous vein *(arrows)* that will eventually empty into the superior vena cava. Also, note the reconstitution of the suprahepatic segment of the IVC *(arrowhead)* from the hepatic veins.

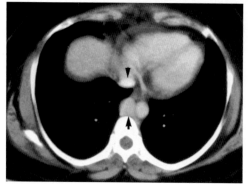

veins will coalesce and empty directly into the right atrium.

Suprarenal IVC anomalies can be suspected because of the absence of the IVC shadow on a lateral chest x-ray. A prominent azygous vein can be seen on a frontal chest radiograph and mistaken for a mediastinal mass. These anomalies are associated with congenital heart disease, polysplenia, and aspenia.

PORTOSYSTEMIC COLLATERAL VEINS

Portosystemic collateral veins usually occur in the setting of portal hypertension. These can take the appearance of a recanalized paraumbilical vein (Fig. 21.20). In an unenhanced scan, a prominent or enlarged paraumbilical vein will be seen as a low-density tubular structure in the area of the falciform ligament, which can then be traced down to the umbilicus, taking a course just deep to the abdominal wall. After the administration of intravenous contrast, this structure enhances similar to the other venous structures of the abdomen. The paraumbilical vein arises in the left sagittal fissure but can enlarge significantly and take a very tortuous course when portal hypertension becomes advanced. In these cases, the paraumbilical vein can present as a "liver" mass usually within the medial segment of the left lobe (15). Other portosystemic shunts may also mimic a liver lesion. The diagnosis should be suspected once intravenous contrast is given

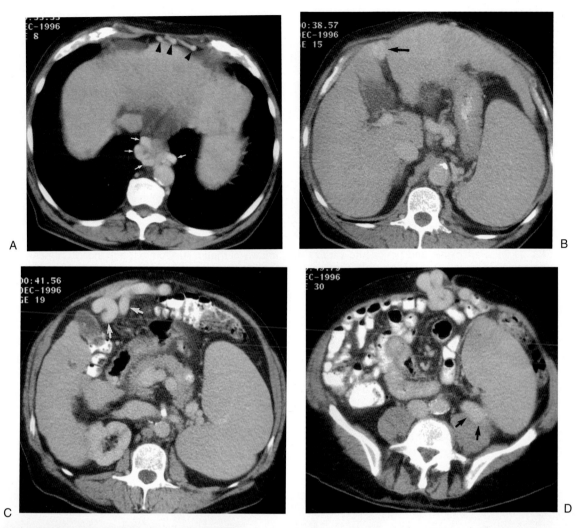

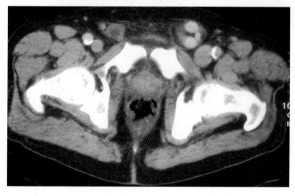

FIG. 21.20. Cirrhosis with prominent venous collaterals. Patient has end-stage liver disease from cirrhosis and splenomegaly. **A:** Collateral venous structures include paraesophageal varices *(arrows)* as well as ascending perihepatic venous collaterals *(arrowheads).* **B:** At a somewhat lower level, one can identify a recanalized paraumbilical vein *(arrow)* within the ligamentum teres as well as gastrohepatic varices. **C:** More caudally, prominent tortuous abdominal wall varices *(arrows)* descend toward the umbilicus; splenic varices are seen at the splenic hilum. **D:** At the level of the umbilicus, paraumbilical varices (Caput Medusa) can be seen as well as a large parasplenic vein *(arrows),* which contributes to a splenorenal shunt in this patient. **E:** Bilateral inguinal varices are present. All of these varices can potentially be mistaken for adenopathy or bowel when nonenhanced or poorly enhanced.

and the entire portosystemic collateral vein enhances to a similar degree as the main portal trunk. This will be seen in contrast to the characteristic enhancement pattern of a cavernous hemangioma or hepatocellular carcinoma.

Other examples of collateral venous structures that can stimulate pathology include esophageal varices (Fig. 21-20A), caput Medusa (serpiginous collaterals in the paraumbilical location), splenorenal shunts, and perisplenic and perigastric varices (Fig. 21.21). All of

these can be correctly diagnosed by careful attention to the enhancement pattern after the administration of the IV bolus and also adequate bowel opacification.

Prominent or tortuous vessels can lead to confusion and misdiagnosis. Prominent venous structures can simulate adenopathy (Fig. 21.22). This is especially the case within the pelvis, involving the internal, external, or common iliac veins. Periprostatic or parametrial varices can simulate pathology, particularly in the setting of a pelvic

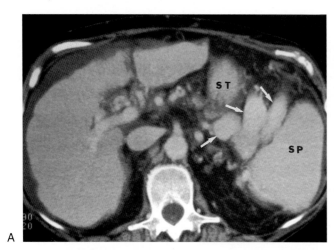

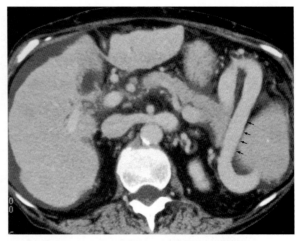

FIG. 21.21. Perisplenic and perigastric varices in a known cirrhotic. **A:** Contrast-enhanced CT scan demonstrates large venous collaterals *(arrows)* between the stomach (ST) and spleen (SP). Note the scalloped liver margin and the presence of ascites. **B:** A slightly more caudal CT scan shows a tortuous large-caliber collateral vein *(arrows)* medial to the spleen.

malignancy. Pelvic sidewall extent of tumor or internal obturator adenopathy can be difficult to differentiate from these types of varices. A rapid bolus of IV contrast and delayed scanning may be necessary to ensure sufficient enhancement of these venous structures.

Arterial structures are prone to atherosclerotic changes and tortuosity. Unusual locations of the arteries because of their tortuous nature can sometimes cause a diagnostic dilemma. Tortuous splenic arteries are often seen in older individuals and, as a result, will course in and out of plane on CT scans. External and internal iliac arteries also can follow a serpiginous path and take unexpected locations, sometimes simulating an appendicolith or appendicitis (Fig. 21.23).

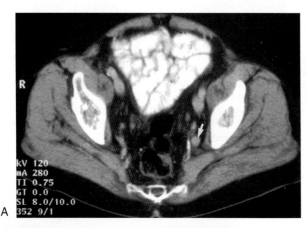

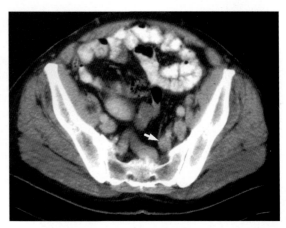

FIG. 21.22. Prominent internal iliac venous branches simulating adenopathy. **A:** Contrast-enhanced CT scan below the level of the iliac vessel bifurcation. The left internal iliac vein *(arrow)* is much more prominent than the right and, if not well enhanced, can be confused for a lymph node in this prostate cancer patient. **B:** Postcontrast CT scan in a different patient than **A**. A prominent left internal iliac vein *(arrow)* is seen without obvious enhancement and is suspicious for a lymph node. **C:** Same patient as in **B** at a lower level and with better enhancement confirms this structure *(arrow)* to be venous in origin.

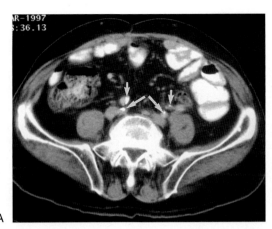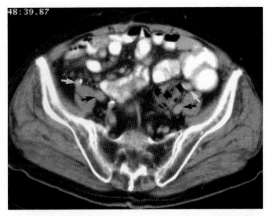

FIG. 21.23. Tortuous right external iliac artery simulating an appendicolith. **A:** The common iliac arteries bifurcate at a higher level, and on this image, external iliac arteries *(short arrows)* and the internal iliac arteries *(long arrows)* are labeled. **B:** Computed tomography scan at a slightly lower level shows both external arteries *(white arrows)* quite lateral to their normal position and relatively distant from their corresponding veins *(black arrows)*. The calcification associated with the right external iliac artery could mimic an appendicolith in the appropriate clinical situation.

There is a fair amount of variability in the branching of the arterial supply of the gut. The common and right hepatic arteries have several unusual but still normal origins. The common hepatic artery, which usually is a branch of the celiac axis, can arise directly from the aorta (Fig. 21.24). A replaced right hepatic artery occurs in approximately 18% of patients and arises as a branch vessel from the superior mesenteric artery (SMA). This variant can be detected by its characteristic course between the IVC and portal vein, the only vascular structure to do so. This must be differentiated from a small tongue of liver tissue at this location or adenopathy.

Malrotation of the gut and resultant reversal of the normal SMA/SMV relationship will be seen in a small number of patients. Normally, the SMV is larger, anterior, and to the right of the SMA. With malrotation, the SMA will be situated to the right and often anterior to the SMV (Fig. 21.25). It may be difficult to determine which of these two vessels is an artery on a CT scan, although calcification of a wall, when present, helps to identify the SMA. Also, each vessel can be traced back to its origin or destination: the SMV will merge with the splenic vein to form the portal confluence, whereas the SMA can be followed back to its origin directly from the aorta or its common origin with the celiac trunk.

Lumbar veins (Fig. 21.26) are not commonly seen on routine scanning unless specifically looked for. They can be identified by their draining point to the posterior wall of the IVC and their course on either side of the lumbar spine.

Iatrogenic or postsurgical changes to the vascular anatomy can be identified on CT scans. Axillary–femoral arterial shunts will be seen along the ipsilateral abdominal wall. The graft can be identified by its course and relatively dense wall. A femoral–femoral bypass shunt (Fig. 21.27) will have a similar appearance although located within the anterior lower abdominal wall or the pelvis. Aortobifemoral grafting can be seen with some frequency on CT scanning.

Adjacent bowel loops, such as the duodenum, can result in a pitfall, simulating either an aneurysm or a rupture of abdominal aneurysm (16). The bowel loop, when poorly opacified or nonopacified, and abutting the aorta would appear as a soft tissue mass, possibly representing thrombus or adjacent hematoma.

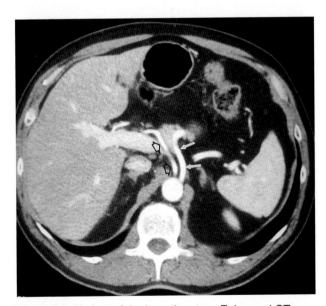

FIG. 21.24. Variant of the hepatic artery. Enhanced CT scan at the level of the common hepatic and splenic arteries. The common hepatic artery *(open arrows)* has a separate origin from the aorta in this patient (instead of arising as a branch of the celiac axis as is the normal case). The splenic artery *(white arrow)* is seen as a separate vessel.

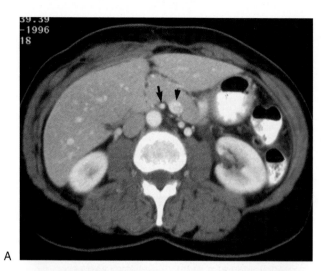

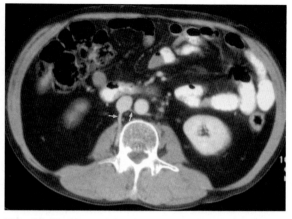

FIG. 21.26. Normal lumbar veins. Contrast-enhanced CT scan at the level of the fourth portion of the duodenum. The IVC is well opacified with demonstration of two lumbar veins *(arrows),* which will course at both sides of the lumbar spine. These veins typically drain into the posterolateral wall of the IVC.

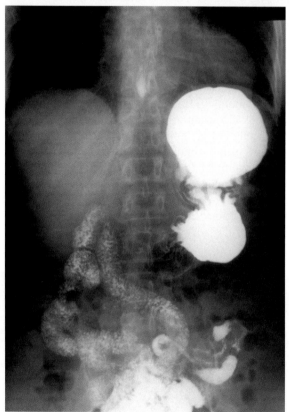

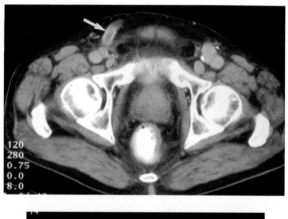

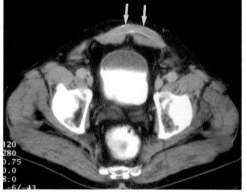

FIG. 21.25. Malrotation of the gut with reversal of the SMA–SMV relationship. **A:** Contrast-enhanced CT scan at the level of the pancreas shows the smaller SMA *(arrow)* to be to the right of the SMV *(arrowhead),* which is opposite of the normal situation regarding these two vascular structures. **B:** Upper GI study demonstrating the proximal small bowel loops to be located in the right of the midline.

FIG. 21.27. Femoral–femoral arterial bypass shunt. Contrast-enhanced CT scan at the level of the symphysis pubis shows an unusual tubular structure *(arrow)* within the right groin relating to a femoral–femoral bypass shunt. Note the typical hyperdense walls of the graft. **B:** On a more cephalad CT scan, the horizontal portion of the shunt *(arrows)* is seen superficial to the rectus muscles.

REFERENCES

1. Fagelman D, Lawrence LP, Black KS, et al. Inferior vena cava pseudothrombosis in computed tomography using a contrast medium power injector: a potential pitfall. *J Comput Assist Tomogr* 1987;11(6): 1042–1043.
2. Glazer GM, Callen PW, Parker JJ. CT diagnosis of tumor thrombus in the inferior vena cava: avoiding the false-positive diagnosis. *Am J Roentgenol* 1981;137:1265–1267.
3. Herts BR, Einstein DM, Paushter DM. Spiral CT of the abdomen: artifacts and potential pitfalls. *Am J Roentgenol* 1993;161;1185–1190.
4. Fox RH, Turner MJ, Gardner AMN. Pseudothrombosis of the infrarenal IVC during helical CT—What causes this pitfall? *Clin Radiol* 1996;51:741.
5. Silverman PM, Cooper CJ, Weltman DI, et al. Helical CT: Practical considerations and potential pitfalls. *RadioGraphics* 1995;15:25–36.
6. Cranston PE, Hamrick-Turner J, Morano JV. Pseudothrombosis of the right ovarian vein—pitfall of abdominal spiral CT. *Clin Imag* 1995;19: 176–179.
7. Hines J, Katz DS, Goffner L, et al. Fat collection related to the intrahepatic inferior vena cava on CT. *Am J Roentgenol* 1999;172: 409–411.
8. Han BK, Im J-G, Jung JW, et al. Pericaval fat collection that mimics thrombosis of the inferior vena cava: demonstration with use of multidirectional reformation CT. *Radiology* 1997;203:105–108.
9. Miyake H, Suzuki K, Ueda S, et al. Localized fat collection adjacent to the intrahepatic portion of the inferior vena cava: a normal variant on CT. *Am J Roentgenol* 1991;158:423–425.
10. Chuang VP, Mena EC, Hoskins PA. Congenital anomalies of the inferior vena cava. Review of embryogenesis and presentation of a simplified classification. *Br J Radiol* 1974;47:206–213.
11. Trigaux J-P, Vandroogenbroek S, DeWispelaere J-F, et al. Congenital anomalies of the inferior vena cava and left renal vein: evaluation with Spiral CT. *J Vasc Interventional Radiol* 1998;9:339–345.
12. Mayo J, Gray R, St. Louis E, et al. Anomalies of the inferior vena cava. *Am J Roentgenol* 1983;140:339–345.
13. Royal SA, Callen PW. CT evaluation of anomalies of the inferior vena cava and left renal vein. *Am J Roentgenol* 1979;132:759–763.
14. Walsh PC, Gittes RF, Perlmutter AD, et al. *Campbell's urology, 5th ed.* Philadelphia: WB Saunders 1986;1743.
15. Yamauchi T, Itai Y, Furui S, et al. Prominent collateral vein in portal hypertension mimicking liver tumours: a pitfall in computed tomography. *Br J Radiol* 1987;60:531–533.
16. Gale ME, Johnson WC, Gerzof SG, et al. Problems in CT diagnosis of ruptured abdominal aortic aneurysms. *J Comput Assist Tomogr* 1986; 10(4):637–641.

Variants and Pitfalls in Body Imaging,
edited by Ali Shirkhoda.
Lippincott Williams & Wilkins, Philadelphia, © 2000.

CHAPTER 22

Doppler Imaging

Beatrice L. Madrazo and Donovan M. Bakalyar

By incorporating the Doppler principle, diagnostic ultrasound can be used to image not only anatomic structures, but blood flow as well. Unfortunately, electronic processing of the Doppler signal along with the nature of sound interaction with tissue can give rise to artifacts that, if not clearly understood and appropriately identified, could lead to misdiagnosis.

This chapter presents a comprehensive explanation of the causes of Doppler artifacts. Whenever possible we will elaborate on the contribution that properly identified artifacts can make to the diagnostic process in conventional Doppler, color Doppler imaging (CDI), and most recently, power Doppler imaging (PDI). Emphasis is placed on the abdomen and pelvic vessels. However, occasional examples of carotid arteries are used to illustrate some examples of Doppler artifacts.

BASIC PRINCIPLES

The echo from a reflector moving directly away from an ultrasonic transducer is stretched in time by the factor

$$\frac{\left(1 + \dfrac{v}{c}\right)}{\left(1 - \dfrac{v}{c}\right)} \; which \; is \; approximately \; 1 + \frac{2v}{c}, \; if \; \frac{v}{c} \ll 1$$

where v is the speed of the reflector and c is the speed of sound (about 154,000 cm/s). (For the reflector moving toward the transducer, v has a negative sign and the echo is compressed in time.)

The transmitted signal may be a sinusoidal oscillation of frequency f_0 that is either a continuous wave (CW) or switched on for a few cycles and then off again (pulse). Only the component of velocity that is collinear with the

ultrasound beam contributes to the Doppler shift, which thus becomes $2 f_0 \frac{v}{c} \cos \theta$ where θ is the angle between the beam and direction of flow. Although the Doppler shift of the transmitted frequency is minuscule (about 0.1% for blood moving at 75 cm/s), it can be measured with great precision by referencing the echo to the frequency of the original signal f_0. Indeed, the spectrum of velocities emanating from a collection of reflectors moving at slightly different speeds can be determined from its composite echo using Fourier analysis or a related method.

TRANSITION OF FOCAL ZONES (BANDING)

Tissue lying within the focal zone of a transducer returns a higher signal strength. Newer transducers will offer multiple focal zones, and the intention of the manufacturers is to provide a uniform transition (seamless) between them. Most often this is the case; however, a horizontal band of increased echogenicity may become perceptible due to a poor transition between focal zones. It can appear in gray scale as well as color Doppler images (Figs. 22.1 and 22.2) The clue to its appropriate recognition on a gray scale image is the straight margins. On the color Doppler image, this band exhibits artifactual color encoding, suggesting the presence of flow; however, the area of presumed flow portrays chaotic pixels of different hues and no perceptible vessels are present.

ALIASING

With pulsed Doppler a single point (sample) from the echo signal is recorded once per pulse at a time corresponding to the round-trip distance to the region of interest. With stationary reflectors, each sample will be at the same voltage, resulting in a flat response with time. (There will always be random fluctuations from noise.) If the reflectors are moving, however, the samples will progress down the pulse shape as shown in Fig. 22.3 (1).

B.L. Madrazo and D.M. Bakalyar: Department of Diagnostic Radiology, William Beaumont Hospital, Royal Oak, Michigan 48073-6769.

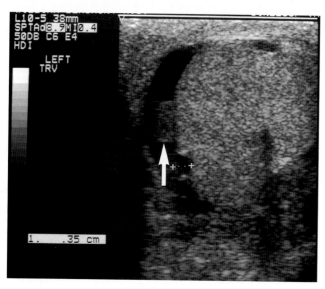

FIG. 22.1. Focal zone banding—gray scale. Gray scale images of the scrotum demonstrate a band of artifactual echoes superimposed both over the hydrocele and the testes *(arrow)*.

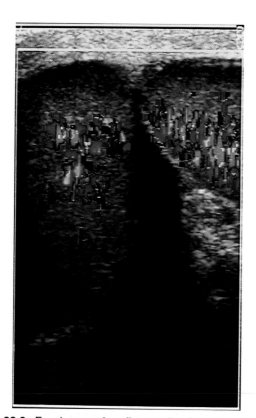

FIG. 22.2. Focal zone banding—color Doppler. Straddle view of both hemiscrotums demonstrating areas within the testis with color-encoded pixels of varying hues.

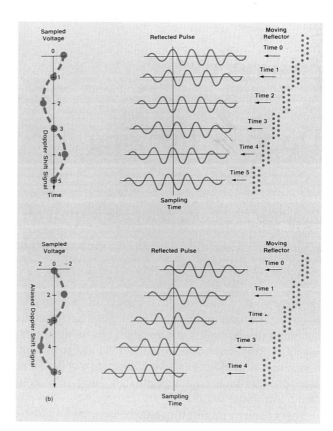

FIG. 22.3. Schematics of aliasing. Origin of aliasing in Doppler ultrasound. The voltage is sampled at the position of the vertical line labeled "Sampling Time." The wall is moving slowly enough to ensure that every cycle is sampled at least once *(top)*. The wall is moving so rapidly that cycles are missed between samples *(bottom)*. The frequency shift is aliased to a lower frequency. (From Reference 1, with permission.)

As long as the resultant shift in the echo-to-echo position is less than half a cycle, the time dependence of the samples will oscillate at the Doppler frequency shift. If the reflectors are moving so fast or if the pulse repetition frequency (PRF) is so low that more than half a cycle occurs between pulses, the Nyquist criterion will be violated and the frequency shift will be aliased to a lower or even a negative frequency (indicating flow in the opposite direction) by an integer multiple of the PRF (2).

Spectral waveforms with aliasing exhibit a truncated appearance, with the peak of the spectrum appearing below baseline (in the opposite direction of flow), whereas CDI portrays aliasing as a multicolored region representing the wrapping around of the signal on the edge of the color spectrum, with an abrupt change in color through a bright band (i.e., the colors appear to indicate infinite velocity before changing direction). Aliasing is illustrated in Figs. 22.4, 22.5, and 22.6.

In the case where there is actual flow reversal, the colors indicate a continuous change through zero flow where the color is black (Figs. 22.7 and 22.8.)

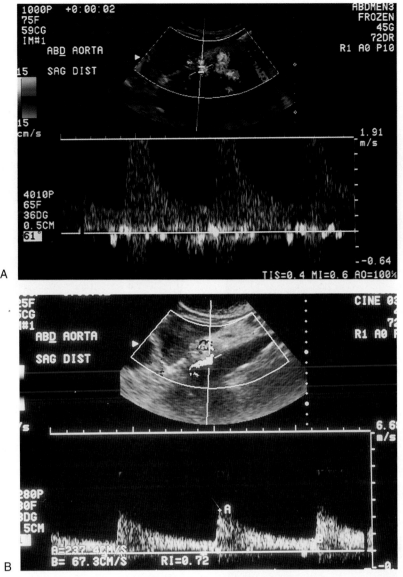

FIG. 22.4. Aliasing—spectral Doppler. **A:** Spectral and color Doppler images of the aorta/celiac artery reveals a truncated appearance to the waveform *(arrow)*. Note the peaks of spectrum portrayed below the baseline *(arrowhead)*. **B:** The velocity scale has been increased to 668 m/s by changing the pulse repetition frequency to 8,280 p/s; this corrects for aliasing by expanding the range of frequencies.

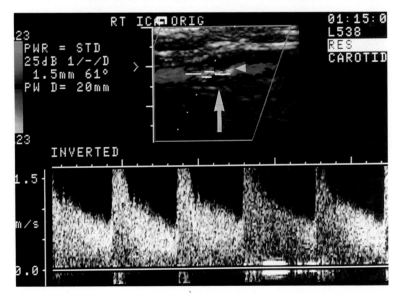

FIG. 22.5. Aliasing—color/spectral Doppler. Sagittal color Doppler image of the internal carotid artery demonstrates an area of stenosis due to a plaque *(arrow)*. Note the multicolored appearance (mosaic) due to the increased velocity and resultant aliasing. Spectral waveforms display significant spectral broadening and truncated peaks.

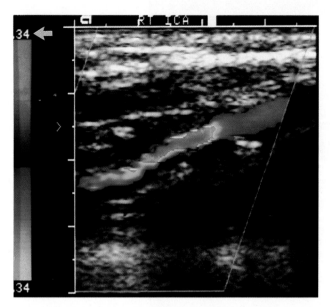

FIG. 22.6. Aliasing-color mosaic. Sagittal sonogram of the internal carotid artery demonstrates typical color changes from deep hues of red, through yellow, cyan, and blue. Notice the color bar at the edge of the image with the Nyquist limit printed on its edges (arrow).

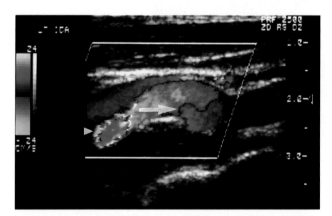

FIG. 22.7. Flow reversal—color Doppler. On this sagittal image of the internal carotid we have the opportunity of analyzing flow reversal with color changes portrayed from deep red to deep blue through the zone of zero Doppler shift—black (arrow). Note also aliasing distally (arrowhead).

CORRECTING FOR ALIASING (3)

Aliasing can be corrected in the following ways:

Decrease the transducer frequency
Shift the baseline (a "cut and paste" method)
Expand the range of frequencies by increasing the PRF
Increase the Doppler angle (thereby decreasing Doppler shifts)
Apply continuous wave sampling

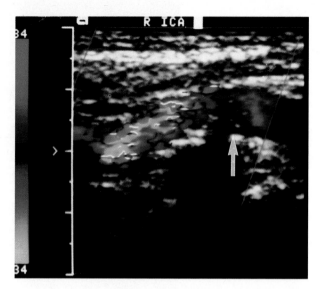

FIG. 22.8. Color Doppler—aliasing flow reversal. Sagittal color image of the internal carotid demonstrates a large soft plaque (arrow). Distal flow demonstrates both flow reversal and aliasing.

Increasing the PRF reduces the possibility of aliasing but increases the likelihood of range ambiguity (2). The optimal compromise depends on the clinical situation. For CW Doppler (which is, in principle, an infinite PRF), the velocity is unambiguous but the region of origin becomes indeterminate.

RING-DOWN ARTIFACT/ COMET TAIL ARTIFACT

A trail of echoes resembling the shape of a comet tail can be found beyond highly reflective objects such as calcifications, surgical clips, nasogastric tubes, hollow structures, etc. The acoustic mismatch between the front and back of such objects gives origin to these reverberant echoes. They are closely spaced, of decreasing intensity, and of a linear configuration. The delayed return of the secondary echoes from the same object can mimic motion, which can result in color encoding in either color Doppler or power Doppler imaging.

We have observed color encoding of the comet tail artifact of the gallbladder in a case of adenomyomatosis (Fig. 22.9) as well as while imaging prostate glands and the signal interacting with corpora amylacea (Fig. 22.10). These color-encoded areas can simulate areas of flow; therefore, their appropriate recognition is paramount. Figures 22.11 and 22.12 illustrate additional artifactual color/power Doppler images of the ringdown artifact.

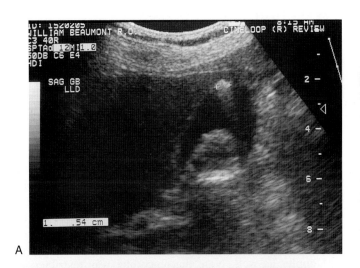

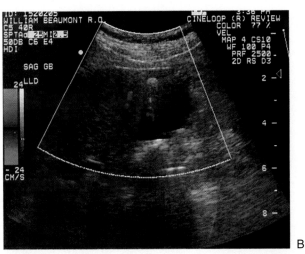

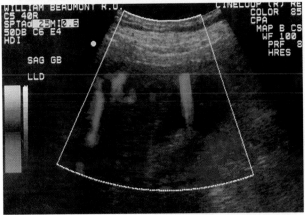

FIG. 22.9. Ring-down artifact. **A:** Sagittal display of the gallbladder demonstrates a high-amplitude area related to gallbladder wall. This is secondary to an adherent calculus and/or an area of adenomyomatosis. We note beyond this highly reflective interface a group of echoes of decreasing intensity. This is consistent with reverberation of the sound waves between the front and back interfaces of this object and the adjacent tissue. **B:** Color Doppler image of the same gallbladder demonstrates color comet tail artifact. **C:** Sagittal display of the same gallbladder demonstrating coloring with power Doppler of this comet tail artifact.

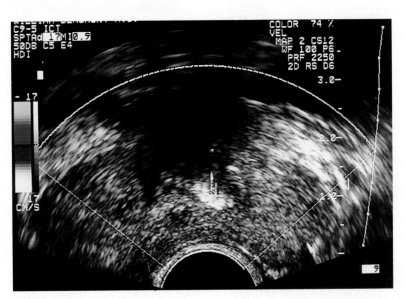

FIG. 22.10. Ring-down artifact—color Doppler. Axial image of the prostate displays a trail of color-encoded signals beyond an area of corpora amylacea.

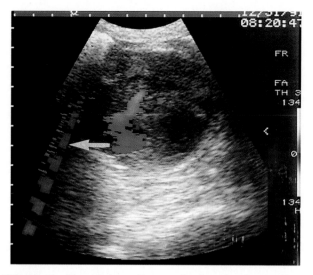

FIG. 22.11. Ring-down artifact—color Doppler. A gas pocket adjacent to a mass has resulting ring-down artifact in color *(arrow)*.

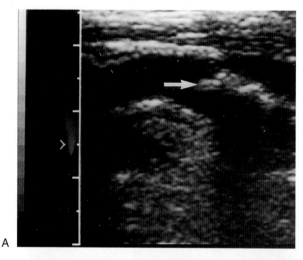

A

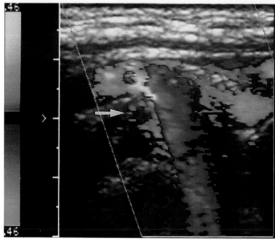

B

FIG. 22.12. Flail plaque. **A:** Gray scale sagittal image of the carotid demonstrates a flail calcified plaque that projects into the vessel lumen *(arrow)*. **B:** The motion of this flail plaque during the cardiac cycle results in a colored ring-down artifact *(arrow)*.

ANECHOIC SPACE COLOR ARTIFACT

Anechoic spaces may fill in with color due to the color/gray scale write priority setting (4–6). When using color priority setting in a low sensitivity, color encoding of anechoic spaces due to noise may result. We have experienced this artifact in cases of hydroceles, cystic masses, and in one case of an abscess with floating debris.

Confusing examples of color encoding of anechoic spaces may be seen with liver cysts (Figs. 22.13 and 22.14). This is likely the result of transmitted pulsations from the adjacent heart. Of interest is the fact that only the fluid compartment becomes color encoded, which implies that it was the result of fluid shift. The presence of motion in the cysts was demonstrated by power Doppler as well. Note that encoding was restricted to

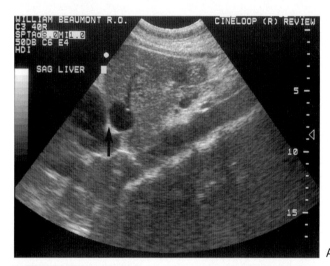

A

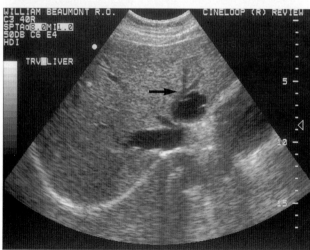

B

FIG. 22.13. Anechoic space. **A:** Sagittal gray scale study of the mid-abdomen demonstrates the abdominal aorta and, within the liver abutting the diaphragm, we note a 3 × 2.8 cm anechoic area. A vascular structure is coursing just anterior to it. Note the close proximity of the cyst to the heart *(arrow)*. **B:** Transverse image of the liver demonstrates the cyst and the left hepatic vein *(arrow)* coursing anterior and to the right.

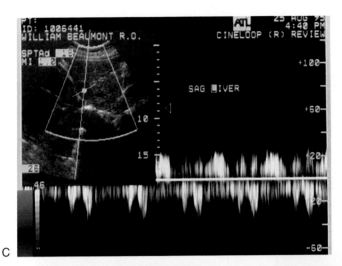

C

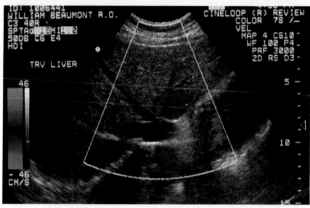

D

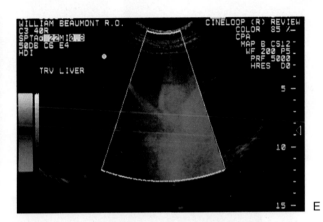

E

FIG. 22.13. *Continued.* **C:** Color Doppler image of the cyst in the sagittal plane demonstrates the adjacent heart with color encoding as well as the cyst *(arrow)*. Spectral waveform of the cyst reflects the transmitted pulsations from the heart (arterial signal). **D:** Transverse color Doppler sonogram of the liver displays color encoding of the liver cyst and hepatic veins. **E:** Transverse image of the liver utilizing power Doppler demonstrates color encoding of the liver cyst, and of the middle left and hepatic veins.

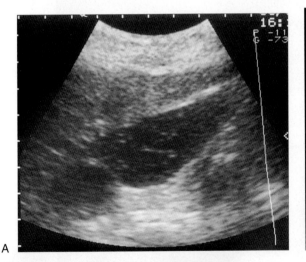

A

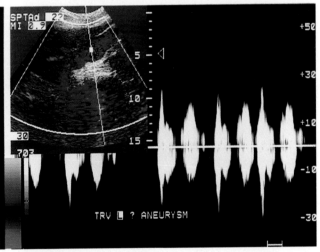

B

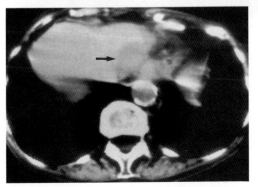

C

FIG. 22.14. Liver cyst. **A:** Transverse image of the liver demonstrates an elliptical cystic area adjacent to the liver, between it and the hemidiaphragm. Internal echoes are present within this predominantly anechoic area. **B:** Transverse image of the same cystic area demonstrating color encoding of the cystic mass. Doppler signal was also obtained due to its proximity to the heart. **C:** Computed tomography (CT) image of the same cyst demonstrating a low-density area adjacent to the heart *(arrow)*.

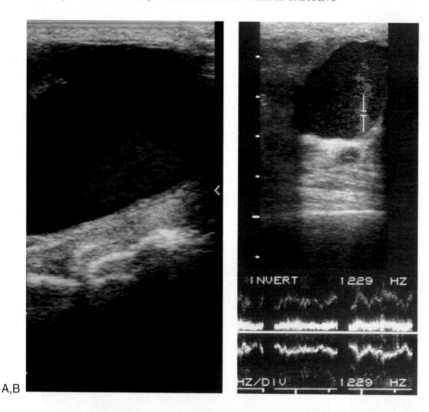

FIG. 22.15. Hydrocele. **A:** Sagittal display of a hydrocele demonstrating partial color encoding. Note the noise within the fluid collection and color encoding in blue of some of the signals. **B:** Transverse image of the same hydrocele now exhibiting an area of greater color encoding. Spectral waveform of the area reveals just electronic noise rather than physiologic spectral waveforms.

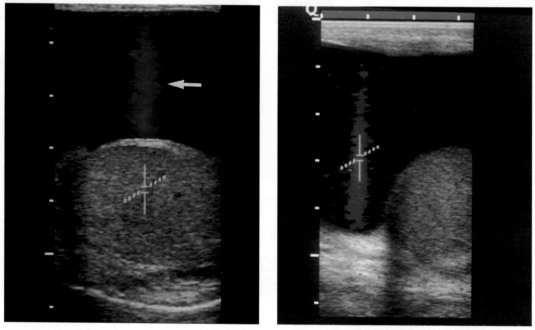

FIG. 22.16. Hydrocele. **A:** Sagittal display of the testes and of a hydrocele demonstrating arterial flow within the testes. Adjacent and anterior to it, within the hydrocele, note the apparent vessel *(arrow)*. **B:** Sagittal display of the hemiscrotum demonstrates a vessel within a hydrocele. Spectral waveform analysis reveals electronic noise. The apparent vessel merely represents areas of color encoding within this fluid compartment, the result of fluid shifting (motion) within the hydrocele.

the cyst itself without any flash artifacts in the surrounding tissues. In the case of the cysts adjacent to the heart, pulsations were transmitted into the cyst itself, giving it an arterial signal on spectral Doppler (Fig. 22.13). Wu et al. (3) reported on the value of color Doppler in discriminating effusion from pleural thickening (fluid-color sign). Additional cases of a series of fluid-filled compartments that portray artifactual partial and/or complete color encoding are illustrated in Figs. 22.15 and 22.16.

DUPLICATION/MIRROR IMAGE ARTIFACTS

Duplication and mirror image artifacts occur not only in gray scale imaging but also in color Doppler and power Doppler examinations. A vascular structure can be mirrored if it lies near a strong specular reflector that redirects the ultrasound beam to make it appear as if it came from a different location (Fig. 22.17). The equipment software assumes that another structure similar to the true vessel lies nearby and, because of the flow within it, is portrayed in color (5,7–9). The effect is particularly noticeable in color flow Doppler where the mirror image can, oddly enough, show flow in either the same or opposite direction of the actual vessel.

The physical principle for such artifact is due to the fact that the real blood vessel is at angle α relative to the ultrasound beam, and the reflector, which acts like a mirror, is at angle β. Just as in optics, the angle between the vessel reflection and the mirror is the same as the angle

between the real vessel and the mirror. Thus, the vessel reflection will be oriented at $\gamma = 2\beta - \alpha$ to the blood flow direction. The critical angle is $\gamma = 90°$. For $\gamma < 90°$, the direction of flow for the reflection will be the same as for the real vessel; for $\gamma > 90°$, however, the flow direction will be opposite and the color will change accordingly. There are two special cases of interest:

1. The vessel and mirror are parallel (as in the carotid ghost, which is discussed below). Then $\gamma = \alpha = \beta$ and the flow directions are always the same.
2. The mirror is perpendicular to the beam. Then $\beta = 90°$ and the flow directions (and colors) of the vessel and its reflection are always opposite. In such a situation, when α is also close to $90°$, the vessel and its reflection will be close to parallel but opposite in color. Then the reflection can easily be mistaken for the real vessel's companion. Also, when α and β are both near $90°$, small fluctuations in transducer angle can flip the mirror image artifact flow direction back and forth between the same and opposite direction of the flow direction in the actual vessel, with the colors alternating accordingly.

Sites where these artifacts are common include the scrutum (Fig. 22-18), the inferior vena cava, either on the sagittal or transverse plane (Fig. 22.19); the subclavian artery and/or vein (Fig. 22.20), due to the highly reflective areas of the apex of the lung; and the femoral and the carotid vessels (Fig. 22.21). The latter has been

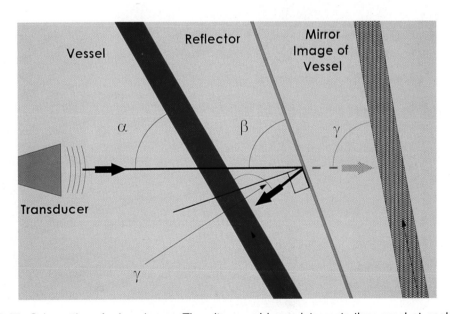

FIG. 22.17. Schematics of mirror image. The ultrasound beam intersects the vessel at angle α and strikes the acoustic mirror at angle β. As in optics, the angle of incidence equals the angle of reflection. The reflected beam intersects the vessel at angle $\gamma = 2\beta - \alpha$ resulting in a second image of the vessel that appears to be at the position labeled "Mirror Image of Vessel." (From reference 1, with permission.)

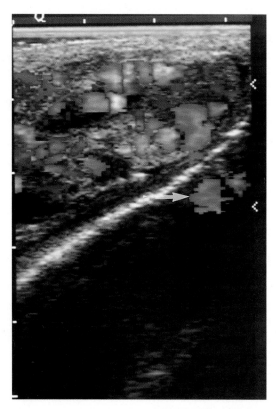

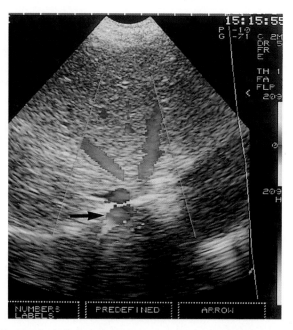

FIG. 22.18. Varicoceles—mirror-image artifact. Sagittal display of the left hemiscrotum demonstrating varicoceles and mirror images of these varicoceles beyond the scrotal skin *(arrow).*

FIG. 22.19. Inferior vena cava—mirror-image artifact. Transverse image of the liver demonstrating the hepatic veins almost at their entry site into the inferior vena cava. The inferior vena cava is noted adjacent to the hemidiaphragm, and a mirror image of the inferior vena cava exhibits opposite flow direction *(arrow).*

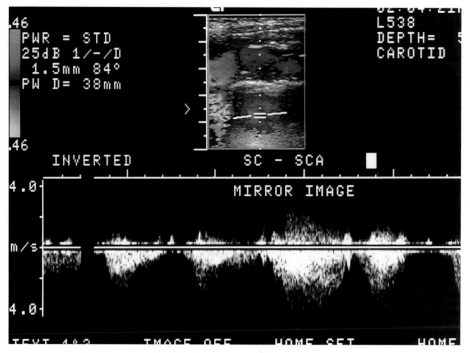

FIG. 22.20. Subclavian vein—mirror-image artifact. Sagittal display of the subclavian vein demonstrating a mirror image projecting over the surface of the apex of the lung. Spectral waveform can be obtained from the artifactual vessel.

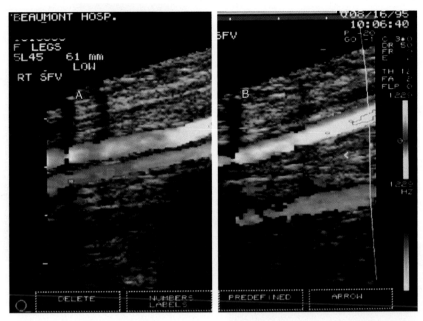

FIG. 22.21. Femoral vein. Two images of the superficial femoral vessels of the right leg are portrayed. **A:** The artery and vein have a parallel and close relationship as would be expected from normal vascular anatomy. **B:** There is a wide separation between the superficial femoral artery and the presumed superficial femoral vein. In reality, a specular reflector (likely the femur) must have generated a mirror image of the superficial femoral artery (flow in the opposite direction due to its inverted nature). Care should be exercised not to mistake it for the superficial femoral vein and presume that the vein is patent.

called the carotid ghost artifact (10) where the reflector is the vessel wall itself.

A phenomenon that has a similar spectral appearance to a mirror-image artifact can occur when the ultrasound beam axis is 90° to the imaged vessel (9,11). Since the beam diverges as it emerges from the transducer, one edge of the beam sees blood flow slightly toward the transducer, while the opposite edge sees blood moving away (12). On spectral analysis, both directions are shown simultaneously and the spectrum appears to mirror itself about the baseline. In color Doppler, the dominant direction is selected by an auto correlation algorithm based on relative power. This technique derives the mean Doppler shift at each gate location and, therefore, assigns each pixel a positive or negative frequency shift (Fig. 22.22) (8).

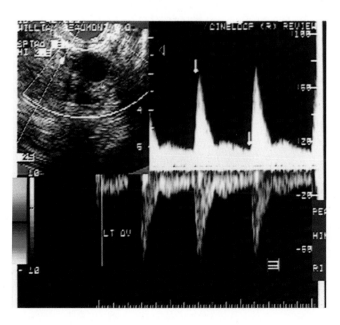

FIG. 22.22. Spectral Doppler—mirror-image artifact. Spectral mirror-image artifact is portrayed in this left adnexal region. The spectral waveform has been portrayed both above and below baseline due to slight angulation of the vessel and the presence of a reflector along the path of beam.

CAROTID GHOST

This artifact was elegantly described by Middleton and Melson (10). It represents a mirror image of the carotid vessels, most commonly of the common carotid. It is the result of a strong reflection being generated from the deep wall of the carotid, resulting in a mirror image of the walls of the carotid, the lumen, and flow within the lumen (Fig. 22.23). Therefore, the artifact portrays color within it. The artifact exhibits these additional characteristics:

1. Signal intensity is lower than that of the true vessel.
2. As the power output is increased, the artifact is better visualized.

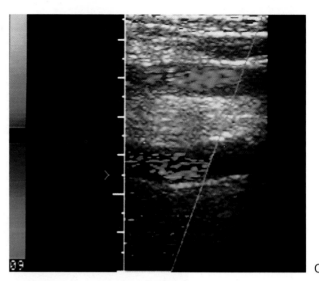

FIG. 22.23. *Continued.* **C:** Sagittal sonogram of the common carotid at a later date reveals a greater distance between the true vessel and its artifact.

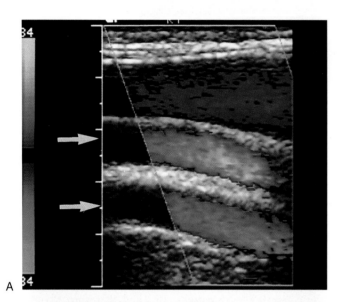

A

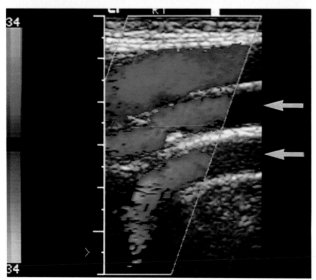

B

FIG. 22.23. Carotid ghost artifact. **A:** Sagittal display of the common carotid demonstrates the artifactual carotid parallel and deep to it. Note the gray scale image of both the true and artifactual vessel beyond the color box *(arrows)*. **B:** Sagittal image of the internal carotid and its ghost is portrayed in color and gray scale *(arrows)*.

3. The ghost artifact is portrayed immediately deep to the carotid in either the sagittal or transverse plane.
4. A corresponding gray scale image of this artifact is not noticed on the images.
5. Spectral waveform analysis of both the true carotid and the ghost carotid demonstrate similar flow patterns; however, a weaker spectral waveform is obtained from the artifact. This is felt to be related to attenuation of the beam due to its deeper location. In our case of carotid ghost the corresponding gray scale image was portrayed.

In the case illustrated in Fig. 22.23, rescanning of the patient at a later date still demonstrated the carotid ghost; however, the distance between the carotid and the artifact (fundamental distance) was increased.

TISSUE VIBRATIONS

Adjacent to areas of stenosis, arteriovenous fistula, or increased pulsations, we may observe perivascular areas of color encoding (13). This represents transmission to the adjacent tissues of motion, secondary to the hemodynamic events of high flow. The color encoding is with deep hues of either red or blue (well-saturated pixels), giving it a staccato appearance (Figs. 22.24 and 22.25). The perivascular tissue vibrations do obscure underlying detail, not allowing for identification of the cause of the tissue vibrations. Indeed, we resort to changing to gray scale imaging to visualize the underlying vessels. Tissue vibrations are not visible on gray scale images.

We have noticed the presence of tissue vibrations adjacent to arteriovenous fistulas in postbiopsy patients (renal transplant recipients). These were occurring more with the 14-gauge needles used for biopsies in the past. Arte-

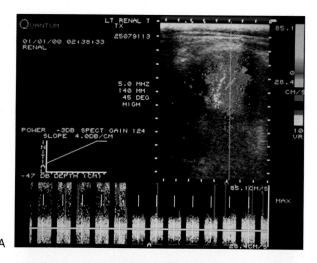

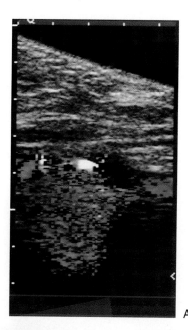

A

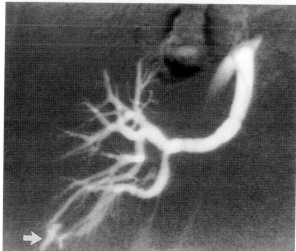

B

FIG. 22.24. Arteriovenous fistula—tissue vibrations. **A:** Sagittal image of the allograft displays a large area, in its lower pole, of randomly assigned colored pixels in red or blue. Detail of the underlying vasculature is obscure by this area of tissue vibration. **B:** Allograft angiogram demonstrating an arteriovenous fistula in the lower pole *(arrow).*

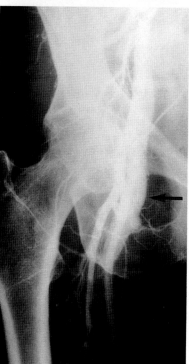

B

FIG. 22.26. Femoral arteriovenous fistula—tissue vibrations. **A:** Sagittal display of the right superficial femoral artery exhibits a large area of perivascular color encoding (tissue vibrations). **B:** Right common iliac artery injection from a left femoral entry site, demonstrates filling of the right superficial femoral vein due to a fistula *(arrow).*

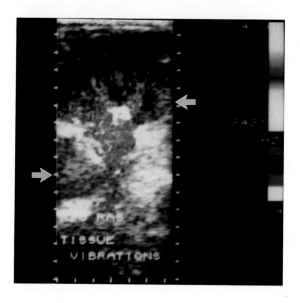

FIG. 22.25. Renal artery stenosis—tissue vibrations. Sagittal sonogram of the allograft at the level of the hilum demonstrating exuberant tissue vibrations due to renal artery stenosis. Impaired renal function existed and areas of increased echogenicity due to vascular compromise are noted in the renal parenchyma *(arrows).*

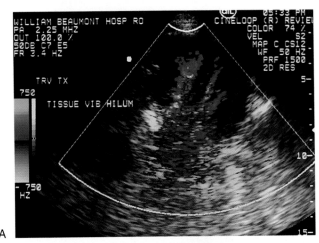

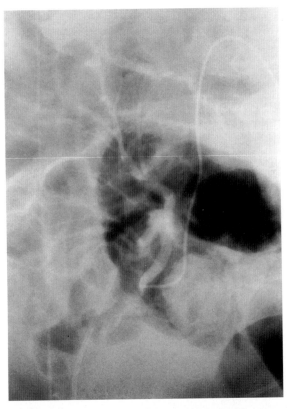

FIG. 22.27. Renal artery vasospasm—tissue vibrations. **A:** Transverse sonogram of the allograft of a recently transplanted kidney. Note large area of color encoding due to tissue vibrations. This was suggestive of an arteriovenous fistula. **B:** Angiography revealed a normal renal artery. Spasm of the renal artery of this recently transplanted kidney may have generated a thrill and consequently areas of perivascular tissue vibrations.

riovenous fistulas, secondary to catheterizations at the level of the femoral vessels (Fig. 22.26), exhibit tissue vibrations, and often associated jets of arterial flow into the adjacent vein are appreciated as well. We caution that recently transplanted patients may have, at the level of the hilum, tissue vibrations that are merely due to an element of spasm of the renal artery subsequent to transplantation. This can be observed in the first 24 to 48 hours subsequent to transplantation and it should not be considered an area of arteriovenous fistula (Fig. 22.27), especially considering the fact that most cadaveric transplants are performed with a Carrel patch. Living-related transplants are performed with end-to-end anastomosis.

CLUTTER ARTIFACT

Pulsations of stationary structures (vessel wall, perivascular tissues, etc.) generate strong low-frequency Doppler shifts. This clutter artifact is portrayed as areas both above and below baseline on spectral waveforms. It can be misconstrued as spectral broadening, and/or flow reversal. Wall filters are used to eliminate clutter. High-pass filters are needed during arterial sampling, while low-pass filters

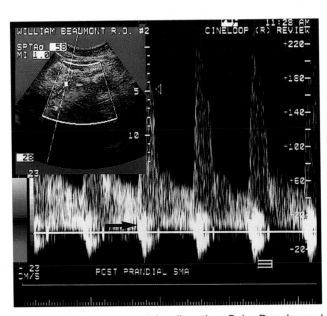

FIG. 22.28. Clutter—arterial wall motion. Color Doppler and spectral waveforms of the superior mesenteric artery demonstrate clutter artifact (arrow). Note the low frequency of clutter that results from motion of stationary structures due to pulsations.

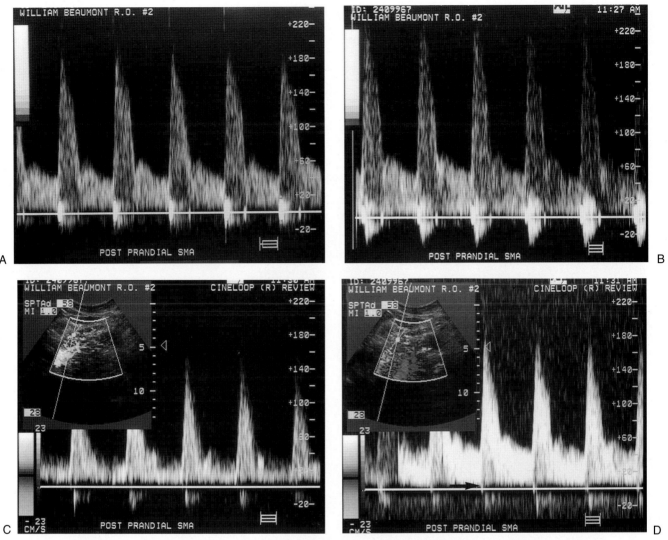

FIG. 22.29. Clutter suppression—wall filtering. This set of four images illustrates the elimination of the clutter artifact by raising the wall filter. **A:** Waveforms demonstrate the clutter artifact at the onset of systole. Wall filter is set at 50 Hz. **B:** Closer to the arterial wall, there is a broader clutter artifact giving even a greater impression of flow reversal. **C:** Setting the wall filter to 100 Hz reduces the clutter artifact to the point where it is barely noticeable. **D:** Clutter artifact has been eliminated leaving only a small amount visible at the onset of systole *(arrow)*.

allow the recording of small Doppler frequency shifts that occur in the venous side of the circulation (Figs. 22.28 and 22.29). These electrical filters are to be used wisely so that true flow is not eliminated (6).

As reported by Burns (14), harmonic imaging has an advantage over Doppler imaging as it greatly reduces clutter.

LINE FREQUENCY INTERFERENCE

The 60-Hz (50-Hz in Europe) interference from incoming power can be portrayed on spectral waveforms as a straight line adjacent and/or parallel to the spectral waveform baseline (8). When these lines are seen a distance away from the baseline they do not mimic flow. However, when portrayed either immediately above or below baseline, they can be mistaken for flow. Often, because of their low amplitude, they mimic either venous flow or diastolic flow. They do exhibit a monotonous pattern without the gradual, diminished volume that is seen with diastolic flow. They don't exhibit respiratory modulation, as would be expected with venous flow. Therefore, one way to recognize this artifact is to note its lack of physiologic variation (Figs. 22.30 and 22.31).

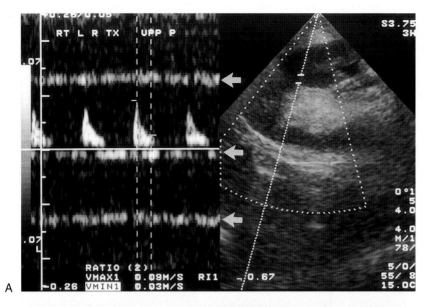

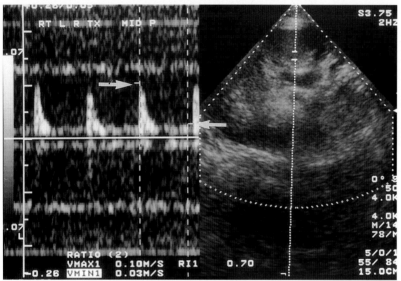

FIG. 22.30. 60-Hz interference. **A:** There are three bands of echoes portrayed on this spectral waveform due to the 60-Hz interference *(arrows).* On this particular image, we note that true information related to the allograft demonstrates absence of flow in diastole. The band of 60-Hz interference is portrayed below baseline, and does not interfere with the analysis of the arterial waveform. **B:** Images from the same allograft now demonstrating four or more bands of 60-Hz interference. Notice that there is a band above and below the baseline, which has resulted in erroneous measurements of the resistivity index of the allograft *(arrows).*

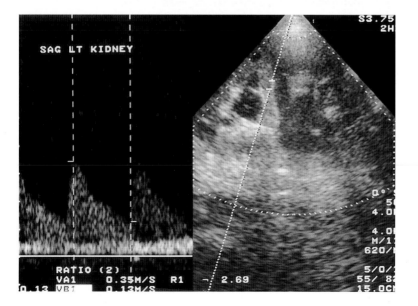

FIG. 22.31. 60-Hz interference superimposed on spectral waveforms. Images of another allograft demonstrating arterial flow with superimposed 60-Hz interference above baseline. Here the systolic and diastolic flows are far greater than the 60-band interference and do not cause erroneous measurements.

EDGE OF COLOR BOX

Signal processing in color requires tremendous computer capabilities. To maintain a high frame rate, a color box and/or color window can be utilized, which will allow tailoring of flow information to a designated area and faster signal processing by the computer. The color box demarcates the boundaries where flow information will be obtained (Fig. 22.32).

UPDATE OF THE IMAGE ON DUPLEX SCANNERS

While obtaining spectral information, we note an absence of information when the scanner updates the image (6). Such gaps on the spectral waveform have to be appropriately recognized and not mistaken for the end of a cardiac cycle. Therefore, care should be exercised to avoid confusing incomplete waveforms (Fig.22.33).

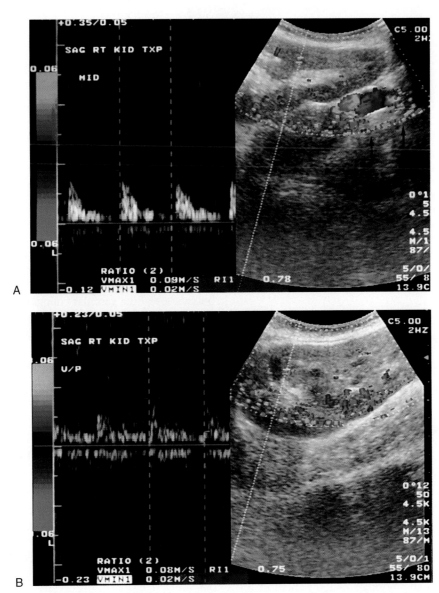

FIG. 22.32. Edge of color box. **A:** Notice that along the edge of the color box, the spurious echoes come to an abrupt end, which can be visually misleading *(arrows)*. However, these echoes lie predominantly outside of the area of interest, which is, in this case, the renal transplant. **B:** Sagittal sonogram demonstrates color encoding along the edge of the color box, which projects over the upper pole of the allograft and simulates flow in this region.

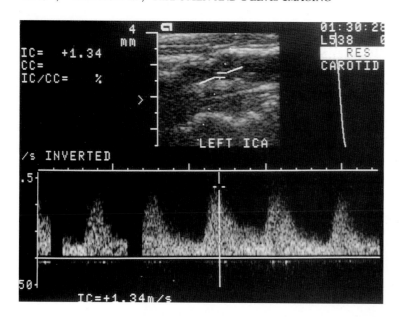

FIG. 22.33. Update of duplex image. Spectral waveform of the left internal carotid artery demonstrates two gaps on the spectral waveform secondary to image updating. One is occurring in the early part of diastole and the second on the end of diastole. When determining indices such as resistivity and/or pulsatility, care should be taken not to assume that there is a complete cardiac cycle when these image updates are occurring.

ARTIFACTS AND PITFALLS RELATED TO ULTRASOUND CONTRAST AGENTS

The configuration of ultrasound scanners has changed over the years as newer clinical applications became identified. The most recent challenge to equipment manufacturers is to prepare the scanners so that they could capitalize on the signals generated by ultrasound contrast without either registering artifacts or introducing inaccuracies in velocity estimates.

The authors have not yet used contrast agents; however, sonographic contrast agents may bring possible artifacts and pitfalls to image analysis.

RATIONALE FOR ULTRASOUND CONTRAST AGENTS

The conventional ultrasound image results from the signals returning from tissue interfaces with mismatched acoustic impedances while the Doppler image is constructed from the differences between emitted and received frequencies. Power Doppler takes advantage of both types of image formation, offering an advantage over color Doppler in flow detection but having the disadvantage of not allowing flow direction to be established. These Doppler imaging techniques make spectral Doppler more robust than duplex Doppler methods.

Unfortunately, just as in any other imaging method, a combination of true signal mixed with noise is persistently present. Recently, harmonic imaging, a method with an improved signal-to-noise ratio has been developed. Based on the nonlinear oscillation properties of the contrast bubbles, harmonic imaging can be refined to exclusively record specific harmonics (signature). This allows the recording of harmonics emitted by a specific contrast agent while greatly reducing the unwanted tissue signals.

COLOR BLOOMING

The effect of the contrast agents on both the axial and lateral resolution of the beam, especially when color Doppler is being used, is to augment the signal to the point of artificially causing the appearance of flow beyond the boundaries of the vascular compartment or the suggestion of smaller vessels where none exists. This results in loss of the spatial resolution as well as individual vessels becoming incorporated into a broad area of color blooming. The best method for overcoming this artifact may be to decrease the ensemble length of the color detection scheme so that more lines could be acquired in a shorter time, increasing the resolution (15).

ARTIFACTUAL INCREASED VELOCITY ON SPECTRAL DOPPLER

In reality, the velocity of flow does not increase with the administration of ultrasound contrast agents, but the backscatter caused by these agents allows the recording of previously below threshold frequency shifts in high ranges of the velocity spectrum. This has been corrected in the newer systems by expanding the dynamic range of the units. Commercially available scanners now have dynamic ranges of 90 to 100 Db compared to older systems with top dynamic ranges of 60 Db.

ACKNOWLEDGMENT

This work would be incomplete without the knowledgeable input of our colleague Lance Hefner, M.S.

REFERENCES

1. Magnin PA. Doppler effect: history and theory. *Hewlett-Packard J* 1986;37:26.
2. Kremkau FW. Doppler principles. *Semin Roentgenol* 1992;27:6.
3. Wu RG, Yang PC, Kuo SH, Luh KT. Fluid color sign: a useful indicator for discrimination between pleural thickening and pleural effusion. *J Ultrasound Med* 1995;14:767.
4. Mitchell DG, Burns P, Needleman L. Color Doppler artifacts in anechoic regions. *J Ultrasound Med* 1990;9:255.
5. Mitchell DG. Color Doppler imaging: principles, limitations and artifacts. *Radiology* 1990;177:1.
6. Kremkau FW. *Doppler ultrasound:* principles and instruments, 2nd ed. Philadelphia: WB Saunders, 1995.
7. Pozniak MA, Zagzebski JA, Scanlan KA. Spectral and color Doppler artifacts. *Radiographics* 1992;12:35.
8. Kremkau FW. Principles of color flow imaging. *J Vasc Technol* 1991; 15:104.
9. Burns PN. Doppler artifacts. In: Taylor KJW, Burns P, Wells PNT, eds. *Clinical applications of Doppler ultrasound.* New York: Raven Press, 1995:14.
10. Middleton WD, Melson GL. The carotid ghost—a color Doppler ultrasound duplication artifact. *J Ultrasound Med* 1990;9:487.
11. Taylor KJ, Holland S. Doppler US I—basic principles instrumentation and pitfalls. *Radiology* 1990;174:297.
12. Reading CC, Charboneau JW, Allison JW, Cooperberg PC. Color and spectral Doppler mirror image of the subclavian artery. *Radiology* 1990;174:41.
13. Middleton WD, Erickson S, Melson GL. Perivascular color artifact: pathologic significance and appearance on color Doppler US images. *Radiology* 1989;171:647.
14. Burns PN. Harmonic imaging adds to ultrasound capabilities. *Diagn Imaging* 1987;15:567.
15. Burns PN. Contrast agents for ultrasound imaging and Doppler. In: Rumack CM, Wilson SR, Charboneau JW, eds. Diagnostic ultrasound. St. Louis: Mosby-Year Book, Inc., 1998:65.

Variants and Pitfalls in Body Imaging,
edited by Ali Shirkhoda.
Lippincott Williams & Wilkins, Philadelphia, © 2000.

CHAPTER 23

Magnetic Resonance Angiography: Imaging Methods and Artifacts in the Abdomen

Anil N. Shetty, Suzanne Marre, Kostaki G. Bis, and Ali Shirkhoda

One of the significant advances in magnetic resonance technology is the ability to visualize moving blood signal. This has been accomplished without the need of interventional technique. Today, magnetic resonance angiography (MRA) has been widely accepted as a valuable diagnostic technique. In contrast to conventional x-ray angiography, MRA offers multiple views of vascular anatomy, with virtually no systemic reaction from the MR contrast agent and relative ease in performing the examination (1–3). The vascular signal in MRA is based primarily on increased blood signal against surrounding background tissue. Therefore, improving the signal of blood against the signal of the background tissue forms the basis of generating contrast in MRA (4,5). However, there are a number of artifacts and pitfalls associated with data acquisition and postprocessing that at times may lead to erroneous results in inexperienced hands. This chapter discusses angiographic methods and associated artifacts.

MAGNETIC RESONANCE ANGIOGRAPHY METHODS

Signal characteristics in blood flow imaging greatly depend on the type of pulse sequences used as well as flow characteristics. For example, in a conventional spin echo, when a slice is placed perpendicular to a blood vessel the blood will appear dark. This is due to the so-called washout phenomenon based on the flow velocity and imaging parameters in which spins excited by a 90-degree radiofrequency (RF) pulse in a slice will exit that slice

A. N. Shetty, K. G. Bis, and A. Shirkhoda: Department of Diagnostic Radiology, Wayne State University School of Medicine, Detroit, Michigan, and William Beaumont Hospital, Royal Oak, Michigan 48073-6769.
S. Marre: Institute of Diagnostic Radiology, Inselspital, University of Berne, CH-3010 Berne, Switzerland.

during the next 180-degree RF pulse (6). It is for this reason that most MRA methods use gradient recalled echo (GRE) pulse sequences, in which blood signal is always bright due to the so-called inflow enhancement (7–9). In addition to changes in flow velocity, another parameter that governs the overall signal is the spin phase effect. Currently, all GRE techniques available for imaging blood vessels fall into two main classes: time-of-flight (TOF) technique (7–9) and phase contrast (PC) technique (10,11). Today, there is a more robust technique in which 3D-MRA with gadolinium contrast injection has been routinely used (12,13).

Time of Flight

The TOF is the most widely prescribed GRE technique to answer a wide variety of clinical questions concerning vascular anatomy and pathology. The basic principle behind this technique is inflow enhancement, in which the blood flowing into an imaging section has higher magnetization than that of the stationary surrounding tissue. The stationary tissue magnetization in the same section is saturated by the repeated application of RF pulse with a repetition time (TR) that is much shorter than the longitudinal relaxation time (T1) of that tissue. On the other hand, the flowing blood in that section is constantly replaced by unsaturated and fully magnetized blood, thus acquiring a higher magnetization (Fig. 23.1).

The appearance of blood signal in a vessel significantly varies due to the variable nature of inherent parameters such as T1, T2, and the velocity of protons in the blood, as well as other parameters such as TR, flip angle, and slice thickness. Given the flow velocity, TR, and T1, the section of blood excited by an RF pulse is partially replaced by the inflow of unsaturated blood as shown in Fig. 23.1. The stationary tissue magnetization, on the

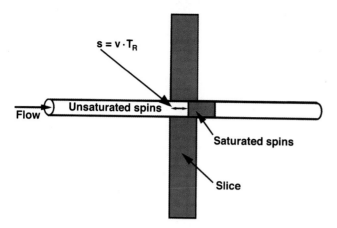

FIG. 23.1. Inflow effects in a gradient recalled echo (GRE) sequence. Here the excited spins will exit the slice but are replaced by fresh unsaturated spins, fully magnetized spins. The result is to provide higher initial magnetization before each radiofrequency (RF) pulse. The fraction of inflow depends on the distance traveled by the excited bolus, TR, and the flip angle.

other hand, is progressively reduced. After a certain number of RF-pulse repetitions, the signal in blood and tissue reach a steady state beyond which there is no further saturation effect from the RF pulse. This steady state in the tissue and blood is attained at a different magnitude and at different times. The goal of the MRA technique is to exploit the difference in steady-state signals between blood and tissue by optimizing other extrinsic parameters such as the flip angle, TR, and slice thickness and orientation.

Two-Dimensional Time-of-Flight MRA

In a two-dimensional (2D) TOF MRA, the slices are placed perpendicular to flow direction to increase the flow signal. Due to the complex nature of blood flow, the net movement of protons in the blood may include components from linear, acceleration, and jerk motions. Each of these components in flow gives rise to phase dispersion, eventually leading to a decreased signal. Applying the same magnetic field gradient in the opposite direction (bipolar) can reverse phase change. While such a bipolar gradient restores the phase of the stationary spins, it does not work for flowing spins (Fig. 23.2). At least three gradients are required to correct the effects of the first-order component of flow (Fig. 23.2) (14). The need for the number of gradients increases as we try to compensate higher order components in flow. However, by increasing gradients, the echo time (TE) is also prolonged, causing more dephasing during TE. Therefore, higher order components are best handled with the shortest possible TE. This is why most of the TOF techniques use GRE pulse sequences with a first-order flow compensation and with the shortest TE possible.

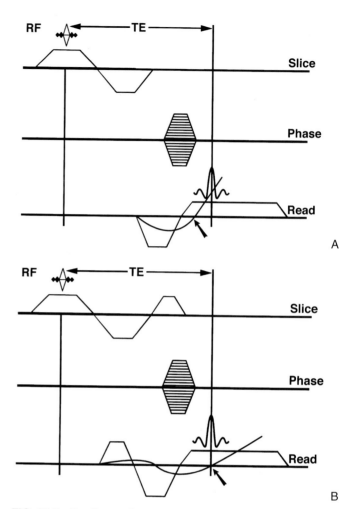

FIG. 23.2. Gradient-echo pulse sequences without and with a first-order flow compensation. **A:** In a conventional gradient-echo pulse sequence, the flow spin phase (arrow) is significantly off-center of the echo. As a result, phases of stationary and moving spins will be incoherent at the echo, resulting in a loss of signal. **B:** Same pulse sequence is shown with a three-lobe gradient structure to indicate first-order (linear velocity of flow) compensation at the echo (arrow). The phase of constant velocity spins are made to pass through the center of the echo, resulting in phase coherence and a higher signal.

Three-Dimensional Time-of-Flight MRA

A significant drawback in a 2D TOF is the increased slice thickness (to cover larger vascular anatomy) and a long TE, resulting in lower spatial resolution and pixel dephasing. By performing a three-dimensional (3D) MRA, one can reduce the voxel dimension because of inherently higher signal. Also, a very short TE can be used with a flow compensation technique (15). However, due to the large coverage, most 3D-TOF techniques suffer signal loss when blood has to travel a long distance within the 3D slab. The progressive saturation is evident when images show relatively bright signal in a vessel among a few partitions at the entry site and a progressively lower signal further into the slab. This effect is more pronounced with small vessels and among vessels with slow-flowing blood.

Phase Contrast

Phase contrast (PC) MRA is based on exploiting the relative phase differences between moving and stationary spins. The phase change among spins is a result of their movement during the presence of an active gradient. The net accumulated phase is dependent on the gradient amplitude and duration. This effect can be reversed for stationary spins by applying the gradient with the same amplitude in the opposite direction (bipolar) for the same duration. Thus, by using a bipolar gradient, moving spins will acquire a net phase shift while stationary spins will not.

Since the vessels are tortuous, to acquire an MR angiogram one has to sensitize the gradient in each of the three orthogonal directions and repeat the measurement along each direction. To acquire a 3D view of vessels, at least four measurements are required. The first is obtained without any flow sensitive gradient and is used as a mask for subtraction (16). The remaining three measurements are obtained by using a flow-sensitizing gradient along the slice, read, and frequency directions. The total scan time in some cases can exceed 12 to 15 minutes, which is long compared to most TOF techniques. Since the relative phase shift depends on movement of spins during an active gradient, unlike in TOF, it is sensitive to very slow flow, and therefore is useful for evaluating vessels with slow-flowing blood. Also, one can estimate the velocity of flowing spins knowing the amount of accumulated phase shift (17,18).

GADOLINIUM-ENHANCED
FIRST-PASS 3D-MRA

Recent advances in gradient technology have dramatically changed the way MRA is performed (19–21). Images can be acquired during the first pass of gadolinium contrast following a bolus injection. The technique uses 3D GRE in which short TR, TE, and RF flip angle are used so that the entire 3D set of data can be acquired in a single breath hold. Such a contrast-enhanced 3D MRA, combined with gadolinium injection, requires very high gradient amplitudes and shorter gradient rise times. A measurement time as short as 8 to 10 seconds with good spatial resolution is easily achieved with these techniques. One of the advantages of this technique is that, unlike conventional TOF MRA or PC MRA, where the signal is dependent on inflow or phase characteristics, contrast-enhanced MRA is based on T1-shortening effects of gadolinium during the first pass (21,22). This has a significant effect on how one prescribes imaging volume. At a very short TR, the relative contrast between blood and tissue is nearly zero. This is due to the fact that ultrashort TR does not allow for sufficient magnetization recovery in both blood and tissue on account of their relatively long T1. Under these conditions, administration of paramagnetic contrast allows for rapid recovery of blood magnetization due to the rapid T1 shortening effect of contrast. However, the tissue signal remains low due to the lack of paramagnetic contrast agent in the tissue. In a typical imaging method, the contrast is injected as a rapid bolus and the measurement is commenced so that the central k-space of data (which refers to signal content) coincides with the arrival of contrast bolus at the region of interest during first pass. The knowledge of bolus arrival time is crucial for obtaining complete arterial or venous flow without an overlap. Due to a short data acquisition window for the best contrast, one must be sure that the central portion of data acquisition (k-space) coincides with the signal peak. The transit time varies from patient to patient and depends on the patient's circulation time and cardiac output. One method to estimate transit time is the use of the test bolus technique (23,24).

MAXIMUM INTENSITY PROJECTION (MIP)

Maximum intensity projection is a useful processing tool that allows construction of a vessel based on information from each of the 2D slices or 3D partitions. Using a postprocessing MIP tool, contiguous 2D or single 3D slab data allow for visualization of vessels in a single 2D plane. The MIP is based on using a ray-tracing algorithm to cast the maximum intensity pixel projection using a stack of images (25). In the MIP method, by stacking all the slices together, a single ray or a line of view is cast through a user-selected direction and a single maximum intensity is projected. The contrast between blood and the background tissue is excellent due to MIP, rather than to the summation of pixels across the entire projected volume. For a reliable projection of any vascular segment, the signal in the vessel must be at least two standard deviations above the background signal (26). In many cases, a subset of volume or targeted volume is used to confine the image projection. This reduces the processing time and prevents the unnecessary portion of tissue from projecting into the image plane.

In addition, multiplanar reconstruction (MPR) and digital image subtraction may be useful in improving vessel detectability in MIP. For most gadolinium-enhanced studies, the subtraction technique, in which images from a precontrast study are subtracted from the corresponding postcontrast study, is routinely used. The subtraction allows for removing unenhanced background signal from the MIP data. This may prove useful in MIP, as it will increase the signal variance to well above the background. MPR is also used in cases where multiple overlapping vessels present a problem in MIP. In fact, with MPR, the individual slice can be viewed without any change in the relative mean intensities in the vessel and background.

PITFALLS AND ARTIFACTS IN MRA

In-Plane Saturation

In a sequential 2D or 3D TOF, the orientation of the plane of acquisition is crucial in determining the effects of inflow. If the vessel courses in-plane, the spin magnetization may not recover sufficiently between RF pulses. Although to some extent a large flip angle may be useful, it will have a negative effect on contrast due to the decreased saturation of surrounding tissue signal. Because of the tortuous nature of vessels, one will always encounter a section of vessel that may be parallel to the plane of excitation. This is true in the case of abdominal and iliac vessels. The problem of in-plane saturation arises when T1 is larger than TR. When the flow is in plane, the distance traveled is considerably long, and

therefore under a repeated application of RF pulse, magnetization does not have enough time to recover back to the magnetic field direction. This situation does not arise when we perform contrast-enhanced 3D TOF MRA. As discussed earlier, the contrast in these techniques is based on T1 reduction by gadolinium and not inflow effects (Fig. 23.3). In Fig. 23.3A, a sequential 2D TOF is performed using a body-phased array coil, and the slices are placed perpendicular to the flow direction to obtain maximum inflow effects. However, due to the anatomic course of the iliac vessels at their origin, the sections of vessel course parallel to the imaging plane, and because of the in-plane saturation, the signal is reduced. In Fig. 23.3B, the same patient is studied with contrast-enhanced MRA. The reduction of signal as observed with 2D TOF in Fig. 23.3A is absent.

Another artifact in 2D TOF that is seen routinely is the pixel misregistration between acquired images due to inconsistent breath holding (Fig. 23.4). In Fig. 23.4A, a

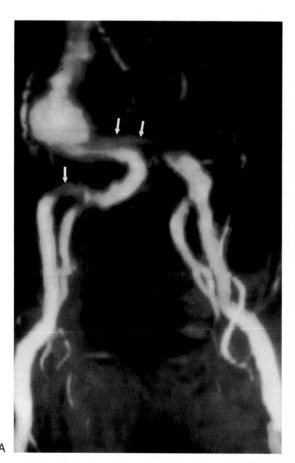
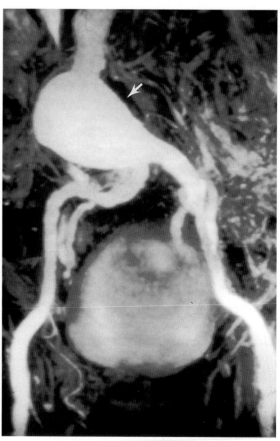

A
B

FIG. 23.3. In-plane saturation. **A:** Coronal projection using maximum intensity projection (MIP) is obtained from axially acquired two-dimensional time of flight (2D TOF) with a traveling saturation band. In-plane saturation effects are seen involving the common iliac arteries *(arrows)*. The signal loss in the abdominal aortic aneurysm is likely from a combination of in-plane flow and from saturation of retrograde flow. **B:** A coronal MIP image from a contrast-enhanced (0.2 mmol/kg, gadoteridol) magnetic resonance angiography (MRA) of the same region shows no in-plane saturation and a large distal abdominal aortic aneurysm *(arrow).* (Reproduced with permission from Reference 22.)

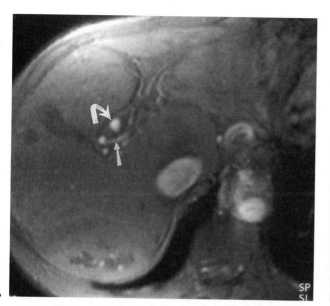

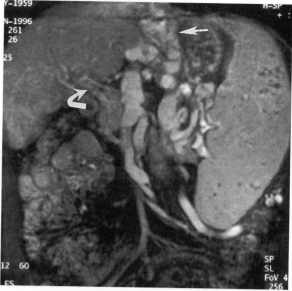

FIG. 23.4. Pseudopatency of the main portal vein on time-of-flight imaging. **A:** A transverse 2D TOF gradient echo sequence reveals the hepatic artery *(arrow)* as well as an additional larger vessel ventral to it *(curved arrow)*. This could be mistaken for a patent portal vein. **B:** On the coronal 3D contrast-enhanced MRA, the larger vessel *(curved arrow)* represented a mesenteric collateral vessel in this patient with portal vein occlusion and cavernous transformation. The esophageal varices and splenomegaly are demonstrated, due to portal venous hypertension.

transverse 2D TOF GRE sequence reveals the hepatic artery as well as an additional larger ventral vessel. This could be mistaken for a patent portal vein; however, in this patient with portal vein occlusion and cavernous transformation, in the coronal 3D contrast-enhanced MRA shown in Fig. 23.4B, the larger vessel represented a mesenteric collateral. The anatomy is best depicted on the coronal 3D contrast-enhanced MRA sequence. The MIP of the 2D TOF source data was sub-optimal due to the misregistration between several breath-hold data sets that were required to evaluate the entire volume.

Stenosis: Overestimation Artifact

Overestimation of stenosis has been a consistent problem with 2D as well as 3D TOF, usually due to the way MIP is performed. The MIP algorithm is designed to reduce the noise by adjusting the threshold for data inclusion. In doing so, the variances of the low-intensity background signal as well as portions of low-signal vessels are removed from projecting into the final plane. For a good MIP, the vessel signal must be at least two standard deviations above the mean background signal intensity (26). In the case of stenosis, the blood flow pattern is suddenly changed due to different components. As a result, two important changes take place affecting the outcome. First, the severe intravoxel dephasing due to various velocity components can lead to signal loss. Second, the MIP may not project low intensity (from intravoxel dephasing) because the projected intensity of the background is in fact more than that of the vessel (Fig. 23.5). In Fig. 23.5, the 2D TOF image shows severe dephasing and subsequent loss of signal in MIP. The effect is somewhat removed when a 3D TOF is performed using a bolus contrast agent. A corresponding x-ray angiogram shows contrast washout at the area of interest, which prompted for an MRA. Even with sufficiently small pixels, the intravoxel dephasing still exists. In Fig. 23.6, contrast-enhanced 3D MRA shows the effect of signal loss at the origin of the right renal artery. However, the MIP shows focal loss of signal, indicating occlusion.

The intravoxel phase dispersion can be minimized by improving spatial resolution with increased matrix size and reduced partition thickness. However, that will not solve completely the problem of intravoxel dephasing at the site of the vascular junction as in the case of renal artery origin. In such instances, viewing the individual source image is very important to confirm the results obtained in MIP.

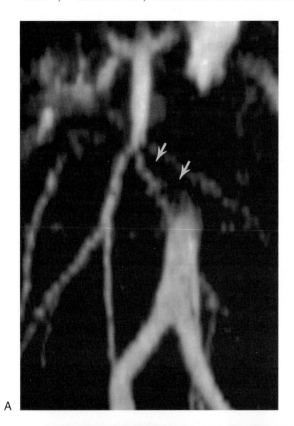

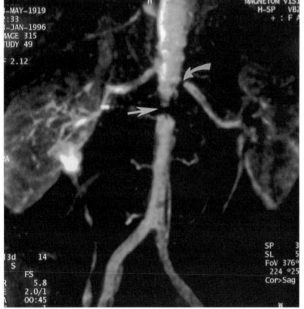

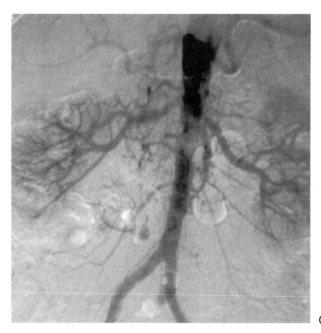

FIG. 23.5. Intravoxel dephasing. **A:** A coronal MIP with data acquisition using axial sequential 2D TOF with a traveling saturation band. The resulting MIP demonstrates severe dephasing at the level of the aortic stenosis due to spin dephasing effects in areas of turbulent flow *(arrows)*. **B:** Contrast-enhanced (0.2 mmol/kg, gadoteridol) 3D MRA shows a coronal MIP from a coronal slab position. The resulting MIP shows severe narrowing involving the left renal artery (curved arrow) as well as infrarenal abdominal aorta *(straight arrow)*. Signal loss from dephasing is not identified at the two sites of severe stenoses. Focal signal loss is caused by a protruding calcified plaque. **C:** A frontal digital subtraction x-ray angiogram is shown for correlation. The contrast-injected conventional angiogram does not depict the stenosis well due to contrast dilution effects. (Reproduced with permission from Reference 22.)

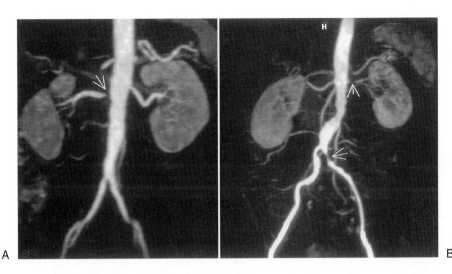

A   B

FIG. 23.6. MIP artifact. **A:** The right renal artery shows occlusion while both kidneys are perfused symmetrically. This was verified by performing a perfusion study using time-intensity curves. **B:** In this patient the origin of the left renal artery shows critical stenosis while the kidneys show normal perfusion.

Maximum Intensity Projection Artifact: Saturation Banding

In a 2D TOF, sequence parameters such as slice and traveling saturation band placement are critical, especially when imaging the normal triphasic arterial waveform in the peripheral circulation. Masui and co-workers (27) first noticed the effect of these parameters while imaging popliteal arteries. A series of horizontal bands throughout the course of the lower extremity artery was observed, and their appearance varied with the distance between the RF and saturation pulses. When the pulses are sufficient and robust, during the early diastolic phase,

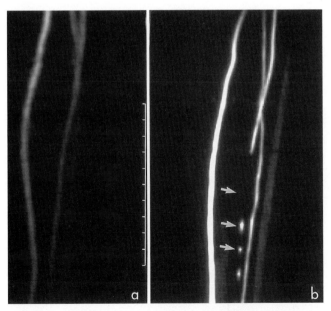

FIG. 23.7. Artifact from retrograde flow. **A:** Normal flow in the posterior tibial artery with contrast-enhanced 3D MRA. **B:** The effects of retrograde flow when performed with sequential 2D TOF with traveling saturation band (arrows). The position of the saturation band is crucial when flow changes its course due to biphasic modes in the flow.

they enter the saturation band before entering the imaging slice. In such instances the saturation pulse intended for the saturating flow in the opposite direction also saturates the normal flow (Fig. 23.7).

Another similar artifact occurs when multiple overlapping slabs are used in 3D TOF imaging. With incorrect overlapping, one observes nonuniform intensities at the edges, causing an artifact, termed the venetian-blind artifact, that is commonly seen in intracranial MRA.

MAXIMUM INTENSITY PROJECTION (MIP): POSTPROCESSING ARTIFACT

MIP displays images of different intensities when viewed at oblique angles. This happens when the signal intensity in the oblique projection falls below the source images by at least two standard deviations from the background (26,28). To acquire optimal MIP images, it is important to ensure the homogeneity of the background tissue. This may not be achievable when viewing small vessels or vessels with slow-flowing blood. In such cases, one either relies on source images or performs MPR on the data. On the other hand, one can perform a targeted MIP to improve vessel contrast. For example, by targeting a smaller region of interest from the acquired image field of view (FOV), one has the ability to remove overlapping vessels and unwanted vessels from the FOV. Overall, targeted MIP improves contrast as well as reduces the processing time considerably and reduces the missing vessel artifact as observed on a full MIP (Fig. 23.8). In cases of tortuous arteries, such as transplant renal arteries or splenic arteries, MIP may show many overlapping loops. Sometimes it is impossible to find the appropriate orientation for the MPR images to document a stenosis (Fig. 23.9).

Occasionally, the presence of foreign objects such as a filter may obscure MIP. Once again, the use of source data is critical in the diagnosis in patients presented with filters (Fig. 23.10).

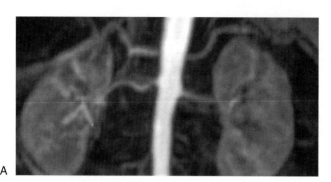

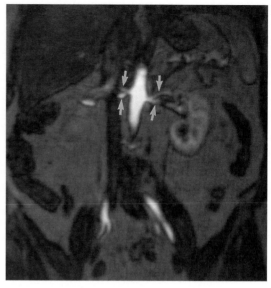

A

B

FIG. 23.8. Targeted MIP. **A:** Normal MIP of a 3D set of coronal images presented in the entire FOV. Note the lack of visibility of the accessory renal arteries when their signal falls two standard deviations below that of the surrounding background signal intensity. **B:** A targeted MIP, performed by eliminating unwanted outer regions, shows the existence of bilateral accessory renal arteries *(arrows)*.

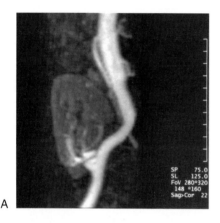

A

FIG. 23.9. Vascular overlapping. **A:** MRA in an oblique orientation of a tortuous renal transplant artery. Neither thin axial MIP and MPR images nor the analysis of the source images was sufficient to depict the stenosis located distal to the anastomosis within a loop of the renal artery. **B,C:** An angiography using the digital subtraction arteriography (DSA) technique has to be performed to confirm the diagnosis.

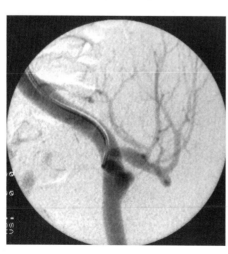

B

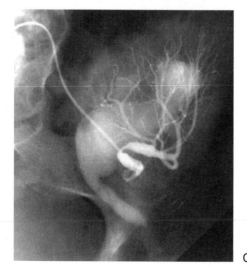

C

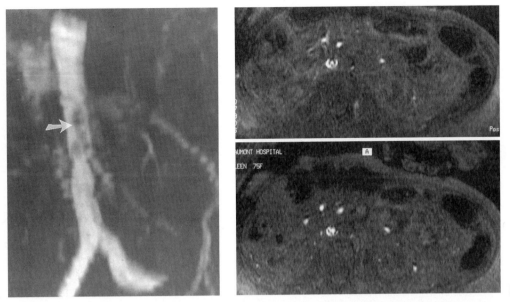

FIG. 23.10. Nonspecificity of defects seen on MIP venography. **A:** A coronal MIP image of the inferior vena cava and common iliac veins performed with a transverse 2D TOF sequence employing arterial traveling saturation. A defect is identified in the inferior vena cava *(arrow)*. **B:** Upon further evaluation of the source data, the nature of this defect is better appreciated. It represents a Greenfield/Ward filter, and its morphology is best depicted on the source data. This should not be confused with a thrombus on the MIP images.

Incorrect Bolus Timing in Contrast-Enhanced 3D MRA

In a contrast-enhanced 3D MRA, the optimal contrast-to-noise ratio between the vessel and surrounding tissue requires an accurate bolus timing based on the flow characteristics and circulation time, which varies from patient to patient. The concentration of gadolinium in the vessel of interest should be at its peak during the acquisition of the central k-space data (29). Based on the input characteristics of the bolus, the first-pass concentration peak may have an appearance of a bell shape. The data acquisition window is timed to coincide with the shape of the concentration time curve. In doing so, the central portion of the data acquisition window correctly coincides with the peak flow. Otherwise, a severe ringing artifact may occur at the edges of the vessel. Also, if the contrast arrives late, the result will be poor assessment of vascular pathology. On the other hand, if the contrast arrives too quickly the surrounding venous structure might overlap the arterial vessels. Therefore, to acquire an optimal image, one may (a) establish the transit time prior to data acquisition in each patient, or (b) minimize misregistration artifacts by acquiring contiguous scans in a single breath hold period. Figure 23.11 demonstrates the lack of signal due to inappropriate timing in which the data acquisition window did not match the peak symmetrically. However, with the appropriate scan delay, the contrast arrives on time during the acquisition of central k-space data. A similar problem is also illustrated in Fig. 23.12. The true T1 of blood at the time of data

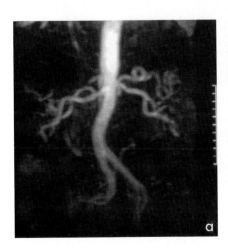
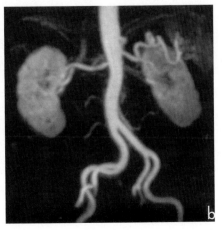

FIG. 23.11. Incorrect bolus timing. **A:** Incorrect bolus timing may lead to a mismatch of the central k-space with the center of the peak bolus signal. In this case the sequence was initiated during the filling of the superior aspects of the abdominal aorta. **B:** In the same patient the study was repeated, properly adjusting the start of the scan with respect to the start of the injection.

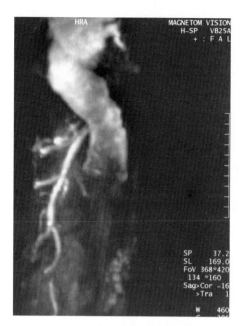

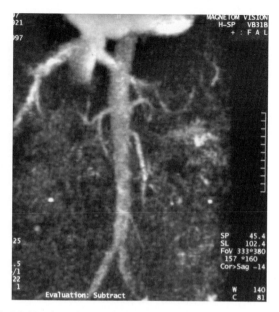

FIG. 23.12. Incorrect scan delay. A patient with an aneurysm of the abdominal aorta. An MIP projection of the first sequence was acquired 12 seconds after the start of the injection. The peak gadolinium concentration was reached shortly after the acquisition of the central k-space data, resulting in poor contrast in the inferior part of the aorta and an artifact at the edge of the vessel wall, due to rapid changes of gadolinium concentration during the acquisition of central k-space data.

FIG. 23.13. A patient with cardiac failure and renal insufficiency. MRA was performed to verify aneurysm and renal artery stenosis in a female patient with cardiac failure and renal insufficiency. The first sequence initiated 15 seconds after the beginning of the bolus injection. Little contrast in the proximal aorta but high signal in the intrahepatic segment of the inferior vena cava and the central liver veins was found, caused by a heart insufficiency with impaired cardiac output and lengthened circulation time.

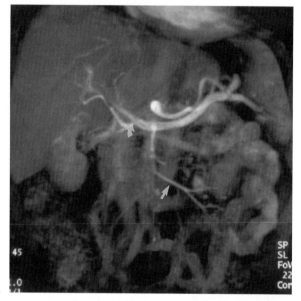

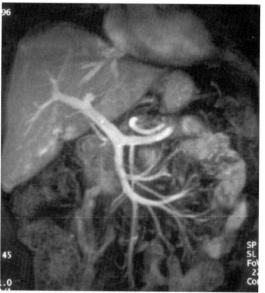

FIG. 23.14. Pseudo-occlusion of the superior mesenteric vein and portal vein on 3D contrast-enhanced MRA: incorrect timing. **A:** The early post–contrast-enhanced 3D acquisition reveals a portion of the superior mesenteric artery *(arrow)* as well as enhancement of the portal vein *(curved arrow).* The superior mesenteric vein and portal vein are not enhancing completely at this time, which is related to the timing of data acquisition and should not render a diagnosis of mesenteric and/or portal venous occlusion. **B:** The subsequent 3D data set reveals enhancement of the superior mesenteric venous and portal venous system. In performing contrast-enhanced sequences, it is imperative to obtain several data sets over time to image the veins during their enhancement.

acquisition is based on the first-pass concentration of blood following the injection. The first-pass concentration and the bolus arrival time depend on the patient circulation time and cardiac output (Fig. 23.13).

Improper timing can lead to either incompletely enhanced arteries or the presence of venous signal (Fig. 23.14). In performing contrast-enhanced sequences, it is imperative to obtain several data sets obtained over time to image the veins during their enhancement. With the proper bolus timing and injection rate, the images provide optimal contrast in both the arterial and venous phases (Fig. 23.15).

Artifacts from Improper Positioning of the 3D Slab

In contrast-enhanced 3D MRA of the abdomen, the coronal plane is to include most of the thoracic and the entire abdominal aorta. Since the technique is independent of vessel geometry, coronal imaging is the best-suited method in that the vessel is projected parallel to the imaging plane, and minimum number of partitions are acquired. A concomitant savings in time is used to increase the spatial resolution. However, correct positioning of the 3D slab may be difficult in patients with elongation or aneurysm of the aorta or with elongated tortuous iliac arteries. If parts of a vessel are projecting outside the imaging slab, then the corresponding MIP image in the coronal or oblique orientation will show falsely an occluded or stenotic vessel (Fig. 23.16). How-

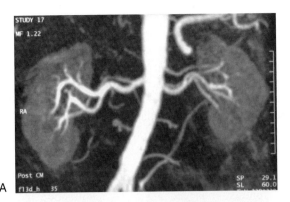
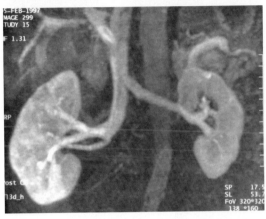

FIG. 23.15. Correct bolus time and scan delay. **A,B:** The correct start of the sequence following the injection shows the arterial and venous phases without overlapping signals.

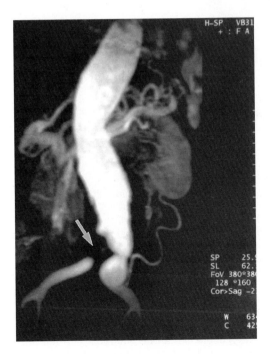

FIG. 23.16. Vascular kinking. Noninclusion of the vessel in the FOV. A 41-year-old patient with Marfan's syndrome and thoracic aortic ectasia was referred for MRA to depict aneurysm of the aorta abdominalis. Coronal MIP demonstrates normal renal arteries, but the common iliac artery on the right side seems to be occluded *(arrow)*. This part of the iliac artery was not completely included in the slab because of elongation and kinking as was proven on the angiogram to be normal.

ever, with a sagittal projection, the apparent occlusion is often proven to be an artifact. This is due in part to the fact that the iliac artery is not being included in the slab. It is very important to check the sagittal view of MIP or the source images to ascertain whether or not the vessel or aneurysm is entirely included in the coronal slab. This artifact can be assumed when the distal segment behind the suspected occlusion has the same signal intensity as the proximal segment and when there are no collaterals. This pitfall can be avoided by increasing the slab thickness to include all segments of the vessel in the MIP. Extended slab thickness also increases scan time when spatial resolution is kept the same. Thus, shortening TR (which requires high-performance gradients) would be helpful in reducing the scan time and allowing a larger slab thickness without the loss of spa-

tial resolution. Increasing the slab thickness without increasing the number of partitions achieves greater coverage within the same scan time and a better signal-to-noise ratio (SNR), but with reduced spatial resolution. Sometimes it may be helpful to change the orientation of the slab from the coronal to the sagittal plane, especially when imaging large aneurysms of the thoracic aorta.

Artifact from Inconsistent Breath Holding

In contrast-enhanced 3D MRA, subtraction methods are frequently employed to further decrease the background signal and to improve the effect of MIP. This requires no pixel displacement between the same image partitions. However, if breath holding is inconsistent, as

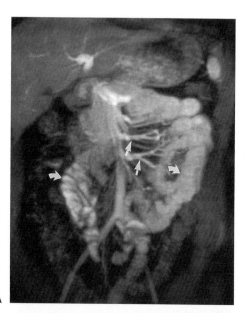

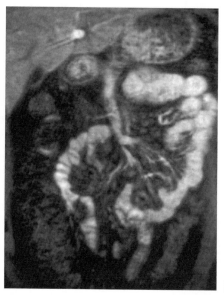

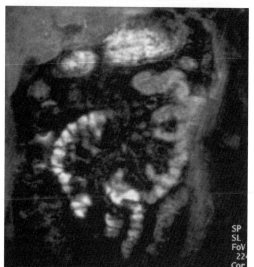

FIG. 23.17. High signal intensity of the GI tract on mesenteric MRA: use of the subtraction technique. **A:** A coronal MIP image reveals the mesenteric arterial circulation *(arrows)* as well as high signal intensity of the small and large bowel loops *(curved arrows)*. **B,C:** The high signal intensity of the fluid within the gastrointestinal tract is also seen on the postcontrast individual partition (**B**), as well as on the precontrast individual partition (**C**). The high signal is related to the mucoproteinacious fluid content within the gastrointestinal tract, which results in a reduction of the fluid T1-relaxation time and an associated increase in its signal. This can be problematic in that it could obscure the underlying vasculature. If a subtraction technique is employed, whereby the precontrast evaluation is used as a mask, the high signal gastrointestinal tract contents can be subtracted on the postcontrast evaluation. Alternatively, negative oral contrast agents may be employed to reduce the gastrointestinal signal. A subtraction technique would require that the mask be obtained during the same breath-hold period following the injection of contrast.

in the case of multiple 2D-TOF sets, the signal subtraction between identical pixels may not completely eliminate the background signal. Even with 3D contrast-enhanced techniques, it is important that scan time be held very short so that multiple measurements can be performed in a single long breath hold. With slice interpolation, it is possible to reduce the scan time for a single measurement to 6 to 8 seconds. Thus, three to four measurements can be performed by having patients sufficiently hyperventilate and then holding their breath during the measurements. This results in an optimal subtraction of the background signal (Fig. 23.17).

Wraparound Artifact (Aliasing)

Aliasing may occur when the FOV does not include the whole circumference of the body. The anatomic structures excluded by the FOV but excited by the RF pulse project over to the opposite side of the image. In the MRA examination, patients are positioned in a supine position with their arms beside their body. When the arm with the venous line is not included in an operator-selected rectangular FOV, it will wrap around to the opposite side of the image. In most cases image quality will not be compromised because the region of interest is centrally located and the wraparound occurs in the periphery of the image (Fig. 23.18). Aliasing may sometimes lead to the misdiagnosis of aberrant vessels, such as an accessory artery to the lower pole of the kidney. When structures with high signal (subcutaneous fat of the thoracic wall) have wrapped around and are in the same plane as the vessel of interest in the frequency-encoding direction, they may erase the signal of the vessel, resulting in false diagnosis of a stenosis or occlusion.

This artifact can be reduced or eliminated by increasing the FOV. However, with the increase in FOV, the spatial resolution may suffer, which could cause other problems such as nonvisualization of smaller vessels. Sometimes, patient position may be changed by placing the arm with the injection site over the head.

Metal Stent Artifact

A stent made up of knitted titanium wire has been routinely imaged using magnetic resonance imaging (30,31). These stents are designed to produce a very low-level MR artifact near the placement. GRE pulse sequences, due to a lack of 180-degree refocusing RF pulse (32), have been known to produce susceptibility artifact at the site of the stent placement. However, MRA can be successfully used to investigate the flow distal to the stent placement. The majority of MRA techniques use gadolinium-enhanced studies to reliably identify the placement of stents. The source images show focal loss of signal at the site of the stent. In evaluating patients with stents in vessels such as in renal arteries, the loss of signal in TOF imaging appears exaggerated due to susceptibility effects, often resulting in an artifact that can mimic stenosis. It is important to rely on source images along with MIP images (Fig. 23.19).

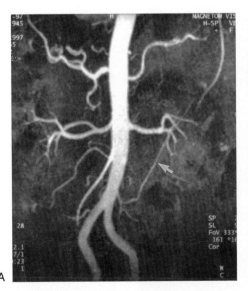 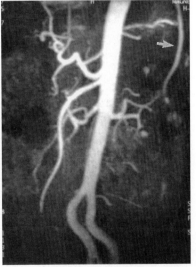

FIG. 23.18. Aliasing or wraparound artifact. The coronal (**A**) and oblique coronal (**B**) MIP of the aorta abdominalis demonstrate aliasing. The right antecubital vein with high signal after gadolinium injection is wrapped around to the left side of the image (*arrow* in **B**). In this case the image quality and diagnostic efficacy is not compromised because the artifact does not overlap the region of interest (renal arteries). *Arrow* in **A**; left colic artery.

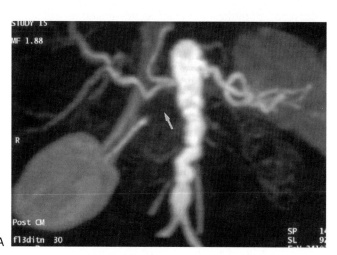
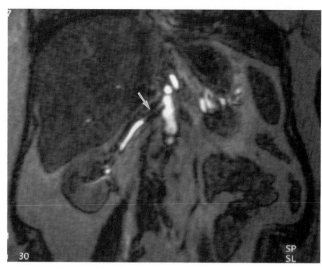

FIG. 23.19. Vascular stent artifact. **A:** MIP performed using contrast-enhanced 3D MRA data in a coronal plane. There is a severe loss of signal around the placement of the stent, indicating occlusion of the right renal artery *(arrow)*. **B:** On the source image the placement and flow within the stent is clearly visible. The loss of signal (**A**) is due to a susceptibility change around the stent and the use of gradient recalled echo sequences without refocusing 180-degree RF pulse *(arrow)*. The right kidney is normally perfused.

PULSE SEQUENCE–RELATED ARTIFACT

Performing MRA requires optimizing pulse sequence parameters based on intrinsic conditions of the tissue and blood. The proper choice of sequence is important to achieve the desired contrast in a reasonable time. For example, sometimes it helps to use black blood techniques to differentiate flow from other bright structures (Fig. 23.20). Notice the signal appearance in the lumen when imaging is performed axially at the level of the abdominal aorta. The separation of regions within the lumen is due to incomplete nulling of the blood because of varying degrees of flow velocity (Fig. 23.20A). Blood nulling based on a fixed velocity is not useful in this instance. Figure 23.21 shows the effects of laminar flow, in which pulse sequence without an adequate flow com-

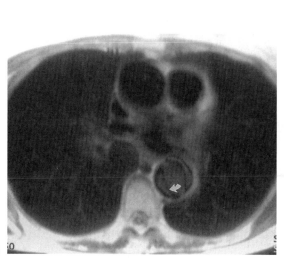
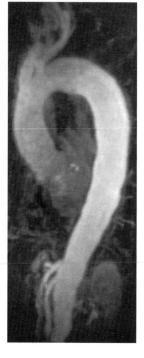

FIG. 23.20. Incomplete nulling of blood signal. **A:** When a half-Fourier single-shot turbo spin echo (HASTE)-type pulse sequence with black blood preparation pulses is used in the area of descending aorta, due to a complex blood flow pattern downstream, the signal is not completely nulled *(curved arrow)*. As a result, image shows remarkable boundaries separating different flow regions. **B:** With contrast-enhanced MRA, there is no indication of dissection.

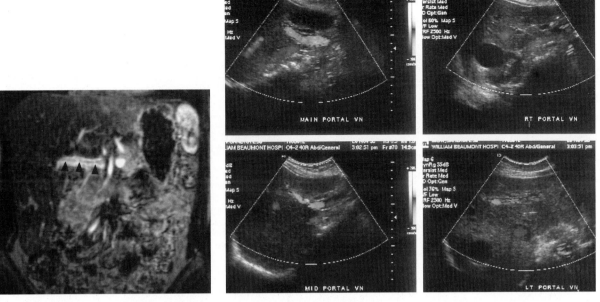

FIG. 23.21. Vascular flow variation. **A:** Laminar flow and absence of flow compensation in the sequence leads to a streak of low signal along the center of the vessel as shown *(arrowheads)*. **B:** The corresponding Doppler ultrasound reveals normal vascular anatomy.

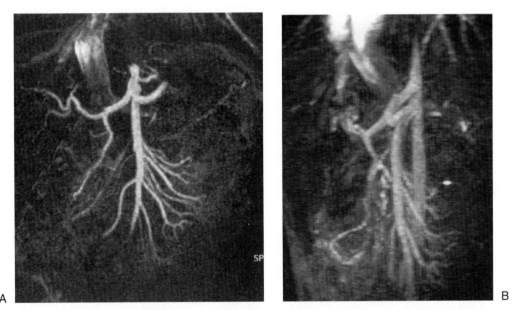

FIG. 23.22. Improved spatial resolution of MIP images due to the slice interpolation technique and removal of bowel contents through the subtraction technique. **A:** A 3D contrast-enhanced MRA in this patient was performed with a coronal acquisition employing a slice interpolation technique, as well as subtraction of the precontrast data from the postcontrast data. The coronal MIP image reveals the mesenteric circulation. **B:** The spatial resolution is preserved on the lateral projection where the celiac and superior mesenteric artery origins are delineated with good spatial resolution due to the slice interpolation technique. Here, the 3D data is in sync and interpolated in the Fourier domain with reconstruction of partitions at a 50% overlap, thus resulting in duplication of the initial partition number. Furthermore, since the subtraction technique was employed, whereby the 3D partitions obtained prior to intravenous contrast were subtracted from the 3D partitions obtained following intravenous contrast, not only are the muscle and fat subtracted from the postcontrast partitions, but so is the high signal of mucoproteinacious fluid within the gastrointestinal tract. This may obviate the need of using negative oral contrast agents to eliminate the signal from the GI tract; however, the mask data should be acquired during the same breath-hold period following contrast administration. This typically requires a high gradient performance system, which allows for a short scanning time of 3D sequences due to the reduction of the repetition time (TR).

pensation scheme was used. A central dark line that follows the entire vessel can be seen in Fig. 23.21A.

Currently, the spatial resolution in 3D sequences is increased by employing slice interpolation techniques in which interleaved slices are obtained, thus reducing the overall slice thickness. This is essential if one is to reduce intravoxel dephasing. In addition, by improving temporal resolution, multiple measurements of a single 3D sequence can be performed during the breath hold. In doing so, there is greater consistency between the location of the same pixels and between the same partitions of different 3D data sets. This allows for superior results from subtraction of non–contrast-enhanced partitions from contrast-enhanced partitions between 3D data sets (Fig. 23.22).

REFERENCES

1. Edelman RR. Basic principles of magnetic resonance angiography. *Cardiovasc Intervent Radiol* 1992;15:3.
2. Chien D, Anderson CM, Lee R. MR angiography: basic principles. In: Edelman RR, Hesselink JR, Zlatkin MB, eds. *Clinical magnetic resonance imaging.* Philadelphia: WB Saunders, 1994:271.
3. Spritzer CE, Blinder RA. Vascular applications of magnetic resonance imaging. *Magn Reson Q* 1989;5(3):205.
4. Haacke EM, Masaryk TJ, Wielopolski PA, et al. Optimizing blood vessel contrast in fast three-dimensional MRI. *Magn Reson Med* 1990;14:202.
5. Sattin W, Haacke EM. Fast imaging and vessel contrast. In: Potchen EJ, Siebert JE, Haacke EM, et al., eds. *Magnetic resonance angiography. Concepts and applications.* St. Louis: Mosby, 1993:35.
6. Bradley WG. Basic flow phenomena. *MRI Clin North Am* 1995;3:375.
7. Anderson CM, Lee RE. Time-of-flight angiography. In: Anderson CM, Edelman RR, Turski PA, eds. *Clinical magnetic resonance angiography.* New York: Raven Press, 1993:11.
8. Keller PJ, Saloner D. Time of flight flow imaging. In: Potchen EJ, Siebert JE, Haacke EM, et al., eds. *Magnetic resonance angiography. Concepts and applications.* St. Louis: Mosby, 1993:146.
9. Keller P. Time of flight magnetic resonance angiography. *Neuroimaging Clin North Am* 1992;4:639.
10. Dumoulin CL. Phase-contrast magnetic resonance angiography. In: Yucel EK, ed. *Magnetic resonance angiography: a practical approach.* New York: McGraw-Hill, 1995:19–34.
11. Dumoulin CL, Yucel EK, Vock P, et al. Two and three dimensional phase contrast MR angiography of the abdomen. *J Comput Assist Tomogr* 1990;14:779.
12. Steffens JC, Link J, Grassner J, et al. Contrast-enhanced, k-space-centered, breath-hold MR angiography of the renal arteries and the abdominal aorta. *J Magn Reson Imaging* 1997;7:617.
13. Boos M, Lentschig M, Scheffler K, Bongartz GM, Steinbrich W. Contrast enhanced magnetic resonance angiography of peripheral vessels:
    different contrast agent applications and sequence strategies: a review. *Invest Radiol* 1998;33(9):538.
14. Laub GA, Kaiser WA. MR angiography with gradient motion refocussing. *J Comput Assist Tomogr* 1988;12:377.
15. Lewin JS, Laub G, Hausmann R. Three-dimensional time-of-flight MR angiography: applications in the abdomen and thorax. *Radiology* 1991;179:261.
16. Edelman RR, Chien D, Atkinson DJ, Sandstrom J. Fast time-of-flight magnetic resonance angiography with improved background suppression. *Radiology* 1991;179:867.
17. Firmin DN, Naylor GL, Kilner PJ, Longmore DB. The application of phase shift in NMR for flow measurements. *Magn Reson Med* 1990;14:230.
18. Walker MF, Souza SP, Dumoulin CL. Quantitative flow measurement in phase contrast MR angiography. *J Comput Assist Tomogr* 1988;12:304.
19. Maki JH, Prince MR, Chenevert TC. Optimizing three-dimensional gadolinium-enhanced magnetic resonance angiography. *Invest Radiol* 1998;33(9):528.
20. Kouwenhoven M. Contrast-enhanced MR angiography: methods, limitations and possibilities. *Acta Radiol* 1997;38(suppl 412):57.
21. Earls JP, Rofsky NM, Decorato DR, Krinsky GA, Weinreb JC. Breath-hold single-dose gadolinium-enhanced three-dimensional MR angiography: usefulness of a timing examination and MR power injector. *Radiology* 1996;201:705.
22. Shetty AN, Bis KG, Vrachliotis TG, et al. Contrast-enhanced 3D MRA with centric ordering in k space: a preliminary clinical experience in imaging the abdominal aorta and renal and peripheral arterial vasculature. *J Magn Reson Imaging* 1998;8:603.
23. Kopka L, Vosshenrich R, Rodenwaldt J, Grabbe E. Differences in injection rates on contrast-enhanced breath hold three-dimensional MR angiography. *AJR* 1998;170:345.
24. Westenberg JJM, Wasser MNJM, Geest RJV, et al. Scan optimization of gadolinium contrast-enhanced three-dimensional MRA of peripheral arteries with multiple bolus injections and in vitro validation of stenosis quantification. *Magn Reson Imaging* 1999;17(1):47.
25. Anderson CM. Post processing and display. In: Anderson CM, Edelman RR, Turski PA, eds. *Clinical magnetic resonance angiography.* New York: Raven Press, 1993:83.
26. Anderson CM, Saloner D, Tsuruda JS, Shapeero LG, Lee RE. Artifacts in maximum intensity projection display of MR angiograms. *AJR* 1990;154:623.
27. Masui T, Caputo GR, Bowersox JC, Higgins CB. Assessment of popliteal arterial occlusive disease with 2D-TOF MRA. *J Comput Assist Tomogr* 1995;19(3):449.
28. Brown DG, Riederer SJ. Contrast-to-noise ratios in maximum intensity projection images. *Magn Reson Med* 1992;23:130.
29. Maki JM, Prince MR, Londy FJ, Chenevert TL. The effects of time varying intravascular signal intensity and k-space acquisition order on three dimensional MR angiography image quality. *J Magn Reson Imaging* 1996;6:642.
30. McCarty M, Gedroyc WMW. Surgical clip artifacts mimicking arterial stenosis: problem with magnetic resonance angiography. *Clin Radiol* 1993;48:232.
31. Matsumoto AH, Teitelbaum GP, Carvlin MJ, et al. Gadolinium enhanced MR imaging of vascular stent. *J Comput Assist Tomogr* 1990;14(3):357.
32. Czervionke LF, Daniels DL, Wehrli FW, et al. Magnetic susceptibility artifacts in gradient-recalled echo MR imaging. *AJNR* 1987;9:1149.

Variants and Pitfalls in Body Imaging,
edited by Ali Shirkhoda.
Lippincott Williams & Wilkins, Philadelphia, © 2000.

CHAPTER 24

Abdomen and Pelvis: Postoperative Changes on CT

Ali Shirkhoda

Complete medical histories of the patients, including those of any prior surgeries, are often unavailable for the radiologist at the time of CT examination. However, in order to properly plan such studies and be able to optimally interpret the images, information regarding the patient's current condition and previous surgical procedures is often important. Previous surgeries or procedures of any type within the abdomen and pelvis may affect the normal orientation of the solid and hollow viscera as seen on cross-sectional imaging. It is the objective of this chapter to illustrate the anatomic and morphologic changes in the abdomen and pelvis that occur as the result of surgery, whether from organ removal or transplant or as a result of an erroneously implanted foreign object. Because these changes have the potential of causing erroneous CT interpretation, guidelines are provided as to how one can avoid such pitfalls.

Postsurgical anatomic variations and pitfalls are presented in the following five categories: (a) pitfalls as the result of organ removal; (b) pitfalls as the result of implantation of tissue or a prosthesis; (c) pitfalls as the result of organ transplant; (d) pitfalls as the result of foreign objects; and (e) pitfalls as the result of recent procedures, pouches, and ostomies.

PITFALLS AS THE RESULT OF ORGAN REMOVAL

The nature of surgery may be such that a solid viscus such as one kidney, spleen, a lobe of the liver, or a hollow viscus such as the rectum is removed. Therefore, as a

---

A. Shirkhoda: Department of Diagnostic Radiology, William Beaumont Hospital, Royal Oak, Michigan 48073.

result, other organs such as bowel loops, pancreas, gallbladder, or uterus may fall into the vacant space. Therefore, because of their unusual anatomic orientation on axial images, they may become a source of diagnostic pitfall in the interpretation of abdominal or pelvic CT scans. In patients with partial hepatectomy, the remaining liver will progressively regenerate. Irregularity at the site of resection is common along with displacement of portal veins and other vessels (1). Such changes should not be mistaken for an abnormality.

In the pelvis, the common surgical procedures that involve organ removal include abdominoperineal resection (APR), pelvic exenteration, cystectomy, hysterectomy, and prostatectomy. Any one of these operations can result in displacement of adjacent organs into an unfamiliar location (2–4). Small bowel loops tend to descend after removal of solid pelvic viscera. When these loops are not opacified with oral contrast, they often become a source of pitfall on CT images, mimicking a mass or an abscess.

Postnephrectomy Pitfalls

As the result of right nephrectomy, bowel loops (Fig. 24.1), gallbladder (Figs. 24.2 and 24.3), or the liver and pancreas (Fig. 24.4) each may occupy the vacant renal fossa. On the left side, it is usually the bowel, pancreas (Fig. 24.5), or spleen that falls back into the renal space. On abdominal CT, these structures can mimic tumor recurrence or simulate an abscess, occasionally resulting in unnecessary intervention (5) (see Figs. 24.2 and 24.4). A posteriorly displaced pancreas with pancreatitis and pseudocyst may also mimic an abscess (Fig. 24.6). The unopacified bowel loops are the most common structures

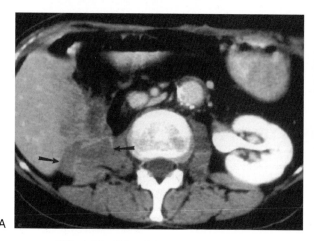

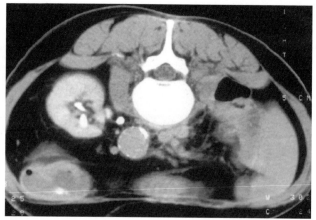

FIG. 24.1. Prior right nephrectomy, rule out tumor recurrence. **A:** This patient had a right nephrectomy for renal cell carcinoma, and now the follow-up CT shows a hypodense soft tissue mass in the right renal fossa *(arrows),* which did not opacify on this delayed image and can be mistaken for local recurrent tumor. **B:** To rule out this possibility, the patient is rescanned in prone position. The unopacified small bowel loops are now delineated by gas, and there is no abnormality.

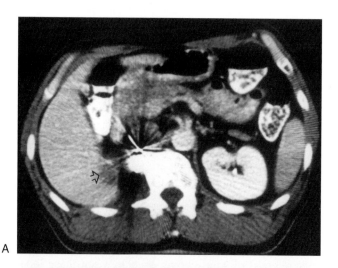

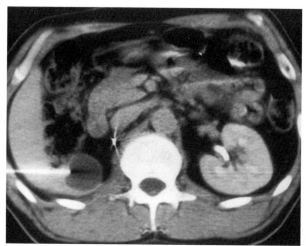

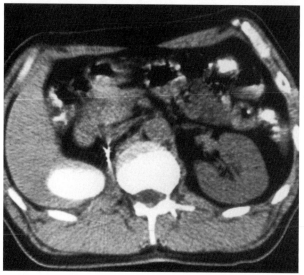

FIG. 24.2. Prior right nephrectomy, rule out abscess. **A:** In this febrile patient, a CT scan was done 3 weeks after right nephrectomy and was interpreted as possible abscess medial to the right hepatic lobe in the renal fossa *(arrow).* **B:** He was scheduled for percutaneous aspiration, at which time the fluid collection was found to be larger. However, the result of aspiration was sterile bile. **C:** A normally displaced gallbladder was better illustrated by repeating CT after overnight ingestion of tablets for oral cholecystography. (Reproduced with permission from reference 5.)

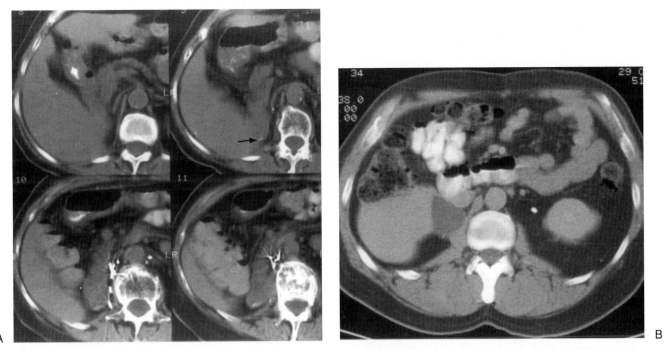

A   B

FIG. 24.3. Prior right nephrectomy, gallbladder in adrenal fossa. **A:** Four sequential images show gallbladder with a tiny stone *(arrow)* in the right adrenal fossa. **B:** Another similar patient with the gallbladder behind the IVC. (Reproduced with permission from reference 5.)

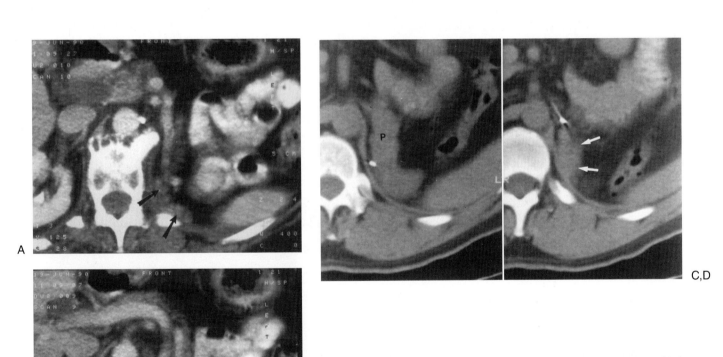

C,D

FIG. 24.4. Prior left nephrectomy. **A,B:** In this patient with history of left nephrectomy for renal cell carcinoma, a tail of the pancreas *(arrows)* (A) has occupied the left renal fossa and could be mistaken for abnormal soft tissue such as tumor recurrence. Generally, repeat scanning with thinner slices will illustrate continuity of tissue with the pancreas. Also, an image in the prone position occasionally helps to move the pancreas away from the renal fossa. (Reproduced with permission from reference 5.) **C,D:** Another patient with similar history showing the body of the pancreas *(arrows)* (D) mimicking a mass.

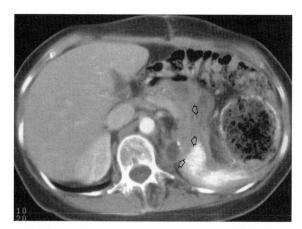

FIG. 24.5. Prior left nephrectomy, rule out abscess. This patient, who had prior left nephrectomy, presented with low-grade fever, and the CT scan was obtained. On this image, the patient has pancreatitis with the body and tail of the pancreas *(arrows)* containing a small pseudocyst in the left renal fossa. This should not be mistaken for a necrotic recurrent tumor.

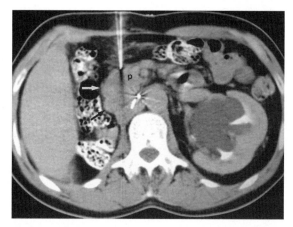

FIG. 24.6. Prior right nephrectomy. This patient had a prior right nephrectomy and adrenonectomy for adrenal cortical carcinoma. A follow-up CT scan shows a soft tissue mass anterior to the cava for which a percutaneous aspiration biopsy was performed. There is slight posterior displacement of the normal head of the pancreas (P). Unopacified duodenum behind the pancreas *(arrows)* mimics a mass. The biopsy result was normal pancreas.

filling the vacant space and can mimic recurrent tumor or abscess. Therefore, delayed imaging following oral administration of contrast material is very important in these patients to see the opacified bowel loops.

Post–Hepatic Lobectomy Pitfalls

Based on the hepatic arterial anatomy, the liver is composed of two lobes, the right and the left. The caudate lobe, a surface projection, is supplied by both the right and left hepatic arteries. Each lobe is subdivided into two segments: the right lobe into the anterior and posterior segments and the left into the medial (quadrate) and lateral

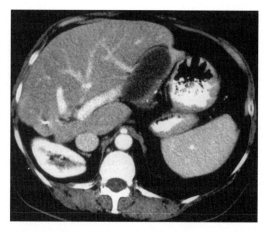

FIG. 24.7. Prior hepatic trisegmentectomy. Displacement of portal vein and hypertrophy of caudate and remaining left lobe are seen.

segments. Each segment has superior and inferior subsegments. A plane along a line drawn between the gallbladder bed and the inferior vena cava topographically separates the right lobe from the left lobe. The left lobar intersegmental plane is located along the umbilical fissure, delineated by the falciform ligament and ligamentum teres.

Partial hepatic resection generally modifies the anatomy of the liver, which can be defined by different diagnostic modalities, particularly CT scanning (1).

Regeneration of the remaining liver by hypertrophy or hyperplasia or both takes place immediately following lobectomy or segmentectomy and at times even preoperatively, depending on the amount of tissue replacement involved and the status of the remaining liver (Fig. 24.7). Only 10% to 15% of the liver is necessary for patient survival as long as the residual liver is healthy. In experi-

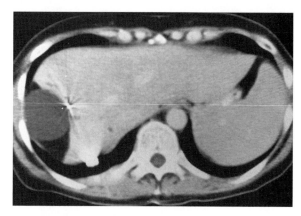

FIG. 24.8. Prior right hepatic lobectomy. This patient with prior right hepatic lobectomy for metastatic colon carcinoma had a follow-up CT scan. A well-defined low-density collection is seen lateral to the remaining liver. Surgical history proved that the patient did not have a cholecystectomy. This collection represented a normal displaced gallbladder, which was later proven by sonography. (Reproduced with permission from reference 5.)

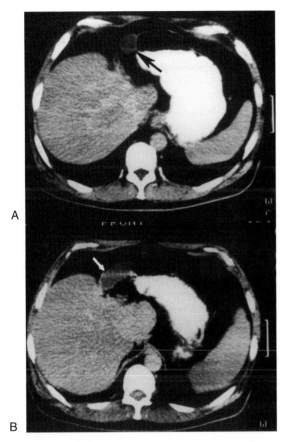

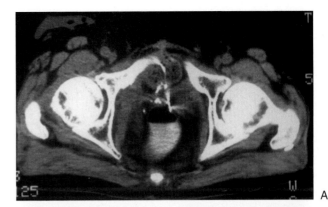

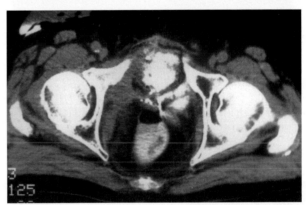

FIG. 24.9. Prior left hepatic lobectomy. **A,B:** This CT scan was done as a follow-up in a patient who had a left hepatic lobectomy for metastatic colon carcinoma. There is a tubular structure near the gastric antrum *(arrows)* that mimics a diverticulum or other abnormal fluid collection. Because the history indicated that the gallbladder was not removed, sonography was done, and this proved to be a normally displaced gallbladder. (Reproduced with permission from reference 5.)

FIG. 24.10. Prior cystectomy, rule out abscess. This patient with recent history of cystectomy underwent CT examination because of low-grade fever. **A:** The CT scan that was done following oral and rectal contrast reveals a collection near the symphysis pubis containing small air bubbles. This was suspected to be an abscess. **B:** A repeat examination done about 1 hour later with additional rectal contrast reveals that the presumed abnormal collection is now opacified with oral contrast and therefore represents unopacified bowel loops and not an abscess.

ments with animals, McDermott et al. found that regeneration of the total liver volume is progressive and takes over 4 months after an 80% to 85% resection (6). On CT, this regeneration is recognized by progressive enlargement and change in contour of hepatic parenchyma over a period of 6 months to 1 year after surgery. As a result of hepatic lobectomy, along with reconfiguration of the remaining liver, the gallbladder will often be displaced to unfamiliar locations, mimicking other pathologic conditions (Figs. 24.8 and 24.9).

Postcystectomy or Postvaginectomy Pitfalls

Radical cystectomy is done for treatment of invasive bladder carcinoma, and the vacant space usually is filled by intestinal loops. Immediate postoperative CT may be obtained to rule out an abscess, and follow-up CT is often requested to rule out any recurrent neoplasm. Adequate oral contrast before CT is important in such patients, and delayed images should be obtained to avoid any pitfall (Fig. 24.10). Ileostomy, particularly when identified with

opacified urine, is recognizable on CT. However, a nonopacified continent ileostomy can be mistaken for an abscess or other collections (2). After vaginal resection, a reconstructed neovagina has typical characteristics (Fig. 24.11).

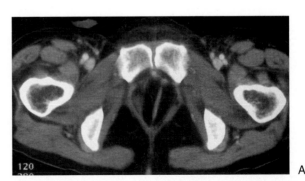

FIG. 24.11. Neovagina. **A:** This patient with history of invasive cervical carcinoma underwent pelvic exenteration and total vaginectomy. This CT image shows typical features of neovagina as a result of reconstructive surgery. *Continued on next page.*

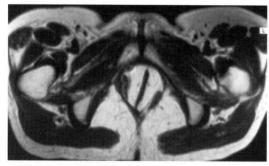

FIG. 24.11. *Continued.* **B:** Corresponding T$_1$-weighted MR image.

Pitfalls as a Result of Abdominoperineal Resection

Despite aggressive surgical treatment of advanced rectal carcinoma by abdominoperineal resection (APR), along with postoperative radiation, there is still a relatively high incidence of recurrent tumor. In fact, Phil et al. (7) observed that after potentially curative resection, therapeutic failures in the form of only local recurrence tend to be more common in rectal than colonic tumors. It has been shown that 57% of recurrences after resection are pelvic alone or pelvic along with other sites. The pelvic recurrence usually is in the form of presacral soft tissue. However, after APR, in addition to recurrent tumors, the differential diagnosis of a presacral soft tissue mass should include such entities as unopacified bowel loops, relocated pelvic organs such as seminal vesicles (Fig. 24.12) or uterus (Fig. 24.13), and postoperative fibrosis (3). Although the recurrent tumor often needs to be proven by biopsy, recognition of the other conditions is important to prevent an unnecessary intervention or additional imaging studies (see Fig. 24.12C,D). Generally, in a man the configuration of seminal vesicles, and in a woman lack of a history of hysterectomy, helps to recognize these organs. However, fibrosis is often difficult to differentiate from tumor, and other exams or a biopsy may be needed. Also, the urinary bladder is occasionally displaced into the rectal fossa and, therefore, if unopacified can mimic abnormal fluid collection (Fig. 24.14).

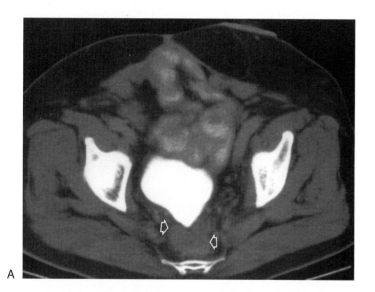

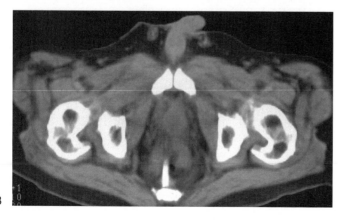

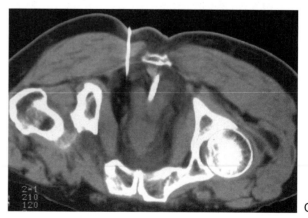

FIG. 24.12. Displaced seminal vesicles after APR. **A:** This man with history of rectal carcinoma had an APR, and a follow-up CT in 6 months demonstrates two midline small soft tissue structures *(arrows)*. This is a normal descent of the seminal vesicles after removal of the rectum and should not be mistaken for tumor recurrence. **B,C:** In another man with prior APR for rectal carcinoma, the two seminal vesicles were mistaken for nodes (**B**), and an attempt at biopsy (**C**) was aborted.

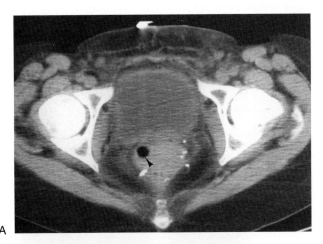

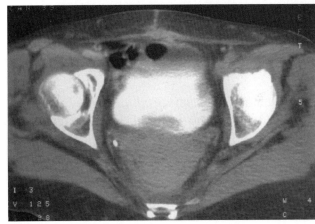

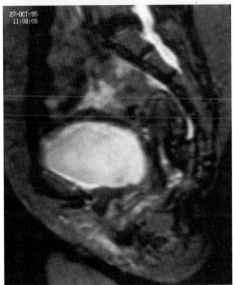

FIG. 24.13. Displaced uterus after APR. **A:** This woman with previous APR shows a well-defined soft tissue density in the rectal fossa. This is a normal descent of uterus after removal of the rectum and should not be mistaken for local recurrent neoplasm. Note that there is a tampon placed within the vagina *(arrowhead).* **B,C:** This woman with prior APR needed MRI to confirm posterior displacement of the uterus as shown in **C** (sagittal T₂ image).

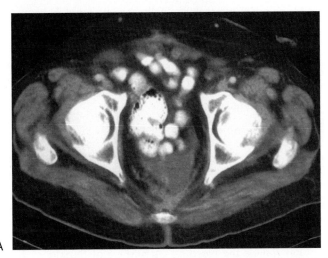

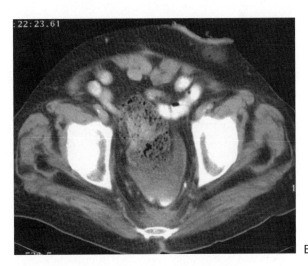

FIG. 24.14. Displaced bladder after APR. **A:** The urinary bladder is displaced inferiorly and posteriorly in this patient. Notice the change in its normal smooth posterior borders. To avoid a pitfall for abscess, a delayed scan should be obtained. **B:** Partial opacification on delayed CT is present. Notice presacral fibrosis as a result of APR.

PITFALLS AS THE RESULT OF IMPLANTATION OF TISSUE AND PROSTHESES

In addition to organ removal, implantation of tissues and prostheses within the abdomen or pelvis, which may be done in oncologic patients, can be misinterpreted by the radiologist. Whenever postoperative radiation therapy is contemplated in the pelvis, one of the limiting factors in optimizing its effects is the low level of radiation tolerance of the small intestine. From the surgeon's prospective, a method of excluding loops of small bowel from the pelvic critical treatment volume should be easy to perform, consistent, and not itself associated with complications (8). Omental fat (Fig. 24.15) or synthetic absorbable mesh and occasionally breast implants (Fig. 24.16) have been utilized at the time of exploration or definitive surgery aimed at sustaining the loops of small bowel out of the radiation field in patients treated for gynecologic or colonic malignancies. The omental lid is formed into a pedicle flap based on either the left or the right gastroepiploic artery and is usually swung down to the left pericolic gutter to cover the denuded pelvic wall (omentopexy). Such a flap serves both as a vascular bed to absorb the serous drainage and as an x-ray barrier for the bowel loops. Without the knowledge of such operations, the radiologist is at a disadvantage and may potentially make an erroneous interpretation of the

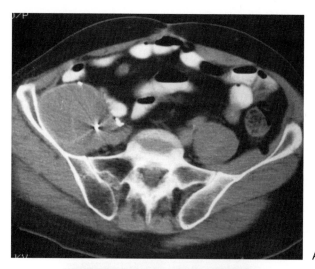

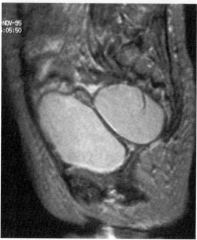

FIG. 24.16. Breast prosthesis in cecal and rectal fossa. **A:** This patient with cecal carcinoma was planned at the time of surgery to undergo postoperative irradiation. However, in preparation, the surgeon chose to displace the small bowel loops out of the radiation field by using a breast prosthesis, implanting that into the right iliac fossa. Without such history, the low-density mass (53 HU) seen on CT can easily be mistaken for an abnormal fluid collection. **B:** This patient with history of rectal carcinoma had surgery, and a breast prosthesis was placed in the rectal fossa to displace the bladder out of the radiation field. T_2 sagittal image shows the prosthesis with radial fold.

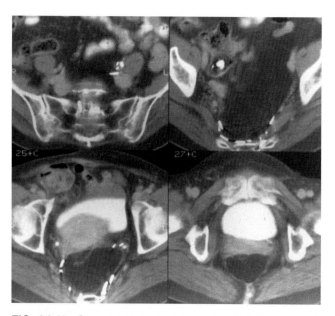

FIG. 24.15. Omental transplant (omentopexy). This patient with rectal carcinoma was discovered at the time of surgery to need postoperative radiation to the pelvic floor for control of the local malignancy. After removal of tumor, the surgeon brought down the omentum along the left side of the pelvis and implanted it within the pelvic floor in order to keep the small bowel loops out of the radiation field. This will enable the radiation oncologist to deliver the maximum radiation with minimum side effects to the small intestine. Without the knowledge of such an operation, the radiologist will have difficulty explaining the abnormal fatty mass in the pelvis as seen in these four sequential CT images.

CT images. Other prosthetic devices such as a penile prosthesis, erection pumps, or vascular grafts are usually recognizable on CT images.

After localized resection of a renal lesion such as a cyst, stone-filled caliceal diverticulum, or a small renal cell carcinoma, perinephritic fat has been used by surgeons to tamponade the bleeding cut surface of the kidney before closing the renal capsule over the cortical defect (9). Such fat can be a source of pitfall in the interpretation of renal CT or ultrasound done after such operation (Fig. 24.17). Similar surgery (omentopexy) is occasionally done in a patient with hydatid cyst of the liver (Fig. 24.18).

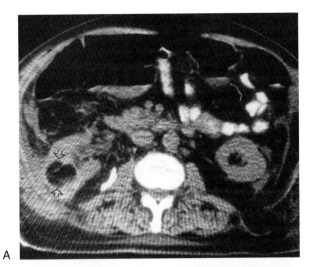

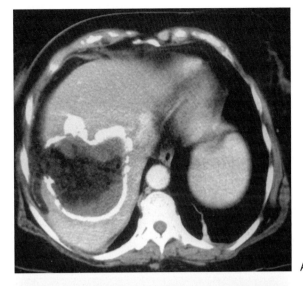

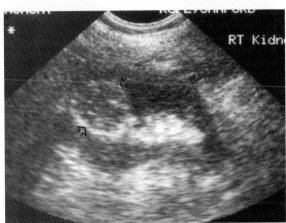

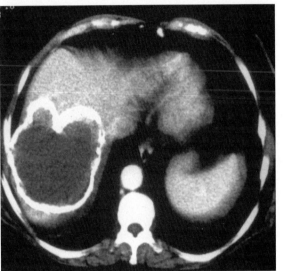

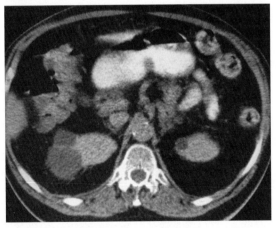

FIG. 24.17. Fat implant in place of renal cyst. **A:** The abdominal CT scan in this febrile patient shows a soft tissue mass with fatty density in the right kidney. **B:** Sonograms demonstrate the echogenic nature of this mass, which measures 2.9 cm. Without appropriate surgical history, it can erroneously be called a fatty renal tumor such as angiomyolipoma. **C:** However, this patient with previous septated renal cyst was explored, and the surgeon, after removal of the cyst, chose to tamponade the surgical area with perirenal fat before closing the renal capsule over the cortical defect.

FIG. 24.18. Omentoplexy for hydatid cyst. **A:** After evacuation of this hydatid cyst, omentum was mobilized, and the cystic cavity was packed. **B:** Hydatid cyst before surgery.

PITFALLS AS THE RESULT OF ORGAN TRANSPLANT

The common organs that are transplanted in the abdomen include kidney, pancreas, and liver. Ovaries may be transplanted for the purpose of radiation therapy.

Renal Transplant

Renal transplant is a common surgical procedure, and the transplanted kidney is easily recognized by its shape and location, usually in the upper portion of iliac fossa. However, postoperative complications such as infarction (Fig. 24.19), abscesses, or complete necrosis and calcification (Fig. 24.20) may be difficult to diagnose if proper history is not available.

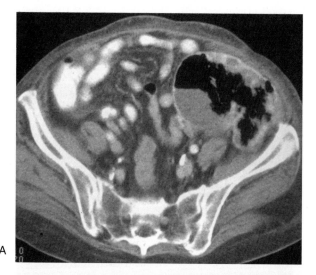

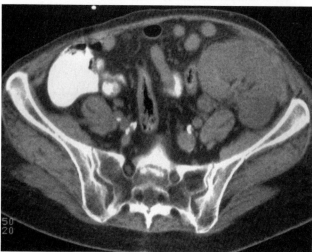

FIG. 24.19. Infarcted renal transplant. **A:** Six months after renal transplant, contrast-enhanced CT shows the infarcted kidney, which is difficult to diagnose if proper history is not available. **B:** Nonenhanced CT 2 months before infarction.

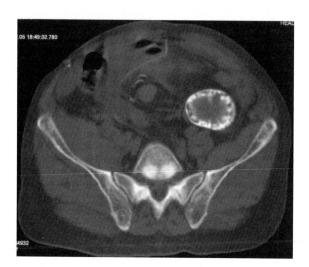

FIG. 24.20. Calcified transplant. The calcified mass in the left lower quadrant represents the infarcted and calcified renal transplant.

Pancreatic Transplant

More than 50% of patients with insulin-dependent diabetes have nephropathy, retinopathy, or neuropathy within 20 years of the onset of their disease. Pancreatic transplantation is undertaken in selected patients in an attempt to prevent, arrest, or reverse progression of these complications (10). For such a procedure, a whole or segmental graft may have been obtained from a cadaver, and the transplantation takes place in the pelvis, where the transplanted pancreas is drained into the small bowel or bladder. The whole pancreas is preferred because of the theoretically lower risk of thrombosis and also because of the larger beta-cell mass available. Without clinical information, a transplanted pancreas, which appears as a soft tissue mass (Fig. 24.21), can become a source of pitfall in pelvic or abdominal CT.

Oophoropexy

At the time of radical hysterectomy for early-stage cervical carcinoma, the decision to remove or retain grossly normal ovaries in premenopausal patients involves several competing factors (11). Ovarian conservation and lateral ovarian transplantation is a technique that may be used in treating such patients. In these patients who are planned to have pelvic irradiation, the ovaries are mobilized at the time of surgery. Then, with their vascular pedicle, they are transplanted near the peritoneum in each pericolic gutter (oophoropexy) and, therefore, will remain out of the radiation field (Fig. 24.22). This information is vital to the radiologist so such normal ovaries will not be mistaken for an abnormal mass.

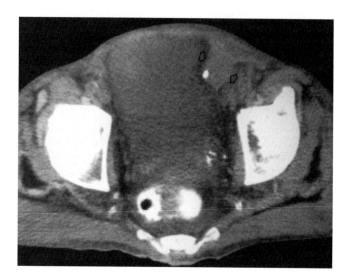

FIG. 24.21. Pancreatic transplant. The soft tissue mass that is seen in the left side of the pelvis (arrows) can be correctly diagnosed only if proper clinical history is available. This patient with long-standing insulin-dependent diabetes had undergone a segmental pancreatic transplant 6 months before the CT study.

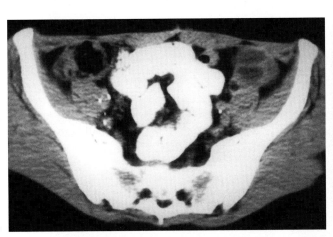
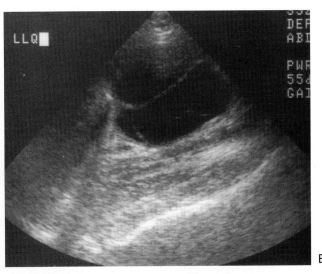

A   B

FIG. 24.22. Oophoropexy. A: Pelvic CT shows a 5-cm complex cystic mass in the left iliac fossa. B: Sonogram demonstrates presence of septations within the fluid-filled structures. Transplantation of the ovary out of the pelvis was done in this 34-year-old woman because, at the time of surgery for cervical carcinoma, the gynecologist decided that she will need postsurgical pelvic radiation. With proper history, the CT scan was reported as showing a few peripheral cysts or follicles within the ovary in the left side of the pelvis. Without appropriate clinical history, such diagnosis will be difficult.

PITFALLS AS THE RESULT OF FOREIGN OBJECTS

During abdominal surgery, topical hemostatic materials are widely used to control bleeding at sites such as kidneys, pancreas, bowel, or the biliary system. They are often oxidized regenerated cellulose and are locally absorbed without tissue reaction. However, they can mimic an abscess when a follow-up CT is done in a febrile postoperative patient (12). Generally, the diagnosis of retained surgical foreign bodies will continue to be a problem as long as nonabsorbable materials are used.

Cotton sponges are inert and do not undergo any specific decomposition or biomedical reaction (13). Pathologically, however, two types of foreign body reactions develop. One is an aseptic fibrinous response that creates adhesions and encapsulation, which results in a foreign body granuloma. The second is exudative in nature and leads to abscess formation with or without secondary bacterial invasion. This type of reaction happens far earlier than the first one, usually within a few months. However, the first type is often discovered on CT done several years later and can be misinterpreted as an abnormal collection or abscess (Fig. 24.23). A retained surgical

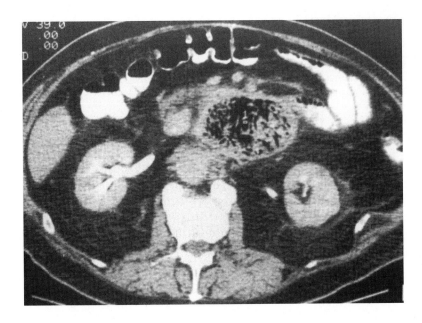

FIG. 24.23. Towel left at surgical site. This patient with previous surgery for abdominal aortic aneurysm continued to have pain several months later when a CT scan was done showing an unusually walled off collection of gas with streaky densities in the midabdomen extended to the right lower quadrant. Barium examination of the small and large bowel proved this to be extraluminal, and at surgery a large encapsulated towel was removed from the operative site.

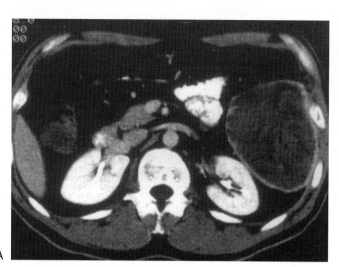 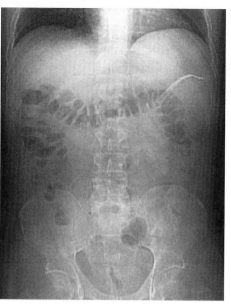

FIG. 24.24. Retained sponge at remote surgical site. This patient with a remote history of abdominal surgery done approximately 10 years ago presented with pain in the left upper quadrant. **A:** Enhanced CT shows a well-defined encapsulated low-density mass in the left upper quadrant below the spleen. **B:** Proper history along with the presence of an opacified marker in the surgical sponge better seen on topogram (was also seen on CT) led to the diagnosis of foreign body granuloma which was surgically removed.

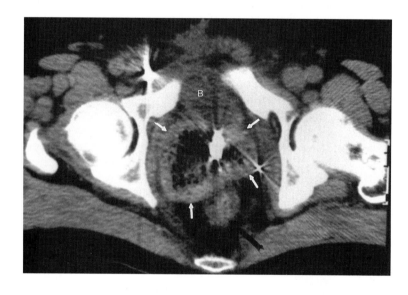

FIG. 24.25. Retained sponge at recent surgical site. This patient with recent prostatectomy continued to have a fever, and the CT shows a sponge with a marker *(arrows)* behind the bladder (B) in the prostate fossa. It was surgically removed.

sponge, which may be referred to as gossypiboma (14), generally has radiopaque markers readily visible on plain radiograph or CT topogram (Figs. 24.24 and 24.25). However, those used in previous years may lack the marker, and without proper history the correct diagnosis will be difficult.

PITFALLS AS THE RESULT OF RECENT PROCEDURES, POUCHES, AND OSTOMIES

Surgical procedures such as gastroduodenostomy (Biliroth I), gastrojejunostomy (Biliroth II), ileo-colostomy, and other types of anastomosis in the GI tract, including those done on the biliary system, are not generally sources of pitfalls. However, in patients with Biliroth II surgery, an unopacified duodenal loop can cause confusion in the evaluation of the head of the pancreas for mass lesions (2). Ileostomies and colostomies, particularly when opacified by intravenous or oral contrast, are easily recognizable on CT. However, a nonopacified continent ileostomy (Fig. 24.26) or the reservoir from ileocystostomy can become a confusing source for diagnosing abscesses and other abnormal fluid collections.

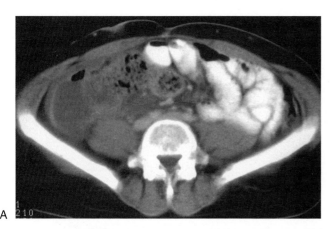 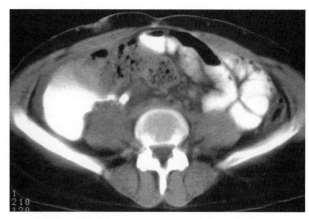

A   B

FIG. 24.26. Prior cystectomy and continent ileostomy. **A:** The fluid-containing structure in the right side of the abdomen represents an unopacified continent ileostomy. **B:** Delayed CT establishes communication with the ureters and proves the nature of collection.

REFERENCES

1. Couanet D, Shirkhoda A, Wallace S. Computed tomography after partial hepatectomy. *J Comput Assist Tomogr* 1984;8:453–457.
2. Shirkhoda A. Diagnostic pitfalls in abdominal CT. *RadioGraphics* 1991;11:969–1002.
3. Lee JKT, Stanley RJ, Sagel SS, et al. CT appearance of the pelvis after abdominoperineal resection for rectal carcinoma. *Radiology* 1981;141:737.
4. Pan G, Shirkhoda A. Pelvic exenteration: Role of CT in follow-up. *Radiology* 1987;164:665–670.
5. Shirkhoda A. Diagnostic pitfalls in abdominal CT relevant to percutaneous interventions. *Semin Intervent Radiol* 1995;12(2):146–162.
6. McDermott WV Jr, Greenberger NJ, Isselbacher KJ, et al. Major hepatic resection: diagnostic techniques and metabolic problems. *Surgery* 1963;54:56–66.
7. Phil E, McDermott FT, Price AB. Disease free survival and recurrence after resection of rectal carcinoma. *J Surg Oncol* 1981;152:131–136.
8. Bakare SC, Shafir M, McElhinney AJ. Exclusion of small bowel from pelvis for postoperative radiotherapy for rectal cancer. *J Surg Oncol* 1987;35:55–58.
9. Papanicolaou N, Harbury OL, Pfister RC. Fat-filled postoperative renal cortical defects: sonographic and CT appearance. *Am J Roentgenol* 1988;151:503–505.
10. Low RA, Kuni CC, Letourneau JG. Pancreas transplant imaging: an overview. *Am J Roentgenol* 1990;155:13–21.
11. Parker M, Bosscher J, Barnhill D, Park R. Ovarian management during radical hysterectomy in the premenopausal patient. *Obstet Gynecol* 1993;82:187–190.
12. Young ST, Paulson EK, McCann RL, et al. Appearance of oxidized cellulose (Surgicel) on post-operative CT scans: similarity to postoperative abscess. *Am J Roentgenol* 1993;160:275–277.
13. Sturdy JH, Baird RM, Gerein AN. Surgical sponges: a cause of granuloma and adhesion formation. *Ann Surg* 1967;165:128–134.
14. Apter S, Hertz M, Rubinstein ZJ, Zissin R. Gossypiboma in the early postoperative period: a diagnostic problem. *Clin Radiol* 1990;42(2):128–129.

SECTION III

Variants of Normal Anatomy and Diagnostic Pitfalls in Imaging of the Musculoskeletal System

Variants and Pitfalls in Body Imaging,
edited by Ali Shirkhoda.
Lippincott Williams & Wilkins, Philadelphia, © 2000.

CHAPTER 25

Thoracoabdominal and Pelvic Musculoskeleton in Adults

Ali Shirkhoda, Steven Morgan, and Georges Y. El-Khoury

In routine CT and MR examinations of the thorax, abdomen, and pelvis, the muscular and osseous structures are frequently underevaluated and occasionally neglected. Computed tomography (CT) is a useful method for demonstrating normal anatomy and many of the osseous pathologic processes, whereas magnetic resonance imaging (MRI) has a better spatial resolution for soft tissue abnormalities. The recognition of anatomic variants and diagnostic pitfalls remains an essential part of a complete imaging evaluation of the thorax, abdomen, and pelvis. Potential errors in diagnostic interpretation can be avoided with a thorough understanding of normal anatomy and recognition of nonpathologic and often normal variants.

In this chapter, the anatomy of the muscles and bones in the thorax and abdomen is briefly explored, and the common normal anatomic variants and sources of diagnostic pitfalls are discussed.

THORACIC CAGE

The thoracic cage is an interconnected network of muscles, lymphatics, and neurovascular and osseous structures (1,2). The anatomy of muscles and bones in the chest wall on CT may be briefly examined in four different areas of (a) thoracic inlet, (b) anterior group, (c) paracapsular group, and (d) paraspinal group.

Thoracic Inlet

The superior aperture of the thorax is called the thoracic inlet, through which pass the viscera and blood ves-

sels from the head, neck, and the upper extremity. The scalenes and sternocleidomastoids are the muscles of major interest in this region (Fig. 25.1). It is important to recognize these vessels and muscles, as their size and symmetry can be variable in different patients and even at different positions of arms while the patient is within the CT gantry (Fig. 25.2). For example, when rapid acquisition of spiral CT data is coupled with higher IV contrast medium flow rates in a patient who has both arms above the head, occasionally the CT image may show diversion of contrast medium into collateral routes (3), mimicking soft tissue calcifications. It can also give the impression of central venous obstruction (Fig. 25.3). Hypertrophy of the sternocleidomastoid could develop in conditions such as COPD, when they are used as accessory muscles of respiration (Fig. 25.4). In addition, the attachment site of this muscle on the medial aspect of the clavicle can be a source of volume averaging on CT, mimicking a bone lesion (Fig. 25.5). The sternocleidomastoid receives nerve supply from the 11th cranial nerve. The scalenes are composed of anterior, middle, and posterior and are innervated by C3 to C8 cervical nerves (4). The posterior and middle scalenes are collectively called scalene mass.

The osseous structures in the thoracic inlet include clavicles, ribs, and sternum. The sternum has three parts: manubrium, body, and xiphoid. The manubrium is the site of attachment of the clavicles and first and second ribs. It joins with the body at the manubriosternal junction (angle of Luis). Computed tomography scans of the sternum, sternoclavicular articulations, and the adjacent soft tissues possess several normal variants that may be confused with a pathologic condition (4). Failure of fusion of the sternal ossification centers leads to various congenital anomalies. Midline fusion defects (Fig. 25.6) vary from completely cleft sternum to lesser clefts, midline foramina (5), and bifid xiphoid. Other

A. Shirkhoda: Department of Diagnostic Radiology, William Beaumont Hospital, Royal Oak, Michigan 48073.

S. Morgan: The St. Luke Hospitals Health Alliance, Ft. Thomas, Kentucky 41075.

G. Y. El-Khoury: Departments of Radiology and Orthopaedics, The University of Iowa Hospitals and Clinics, Iowa City, Iowa 52242.

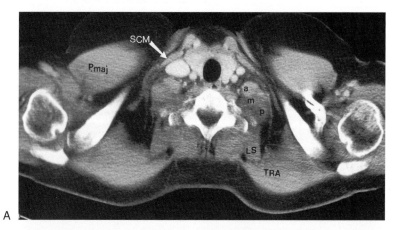

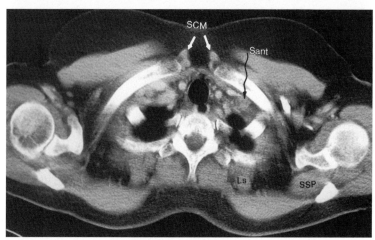

FIG. 25.1. Thoracic inlet muscles. **A:** At this level, the pectoralis major (P.maj), trapezius (TRA), levator scapularis (LS), and the three scalenus muscles (a, anterior; m, middle; p, posterior) and the sternocleidomastoid (SCM) are seen. **B:** At a level 10 mm below **A,** sternocleidomastoid (SCM) near its attachment, scalenus anterior (S. ant), levator scapularis (L), and the supraspinatus muscles (ssp) are seen. The scalenus anterior muscle should not be mistaken for a lymph node at this level.

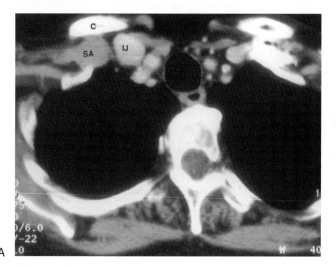

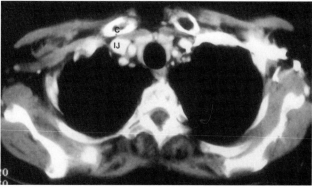

FIG. 25.2. Asymmetry of scalene muscles. **A:** The right anterior scalenus muscle (SA) is seen because the right arm has not been raised above the head. **B:** Repeat follow-up CT scan at a similar level with both arms above the head, showing that the muscle is no longer visible. C, Clavicle; IJ, internal jugular vein.

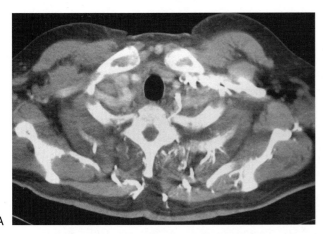
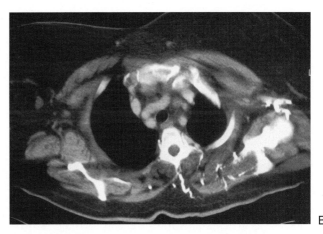

FIG. 25.3. Opacification of the collaterals. **A:** With both arms above the head, the upper extremity venous return to the thorax is minimally compromised, and with left arm injection there is visualization of numerous venous collaterals around the left scapula as well as the upper thoracic vertebrae and the ribs. The left subclavian vein is opacified. **B:** In a different patient, the image at the level of the thoracic inlet reveals smaller collaterals in the posterior muscle groups including the infraspinatus and paraspinal muscles. These collaterals seen in **A** and **B** should not be mistaken for calcifications.

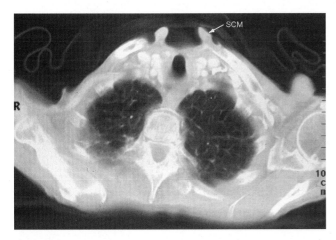

FIG. 25.4. Prominent sternocleidomastoid muscles in a patient with emphysema. Both sternocleidomastoids (SCM) are seen to be slightly prominent in this patient, who has pulmonary emphysema.

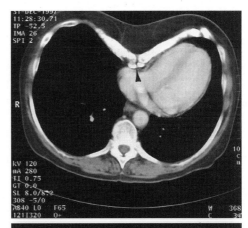
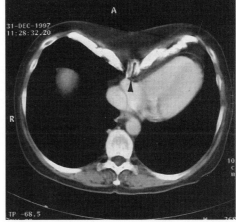

FIG. 25.6. Sternal fusion defect. In this patient with pectus excavatum, there is a fusion defect in the lower aspect of the sternum *(arrowheads).* This has resulted in a partial sternal cleft.

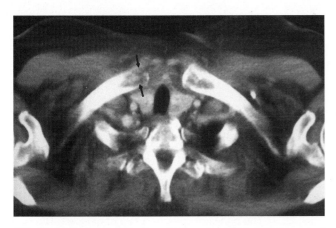

FIG. 25.5. Pseudolytic lesion. At the site of the attachment of the right sternocleidomastoid on the clavicle, volume averaging can result in a pseudolytic lesion of the distal clavicle *(arrows).*

variants include separate or fused episternal ossicles (6), a low manubriosternal junction (at the level of the third rib), or ribs that articulate with the sternum alternately rather than as pairs. Suprasternal or episternal ossicles occur in pairs or singly, may be united to the manubrium by a synchondrosis, and are more common in women. They should not be confused with vascular calcifications or calcified lymph nodes. Other variants of sternum include pectus excavatum (Fig. 25.7), pectus carinatum, sternal tilt, and sternal agenesis (7). Cortical unsharpness is frequently noted at the posterior aspect of the manubrium or lateral surfaces of the body. The latter is probably a result of the shallow sternal notches that serve as articulations for the costal cartilage. Cortical unsharpness is slightly more frequent in women and is mainly found in patients above the age of 40 years (8). The unsharpness seen in the posterior manubrial cortex results in part from true variations in the thickness of the cortex and in part from the slope of the manubrium in relation to the axial plane of CT. It can mimic either an intrinsic bone disease or invasion from adjacent pathologic conditions. In addition, it is not uncommon to see asymmetric sternoclavicular junction in patients over 50 years of age (4).

Anterior Group

The principal muscles of interest in this group include pectoralis major, pectoralis minor, serratus anterior, deltoid, and intercostal muscles (Fig. 25.8). Pectoralis muscle innervations originates from the C5 to C8 cervical and T1 thoracic nerves. The long thoracic nerve (C5 to C7) innervates the serratus anterior muscle. The pectoralis muscles are usually symmetric; however, they can be small on one side (Fig. 25.9) or even be absent (Fig. 25.10). Absence of the pectoralis muscles is usually congenital, presenting as a componant of Poland syndrome (9). In this syndrome, congenital muscle agenesis often affects the pectoralis major and minor muscles. Partial agenesis of the pectoralis major is most common, with complete agenesis being a rare event (10,11). History of prior surgery, particularly radical mastectomy, must be excluded. The anterior group of muscles participate in the formation of axilla, which has its own anatomic landmarks consisting of four walls: anterior, posterior, lateral, and medial (1). The anterior wall is made of pectoralis major muscle, and the posterior wall is made from subscapularis, teres minor, and latissimus dorsi muscles (see Figs. 25.8 and 25.10). The lateral wall is made of humeral bicipital groove, and the medial wall is made from upper second through the sixth ribs, and also the serratus anterior muscle. The intercostal muscles are arranged in a similar manner to the muscles of the anterior abdominal wall. Three layers of flattened muscles attach to the ribs and cartilage consisting of external, internal and inner intercostals. These costal cartilages and their muscular attachment can be quite prominent in the anterior lower thorax and the upper abdomen (Fig. 25.11).

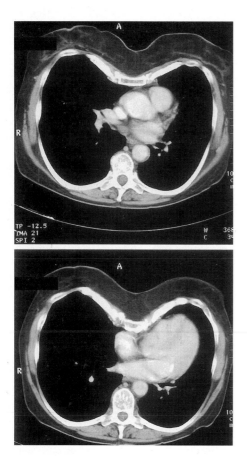

FIG. 25.7. Pectus excavatum. In this 65-year-old woman, there is a relatively severe degree of pectus excavatum.

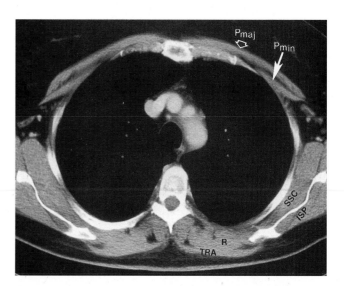

FIG. 25.8. The principal anterior group of muscles. The pectoralis major (P.maj) and pectoralis minor (P.min) are seen. Subscapularis (SSC), infraspinatus (ISP), rhomboid (R), and trapezius (TRA) muscles are also seen.

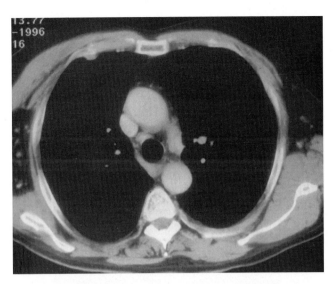

FIG. 25.9. Small left pectoralis muscles. The pectoralis muscles on the left side, particularly the pectoralis major, are remarkably smaller than those on the right side. There was no history of thoracic surgery, and this appearance was stable over many years.

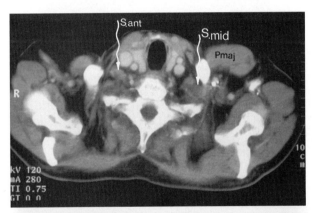

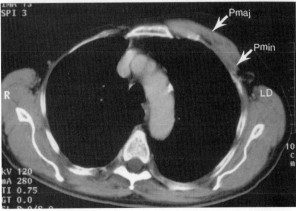

FIG. 25.10. Poland syndrome. In this patient, there is complete absence of both pectoralis muscles in the right side. Notice presence of both pectoralis major (P.maj) and minor (P.min) muscles on the left side. S.ant, anterior scanlene muscle; S.mid, middle scalenus muscle; LD, latissimus dorsi muscle.

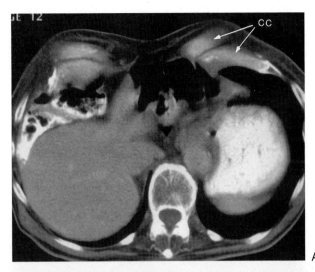

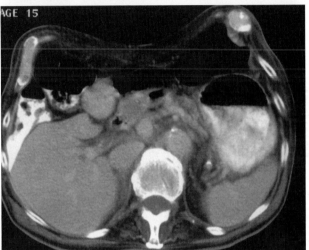

FIG. 25.11. Prominent costal cartilage. **A:** Bilateral prominence of the costochondral cartilage (CC) is seen but should not be mistaken for a mass. **B:** The costal cartilage in the left side is prominent with nodular appearance and calcification. This patient has pectus excavatum, which has resulted in continuous concavity of the upper abdominal wall.

Parascapular Group

The most anterior muscle in this group is subscapularis, which originates from the subscapular fossa. The posterior and superior groups are infraspinatus, supraspinatus, and teres minor (see Fig. 25.8). These three muscles along with the subscapularis make up the rotator cuff. The subscapularis tendon inserts on the lesser tuberosity, and the tendons of the other three muscles insert on the greater tuberosity. The teres major muscle originates from the lower lateral border of the inferior angle of the scapula. The suprascapular nerve (C5-6) innervates supra- and infraspinatus muscles, and the axillary nerve (C5) innervates the teres minor (1). The subscapularis muscle is innervated by the upper and lower subscapular nerves (C5-6). Injury to the nerve or tendon of the rotator cuff muscles can result in fatty infiltration and atrophy. One of the common findings in the

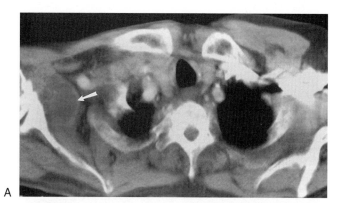

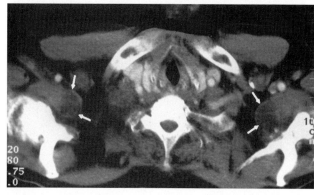

FIG. 25.12. Paralabral cyst. **A,B:** The low-density masses that are seen in the vicinity of the scapula *(arrow),* more prominent on the right (**A**), result from the presence of paralabral cysts and should not be mistaken for cystic nodes or masses.

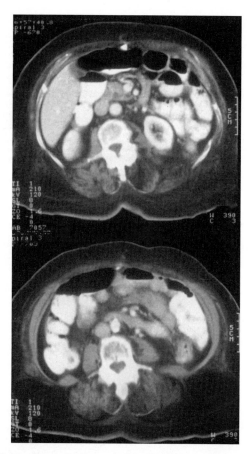

FIG. 25.13. Paraspinal muscle fatty filtration. In this patient with scoliosis, there is a significant degree of fatty infiltration in the left paraspinal muscle groups, resulting in marked asymmetry. There is also minimal atrophy of the left psoas muscle.

shoulder is paralabral ganglion, which is often associated with labral tear (12). They might be occasionally discovered on thoracic CT and should not be mistaken for necrotic nodes (Fig. 25.12). If these ganglia are in the suprascapular and spinoglenoid notches, they can lead to entrapment of the suprascapular nerve with resultant atrophy and weakness of supraspinatus or infraspinatus muscles.

Paraspinal Group

The muscles of the back are arranged in superficial, intermediate, and deep groups (see Fig. 25.8). The most superficial group acts on the upper extremity, and those of the intermediate group have a respiratory function. The deep group of muscles act in extending the spine.

The superficial group include trapezius, latissimus dorsi, levator scapulae, and rhomboid major and minor (see Figs. 25.1 and 25.8). The intermediate group includes serratus posterior. The deep group, the erector spinae muscles (from medial to lateral), consist of the multifidus, semispinalis, and longissimus. These muscles are innervated by branches from cervical, upper thoracic, and 11th cranial nerves. Asymmetry of these muscles usually results from scoliosis of the spine and is often associated with fatty infiltration (Fig. 25.13). Unilateral atrophy of latissimus dorsi muscle (Fig. 25.14) has been

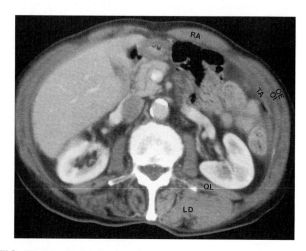

FIG. 25.14. Abdominal wall muscle groups. The major muscle groups of the abdominal wall include the rectus abdominis (RA) in the anterior portion, the external and internal oblique muscles (OE, OI) and transverse abdominis muscle (TA) in the lateral group, and, finally, the longissimus dorsi (LD) and quadratus lumborum (QL) in the posterior portion. Notice minimum fatty infiltration of the paraspinal muscle groups in the right side with smaller right rectus abdominis muscle.

described in patients with prior history of posterolateral thoracotomy (13). In such patients, atrophy can affect the serratus anterior muscle.

ABDOMEN AND PELVIS

The abdominal wall is composed of several muscles, which can be divided into three groups (2). They include the anterior group (rectus abdominis), anterolateral group (external and internal oblique muscles as well as transversus abdominis muscle), and posterior group (latissimus dorsi, quadratus lumborum, and paraspinous muscles) (5,14).

The rectus abdominis is a paired muscle that extends from the fifth to the seventh costal cartilages and xiphoid process down to the pubic bone and is innervated by the lower thoracic nerves (T6 to T12). The rectus sheath is

formed by the aponeurosis of the anterolateral group of muscles. The upper two-thirds of the sheath encloses the muscle both anteriorly and posteriorly while the lower one-third is deficient posteriorly. The rectus abdominis muscles are usually symmetric and become thinner as they descend. However, they can be asymmetric (Figs. 25.15 and 25.16) or segmented more inferiorly (see Figs. 25.16 and 25.17). The rectus abdominis muscles can be widely separated by the rectus sheet (Fig. 25.18).

The internal and external oblique muscles extend from the lower rib cage to the iliac crest and are innervated by the lower thoracic nerves (T7 to T12). On CT scan, they are seen often to be symmetric with a small amount of fat separating each muscle (see Fig. 25.14). However, like the rectus abdominis muscles, their size, configuration (Figs. 25.19 and 25.20) and symmetry can vary (Fig. 25.21). Occasionally, atrophy of the abdominal wall muscle results from surgical incisions and, therefore, are secondary to denervation injury (15–17).

The transversus abdominis muscle spans the iliac crest, thoracolumbar fascia, and undersurface of the lowest six

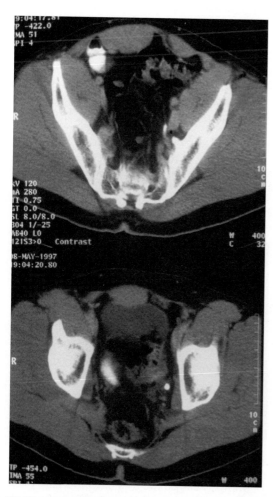

FIG. 25.15. Asymmetric rectus muscles. There is a significant difference in size of the right and left rectus abdominis muscles, the left being markedly smaller. There is no indication of atrophy of any other muscles, and there has not been any prior surgical procedure on the abdominal wall. This probably is a normal variance, and the right should not be considered pathologically enlarged.

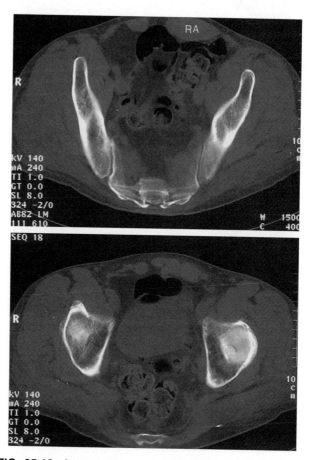

FIG. 25.16. Asymmetric rectus abdominis muscles. In this elderly patient, the right rectus abdominis is smaller than the left, and the distal aspect of the left muscle has a lobulated appearance as seen on the **lower image.** That should not be mistaken for nodes or masses.

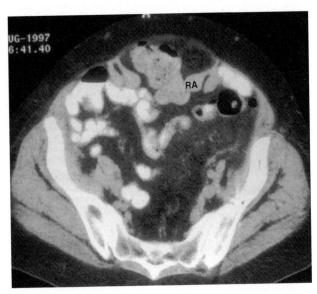

FIG. 25.17. Separation and lobulation of rectus muscles. There is marked separation of the rectus muscles, which have a lobulated appearance in the lower portion.

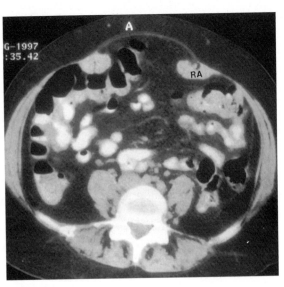

FIG. 25.18. Separated rectus muscles. There is wide separation of the two rectus muscles (RA), which are connected by a rectus sheath.

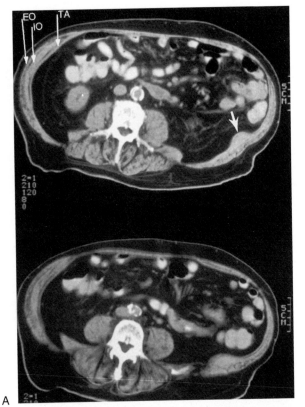

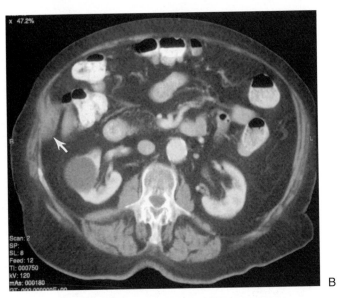

FIG. 25.19. Lobulated lateral wall muscles. **A:** The three muscles in the right side of the abdomen (external oblique, EO; internal oblique, IO; and transverse abdominis, TA) are smoothly outlined. However, on the left side, there is lobulation of the muscle *(arrow)*, which is seen on two different levels and should not be mistaken for a mass. This is a normal variation. **B:** In a different patient, this phenomenon is seen in the right side *(arrow)*.

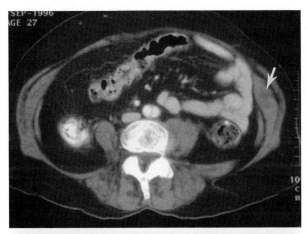

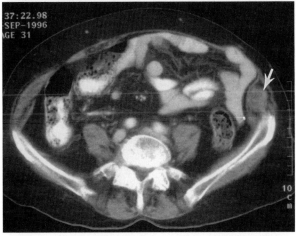

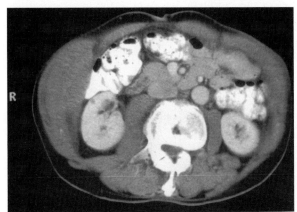

FIG. 25.20. Lobulated oblique muscle. The left internal oblique muscle is selectively prominent and lobulated, as seen on two different levels. This lobulation is particularly prominent near its inferior attachment *(arrow)* on the iliac crest. This should not be mistaken for mass.

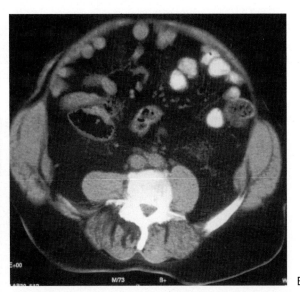

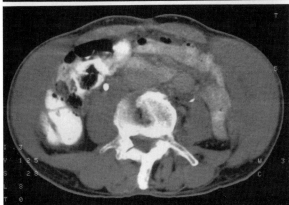

FIG. 25.21. Prominent lateral abdominal muscles. **A:** In this 68-year-old man, there is prominence of the three lateral abdominal wall muscles. This relatively symmetric prominence was noted throughout the entire length of these muscles. (The two images are 4 cm apart.) **B:** A different pattern for prominence of the oblique muscles near their inferior attachment on the iliac crests. Note that in neither of the above cases is there associated prominence of other muscular groups including the rectus abdominis or the psoas muscles. Clear fat plane between these muscles and homogeneous density rule out conditions such as hematoma or tumor infiltrate.

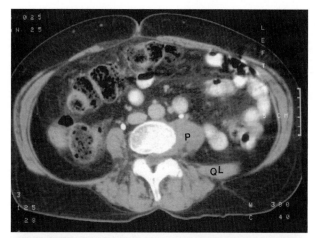

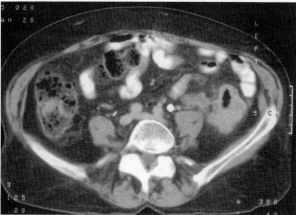

FIG. 25.22. Atrophy of paraspinal muscles. The right quadratus lumborum muscle is not seen. This muscle on the left side (QL) is normal. There is also an associated mild degree of atrophy of the right psoas muscle.

ribs. It attaches inferiorly to the pubis, forming the conjoined tendon, and is innervated by T7 to L1 nerve roots.

The paraspinous, latissimus dorsi, and quadratus lumborum muscles make the posterior abdominal group. Quadratus lumborum originate from the 12th rib and transverse processes of L1 to L4 and inserts on iliolumbar ligament and iliac crest (18). Disuse atrophy is not uncommon in these muscles and can result in marked asymmetry (Fig. 25.22). Muscle atrophy is frequently associated with fatty infiltration (Fig. 25.23) (19). These muscular changes are often seen in several unilateral conditions resulting from limited or lack of lower extremity motility such as osteoarthritis of hip or knee joint (Fig. 25.24), or in patients with lower limb amputation.

In the pelvis, the muscles of the lower abdominal wall contribute supporting the anterior and superolateral aspects of the pelvic cavity. The posterior pelvic musculature includes the gluteals (maximus, minimus, and medius), erector spinae, iliopsoas, piriformis, and obturator internus and externus muscles (Fig. 25.25).

The gluteus maximus muscle has a broad origin along the outer surface of the ilium and the iliac crest, coccyx, and sacrotuberous ligament (1,2). It inserts distally along the gluteal tuberosity of the femur and iliotibial band and is innervated by the inferior gluteal nerve (L5, S1, S2). The gluteus medius and minimus originate from the external surface of the ilium and insert on the greater trochanter. Their nerve supplies come from superior gluteal nerve (L4, L5, S1). Although these muscles are typically symmetric, they can be atrophic on one side, usually because of abnormalities of the ipsilateral hip joint or the lower extremity (Figs. 25.26–25.28). Asymmetric atrophy can be seen in one or all gluteal muscles, and, if associated with fatty infiltration, it should not be mistaken for fat-containing tumors (Fig. 25.29).

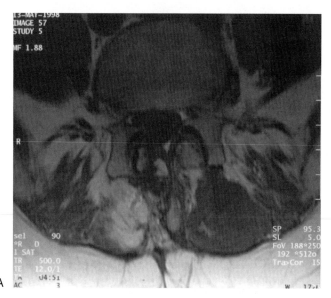

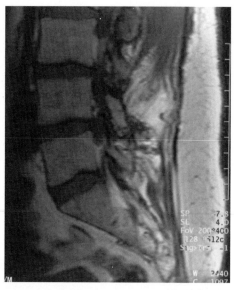

FIG. 25.23. Fatty infiltration of paraspinal muscle. **A:** There is fatty infiltration of the right paraspinal muscle as noted on this axial T1-weighted MR image (TR/TE, 500/12). **B:** The sagittal T1-weighted image shows the longitudinal extent of fatty infiltration. This patient had degenerative changes of the spine. There is minimal fatty infiltration in the left side.

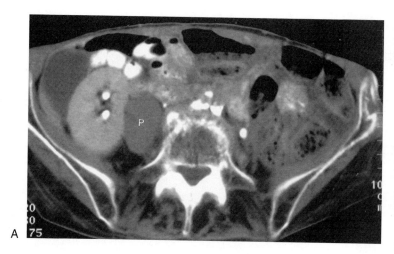

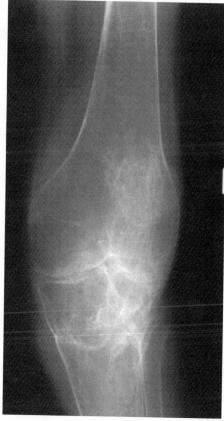

FIG. 25.24. Severe atrophy of paraspinal muscles. **A:** The CT scan at the midpelvic level shows almost complete atrophy of the left psoas muscle. The right psoas (P) is normal. There is also diffuse fatty infiltration of the paraspinal muscles. **B:** The left knee radiograph shows diffuse osteoarthritis being responsible for muscular atrophy.

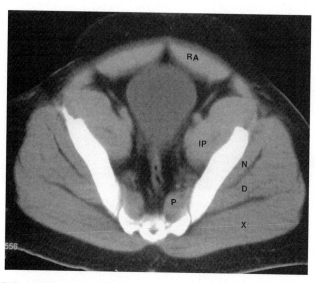

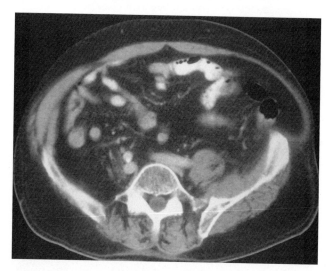

FIG. 25.25. Prominent muscular groups. There is symmetric prominence of all the muscles of the lower abdominal wall and the pelvis in this 37-year-old athletic man. The rectus abdominis (RA), iliopsoas (IP), gluteus maximus (X), gluteus medius (D), gluteus minimus (N), and piriformis (P) muscles are all prominent.

FIG. 25.26. Atrophy of the left muscle groups. There is almost complete atrophy of the right gluteal as well as the iliacus and psoas muscles. There is some degree of fatty infiltration of the right psoas muscle. Interestingly, the oblique muscles are also asymmetric, with the left side being atrophic. This patient had amputation of the right foot because of the diabetes.

The psoas major is a fusiform muscle that arises from the transverse processes of T12 and the upper four or five lumbar vertebrae (20,21), descends lateral to the lumbar spine and along the anterior margin of the pelvic brim, and, after merging with iliacus muscle, it passes underneath the inguinal ligament to insert on the lesser trochanter of the femur (22–24). The size of the psoas muscles depends on the patient's age and degree of physical activity (see Fig. 25.25), but it attains its greatest bulk in the L5 to S1 region. In those areas in which the psoas assumes a somewhat rounded configuration (L3 to S1), a potential recess is formed between the

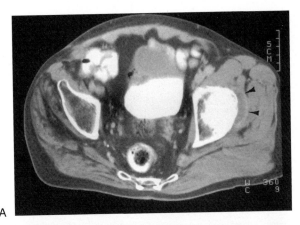

A

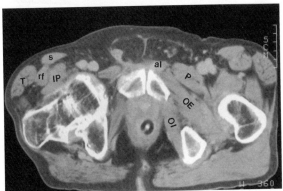

B

FIG. 25.27. Muscle atrophy caused by degenerative hip disease. There is a mild degree of atrophy of the right pelvic muscles caused by degenerative joint disease involving the right hip, which is associated with subluxation. Notice the atrophy of the right obturator internus (OI), obturator externus (OE), pectineus (p), abductor longus (AL), iliopsoas (IP), sartorius (S), rectus femoris (RF), and tensor of fascia lata (T). There is prominence of the left trochanteric bursa on the upper image (arrowheads). Also, the gluteal muscles in the right side are all atrophic with fatty infiltration.

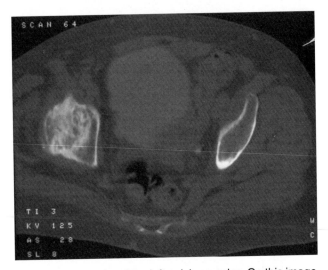

FIG. 25.28. Atrophy of the left pelvic muscles. On this image with bony windows, a significant degree of osteoarthritis of the right hip is noted along with diffuse atrophy of the surrounding muscles.

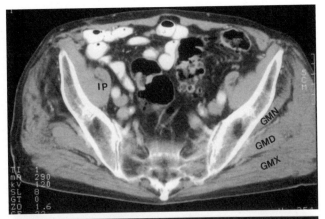

A

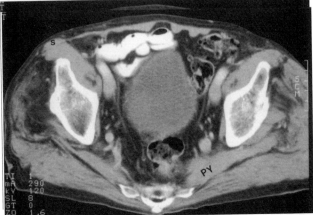

B

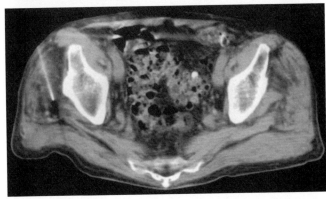

C

FIG. 25.29. Fatty infiltration mimicking tumor. **A,B:** Two images of the pelvis reveal diffuse fatty infiltration of the right gluteus medius and minimus muscles. The normal gluteal muscles on the left (gluteus maximus, GMX; gluteus midius, GMD; and gluteus minimus, GMN) are seen along with piriformis (P), ileopsoas (IPip), and sartorius (S) muscles. This fatty infiltration in the right side along with the patient's pain was misinterpreted as tumor, and to rule out a liposarcoma, a biopsy was done. **C:** A needle biopsy of the right fatty infiltrated gluteal muscles revealed normal fat and muscle fibers, and there was no indication of neoplasm.

psoas muscle anteriorly and the more posterior quadratus lumborum, or the iliacus, more inferiorly. In the majority of individuals, this potential recess is filled with fat within the posterior pararenal space. However, in individuals with very little retroperitoneal fat, the peritoneal cavity may extend posteromedially into this space forming the retropsoas recess (21). The small bowel can invaginate into the space. The iliacus muscle, which arises in the iliac fossa, descends along the lateral edge of the psoas muscle. It is innervated by branches of the upper four lumbar nerves. Because the psoas passes beneath the arcuate ligament of the diaphragm superiorly (see Chapter 5), there is a potential channel from the mediastinum to the thigh (23). Atrophy of the psoas muscle is encountered in adults with hip surgery (Fig. 25.30) or osteoarthritis (see Figs. 25.24 and 25.31). When it is completely atrophic, the normal or the atrophic muscle should not be mistaken for a mass (see Figs. 25.24 and 25.30). Various degrees of fatty infiltration can also occur in the psoas muscle, which can be a source of diagnostic pitfalls (Fig. 25.32).

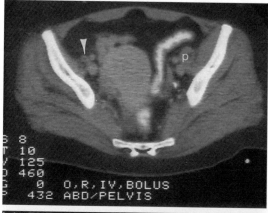

FIG. 25.30. Psoas atrophy. This patient, who had above-knee amputation 5 months earlier, reveals a very small right psoas muscle (P). This atrophic psoas muscle should not be mistaken for a lymph node.

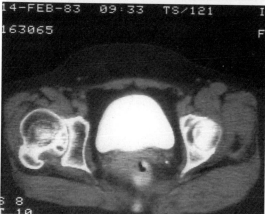

FIG. 25.31. Atrophy of the right psoas muscle. In these two images, the osteoarthritis of the right hip joint is seen as the cause of a very small right psoas muscle seen on the **upper image** (arrowhead). The normal left psoas muscle is seen (P).

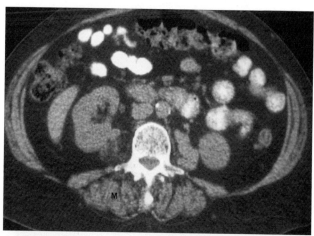

A

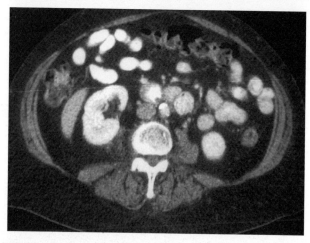

B

FIG. 25.32. Fatty infiltration of the psoas muscle. **A:** On this unenhanced CT scan, the right psoas muscle has fatty infiltration; initially it was thought to represent an exophytic fat-containing right renal mass. **B:** The contrast-enhanced CT reveals the normal right kidney and sharp delineation between that and the fatty infiltrated right psoas muscle.

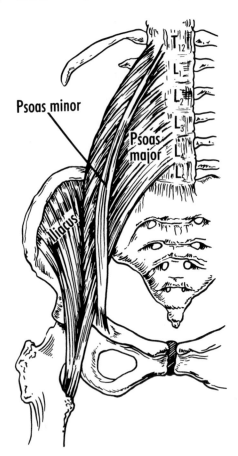

The psoas minor arises from the lateral aspect of T12 and L1 vertebrae and lies immediately anterior to the psoas major (25). However, it rapidly turns into a long flattened tendon that inserts on the iliopectineal eminence (Fig. 25.33). This muscle can be seen on one or in both sides (Figs. 25.34—25.36) and is present in approximately 40% of individuals. On CT images, occasionally it is seen on only a few axial images separate from psoas major and can be mistaken for a retroperitoneal node (Figs. 25.37 and 25.38).

The piriformis muscle arises from the anterior surface of the sacrum and sacrotuberous ligament (see Fig. 25.25) and inserts on the greater trochanter. Diagnostic pitfalls related to this muscle are generally related to its asymmetric appearance on axial images (Fig. 25.39). This can result from the patient's positioning within the CT gantry (Fig. 25.40) or unilateral atrophy of the muscle (Fig. 25.41).

The obturator internus muscle arises from the entire inner surface of the obturator foramen and inserts on the medial surface of the greater trochanter. These muscles are usually symmetric and can be large particularly in athletes (Fig. 25.42).

FIG. 25.33. Drawing of the psoas muscles. The right psoas minor is seen extending from the lateral aspect of T12 down to its inferior attachment on the iliopectineal eminence. It lies anterior to the psoas major.

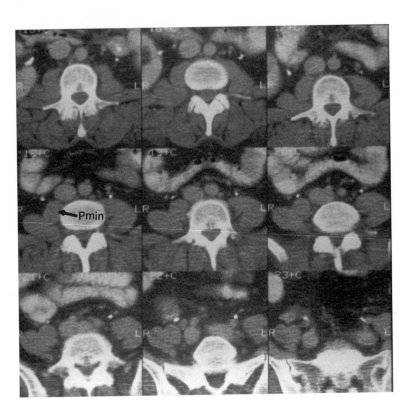

FIG. 25.34. Psoas minor. Nine sequential images of the lower lumbar spine reveal presence of right psoas minor (Pmin), which lies anterior to the right psoas major. The left psoas minor, except for its most proximal portion, is not well seen on the lower images.

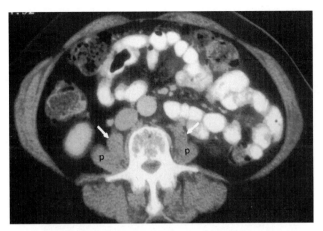

FIG. 25.35. Bilateral psoas minor. The psoas minors are seen as prominent muscles in both sides *(white arrows)*, which are lying anterior to the psoas major (P).

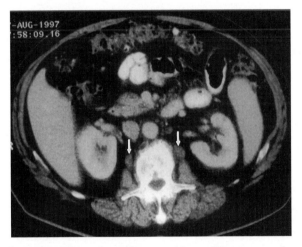

FIG. 25.36. Bilateral small psoas minors. The psoas minors in this patient *(white arrows)* are quite separate from the psoas majors and should not be mistaken for adenopathy.

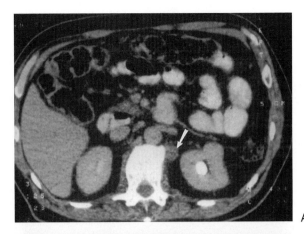

A

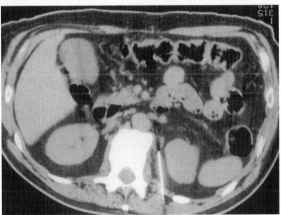

B

FIG. 25.38. Psoas minor mimicking node. **A:** This patient with a history of bladder carcinoma was thought to have a left-sided lymph node *(white arrow)* just below the level of the left renal vein. **B:** Biopsy was done by posterior approach and revealed muscle fibers. Retrospective analysis of the images showed that the left psoas minor appeared prominent at its most superior attachment and then blended into the psoas major on the inferior images.

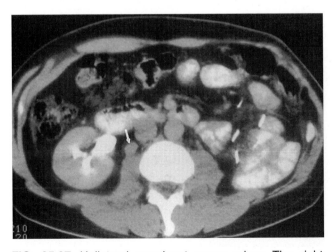

FIG. 25.37. Unilateral prominent psoas minor. The right psoas minor *(white arrows)* is prominent and somehow separate from the psoas major. In this patient with prior left nephrectomy, it should not be mistaken for a node.

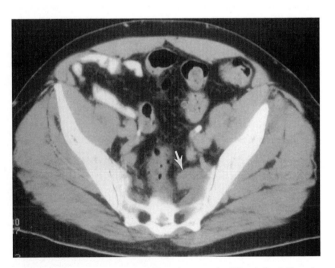

FIG. 25.39. Asymmetric piriformis muscle. The left piriformis muscle *(arrow)* is slightly more prominent on its superior attachment on the sacrum. This should not be mistaken for a mass or node.

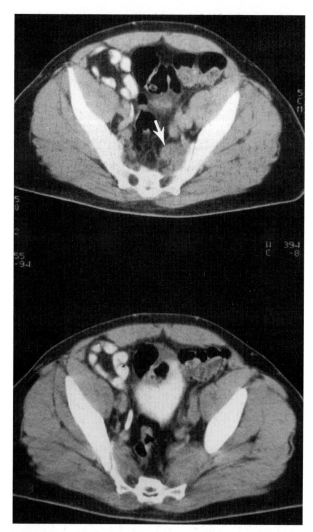

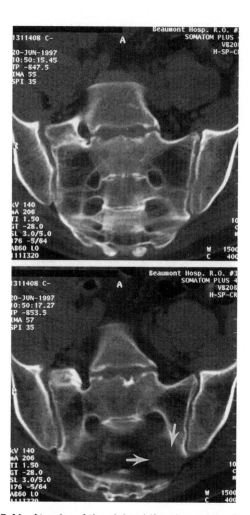

FIG. 25.40. Apparent prominence of piriformis as a result of positioning. This patient, who is not symmetrically positioned within the CT gantry, shows the left piriformis muscle *(arrow)* apparently more prominent than the right one. This is a normal variation.

FIG. 25.41. Atrophy of the right piriformis muscle. On these images, which were obtained in an oblique coronal plane for evaluation of sacrum, the left piriformis muscle *(arrows)* appears to be slightly more prominent, mimicking a mass in the midsacrum. Axial images show a moderate degree of atrophy of the right piriformis and a normal left side.

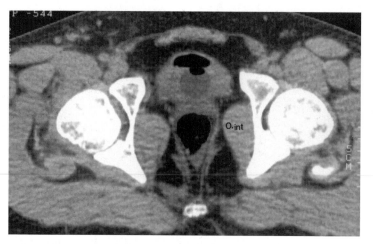

FIG. 25.42. Prominent obturator muscles. There is significant prominence of the obturator internus (O.int), which is noted on both sides.

Trochanteric and Iliopsoas Bursa

There are three bursae around the greater trochanter of the femur. The gluteus medius and minimus bursae separate the tendons of these muscles from the greater trochanter anteriorly, and the gluteus maximus bursa is a large bursa separating this muscle from the greater trochanter posteriorly. A nondistended bursa is not seen on CT images. Bursal distention is seen in patients with bursitis (Fig. 25.43), but it can also be present in asymptomatic patients (26). In such cases, it should not be mistaken with cystic neoplasm, lymphadenopathy, hematoma, abscess or lymphocele (27).

The iliopsoas bursa is the largest bursa around the hip joint and is located beneath the musculotendinous portion of the iliopsoas muscle in front of the hip joint and lateral to the femoral vessels (Fig. 25.44 and 25.45) (14,26). On CT or MRI, distension of iliopsoas bursa can mimic inguinal or femoral hernia, neoplasm, nodes, hematoma, abscess, or aneurysm (Fig. 25.46).

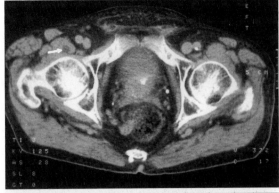

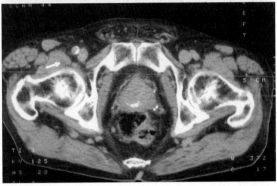

FIG. 25.44. Prominent right iliopsoas bursa. **A,B:** In this patient, there is a well-defined low-density area *(arrows)* posterior to the right iliopsoas muscle. This is one of the manifestations of iliopsoas bursa containing fluid. This patient did not have any symptoms related to the hips.

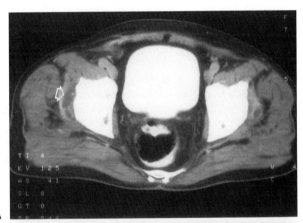

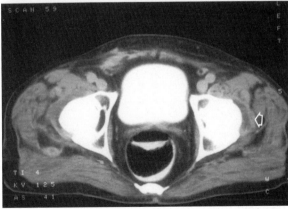

FIG. 25.43. A,B: Trochanteric bursa. There is indication of distention of bilateral trochanteric bursa *(open arrows).* This patient did have hip pain, and there is slight enhancement of the bursa, probably because of underlying bursitis.

FIG. 25.45. A,B: Prominent and lobulated left iliopsoas bursa. The iliopsoas bursa is markedly prominent on the left side. Typically, this is located behind the femoral vessels and posterior or medial to the iliopsoas muscles.

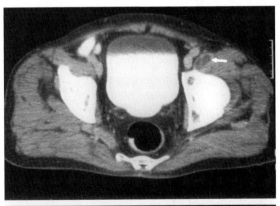

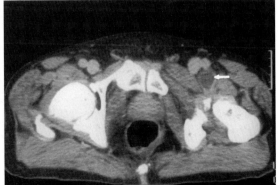

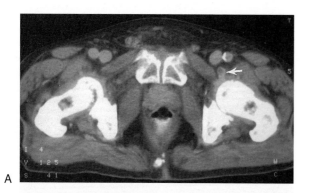

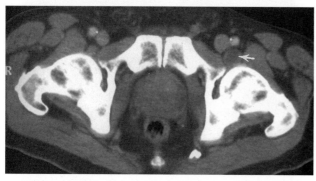

FIG. 25.46. Prominent iliopsoas bursa. **A:** The thick-walled left iliopsoas bursa *(arrow)* should not be mistaken for a necrotic lymph node. **B:** At the lower level, the left iliopsoas bursa is seen as a more prominent cystic structure *(arrow).*

REFERENCES

1. Clemente CD. *Anatomy, a regional atlas of the human body, 4th ed.* Baltimore: Williams & Wilkins, 1997.
2. Basmajian JV, Slonecker CE. *Grant's method of anatomy: a clinical problem solving approach, 11th ed.* Baltimore: Williams & Wilkins, 1989.
3. Gosselin MV, Rubin GD. Altered intravascular contrast material flow dynamics: Clues for refining thoracic CT diagnosis. *Am J Roentgenol* 1997;169:1597–1603.
4. Goodman LR, Teplick SK, Kay H. Computed tomography of the normal sternum. *Am J Roentgenol* 1983;141:219–223.
5. Stark P. Midline sternal foramen: CT demonstration. *J Comput Assist Tomogr* 1985;9(3):489–490.
6. Stark P, Watkins Ge, Hildebrandt-Stark HE, Dunbar RD. Episternal ossicles. *Radiology* 1987;165:143–144.
7. Stark P, Jaramillo D. CT of the sternum. *Am J Roentgenol* 1986;147:72–77.
8. Hatfield MK, Gross BH, Glazer GM, Martel W. Computed tomography of the sternum and its articulation. *Skel Radiol* 1984;11:197–203.
9. Perez-Aznar JM, Urbano J, Laborda EG, et al. Breast and pectoralis muscle hypoplasia: a mild degree of Poland's syndrome. *Acta Radiol* 1996;37:759–762.
10. Hodgkinson DJ. Chest wall implants: their use for pectus excavatum, pectoralis muscle tears, Poland's syndrome and muscular insufficiency. *Aesth Plast Surg* 1997;21:7–15.
11. Wright AR, Milner LH, Bainbridge C, et al. MR and CT in the assessment of Poland syndrome. *J Comput Assist Tomogr* 1992;16:442–445.
12. Steiner E, Steinbach LS, Schnarkowski P. Ganglia and cysts around joints. *Radiol Clin North Am* 1996;34:395–425.
13. Goodman P, Balachandran S, Guinto FC Jr. Postoperative atrophy of posterolateral chest wall musculature: CT demonstration. *J Comput Assist Tomogr* 1993;17(1):63–66.
14. Varma DG, Richli WR, Charnsangavej C, Samuels B, Kim EE, Wallace S. MR appearance of the distended iliopsoas bursa. *Am J Roentgenol* 1991;156:1025–1028.
15. Goodman P, Balachandran S. CT evaluation of the abdominal wall. *Crit Rev Diag Imag* 1992;33:461–493.
16. Shirkhoda A. Postsurgical anatomic variations and diagnostic pitfalls in abdominal and pelvic computed tomography. *Postgrad Radiol* 1996;16:59–71.
17. Goodman P, Balachandran S. Postoperative atrophy of abdominal wall musculature: CT demonstration. *J Comput Assist Tomogr* 1991;15(6):989–993.
18. Wechsler RJ. *Cross-sectional analysis of the chest and abdominal wall.* St. Louis: CV Mosby, 1989.
19. Hadar H, Gadoth N, Heifetz M. Fatty replacement of lower paraspinal muscles: Normal and neuromuscular disorders. *Am J Roentgenol* 1983;141:895–898.
20. King AD, Hine AL, Abrahams P. The ultrasound appearance of the normal psoas muscle. *Clin Radiol* 1993;48:316–318.
21. Kelly RB, Mahoney PD, Frick MP. The retropsoas recess: demonstration using computed tomography. *Invest Radiol* 1987;22:550–555.
22. Donovan PJ, Zerhouni EA, Siegelman SS. CT of the psoas compartment of the retroperitoneum. *Seminars in Roent* 1986;16:241–250.
23. Feldberg MA, Koehler PB, Van Waes PF. Psoas compartment disease studied by computed tomography. *Radiology* 1983;148:505–512.
24. Lenchik L, Dovgan DJ, Kier R. CT of the iliopsoas compartment: valve in differentiating tumor, abscess, and hematoma. *Am J Roentgenol* 1994;162:83–86.
25. Fritz RC, Helms CA, Steinbaach LS, et al. Suprascapular nerve entrapment: Evaluation with MR imaging. *Radiology* 1992;182:437.
26. Peters JC, Coleman BG, Turner ML, et al. CT evaluation of enlarged iliopsoas bursa. *Am J Roentgenol* 1980;135:392–394.
27. Varma DG, Parihar A, Richli WR. CT appearance of the distended trochanteric bursa. *J Comput Assist Tomogr* 1993;17:141–143.

Variants and Pitfalls in Body Imaging,
edited by Ali Shirkhoda.
Lippincott Williams & Wilkins, Philadelphia, © 2000.

CHAPTER 26

The Thoracoabdominal and Pelvic Musculoskeleton in Pediatrics

Alexander A. Cacciarelli and Donald P. Gibson

Until the pediatric musculoskeletal system reaches adult maturity, there exist a number of normal anatomic developments and variations that may be confused with pathology. We have assembled these normal findings in atlas form to be used as a reference when one is reviewing pediatric body computed tomography (CT) imaging.

This material has been collected from patients undergoing CT imaging for various reasons that primarily include trauma, abdominal pain, and oncologic follow-up. Clinical information as well as anatomic and embryologic references are included where necessary.

THE SPINE

The Neurocentral Synchondrosis

This developmental variant can be explained by understanding the embryology of the vertebrae (1). The centrum, which encloses the notochord and gives rise to the main portion of the vertebral body, is separated from the adjacent neural arch on each side by the neurocentral growth cartilage. Although progressive ossification and fusion occur in infancy, remnants of the neurocentral synchondrosis can be seen as oblique symmetric lucencies at the vertebral body/pedicular junction. These lucencies can be seen even in older children and may have a sclerotic border (Figs. 26.1–26.3).

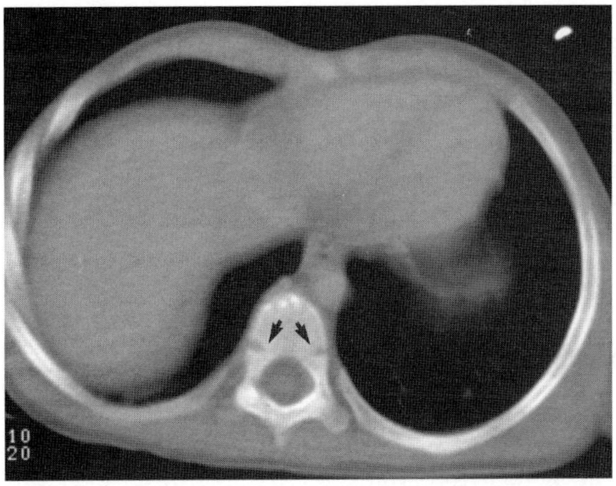

A. A. Cacciarelli and D. P. Gibson: Department of Diagnostic Radiology, William Beaumont Hospital, Royal Oak, Michigan 48073-6769.

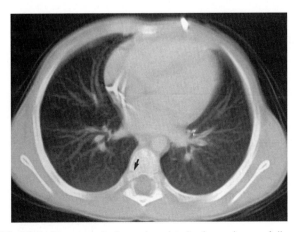

FIG. 26.1. Neurocentral synchondrosis. Abdominal CT scan of a 4-year-old boy who fell two stories. The neurocentral synchondrosis *(arrows)* could be seen in multiple vertebrae.

FIG. 26.2. Neurocentral synchondrosis *(arrow)* on a follow-up CT scan in a 3-year old girl with a previous abdominal neuroblastoma.

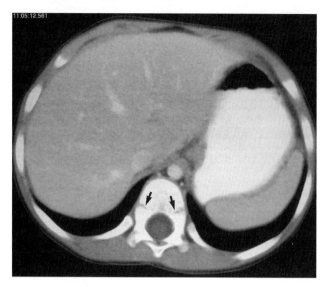

FIG. 26.3. Neurocentral synchondrosis *(arrows)* in a 4-year-old boy being evaluated for an abdominal mass.

The Posterior Vertebral Body Vascular Channel

An area of decreased attenuation can be seen in the posterior aspect of vertebral bodies related to the entrance and exit of nutrient arteries and veins (2). These areas can mimic a lytic vertebral body lesion (Fig. 26.4).

The Epidural Venous Plexus

The epidural space contains fatty areolar tissue, which contains a rich venous plexus (3). The lower attenuation of the fatty tissue allows these veins to be seen and to mimic mass lesions in the spinal canal. They enhance with intravenous contrast similar to other surrounding vascular structures (Fig. 26.5).

The Sacral Segments Synchondrosis

Maturation of the sacrum and coccyx is a complex process that has been well described (4). It involves the fusion of 50 to 60 sacral and eight coccygeal ossification centers and may not be complete until age 30. Fusion of the growth plates between these ossification centers can be asymmetric and mimic fracture lines during cross-sectional imaging (Figs. 26.6—26.8).

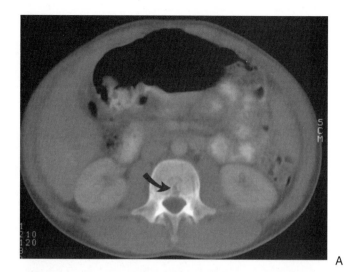

A

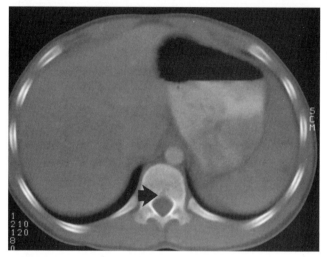

B

FIG. 26.4. Normal vascular channel. Posterior vertebral body vascular channel *(arrows)* in a 13-year-old boy who was evaluated for splenic trauma.

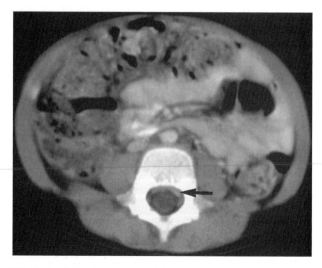

FIG. 26.5. Epidural venous plexus *(arrow)* in a 3-year-old girl who was previously treated for an adrenal neuroblastoma.

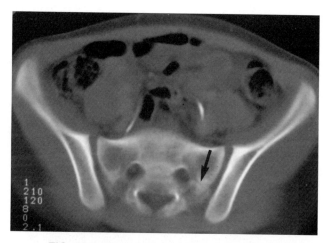
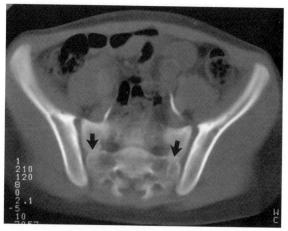

FIG. 26.6. Sacral segment synchondrosis in a 9-year-old boy who sustained blunt abdominal trauma. **A:** Growth plate *(arrow)* between sacral alar ossification centers mimics a fracture line. **B:** Growth plate *(arrows)* between sacral centrum ossification centers.

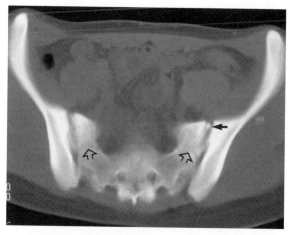
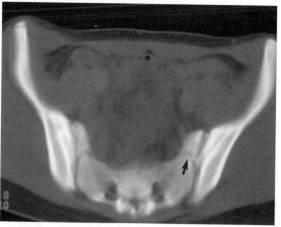

FIG. 26.7. Sacral segment synchondrosis in a 14-year-old girl who was involved in a motor vehicle accident. **A:** Growth plate *(open arrows)* between sacral centrum ossification centers. Also shown is an anterior costal ossification center *(arrow)*. **B:** Growth plate *(arrow)* between sacral alar ossification centers.

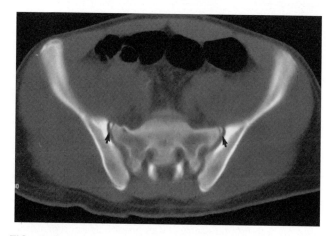

FIG. 26.8. Sacral ossification center. Sacral anterior costal ossification center *(arrows)* in a 17-year-old girl who sustained abdominal trauma.

THE CHEST

Paired Sternal Ossification Centers

There is wide variation in the number and pattern of sternal ossification centers. Ossification centers in the third and fourth sternal segments are often paired (5,6). Failure of fusion of these paired centers may result in varying degrees of sternal cleft and midline foramina later in life (7) (Fig. 26.9).

Normal Dense Humeral Head Ossification

The proximal humeral physeal line is formed by the junction of ossification centers of the greater tuberosity and the humeral head with the main shaft of the humerus.

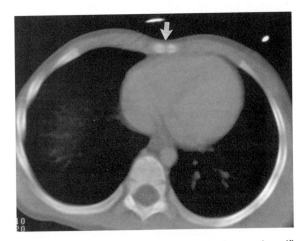

FIG. 26.9. Sternal ossification center. Paired sternal ossification centers *(arrow)* in a 4-year-old girl with a history of trauma.

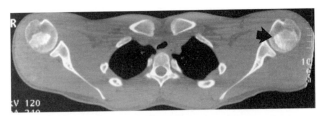

FIG 26.10. Physeal lines. Normal fused proximal humeral physeal lines *(arrows)* mimicking blastic bone lesion in a 15-year-old boy being evaluated for shoulder pain.

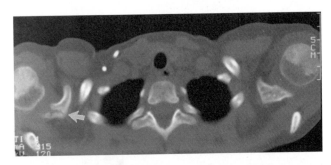

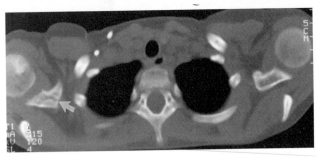

FIG. 26.11. Coracoid synchondrosis. Synchondrosis *(arrows)* at the base of the coracoid process simulating a fracture in an 8-year-old girl who had this CT scan as a follow-up after treatment for an abdominal neoplasm.

This closed physeal line in older adolescents can mimic a blastic lesion of bone (8) (Fig. 26.10).

Synchondrosis at the Base of the Coracoid Process

The junction of the base of the coracoid secondary ossification center with the remainder of the scapula produces a synchondrosis that may simulate a fracture on plain films and CT scans (9,10) (Fig. 26.11). Symmetry and comparison with the opposite side aid in correct interpretation.

Anomalous First Rib Articulations

Congenital anomalous first rib articulations may simulate acute or healing fractures (Fig. 26.12). Symmetry and lack of supportive history and physical findings as well as lack of new bone formation or change on follow-up imaging studies will confirm the congenital nature of these findings. The appearance of these articulations may be smooth and corticated or irregular, sclerotic, and fragmented (11).

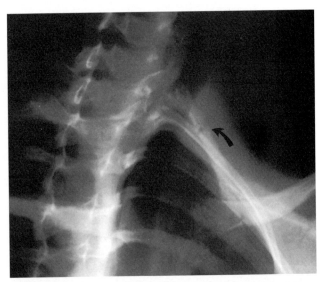

A

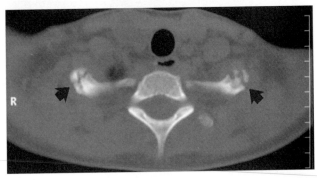

B

FIG. 26.12. Rib synchondrosis. **A:** Plain film from a rib exam on a 13-year-old female gymnast with back pain. A lucent area on both first ribs *(arrow)* was previously seen bilaterally on spine x-rays. **B:** A CT scan of the same patient 3 weeks later showed the lucent lines bilaterally *(arrows)*. Follow-up plain films at that time and 3 months later showed no change and no evidence of periosteal new bone formation.

Prominent Rhomboid Fossae

Rhomboid fossae are broad areas of depression on the medial aspect of the clavicles (Fig. 26.13). These fossae represent the insertion of the costoclavicular ligament (rhomboid ligament). These depressions may be signifi-cantly asymmetric and can mimic a destructive process in the medial aspect of the clavicle (12,13).

THE PELVIS

Wide-Appearing Sacroiliac Joints in the Pediatric Patient

Compared to the adult patient, the normal sacroiliac joint in children appears relatively wider. This apparent widening can simulate traumatic diastasis. Symmetry, the lack of associated pelvic fractures elsewhere, the lack of soft tissue hematoma, and clinical history all aid in cor-rect interpretation (Figs. 26.14 and 26.15).

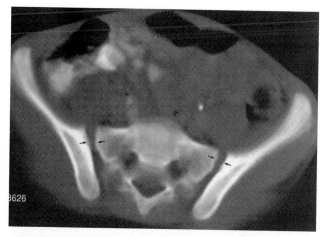

FIG. 26.14. Sacroiliac joint variant in a child. Normal rela-tively wide appearing sacroiliac joints *(arrows)* in a CT scan of a 9-year-old boy who sustained a splenic contusion.

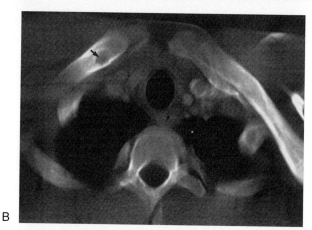

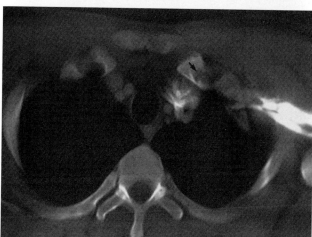

FIG. 26.13. Rhomboid fossa. Computed tomography scan of a 20-year-old man who is being followed for metastatic dis-ease from a previously resected synovial sarcoma. The CT scan of the chest with soft tissue **(A)** and bone windows **(B, C)** shows prominent rhomboid fossae mimicking a destruc-tive process in the medial aspect of the clavicles *(arrows)*.

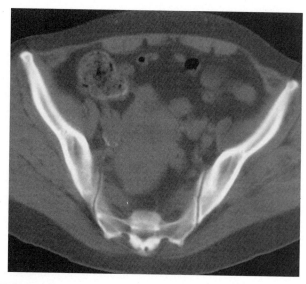

FIG. 26.15. Normal SI joint in an adult. Computed tomogra-phy scan of a 55-year-old adult for comparison. The normal sacroiliac joints appear relatively narrower.

Secondary Ossification Centers of the Pelvis

Secondary ossification centers for the iliac crest (Fig. 26.16) and the ischial tuberosity (Fig. 26.17) appear about puberty and fuse with the primary bone between the age of 15 and 25 years (14). Before fusion, these centers can mimic avulsion fractures. Symmetry in general is helpful in excluding fractures.

Acetabular roof (Figs. 26.18—26.20) and acetabular rim (Figs. 26.21—26.23) ossifications appear around 8 to 9 years of age. During puberty, these centers expand and produce irregular areas of ossification in the acetabulum, which may simulate fractures on axial imaging. Fusion between these centers occurs between 16 and 18 years (14).

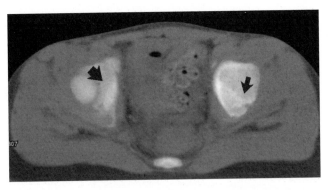

FIG. 26.18. Acetabular ossification center. Computed tomography scan through the acetabular roofs in a 5-year-old girl who fell 10 feet. Injury was primarily to the head and neck. Note normal irregular ossification in acetabular roofs simulating fractures *(arrows)*.

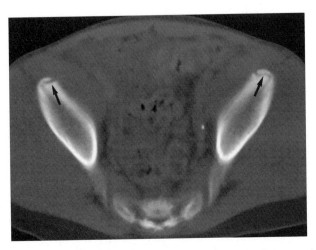

FIG. 26.16. Iliac secondary ossification centers. Computed tomography scan of a 13-year-old boy with a splenic laceration. Iliac secondary ossification centers appear on symmetric separate ossifications *(arrows)*.

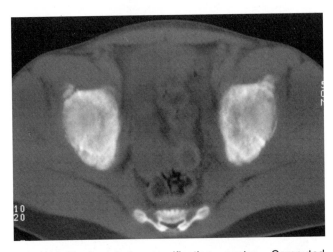

FIG. 26.19. Acetabular ossification center. Computed tomography scan of a 13-year-old boy with blunt abdominal trauma. Note irregular normal acetabular roof ossification similar to Fig. 26.18.

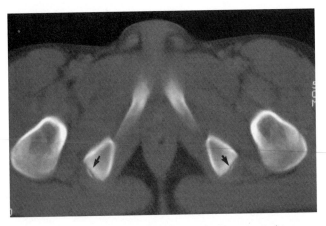

FIG. 26.17. Ischial apophysis. Computed tomography scan of another 13-year-old boy with abdominal trauma. Ischial apophyses also appear symmetric *(arrow)*.

The Acetabular Notch

A central mild depression in the inferior acetabular ossification (the acetabular notch) is seen normally on cross-sectional imaging of the pelvis (14,15) (Fig. 26.24). This depression is symmetric and should not be mistaken for a depressed fracture segment. This anatomic finding is also seen in adults.

Cartilaginous Growth Plates

The triradiate cartilage originates from the junction of the ossification centers for the ilium, ischium, and pubis. This junction produces a Y-shaped cartilage in the medial acetabulum (14). This cartilaginous plate is typically obliterated between 16 and 18 years of age. Before this

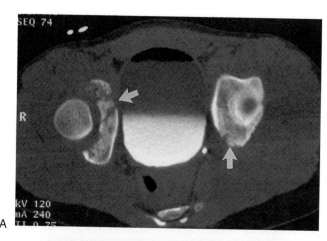

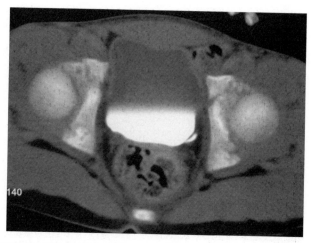

FIG. 26.22. Acetabular rim ossifications. Pelvic CT of a 9-year-old boy who had abdominal trauma. Note normal irregular anterior and posterior acetabular rim ossifications.

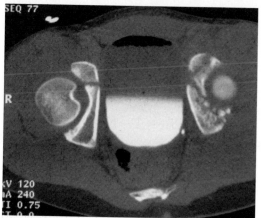

FIG. 26.20. A,B: Acetabular pseudofracture. Pelvic CT scans of an 11-year-old boy who was hit by a car and sustained a femoral shaft fracture. Note irregular ossification of acetabular roofs *(arrows)*, which is a normal finding. There was no evidence of any pelvic fractures.

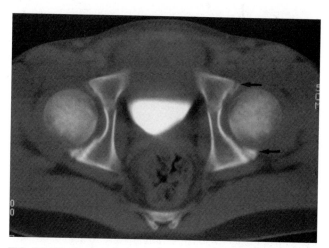

FIG. 26.23. Acetabular pseudofracture. Computed tomography scan through the acetabulum of a 13-year-old boy with abdominal trauma. Anterior and posterior acetabular rim ossifications *(arrows)* mimic fractures.

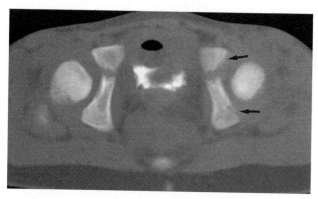

FIG. 26.21. Acetabular rim ossifications. Pelvic CT of a 5-year-old girl. Note normal early anterior and posterior secondary acetabular rim ossifications *(arrows)*.

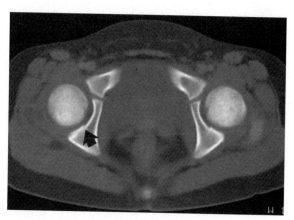

FIG 26.24. Acetabular pseudofracture. Pelvic CT of an 8-year-old girl being followed for a neuroblastoma. Note the symmetric notched appearance to the acetabulum *(arrow)* simulating the step-off of a depressed fracture.

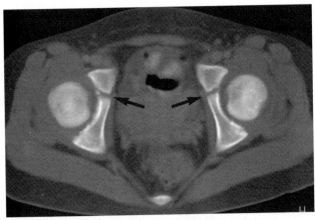

FIG. 26.25. Triradiate cartilage. Pelvic CT of the same patient as in Fig. 26.24. Note normal triradiate cartilage growth plates *(arrows)*.

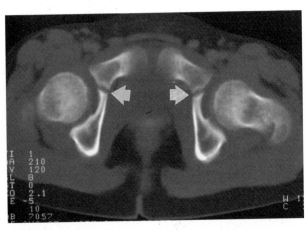

FIG. 26.26. Triradiate cartilage. A 9-year-old boy who had CT scan for blunt abdominal trauma. Note triradiate cartilage growth plates *(arrows)*.

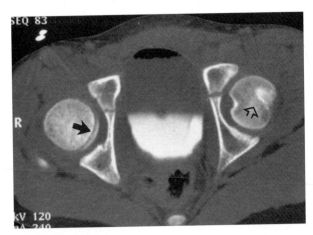

FIG. 26.27. Femoral head pseudofracture. Computed tomography scan through the hips of an 11-year-old boy. The patient is positioned asymmetrically in the scanner. Note the physeal plate on the patient's right simulating a fracture line *(arrow)* and on the patient's left simulating a blastic lesion *(open arrow)*.

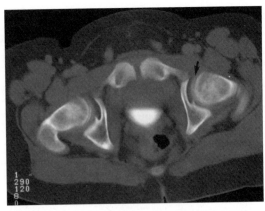

FIG. 26.28. Femoral physeal line. Computed tomography scan of a 13-year-old boy where the proximal femoral physeal line on the patient's left also simulates a fracture *(arrow)*. However, the appearance on the right is more easily recognizable as the physis.

point it should be recognized as a normal structure and not mistaken for a fracture (Figs. 26.25 and 26.26).

The femoral head ossification center appears in the first year of life and enlarges so that during puberty a radiographically apparent physeal line is formed at the junction with the femoral shaft and neck ossification. This physis closes around the 18th or 19th year of life (16). Before this closure, the physeal line can mimic a fracture on axial scans. Also axial scans tangential to the physeal line may produce an apparent sclerotic area mimicking a blastic lesion of the femoral head (Figs. 26.27 and 26.28).

A secondary ossification center appears for the greater trochanter of the femur during the fourth year of life and for the lesser trochanter during puberty. These centers unite with the shaft of the femur around 18 to 19 years of age (16). Although avulsion fractures can occur at these centers (17), the normal growth plates (Figs. 26.29–26.31) should not be mistaken for fractures.

The ischiopubic synchondrosis occurs at the junction of the ischial and pubic ossifications in the inferior pubic

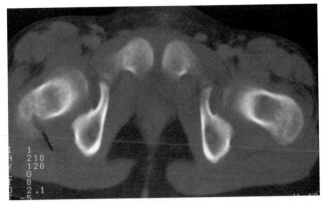

FIG. 26.29. Femoral neck pseudofracture. Cartilaginous plate *(arrow)* separating the greater trochanteric ossification from the femoral shaft mimicking fracture in a CT of a 9-year-old boy.

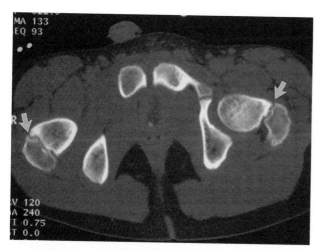

FIG. 26.30. Normal femoral cartilaginous plates. Cartilaginous plate *(arrows)* separating the greater trochanter in an 11-year-old boy.

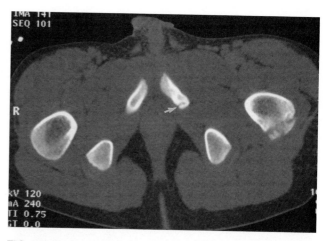

FIG. 26.33. Ischiopubic synchondrosis. Normal asymmetric fusion of the ischiopubic synchondrosis (with the left side unfused) simulating a lytic area *(arrow)*. The CT scan is of an 11-year-old boy with abdominal trauma.

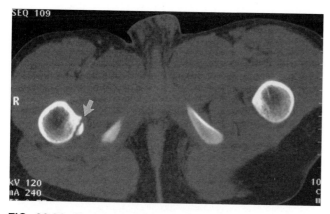

FIG. 26.31. Pseudofracture of the femoral neck. Cartilaginous plate *(arrow)* separating the lesser trochanter from the femoral shaft in an 11-year-old boy. The plane of the scan is not symmetric.

ramus. Fusion to form a continuous ramus occurs at the seventh or eighth year (14). Before fusion, a well-defined line can be seen at the synchondrosis on axial imaging (Fig. 26.32). Asymmetric fusion of this synchondrosis occurs (18) and may simulate a lytic lesion with surrounding sclerosis (Fig. 26.33).

The Fovea of the Femoral Head

The fovea is a small depression posteroinferior to the center of the femoral head articular surface. The ligament of the femoral head is attached to the fovea (19). This depression can be mistaken for an area of osteochondritis or a lytic lesion in the femoral head (Fig. 26.34).

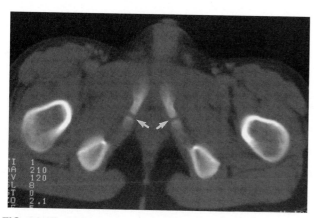

FIG. 26.32. Ischiopubic synchondrosis. Normal, symmetric, unfused ischiopubic synchondrosis *(arrows)* on a CT scan of a 9-year-old boy.

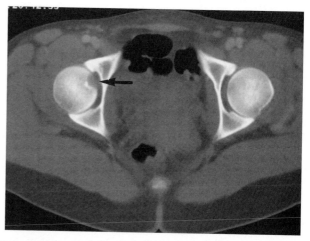

FIG. 26.34. Femoral head fovea. Pelvic CT of a 16-year-old girl who was in a motor vehicle accident. The normal fovea of the right femoral head *(arrow)* seen here can be mistaken for a lytic lesion or area of osteochondritis dissecans, especially when the plane of the scan is not symmetric, as in this case.

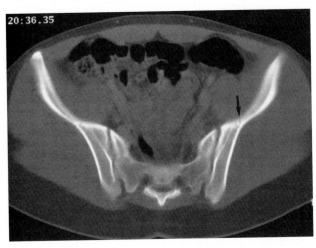

FIG. 26.35. Iliac pseudofracture. Normal vascular channel in the middle of the left iliac bone *(arrow)* in a 16-year-old girl, which can be seen bilaterally. If unilateral, it can be mistaken for a fracture.

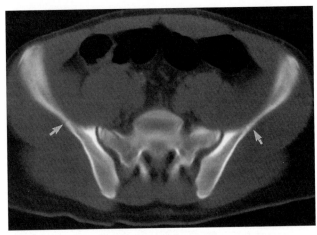

FIG. 26.37. Bilateral iliac vascular channels. Pelvic CT of a 17-year-old boy with abdominal trauma. The normal vascular channels of the iliac bone *(arrows)* simulate fracture lines.

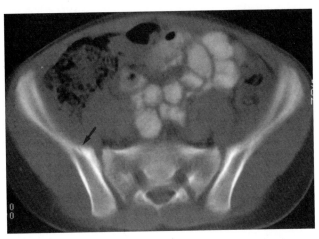

FIG. 26.36. Iliac pseudofracture. Pelvic CT of a 13-year-old boy with abdominal trauma. Note the normal vascular channel in the right iliac bone *(arrow)* simulating a small lytic area with surrounding sclerosis.

Vascular Channels in the Iliac Bone

Vascular foramina on the gluteal surface of the iliac bone lead to large vascular channels within the bone (20,21). Seen on axial imaging, these channels can simulate small lytic areas (Figs. 26.35 and 26.36) or fracture lines (Fig. 26.37).

REFERENCES

1. Collins P. Embryology and development. In: *Gray's anatomy.* New York: Churchill Livingstone, 1995;269.
2. Silverman FN, Byrd SE, Fit CR. The skull, spine, and central nervous system. In: *Caffey's pediatric x-ray diagnosis, 9th ed.* St Louis: CV Mosby, 1993;119.
3. Shapiro R. *Myelography.* Chicago: Yearbook, 1975;90–91.
4. Broome DR, Hayman LA, Herrick RC, et al. Postnatal maturation of the sacrum and coccyx: MR imaging, helical CT, and conventional radiography. *Am J Roentgenol* 1998;170:1061–1066.
5. Soames RW. Skeletal system. In: *Gray's anatomy.* New York: Churchill Livingstone, 1995;539.
6. Kuhn JP, Slovis TL, Silverman FN, Kuhns LR. The neck and respiratory system. In: *Caffey's pediatric x-ray diagnosis, 9th ed.* St Louis: CV Mosby, 1993;391.
7. Goodman LR, Teplick SK, Kay H. Computed tomography of the normal sternum. *Am J Roentgenol* 1983;141:219–223.
8. Keats TE. *Atlas of normal variants that may simulate disease, 5th ed.* St Louis: Mosby-Year Book, 1992;385.
9. Swischuk LE. *Emergency imaging of the acutely ill or injured child, 3rd ed.* Baltimore: Williams & Wilkins, 1994;396.
10. Keats TE. *Atlas of normal variants that may simulate disease, 5th ed.* St Louis: Mosby-Year Book, 1992;323–324.
11. Keats TE. *Atlas of normal variants that may simulate disease, 5th ed.* St Louis: Mosby-Year Book, 1992;364.
12. Keats TE. *Atlas of normal variance that may simulate disease, 5th ed.* St Louis: Mosby-Year Book, 1992;344–348.
13. Taveras JM, Ferrucci JT. *Radiology diagnosis–imaging–intervention.* Philadelphia: Lippincott-Raven, 1998;9.
14. Soames RW. Skeletal system. In: *Gray's anatomy.* New York: Churchill Livingstone, 1995;668–670.
15. Christoforidis AJ. *Atlas of axial, sagittal, and coronal anatomy.* Philadelphia: WB Saunders Company, 1988;310.
16. Soames RW. Skeletal system. In: *Gray's anatomy.* New York: Churchill Livingstone, 1995;684.
17. Fernbach SK, Wilkinson RH. Avulsion injuries of the pelvis and proximal femur. *Am J Roentgenol* 1981;137:581–584.
18. Ozonoff MB. *Pediatric orthopedic radiology.* Philadelphia: WB Saunders, 1992;168.
19. Soames RW. Skeletal system. In: *Gray's anatomy.* New York: Churchill Livingstone, 1995;681.
20. Soames RW. Skeletal System. In: *Gray's anatomy.* New York: Churchill Livingstone, 1995;665.
21. Keats TE. *Atlas of normal variants that may simulate disease, 5th ed.* St Louis: Mosby-Year Book, 1992;293.

Variants and Pitfalls in Body Imaging,
edited by Ali Shirkhoda.
Lippincott Williams & Wilkins, Philadelphia, © 2000.

CHAPTER **27**

The Spine: CT and MRI

Jamshid Tehranzadeh, George Rappard, Arash Anavim, and Henry Pribram

A sound knowledge of the normal spine is required to interpret spinal images. Unfortunately, the definition of normal depends on the imaging modality and the particulars of each patient. For example, normal anatomic variants on MRI and CT have a characteristic appearance. In addition, this appearance may differ depending on the type of MRI sequence used or on whether one is viewing axial, reformatted sagittal, coronal, or three-dimensional (3-D) CT images. One must be familiar with artifacts peculiar to each type of spinal imaging modality. Finally, patients occasionally may have benign, static conditions that mimic the imaging appearance of a lesion.

We briefly review spinal embryology and development. Next, we discuss normal variants of the spine and their appearance on CT and MRI. Conditions affecting radiographic interpretation, such as postoperative changes and spinal instrumentation, are also reviewed. Imaging-related artifacts and their manifestations and potential pitfalls are also covered.

EMBRYOLOGY AND DEVELOPMENT

Development of the spinal cord begins in the third week of fetal life, when the ectodermal layer thickens, giving rise to the neural plate. This is followed by neurulation. In the process of neurulation, the neural folds fuse at the midline. Fusion occurs first in the cervical region

---

J. Tehranzadeh: Departments of Radiology and Orthopaedics, Section of Musculoskeletal Radiology, University of California at Irvine Medical Center, Orange, California 92868.

G. Rappard and A. Anavim: Department of Radiological Sciences, University of California at Irvine Medical Center, Orange, California 92868.

H. Pribram: Departments of Radiological Sciences and Neurology, University of California at Irvine Medical Center, Orange, California 92868.

and then irregularly in the cephalic and caudal directions (1,2). Neuroepithelial cells then give rise to primitive nerve cells, called neuroblasts, which form a mantle layer around the neuroepithelial layer. The mantle layer gives rise to the gray matter of the spinal cord. The outermost layer contains nerve fibers emanating from the neuroblast; this is called the marginal layer. The marginal layer eventually becomes myelinated and gives rise to the white matter of the spinal cord. Myelination does not begin until the fourth month of life. In general, nerve tracts in the central nervous system (CNS) do not become myelinated until they start to function. Some are not myelinated until the end of the first year of postnatal life (3).

Development of the spinal column begins in the fourth week of gestation, when cells of the sclerotomes surround the spinal cord and notochord. These form a mesenchymal column, which retains its segmental origin, and its blocks are separated by less dense areas (4). This is followed by proliferation and condensation of the sclerotomal segments and extension into subjacent intersegmental tissue, binding the caudal half of one sclerotome to the cephalic half of the superior sclerotome. Thus, the vertebral body is intersegmental in origin.

A number of abnormalities arise from anomalous intersegmental origin of the vertebral bodies. Asymmetric fusion of a sclerotomal segment may lead to a hemivertebra. Symmetric abnormalities in intersegmentation probably lead to either an increase or a decrease in an individual's number of vertebrae. Normal segmentation of the spine should not be mistaken for fracture (Figs. 27.1 and 27.2), or vice versa (Fig. 27.3).

The intervertebral disk is mesenchymal in origin and is derived from the tissue between the cephalic and caudal portions of the original sclerotome. This tissue does not proliferate like the caudal and cephalic portions of the sclerotome. Rather, it fills the space between and will

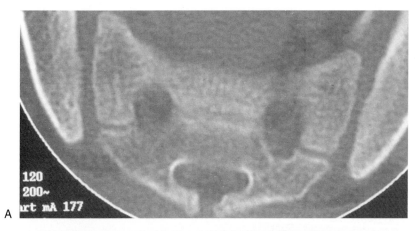

A

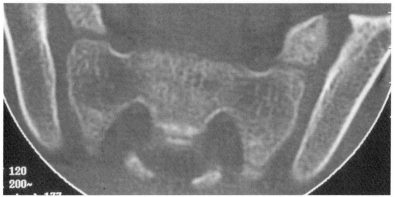

B

FIG. 27.1. Normal sacral segmentation. Axial CT of the sacrum in an 8-year-old boy shows normal segmentation.

eventually become two precartilaginous vertebral bodies. Though the notochord regresses in the region of the vertebral body, it persists and enlarges in the region of the intervertebral disk. When the persistent notochord later undergoes mucoid degeneration, it becomes the nucleus pulposus and is surrounded by the circular fibers of the annulus fibrosus.

Failure of the posterior elements to fuse leads to spina bifida operta (meningocele, myelocele, or myelomenin-

gocele) and spina bifida occulta (5). Spina bifida occulta at the S1 level is quite common and may be considered a normal variant.

The position of the spinal cord changes with age; the vertebral canal and dura lengthen to a greater degree than the spinal cord. The result is that the terminal end of the spinal cord shifts to a higher level. At birth, the spinal cord ends at approximately L1 to L3. Because of the disproportionate growth between the spinal cord and verte-

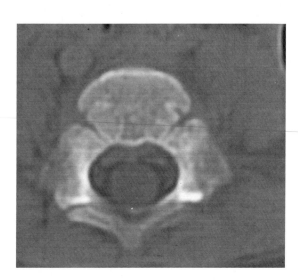

FIG. 27.2. Normal segmentation of the vertebra. Axial CT of the lumbar spine in an 18-month-old boy. These separate ossification centers will coalesce later to create a solid vertebra.

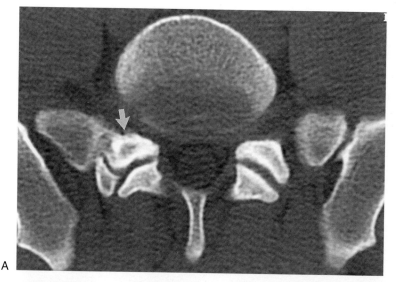

A

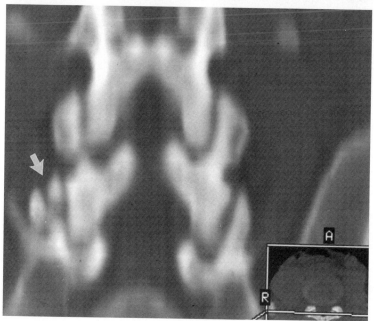

B

FIG. 27.3. Old fracture of the superior articular process simulating segmentation. Axial **(A)** and coronal **(B)** CT reconstruction of lumbosacral spine (L5 to S1) showing fragmentation of the right superior articular process of S1 *(arrows)* mimicking segmentation.

bral canal, the spinal nerves course obliquely from their origin to exit at the correct vertebral level.

Paraspinal musculature is derived from the myotomal segments found adjacent to the sclerotomes. Because of the intersegmental origin of the vertebral bodies, the myotomes now bridge the intervertebral disk. Once the myotomal segments have matured into skeletal muscle, this bridging allows movement of the spine.

DEVELOPMENT AND RELATED IMAGING PROBLEMS

The intervertebral disks are prominent during infancy (6). They progressively decrease in volume with age. The normal adult disk has intermediate signal on T_1-weighted images (T1WI) and high signal on T_2-weighted images (T2WI). With age, there is progressive volume loss and decreased signal intensity on T2WI. This disk change can be observed in children as well as in adults (7). Disk degeneration in the pediatric age group is not normal and may be posttraumatic. A central, linear focus of decreased signal intensity with the appearance of an internuclear disk cleft is seen on MRI (Fig. 27.4). This represents a fibrous remnant of the notochord (8). Absence of this cleft might be a secondary sign of disk space infection (9), but it could be a normal variant or a sign of degenerative disk disease.

Hematopoietic bone marrow is prominent in the vertebral bodies of infants and children. On MRI, hematopoietic marrow is of low signal intensity on T1WI and T2WI. Enhancement of normal marrow can be seen in children after administration of gadolinium (10). There is a change in signal intensity of the vertebral bodies with age (Fig. 27.5). In the first month of life, the vertebral bodies are

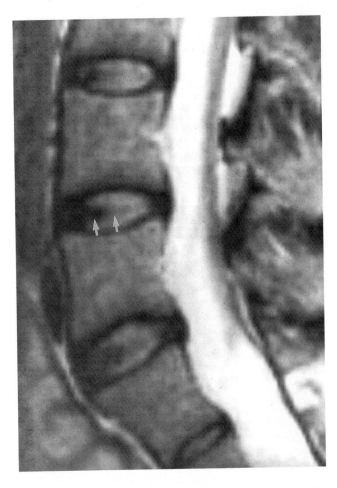

FIG. 27.4. Normal intranuclear cleft of intervertebral disks. Sagittal T2WI (3,000/96) in a 38-year-old woman shows normal horizontal dark signal line *(arrows)* inside the bright nuclear disk substance.

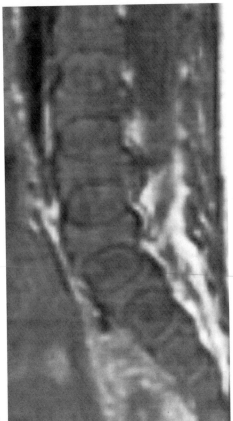

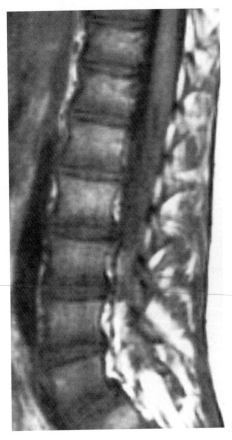

FIG. 27.5. Evolution of hematopoietic to fatty marrow in a growing skeleton. **A:** Sagittal T1WI (850/23) of the spine in a 4-month-old infant showing hematopoietic low signal marrow. Note prominent disks at infancy. **B:** Sagittal T1WI (650/19) of the spine in a 6-year-old boy showing intermediate to low signal intensity in bone marrow, indicating partial fatty replacement of hematopoietic marrow.

A,B

hypointense on T1WI and T2WI, except for linear hyperintensity along the course of the basivertebral vein on T2WI (11). Surrounding the vertebral body ossification center is hyaline cartilage, which is of high signal on T1WI and T2WI (11). Hyaline cartilage also enhances with the administration of gadolinium (11). Between 1 and 6 months of age there is an increase in vertebral body signal intensity that starts at the endplates and progresses centrally. Relative isointensity between the vertebral body and cartilage is achieved by 7 months of age (11).

Lap-belt injuries in children tend to occur in the midlumbar area because of their unique anthropomorphic characteristics. Children have a higher center of gravity than adults, a larger head size relative to body length, and incompletely developed iliac crests. These factors cause hyperflexion of the midlumbar spine and riding up of the lap belt above the pelvis, leading to spinal and visceral injury. Spinal fractures in restrained children tend to occur in the midlumbar area, tend to be oriented in an axial plane, and may be missed on transaxial images. Transaxial imaging may also fail to detect dislocations in the axial plane (12). Spiral CT, with sagittal and coronal reformatted images, may prevent this potential pitfall. In restrained pediatric trauma patients undergoing CT imaging of the abdomen and pelvis, one might consider obtaining the entire examination in spiral mode, allowing sagittal and coronal reconstructions.

NORMAL VARIANTS

Spinal Column and Paravertebral Soft Tissues

The spinous processes of the cervical spine are often bifid and may or may not have lateral tubercles at the lower cervical levels (13). The foramen transversarium is subject to variation (Fig. 27.6). It is larger on the side of the dominant vertebral artery. At C7 it may be absent. There may also be accessory foramina transversaria (13). The dens can undertake a variety of forms. The dens may originate from the anterior arch of the atlas. Also, the dens may not be united with the axis, simulating a fracture (os odontoideum) (Fig. 27.7). The dens may even be absent (13). Posterior inclination of the odontoid process is not uncommon (Fig. 27.8). Abnormalities of fusion may occur, with the atlas partially or wholly fused to the occipital bone or fused to the axis. Atlanto-occipital fusion may be associated with atlantoaxial subluxation and C2–C3 fusion. Normal synchondrosis of the arch of the atlas in infancy and early childhood should not be mistaken for a Jefferson fracture (Fig. 27.9). Partial or complete fusion of cervical vertebrae (Fig. 27.10) may predispose to injury above or below the level of fusion because of a lack of physiologic movement at this level in response to external stresses (i.e., sudden deceleration). Other variants in the anatomy of the atlas include incomplete ossification of the anterior or posterior arches (13). There is much variability in the prominence of the transverse and costal processes of the cervical vertebrae. Occasionally, cervical ribs arise from the lower cervical vertebrae (9).

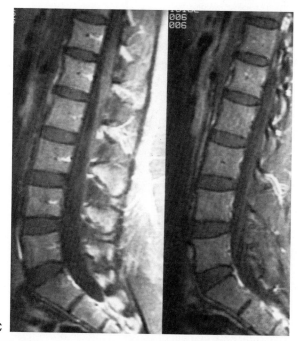

FIG. 27.5. *Continued.* **C:** Sagittal T1WI (400/19) of the spine in a 29-year-old woman showing further fatty replacement of bone marrow.

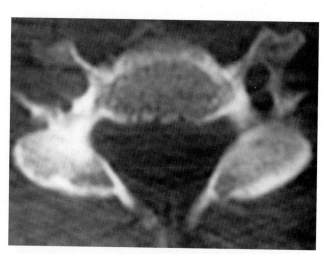

FIG. 27.6. Bifid foramen transversarium. Axial CT of the cervical spine shows bony septation at the left foramen transversarium.

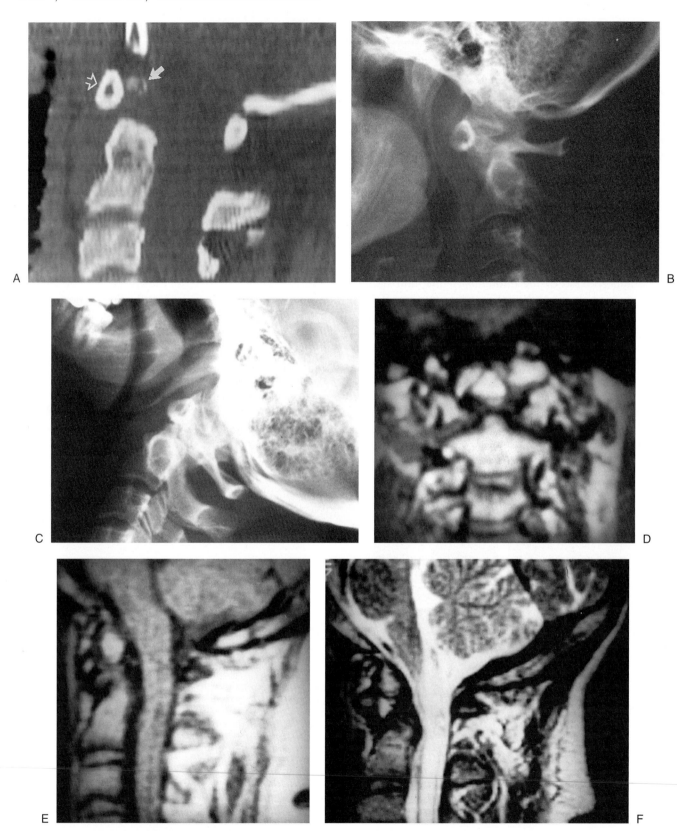

FIG. 27.7. Os odontoideum. **A:** Sagittal CT reconstruction of C-spine in a 45-year-old woman with os odontoideum *(arrow)* and absence of fusion with body of axis. Note enlargement of anterior tubercle of the atlas *(open arrow)*. **B:** Lateral flexion plain radiograph shows atlantoaxial subluxation. **C:** Lateral extension plain radiograph shows subluxation and instability of the atlantoaxial joint. **D:** Coronal T1WI (500/23) shows absence of normal odontoid and convex odontoid base. Sagittal T1WI (750/19) **(E)** and sagittal T2WI (3,000/102) **(F)** shows an ossicle above the hypoplastic odontoid process.

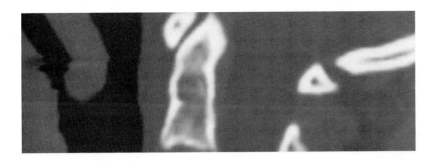

FIG. 27.8. Normal posterior inclination of the odontoid process. Sagittal CT reconstruction of the odontoid process displays normal posterior inclination of the odontoid process.

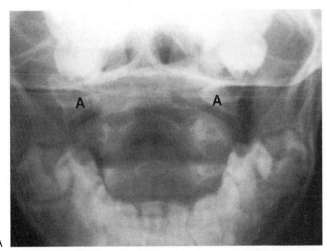

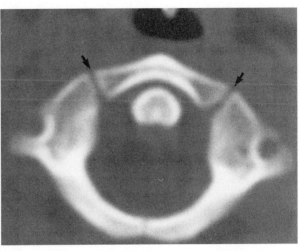

FIG. 27.9. Normal synchondrosis of the atlas. **A:** Plain radiograph of open-mouth view of the odontoid process shows bilateral symmetric increased distance of lateral masses of the atlas (A) from the odontoid process. This results from nonfused synchondrosis of the anterior arch of the atlas. **B:** Axial CT of the atlas in a 2-year-old girl shows normal synchondrosis of the anterior arch of the atlas *(arrows).*

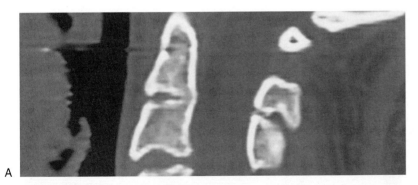

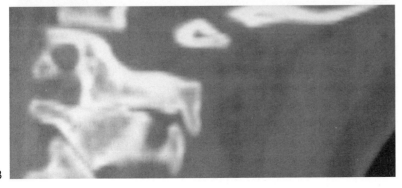

FIG. 27.10. Congenital fusion of C2-3. **A:** Sagittal reconstruction CT at the C2-3 level shows partial fusion of C2 (axis) to C3. **B:** Oblique parasagittal reconstruction CT along the right laminae of C2 and C3 shows partial fusion of C2 and C3.

Hemivertebrae may be found throughout the spinal column, and they may be fused with adjacent vertebrae (9) (Fig. 27.11). Other congenital anomalies include butterfly vertebra and hypoplastic or absent pedicle and lamina (Figs. 27.12 and 27.13). Unilateral arch hypertrophy may occur and results from the increased stress placed on the arch to compensate for a hypoplastic pedicle or lamina on the opposite side. On plain radiographs this hypertrophy may appear as a dense pedicle, thus mimicking metastatic disease (14). Sacrococcygeal elements may be of varied

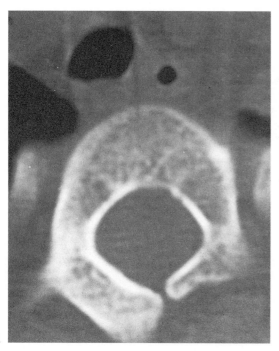
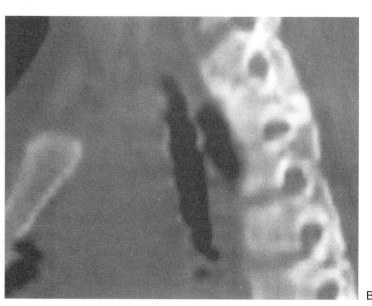

A   B

FIG. 27.11. Congenital anomaly of the thoracic spine. **A:** Axial CT of the thoracic spine in a 13-year-old boy shows spina bifida occulta and asymmetry of the laminae. **B:** Parasagittal reconstruction CT of the thoracic spine shows fusion anomaly.

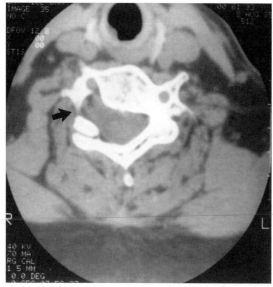
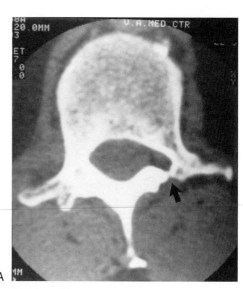

FIG. 27.12. Congenital absence of the pedicle. Axial CT of cervical spine shows congenital absence of the right pedicle *(arrow)*.

FIG. 27.13. Congenital hypoplastic pedicle and lamina of the lumbar spine. **A:** Axial CT shows hypoplasia of the left pedicle and defect in the left lamina of the lumbar spine *(arrow)*.

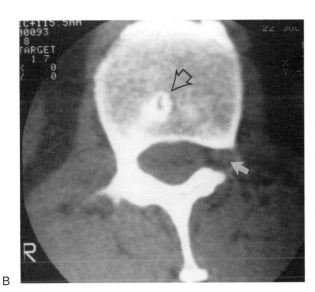

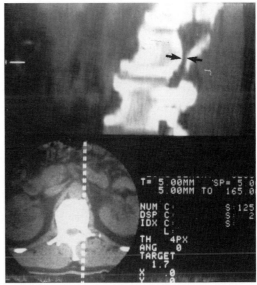

B

C

FIG. 27.13. *Continued.* **B:** Axial CT of the lumbar spine. Same vertebra as **A** shows absent left pedicle *(arrow).* Incidentally noted Schmorl node of the vertebral endplate *(open arrow).* **C:** Sagittal reconstruction CT of the lumbar spine at the level of the pedicular defect shows the absence of the pedicle *(arrows).*

number and size (9). Schmorl nodes (Fig. 27.14) represent disk material herniated into the vertebral endplate and are enhanced on MRI (15). They may be mistaken for a metastasis. Metastasis can be differentiated from a Schmorl node based on the typical location of the latter adjacent to the disk space and by its well-defined sclerotic border surrounding a zone of variable lucency (14). A case of "tunneling Schmorl node" of lumbar vertebra with communicating superior and inferior Schmorl nodes, creating a longitudinal tunnel through the vertebral body, has been reported (16). In Scheuermann's disease (juvenile kyphosis) abnormal softening of the endplates leads to development of multilevel Schmorl nodes and vertebral compression (Figs. 27.15 and 27.16).

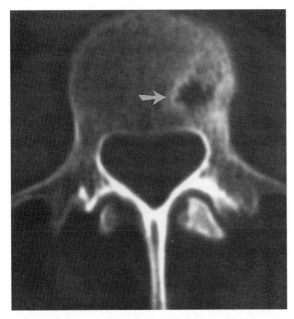

FIG. 27.14. Schmorl node. Axial CT of the lumbar spine shows a Schmorl node *(arrow).* Schmorl node represents focal herniation of the intervertebral disk into the endplate.

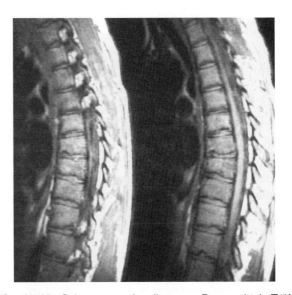

FIG. 27.15. Scheuermann's disease. Parasagittal T1WI (700/19) of the thoracic spine shows exaggeration of the thoracic kyphosis with multiple wedging of midthoracic vertebra in a 13-year-old girl with Scheuermann's disease presenting with juvenile kyphosis.

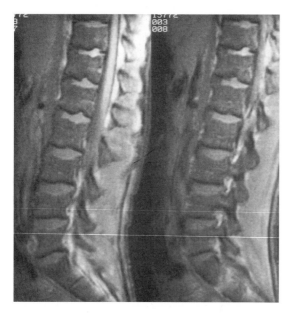

FIG. 27.16. Scheuermann's disease. Parasagittal T1WI (650/19) in a 34-year-old man shows multiple thoracolumbar Schmorl nodes indicating Scheuermann's disease.

Occasionally, it is difficult to number the vertebral bodies on axial images. One method is to refer to a reference image in which numbered lines, corresponding to the axial images, are superimposed on either a CT scout film or an MR sagittal image. However, if the patient has moved between the time of the scout film and the axial images, the vertebral body level may be misinterpreted. There are other pitfalls; for example, in CT, scanning from the mid- or low cervical area to the cervicothoracic junction, the convention is to count up from the first rib-bearing vertebra as being T_1. However, a cervical rib can lead to misnumbering of the vertebrae. This can be avoided by carefully reviewing the AP plain film or the scout image for the presence of a cervical rib. In the lumbar spine, abnormalities of fusion can lead to assigning incorrect vertebral body levels. Transitional vertebrae occur with partial or complete lumbarization of a sacral vertebra or partial or complete sacralization of a lumbar vertebra. Transitional vertebrae can lead to mistakes in assigning vertebral body levels to lesions in the lumbosacral spine, including the bodies themselves or the intervertebral disks (17).

Mirowitz makes several recommendations for determining the correct level in an MRI of the spine (9). The correct level may be determined if a large field of view encompassing the odontoid process is available. The position of each vertebral body can be noted by determining its position relative to anatomic structures, such as the pulmonary artery. However, such structures may be obscured if one uses an anterior presaturation band to decrease pulsation artifact (9). With a large-field-of-view MRI body coil, one may localize vertebral bodies on sur-

face coil images by placing an external marker (vitamin E capsule) over a particular vertebral body and then using an electronic cursor (18). The right renal artery interposed between the crus of the diaphragm and the inferior vena cava on parasagittal images can indicate the L1-2 disk level 86% of the time (19). Some sources consider this method unreliable (20). It is important to state in a report how one has numbered the vertebrae.

Posterior Elements

Spina bifida occulta results from incomplete fusion of the posterior elements. In the sacral spine it is common and may be considered a normal variant. Other variants include pseudoarthrosis between the transverse processes of L5 and S1, often associated with transitional vertebra. There may also be variations in the diameter of the spinal canal. For example, the AP diameter of the cervical spine canal at the C4 level ranges from 13 to 22 mm; below 13 mm is considered narrow (21). Spinal canal narrowing can occur when congenitally short pedicles are present (21). Defects in the pars interarticularis (spondylolysis) or fracture in the lamina can result in vertebral subluxation (spondylolisthesis) (Figs. 27.17–27.19). This may not be evident on axial MR images (22). On CT, axial views are diagnostic for spondylolysis; otherwise one should refer to the sagittally reconstructed images. Often, one can identify spondylolisthesis on the scout images. On MRI, these defects are best appreciated on the sagittal and parasagittal images. A false diagnosis of spondylolisthesis can occur with partial volume averaging of facet osteophytes (23). In addition, sclerosis involving the pars may also give the false appearance of a defect (23,24).

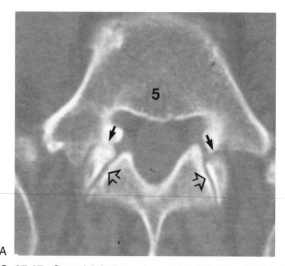

A

FIG. 27.17. Spondylolysis and spondylolisthesis of L5 to S1. A: Axial CT at the L5 vertebral body shows bilateral pars interarticularis (isthmus) defects (horizontal orientation) (solid arrows). It should not be mistaken for facet joints oblique orientation (open arrows). Note that the spinal canal size is not narrowed in true spondylolysis.

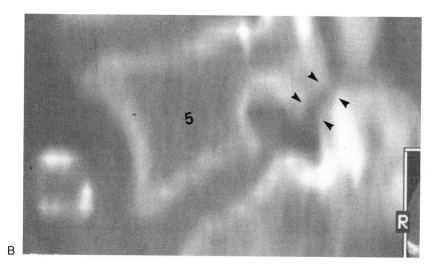

FIG. 27.17. *Continued.* **B:** Sagittal reconstruction CT of L5 to S1 shows isthmus defect *(arrowheads)* with grade I spondylolisthesis.

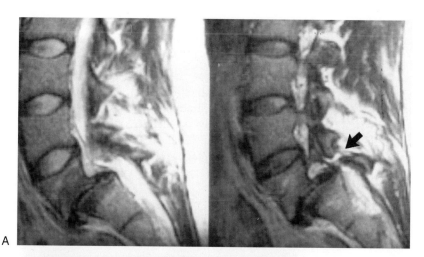

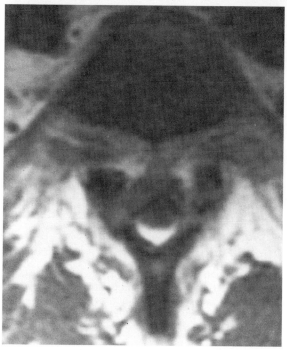

FIG. 27.18. Spondylolysis and spondylolisthesis. **A:** Parasagittal T2WI (3,000/96) shows pars interarticularis defect at the L5 to S1 level *(arrow)* with grade I spondylolisthesis. **B:** Axial T1WI (700/14) at the L5 to S1 level shows spondylolysis. Note the canal size does not appear small. Rather, it appears larger than normal.

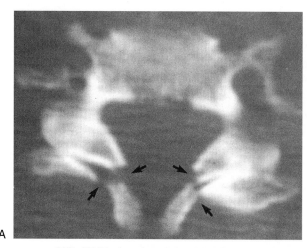

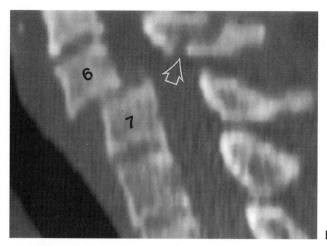

FIG. 27.19. Laminar fracture of C6 and C7 and spondylolisthesis. **A:** Axial CT of the cervical vertebrae showing bilateral laminar fracture of C6 and C7 *(arrows)*. Double lamina is caused by subluxation and not partial volume averaging. Note that the spinal canal appears larger than normal. **B:** Sagittal reconstruction CT of the cervical vertebrae shows laminar fracture *(open arrow)* with subluxation of C6 on C7.

Differentiation of Degenerative Subluxation from Spondylolisthesis

In a degenerative subluxation, so-called pseudospondylolisthesis, the canal depth is usually decreased (Fig. 27.20). However, in spondylolisthesis, because of the pars interarticularis defect, there is preservation of the canal depth (see Figs. 27.17 and 27.18), but there is narrowing of the neural foramen on sagittal views (25).

Marrow Space

Hematopoietic marrow is of low signal intensity on both T1WI and T2WI in children and young adults. With age, the marrow signal gradually increases in intensity. In adults, the red marrow is changed to yellow marrow, which shows increased signal on T_1 with less bright signal on T_2-weighted images (T_2 appearance may vary according to the pulse sequences). In myeloproliferative

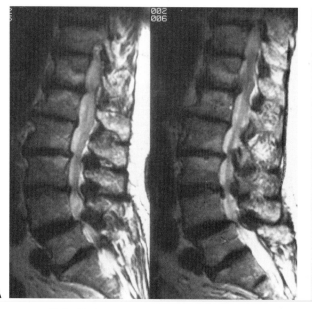

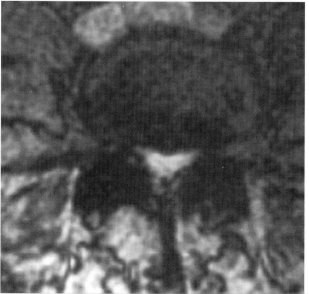

FIG. 27.20. Degenerative pseudospondylolisthesis at L4-5. **A:** Parasagittal T2WI (3,000/96). In this case, subluxation of L4 over L5 is related to facet arthritis and ligamentous laxity and not to pars interarticularis defect. Note that the spinal canal is consequently narrowed. Thickening of ligamentous flavum is also noted. **B:** Axial multiplanar gradient-echo (316/17) image shows that subluxation has resulted in small spinal canal. Subluxation in pseudospondylolisthesis is related to degenerative process rather than pars interarticularis defect.

diseases, anemia and hypoxemia due to conditions such as obesity and Pickwickian syndrome, congenital cyanotic heart diseases and COPD, and in patients with AIDS (Fig. 27.21) there is a reconversion of yellow marrow to red marrow with low signal intensity on MR images (26,27). There is also decreased signal intensity on both T_1 and T_2 images with fibrotic changes in the bone marrow. In patients following radiation therapy, replacement of the bone marrow with fatty marrow results in increased signal intensity in the vertebral bodies (Fig. 27.22). Marrow of low signal intensity on T1WI and T2WI can be seen in women of reproductive age secondary to physiologic anemia (9). It may also be seen in anemia of any cause, where the vertebral body marrow has had an opportunity to compensate with hematopoiesis. This condition may also be seen in infiltrative marrow disorders, where normally dormant vertebral marrow is seen to undergo compensatory hematopoiesis. Normal marrow in adults has bright signal intensity on T1WI. STIR and fat-saturation sequences are sensitive to abnormal marrow changes.

Marrow of low signal intensity on T1WI may be mistaken for diffuse tumor involvement (9). If edema or necrosis is present, as in the case of many neoplasms, it will be of increased signal intensity on T2WI. Some spinal tumors, however, are mostly fibrotic and will thus appear hypointense on T2WI (9). A further confusing

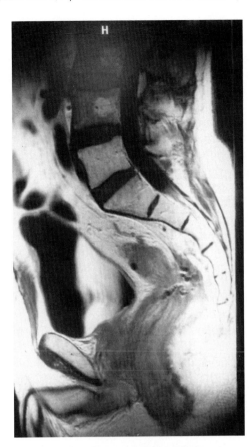

FIG. 27.22. Fatty marrow changes after radiation therapy. Parasagittal proton density (900/12) image of lumbosacral spine in a patient with rectal carcinoma who received radiation with a port extending from L5 to sacrum and coccyx. Note bright signal (fatty changes) at L5 and sacral levels.

matter is the fact that on fat-suppressed T2WI or STIR images, hematopoietic marrow may appear relatively hyperintense, mimicking a tumor. Further distinction between tumor and hematopoietic marrow can be made by comparing the vertebral body signal intensity to that of the intervertebral disk. With hematopoietic marrow, the vertebral bodies have a higher signal intensity than the adjacent disk on T1WI. This relationship is reversed in the case of neoplasm (9), where on T1WI the disk will be of increased signal intensity compared to the vertebral body. This has been termed the hyperintense disk sign (28). The hyperintense disk sign is not always sensitive. The disks may become hyperintense relative to the vertebral body in cases of iron overload or severe anemia when hyperplastic marrow is present (9). In equivocal cases, gadolinium can be administered before the acquisition of T1WI. The disks will be noticeably hypointense adjacent to the enhancing neoplasm. The contrast will be even more evident on fat-suppressed images. It is important always to precede a contrast scan with a noncontrast examination.

Fatty vertebral bone marrow is normally present later in life. The MR characteristics of fatty marrow are high signal intensity on T1WI and moderately decreased sig-

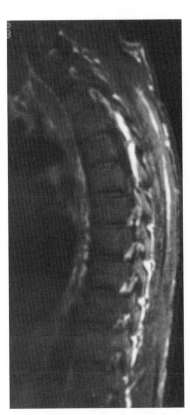

FIG. 27.21. Parasagittal T_1-weighted gradient-echo image of the thoracic spine in a 30-year-old man with AIDS showing diffuse low signal intensity of bone marrow.

nal intensity on T2WI. Also, there is decreased signal intensity on fat-suppressed T1WI versus regular T1WI. Although diffuse fatty marrow will normally be identified as age related, focal vertebral body fat may be mistaken for benign and malignant tumors and hemangioma. This may also occur following radiation therapy (29–32), where fatty marrow will be sharply demarcated along the extent of the radiation port (see Fig. 27.22). The appearance of vertebral body signal alterations after radiation therapy is variable. The appearance of these changes is dependent on dose of radiation as well as the elapsed time (29). These fatty changes could be seen as soon as 9 days following completion of radiotherapy with a radiation dose of at least 800 rads (8 Gy) (29) and could remain unchanged for more than 10 years (32). The use of fat-suppressed images may be helpful, as tumor should not change in appearance. The use of gadolinium may be confusing because postradiation fibrosis has a variable pattern of enhancement.

Hematopoietic bone marrow is of low signal intensity on T1WI and T2WI but may also be of moderately increased signal intensity on T2WI or short-tau inversion recovery (STIR) imaging. At times it may be difficult to distinguish hematopoietic marrow from tumor (33). Tumor is usually of moderately increased signal intensity on T2WI. Tumor necrosis will be of increased signal on T2WI, whereas tumor fibrosis will be of decreased signal intensity on T2WI (9). The hyperdense disk sign is used to distinguish hematopoietic marrow from tumor involvement. The presence of this sign is not always associated with pathology.

Marrow heterogeneity is another variant of normal that could be mistaken for a pathologic condition. Heterogeneous vertebral body bone marrow may also be seen in Waldenstrom's macroglobulinemia, metastatic disease, multiple myeloma, or other infiltrative conditions (34,35). Marrow heterogeneity is more conspicuous in high-field-strength MR systems and in older adults (9,36). Clinical information and other laboratory findings or even bone biopsy may be necessary to reach the diagnosis.

Significance of Focal Bright Marrow in Vertebrae

Focal bright marrow in the vertebral body may represent veins, focal fat, endplate fat such as type II degeneration, or hemangioma (Fig. 27.23). Generally, the presence of a focal bright spot in the T1WI indicates a benign process. The only exception is the rare appearance of metastatic melanoma. Vertebral hemangiomas are of increased signal intensity on T1WI. This is because of fat

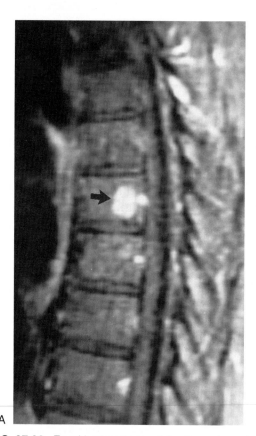
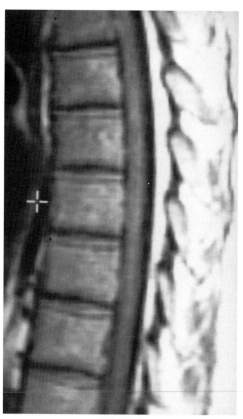

A   B

FIG. 27.23. Focal hemangioma of the thoracic vertebral body mimicking metastasis. **A:** Sagittal fat-saturated T1WI (433/19) in a 37-year-old woman with a history of melanoma shows focal bright signal at T7 vertebra *(arrow)*, which was also bright on T2WI (not shown). **B:** Sagittal spin-echo T1WI (633/19) of the thoracic spine. The lesion is isointense at T7 level.

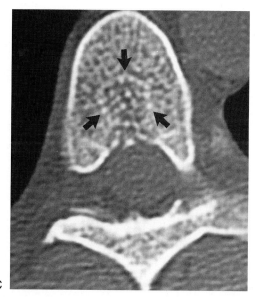

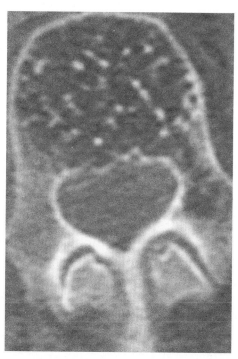

FIG. 27.23. *Continued.* **C:** Axial CT of the thoracic spine at T7 level shows focal vertebral hemangioma with typical polkadot pattern *(arrows).*

FIG. 27.25. Hemangioma of the vertebral body. Axial CT of the spine shows scant vertical bony trabeculae.

interspersed within the trabeculae of the hemangioma (37,38). They have decreased signal intensity on fat-saturated T1WI and T2WI. Hemangioma may even present as isointense foci on T1WI. On CT, the vertebral hemangioma has a typical polkadot appearance within a low-density area (Figs. 27.24–27.26). Other lesions in the spine such as metastases or myeloma may be mistaken for hemangioma (37) (Fig. 27.27), and occasionally, a small polkadot pattern is seen as a result of localized hypertrophied struts (14,37) (see Figs. 27.23 and 27.26). The polkadot pattern in hemangioma is symmetric and homo-geneous, whereas those of myeloma and metastasis often have inhomogeneous and asymmetric aggregations of bone trabeculae.

Occasionally, lipid rests are found in the spine. These also occur as foci of increased signal intensity on T1WI (39). The basivertebral venous complex has a horizontal striated appearance with a predilection for fat along its course (9).

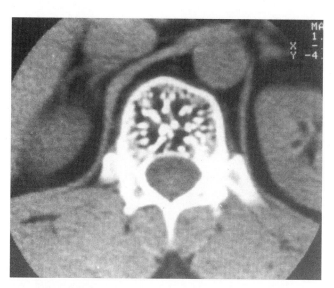

FIG. 27.24. Hemangioma of the thoracic spine. Axial CT of the thoracic vertebra shows radiating polkadot appearance indicating vertebral body hemangioma. (From reference 28, with permission.)

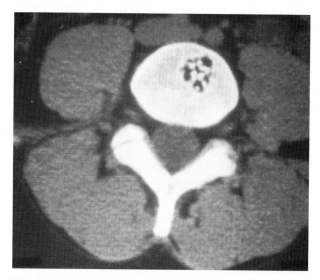

FIG. 27.26. Focal vertebral body hemangioma. Axial CT of the spine shows a focal lytic lesion with polkadot appearance inside indicating focal hemangioma. (From reference 9, with permission.)

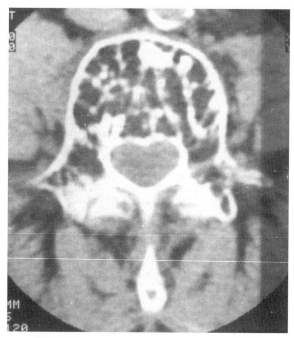

FIG. 27.27. Myeloma of the spine. Axial CT of the spine showing lytic lesion of the vertebral body mimicking hemangioma. However, this does not have the typical polkadot appearance of hemangioma. (From reference 28, with permission.)

Discrete fatty marrow changes may simulate hemorrhagic (subacute hemorrhage) or proteinaceous lesions (tumor) of the spine. Fat-suppression techniques may be of some benefit in distinguishing these entities from one another.

Paraspinal Soft Tissues

Hiatal hernias can simulate cystic or necrotic masses of the anterior thoracic spinal column (9). Inferior lumbar space hernias can simulate paravertebral mass lesions (40). Paraspinal soft tissue inflammatory processes can simulate neoplastic lesions in this region. Tuberculosis is certainly known to simulate neoplasm. Soft tissue pseudotumors of the cervical spine sometimes consist of pannus material in rheumatoid arthritis (9). Pseudotumors comprised of reactive inflammatory tissue are sometimes seen with chronic vertebral subluxation (41).

Normal paravertebral soft tissues can be mistaken for masses. One example is a prominent ascending lumbar vein. These are of intermediate signal intensity, similar to soft tissue, because of slow flow within the vein. Flow-sensitive gradient-echo imaging is helpful in confirming the presence of flowing (moving) blood. Similarly, a prominent azygos or hemizygous vein can also simulate a mass or lymphadenopathy (9). A cervical prevertebral mass may be simulated by the collapsed esophagus and prevertebral fat stripe on plain radiograph. On MR, fibro-fatty tissue seen surrounding the superior dens may be interpreted as a prevertebral soft tissue abnormality (42).

Fatty changes may occur in the paraspinal soft tissues and are present as focal or diffuse increased signal intensity on T1WI. One cause is fatty replacement in paraplegia, quadriplegia, or chronic disuse (9). Paraspinal lipomatosis is seen in cases undergoing chronic steroid treatment, in adrenal tumors, or in cases of adrenal hyperplasia (43).

The Intervertebral Disk

The intervertebral disk changes in size with age. It is prominent during infancy (6) (see Fig. 27.5A) and decreases in volume with age. The intervertebral disk also has changing signal characteristics. Normally the disk is of decreased signal intensity on T1WI and increased signal intensity on T2WI. There is loss of signal on T2WI with disk degeneration caused by loss of hydration and alteration in the connective tissue components of the disk. These changes are accentuated in sequences with long echo times such as T_2-weighted gradient-echo imaging or fast spin-echo sequences (9). Disk degeneration occurs in older individuals but may also be seen in children (7). Degenerative changes do not always correlate with symptoms (44) and may be seen in asymptomatic patients.

Extradural Space

The basivertebral vein appears dark on T1WI and bright on T2WI (Fig. 27.28). A focal prominence of the basivertebral vein may simulate a small disk herniation

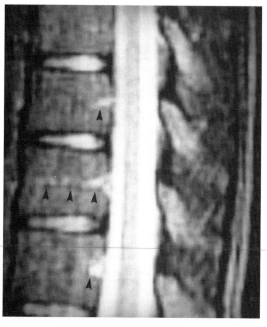

FIG. 27.28. Basivertebral vein. Sagittal T2WI (3,000/96) of thoracic spine shows basivertebral veins in the middle of the vertebral body *(arrowheads)*.

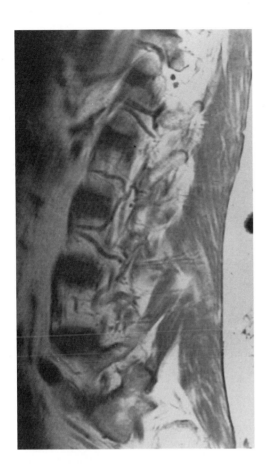

FIG. 27.29. Normal lumbar vessels. Lateral parasagittal T1WI (510/15) shows normal lumbar vessels that hug the periphery of vertebral bodies.

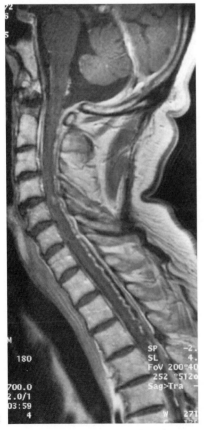

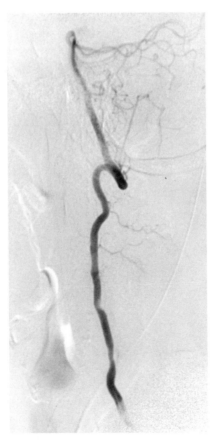

A,B

FIG. 27.30. Epidural vessels mimicking arteriovenous malformation (AVM). A: Sagittal T1WI (700/12) of the cervical spine showing serpiginous linear bright signal in posterior epidural space mimicking AVM. This probably represents the varices or prominent epidural venous plexus. B: Vertebral artery angiogram showing normal appearance and absence of AVM. (Case courtesy of Ay-Ming Wang, M.D., William Beaumont Hospital.)

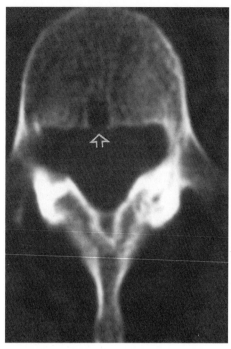

FIG. 27.31. Basivertebral vein. Axial CT of the lumbar spine shows normal basivertebral vein *(open arrowhead).*

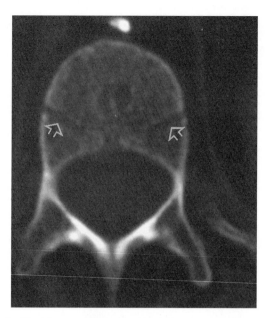

FIG. 27.32. Venous channels. Axial CT of the thoracic vertebra shows normal intrasomatic venous channels *(open arrowheads).*

on sagittal or transaxial images. Because the venous plexus enhances with gadolinium, further confusion with a mass may occur (45). Lumbar veins at the periphery of the spine should not be confused with a basivertebral vein. Basivertebral veins are noted on midsagittal images, whereas lumbar veins are at the periphery of the vertebral bodies (Fig. 27.29). A prominent epidural venous plexus may simulate a herniated disk (46–48) or arteriovenous malformation (AVM) (Fig. 27.30). Relative increased signal intensity on T1WI and T2WI can be observed in these veins because of slow flow and second echo rephasing (9). On CT examination, the basivertebral vein within

the bony column should not be mistaken for a lytic lesion (Fig. 27.31). The basivertebral plexus has distinct margins. Occasionally, a small amount of calcification may be seen within the plexus, and in some instances a calcific spur can be seen protruding posteriorly from the plexus. Venous channels may simulate fractures (Figs. 27.32 and 27.33), and, alternatively, fractures may mimic venous channels (Fig. 27.34). Venous channels present as linear lucent lines, identified exclusively in the midportion of the vertebral body and extending to the basivertebral plexus (14). Conjoined nerve roots may simulate disk herniation. These conjoined nerve roots can be seen to divide on consecutive images (9).

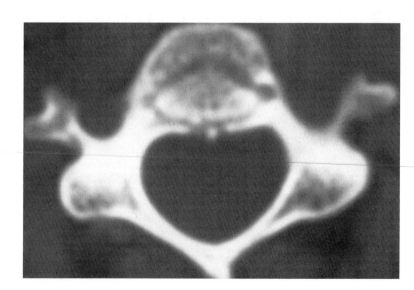

FIG. 27.33. Venous channels inside the vertebral body simulating fracture. Axial CT of the cervical spine in a 51-year-old man showing normal venous channels inside the vertebral body.

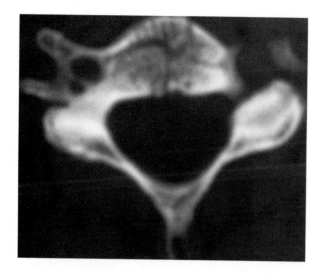

FIG. 27.34. Linear fractures in the vertebral body simulating vascular channels. Axial CT of the cervical spine shows fractures simulating vascular channels. Note normal bifid foramen transversarium on the right side.

Epidural Soft Tissues

The ligamentum flavum has increased signal intensity on T1WI compared with other ligamentous structures. This is because of the heavy concentration of elastin (9). Ligamentous ossification is usually associated with decreased signal intensity on all sequences and may be difficult to distinguish from ligamentous hypertrophy, but there may be increased signal intensity on T1WI because of marrow fat (22,49–54). When axial forces are applied to the spine, the ligamentum flavum may appear to bulge (50). Focal globular calcifications can give the appearance of a mass, similar to a synovial cyst (51). Figure 27.35 shows an air-filled calcified synovial cyst on both CT and MRI. The air

resulting from vacuum phenomena from a degenerative disk or facet joint may diffuse into the epidural space and be a source of diagnostic pitfall (Fig. 27.36).

A redundant or prominent posterior longitudinal ligament may resemble a vertebral osteophyte (52). This is most likely to occur on gradient-echo images when the ligament is calcified (9). On CT examination, the presence of a dividing cleft between the vertebral body and a calcified posterior longitudinal ligament (Fig. 27.37) can differentiate this condition from a bony ridge arising from the vertebral endplate.

Epidural masses may be simulated by hypertrophy of the posterior elements (22) or by synovial cysts arising from the facet joints and projecting into the spinal canal (55).

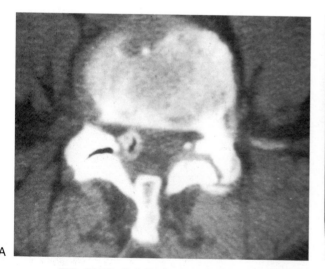

A

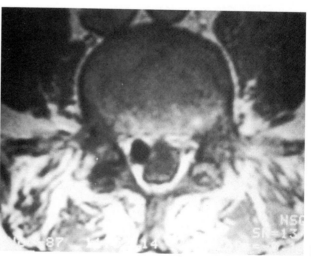

B

FIG. 27.35. Calcified synovial cyst with vacuum air in the facet joint and in the cyst. (Courtesy of Clyde Helms, Durham, NC.) **A:** Axial CT of the lumbar spine showing calcified synovial cyst filled with air that has leaked from degenerative facet arthrosis on the right side. **B:** Axial T1WI MR of the lumbar spine showing calcified synovial cyst with air presenting as low-signal-intensity mass. Right facet arthrosis shows low signal from sclerosis and presence of air in the facet joint.

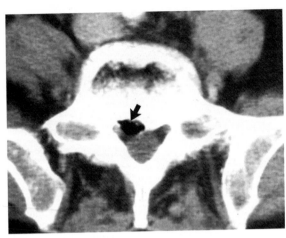

FIG. 27.36. Vacuum air in the intervertebral disk and inside the spinal canal. Axial CT of L5 to S1 level shows volume averaging of a degenerated intervertebral disk and vertebral endplate with vacuum air inside the disk diffused to appear in the anterior epidural space *(arrow).*

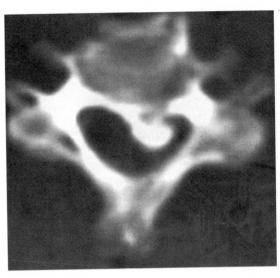

FIG. 27.37. Ossification of the posterior longitudinal ligament. Axial CT of the cervical spine shows ossification of posterior longitudinal ligament.

Neuroforamina

The dorsal root ganglia may enhance after the administration of gadolinium (56–58). The cervical spine foraminal venous plexus also enhances, aiding in the diagnosis of small foraminal disk herniations. Synovial cysts may extend into the neuroforamina (58). A tortuous vertebral artery may erode into the neural foramen (9).

Spinal Cord

The thecal sac has a variable caudal termination. Usually, it ends at the level of the second sacral vertebra; however, in many individuals it terminates at higher levels (13) such as L5. The spinal subarachnoid space varies in prominence. Cystic dilation of the thecal sac can be seen, especially in the lower lumbar and sacral areas (9). Sacral meningeal cysts are rarely associated with neurologic symptoms (59). Prominence of the subarachnoid space can be seen in patients with spinal cord atrophy, simulating an arachnoid cyst (60), and in patients with a tethered cord. Tarlov cysts may mimic an expansile lesion or even metastasis (Fig. 27.38).

The conus medullaris is usually at L1 but may be at T12 or L3 (13). Early in development the conus is low lying, ascending with maturity (61,62). On sagittal

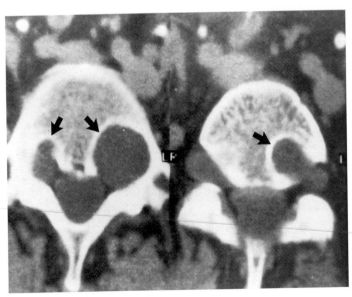

FIG. 27.38. Tarlov cysts simulating tumor or metastasis. Axial CT of the lumbar spine shows Tarlov cysts simulating tumor or metastasis. (Courtesy of Clyde Helms, Durham, NC.)

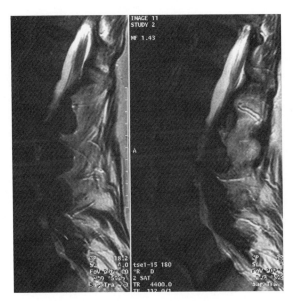

FIG. 27.39. Scoliosis. Parasagittal T2WI (4,400/112) shows the upper lumbar region close to midline and the lower lumbar area more lateral, close to the neural foramina, indicating scoliosis at this level.

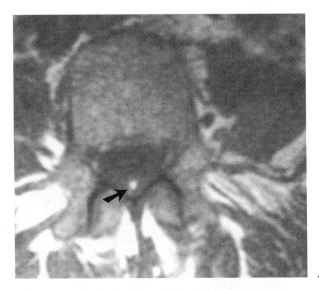

A

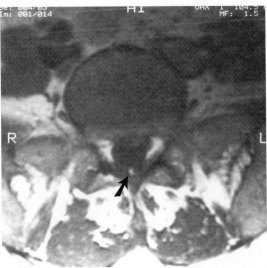

B

FIG. 27.40. Filum lipoma. **A:** Axial T1WI (650/14) at the body of L4 vertebra shows small focal fatty bright area that extends at multiple levels superiorly and inferiorly, indicating filum lipoma *(arrow)*. Note the normal thin layer of epidural fat. **B:** Axial T1WI (650/14) at L5 to S1 level shows extension of the filum lipoma *(arrow)* down to the sacral level. Note more epidural fat presence at L5 to S1 level.

images, the exact location of the conus can be difficult to determine because of clustering of the proximal cauda equina nerve roots (9,61–63), and this may be mistaken for an intradural mass on axial images (9). Clustering of the nerve roots may be caused by spinal stenosis or arachnoiditis (63).

Scoliosis can present difficulties in spinal imaging because the spine comes into and out of the plane of imaging (Fig. 27.39). The spine is thus imaged segmentally. It is also subject to partial volume averaging effects (9). Mirowitz recommends imaging the spine by reformatting sagittal images along oblique or curved planes, allowing continuous visualization of the spinal cord (64); alternatively, a coronal image may help.

Spinal Nerves and Ganglia

There are numerous variations of the spinal nerve roots and associated ganglia. The dorsal root ganglia may be larger in size than the corresponding ventral roots, and there may be duplication of the dorsal root ganglia at the lumbar and upper sacral levels. The L5 through S4 ganglia are located in the spinal canal and not the neural foramen. Some ganglia, usually sacrococcygeal, are located in the dural sac (13). A filum lipoma may be seen at several levels parallel to the cauda equina (Fig. 27.40).

Vertebral Bodies

Degenerative discogenic vertebral changes can be noted on the endplates bordering the intervertebral disks. There are three phases of degenerative disease on MR imaging of the spine (33,65). Type I results in decreased signal intensity on T1WI and increased signal intensity on T2WI (Fig. 27.41), and there is increased signal intensity with gadolinium. These changes are caused by edema and/or granulation tissue (58,66,67). It is not easy to distinguish this type

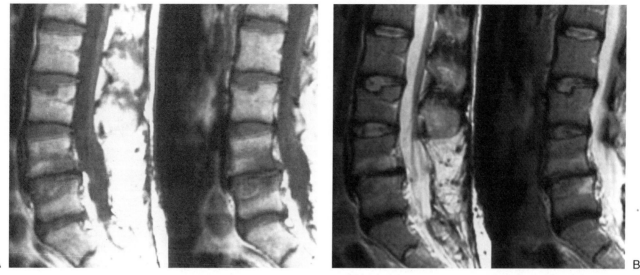

FIG. 27.41. Type I endplate changes (edema). **A:** Parasagittal T1WI (583/19) of the lumbar spine shows eroded L4-5 endplate with low signal intensity and narrowed disk, suggesting marrow edema and infection. **B:** Parasagittal T2WI (3,000/96) shows bright signal at L4-5 endplate with disk narrowing and endplate erosion suggesting marrow edema and infection.

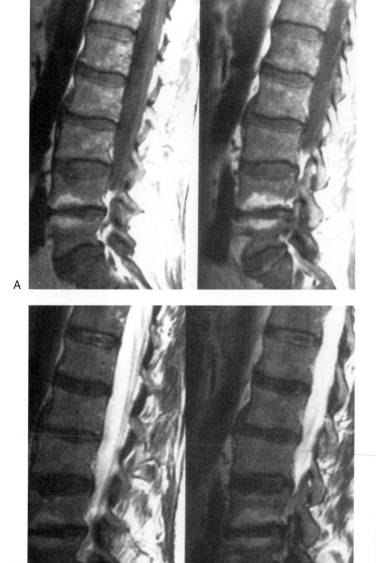

FIG. 27.42. Type II endplate changes (fatty degeneration). **A:** Sagittal T1WI (650/19) of the lumbar spine shows bright signal intensity of endplates at L5 to S1 level representing fatty degeneration. **B:** Sagittal T2WI (3,000/96) of the lumbar spine shows the fatty changes at the endplate representing intermediate signal intensity.

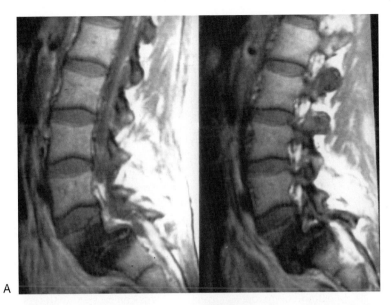

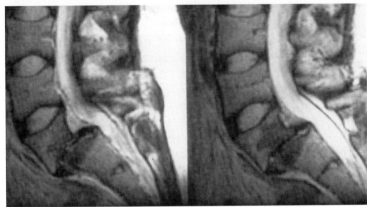

FIG. 27.43. Type III endplate changes (sclerosis). **A:** Sagittal T1WI (650/19) of the lumbar spine in a patient with spondylolysis and spondylolisthesis. Discogenic endplate sclerosis at the L5 to S1 endplate represents type III (sclerotic) marrow changes. **B:** Sagittal T2WI (3,000/96) of the lumbar spine in a patient with spondylolysis and spondylolisthesis. The sclerotic endplate changes at the L5 to S1 level remain with low signal intensity.

of degenerative disease from infection. Type II changes are secondary to fatty change with increased signal intensity on T1WI and mildly increased (less than T_1) signal intensity on T2WI (9) (Fig. 27.42). Type III changes result from sclerosis and lead to hypointensity on all sequences (Fig. 27.43). These changes are distinguished from more serious conditions by serial examinations or by the presence of associated disk degeneration or disk protrusion (9).

Summary of Marrow Changes at Endplates

1. Type 1: Edema. Decreased signal intensity on T1 and increased signal intensity on T2.
2. Type 2: Fatty changes. Increased signal intensity on T1- and increased (but less than T1) signal intensity on T2-weighted images.
3. Type 3: Sclerotic changes. Decreased signal intensity on T1- and T2-weighted images.

There are a multitude of other vertebral pathologic conditions with overlapping features. Occasionally, conditions

as diverse as vertebral neoplasm, infection, avascular necrosis, Paget's disease, and fracture are difficult to distinguish (68). Tuberculosis or coccidiomycosis commonly spares the adjacent disk (69). This may lead one to diagnose neoplasm, especially if there is an associated soft tissue mass. Vertebral osteomyelitis typically involves two contiguous vertebral bodies and the intervertebral disk. Many disease processes such as metastatic disease and low-grade pyogenic infections such as brucellosis, fungal infections, and sarcoidosis have imaging findings similar to TB of the spine. Characteristic features of brucellar spondylitis include gas within the disk, minimal associated paraspinal soft tissue mass, absence of gibbus deformity, and predilection for the lower lumbar spine (70).

Vertebral compression fractures may be secondary to insufficiency or may be pathologic. Insufficiency fractures have been distinguished from pathologic fractures by the preservation of vertebral marrow signal on MRI in association with fracture. However, with acute insufficiency fractures, the presence of edema and hemorrhage may simulate tumor or infection (71–73). Chronic insufficiency fractures may have relative decreased signal intensity on T1WI because of fibrosis or sclerosis, resembling tumor (71). Sacral insufficiency fractures may also simulate neoplasm (9). Pathologic fractures are characterized by marrow replacement as well as decreased vertebral body height (9). There may be enhancement after gadolinium in both insufficiency and pathologic fractures (34,35). There may be enlargement of the intervertebral disk adjacent to a fractured vertebra as well as increased signal intensity on T2WI. These changes reflect increased disk hydration in an effort to occupy the volume lost by a vertebral compression fracture (9).

Differentiation of Compression Fracture from Pathologic Fracture on MRI

In this situation, if the marrow is normal, the lesion may represent an old process. However, if the marrow is abnormal, this may represent either a new (acute) fracture, tumor, or metastasis. It is important to decide whether the lesion is focal and caused by a neoplasm or a lesion in the endplate, which may represent a traumatic fracture. If the lesion extends into the pedicle or affects several levels (multiple foci) in the spine, it is most probably metastatic. If this differentiation cannot be made on the basis of MRI, a plain film, CT, or possibly a bone scan may be helpful. If there is clinical concern, a follow-up or a bone biopsy may be performed.

The intravertebral vacuum cleft seen on plain films in avascular necrosis (Kummel disease) may not be seen on MRI because of the relative insensitivity of MRI to small air collections (9). Occasionally, paradoxic signal alterations may be seen (74). Images that initially show a signal void from air will later show increased signal on T2WI. This is because of fluid in the vacuum cleft accumulating in the supine position. This can mimic infection or neoplasm (9). Rarely, the presence of air in the intervertebral disk may be a sign of infection; such findings have been described in spinal brucellosis (70).

THE POSTOPERATIVE SPINE

Postoperative Changes

Postoperative changes include spondylolisthesis, central stenosis, foraminal stenosis, arachnoiditis, infection, hemorrhage, nerve injury, epidural fibrosis, recurrent disk herniation, pseudomeningocele, and wrong operation.

Chemonucleolysis

Chymopapain injection for chemonucleolysis results in characteristic changes on MRI. The treated disk will have a very low signal intensity on T2WI (75) as well as

decreased height (76). Decreased signal intensity can be seen 2 weeks following treatment, with a return to baseline appearance approximately 2 years later, as a result of scar formation (76).

Discectomy

Diffusely decreased signal intensity of the disk is usually observed after discectomy (9), as well as increased signal intensity on T2WI within the posterior disk margin. In the immediate postoperative period, this is caused by fluid at the site of disk curettage (77). This is later replaced by granulation tissue, which undergoes enhancement after contrast (9). This is distinguished from postoperative discitis, where there is increased disk signal intensity on T2WI and enhancement of the adjacent vertebral endplates (78). Comparison with previous studies should be made, as similar changes can be seen with type I degenerative changes in the vertebral endplates (9).

In the immediate postoperative period, the configuration of the interspace may be identical to its preoperative appearance for at least 1 month postsurgery. Between 2 and 6 months following surgery, false-positive appearance would decrease (77–79). The appearance of apparent herniated disk material results from the presence of postoperative edema and/or hemorrhage (9). As a result, the utility of MRI in detecting residual disk material in the immediate postoperative period is limited but is important as a baseline study.

Bone Marrow Transplantation

In individuals who have undergone bone marrow transplantation, increased marrow signal intensity on T1WI will occur (48). Like other discrete high signal foci, this may mimic infection or neoplasm.

Persistent Appearance of Pseudoherniation Following Surgery

Patients with relief following surgery may have imaging evidence of persistent herniation in the immediate postoperative period in 20% of cases. This is because early on there are changes such as granulomatous reactions that may mimic disk protrusion but in fact are a pseudoherniation. In 10% of patients, following surgery, postenhancement images may still be abnormal and resemble type II endplate changes despite the fact that the patient did well (80).

Pseudodisk Appearance

The conditions that may produce a pseudodisk appearance include scar, spur, posterior longitudinal ligament calcification, spondylolisthesis, conjoined nerve root, neuroma, schwannoma, Tarlov cyst, synovial cyst (see Fig. 27.35), epidural abscess, and epidural hematoma. Tarlov cyst may simulate an expansile lesion or metastasis (see Fig. 27.38).

Long after spinal surgery, epidural soft tissue masses are frequently seen; these represent herniated disk material, granulation tissue, fibrosis, or a combination of these (9). There are certain general principles that may aid in distinguishing these entities. However, there are exceptions to each of these principles, and the patient's clinical condition must be taken fully into account before arriving at any conclusion. On T2WI, granulation tissue and fibrosis usually are of greater signal intensity than herniated disk material (9), but extruded disk fragments may appear hyperintense on T2WI, similar to inflammatory tissue (46). Mature fibrosis may develop decreasing signal intensity on T2WI because of the declining proportion of extracellular space (81). Herniated disk fragments are usually associated with mass effect, whereas epidural fibrosis either does not or is characterized by retraction of adjacent tissues (9). Mass effect, however, can be associated with epidural granulation tissue or fibrosis (64,66,82). Because disk material is avascular, it does not enhance, whereas postoperative inflammatory tissue is very vascular and will enhance prominently (9). Enhancement of herniated disk material can occur if MR imaging is delayed 20 minutes or more following the administration of gadolinium (58,66). Areas of epidural fibrosis have been known to enhance up to 20 years following surgery (82). Enhancement is most intense in the 9 months following surgery and declines thereafter (83) and may lead to confusion with recurrent disk herniation. Subtle enhancement of epidural fibrosis may be recognized by using contrast-enhanced T1WI with fat suppression (64,84). Region-of-interest measurements can be obtained and compared with the precontrast scan. Noncontrast scans should always precede contrast scans because failure to do so may lead to serious errors of diagnosis (9).

Summary: How to Differentiate Scar from Recurrent Disk

Following injection of the contrast agent, scar tissue reveals homogeneous enhancement (Figs. 27.44 and 27.45), whereas the recurrent disk shows peripheral enhancement (Fig. 27.46). The anterior scar remains vascular and enhances for many years. The posterior scar becomes fibrotic, and after a few months there is diminished enhancement. Scar consistently enhances, causing

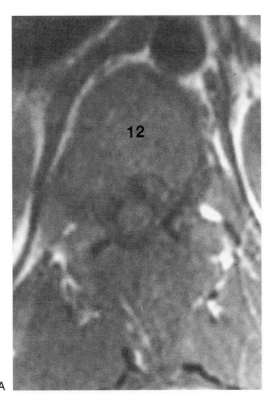
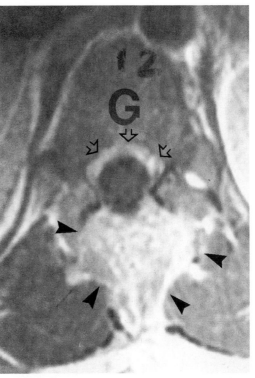

FIG. 27.44. Postoperative scar tissue. **A:** Axial T1WI (583/11) shows low-signal-intensity area around the dural sac. **B:** Axial T1WI (583/11) postgadolinium. Low-intensity area around the dural sac *(open arrowheads)* shows high enhancement indicating scar tissue rather than recurrent disk. Note large area of posterior scar at laminectomy site *(arrowheads)*.

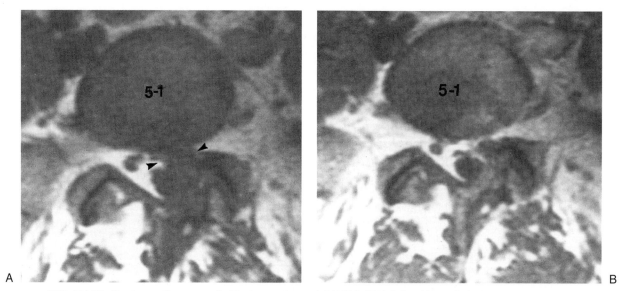

FIG. 27.45. Postoperative scar. **A:** Postoperative axial T1WI (700/14) without Gd shows a low-signal focal area *(arrowheads)* near the left lateral nerve root mimicking a recurrent disk protrusion. **B:** Axial T1WI (700/14) post-Gd shows enhancement of low-signal area indicating postoperative scar tissue. Note enlarged left nerve root ganglion as a result of edema.

retraction of the thecal sac, and may even show mass effect or may be contiguous with the disk space.

A scar may even be noted in unoperative spine surrounding disk herniation, also seen at operative spine, surgical curettage site, intervertebral disk in diffuse, spotty, or linear form, and in type I endplate changes.

The recurrent disk does not enhance within 20 minutes postinjection, and it is expected to enhance on delayed images. Therefore, it is important that imaging is done within 20 minutes of injection. In general, all disks, whether operated or not operated, are surrounded by some scar.

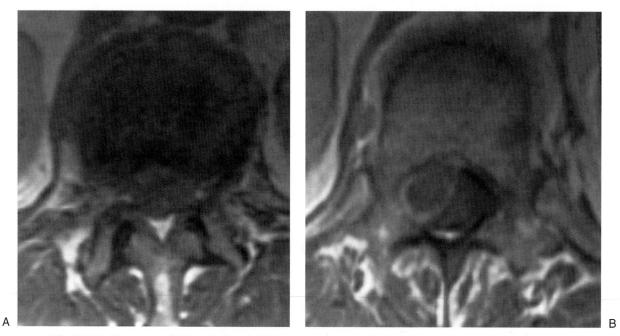

FIG. 27.46. Recurrent disk herniation. **A:** Noncontrast axial T1WI (700/14) MRI at the T12 to L1 disk level shows focal abnormal low signal mass at the epidural space. **B:** Axial T1WI (800/11) post-Gd injection shows peripheral enhancement around the recurrent disk herniation at the T12 to L1 level.

Imaging differentiation of scar from recurrent disk has improved from 83% (CT myelogram) in 1983 to almost 100% in 1993 with high-resolution enhanced MR imaging.

Failure of Differentiation of Disk from Scar

This may be the result in part from partial volume averaging; for example, a small amount of disk or a large amount of scar, vascularization of the disk, and the timing after injection.

Postoperative Epidural and Paraspinal Soft Tissue Changes

There may be a postoperative pseudomeningocele. If fat packing is performed at the operative site, collections of fat will be seen within the epidural space (77). This can simulate the T1 shortening effects of methemoglobin within an epidural hematoma (9). Gelfoam or methyl-methacrylate may result in heterogeneous signal intensity and simulate an abscess (77) at the laminectomy site (9). The paraspinal musculature will have an abnormal post-operative appearance. Air within the tissues will show a signal void. Increased signal intensity on T2WI resulting from edema and hemorrhage may be noted. Not only does the postoperative paraspinal musculature appear distorted in the postoperative state, it may also show abnormal contrast enhancement (77).

Myelography

Retained iophendylate (Pantopaque) in patients who have undergone previous myelography presents as increased signal intensity on T1WI because of the lipid composition of iophendylate (9). This may simulate intradural lesions such as lipomas, hemorrhage, or dermoid (85–91). Chemical shift misregistration may surround the retained iophendylate because of its lipid composition (9). Retained iophendylate is hypointense to CSF on gradient-echo imaging and, hence, may simulate intra- or extradural lesions, magnetic susceptibility, or flow artifact (89).

IMAGING ARTIFACTS

Magnetic Resonance Imaging Artifact Caused by Nonuniform Magnetic Field

Artifacts occur when the "read gradient" cannot create an orderly change in the magnetic field.

Tissue Interfaces

Bone–tissue interfaces cause variation in the magnetic field, which can change the frequency of tissue signal. In the spine, magnetic susceptibility variation occurs within the trabecular bone. This causes rapid dephasing of the signal and a mottled hypointense appearance on gradient-echo scan. A T1-weighted spin-echo image of bone appears brighter than a gradient-echo image because it is much less sensitive to magnetic field inhomogeneities.

Incomplete Fat Saturation

An air–fat interface causes variation in the magnetic field, which causes lipid protons to have a Larmour frequency that does not match that of the saturation pulse. Thus, the lipid will appear bright.

Ferromagnetic Artifact

Ferromagnetic artifact is caused by the large magnetic susceptibility of ferromagnetic material. Magnetic susceptibility is the ratio of intensity of magnetization produced in a substance to the intensity of the applied external magnetic field (92,93). This large magnetic susceptibility causes gross local static magnetic field inhomogeneities (92). This kind of artifact results in spatial and signal distortion displayed along the frequency-encoding axis, usually presenting as a signal void associated with peripheral signal hyperintensity (9) (Figs. 27.47 and 27.48). Stainless steel produces severe artifact compared to titanium (94) (Fig. 27.49). Ferromagnetic arti-

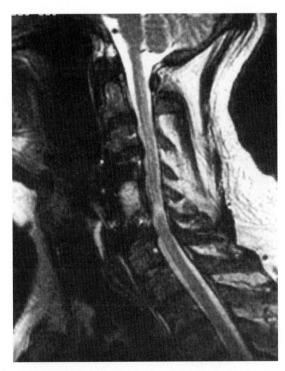

FIG. 27.47. Magnetization susceptibility artifact. Sagittal fat-saturated FSE T2WI (3,000/102) of the cervical spine shows fusion of C3 to C6 with titanium plate. Note low-signal magnetic susceptibility artifact.

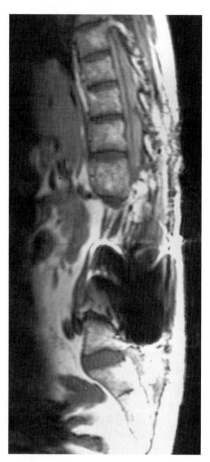

FIG. 27.48. Magnetization susceptibility artifact. Parasagittal T1WI of the lumbar spine (510/15) shows metallic artifact caused by spine fusion.

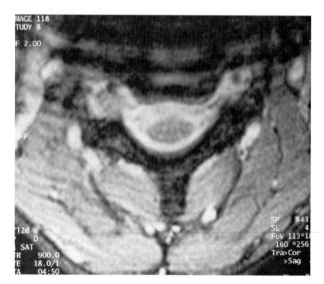

FIG. 27.49. Magnetization susceptibility artifact. Axial gradient echo (900/18) with flip angle of 12 degrees shows curvilinear multilayer low-signal-intensity metal artifact arising from the dental brace.

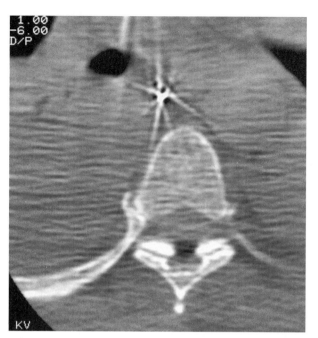

FIG. 27.50. Beam-hardening artifact from a nasogastric (NG) tube. Axial CT of the thoracic spine showing starburst radiating artifact created by the NG tube.

fact is greater with gradient-echo imaging than it is with both conventional and fast spin-echo imaging. It is also worse with reduced-bandwidth imaging (92), large voxel sizes, long echo times, and high-field-strength magnets (57,95). Apart from causing artifacts, ferromagnetic objects can be hazardous during MR examination and should be removed, if possible. However, a number of nonremovable metallic objects will still be encountered. Spinal fixation rods are a common problem. Others may be shrapnel or inferior vena cava filters. Nonferrous devices can cause similar artifacts through the generation of Eddy currents (96–99). On CT examination, metallic artifact results in a beam-hardening phenomenon causing image deterioration (Fig. 27.50).

Chemical Shift

Chemical shift is the difference in Larmour frequency of hydrogen nuclei bound into a different chemical compound (92). Chemical shift misregistration artifact is caused by differences in precessional frequencies of fat and water protons, causing an artifactual shift in signal intensity along fat–water interfaces in the frequency-encoding direction of an image (9). This causes spatial mismapping of one of the two, fat or water, in an MR image (100–105). Because MR systems are tuned to the frequency of water, fat will be mismapped on the image (92). Misregistration artifact increases with reduced-bandwidth imaging and high-field-strength magnets (9,92). Fat-suppression methods can be combined with reduced bandwidth to decrease chemical shift misregistration artifact. The discovertebral junction represents a fat–water interface. Thus, chemical shift misregistration can cause an artifactual shift in signal intensity from one vertebral endplate to the opposite endplate on sagittal images of the spine (103). The posterior longitudinal ligament can be obscured by chemical shift misregistration, suggesting a tear (66). This problem can be avoided by swapping phase and frequency axes.

Fat-Induced Chemical Shift Artifact

This occurs when the read gradient cannot create an orderly change in the magnetic field because all tissues are not responding in the same way (some are less magnetized). Because the computer assumes predictable changes in radiowave frequency, some tissues will be spatially shifted. Fat gives rise to a common artifact, called chemical shift or misregistration effect. Protons in the lipid resonate at a lower frequency than protons in water. The slower lipid protons are mismapped relative to the water in the frequency-encoding direction, resulting in an appearance of a signal void where the lipid is displaced from water protons and a hyperintense region where lipid and water protons overlap. The artifact tends to be more prominent on images made with higher-field-strength machines. In the spine, fat in the vertebral body can give rise to chemical shift artifacts. When the frequency-encoding direction is anterior–posterior, the disk boundaries appear normal. However, when the frequency-encoding direction is inferior–superior, the fat image of the vertebra shifts, causing a thickened dark band on the lower vertebral endplate and almost complete obliteration of the upper endplate (Figs. 27.51 and 27.52).

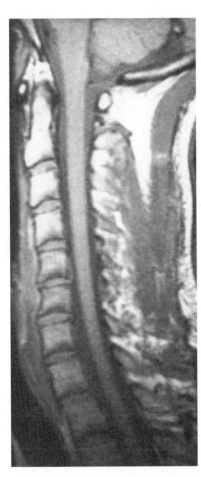

FIG. 27.51. Chemical shift misregistration artifact. Sagittal T1WI of the cervical spine. Note that when the frequency-encoding direction is inferior-superior, the fat image of the vertebra shifts, causing a thickened dark band of the inferior endplates of vertebrae and almost completely obliterates the cortex of the superior vertebral endplate.

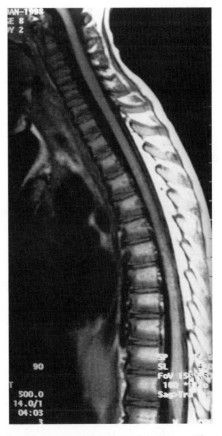

FIG. 27.52. Chemical shift misregistration artifact. Sagittal T1WI (500/14) shows chemical shift artifact caused by inferior-superior frequency-encoding direction axis. Note low-signal bands at the inferior endplate of the vertebral bodies. This was normal on T2WI (not shown). (Courtesy of Zehava S. Rosenberg, New York, NY.)

Motion Artifact

This can cause artifactually increased or decreased signal intensity (9). Motion artifact occurs in the phase-encoding direction and can lead to blurring or ghosting of structures (9,92) (Fig. 27.53). Blurring may occur in any direction, causing spatial dispersion of signal (99,106). Blurring occurs when an object changes location between phase-encoding views (107). The signal of the structure is displayed over its range of motion, causing decreased edge definition (108–110). Ghost artifact is structured noise (108) caused by periodic signal intensity or phase shift variations (108–110). With a constant frequency of the periodicity, the effect is to display copies or ghosts across the phase-encoding axis. Ghost artifact propagates across the entire image (92). With a variable frequency of periodic motion, there will be mismapped signal along the phase-encoding axis appearing as streak artifact (107,110). Motion artifact in the cervical spine is usually caused by swallowing (see Fig. 27.53). In the thoracolumbar region, motion artifact results from respiratory motion and vascular pulsations from the heart and aorta. Motion artifacts are expressed along the phase-encoding axis of an image, which in the spine is usually anteroposterior (9,99). On CT examination, motion misregistration artifact can lead to significant deterioration on reconstructed images (Fig. 27.54A) and may be misleading on axial images (Fig. 27.54B).

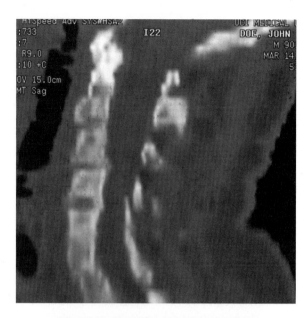

A

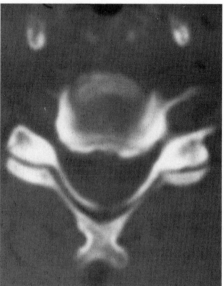

B

FIG. 27.54. Motion misregistration artifact. **A:** Sagittal reconstruction CT shows motion misregistration artifact. Note step-like irregularity of the posterior cervical spine. **B:** Axial CT of the cervical spine shows double lamina appearance because of motion artifact rather than dislocation.

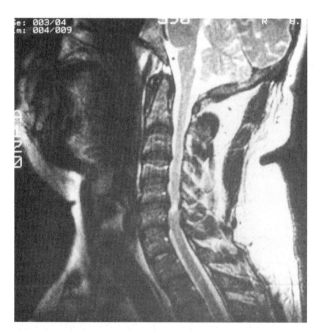

FIG. 27.53. Swallowing (motion) artifact. Sagittal T2WI (3,000/102) MRI of the cervical spine shows a series of artifactual bands overlying the vertebral bodies, creating longitudinal parallel lines related to swallowing or esophageal motion.

Vascular Artifact

In the normal patient, the aorta has fast pulsatile laminar arterial flow. Multiple ghost images of this flow create a complex multilayered horizontal band artifact, often referred to as phase shift within the image. This artifact becomes more prominent when a contrast agent is administered unless the ghost artifacts are minimized with inferior and superior saturation pulses, which prevent contrast media from exaggerating the vascular artifacts from flowing blood.

Cerebrospinal Fluid Pulsation Artifact

Pulsatile motion of CSF (up and down the spinal canal) can cause ghost images propagating parallel to the phase-encoding direction (Figs. 27.55 and 27.56) and may mimic a vascular malformation.

Motion artifact can be reduced by respiratory gating (9,99,106), pseudogating, breath-hold technique, and restraints (99,106). In addition, presaturation bands can be positioned over moving structures (49,99,111). Last, sagittal images can be acquired with the phase-encoding gradient aligned along the craniocaudal direction to prevent motion artifacts traversing the spinal canal (112). The CSF signal may vary depending on the location of CSF in the spinal canal. In cases of spinal stenosis, the free flow of CSF above the level of stenosis creates mild loss of signal, whereas below the level of stenosis stagnation of CSF would result in a brighter signal intensity of CSF (110) (Fig. 27.57).

Saturation artifact may occur when angled images of the lumbar intervertebral disks are obtained. In patients with accentuated lumbar lordosis, oblique slices may overlap posteriorly. This results in saturation effects, represented as a series of linear areas of decreased signal

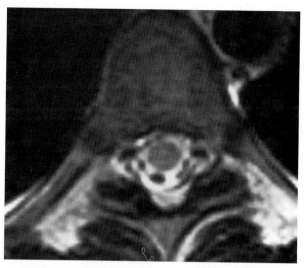

FIG. 27.56. Cerebrospinal fluid flow void artifact. Axial fat-saturated FSE T2WI (3,466/108) shows a ring of focal, small black signal artifacts in the bright CSF, palisading around the spinal cord. These represent CSF flow artifacts.

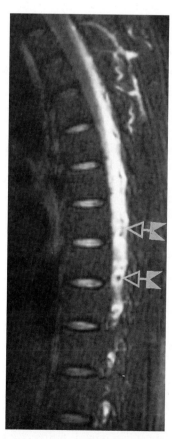

FIG. 27.55. Cerebrospinal fluid flow void artifact simulating AVM. Parasagittal fat-saturated FSE T2WI (3,000/96) shows serpiginous black artifacts *(arrows)* in CSF representing CSF flow artifact simulating AVM. Angiogram proved normal.

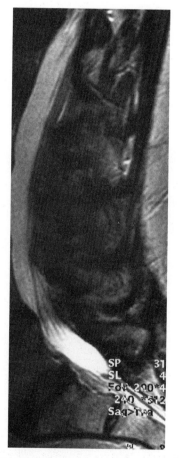

FIG. 27.57. Cerebrospinal fluid signal variation related to slow CSF flow. Sagittal T2WI (4,400/112) MRI of lumbosacral spine shows very bright signal of CSF at the sacral region because of decreased CSF flow there.

intensity overlying the posterior paraspinal soft tissues. This artifact may even obscure intraspinal lesions. A less acute oblique angle or transaxial images can solve this problem (9).

Paradoxic enhancement results in flow-related increased signal intensity. Because routine pulse sequences use multiple repetitions at an interval that does not allow complete recovery of longitudinal magnetization, the net signal from stationary spins is less than if complete recovery of magnetization were allowed. The flowing spins from outside the imaging volume have not been exposed to radiofrequency excitation pulses, so that their full magnetization leads to a greater signal intensity than stationary spins (92). Moving spins are saturated, then quickly replaced by inflowing fully magnetized spins (111). Thus, there is a greater signal intensity of moving fluids than stationary tissue in an image (108–110,113). Flow-related enhancement causes signal gain for both blood and CSF (92). Flow-related enhancement is most conspicuous on short-T_R and short-T_E images because of the hypointensity of stationary CSF on this sequence. Under these conditions, flow-related enhancement may mimic extramedullary pathology and reduce CSF cord contrast (114). To avoid paradoxic enhancement, one should send upstream presaturation pulses.

Partial volume averaging occurs when two structures or an anatomic interface with different signal intensities is included within the same voxel (99,113). This leads to an averaging of signal intensity within the voxel (113). Artifactually increased or decreased signal intensity may obscure or simulate pathology (Fig. 27.58). The results of

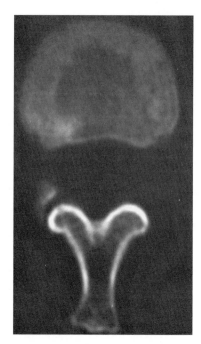

FIG. 27.59. Partial volume averaging of the intervertebral disk and bony vertebral body. Axial CT of the lumbar vertebral endplate shows low density of the body because of volume averaging with the disk.

partial volume averaging may cause the appearance of pseudomasses or may decrease the visibility of objects that are of low contrast (99). Partial volume averaging is more likely with increased slice thickness and interslice gaps (113); thus, selecting a thinner slice will reduce the amount of artifact present. Decreasing the voxel size will also be of help (92). Partial volume averaging between the vertebral body and intervertebral disk may simulate vertebral marrow replacement, and vice versa (81). The scoliotic spine is subject to increased partial volume effects (9). On CT examination, partial volume averaging results in an image that has the average density of two different adjacent structures (Fig. 27.59).

Artifact Secondary to Protocol Error

1. Coherence artifact. See Saturation Artifact.
2. Radiofrequency interface artifact. Static electricity from an electric blanket would lead to an artifact.
3. Shading artifact. Radiofrequency fields fall off rapidly away from the coil, causing gradual image loss of brightness (Fig. 27.60).
4. Leakage of radiowaves. This involves leakage of radiowaves from the transmitter to the receiver (zipper artifact) through the center of the image parallel to the phase-encoding direction.
5. Aliasing, or wraparound artifact, occurs through excitation of tissue outside the field of view, resulting in a mismapping of the signal intensity of the tissue into the field of view (9). This occurs on the

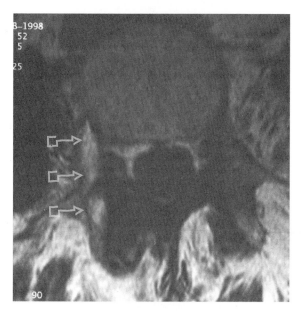

FIG. 27.58. Partial volume-averaging artifact. Axial T1WI (525/12) shows a band of bright signal intensity projecting over the right pedicle and lamina of the lumbar spine *(arrows)*, representing partial volume averaging of paraspinal fat at adjacent sections.

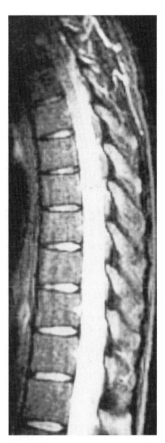

FIG. 27.60. Shading artifact. Sagittal T2WI (3,000/96) of the thoracic spine. Note that the radiofrequency field falls off rapidly away from the coil, causing gradual loss of image brightness in the upper thoracic levels.

opposite side of the image (99,106,108,113,115). Aliasing occurs when the field of view is smaller than the dimensions of the object being imaged in that selected plane (92). This causes an error during analog-to-digital conversion of the MR signal (113). Undersampling of the out-of-view tissue occurs, and, as a result, high-frequency signal will be digitized to low-frequency components of opposite-phase polarity (92,108). When a small field of view is selected, oversampling techniques available on current scanners can reduce the incidence of this artifact. Aliasing artifact occurs on the slice selection and the phase-encode direction (in 2-D acquisitions) as well as the slice partition direction (for 3-D acquisitions) (116, 117). With aliasing, images of the upper spine can be represented on images of the lower spine (9). Obviously, this has the potential to obscure lesions of the spine and adjacent tissues. The aliasing artifact can be avoided by increasing the field of view and phase-encoding steps.

6. Truncation artifact (Gibbs phenomenon) is seen at high-tissue-contrast interfaces such as the discovertebral junction and CSF–cord interface (118,119). This artifact presents as a linear focus of alternating high and low signal intensity that propagates along the phase-encoding direction from both sides of a high contrast interface. These signal intensity changes will diminish in amplitude with increasing distance from the high-contrast interface (92). Truncation artifacts are caused by the inability of two-dimensional Fourier transformation to reproduce signal intensity changes at high-contrast interfaces accurately (118, 120–123). There is a resultant fluctuating underestimation and overestimation of true signal intensity. Truncation artifact may result in a syrinx-like artifact of the cervical spine (Fig. 27.61). This artifact is the result of the summation of overshoot and undershoot signal intensity changes from the high-contrast spinal cord–CSF interface (120–122). Underestimation of signal intensity in the center of the cord on T1WI and overestimation on T2WI results in a hyperintense and hypointense signal traversing the cord in the craniocaudal direction on sagittal images. Thus, the pseudosyrinx artifact is similar in appearance to a true syrinx on T1WI and T2WI. Truncation artifact can be reduced by decreasing the pixel size (by either increasing the number of phase-encoding steps or by

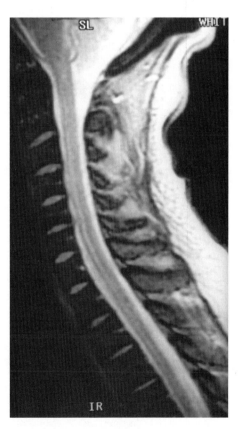

FIG. 27.61. Truncation artifact (Gibbs phenomenon). Sagittal gradient echo (450/15) with flip angle of 25 degrees shows a longitudinal bright signal in the spinal cord, which may mimic syringomyelia. This is caused by use of too few phase-encoding steps. Truncation artifact can be minimized by using higher gradient or phase-encoding steps.

decreasing the field of view), switching the phase- and frequency-encoding directions, filtering raw data before image reconstruction, or using alternative methods of image reconstruction (120–123).

Other Artifacts

Flair

Sometimes an unusual bright artifact is produced because of an unexplained technical reason.

Incomplete Fat Saturation at Edge of a Large Field of View

In a large field of the spine, fat in vertebrae may not be suppressed at the top edge of the field. In this area, water being saturated instead of fat causes loss of signal from spinal cord.

ACKNOWLEDGMENT

We would like to thank Drs. Ay-Ming Wang, Mauricio Castillo, and James Mastromatteo for reviewing the chapter and for their constructive comments. Also, the efforts of Mrs. Betty Trent for preparation of the manuscript are appreciated.

REFERENCES

1. Geelen JAG, Langman J. Closure of the neural tube in the cephalic region of the mouse embryo. *Anat Rec* 1977;189:625.
2. Waterman RE. Topographical changes along the neural fold associated with neurolatism in the hamster and the mouse. *Am J Anat* 1976;146:151.
3. Jacobson M, ed. *Developmental neurobiology, 2nd ed.* New York: Plenum Press, 1978.
4. Sadler TW. *Langman's medical embryology, 6th ed.* Baltimore: Williams & Wilkins, 1990;139–156.
5. Naidich TP, Zimmerman RA, McLone DQ, et al. Congenital anomalies of the spine and spinal cord. In: Atlas SW, ed. *Magnetic resonance imaging of the brain and spine, 2nd ed.* Philadelphia: Lippincott-Raven, 1996;1265–1337.
6. Yu S, Haughton VM, Ho PSP, et al. Progressive and regressive changes in the nucleus pulposus. II. The adult. *Radiology* 1988;169:93–97.
7. Tertti MO, Salminen JJ, Paajanen HEK, et al. Low-back pain and disc degeneration in children: a case-control MR imaging study. *Radiology* 1991;180:503–507.
8. Pech P, Haughton VM. Lumbar intervertebral disc: correlative MR and anatomic study. *Radiology* 1985;156:699–701.
9. Mirowitz SA. *Pitfalls, variants and artifacts in body MR imaging.* St Louis: Mosby-Year Book, 1996;411–497.
10. Sze G, Bravo S, Baierl P, et al. Developing spinal column: gadolinium-enhanced MR imaging. *Radiology* 1991;180:497–502.
11. Sze G, Baierl P, Bravo S. Evolution of the infant spinal column: evaluation with MR imaging. *Radiology* 1991;181:819–827.
12. Taylor GA, Eggli KD. Lap-belt injuries of the lumbar spine in children: a pitfall in CT diagnosis. *Am J Roentgenol* 1988;150:1355–1358.
13. Bergman RA, Thompson SA, Afifi AK, et al. *Compendium of human anatomic variation: text, atlas and world literature.* Baltimore: Urban & Schwarzenberg, 1988;131.
14. Major NM, Helms CA. Normal variants and pitfalls in CT of the lumbar spine. *Contemp Diagn Radiol* 1993;16(11):1–6.
15. Stabler A, Bellan M, Weiss M, Gärtner C, Brossmann J, Reiser MF. MR imaging of enhancing intraosseous disc herniation (Schmorl's node). *Am J Roentgenol* 1997;168:933–938.
16. Leibner ED, Floman Y. Tunnelling Schmorl's node. *Skel Radiol* 1998;27:225–227.
17. Hahn PY, Strobel JJ, Hahn FJ. Verification of lumbosacral segments on MR images: identification of transitional vertebrae. *Radiology* 1992;182:580–581.
18. Tien R, Newton TH, Dillon WP, et al. A simple method for spinal localization in MR imaging. *Am J Neuroradiol* 1989;10:1232.
19. Ralston MD, Dykes TA, Applebaum BI. Verification of lumbar vertebral bodies (letter). *Radiology* 1992;185:615–616.
20. Hahn PY, Strobel JJ, Hahn FJ. Verification of lumbar vertebral bodies: response to letter to editor. *Radiology* 1992;185:616.
21. Keats TE, Lusted LB. *Atlas of roentgenographic measurement, 5th ed.* Chicago: Year Book Medical Publishers, 1985;121–122.
22. Grenier N, Greselle J-F, Vital J-M, et al. Normal and disrupted lumbar longitudinal ligaments: correlative MR and anatomic study. *Radiology* 1989;171:197–205.
23. Jinkins JR, Matthes JC, Sener RN, et al. Spondylolysis, spondylolisthesis, and associated nerve root entrapment in the lumbosacral spine: MR evaluation. *Am J Roentgenol* 1992;159:799–803.
24. Johnson DW, Farnum GN, Latchaw RE, et al. MR imaging of the pars interarticularis. *Am J Roentgenol* 1989;152:327–332.
25. Ulmer JL, Elster AD, Mathews VP, King JC. Distinction between degenerative and isthmic spondylolisthesis on sagittal MR images: importance of increased anteroposterior diameter of the spinal canal (wide canal sign). *Am J Roentgenol* 1994;163:411–416.
26. Geremia GK, McCluney KW, Adler SS, et al. The magnetic resonance hypointense spine of AIDS. *J Comput Assist Tomogr* 1990;14:785–789.
27. LeBlanc AD, Schonfeld E, Schneider VS, et al. The spine: changes in T_2 relaxation times from disuse. *Radiology* 1988;169:105–107.
28. Castillo M, Malko JA, Hoffman JC Jr. The bright intervertebral disc: an indirect sign of abnormal spinal bone marrow on T1-weighted MR images. *Am J Neuroradiol* 1990;11:23–26.
29. Remedios PA, Colletti PM, Raval JK, et al. Magnetic resonance imaging of bone after radiation. *Magn Reson Imag* 1988;6:301–304.
30. Rosenthal DI, Hayes CW, Rosen B, et al. Fatty replacement of spinal bone marrow due to radiation: demonstration by dual energy quantitative CT and MR imaging. *J Comput Assist Tomogr* 1989;13:463–465.
31. Yankelevitz DF, Henschke CI, Knapp PH, et al. Effect of radiation therapy on thoracic and lumbar bone marrow: evaluation with MR imaging. *Am J Roentgenol* 1991;157(1):87–92.
32. Ramsey RG, Zacharias CE. MR imaging of the spine after radiation therapy: easily recognizable effect. *Am J Neuroradiol* 1995;6:247–251.
33. de Roos A, Kressel H, Spritzer C, et al. MR imaging of marrow changes adjacent to end plates in degenerative lumbar disc disease. *Am J Roentgenol* 1987;149:531–534.
34. Mouloupoulos LA, Dimopoulos MA, Varma DGK, et al. Waldenstrom macroglobulinemia: MR imaging of the spine and CT of the abdomen and pelvis. *Radiology* 1993;188:669–673.
35. Mouloupoulos LA, Varma DGK, Dimopoulos MA. Multiple myeloma: spinal MR imaging in patients with untreated newly diagnosed disease. *Radiology* 1992;185:833–840.
36. Ricci C, Cova M, Kang YS, et al. Normal age-related patterns of cellular and fatty bone marrow distribution in the axial skeleton: MR imaging study. *Radiology* 1990;177:83–88.
37. Helms CA, Volger JB III, Genant HK. Characteristic CT manifestation of uncommon spinal disorder. *Orthoped Clin North Am* 1985;16(3):445–459.
38. Ross JS, Masaryk TJ, Modic MT, et al. Vertebral hemangiomas: MR imaging. *Radiology* 1987;165:165–169.
39. Hajek PC, Baker LL, Goobar JE, et al. Focal fat deposition in axial bone marrow: MR characteristics. *Radiology* 1987;162:245–249.
40. Siffring PA, Forrest TS, Frick P. Hernias of the inferior lumbar space: diagnosis with US. *Radiology* 1989;170:190.
41. Sze G, Brant-Zawadzki MN, Wilson CR, et al. Pseudotumor of the craniovertebral junction associated with chronic subluxation: MR imaging studies. *Radiology* 1986;161:391–394.
42. Ellis JH, Martel W, Lillie JH, et al. Magnetic resonance imaging of the normal craniovertebral junction. *Spine* 1991;16:105–111.
43. Glickstein MF, Miller WT, Dalinka MK, et al. Paraspinal lipomatosis: a benign mass. *Radiology* 1987;163:79–80.

44. Isherwood I, Prendergast DJ, Hickey DS, et al. Quantitative analysis of intervertebral disc structure. *Acta Radiol Suppl (Stockh)* 1986;369: 492–495.

45. Gelber ND, Ragland RL, Knorr JR. Gd-DTPA enhanced MRI of cervical anterior epidural venous plexus. *J Comput Assist Tomogr* 1992; 16:760–763.

46. Bundschuh CV, Modic MT, Ross JS, et al. Epidural fibrosis and recurrent disc herniation in the lumbar spine: MR imaging assessment. *Am J Roentgenol* 1988;150:923–932.

47. Flannigan BD, Lufkin RB, McGlade C, et al. MR imaging of the cervical spine: neurovascular anatomy. *Am J Roentgenol* 1987;148: 785–790.

48. Parizel PM, Rodesch G, Baleriaux D, et al. Gd-DTPA-enhanced MR in thoracic disc herniations. *Neuroradiology* 1989;1:75–79.

49. Sugimura H, Kakitsubata Y, Suzuki Y, et al. MRI of ossification of ligamentum flavum. *J Comput Assist Tomogr* 1992;16:73–76.

50. Nowicki BH, Yu S, Reinartz J, et al. Effect of axial loading on neural foramina and nerve roots in the lumbar spine. *Radiology* 1990;176: 433–437.

51. Grenier N, Grossman RI, Schiebler ML, et al. Degenerative lumbar disc disease: pitfalls and usefulness of MR imaging in detection of vacuum phenomenon. *Radiology* 1987;164:861–865.

52. Russell EJ. Cervical disc disease. *Radiology* 1990;177:313–325.

53. Otake S, Matsuo M, Nishizawa S, et al. Ossification of the posterior longitudinal ligament: MR evaluation. *Am J Neuroradiol* 1992; 13:1059.

54. Yomashita Y, Takahashi M, Matsuno Y, et al. Spinal cord compression due to ossification of ligaments: MR imaging. *Radiology* 1990;175: 843–848.

55. Jackson DE Jr, Atlas SW, Mani JR, et al. Intraspinal synovial cysts: MR imaging. *Radiology* 1989;170:527–530.

56. Breger RK, Williams AL, Daniels DL, et al. Contrast enhancement in spinal MR imaging. *Am J Neuroradiol* 1989;10:633–637.

57. Czervionke LF, Daniels DL, Ho PSP, et al. Cervical neural foramina: correlative anatomic and MR imaging study. *Radiology* 1988;169: 753–759.

58. Ross JS, Modic MT, Masaryk TJ, et al. Assessment of extradural degenerative disease with Gd-DTPA-enhanced MR imaging: correlation with surgical and pathologic findings. *Am J Neuroradiol* 1989;10: 1243–1249.

59. Davis SW, Levy LM, LeBihan DJ, et al. Sacral meningeal cysts: evaluation with MR imaging. *Radiology* 1993;187:445–448.

60. Sklar E, Quencer RM, Green BA, et al. Acquired spinal subarachnoid cysts: evaluation with MR, CT myelography, and intraoperative sonography. *Am J Roentgenol* 1989;153:1057–1064.

61. Raghavan N, Barkovich AJ, Edwards M, et al. MR imaging in the tethered spinal cord syndrome. *Am J Roentgenol* 1989;152:843–852.

62. Wilson DA, Prince JR. MR imaging determination of the location of the normal conus medullaris throughout childhood. *Am J Neuroradiol* 1989;10:259–262.

63. Ross JS, Masaryk TJ, Modic MT, et al. MR imaging of lumbar arachnoiditis. *Am J Roentgenol* 1987;149:1025–1032.

64. Mirowitz SA, Shady KL. Gadopentetate dimeglumine-enhanced MR imaging of the postoperative lumbar spine: comparison of fat-suppressed and conventional T_1-weighted images. *Am J Roentgenol* 1992; 159:385–389.

65. Modic MT, Steinberg PM, Ross JS, et al. Degenerative disc disease: assessment of changes in vertebral body marrow with MR imaging. *Radiology* 1988;166:193–199.

66. Hueftle MG, Modic MT, Ross JS, et al. Lumbar spine: postoperative MR imaging with Gd-DTPA. *Radiology* 1988;167:817–824.

67. Sether LA, Yu S. Intervertebral disc: normal age-related changes in MR signal intensity. *Radiology* 1990;177:385–388.

68. Smith AS, Weinstein MA, Mizushima A, et al. MR imaging characteristics of tuberculous spondylitis vs. vertebral osteomyelitis. *Am J Roentgenol* 1989;153:399–405.

69. Ahmadi J, Bajaj A, Destian S, et al. Spinal tuberculosis: atypical observations at MR imaging. *Radiology* 1993;189:489–493.

70. Yao DC, Sartoris DJ. Musculoskeletal tuberculosis. *Radiol Clin North Am* 1995;33(4):679–689.

71. Baker LL, Goodman SB, Perkash I, et al. Benign versus pathologic compression fractures of vertebral bodies: assessment with conventional spin-echo, chemical-shift, and STIR MR imaging. *Radiology* 1990;174:495–502.

72. Frager D, Elkin C, Swerdlow M, et al. Subacute osteoporotic compression fracture: misleading magnetic resonance appearance. *Skel Radiol* 1988;17:123–126.

73. Yuh WTC, Zachar CK, Barloon TJ, et al. Vertebral compression fractures: distinction between benign and malignant causes with MR imaging. *Radiology* 1989;172:215–218.

74. Malghem J, Maldague B, Labaisse M-A, et al. Intravertebral vacuum cleft: changes in content after supine positioning. *Radiology* 1993; 187:483–487.

75. Masaryk TJ, Boumphrey F, Modic MT, et al. Effects of chemonucleolysis demonstrated by MR imaging. *J Comput Assist Tomogr* 1986; 10:917–923.

76. Kato F, Mimatsu K, Kawakami N, et al. Changes seen on magnetic resonance imaging in the intervertebral disc space after chemonucleolysis: a hypothesis concerning regeneration of the disc after chemonucleolysis. *Neuroradiology* 1992;34:267–270.

77. Ross JS, Masaryk TJ, Modic MT, et al. Lumbar spine: postoperative assessment with surface-coil MR imaging. *Radiology* 1987;164: 851–860.

78. Boden SD, Davis DO, Dina TS, et al. Contrast-enhanced MR imaging performed after successful lumbar disc surgery: prospective study. *Radiology* 1992;182:59–64.

79. Boden SD, Davis DO, Dina TS, et al. Postoperative discitis: distinguishing early MR findings from normal postoperative disc space changes. *Radiology* 1992;184:765–771.

80. Winkler ML, Modic MT. *MRI of the spine.* Paper presented at the Magnetic Resonance Imaging National Symposium, Las Vegas, Nevada, 1997.

81. Bundschuh CV, Stein L, Slusser JH, et al. Distinguishing between scar and recurrent herniated disc in postoperative patients: value of contrast-enhanced CT and MR imaging. *Am J Neuroradiol* 1990; 11:949–958.

82. Ross JS, Masaryk TJ, Schrader M, et al. MR imaging of the postoperative lumbar spine: assessment with gadopentetate dimeglumine. *Am J Neuroradiol* 1990;11:711–776.

83. Glickstein MF, Sussman SK, et al. Time-dependent scar enhancement in magnetic resonance imaging of the postoperative lumbar spine. *Skel Radiol* 1991;20:333–337.

84. Bobman SA, Atlas SW, Listerud J, et al. Postoperative lumbar spine: contrast-enhanced chemical shift MR imaging. *Radiology* 1991;179: 557–562.

85. Barsi P, Kenez J, Varallyay G, et al. Unusual origin of free subarachnoid fat drops: a ruptured spinal dermoid tumour. *Neuroradiology* 1992;34:343–344.

86. Braun IF, Malko JA, Davis PC, et al. The behavior of pantopaque on MR: *in vivo* and *in vitro* analyses. *Am J Neuroradiol* 1986;7:997–1001.

87. Gupta RK, Jena A, Kumar S. Iophendylate or spillage from epidermoid—a diagnostic dilemma on cranial MR imaging. *Magn Reson Imag* 1989;7:293–295.

88. Hackney DB, Grossman RI, Zimmerman RA, et al. MR characteristics of iophendylate (Pantopaque). *J Comput Assist Tomogr* 1986;10: 401–403.

89. Jack CR Jr, Gehring DG, Ehman RL, et al. Cerebrospinal fluid–iophendylate contrast on gradient-echo MR images. *Radiology* 1988; 169:561–563.

90. Mamourian AC, Briggs RW. Appearance of Pantopaque on MR images. *Radiology* 1986;158:457–460.

91. Suojanen J, Wang AM, Winston KR. Pantopaque mimicking spinal lipoma: MR pitfall. *J Comput Assist Tomogr* 1988;12:346–348.

92. Hendrick RE, Russ PD, Simon JM. *MRI: principles and artifacts.* New York: Raven Press, 1993.

93. Czervionke LF, Daniels DL, Wehrli FW, et al. Magnetic susceptibility artifacts in gradient-recalled echo MR imaging. *Am J Neuroradiol* 1988;9(6):1149–1155.

94. Mirvis SE, Geisler F, Joslyn JN, et al. Use of titanium wire in cervical spine fixation as a means to reduce MR artifacts. *Am J Neuroradiol* 1988;9:1229–1231.

95. Young IR, Cox IJ, Bryant DJ, Bydder GM. The benefits of increasing spatial resolution as a means of reducing artifacts due to field inhomogeneities. *Magn Reson Imag* 1988;6(5):585–590.

96. Malko JA, Hoffman JC, Jarrett PJ. Eddy-current-induced artifacts caused by an MR-compatible halo device. *Radiology* 1989;173: 563–564.

97. Farahani K, Sinha U, Sinha S, et al. Effect of field strength on sus-

ceptibility artifacts in magnetic resonance imaging. *Comput Med Imag Graphics* 1990;14:409–413.

98. Schick RM, Wismer GL, Davis KR. Magnetic susceptibility effects secondary to out-of-plane air in fast MR scanning. *Am J Neuroradiol* 1988;9(3):439–442.

99. Wesbey G, Edelman RR, Harris R. Artifacts in MR imaging: description, causes, and solutions. In: Edelman RR, Hesselink JR, eds. *Clinical magnetic resonance imaging.* Philadelphia: WB Saunders, 1990; 74–108.

100. Szumowski J, Simon JM. Proton chemical shift imaging. In: Stark DD, Bradley WG Jr, eds. *Magnetic resonance imaging, 2nd ed.* St Louis: CV Mosby, 1991;471–521.

101. Babcock EE, Brateman L, Weinreb JC, Horner SD, Nunnally RL. Edge artifacts in MR images: chemical shift effect. *J Comput Assist Tomogr* 1985;9(2):252–257.

102. Simon JH, Szumowski J, Totterman S, et al. Fat-suppression MR imaging of the orbit. *Am J Neuroradiol* 1988;19(5):961–968.

103. Dwyer AJ, Knop RH, Hoult DI. Frequency shift artifacts in MR imaging. *J Comput Assist Tomogr* 1985;9(1):16–18.

104. Brateman L. Chemical shift imaging: a review. *Am J Roentgenol* 1986;146:971–980.

105. Daniels DL, Kneeland JB, Shimakawa A, et al. MR imaging of the optic nerve and sheath: correcting the chemical shift misregistration effect. *Am J Neuroradiol* 1986;7(2):249–253.

106. Edelman R, Shellock FG, Ahladis J. Practical MRI for the technologist and imaging specialist. In: Edelman RR, Hesselink J, eds. *Clinical magnetic resonance imaging.* Philadelphia: WB Saunders, 1990;39–67.

107. Hinks RS, Quencer RM. Motion artifacts in brain and spine MR. *Radiol Clin North Am* 1988;26(4):737–753.

108. Johnson BA, Kelly WM. Common MRI artifacts: an overview (concluded). *MRI Decisions* 1989;3:26–32.

109. Axel L, Summers RM, Kressel HY, et al. Respiratory effects in two-dimensional Fourier transform MR imaging. *Radiology* 1986;160: 795–801.

110. Rubin JB, Enzmann DR. Harmonic modulation of proton MR precessional phase by pulsatile motion: origin of spinal CSF flow phenomena. *Am J Neuroradiol* 1987;8:307–318.

111. Edelman RR, Rubin JB, Buxton RB. Flow. In: Edelman RR, Hesselink JR, eds. *Clinical magnetic resonance imaging.* Philadelphia: WB Saunders, 1990;109–182.

112. Holtas SL, Plewes DB, Simon JH, et al. Technical aspects on magnetic resonance imaging of the spine at 1.5 tesla. *Acta Radiol* 1987;28: 375–381.

113. Clark JA II, Kelly WM, et al. Common artifacts encountered in magnetic resonance imaging. *Radiol Clin North Am* 1988;26(5):893–920.

114. Rubin JB. Basic principles of CSF flow. In: Enzmann DR, DeLaPaz RL, Rubin JB, eds. *Magnetic resonance of the spine.* St Louis: CV Mosby, 1990;1–63.

115. Henkelman RM, Bronskill MJ. Artifacts in magnetic resonance imaging. *Rev Magn Reson Med* 1987;2:1–126.

116. Tsuruda JS, Norman D, Dillon W, et al. Three-dimensional gradient-recalled MR imaging as a screening tool for the diagnosis of cervical radiculopathy. *Am J Roentgenol* 1990;154:375–383.

117. Yousem DM, Atlas SW, Goldberg HI. Degenerative narrowing of cervical spine neural foramina. *Am J Roentgenol* 1991;156:1229–1236.

118. Breger RK, Czervionke LF, Kass EG, et al. Truncation artifact in MR images of the intervertebral disc. *Am J Neuroradiol* 1988;9:825–828.

119. Modic MT, Masaryk TJ, Ross JS, et al. Imaging of degenerative disc disease. *Radiology* 1988;168:177–186.

120. Czervionke LF, Czervionke JM, Daniels DL, et al. Characteristic features of MR truncation artifacts. *Am J Neuroradiol* 1988;9:815–824.

121. Bronskill MJ, McVeigh ER, Kucharczyk W, et al. Syrinx-like artifacts on MR images of the spinal cord. *Radiology* 1988;166:485–488.

122. Levy LM, DiChiro G, Brooks RA, et al. Spinal cord artifacts from truncation errors during MR imaging. *Radiology* 1988;166:479–483.

123. Yousem DM, Janick PA, Atlas SW, et al. Pseudoatrophy of the cervical portion of the spinal cord on MR images: a manifestation of the truncation artifact? *Am J Neuroradiol* 1990;11(2):373–377.

Variants and Pitfalls in Body Imaging,
edited by Ali Shirkhoda.
Lippincott Williams & Wilkins, Philadelphia, © 2000.

CHAPTER 28

The Shoulder: MRI

Vamsidhar R. Narra and Scott A. Mirowitz

Conventional radiographic techniques demonstrate the osseous structures of the shoulder girdle, but provide limited evaluation of the soft tissues and rotator cuff. Magnetic resonance imaging (MRI) has made significant contributions to shoulder imaging, since it affords superb visualization of both soft tissue and osseous pathology. This chapter discusses imaging techniques, normal variations, artifacts, and diagnostic pitfalls that are involved in the acquisition and interpretation of shoulder MRI.

TECHNIQUE

When imaging the shoulder a number of factors must be considered so that optimal images of the rotator cuff, joint space, labrum, osseous structures, and soft tissues are obtained. Since most patients undergoing shoulder MRI present with shoulder pain, they may not tolerate long imaging times. Consequently, it is important that imaging protocols be appropriately tailored so as to keep the imaging time as brief as possible.

Coil

Improvements in surface coil design and development of dedicated shoulder coils based on quadrature and phased array technology permit the acquisition of high spatial resolution images with adequate signal-to-noise ratio. The combination of adequate signal-to-noise ratio, small field of view, thin slices, high spatial resolution matrices, and effective artifact control generally contributes to good image quality. Surface coils should be positioned in a coronal oblique plane over the shoulder, rather than a true anteroposterior plane, to maximize signal-to-noise ratio in the region of the rotator cuff (1).

Once the surface coil is positioned, it must be restrained with bands so that it does not move with patient respiration. The size of the surface coil should be concordant with the size of the shoulder being examined, since the coil's sensitive range is directly proportional to its diameter. Hence, larger coils are more successfully used for larger patients (2). Signal intensity is increased in close proximity to the surface coil. Such near coil "burnout" can result in a very bright signal in tissues located close to the coil (Fig. 28.1). This can be mistaken for fluid in the acromioclavicular (AC) joint and can mimic or obscure soft tissue abnormalities.

Patient Positioning

Images of the shoulder are obtained with the patient in the supine position. In addition to routine measures intended to make the patient as comfortable as possible, some additional precautions are recommended for shoulder imaging. These include placing the patient's upper extremity in a neutral to mildly externally rotated position. The patient's arm is positioned by the side of the body and appropriately supported for comfort and stability. It is important that the patient's forearm not be placed on the abdomen, since this position would internally rotate the shoulder and result in transmitted shoulder motion with respiratory movement. Excessive internal rotation of the shoulder causes the anterior capsular structures to appear lax and ill-defined, and can simulate pathology (3) (Fig. 28.1).

Imaging Planes and Sequences

In general, a relatively small field of view should be prescribed, usually no greater than 16 cm. Reducing the field of view results in a statistically significant improvement in sensitivity of MRI for diagnosing rotator cuff tears (4). A matrix size of 192 (phase)×256 (frequency) is often used, though many centers now employ higher

V. R. Narra and S. A. Mirowitz: Mallinckrodt Institute of Radiology, Washington University School of Medicine, St. Louis, Missouri 63110.

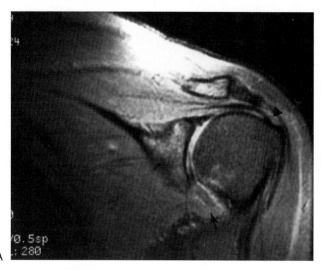

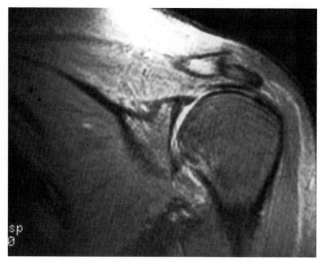

A

B

FIG. 28.1. Internal and external rotation. Coronal oblique proton density–weighted fat saturated images of the shoulder were acquired with the patient's arm in relative internal **(A)** and external **(B)** rotation. Notice increased signal intensity (burnout) in proximity to the surface coil. In **A**, relative increased signal intensity is present along the superior aspect of the distal supraspinatus tendon *(arrowhead)* due to overlapping muscle fibers. (From ref. 2, with permission.)

resolution matrices such as 224×512, at least for portions of the examination. Images are generally acquired using a 3-mm section thickness and a 0.5-mm intersection gap.

Gradient echo images can be obtained using a repetition time (TR) of 300 msec, echo time (TE) of 15 msec, and an excitation flip angle of 30 degrees. We routinely acquire such proton density–weighted gradient echo images in the transaxial plane to evaluate the labrum. These images are supplemented by transaxial T2-weighted fast spin echo (FSE) images, acquired using a TR of 4000 msec, effective TE of 70 msec, and an echo train length of 12 with radiofrequency (RF) fat saturation. The latter images are useful for evaluating the biceps tendon as well as the labral complex. Transaxial images are acquired from the AC joint to the inferior glenoid.

Next, we acquire proton density– and T2-weighted FSE images with RF fat saturation in the coronal oblique plane, parallel to the course of the supraspinatus tendon (Fig 28.2). These images are critical for evaluating the rotator cuff and for assessing the amount of retraction in patients with complete rotator cuff tear. Proton density–weighted images provide maximum signal-to-noise ratio because of their relatively long TR and short TE. T2-weighted images provide the contrast necessary for depicting soft tissue edema and fluid collections, and for characterizing signal alterations that are observed within the rotator cuff with other pulse sequences.

Sagittal oblique images are acquired perpendicular to the supraspinatus tendon from the glenoid fossa to the lateral humerus. We generally acquire FSE T1- and T2-weighted images in the sagittal oblique plane, using relatively low echo train lengths to minimize blurring. T1-weighted images are useful for assessing muscle thickness and evaluating for associated fatty atrophy.

Sagittal oblique fat saturated T2-weighted images are important for confirming the presence of a suspected rotator cuff tear and for assessing the thickness of any such tears.

The reduction in image acquisition time afforded by FSE (or turbo spin echo) sequences provides many benefits for rotator cuff imaging. These include the ability to increase spatial resolution, signal-to-noise ratio, and image contrast while maintaining a reasonable imaging time. Consequently, FSE sequences have replaced con-

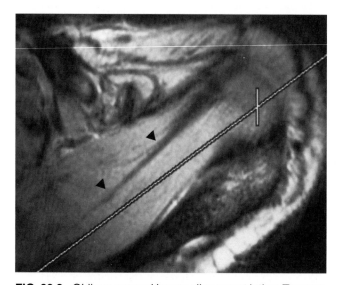

FIG. 28.2. Oblique coronal image slice prescription. Transaxial gradient echo image through the superior aspect of the supraspinatus muscle and tendon is shown. A ray has been prescribed along the long axis of the muscle. Note the divergence in angle between the axis of the tendon *(arrowheads)* and that of the muscle.

ventional spin echo sequences for shoulder imaging in some centers (5–8).

Magnetic Resonance Arthrography

In shoulder magnetic resonance arthrography, paramagnetic contrast material is injected into the glenohumeral joint space. This technique has been used to evaluate the rotator cuff as well as the labral-capsular complex (9). 12 to 20 cc of a dilute gadolinium chelate contrast material solution (1 cc of gadolinium chelate in 250 cc of saline), along with a small amount of iodinated contrast material to confirm intra-articular position, is injected into the joint space under fluoroscopy. T1-weighted images with fat saturation are typically acquired for evaluation of the rotator cuff (10,11).

NORMAL VARIANTS AND DIAGNOSTIC PITFALLS

Rotator Cuff

Signal Intensity Variations

Most normal tendons demonstrate uniformly low signal intensity on all pulse sequences, with any focal increase in their signal regarded as a manifestation of pathology (12,13). However, in the rotator cuff, foci of relatively increased signal intensity are frequently observed in asymptomatic subjects (2). It is important to be aware of these normal signal variations so that they can be distinguished from pathology. These normal signal variations in the rotator cuff are usually demonstrated most prominently on proton density–weighted images. Observation of marked high signal intensity (i.e., similar to that of fluid) within the rotator cuff tendons on T2-weighted images is a reliable indicator of rotator cuff tear. However, foci of relatively increased signal intensity on short TE sequences such as T1- and proton density–weighted images can represent either pathology or normal variation.

Within the supraspinatus tendon, a focus of relatively increased signal intensity is often observed on T1- and proton density–weighted images just proximal to the tendon's insertion on the greater tuberosity of the humerus. This signal variation has been noted in asymptomatic subjects (13,14). It usually appears round or oval in configuration and measures approximately 6 to 8 mm in diameter. This signal variation is typically observed 5 to 10 mm proximal to the insertion of the supraspinatus tendon, and is best appreciated on coronal oblique images (14).

Although the underlying basis for this observation has not been definitively established, several hypotheses have been suggested, as discussed below. It should be noted that these hypotheses are not mutually exclusive. A practical point, which helps avoid misdiagnosis, is that this focus of relatively increased signal intensity closely follows the signal intensity of surrounding skeletal muscle tissue and therefore it does not appear hyperintense on T2-weighted images.

Critical Zone

Based on the observed size and morphology of this signal variation, it has been proposed that it may relate to the critical zone of the supraspinatus tendon (14). The critical zone is a microvascular watershed zone between the anterior circumflex humeral and suprascapular arteries. Chronic ischemia, in addition to impingement, is thought to predispose the rotator cuff to tear at this location. The critical zone is of similar size, shape, and location to the observed signal alteration. It is speculated that the critical zone may have slightly different signal properties than the surrounding rotator cuff, or that subclinical degenerative changes could exist in this location due to the aforementioned causes.

Magic Angle Phenomenon

Another proposed explanation for the focus of relatively increased signal intensity within the distal supraspinatus tendon is the magic angle phenomenon, which is observed when collagen fibers are oriented at approximately 55 degrees with respect to the main magnetic field (14). In this situation, such fibers can display artifactual increased signal intensity on short TE images. Timins et al. (15) showed that altering the position of the subject's arm within the scanner caused changes in the location of the area of hyperintensity, supportive of this hypothesis.

Partial Volume Averaging

Partial volume averaging is a common contributor to artifactual increased signal intensity within the distal rotator cuff on coronal oblique images. Partial volume effects are accentuated by excessive external rotation of the arm (16), due to averaging of fluid in the biceps tendon sheath with the adjacent supraspinatus tendon. Partial volume averaging can also be accentuated by internal rotation of the arm. With the arm internally rotated, the infraspinatus muscle belly is located superior and lateral to the supraspinatus tendon. This can result in partial volume averaging of these two structures, producing relatively increased signal intensity (14,16). Therefore, imaging of the rotator cuff should generally be performed with the arm in a neutral to slightly externally rotated position. Misdiagnosis can also be avoided by closely correlating findings observed on coronal oblique images to those on sagittal oblique T2-weighted images, since increased signal intensity due to partial volume averaging is generally not observed on images acquired in multiple planes (15,17).

Inhomogeneity of Fat and Muscle

Overlap of fat located adjacent to the subacromial-subdeltoid bursa with fibers of the supraspinatus tendon can be mistaken for pathologic signal involving the rotator cuff (Fig. 28.3). The use of fat suppression methods can help distinguish this finding from rotator cuff tear (13,14,18). Similarly, portions of the supraspinatus muscle often extend quite far distally, insinuating between the tendon slips and joint capsule. Because skeletal muscle is of somewhat higher signal intensity than tendon, adjacency of these structures can result in the appearance of diffuse relatively increased tendon signal intensity. This finding can be mistaken for tendon inflammation and/or degeneration, i.e., tendinosis. The key to recognizing this pitfall is to note that the area of increased signal intensity can be followed back toward the supraspinatus muscle belly. Furthermore, the signal intensity of this finding is identical to that of skeletal muscle on all pulse sequences (13,14) (Fig. 28.4).

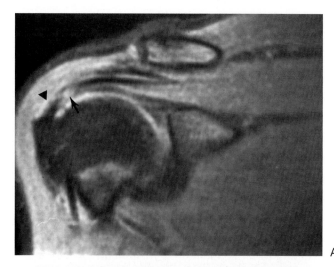

A

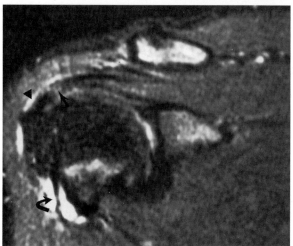

B

FIG. 28.4. Supraspinatus tendon signal variation. Coronal oblique fat saturated proton density– **(A)** and T2-weighted **(B)** images in a normal subject. Note the area of relative increased signal intensity in the distal supraspinatus tendon *(arrows)*. This focus maintains isointensity with skeletal muscle on both proton density– and T2-weighted images. Also noted is a small amount of fluid in the subacromial-subdeltoid bursa *(arrowheads)* and biceps tendon sheath *(curved arrow)*. (From ref. 54, with permission.)

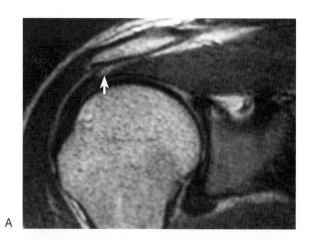

A

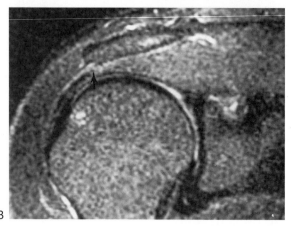

B

FIG. 28.3. Fat interposition. T2-weighted oblique coronal images without **(A)** and with fat saturation **(B)**. Note the focal area of increased signal intensity *(arrow)* overlying the supraspinatus tendon, which is suppressed on the fat saturated image. The latter finding confirms that this represents interposition of fat, as opposed to hemorrhage or other causes of abnormal tendon signal intensity.

Susceptibility Artifact

In patients who have undergone previous arthroscopy or open surgical repair of the rotator cuff, small metallic fragments are often present. These micrometallic fragments produce a focal signal void, with possible associated surrounding increased signal intensity. The latter component can simulate increased signal intensity within the rotator cuff, suggestive of a tear (Fig. 28.5). Susceptibility artifact is minimized when FSE sequences are used, and it is accentuated on gradient echo images, since they lack a 180-degree radiofrequency refocusing pulse. Such artifactual signal loss is also increased on T2-weighted images, compared to proton density–weighted images,

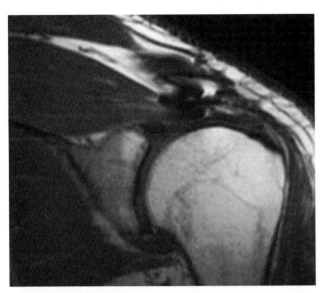

FIG. 28.5. Susceptibility artifact. Multiple foci of signal void with surrounding hyperintensity are present in this patient with micrometallic fragments resulting from previous acromioplasty and rotator cuff repair. These artifacts obscure visualization of the rotator cuff and cause focal areas of increased signal intensity that can appear similar to that due to injury.

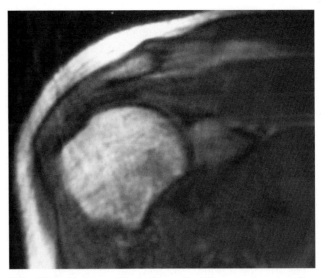

FIG. 28.6. Motion artifact. Coronal oblique proton density–weighted image in a normal volunteer demonstrates a series of curvilinear signal intensity that overlie rotator cuff. These artifacts are due to motion of the shoulder during image acquisition and may either simulate or obscure rotator cuff abnormalities. (From ref. 2, with permission.)

because the longer TE on the former images allows for greater dephasing to occur (19).

Chemical Shift Misregistration Artifact

This artifact occurs at fat–water interfaces, such as the interface between peribursal fat and the rotator cuff. It results in artifactual low signal intensity at one fat–water border and artifactual high signal intensity at the other. Such signal misregistration can be recognized by noting that the increased signal intensity extends beyond the confines of the supraspinatus tendon along the frequency-encoding direction of the image. Chemical shift misregistration can be reduced when small voxel sizes (i.e., high spatial resolution images) are acquired and when fat suppression is used (20). Reorientation of the phase and frequency-encoding gradient directions can displace the artifact to another portion of the image. This maneuver can be useful in confirming the artifactual nature of the signal abnormality and in better visualizing affected structures such as the rotator cuff.

Motion Artifact

As with all MRI examinations, motion artifacts are a significant problem with shoulder MRI. Because patients undergoing shoulder MRI usually present with shoulder pain, they often are uncomfortable and therefore they may be unable to remain still throughout imaging. In addition to gross movement of the shoulder and arm, respiration and vascular pulsation are additional sources of motion artifacts that can degrade image quality (Fig. 28.6).

One practical approach to this problem is to simply acquire the most diagnostically important T2-weighted fat saturated images relatively early in the imaging protocol, before patient fatigue and discomfort set in. In addition, it may become necessary to repeat the acquisition of some pulse sequences if they are rendered nondiagnostic by motion artifacts or when specific questions arise. When repeat images are obtained, it is often useful to do so after reorienting the phase and frequency-encoding gradient directions, so that the artifactual nature of any observed signal abnormalities on prior sequences can be verified.

Another useful method is respiratory ordered phase encoding, although it is not universally available. This technique involves recording the patient's respiratory cycle, with use of a bellows device. Phase-encoding data are retrospectively reordered so as to simulate that of a slow, prolonged respiratory cycle. This method is helpful in reducing the prominence of respiratory motion artifacts without significantly prolonging examination time.

Secondary Signs of Rotator Cuff Injury

Primary diagnostic signs of rotator cuff tear include observation of focal high signal intensity, similar to that of fluid, on T2-weighted images or morphologic disruption of the rotator cuff tendons. For situations in which these findings are not clearly identified, several secondary or ancillary signs of rotator cuff injury have been described. These signs are intended to heighten one's suspicion for rotator cuff injury, though they alone are usually insufficient for diagnosis of a rotator cuff tear. While these observations can serve a useful function, they are also associated with some potential diagnostic pitfalls.

Focal or complete obliteration of the subacromial-subdeltoid peribursal fat plane can be seen in some patients with rotator cuff injury (13,18). In such situations, the peribursal fat plane is obliterated due to edema that is associated with the injury. However, apparent partial or complete absence of the peribursal fat plane on individual images has been observed in many normal subjects (14). Poor visualization of segments of the peribursal fat plane may also be related to limited spatial resolution on MR images, since the fat plane can be quite thin. For these reasons, this sign is of limited diagnostic utility. Furthermore, edema obliterating the peribursal fat plane can occur in patients with subacromial bursitis, and is therefore not definitive for rotator cuff tear.

On oblique sagittal images, the musculotendinous junction of the supraspinatus is normally located between the 11 and 1 o'clock positions, relative to the apex of the humeral head. Proximal retraction of the musculotendinous junction is a very specific sign for full-thickness rotator cuff tear (3,21). However, it is a relatively insensitive sign, since it is not observed in patients with partial-thickness tears and in many patients with full-thickness tears. Some variability in the position of the musculotendinous junction can also be observed in normal subjects with changes in arm position, with increasing abduction of the arm resulting in apparent proximal migration of this anatomic landmark.

The presence of focal calcification within the rotator cuff tendons on plain radiographs is characteristic of calcific tendinitis. Although small foci of calcium are often inapparent on MR images, focal or diffuse signal alterations attributable to associated inflammatory changes are often present. When calcific tendinitis is suspected, gradient echo images can result in improved depiction of signal voids representing calcifications, due to the heightened sensitivity of such images to susceptibility effects (2) (Fig. 28.7).

Atrophy of the rotator cuff musculature, which may be associated with muscular fatty replacement, is another sign associated with full-thickness rotator cuff tear (18). However, it should be recalled that rotator cuff atrophy can also be present in patients with other conditions, such as neuritis, neural impingement due to space-occupying lesions such as ganglia, and quadrilateral space syndrome (3).

The presence of synovial fluid within the glenohumeral joint space, and particularly in the subacromial-subdeltoid bursa, is often associated with full-thickness rotator cuff tear (13,18,22). However, a small amount of fluid can normally be observed in these locations, particularly on fat-suppressed T2-weighted images, which are highly sensitive to depiction of fluid. Even large fluid collections in these locations can be attributed to causes other than rotator cuff tear, such as subacromial bursitis or other inflammatory or infectious conditions.

Iatrogenic Changes

Patients with suspected rotator cuff tear should ideally be imaged prior to any intervention. Prior corticosteroid and/or local anesthetic injection can result in transient foci of increased signal intensity in the rotator cuff and surrounding soft tissues, simulating pathology (23) (Fig. 28.8). Patients who have undergone prior rotator cuff repair with tendon-to-tendon anastomosis frequently demonstrate increased signal intensity within the rotator

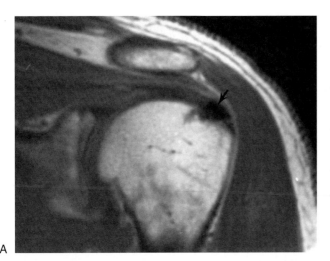 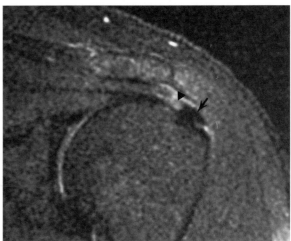

A   B

FIG. 28.7. Calcific tendinitis. Coronal oblique coronal T1- **(A)** and fat-saturated T2-weighted **(B)** images demonstrate a focal area of decreased signal intensity *(arrow)* near the insertion of the supraspinatus tendon. This is secondary to calcific tendinitis, which was confirmed on plain radiograph (not shown). Also note the area of increased signal intensity on the T2-weighted image *(arrowhead)* from associated inflammatory change tendinopathy involving the distal supraspinatus tendon.

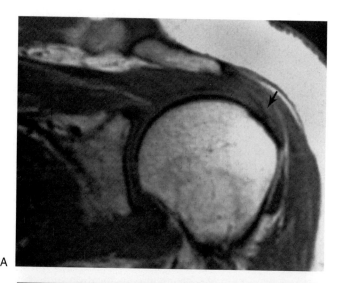

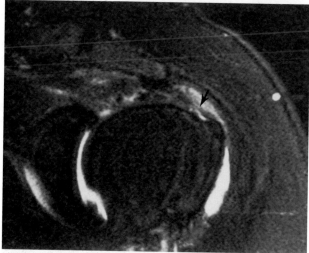

FIG. 28.8. Steroid injection. T1-weighted **(A)** and fast spin echo fat saturated T2-weighted images **(B)** demonstrate abnormal foci of increased signal intensity *(arrow)* involving the supraspinatus tendon, as well as fluid within the overlying subacromial-subdeltoid bursa, in this patient who received local anesthetic and steroid injection 1 day earlier. Follow-up images (not shown) obtained 4 weeks later did not demonstrate any tear. (From ref. 17, with permission.)

cuff on proton density– and T2-weighted images (24). Usually, these areas of increased signal intensity are not as intense as that of fluid on T2-weighted images and can thus be distinguished from most rotator cuff tears. Correlation with surgical records is often useful, and when questions remain MR arthrography can be performed to evaluate the integrity of the rotator cuff (24). When surgery involves only the extracapsular soft tissues, no consistent pattern of signal abnormality is identified (24). Following osseous procedures such as acromioplasty, metallic artifacts, flattening of the undersurface of the acromion process, and decreased acromial marrow signal intensity are common findings (22,24).

Magnetic Resonance Arthrography

Magnetic resonance arthrography has been shown to improve the sensitivity of MRI for detection of labral lesions and rotator cuff abnormalities in patients who have undergone previous surgical repair or reconstruction (23,25). One method for performing MR arthrography is to dilute 1 cc of gadolinium chelate contrast material in 250 cc saline; 10 cc of this solution is then mixed with 5 cc of iodinated contrast material and 5 cc of 1% lidocaine, and 12 to 18 cc of the mixture is injected into the shoulder joint under fluoroscopic guidance.

Care must be taken to avoid injecting air into the joint, since air bubbles can lead to susceptibility artifacts. Injection pressure must also be regulated to avoid overdistending the joint capsule, which can lead to contrast material extravasation into the periarticular soft tissues. In the latter situation, it may be difficult to determine whether the extra-articular contrast material resulted from leakage through a rotator cuff defect or was due to extravasation. Following contrast material injection, T1-weighted images can present a confusing picture, as the high signal intensity of peribursal fat can appear similar to that of extravasated contrast material. Therefore, the use of fat saturation for arthrographic T1-weighted images is recommended. In addition to allowing for improved distinction between fat and gadolinium chelate, fat saturation also heightens the sensitivity for detection of small amounts of extravasated contrast material, due to its favorable effects on the dynamic range for image display.

MR arthrography is very useful in depicting small articular surface partial-thickness tears of the rotator cuff (23,25,26). Of course, the use of intra-articular contrast material confers no diagnostic advantage for detection of intrasubstance or bursal surface partial-thickness tears of the rotator cuff.

Glenoid Labrum-Capsular Complex

The glenoid labrum, joint capsule, and glenohumeral ligaments help to maintain the stability of the glenohumeral joint. There are three glenohumeral ligaments, which are band-like areas of capsular thickening. The inferior and middle glenohumeral ligaments are the major stabilizers of the shoulder in abduction. Labral injury and tears often occur at the insertion sites of the glenohumeral ligaments, in the anterior portion of the labrum. The middle glenohumeral ligament is absent in 30% of normal subjects (27). Although the superior glenohumeral ligament is seen only in 30% of routine shoulder MRI examinations, it is more consistently depicted in the presence of large joint effusions and during MR arthrography (27).

The glenoid labrum is subject to considerable variation in size and morphology. Such variations are not necessarily bilaterally symmetric (28). The labrum classically has a smooth, triangular shape, though variations in labral morphology are frequent. Common variations in labral shape include irregularity, notching, and rounded, cleaved, or blunted configurations (28,29). In a study of normal subjects, Neumann et al. (28) demonstrated the classic triangular shape of the anterior labrum in only 45% and of the posterior labrum in 78% of subjects.

Because these morphologic alterations in labral configuration occur frequently in individuals without glenohumeral instability, they are assumed to represent normal variations. However, it has been suggested that they may increase in prominence with age, and therefore could be partially reflective of degenerative changes (29,30).

There is also considerable variation in labral size among normal subjects. The labrum can be diffusely or focally small in the absence of a tear (29). The posterior labrum is often slightly smaller than the anterior labrum. Complete absence of the labrum, or visualization of its separation from the bony glenoid, usually indicates labral tear (31). An unusually large labrum can also be seen in asymptomatic individuals (28). This finding must be differentiated from a retracted and enlarged anterior superior labrum that occurs secondary to a tear. The latter finding is known as the glenoid labrum ovoid mass (GLOM) sign (31,32).

The labrum is usually well visualized on gradient echo images, where its fibrocartilage appears markedly hypointense relative to adjacent hyaline cartilage. High signal intensity hyaline cartilage that undercuts the fibrocartilaginous labrum must be distinguished from signal alterations due to labral tear (Fig. 28.9). Such distinction can be made by noting that hyaline cartilage appears smooth, continuous, and of uniform thickness, and it parallels the glenoid labrum and does not extend through the substance of the labrum (29,31). One study suggests that increased signal intensity that undercuts the labrum may also represent a transitional zone of fibrocartilage or fibrovascular tissue (33).

Although the labrum is usually devoid of internal signal, foci of relatively increased intrasubstance signal intensity can be observed in the absence of labral tear (28–31) (Fig. 28.10). In such situations, labral configuration should be carefully assessed before a tear is diagnosed. The magic angle phenomenon can result in foci of increased signal intensity in the posterosuperior and anteroinferior labrum, particularly on proton density– and T1-weighted images. In this situation, recognition is assisted by noting the characteristic location and relatively reduced signal intensity of the observed signal alterations on T2-weighted images (34).

Another entity that can simulate labral pathology is focal thickening of the glenohumeral ligaments. The Buford complex refers to a thickened, cord-like middle glenohumeral ligament that attaches directly to the superior labrum anterior to the biceps tendon. It is associated with absence of the anterosuperior labrum (35,36). In patients with this condition, the middle glenohumeral ligament can be as prominent as the biceps tendon, and it can simulate a torn labral fragment (37). A dislocated biceps tendon can also simulate a torn anterior labrum, when the tendon abuts the anterior labrum (31,38) (Fig. 28.11).

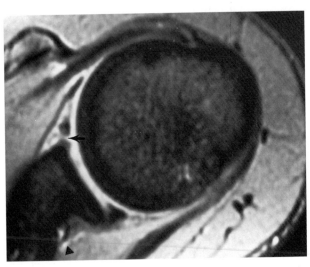

FIG. 28.9. Cartilage undercutting of labrum. Gradient echo transaxial image demonstrates undercutting of the fibrocartilaginous anterior labrum by high signal intensity hyaline cartilage (arrow). This should not be mistaken for labral injury. Also note the focus of increased signal intensity (arrowhead) in the suprascapular notch due to vascular flow, which when prominent can simulate cystic lesions.

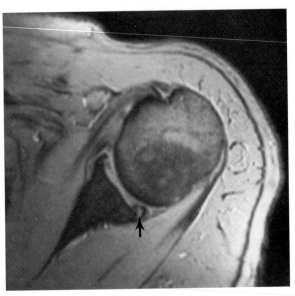

FIG. 28.10. Globular labral signal. Transaxial gradient echo image in a young patient without glenohumeral instability demonstrates a globular focus of increased signal intensity (arrow) within the substance of the posterior labrum, presumed to represent a variation. (From ref. 54, with permission.)

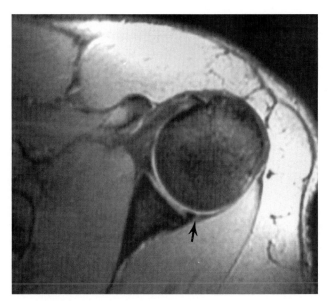

FIG. 28.11. Pseudolabral tear. Transaxial gradient echo image demonstrates interposition of fibro-fatty tissue between the posterior glenoid labrum and the posterior joint capsule *(arrow)* simulating a tear. (From ref. 2, with permission.)

Intra-articular air, resulting from vacuum phenomenon, joint aspiration, or procedures such as arthrography, can cause susceptibility artifacts that simulate labral surface irregularity or discrete defects (39). The posterior joint capsule can appear redundant when the patient's arm is positioned in external rotation; this can simulate a posterior labral tear.

On MR arthrographic images, sublabral foramina can be observed in normal subjects. These foramina occur at the base of the superior labrum, at its junction with the biceps tendon, and at the base of the anterosuperior labrum, between the origins of the middle and superior glenohumeral ligaments, in approximately 10% of subjects (40). They can collect contrast material and simulate a labral tear. One must be cautious when diagnosing tears in these locations, unless there is clear separation of the labrum from the underlying bony glenoid, with extension into the anteroinferior or posterosuperior quadrants of the labrum. With sublabral foramina, the biceps tendon attachment and surrounding labrum appear normal (41,42).

Three types of anterior capsular insertion of glenohumeral ligaments are recognized by the site of their attachment to the glenoid (27,28,43). Type 1 capsules attach at the tip of the labrum. Type 2 capsules insert more medially, but less than 1 cm from the labrum on the glenoid. Type 3 capsules insert more than 1 cm proximal to the labrum on the scapular neck. Although type 3 capsules have been associated with anterior glenohumeral instability, a recent prospective MR arthrography series demonstrated no correlation between type of capsular insertion and the presence of glenohumeral stability (44).

Osseous Structures

The bony structures around the shoulder joint should be routinely evaluated on MR images, since abnormalities involving them may be responsible for shoulder pain. Foci of relative decreased marrow signal intensity are routinely observed in the proximal portion of the humeral metaphysis in adults. These findings correspond to foci of residual or reconverted hematopoietic marrow. Although the epiphyses of most long bones often do not contain hematopoietic marrow in normal adults, these findings have been observed frequently in the proximal humeral epiphysis (45) (Fig. 28.12). In the epiphysis, hematopoietic marrow is most commonly observed along the medial subcortical portion of the humeral head, where it assumes a curvilinear distribution. However, globular or speckled patterns may also be observed. Relative to surrounding fatty marrow, hematopoietic marrow appears hypointense on T1- and T2-weighted images and mildly hyperintense on fat-suppressed T2-weighted or short tau inversion recovery (STIR) images (Fig. 28.13). Residual hematopoietic marrow is more prominent in children and adolescents, and reconverted hematopoietic marrow can be observed in patients with anemia or marrow replacement (46). Distinction between residual or reconverted marrow and marrow lesions is based on the lack of medullary cavity expansion, cortical destruction, or juxtacortical soft tissue mass with hematopoietic marrow, as well as its relatively reduced signal intensity on T2-weighted images and reduced enhancement following intravenous gadolinium chelate contrast material administration.

The normal physeal plate appears as a linear area of low signal intensity on T1-weighted images, with correspond-

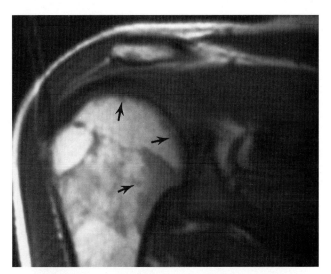

FIG. 28.12. Hematopoietic marrow. Coronal oblique T1-weighted image demonstrates foci of low signal intensity within the proximal humeral epiphysis *(arrows)*, due to hematopoietic marrow. (From ref. 54, with permission.)

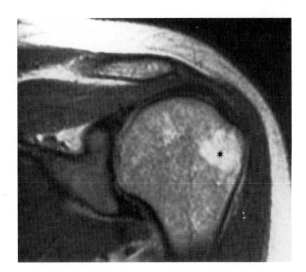

FIG. 28.13. Hematopoietic marrow. A coronal oblique T2-weighted image in a 30-year-old woman demonstrates extensive hematopoietic marrow involving the proximal humeral epiphysis and metaphysis. Focal area of fatty marrow is identified *(asterisk)*.

ing high signal intensity on fat-suppressed T2-weighted images. This appearance can potentially be mistaken for fracture or aggressive lesions, especially on axial images where the physis can undergo partial-volume averaging with adjacent marrow (45). In skeletally immature patients, areas of low signal intensity related to the apophyses can potentially simulate fractures (45). In problematic cases, imaging the contralateral shoulder may be helpful in arriving at the correct diagnosis. Failure of fusion of the secondary ossification center of the acromion can occur as a normal variant, and is termed an os acromiale (Fig. 28.14). It is seen in 5% of individuals (47).

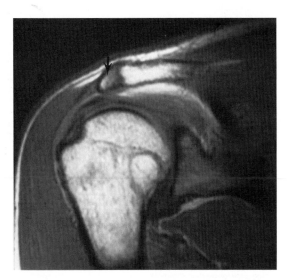

FIG. 28.14. Os acromiale. Coronal oblique T1-weighted image demonstrates an os acromiale *(arrow)*, which can simulate the appearance of the acromioclavicular joint.

Cystic changes are frequently present in the humeral head, near the insertion of the supraspinatus tendon and the greater tuberosity. These findings may be associated with rotator cuff pathology (3). Areas of ill-defined increased marrow signal intensity on T2-weighted images may represent microtrabecular injury in patients who have sustained recent shoulder trauma, and must be differentiated from neoplasm, infection, or infiltrative marrow pathology.

The posterolateral aspect of the humerus demonstrates normal flattening, just proximal to the insertion of the teres minor muscle (48). This can appear to represent a Hill-Sachs impaction deformity (Fig. 28.15). The normal posterolateral depression occurs 20 mm or more caudal to the proximal humeral head, whereas Hill-Sachs lesions occur more proximally. Hill-Sachs injuries are usually observed about 12 mm from the proximal humeral head, at or immediately cephalad to the level of the coracoid process (48).

In patients presenting with shoulder pain and suspected rotator cuff injury, evaluation of acromial morphology and

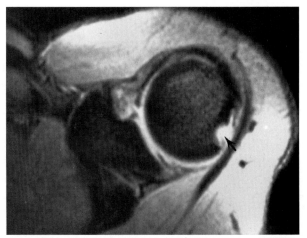

A

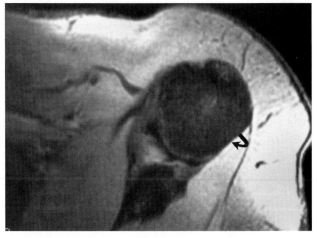

B

FIG. 28.15. Hill-Sachs versus normal flattening. Axial gradient echo images in an 18-year-old man with history of shoulder dislocations. Note the Hill-Sachs deformity *(arrow)* at a superior level **(A)** as compared with the normal flattening seen along the inferior aspect of the humeral head **(B)** *(curved arrow)*.

the acromioclavicular joint has been emphasized, as these structures are implicated in the pathogenesis of rotator cuff impingement. An anteriorly hooked (type 3) acromion has been suggested to be a contributor to shoulder pain (49). The slope of the acromion is best evaluated on sagittal oblique images. An anterior downsloping acromion is diagnosed when the anterior inferior cortex of the acromion is located more caudal relative to its posterior cortex. Lateral downsloping of the acromion process narrows the acromio-humeral distance and can contribute to impingement of the supraspinatus tendon (50) (Fig. 28.16).

Fibrocartilaginous hypertrophy at the insertion site of the coraco-acromial ligament can result in a pseudospur along the undersurface of the acromion process (3). The insertion of tendon slips of the deltoid muscle in this location can also simulate a subacromial osteophyte (3) (Fig. 28.17). A

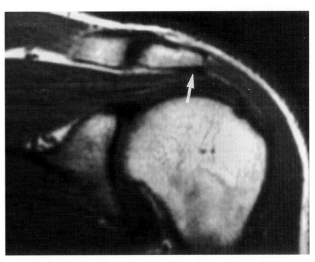

FIG. 28.17. Pseudoacromial spurring. Coronal oblique proton density–weighted image in a normal subject. A focus of decreased signal intensity projects laterally from the undersurface of the acromion process *(arrow)*, simulating the appearance of a subacromial osteophyte. This finding represents a tendinous slip of the deltoid muscle. (From ref. 54, with permission.)

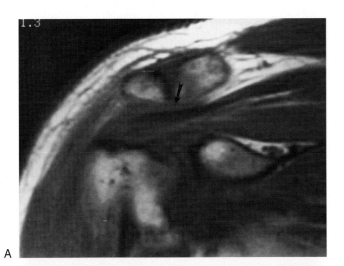

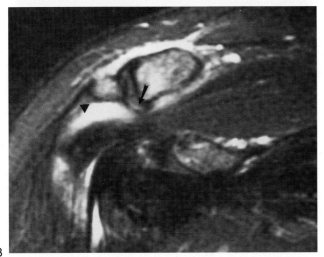

FIG. 28.16. Impingement. Coronal oblique T1-weighted **(A)** and fat-saturated fast spin echo T2-weighted **(B)** images demonstrate degenerative changes along the inferior aspect of the acromioclavicular joint with prominent osteophyte formation *(arrows)*, causing impingement of the supraspinatus muscle and tendon. Also seen is fluid in the subacromial-subdeltoid bursa *(arrowhead)*. There is no disruption of the rotator cuff.

mature osteophyte is verified by the observation of contained marrow fat, which demonstrates high signal intensity on T1-weighted images, though this finding is often absent in immature or sclerotic osteophytes.

Biceps Tendon

The location and signal characteristics of the biceps tendon should also be routinely evaluated on shoulder MRI examinations. T2-weighted fat saturation images in the transaxial plane are useful for evaluating the biceps tendon. The biceps tendon normally appears as a low signal intensity structure on all pulse sequences.

Due to communication between the biceps tendon sheath and the glenohumeral joint (3,13), a small amount of synovial fluid is frequently observed within this space in normal subjects. When fluid completely encircles the biceps tendon, underlying inflammation and/or injury involving the tendon should be suspected (13,51,52).

A rounded focus of increased signal intensity is frequently observed along the lateral aspect of the bicipital groove. This represents flow-related enhancement within branches of the anterior circumflex humeral artery and vein. This finding is usually observed on transaxial gradient echo images, where it can simulate a focal fluid collection or abnormality of the biceps tendon (13).

The magic angle phenomenon can produce foci of relatively increased signal intensity within the substance of the biceps tendon, simulating bicipital tendinitis or partial-thickness tear. As noted previously, magic angle effect is most prominent on short TE images and it is usually not observed on T2-weighted images.

Anatomic variations involving the biceps muscle include the presence of a third head in approximately 12% of individuals (52). The long head of the biceps muscle may be absent, with the bicipital tendon arising within its groove (52).

Joint Space and Bursae

Observation of fluid within the subacromial-subdeltoid bursa is an ancillary finding in patients with full-thickness rotator cuff tear. This bursa does not normally communicate with the glenohumeral joint space. However, bursal fluid collections can be present in patients with subacromial bursitis or in those who have received recent steroid or local anesthetic injection (3). A small amount of fluid can also be observed within the subacromial-subdeltoid bursa in normal subjects, particularly on fat-suppressed T2-weighted images. Due to communication between the subcoracoid and subacromial-subdeltoid bursae, inadvertent injection of contrast material during MR arthrography into the subcoracoid bursa may lead to simulation of rotator cuff tear (3).

Anatomic variations include the potential for additional bursae around the shoulder. These bursae can be located ventral to the subscapularis tendon and between the infraspinatus tendon and the joint capsule (3,13,47) (Fig. 28.18).

The glenohumeral joint space normally contains between 1 and 2 mL and usually less than 5 mL of synovial fluid (25,47). Distention of the joint capsule indicates joint effusion, which is associated with rotator cuff tears, but can also be seen in elderly patients and in those with osteoarthritis (3).

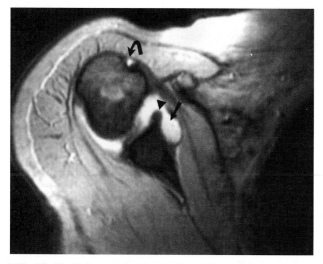

FIG. 28.18. Subscapular bursa. A gradient echo transaxial image demonstrates a large joint effusion extending into the subscapularis bursa *(straight arrow)*. Also note the normal appearance of the anterior glenoid labrum *(arrowhead)* and fluid within the biceps tendon sheath *(curved arrow)*.

Hyaline Cartilage

Accurate assessment of hyaline cartilage about the shoulder with conventional spin echo, gradient echo, and MR arthrography has proven difficult. There is considerable variation in the thickness of articular cartilage in this region. Hodler et al. (53) found it difficult to distinguish hyaline cartilage from overlying muscle in their cadaver study. This problem is frequently encountered over the dorsal aspect of the humerus, where the musculotendinous junction of the infraspinatus muscle may abut the articular surface of the humerus (53). Hence, evaluation of glenohumeral cartilage thickness on MRI should be approached with caution.

CONCLUSION

The use of MRI has made significant contributions to the evaluation of patients with shoulder pain. Familiarity with MRI principles and methods for optimizing the quality and diagnostic content of shoulder MR images is essential. Furthermore, accurate interpretation of shoulder MR images requires a thorough understanding of the many normal variations and diagnostic pitfalls that can simulate pathology.

REFERENCES

1. Glickstein MF. MR imaging of the shoulder: optimizing surface coil positioning [letter]. *AJR* 1989;153:431.
2. Mirowitz SA. *Pitfalls, variants and artifacts in body MR Imaging.* St. Louis: Mosby-Year Book, 1996:317.
3. Stoller DW. *Magnetic resonance imaging in orthopedics and sports medicine,* 2nd ed. New York: Lippincott-Raven, 1997:203.
4. Tuite MJ, Yandow DR, De Smet AA, Orwin JF, Quintana FA. Effect of field of view on MR diagnosis of rotator cuff tears. *Skeletal Radiol* 1995;24:495.
5. Kieft GJ, Bloem JL, Obermann WR, et al. Normal shoulder: MR imaging. *Radiology* 1986;159:741.
6. Sonin AH, Peduto AJ, Fitzgerald SW, Callahan CM, Bresler ME. MR imaging of the rotator cuff: comparison of spin-echo and turbo spin-echo sequences. *AJR* 1996;167:333.
7. Carrino JA, McCauley TR, Katz LD, Smith RC, Lange RC. Rotator cuff: evaluation with fast spin-echo vs conventional spin-echo MR imaging. *Radiology* 1997;202:533.
8. Holder J, Naureth A, Friedburg H. RARE imaging: a fast imaging method for clinical MR. *Magn Reson Med* 1986;3:823.
9. Flannigan B, Kurunoglu-Brahme S, Snyder S, et al. MR arthrography of the shoulder: comparison with conventional MR imaging. *AJR* 1990; 155:829.
10. Loredo R, Longo C, Salonen D, et al. Glenoid labrum: MR imaging with histologic correlation. *Radiology* 1995;196:33.
11. Fritz RC, Stoller DW. Fat-suppression MR arthrography of the shoulder [letter]. *Radiology* 1992;185:614.
12. Iannotti JP, Zlatkin MB, Esterhai JL, et al. Magnetic resonance imaging of the shoulder. Sensitivity, specificity, and predictive value. *J Bone Joint Surg* 1991;73:17.
13. Kaplan PA, Bryans KC, Davick JE, et al. MR imaging of the normal shoulder: variants and pitfalls. *Radiology* 1992;184:519.
14. Mirowitz SA. Normal rotator cuff: MR imaging with conventional and fat-suppression techniques. *Radiology* 1991;180:735.
15. Timins ME, Erickson SJ, Estkowski LD, et al. Increased signal in the normal supraspinatus tendon on MR imaging: diagnostic pitfall caused by the magic-angle effect. *AJR* 1995;165:109.
16. Davis SJ, Teresi LM, Bradley WG, et al. Effects of arm rotation on MR imaging of the rotator cuff. *Radiology* 1991;181:265.

17. Tsao LY, Mirowitz SA. MR imaging of the shoulder: imaging techniques, diagnostic pitfalls and normal variants. *Magn Reson Imaging Clin North Am* 1997;5:683.
18. Quinn SF, Sheley RC, Demlow TA, et al. Rotator cuff tendon tears: evaluation with fat suppressed MR imaging with arthroscopic correlation in 100 patients. *Radiology* 1995;195:497.
19. Elster AD. Sellar susceptibility artifacts: theory and implications. *AJNR* 1993;14:129.
20. Weinreb JC, Brateman L, Babcock EE, et al. Chemical shift artifact in clinical magnetic resonance imaging. *AJR* 1985;145:183.
21. Neuman CH, Holt RG, Steinback LS, et al. MR imaging of the shoulder: appearance of the supraspinatus tendon in asymptomatic volunteers. *AJR* 1992;158:1281.
22. Zlatkin MB, Reicher MA, Kellerhouse LE, et al. The painful shoulder: MR imaging of the glenohumeral joint. *J Comput Assist Tomogr* 1988;12:995.
23. Hodler J, Kursunoglu-Brahme S, Snyder SJ, et al. Rotator cuff disease: assessment with MR arthrography versus standard MR imaging in 36 patients with arthroscopic confirmation. *Radiology* 1992;182:431.
24. Owen RS, Ianotti JP, Kneeland JB, et al. Shoulder after surgery: MR imaging with surgical validation. *Radiology* 1993;186:443.
25. Tirman PFJ, Bost FW, Steinbach LS, et al. MR arthrographic depiction of tears of the rotator cuff: benefit of abduction and external rotation of the arm. *Radiology* 1994;192:851.
26. Chandnani V, Ho C, Gerharter J, et al. MR findings in asymptomatic shoulders: a blind analysis using symptomatic shoulders as controls. *Clin Imaging* 1992;16:25.
27. Massengill AD, Seeger LL, Yao L, et al. Labrocapsular ligamentous complex of the shoulder: normal anatomy, anatomic variation, and pitfalls of MR imaging and MR arthrography. *Radiographics* 1994;14:1211.
28. Neumann CH, Peterson SA, Jahnke AH. MR Imaging of the labral-capsular complex: normal variations. *AJR* 1991;157:1015.
29. McNiesh LM, Callaghan JJ. CT arthrography of the shoulder: variations of the glenoid labrum. *AJR* 1987;149:963.
30. Rafii M, Forooznia H. Variations of normal glenoid labrum [letter]. *AJR* 1989;152:201.
31. McCauley TR, Pope CF, Jokl P. Normal and abnormal glenoid labrum: assessment with multiplanar gradient echo MR imaging. *Radiology* 1992;183:35.
32. Legan JM, Bukhard TK, Goff WB II, et al. Tears of the glenoid labrum: MR imaging of 88 arthroscopically confirmed cases. *Radiology* 1991;179:241.
33. Liou JTS, Wilson AJ, Totty WG, et al. The normal shoulder: common variations that simulate pathologic conditions at MR imaging. *Radiology* 1993;186:435.
34. Monu JUV, Pope TL, Chabon SJ, et al. MR diagnosis of superior labral anterior posterior (SLAP) injuries of the glenoid labrum: value of routine imaging without intraarticular injection of contrast material. *AJR* 1994;163:1425.
35. Williams MM, Snyder SJ, Buford D Jr. The Buford complex the cord-like middle glenohumeral ligament and absent anterosuperior labrum complex: a normal anatomic capsulolabral variant. *Arthroscopy* 1994;10:241.
36. Williams MM, Karzel RP, Snyder SJ. Labral disorders. In: Hawkins RJ, Misamore GW, eds. *Shoulder injuries in the athlete.* New York: Churchill Livingstone, 1991:291.
37. Tuite MJ, De Smett AA, Norris MA, et al. MR diagnosis of labral tears of the shoulder: value of T2*-weighted gradient-recalled-echo images made in external rotation. *AJR* 1995;164:941.
38. Patten RM. Tears of the anterior portion of the rotator cuff (the subscapularis tendon): MR imaging findings. *AJR* 1994;162:351.
39. Shogry MEC, Pope TL Jr. Vacuum phenomenon simulating meniscal or cartilaginous injury of the knee at MR imaging. *Radiology* 1991;180:513.
40. Vhlensieck M, Peterfy CG, Wischer T, et al. Indirect MR arthrography: optimization and clinical applications. *Radiology* 1996;200:249.
41. Palmer WE, Brown JH, Rosenthal DI. Labral ligamentous complex of the shoulder: evaluation with MR arthrography. *Radiology* 1994;190:645.
42. Palmer WE, Caslowitz PL, Chew FS. MR arthrography of the shoulder: normal intraarticular structures and common abnormalities. *AJR* 1995;164:141–146.
43. Zlatkin MB, Dalinka MK, Kressel HY. Magnetic resonance imaging of the shoulder. *Magn Reson Q* 1989;5:3.
44. Palmer WE, Caslowitz PL. Anterior shoulder instability: diagnostic criteria determined from prospective analysis of 121 MR arthrograms. *Radiology* 1995;197:819.
45. Mirowitz SA. Hematopoietic bone marrow within the proximal humeral epiphysis in normal adults: investigation with MR imaging. *Radiology* 1993;188:689.
46. Maniatus A, Vavassoli M, Crosby WH. Factors effecting the conversion of yellow to red marrow. *Blood* 1971;37:581.
47. Bergman RA, Thompson SA, Afifi AK, et al. *Compendium of human anatomic variation:* text, *atlas, and world literature.* Baltimore: Urban & Schwarzenberg, 1988.
48. Richards RD, Sartoris DJ, Pathria MN, et al. Hill-Sachs lesion and normal humeral groove: MR imaging features allowing their differentiation. *Radiology* 1994;190:665.
49. Epstein RE, Schweitzer ME, Frieman BG, et al. Hooked acromion: prevalence on MR images of painful shoulders. *Radiology* 1993;187:479.
50. Ozaki J, Fujimoto S, Nakagawa Y, et al. Tears of the rotator cuff of the shoulder associated with pathological changes in the acromion. A study in cadavers. *J Bone & Joint Surg*–American 1998;70:1224–30.
51. Vahlensieck M, Pollack M, Lang P, et al. Two segments of the supraspinatus muscle: cause of high signal intensity at MR imaging? *Radiology* 1993;186:449.
52. Erickson SJ, Fitzgerald SW, Quinn SF, et al. Long bicipital tendon of the shoulder: normal anatomy and pathological findings on MR imaging. *AJR* 1992;158:1091.
53. Hodler J, Loredo RA, Longo C, et al. Assessment of articular cartilage of the humeral head: MR-anatomic correlation in cadavers. *AJR* 1995;165:615.
54. Mirowitz SA. Imaging techniques, normal variations, and diagnostic pitfalls in shoulder magnetic resonance imaging. *Magn Reson Imaging Clin North Am* 1993;1:19–36.

Variants and Pitfalls in Body Imaging,
edited by Ali Shirkhoda.
Lippincott Williams & Wilkins, Philadelphia, © 2000.

CHAPTER 29

The Wrist and the Hand: MRI

Michael E. Timins

In recent years, magnetic resonance (MR) imaging has become a resourceful tool for imaging the wrist and hand. Developments in imaging software and coil design for obtaining small fields of view have made high-resolution imaging of these structures possible. Current applications include the evaluation of the tendons and ligaments of the wrist and hand, the triangular fibrocartilage (TFC), and the carpal tunnel as well as the assessment of ganglia or other masses, occult fractures, and avascular necrosis of the lunate or proximal scaphoid. Criteria for the evaluation of these entities have been developed, usually involving morphology and signal-intensity characteristics. In this chapter I show how normal variations of the carpal tunnel contents and TFC as well as of the tendons, muscles, ligaments, and bones of the wrist and hand may lead to diagnostic pitfalls if the pathologic criteria are used without knowledge of these variants.

MAGNETIC RESONANCE PROTOCOL

Optimizing image quality in scanning the wrist and hand should be within the means of most MR facilities. Because the signal-to-noise ratio of a scan is proportional to magnetic field strength, magnetic field homogeneity, and coil size commensurate to body part (1), it is ideal to scan the wrist or hand in a 1.5-Tesla magnet at isocenter with a relatively small coil. With a commercially available quadrature wrist coil (Medical Advances), isocenter placement is easily achieved; the patient lies prone with elbow extended and wrist pronated within the coil (Fig. 29.1). A 4-inch single-turn solenoid coil, a research pro-

totype, may also be used because the solenoid design maximizes signal-to-noise ratio (2). For this coil, the patient also lies prone with the wrist pronated in the coil, but the elbow must be flexed 90 degrees because the magnetic vector of the coil (which is parallel to its bore) has to be at 90 degrees to B_0, the main magnetic field vector of the scanner, in order for it to operate (Fig. 29.2). Because the solenoid coil is not readily available, a "poor-man's" solenoid can be fashioned by using a 3- or 5-inch loop coil through which the wrist or hand is placed as through a bracelet (Fig. 29.3). If the patient cannot tolerate a prone position for any of the above situations, a supine position suffices with the patient's palm facing up. If the arm-overhead position is untenable in using any of the coils mentioned above, then the patient should be positioned supine with arm at side and the wrist or hand scanned in a pronated position within the quadrature coil (Fig. 29.4).

An 8-cm field of view for the wrist and a 10-cm field of view for the hand is optimal. It should be noted that the small field of view maximizes spatial resolution. The standard wrist protocol generally consists of (a) spin-density- and T2-weighted images (repetition time msec/echo time msec=2,500/minimum, 80) obtained in the coronal and axial planes, (b) multiplanar gradient-recalled echo (MPGR) images (600+/17; 30-degree flip angle) obtained in the coronal plane, and (c) T1-weighted images (500/17) obtained in the sagittal plane. More recently, the conventional spin-echo long-TR coronal sequence has been replaced with a fast spin-echo T2-weighted coronal sequence (2,000/70, echo train 4) and a 3-D gradient-recalled echo spoiled GRASS (SPGR) coronal sequence (69/15; 20-degree flip angle; 28 partitions). A 3-mm section thickness with a 0.5-mm intersection gap or interleaving (T1-weighted sequence) and an acquisition matrix of 192×256 are used for all sequences.

M. E. Timins: Department of Diagnostic Radiology, Medical College of Wisconsin and Froedtert Memorial Lutheran Hospital, Milwaukee, Wisconsin 53226.

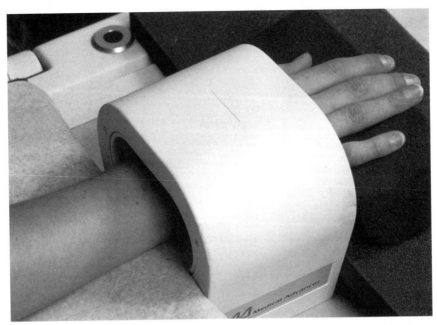

FIG. 29.1. Typical position of the arm for imaging the wrist with the quadrature coil. The patient lies prone with arm overhead, elbow extended, and wrist pronated within the coil.

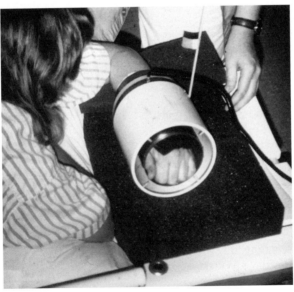

FIG. 29.2. Characteristic position of patient for imaging the wrist with the solenoid coil. The patient lies prone with arm overhead, elbow flexed 90 degrees, and wrist pronated within the coil.

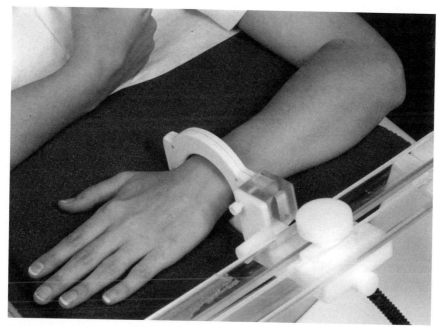

FIG. 29.3. Use of a 3-inch loop coil to simulate a solenoid coil. The patient lies prone with arm overhead, elbow flexed 90 degrees, and wrist through the loop coil as through a bracelet (in a pronated position).

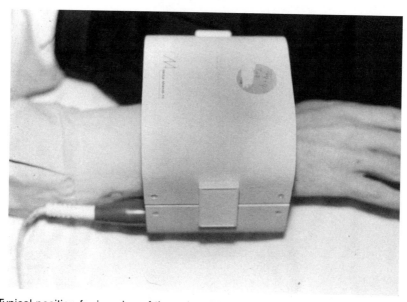

FIG. 29.4. Typical position for imaging of the wrist with arm at side. If the patient is unable to maintain an arm-overhead position, he or she lies supine with elbow extended and wrist pronated within the quadrature coil. Because the wrist is not at the isocenter of the magnet, there is a decrease in the signal-to-noise ratio for this position.

TENDONS

Normal variants of certain tendons at the level of the wrist are important to remember. Figure 29.5 is a drawing of the normal anatomy of the extensor tendons in the axial plane at the level of the distal radius and ulna.

Multiplicity

Although most of the tendons seen at the wrist are single structures, the abductor pollicis longus (APL) in extensor compartment I is a common exception. In as many as 85% of cases, this structure shows multiple tendinous slips

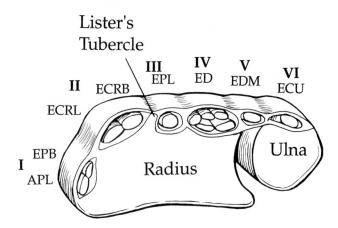

FIG. 29.5. Axial anatomy of the extensor tendons at the level of the wrist. The extensor tendons are organized into six compartments numbered I to VI from radial to ulnar. Compartment I contains the abductor pollicis longus (APL) and extensor pollicis brevis (EPB) tendons; compartment II, the extensor carpi radialis longus (ECRL) and extensor carpi radialis brevis (ECRB) tendons; compartment III, the extensor pollicis longus (EPL) tendon; compartment IV, the extensor indicis proprius and extensor digitorum (ED) tendons; compartment V, the extensor digiti minimi (EDM) tendon; and compartment VI, the extensor carpi ulnaris (ECU) tendon. Lister's tubercle is a bony prominence on the posterior aspect of the distal radius that separates compartments II and III. (Reprinted with permission from reference 3.)

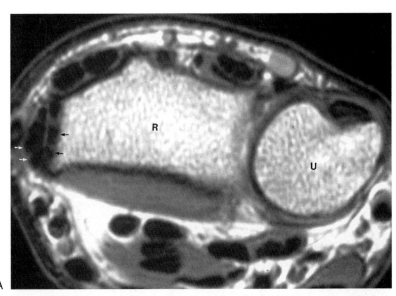

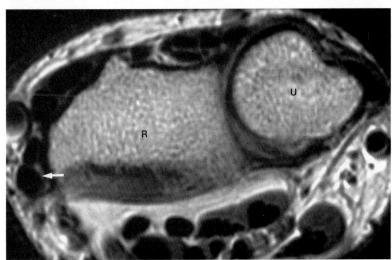

FIG. 29.6. Multiple abductor pollicis longus (APL) tendon slips versus a single APL tendon. **A:** Axial spin-density-weighted MR image shows multiple APL tendon slips *(small arrows)* within the first extensor compartment. R, radius; U, ulna. **B:** Axial spin-density-weighted MR image shows the less common single APL tendon *(arrow)*. R, radius; U, ulna. (Reprinted with permission from reference 3.)

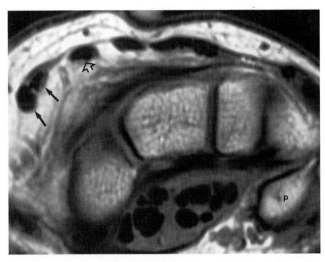

FIG. 29.7. Double tendon slips of the extensor carpi radialis longus (ECRL). Axial spin-density-weighted MR image shows two ECRL tendon slips *(arrows)*. The ECRL and extensor carpi radialis brevis *(open arrow)* comprise extensor compartment II. P, pisiform.

(3) (Fig. 29.6). These accessory tendons may represent ancillary tendinous slips directed not only to the usual insertion site at the base of the first metacarpal but also to the trapezium or flexor retinaculum (4). Occasionally other tendons at the wrist show double tendinous slips; illustrated here are the extensor carpi radialis longus in extensor compartment II (Fig. 29.7) and the flexor carpi radialis, with the latter showing as a doubled musculotendinous unit at the level of the distal radioulnar joint (DRUJ) (Fig. 29.8). Multiple tendinous slips of any of these structures should not be mistaken for longitudinal tears.

Magic Angle Effect

At the level of the distal radius, the extensor pollicis longus tendon lies within the third extensor compartment just ulnar to Lister's tubercle but then passes obliquely across the dorsal aspect of the wrist to insert on the ulnar aspect of the first metacarpal. For its oblique course distal to Lister's tubercle, the tendon invariably demonstrates increased signal intensity and not the normal hypointense appearance characteristic of collagen-containing structures (Fig. 29.9). The physical basis of this phenomenon involves tendon orientation within B_0; such orientation strongly influences tendinous signal. Because of the highly regular structure of collagen, tendons demonstrate increased signal intensity when oriented at or near the magic angle of 55 degrees relative to B_0 (5) (Fig. 29.10). Other tendons in the hand and wrist that demonstrate the magic angle effect include the flexor pollicis longus (Fig. 29.11) and the flexors digitorum profundus and superficialis to the fifth finger (Fig. 29.12), as these tendons angle away from the axis of the wrist and forearm to the first and fifth rays, respectively. The intratendinous increased signal intensity should not be mistaken for a sign of tendinitis.

Extensor Carpi Ulnaris Variants

Like the EPL and flexor tendons just discussed, the extensor carpi ulnaris (ECU) tendon demonstrates increased signal intensity at the level of the wrist in as many as 85% of cases (3). This tendon, however, shows increased signal intensity centrally rather than diffusely (Fig. 29.13). Because the course of the ECU tendon at the level of the wrist roughly parallels the axis of the forearm, implicating the magic angle effect as the cause of its increased signal is difficult, and the etiology of the signal remains unclear. Another ECU tendon variation seen in some individuals is its subluxation out of the ulnar groove with the wrist in pronation (Fig. 29.14). This phenomenon may be explained by variation in the

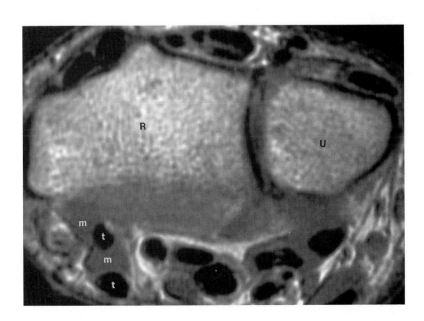

FIG. 29.8. Double flexor carpi radialis. Axial spin-density-weighted MR image shows two flexor carpi radialis musculotendinous units (m, muscle; t, tendon). R, radius; U, ulna.

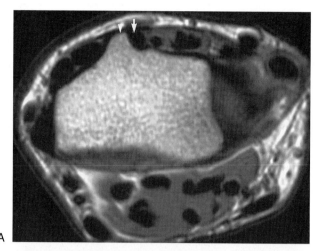

A

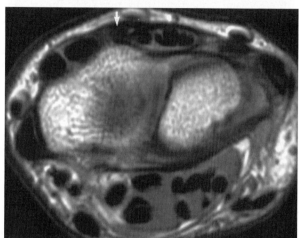

B

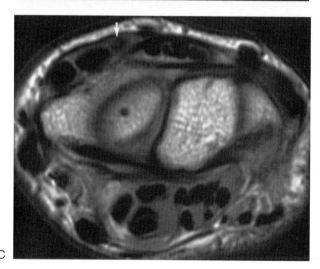

C

FIG. 29.9. Change in signal intensity within the extensor pollicis longus (EPL) tendon secondary to the magic angle effect. **A:** Axial spin-density-weighted MR image shows the normal low signal intensity of the EPL tendon *(arrow)* at its proximal position just ulnar to Lister's tubercle *(arrowhead)*. **B:** Axial spin-density-weighted MR image just distal to **A** shows some increase in signal intensity within the EPL tendon *(arrow)* as it bridges Lister's tubercle. **C:** Axial spin-density-weighted MR image just distal to **B** shows maximal signal intensity within the tendon *(arrow)* as it courses obliquely distal to Lister's tubercle. (Reprinted with permission from reference 3.)

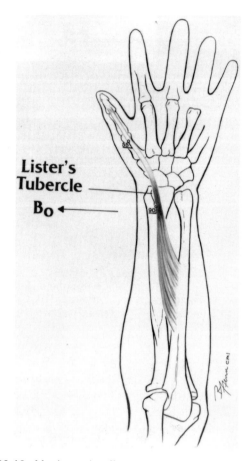

FIG. 29.10. Magic angle effect on the EPL tendon. Diagram shows different signal intensities of portions of the EPL tendon. At the level of Lister's tubercle, where the tendon runs parallel to the forearm, the tendon is at about 90 degrees to B_0, the main magnetic field vector, and low in signal intensity. More distally, for its oblique course at approximately 55 degrees relative to B_0, the tendon has maximal signal intensity because of the magic angle effect. (Reprinted with permission from reference 3).

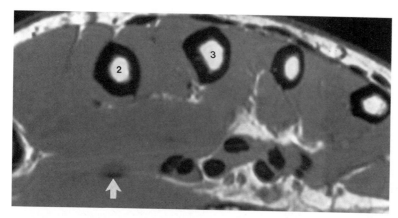

FIG. 29.11. Magic angle effect involving the flexor pollicis longus tendon at the level of the metacarpals. Axial spin-density-weighted MR image shows increased signal intensity within the flexor pollicis longus tendon *(arrow)* secondary to the magic angle effect as the tendon follows an oblique course toward the thumb. 2, second metacarpal shaft; 3, third metacarpal shaft.

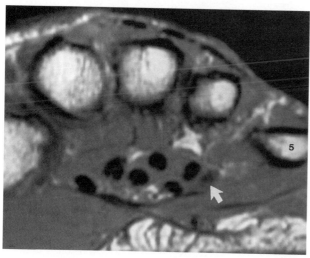

FIG. 29.12. Magic angle effect involving the tendons of the flexors digitorum profundus and superficialis to the fifth finger at the level of the metacarpal bases. Axial spin-density-weighted MR image shows increased signal intensity in the tendons of the flexors digitorum profundus and superficialis to the little finger *(arrow)*. 5, fifth metacarpal base.

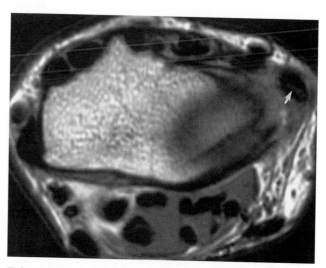

FIG. 29.13. Increased signal intensity within the normal ECU tendon. Axial spin-density-weighted MR image shows increased signal intensity centrally within the ECU tendon *(arrow)*. (Reprinted with permission from reference 3.)

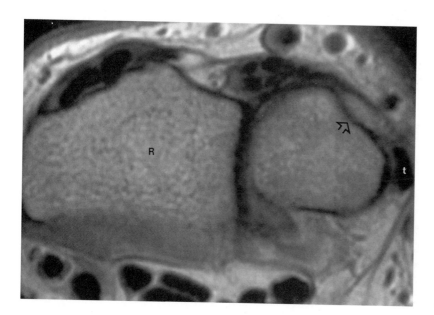

FIG. 29.14. Extensor carpi ulnaris (ECU) tendon subluxation with the wrist pronated. Axial spin-density-weighted MR image shows the ECU tendon (t) subluxed out of the ulnar groove *(arrow)* with the wrist pronated, the standard position for MR imaging of the wrist. Such a finding can occasionally be seen in asymptomatic individuals. R, radius.

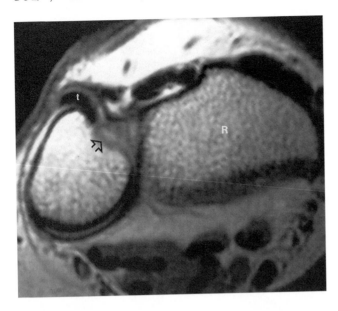

FIG. 29.15. Extensor carpi ulnaris (ECU) tendon subluxation with the wrist supinated. Axial T1-weighted image shows the ECU tendon (t) subluxed out of the ulnar groove *(arrow)* with the wrist supinated, a characteristic finding. It should be noted that the wrist is usually scanned in pronation during MR imaging. R, radius.

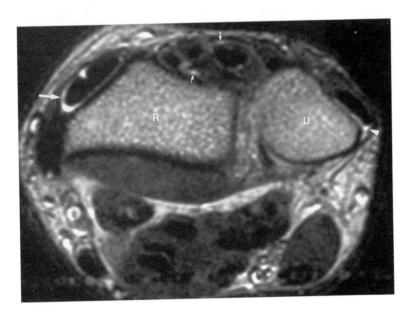

FIG. 29.16. Normal amounts of fluid in the extensor tendon sheaths. Axial T2-weighted MR image of a normal wrist shows a small amount of fluid in the ECRB and ECRL tendon sheaths *(arrow)*. Even smaller quantities of fluid are noted in the ECU tendon sheath *(arrowhead)* and the extensor digitorum tendon sheaths *(small arrows)*. R, radius; U, ulna. (Modified with permission from reference 3.)

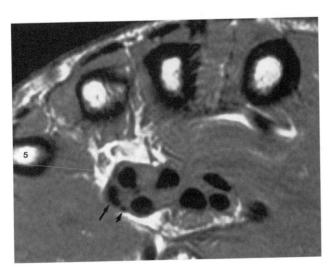

FIG. 29.17. Normally diminutive flexor digitorum superficialis to the fifth finger. Axial spin-density-weighted MR image shows the normally small size of the tendon of the flexor digitorum superficialis to the fifth digit *(small arrow)* relative to the other flexor tendons of the carpal tunnel. The flexor digitorum profundus to the fifth digit *(long arrow)* is also indicated. 5, fifth metacarpal.

attachment site to the ulnar styloid process by the ECU subsheath, the fibrous structure that forms the roof of the ulnar groove, or by variation in its tautness (6). It should be noted that in the supinated wrist, the ECU routinely partially subluxes out of the ulnar grove (Fig. 29.15).

Fluid

Small amounts of fluid are commonly seen in the tendon sheaths of the extensor tendons, particularly the extensors carpi radialis longus and brevis (Fig. 29.16). Although the cause is uncertain, such modest amounts of fluid should not be mistaken for tenosynovitis.

Small Flexor Digitorum Superficialis

There is variation in the appearance of the flexor digitorum superficialis (FDS) to the fifth digit. Although this tendon is always the smallest in cross section of the eight flexor tendons to the fingers seen within the carpal tunnel, often it is remarkably diminutive or even absent (Fig. 29.17).

MUSCLES

Anomalous muscles of the hand and wrist are common and can be detected readily on MR imaging (7). Although they may merely represent incidental anatomic variations, they can be symptomatic, occurring as unexplained mass-like lesions or causing compressive neuropathies. When they are asymptomatic, their correct identification is also important so that they are not mistaken for pathologic conditions or otherwise cause confusion in those unfamiliar with their anatomy.

Accessory Abductor Digiti Minimi

The accessory abductor digiti minimi is a common muscle variation occurring in as many as 24% of all wrists (7). Frequent sites of origin include the antebrachial fascia of the forearm, the palmar carpal ligament, and the palmaris longus tendon. The muscle usually inserts with the abductor digiti minimi on the ulnar aspect of the base of the fifth proximal phalanx (8,9) (Fig. 29.18). The key to its identification is locating on axial images a fusiform mass with the signal characteristics of muscle radial and volar to the pisiform at the level of origin of the abductor digiti minimi (Fig. 29.19). Although usually asymptomatic, the accessory muscle may cause compressive ulnar or median neuropathies, particularly when the muscle is hypertrophied (10).

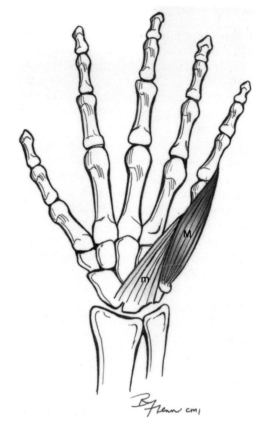

FIG. 29.18. Drawing shows accessory abductor digiti minimi muscle (m), which inserts with the abductor digiti minimi muscle (M) on the ulnar aspect of the base of the fifth proximal phalanx. (Reprinted in modified form with permission from reference 4.)

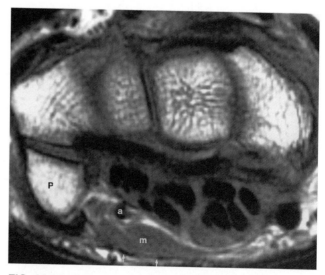

FIG. 29.19. Accessory abductor digiti muscle at level of the proximal carpal row. Axial spin-density-weighted MR image shows accessory abductor digiti minimi muscle (m) volar to the ulnar neurovascular bundle within Guyon's canal. Normally no muscle is seen in this location at the level of the pisiform on axial images. The accessory muscle lies just dorsal to the palmar carpal ligament (arrows), from which it arises in this case. a, ulnar artery; P, pisiform.

Extensor Digitorum Brevis Manus

A dorsal accessory muscle, the extensor digitorum brevis manus muscle, occurs in 1% to 3% of individuals (11,12). Clinically the muscle may be mistaken for a ganglion at the dorsum of the wrist or hand, but it is usually asymptomatic. It typically originates from the distal radius and dorsal radiocarpal ligament and inserts on the index finger, or less commonly, on the long finger (11,12) (Fig. 29.20). To correctly diagnose this variant, it should first be noted that the extensor tendons at or distal to the level of the carpus are unaccompanied by their respective muscle bellies. The extensor digitorum brevis-manus is identified by noting an accessory muscle ulnar to the extensor tendon of the index finger at or distal to the level of the carpus (13) (Fig. 29.21). Its predictable anatomic location and extremely homogeneous appearance on MR should prevent its being mistaken for a giant cell tumor of the tendon sheath or stenosing tenosynovitis of the extensor tendon of the index finger (13). Although it usually accompanies the tendons of both the extensor indicis proprius (EIP) and the extensor digito-

rum to the index finger, in about 40% of cases the EIP is absent or hypoplastic (12).

Flexor Digitorum Superficialis to the Index Finger

An anomalous muscle belly of the flexor digitorum superficialis to the index finger is an unusual variant that has been associated clinically with discomfort related either to a carpal tunnel syndrome or to a palmar mass at the base of the index finger. The accessory muscle belly is interposed within the flexor digitorum superficialis tendon at the level of the second metacarpal or more proximally (Fig. 29.22). The diagnosis is made by following the flexor digitorum superficialis tendon distally from the level of the wrist and noting its replacement by

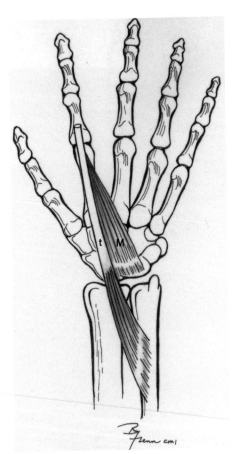

FIG. 29.20. Drawing shows extensor digitorum brevis manus muscle (M) ulnar to the extensor tendon of the index finger (t). Although the extensor indicis proprius and its tendon are illustrated here, this muscle is sometimes absent or hypoplastic in the presence of an extensor digitorum brevis manus muscle, which then coexists with the extensor digitorum to the index finger only (12). (Reprinted in modified form with permission from reference 4.)

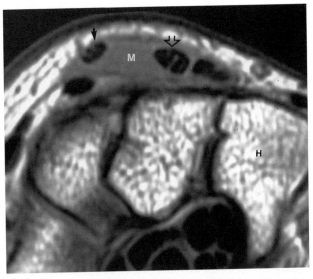

A

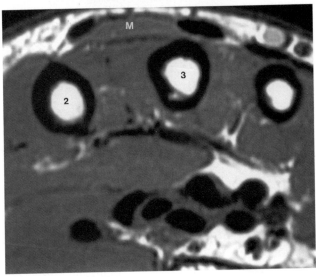

B

FIG. 29.21. Extensor digitorum brevis manus muscle. **A:** Axial spin-density-weighted MR image shows the accessory muscle (M) between the extensor tendons of the index finger *(arrow)* and long finger *(open arrow)*. H, hamate. **B:** Axial spin-density-weighted MR image of same individual shows the muscle (M) more distally at the level of the second (2) and third (3) metacarpals.

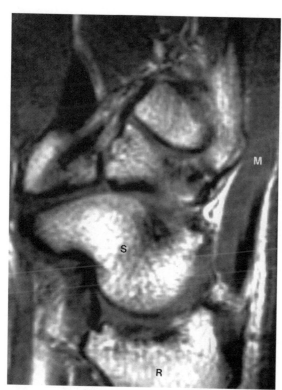

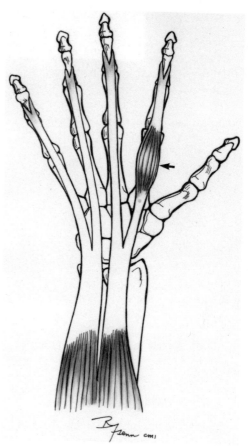

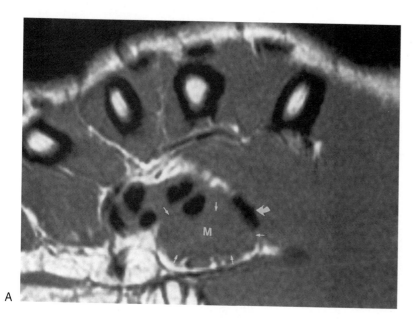

FIG. 29.21. *Continued.* **C:** Sagittal spin-density-weighted MR image of same individual shows the muscle (M) at the dorsum of the wrist. (In all sagittal images, the dorsal aspect is on the right side of the image.) S, scaphoid; R, radius.

FIG. 29.22. Drawing shows anomalous muscle belly *(arrow)* of the flexor digitorum superficialis to the index finger. (Reprinted in modified form with permission from reference 4.)

FIG. 29.23. Anomalous muscle belly of the flexor digitorum superficialis to the index finger. **A:** Axial spin-density-weighted MR image shows anomalous muscle (M) *(arrows)* replacing the flexor digitorum superficialis tendon to the index finger and compressing the adjacent profundus tendon to the index finger *(curved arrow). Continued on following page.*

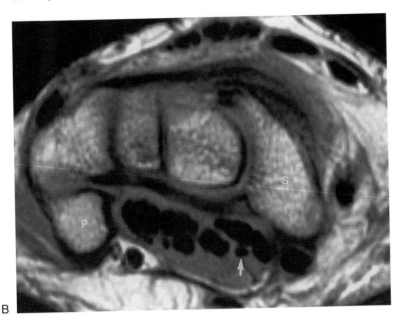

B

FIG. 29.23. *Continued.* **B:** Axial spin-density-weighted MR image more proximally, at the level of the proximal carpal row, shows flexor digitorum superficialis to the index finger as a tendon *(arrow).* S, scaphoid; P, pisiform.

muscular tissue at the level of the carpus or second metacarpal (14,15) (Fig. 29.23).

Palmaris Longus Variants

The palmaris longus muscle arises from the medial epicondyle of the humerus (as part of the common flexor tendon) and inserts on the palmar aponeurosis. In about 13% of individuals the muscle is absent. Normally the structure is fleshy proximally and tendinous distally. However, it may be tendinous proximally and fleshy distally (palmaris longus inversus), fleshy throughout its length, or digastric (16) (Figs. 29.24 and 29.25). Although the diagnosis of these variants is made by not-

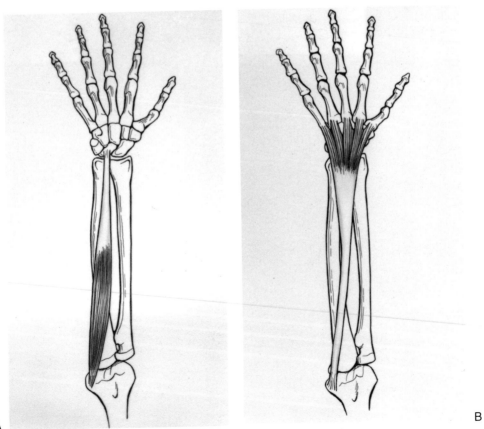

A   B

FIG. 29.24. Drawing shows palmaris longus variants: **A,** normal; **B,** palmaris longus inversus.

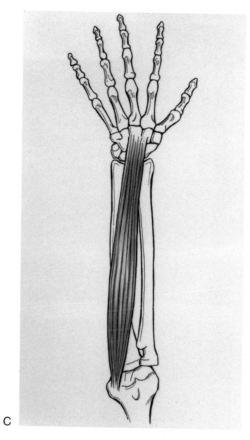

C

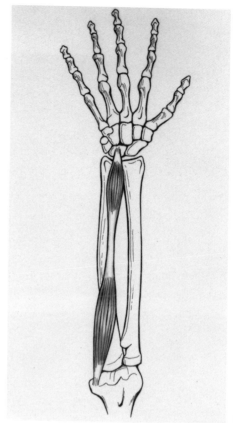

D

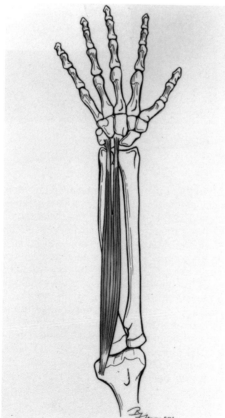

E

FIG. 29.24. *Continued.* **C,** panmuscular; **D,** digastric; **E,** bifid. (Reprinted in modified form with permission from reference 4.)

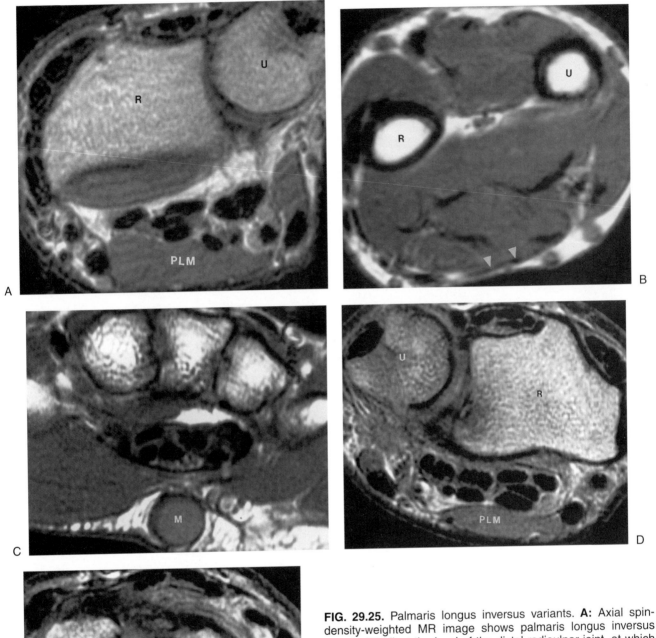

FIG. 29.25. Palmaris longus inversus variants. A: Axial spin-density-weighted MR image shows palmaris longus inversus muscle (PLM) at the level of the distal radioulnar joint, at which level the structure should normally be tendinous only. B: Axial T1-weighted MR image of same individual as in A shows that palmaris longus inversus is tendinous *(arrowhead)* at the mid-forearm level. C: Axial spin-density-weighted MR image at the level of the metacarpal bases shows the palmaris longus inversus muscle (M) at the level of the metacarpals of another individual, in whom the variant has a more rounded appearance. D: Axial spin-density-weighted MR image shows the palmaris longus inversus muscle (PLM) of a third individual at the level of the distal radioulnar joint. R, radius; U, ulna. E: Axial spin-density-weighted MR image of same individual as in D shows that the muscle becomes bifid (m,m) by the level of the proximal carpal row. S, scaphoid; P, pisiform; R, radius; U, ulna.

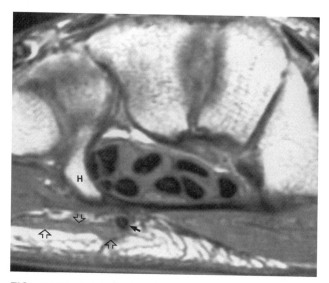

FIG. 29.26. Palmaris brevis muscle. Axial spin-density-weighted MR image shows the palmaris brevis muscle *(open arrows)* forming the volar border of Guyon's canal, which contains the ulnar artery *(solid arrow)*. H, hook of hamate.

mis just palmar to the superficial ulnar neurovascular bundle in Guyon's canal (10) (Fig. 29.26). The palmaris longus inversus variant has been associated with median nerve compression (17).

CARPAL TUNNEL

Carpal tunnel syndrome (CTS) is a compression neuropathy of the median nerve within the carpal tunnel. Based on the presence of typical signs and symptoms, including thumb and finger pain and weakness in the distribution of the median nerve, a diagnosis of CTS is usually made clinically, not radiologically (18). Nevertheless, MR imaging may help determine the anatomic cause of median nerve compression, such as flexor tenosynovitis or the presence of a ganglion cyst or other mass. Also, in clinically equivocal cases, MR imaging may help determine the presence of median nerve neuritis by showing abnormal morphology or signal intensity of the nerve.

ing a midline muscle mass superficial to the flexor retinaculum at the level of the wrist (17), distinguishing between the inversus, panmuscular, and digastric subtypes obviously can be accomplished only by more proximal imaging. It should be noted that the palmaris longus, whether fleshy or tendinous, may be bifid for a portion of its distal course (see Fig. 29.25E). The normally occurring palmaris brevis muscle should not be confused with a palmaris longus variant; the former is a small, thin, ulnar-sided muscle that lies within the dermis just palmar to the superficial ulnar neurovascular bundle.

Normal Median Nerve

Although earlier research suggested that the median nerve normally has signal intensity similar to that of muscle on T1- and T2-weighted images (19), it is now apparent that its signal characteristics on T2-weighted images are similar to those of fat, not muscle (3) (Fig. 29.27). A radiologist unaware of this may make an incorrect diagnosis of neuritis by mistaking normal signal characteristics for those of edematous changes.

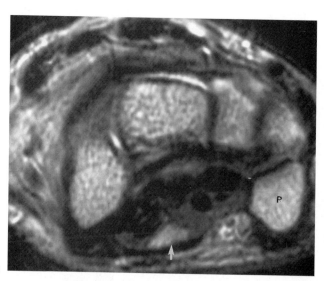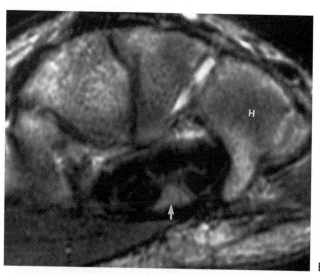

FIG. 29.27. Signal intensity of the normal median nerve. Axial T2-weighted MR image at the level of the proximal **(A)** and distal **(B)** carpal rows demonstrate the signal intensity of the median nerve *(arrow)* to be similar to that of fat. This degree of signal intensity as an isolated finding should not be mistaken for inflammation. P, pisiform; H, hamate. (Reprinted with permission from reference 3.)

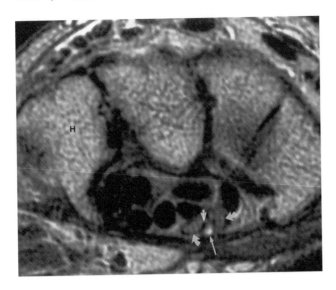

FIG. 29.28. Bifid median nerve. Axial T2-weighted MR image at the level of the distal carpal row shows a bifid median nerve *(curved arrows)* separated by a persistent median artery *(arrow)* and median vein *(long arrow)*. H, hamate.

Bifid Median Nerve

Although the median nerve appears as a single structure at the level of the carpal tunnel in the majority of wrists, it is occasionally seen as a bifid structure; this can occur secondary to a proximal bifurcation of the nerve in the forearm, with the paired nerves usually separated by a persistent median artery (20) (Fig. 29.28).

Persistent Median Artery

Whether accompanying a single or bifid median nerve, the persistent median artery may be seen with one or more venae commitantes (Fig. 29.29). Although the median artery is the dominant blood supply to the hand during fetal growth, it usually involutes by gestation but persists in 2% to 10% of individuals (21). Although a persistent median artery has been implicated as a rare etiology of CTS, a causal relationship is difficult to prove because the

structure is generally an asymptomatic variant, even in the opposite hand of symptomatic individuals (21).

Median Nerve Positions

The median nerve can have a variety of locations within the carpal tunnel, influenced somewhat by wrist and finger positioning. If the wrist is extended, the nerve always lies anterior to the second flexor digitorum superficialis (FDS) tendon; if the wrist is flexed, the nerve usually lies interposed between the flexor pollicis longus and the second FDS tendon with a less common position anterior to the second FDS tendon or interposed between the third and fourth FDS tendons; if the wrist is in neutral position, the nerve usually lies anterior to the second FDS tendon or, much less likely, interposed between the second FDS and the flexor pollicis longus tendons (Fig. 29.30). Finger flexion does not affect median nerve posi-

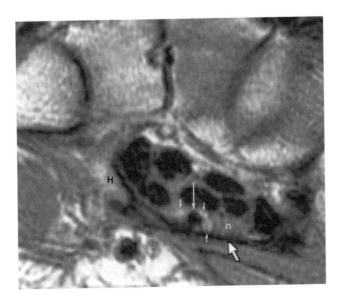

FIG. 29.29. Persistent median artery and veins. Axial spin-density-weighted MR image at the level of the carpometacarpal joints shows a persistent median artery *(long arrow)* with three venae commitantes *(small arrows)* and a single median nerve (n) *(large arrow)*. H, distal portion of hook of the hamate.

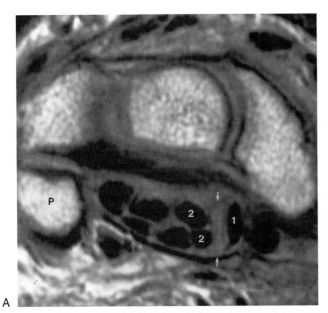
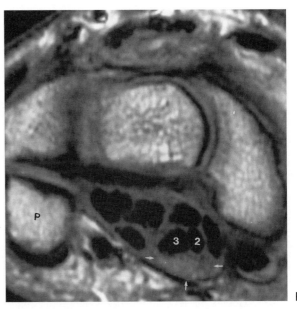

A
B

FIG. 29.30. Change in position of the median nerve within the carpal tunnel for the same patient scanned at two different times. The scans were performed 1 month apart with the wrist and fingers in neutral position at both times. **A:** Axial spin-density-weighted MR image at the level of the proximal carpal row shows the median nerve (arrows) interposed between the flexor pollicis longus tendon (1) and the tendons of the flexors digitorum superficialis and profundus to the index finger (2). P, pisiform. **B:** Axial spin-density-weighted MR image at the same level 1 month later now shows the median nerve *(arrows)* anterior to the second (2) and third (3) flexor digitorum superficialis tendons. P, pisiform.

tion except in the flexed wrist, where it increases the likelihood of an interposed position (22).

TRIANGULAR FIBROCARTILAGE

At MR imaging, the triangular fibrocartilage (TFC) is best identified on coronal images that cover the ulnar and radial styloid processes, where it appears as a band-like structure of low signal intensity that covers the dome of the ulnar head. Arising from the ulnar aspect of the distal radial articular cartilage and inserting on the vessel-rich ulnar fovea and variably along the ulnar styloid process, it acts as a cushion for the ulnar head and lunate during axial loading (23,24).

The thickness of the TFC varies among individuals, and it is important to distinguish a torn structure from one that is thin but intact. A well-known cause of ulnar-sided wrist pain, a TFC tear, is diagnosed at MR imaging by noting a discontinuity in the normally hypointense band. Occasionally, a torn TFC may masquerade as an intact one if, at the site of the tear, the normally hypointense superficial layers of the articular cartilage (25) of the lunate and ulnar head contact each other, thereby simulating the hypointense, band-like TFC at the site of contact (Fig. 29.31). Such a diagnostic pitfall can be distinguished from the correct identification at other times of a very thin, but intact, TFC; in the latter case, the superficial layers of the lunate and ulnar-head articular cartilage can be differentiated as separate structures from the thin

TFC (Fig. 29.32). At the opposite end of the spectrum, a thick TFC may have an unusual appearance to the unwary; this variant occurs in the setting of marked negative ulnar variance (a condition in which the radius extends much more distally than the ulna) (Fig. 29.33).

The normal radial and ulnar attachments of the TFC can be the causes of diagnostic error because they are sites of increased signal intensity, the usual indicator of a TFC

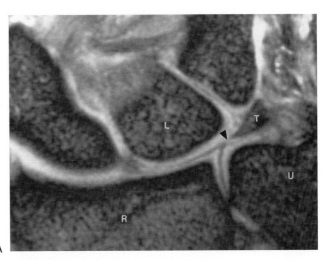

A

FIG. 29.31. Superficial layers of the lunate and ulnar-head articular cartilage obscuring torn TFC. **A:** Coronal gradient-recalled echo MR image shows tear of the TFC evidenced by a defect at its radial aspect *(arrowhead). Continued on following page.*

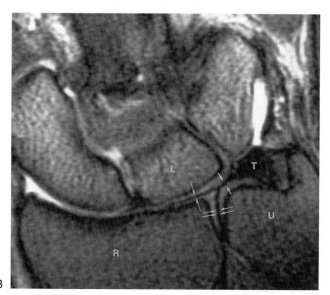

B

FIG. 29.31. *Continued.* **B:** Coronal T2-weighted MR image of the same patient shows that on this sequence the tear is obscured because the normally hypointense superficial layers of the articular cartilage of the lunate and ulnar head are contacting each other and simulating a thin, but intact, midportion of the TFC *(pair of short arrows).* Note a similar hypointense band at the site of contact of the superficial layers of the articular cartilage of the lunate and radius *(pair of long arrows)* and of the radius and ulnar head *(double pair of long arrows).* In this case, evaluation of the T2-weighted sequence alone could lead to the diagnostic pitfall of overlooking the TFC tear. L, lunate; T, triangular fibrocartilage; R, radius; U, ulna.

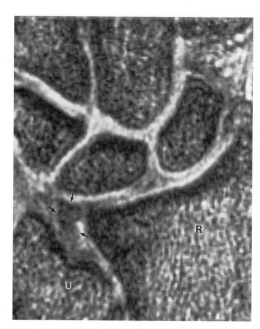

FIG. 29.33. Thick TFC with marked negative ulnar variance. Coronal gradient-recalled echo MR image shows an unusually thick TFC *(arrows)* in this individual with prominent negative ulnar variance. R, radius; U, ulna.

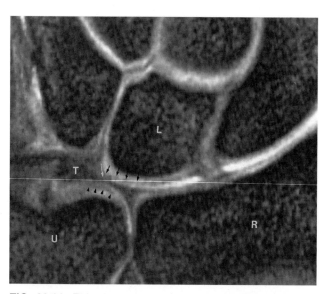

FIG. 29.32. Thin, but intact, TFC as distinguished from the superficial layers of the articular cartilage of the lunate and ulnar head. Coronal gradient-recalled echo MR image shows a thin, but intact, midportion of the TFC *(long arrow)* distinguishable from the superficial layers of the articular cartilage of the lunate *(small arrows)* and of the ulnar head *(arrowheads).* L, lunate; T, triangular fibrocartilage; R, radius; U, ulna.

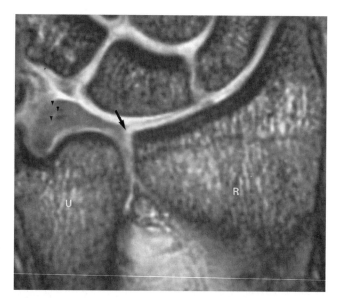

FIG. 29.34. Normal radial and ulnar attachments of the TFC. Coronal gradient-recalled echo MR image shows that the TFC attaches to radial hyaline cartilage *(arrow)* and not to cortex. The ulnar aspect of the TFC near its attachment to the ulnar fovea has a striated appearance *(arrowheads).* These foci of intermediate signal intensity at the TFC attachment sites should not be mistaken for tears. R, radius; U, ulna. (Reprinted with permission from reference 3.)

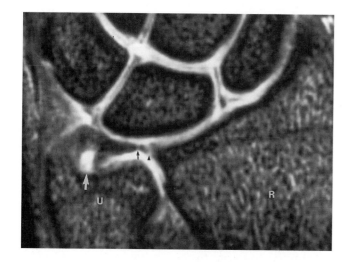

FIG. 29.35. True TFC tears at the radial aspect and ulnar attachment site. Coronal gradient-recalled echo MR image shows a slit-like radial-sided tear of the TFC *(small arrow)* just ulnar to the intermediate-signal-intensity hyaline cartilage of the radial attachment of the TFC *(arrowhead)*. In addition, fluid-intensity signal at the ulnar fovea (which differs from the normal striated intermediate signal intensity) indicates a TFC avulsion at its ulnar attachment site *(large arrow)*. Tears were confirmed at surgery. R, radius; U, ulna. (Modified with permission from reference 3.)

tear. At the radial attachment, the TFC inserts on cartilage, not cortex; as a result, there is a focus of intermediate signal intensity that represents cartilage between the hypointense TFC and the hypointense radial cortex (Fig. 29.34). The striated intermediate signal intensity normally present in the TFC just distal to the ulnar fovea should also not be mistaken for pathology (see Fig. 29.34). Possible explanations for this striated appearance include magic angle effect, decreased collagen content (26), and fibrofatty tissue in the region (27). Actual tears of the TFC at its ulnar and radial attachment sites can be differentiated from these normal findings; a true ulnar-sided tear is evidenced by fluid-intensity signal near the ulnar fovea, not

merely intermediate signal intensity, and a true radial-sided tear usually lies medial to the radial articular cartilage and has a slit-like appearance (Fig. 29.35).

LIGAMENTS

The ligaments of the wrist are either intrinsic or extrinsic. The intrinsic ligaments connect one carpal bone to another, with the scapholunate (SL) and lunotriquetral (LT) ligaments the most important for carpal stability. The extrinsic ligaments are either radiocarpal (connecting the radius to one or more carpal bones) or ulnocarpal (connecting the TFC to the lunate or triquetrum). Two key

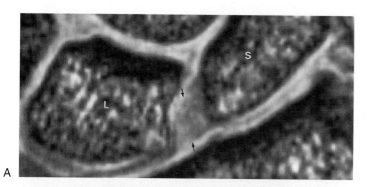

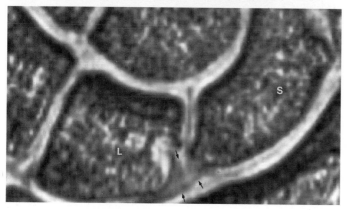

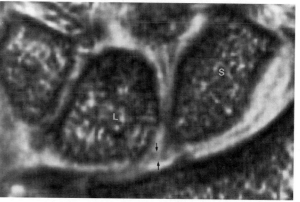

FIG. 29.36. Varying appearance of the SL ligament on coronal gradient-echo recalled images. **A:** At its volar aspect, the ligament *(arrows)* has a trapezoidal appearance with a thicker attachment to the scaphoid than to the lunate. **B:** At its middle portion, the ligament *(arrows)* has a triangular shape. **C:** At its dorsal aspect, the ligament *(arrows)* is bandlike. Note the normal inhomogeneous appearance of the ligament on all sections. S, scaphoid; L, lunate.

radiocarpal ligaments are the radioscaphocapitate and the radiolunotriquetral ligaments. The ulnocarpal ligaments are the ulnolunate and ulnotriquetral ligaments. Both sets of extrinsic ligaments represent sites of focal thickening of the volar wrist joint capsule and are essential for carpal stability (28).

Although the LT ligament is a uniformly thin, horseshoe-shaped structure on coronal images, the SL ligament changes in appearance on coronal sections as one progresses from its dorsal to its volar aspect (29). Awareness of this varied appearance is essential for accurate evaluation of the ligament. Volarly the SL ligament normally has a trapezoidal appearance; at its middle portion the ligament has a triangular shape; and dorsally the ligament has a band-like appearance (29) (Fig. 29.36). On most coronal planes of section, the SL ligament normally has an inhomogeneous, sometimes striated, intermediate-signal-intensity appearance (29); this characteristic is most apparent on gradient-echo images and should not be mistaken for ligamentous injury (see Fig. 29.36).

The radioscaphocapitate is a strong extrinsic ligament that courses obliquely along the waist of the scaphoid (without attachment) to insert on the midportion of the capitate (28). The radiolunotriquetral ligament, the largest ligament of the wrist, originates just ulnar to the radioscaphocapitate ligament from the radial styloid process and also has an oblique course. The radiolunotriquetral ligament attaches to the volar aspects of the lunate and triquetrum (28,30). Both ligaments have a normally striated appearance on coronal MR images that should not be mistaken for pathology (Fig. 29.37).

There is only one important dorsal radiocarpal ligament, and it comprises three parts: a radioscaphoid, a radiolunate, and a radiotriquetral portion (31). Like the other extrinsic ligaments, these three portions actually represent sites of capsular thickening; on sagittal MR images they contribute to the dot–dash appearance of the dorsal capsule that should not be mistaken for discontinuity from injury (Fig. 29.38).

The radioscapholunate ligament (also known as the ligament of Testut) is thought by some to represent a third volar radiocarpal ligament. It arises near the mesial aspect of the distal radial articular surface and inserts into the scapholunate articulation. Although a prominent landmark at arthroscopy, it has been shown to be a neurovascular structure rather than a ligament, with no mechanical function. Instead, it transmits the branch of the anterior interosseous artery and nerve that supplies the scapholunate ligament (32). The radioscapholunate ligament is occasionally seen on MR coronal images, particularly when there is a radiocarpal joint effusion; awareness of its true identity should preclude its being mistaken for a loose body, synovial hyperplasia, or debris (Fig. 29.39).

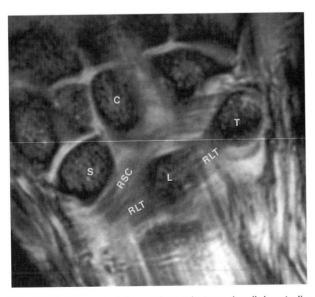

FIG. 29.37. Normal radioscaphocapitate and radiolunate ligaments. Coronal gradient-recalled echo MR image shows the normal striated appearance of the radioscaphocapitate (RSC) and radiolunotriquetral (RTL) ligaments. S, scaphoid; L, lunate; T, triquetrum; C, capitate.

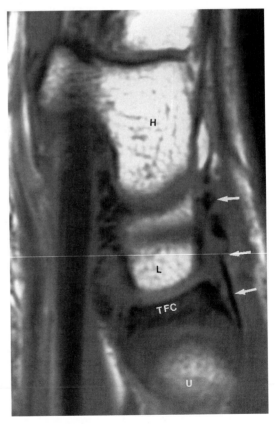

FIG. 29.38. Normal dorsal wrist joint capsule. Sagittal T1-weighted MR image shows the normal dot–dash appearance of the dorsal capsule (arrows). H, hamate; L, lunate; TFC, triangular fibrocartilage; U, ulna.

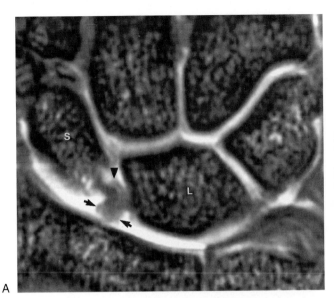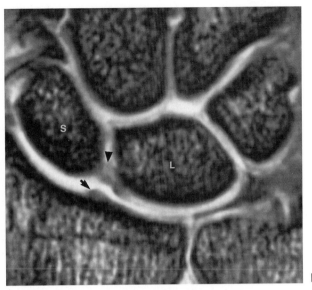

A   B

FIG. 29.39. Normal radioscapholunate ligament (ligament of Testut). Coronal gradient-recalled echo MR images with **A** slightly more volar than **B,** showing the radioscapholunate ligament *(arrows)* outlined by a small amount of fluid in the radiocarpal joint and extending to the scapholunate ligament *(arrowhead).* The radioscapholunate ligament should not be mistaken for a sign of pathology, such as synovial hyperplasia. S, scaphoid; L, lunate.

The ulnolunate and ulnotriquetral ligaments stabilize the lunate and triquetrum to the distal ulna via the TFC. Arising from the volar aspect of the middle third of the TFC, they insert onto the volar aspect of the lunate and triquetrum, respectively. Although the ligaments run in a sagittal plane and are therefore best demonstrated on sagittal images, it should be noted that in about 60% of individuals these structures are not well visualized when conventional spin-echo techniques are used (3) (Fig. 29.40). Reportedly, these ligaments are more consistently visible on three-dimensional Fourier-transform GRE MR imaging (33).

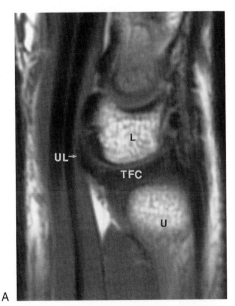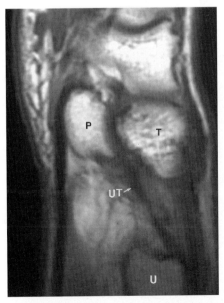

A   B

FIG. 29.40. Inconsistent visualization of the ulnolunate and ulnotriquetral ligaments in normal wrists. **A,B:** Sagittal T1-weighted MR images clearly show the low-signal-intensity ulnolunate (UL) **(A)** and ulnotriquetral (UT) **(B)** ligaments. (Reprinted with permission from reference 3.) *Continued on following page.*

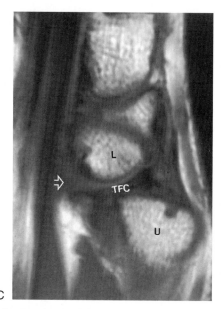
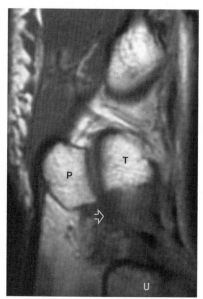

C   D

FIG. 29.40. *Continued.* **C,D:** Sagittal T1-weighted MR images do not clearly show the ulnolunate and ulnotriquetral ligaments. *Arrows* point to their expected locations. L, lunate; P, pisiform; T, triquetrum; U, ulna. (Modified with permission from reference 3.)

OSSEOUS STRUCTURES

Accessory Ossicles

These structures are secondary ossification centers that are distinct from the associated, underlying bone. Although they are generally thought to be congenital in origin, occasionally a posttraumatic or degenerative etiology may be considered (34). Except for these cases, accessory ossicles should not be mistaken for fracture fragments or loose bodies.

According to the classic work of Kohler, there are at least 20 accessory ossicles that can involve the wrist (34). Common accessory ossicles include the lunula as well as the os styloideum, triangulare, epilunate, trapezium secundarium, and os hamuli proprium (34). Their correct identification can be facilitated by an awareness of their typical location in the wrist.

The lunula is an ossification center within the meniscal homologue, a fibrocartilagenous structure that helps link the TFC to the triquetrum and base of the fifth metacarpal (28) (Fig. 29.41). In some individuals, the lunula may be fused to the ulnar styloid process giving the styloid process

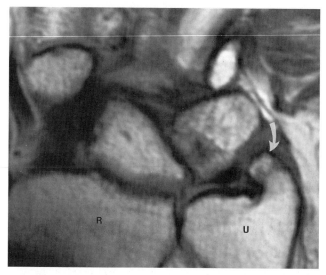

FIG. 29.41. Lunula. Coronal gradient-recalled echo MR image shows lunula *(arrow)* separate from ulnar styloid process. R, radius; U, ulna.

FIG. 29.42. Elongated ulnar styloid process. Coronal spin-density-weighted MR image shows elongated ulnar styloid process *(arrow)* secondary to fusion with lunula. R, radius; U, ulna.

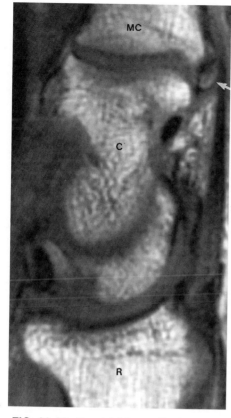

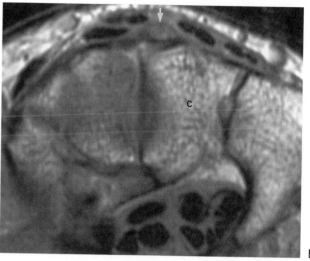

A   B

FIG. 29.43. Os styloideum. Sagittal T1-weighted **(A)** and axial spin-density-weighted **(B)** MR images show the os styloideum *(arrow)* arising from the base of the third metacarpal and overlying the dorsum of the third carpometacarpal joint. MC, third metacarpal base; C, capitate; R, radius.

an elongated appearance (Fig. 29.42). Both the fused and unfused variants are interesting phylogenetically as they are found routinely in certain primates other than man (35).

The os styloideum, also known as a carpal boss, is a bony protuberance at the dorsum of the base of the second or third metacarpal that may or may not be fused (Fig. 29.43). Overlying the carpometacarpal joint, this accessory ossification in some cases may be degenerative, and not congenital, in origin. Although usually asymptomatic, the carpal boss can sometimes limit hand motion, cause pain, or clinically simulate a dorsal ganglion (36).

The triangulare lies just distal to the ulnar fovea and is always considered congenital in origin (Fig. 29.44). The trapezium secundarium occurs at the superomedial aspect of the trapezium (Fig. 29.45). The epilunate lies at the dorsum of the lunate (Fig. 29.46); of the accessory ossicles described here, the epilunate probably has the greatest potential to be misdiagnosed as a loose body (34). The os hamuli proprium is a secondary ossification center of the hook of the hamate (34); its relatively small size and rounded contours help exclude a traumatic etiology (Fig. 29.47). In other cases, the hook of the hamate may appear hypoplastic, perhaps related to deficiency in the appearance or mineralization of the hamulus ossification center; the hook of the hamate may also appear truncated as a result of carpal tunnel release surgery (Fig. 29.48).

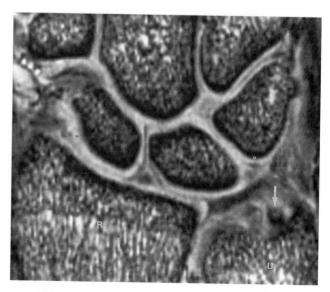

FIG. 29.44. Triangulare. Coronal gradient-recalled echo MR image shows the triangulare ossicle *(arrow)* just distal to the ulnar fovea. R, radius; U, ulna.

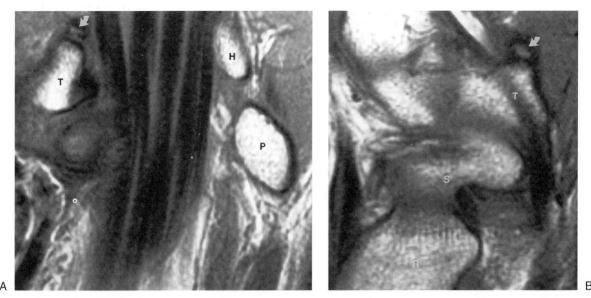

FIG. 29.45. Trapezium secundarium. Coronal spin-density-weighted **(A)** and sagittal **(B)** T1-weighted MR images show the trapezium secundarium ossicle *(curved arrow)* just superior and medial to the tubercle of the trapezium. (On the sagittal image, the volar aspect is on the right side of the image.) T, tubercle of trapezium; H, hook of hamate; P, pisiform; S, scaphoid; R, radius.

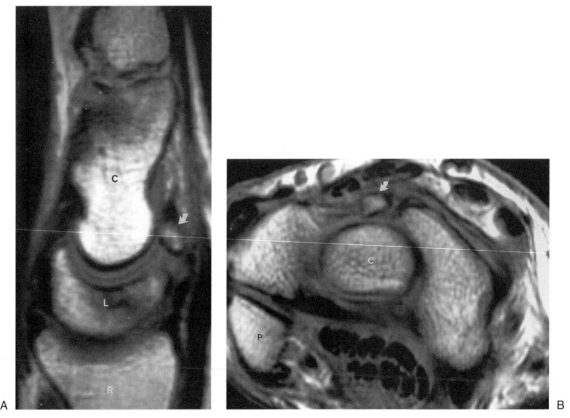

FIG. 29.46. Epilunate. **A:** Sagittal T1-weighted MR image shows the epilunate ossicle *(arrow)* dorsal to the lunocapitate articulation. C, capitate; L, lunate; R, radius. **B:** Axial spin-density-weighted MR image shows the ossicle *(arrow)* posterior to the head of the capitate. P, pisiform; C, head of capitate.

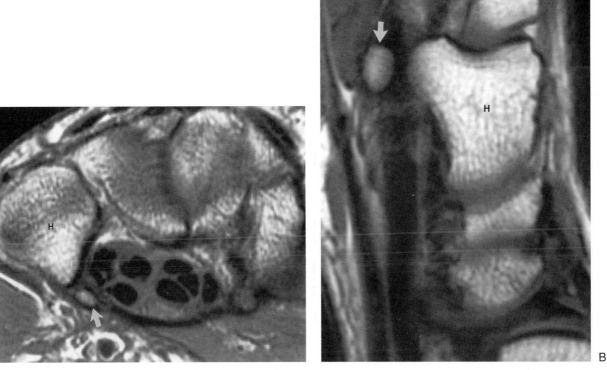

A   B

FIG. 29.47. Os hamuli proprium. Axial spin-density-weighted **(A)** and sagittal T1-weighted **(B)** MR images show the os hamuli proprium *(arrow),* the unfused secondary ossification center of the hook of the hamate. H, hamate.

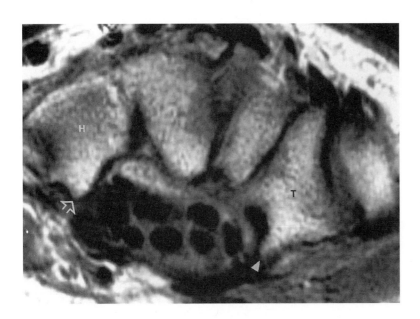

FIG. 29.48. Truncated hook of hamate. Axial spin-density-weighted MR image shows hypoplastic hamulus *(arrow).* In this patient who has had carpal tunnel release surgery, the hook of the hamate is smaller than the tubercle of the trapezium *(arrowhead).* H, hamate; T, trapezium.

Carpal Coalition

A carpal coalition is an osseous fusion between individual carpal bones. Idiopathic coalitions involve adjacent bones in the same carpal row; syndrome-related or postinfectious coalitions usually involve bones in adjacent rows. Idiopathic coalitions are more common in women and African-Americans. By far the most frequent idiopathic cases are lunotriquetral coalitions, whose spectrum has been classified by Minaar (37) (Figs. 29.49–29.51). Although coalitions are normally asymptomatic, fibrous or cartilaginous lunotriquetral coalitions (Minaar type I) may be painful (see Fig. 29.51). Albeit rare, the second most common coalition is the capitohamate (Fig. 29.52) (38,39).

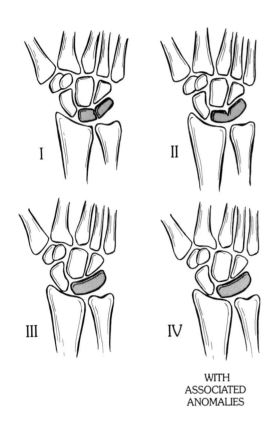

WITH
ASSOCIATED
ANOMALIES

FIG. 29.49. Drawing shows Minaar's classification of lunotriquetral coalition: type I, proximal fibrous or cartilaginous coalition; type II, incomplete osseous fusion with distal notch; type III, complete osseous fusion; type IV, complete osseous fusion with other carpal anomalies. (Reprinted with permission from reference 39.)

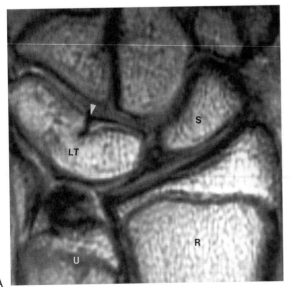
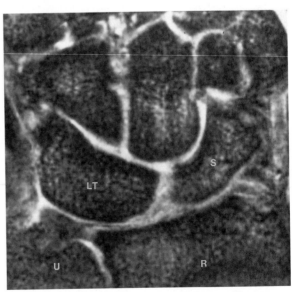

FIG. 29.50. Types II and III lunotriquetral coalitions. **A:** Coronal spin-density-weighted MR image shows incomplete bony fusion of the lunate and triquetral bones. Note distal cleft *(arrowhead)* of this type II coalition. **B:** Coronal gradient-recalled echo MR image shows complete lunotriquetral bony bridging (type III coalition). LT, lunotriquetral coalition; S, scaphoid; R, radius; U, ulna.

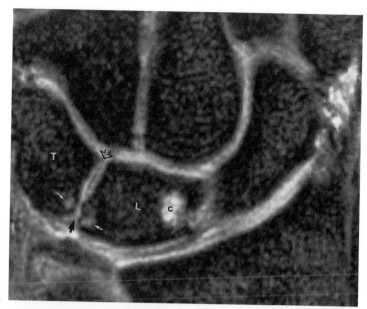

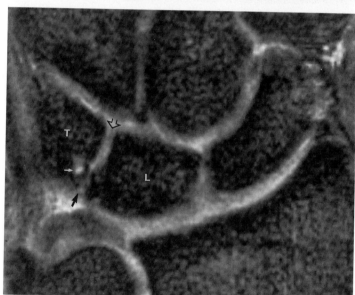

FIG. 29.51. Type I lunotriquetral coalition. **A:** Coronal gradient-recalled echo MR image shows a narrowed interosseous space proximally between the lunate and triquetrum *(black arrow)* consistent with a fibrous or cartilaginous lunotriquetral coalition. Note the normal lunotriquetral articulation distally *(open arrow)* and subcortical edema *(white arrows)* of the affected bones at the site of coalition. An intraosseous cyst (C) of the lunate may be incidental. L, lunate; T, triquetrum. **B:** Coronal gradient-recalled echo MR image 3.5 mm dorsal to **A** shows closer apposition at the site of coalition *(black arrow)*, a subcortical triquetral cyst *(white arrow)* subjacent to the coalition, and the normal lunotriquetral joint space distally *(open arrow)*. L, lunate; T, triquetrum.

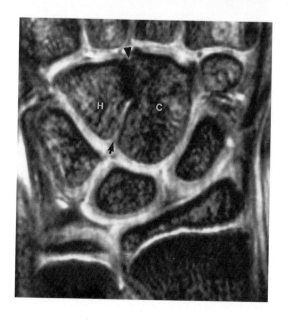

FIG. 29.52. Capitohamate coalition (incomplete). Coronal gradient-recalled echo MR image shows fusion of the capitohamate articulation distally *(arrowhead)*; proximally the interosseous space is narrowed *(arrow)* but not fused. C, capitate; H, hamate.

Lunate Morpology

The morphology of the lunate has been characterized as having two types: a type 1 lunate has a single facet at the midcarpal joint, and a type 2 has an extra medial facet that articulates with the hamate (Fig 29.53). Each type has about equal prevalence (40,41). The type 2 lunate is noteworthy, however, because it can be associated with degenerative changes at the proximal pole of the hamate, which can be the cause of ulnar-sided wrist pain (40,41) (Fig. 29.54). Whereas lunate morphology cannot always

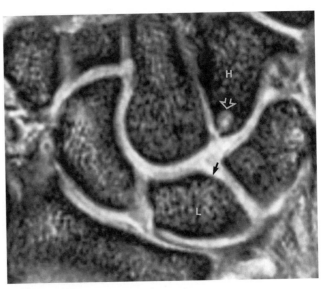

FIG. 29.54. Type II lunate associated with hamate degenerative change. Coronal gradient-recalled echo MR image shows type II lunate with additional midcarpal facet *(arrow)* and associated degenerative subchondral cyst of the hamate *(open arrow)*. L, lunate; H, hamate.

be ascertained reliably from plain film studies (41), MR imaging with its tomographic capability can clearly indicate lunate type (and any coexistent hamate changes) on coronal images.

Pisotriquetral Joint

Aside from lunohamate joint disease, osteoarthritis of the pisotriquetral joint can be another cause of ulnar-sided wrist pain (42). Care should be taken in distinguishing normal lipping of the articular aspects of the pisiform and triquetrum from true degenerative osteophyte formation (Fig. 29.55). The former finding is a commonly seen normal variation.

Distal Radioulnar Joint

Axial MR images of the distal radioulnar joint may be a source of mistaking normal variation for pathology. Normally, in pronation, the ulna lies more dorsal relative to the radius (43). As pronation is the standard position of the wrist for MR scanning, the radiologist must be careful not to overcall this normal alignment as dorsal subluxation; on sagittal images, too, the ulna may appear dorsally subluxed (Fig. 29.56).

Volar Surface of Lunate

Occasionally on sagittal MR images, the volar surface of the lunate may normally have a corrugated appearance that should not be mistaken for injury (Fig. 29.57). This normal variation results from the numerous structures

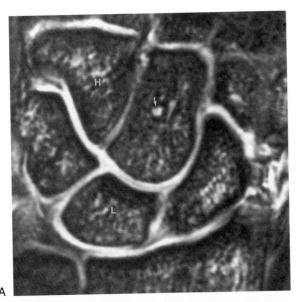

A

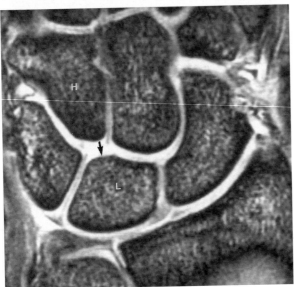

B

FIG. 29.53. Type I and type II lunates. **A:** Coronal gradient-recalled echo MR image shows a type I lunate with a single facet at the midcarpal joint. Note incidental capitate cyst *(arrow).* H, hamate; L, lunate. **B:** Coronal gradient-recalled echo MR image of a different individual shows the lunate with an additional facet *(arrow)* articulating with the hamate. H, hamate; L, lunate.

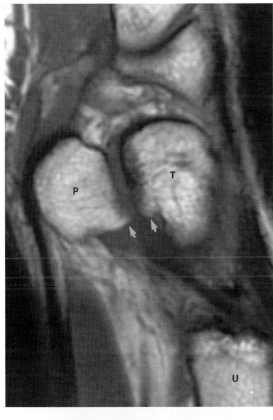

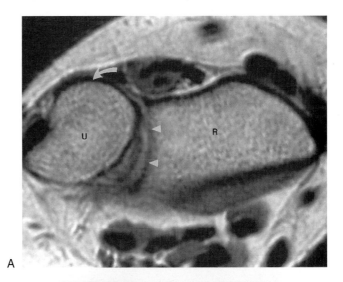

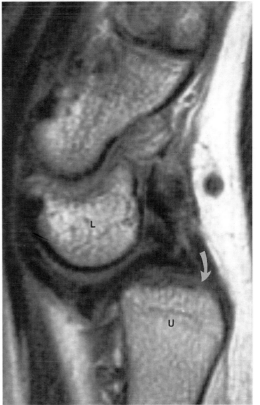

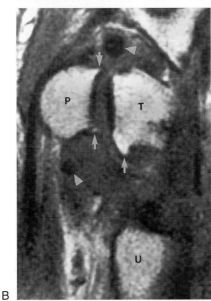

FIG. 29.55. Normal versus osteoarthritic pisotriquetral artic-ulation. Sagittal T1-weighted MR images show **(A)** normal "lipping" *(arrows)* of the articular borders of the pisiform and triquetrum in an asymptomatic volunteer, as opposed to **(B)** degenerative changes of the pisotriquetral joint evidenced by osteophytes *(arrows)* and calcified loose bodies *(arrow-heads)* in a patient with ulnar-sided wrist pain. P, pisiform; T, triquetrum; U, ulna.

FIG. 29.56. Dorsal position of the ulna at the radioulnar joint. **A:** Axial spin-density-weighted MR image shows posterior aspect of the ulnar head *(arrow)* positioned dorsally relative to the radius at the distal radioulnar joint. Note normal lack of congruence of the ulnar head with respect to the sigmoid notch *(arrowheads)*. R, radius; U, ulna. **B:** Sagittal T1-weighted MR image of same individual again shows dorsal pseudosubluxation of the ulna (arrow). L, lunate; U, ulna.

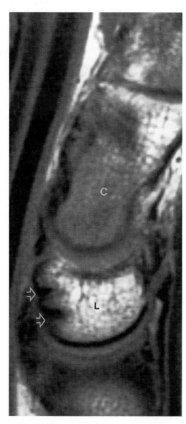

FIG. 29.57. Normal corrugated appearance of the volar surface of lunate. Sagittal T1-weighted MR image shows normal ridges *(arrows)* of the volar aspect of the lunate secondary to ligamentous or vascular insertions. L, lunate; C, capitate.

that insert on the lunate at its palmar aspect, namely, the radiolunotriquetral ligament described earlier as well as the short radiolunate ligament, another important extrinsic ligament, which extends from the volar lip of the radius to the volar aspect of the lunate (44). In addition, multiple nutrient vessels penetrate into the palmar surface of the lunate (45), which may also contribute to its irregular volar surface.

REFERENCES

1. Kneeland JB, Hyde JS. High-resolution MR imaging with local coils. *Radiology* 1989;171:1–7.
2. Erickson SJ. High-resolution imaging of the musculoskeletal system. *Radiology* 1997;205:593–618.
3. Timins ME, O'Connell SE, Erickson SJ, Oneson SR. MR imaging of the wrist: normal findings that may simulate disease. *RadioGraphics* 1996;16:987–995.
4. Tountas CP, Bergman RA. *Anatomic variations of the upper extremity.* New York: Churchill Livingstone, 1993;126–128,176–178.
5. Fullerton GD, Cameron IL, Ord VA. Orientation of tendons in the magnetic field and its effect on T$_2$ relaxation times. *Radiology* 1985;155:433–435.
6. Palmer AK, Skahen J, Werner FW, et al. The extensor retinaculum of the wrist: an anatomic and biochemical study. *J Hand Surg [Br]* 1985;10B:11.
7. Zeiss J, Guilliam-Hadet L. MR demonstration of anomalous muscles about the volar aspect of the wrist and forearm. *Clin Imag* 1996;20:219–221.
8. Warfel JH. *The extremities.* Philadelphia: Lea & Febiger, 1974;56.
9. Zeiss J, Jakab E, Khimji T, Imbriglia J. The ulnar tunnel at the wrist (Guyon's canal): normal MR anatomy and variants. *Am J Roentgenol* 1992;158:1081–1085.
10. Zeiss J, Jakab E. MR demonstration of an anomalous muscle in a patient with coexistent carpal and ulnar tunnel syndrome: case report and literature summary. *Clin Imag* 1995;19:102–105.
11. Gama C. Extensor digitorum brevis manus: a report on 38 cases and a review of the literature. *J Hand Surg* 1993;8:578–582.
12. Ogura T, Hajime I, Tanabe G. Anatomic and clinical studies of the extensor digitorum brevis manus. *J Hand Surg* 1987;12A:100–107.
13. Anderson MW, Benedetti P, Walter J, Steinberg DR. MR appearance of the extensor digitorum manus brevis muscle: a pseudotumor of the hand. *Am J Roentgenol* 1995;164:1477–1479.
14. Sanger JR, Krasniak CL, Matloub HS, Yousif NJ, Kneeland JB. Diagnosis of an anomalous superficialis muscle in the palm by magnetic resonance imaging. *J Hand Surg* 1991;16A:98–101.
15. Smith RJ. Anomalous muscle belly of the flexor digitorum superficialis causing carpal-tunnel syndrome. *J Bone Joint Surg* 1971;53A:1215–1216.
16. Reimann AF, Daseler EH, Anson BJ, Beaton LE. The palmaris longus muscle and tendon: a study of 1600 extremities. *Anat Rec* 1944;89:495–505.
17. Polesuk BS, Helms CA. Hypertrophied palmaris longus muscle, a pseudomass of the forearm: MR appearance case report and review of the literature. *Radiology* 1998;207:361–362.
18. Eversmann WW Jr. Entrapment and the compression neuropathies. In: Green OP, ed. *Operative hand surgery, 2nd ed.* New York: Churchill Livingstone, 1988;1423–1441.
19. Middleton WD, Kneeland JB, Kellman GM, et al. MR imaging of the carpal tunnel: normal anatomy and preliminary findings in the carpal tunnel syndrome. *Am J Roentgenol* 1987;148:307–316.
20. Lanz U. Anatomical variations of the median nerve in the carpal tunnel. *J Hand Surg* 1977;2A:44–53.
21. Zeiss J, Guilliam-Hadet L. MR demonstration of a persistent median artery in carpal tunnel syndrome: case report. *J Comput Assist Tomogr* 1993;17(3):482–484.
22. Zeiss J, Skie M, Ebraheim N, Jackson WT. Anatomic relations between the median nerve and flexor tendons in the carpal tunnel: MR evaluation in normal volunteers. *Am J Roentgenol* 1989;153:533–536.
23. Hagert CG. The distal radioulnar joint. *Hand Clin* 1987;3:41–50.
24. Totterman SMS, Miller RJ. MR imaging of the triangular fibrocartilage complex. *Magn Reson Imag Clin North Am* 1995;3:213–228.
25. Modl JM, Sether LA, Haughton VM, Kneeland JB. Articular cartilage: correlation of histological zones with signal intensity at MR imaging. *Radiology* 1991;181:853–855.
26. Kang SK, Kindynis P, Brahme SK, et al. Triangular fibrocartilage and intercarpal ligaments of the wrist: MR imaging cadaveric study with gross pathologic and histologic correlations. *Radiology* 1991;181:401–404.
27. Zlatkin MB, Chao PC, Osterman AL, et al. Chronic wrist pain: evaluation with high-resolution MR imaging. *Radiology* 1989;173:723–729.
28. Taliesnik J. The ligaments of the wrist. *J Hand Surg* 1976;1(2):110–118.
29. Totterman SMS, Miller RJ. Scapholunate ligament: normal MR appearance on three-dimensional gradient-recalled-echo images. *Radiology* 1996;200:237–241.
30. Mayfield JK, Johnson RP, Kilcoyne RF. The ligaments of the human wrist and their functional significance. *Anat Rec* 1976;186:417–428.
31. Taliesnik J. *The wrist.* New York: Churchill Livingstone, 1985.
32. Berger RA, Kauer JMG, Landsmeer JMF. Radioscapholunate ligament: a gross anatomic study of fetal and adult wrists. *J Hand Surg [Am]* 1991; 16:350–355.
33. Smith DK. Volar carpal ligaments of the wrist: normal appearance on multiplanar reconstructions of three-dimensional Fourier transform MR imaging. *Am J Roentgenol* 1993;161:353–357.
34. Schmidt H, Freyschmidt J. *Borderlands of normal and early pathologic findings in skeletal radiography (Kohler/Zimmer), 4th ed.* New York: Georg Thieme Verlag, 1993;79–93.
35. Lewis OJ, Hamshere RJ, Bucknill TM. The anatomy of the wrist joint. *J Anat* 1970;106(3):539–552.
36. Resnick D. *Bone and joint imaging.* Philadelphia: WB Saunders, 1989;1073.
37. Minaar A. Congenital fusion between the lunate and triquetral bones in the South African Bantu. *J Bone Joint Surg* 1952;34B:45–58.

38. Delaney TJ, Erwar S. Carpal coalitions. *J Hand Surg* 1992;17A(1): 28–31.
39. Simmons BP, McKenzie WD. Symptomatic carpal coalation. *J Hand Surg* 1985;10A(2):190–193.
40. Burgess RC. Anatomic variations of the midcarpal joint. *J Hand Surg* 1990;15A:129–131.
41. Sagerman SD, Hauck RM, Palmer AK. Lunate morphology: can it be predicted with routine x-ray films? *J Hand Surg* 1995;20A:38–41.

42. Paley D, McMurtry RY, Cruickshank B. Pathologic conditions of the pisiform and pisotriquetral joint. *J Hand Surg* 1987;12A:110–119.
43. King GJ, McMurtry RY, Rubenstein JD, Gertzbein SD. Kinematics of the distal radioulnar joint. *J Hand Surg [Am]* 1986;11:798–804.
44. Berger RA, Landsmeer JMF. The palmar radiocarpal ligaments: a study of adult and fetal human wrist joints. *J Hand Surg [Am]* 1990;15:847–854.
45. Lichtman DM. *The wrist and its disorders.* Philadelphia: WB Saunders, 1988;37–39.

Variants and Pitfalls in Body Imaging,
edited by Ali Shirkhoda.
Lippincott Williams & Wilkins, Philadelphia, © 2000.

CHAPTER 30

The Knee: MRI

Vamsidhar R. Narra and Scott A. Mirowitz

Magnetic resonance imaging (MRI) has revolutionized imaging evaluation of the knee. Following clinical examination, MRI is frequently performed to evaluate for suspected internal derangement. MRI has been shown to be highly accurate in demonstrating meniscal and ligamentous abnormalities in and around the knee joint (1,2). However, there are many sources of potential diagnostic error that are commonly encountered on knee MR images. The variety of recognized pitfalls continues to grow with expanded clinical use of MRI and implementation of newer MRI techniques. Such interpretive pitfalls are usually related to one or more of the following factors: (a) the unique physical principles involved with MRI, (b) the ability of MRI to delineate anatomic structures not easily appreciated with other imaging modalities, (c) representation of anatomic structures in unfamiliar planes, and (d) the spectrum of normal anatomic variation. This chapter reviews imaging techniques, normal variations, artifacts, and diagnostic pitfalls involved in the interpretation of knee MRI.

TECHNIQUE

When imaging the knee with MRI, many factors must be considered to provide optimal evaluation of the menisci, ligaments, tendons, cartilage, joint space, osseous structures, and soft tissues. It is ideal to evaluate each of these structures in three planes: axial, sagittal, and coronal. However, this is not always achievable due to practical limitations in total imaging time, since patient compliance, equipment, and the throughput must also be considered.

V. R. Narra and S. A. Mirowitz: Mallinckrodt Institute of Radiology, Washington University School of Medicine, St. Louis, Missouri 63110.

Surface Coil

A circumferential extremity coil using a send-receive, quadrature, or phased array design is commonly used for knee MRI. The coil provides a uniform signal-to-noise ratio throughout the knee. Use of the coil requires that each knee be imaged independently.

Patient Positioning

The knee should be flexed 10 to 15 degrees and positioned in slight external rotation to align the anterior cruciate ligament (ACL) parallel to the sagittal plane. When this cannot be achieved due to patient discomfort or other factors, one can acquire sagittal oblique images parallel to the ACL. Excessive internal rotation of the knee can result in apparent elongation of the anteroposterior dimension of the femoral condyles and may decrease accurate representation of meniscal anatomy (3).

Imaging Planes and Sequences

Numerous protocols are available for knee MRI; however, the menisci are best evaluated on proton density–weighted images. Such images are usually acquired as part of a dual-echo conventional spin echo (CSE) sequence, providing both proton density– (i.e., short echo time, TE) and T2-weighted (i.e., long TE) images. The T2-weighted images are useful for visualizing soft tissue edema and for differentiating fluid and cartilage. A section thickness of 3 to 4 mm is recommended, with a 0 to 0.5 mm intersection gap. CSE sequences are generally considered to be standard for depicting meniscal tears. Fast spin echo (FSE) or turbo spin echo (TSE) sequences have also begun to be used recently for this purpose. It has been shown that by keeping the echo train length less than five on such sequences, it is possible to preserve the high spatial frequency information, resulting in performance similar to that of CSE sequences (4).

Sagittal images are useful to evaluate the cruciate ligaments, extensor mechanism, joint capsule, and patellofemoral joint. Transaxial images (e.g., FSE T2-weighted fat-saturated images), acquired using a section thickness of 3 to 4 mm, and are useful for evaluating the patellofemoral joint, hyaline cartilage, and the collateral ligaments. Meniscal pathology is typically poorly visualized in the transaxial plane. Coronal T1- and proton density–weighted FSE fat saturation images are helpful for evaluating the menisci, collateral ligaments, articular cartilage, and bone marrow. Proton density–weighted images are excellent for demonstrating articular cartilage and underlying bone cortex. The interface between these structures is well visualized using a repetition time (TR) of at least 3,000 msec and an echo time (TE) of 20 msec. The combination of the above sequences allows reasonable evaluation of the soft tissues. The phase-encoding gradient is typically oriented so that vascular pulsation artifacts are directed away from the menisci as much as possible. Intra-articular gadolinium chelate contrast material with acquisition of T1-weighted fat saturation images may be valuable for optimal evaluation of postoperative menisci.

NORMAL VARIANTS AND DIAGNOSTIC PITFALLS

Menisci

The menisci are C-shaped fibrocartilaginous structures that attach to the condylar surface of the tibia. These structures protect the joint articular cartilage and provide joint stability. In adults, the menisci are relatively avascular except for their peripheral 10% to 25% (5). Intact menisci demonstrate uniform low-signal-intensity on T1-, T2- and T2*-weighted images. They are triangular in cross section with an outer convex curve. The apex of these triangular structures is directed toward the intercondylar notch. The meniscus is arbitrarily divided into an anterior horn, body, and posterior horn. The semicircular medial meniscus has

a wide posterior horn and has a more open C-shaped configuration than the more circular lateral meniscus. The medial meniscus is firmly attached to the joint capsule along its entire peripheral circumference. This attachment limits the ability of the meniscus to move adaptively with the femoral condyle and is believed to be a cause of the relatively increased incidence of medial meniscal injury. The lateral meniscus forms a tighter C shape and is more circular than the medial meniscus. The lateral meniscus is separated from the lateral collateral ligament by the popliteal recess, with the popliteal tendon and fibrofatty tissue.

Anatomic Variations

Shape and Size

Peripheral sagittal images through the menisci normally demonstrate a bow-tie configuration, with the central portion corresponding to the meniscal body. When the bow-tie configuration is seen in three or more contiguous slices (3 mm thick), this suggests a discoid meniscus, which is a normal variant (6) (Fig. 30.1). A discoid meniscus is a dysplastic meniscus that has a broad disc-like configuration. Discoid changes more commonly involve the lateral meniscus (1.4% to 15%), than the medial meniscus (0.3%) as demonstrated in a series of meniscectomy specimens (7). Reduced size of the meniscus or a portion of it is usually a normal variant, but can also occur in patients with juvenile rheumatoid arthritis (8). Pseudomeniscal shortening can occur when the knee is positioned in excess external rotation. Correlation of sagittal images with coronal and transaxial images is helpful in making this determination.

Position

Alterations in meniscal position are frequently associated with meniscal injury, though subluxation of an intact meniscus occurs as a normal variant. Meniscal subluxa-

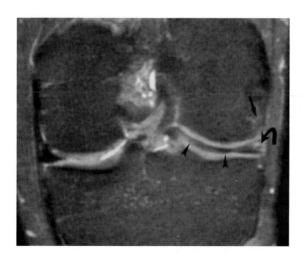

FIG. 30.1. Discoid lateral meniscus. A coronal fat-saturated proton density–weighted image demonstrates a band of meniscal tissue consistent with a discoid lateral meniscus *(arrowheads)*. Also noted is increased signal intensity within the lateral aspect of the discoid lateral meniscus *(curved arrow)* and subchondral marrow edema involving the lateral femoral condyle *(arrow)*.

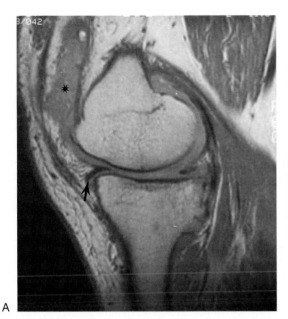

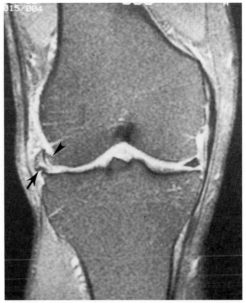

A

B

FIG. 30.2. Meniscal subluxation. **A:** A sagittal proton density–weighted image demonstrates anterior displacement of the medial meniscus *(arrow)*. Also note the small joint effusion *(asterisk)*. **B:** A coronal proton density–weighted fat-saturated image in a different patient demonstrates a medially subluxed medial meniscus *(arrow)* with extensive increased signal consistent with a degenerative type tear. Also note the adjacent osteoarthritic changes with osteophyte formation *(arrowhead)*.

tion is commonly encountered in patients with degenerative arthritis. This entity commonly involves the anterior horns of the menisci, which are displaced anteriorly relative to the tibial plateau (Fig. 30.2).

Diagnostic Pitfalls

Image Acquisition

Proton density–weighted CSE or FSE sequences acquired with an echo train length of four or less are most widely used to evaluate the menisci. FSE sequences acquired using relatively long echo trains or gradient echo pulse sequences can result in alterations in intrameniscal signal, which may result in over- or underestimation of meniscal tears. Gradient echo pulse sequences can produce accentuation of intrameniscal signal alterations causing tears to become obscured or overestimated (9). Optimization of the sequence parameters should be based on controlled studies, with clinical experience providing a template for the range of expected meniscal signal alterations using a given pulse sequence and combination of imaging parameters.

The menisci are usually evaluated on images acquired in a direct sagittal plane. Sagittal oblique or radial images profile the menisci segmentally, resulting in an appearance similar to that obtained during arthrography. However, previous investigation has indicated that radial images do not provide significant improvement over standard orthogonal views, and hence they are not widely utilized at the present time (10).

Image Display

Window level and width settings affect the ability to accurately diagnose and characterize meniscal abnormalities. High contrast, narrow window settings (i.e., meniscal windows) are useful for accentuating intrameniscal signal changes. However, they do carry the potential for causing overestimation of the extent of abnormal meniscal signal. For this reason, findings on meniscal windows should be closely correlated to those obtained using a standard display and other sequences. Buckwalter et al. (11) found no significant improvement in the detection of meniscal tears using meniscal window display settings.

Motion Artifact

The presence of motion during image acquisition results in ghost artifacts, which are partial or complete replications of high signal intensity moving structures. These artifacts are displayed along the phase-encoding direction of the image. To minimize the impact of such artifacts, the phase-encoding direction is usually assigned along the shortest dimension of the anatomic area being imaged. However, when sagittal knee images are acquired, the superoinferior direction, which is the long axis of the knee, is sometimes assigned as the phase-encoding direction. This is done in an attempt to redirect vascular pulsation artifacts arising from the popliteal vessels away from the cruciate ligaments and other structures. One must be aware that with this reoriented gradient configuration, even slight knee motion can produce

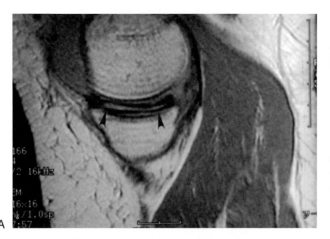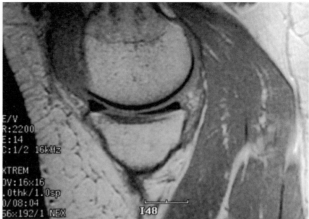

A   B

FIG. 30.3. Motion artifact. **A:** Sagittal proton density–weighted image demonstrates linear increased signal intensity within the medial meniscus *(arrowheads)*, simulating a tear. **B:** Repeat image obtained following reorientation of the phase- and frequency-encoding gradients eliminates the artifact, which is due to subtle patient motion.

high signal intensity replications of the femoral condyles, or overlying hyaline cartilage. The resultant curvilinear phase errors can closely simulate the appearance of a meniscal tear (12) (Fig. 30.3). Clues that help distinguish such motion artifacts from an actual meniscal tear include observation of extension of the increased signal intensity beyond the meniscal confines and recognition that they closely reproduce the contour of the femoral condyle and overlying hyaline cartilage. When uncertainty remains, images can be reacquired using a conventional phase-encoding orientation along the anteroposterior axis of the knee.

Truncation Artifact

Truncation artifact produces a series of curvilinear lines that parallel adjacent high-contrast interfaces. Truncation artifact reflects an inherent limitation of Fourier transformation, which is the method used to reconstruct MR signals into images. In MRI, sampling is restricted to a finite number of frequencies, which approximate the image using only a few harmonics in its Fourier representation. The Fourier series is then cut short or truncated, thus the name for the artifact (13). Truncation artifact occurs in both phase- and frequency-encoding directions. However, since fewer data lines are routinely acquired in the phase-encoding direction, the artifact is more apparent in this axis. Truncation artifact is most apparent when a relatively low spatial resolution, rectangular (128×256) matrix is prescribed. As noted previously, for knee imaging the phase-encoding direction is often assigned along the superoinferior axis in an effort to redirect popliteal artery pulsation artifacts. In this situation, truncation artifacts can appear as foci of curvilinear increased signal intensity. These artifacts correspond to the configuration of the femoral condyle, where there is an abrupt change from

high signal intensity fatty marrow and hyaline cartilage to low signal intensity meniscal tissue. When these artifacts project over the menisci, they can closely simulate the appearance of a meniscal tear (14). Increasing the number of phase-encoding steps can reduce truncation artifact or they can be redirected by orienting the phase-encoding direction along the anteroposterior axis of the knee.

Chemical Shift Misregistration Artifact

Chemical shift misregistration artifact reflects differences in the precessional frequencies of water and lipid protons that coexist in an imaging volume element, or voxel. Lipid protons have a lower resonant frequency than water protons. Therefore, with the receiver frequency set to the water frequency, signal from lipid protons appears to have arisen from water protons located in another part of the field. This is manifested as artifactual decreased signal intensity at one fat–water border, with corresponding increased signal intensity at the opposite fat–water border. This artifact is displayed along the frequency-encoding direction of the image (15). Thus, if the frequency-encoding axis is oriented along the superoinferior direction of the knee on sagittal images, the high signal intensity component of this artifact can potentially overlie the meniscus and simulate a tear (16). Chemical shift misregistration artifact can be reduced by increasing the receiver bandwidth, increasing the number of matrix elements, or by using fat saturation. Furthermore, this artifact can be redirected to another portion of the image by gradient reorientation.

Susceptibility Artifact

Susceptibility artifacts occur at interfaces between substances having different magnetic properties. When two

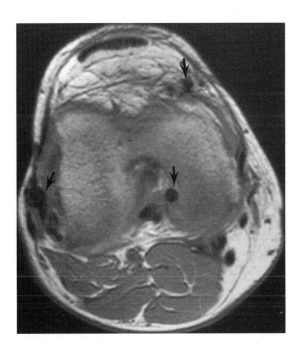

FIG. 30.4. Susceptibility artifact. Gradient echo T1-weighted transaxial image demonstrates multiple round areas of signal void *(arrows)* from metallic microfragments in a patient who underwent previous arthroscopic repair of a meniscal tear.

materials with different magnetic properties are juxtaposed, a local distortion of the magnetic field occurs. This creates dephasing and frequency shifts of nearby protons. Signal void foci resulting from metallic microfragments are commonly encountered in patients who have undergone previous arthroscopy or open knee surgery (Fig. 30.4). Intra-articular air, metal, calcium, and hemorrhage can also result in susceptibility artifacts. These artifacts are seen as foci of low signal intensity, often with surrounding irregular high signal intensity. When these artifacts intersect the meniscus, the high signal intensity component can simulate a meniscal tear (17) (Fig. 30.5). Susceptibility artifacts are more pronounced when imaging is performed at high magnetic field strengths, and when gradient echo and fat saturation imaging techniques are used. The use of FSE pulse sequences, high spatial resolution imaging matrix, and low magnetic field strengths can reduce the prominence of susceptibility effects.

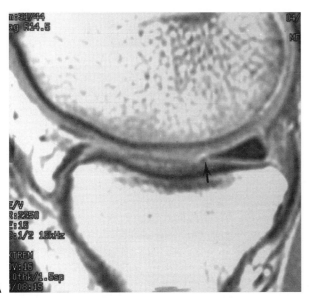
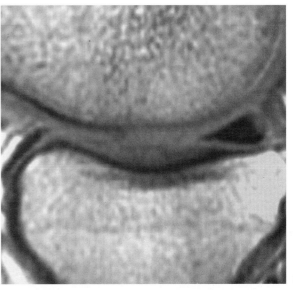

FIG. 30.5. Susceptibility artifact. **A:** Intra-articular air from previous arthrocentesis creates susceptibility artifact as manifested by an area of signal void with surrounding hyperintensity *(arrow)*. This appearance simulates a tear of the posterior horn of the medial meniscus. **B:** Repeat MR examination, performed at a later date, demonstrates a normal appearance of the medial meniscus, with no tear seen. (From ref. 16, with permission.)

Partial Volume Effects

Partial volume averaging is a common cause for diagnostic errors in MRI and other cross-sectional imaging. Volume averaging of the meniscus with adjacent soft tissues can simulate a meniscal tear. This is commonly seen on sagittal images that are acquired through the periphery of the joint. On such images, partial volume averaging of the meniscus can occur with adjacent fibrofatty tissue. Partial volume averaging can also interfere with diagnosis of small tears involving the free edge of the meniscus (18,19). Thin-section transaxial and coronal images are useful in the evaluation of free edge and small vertical tears (20).

Magic Angle Phenomenon

On short TE images the magic angle phenomenon may produce foci of relative increased meniscal signal intensity. This occurs most frequently in the upward-sloping portion or medial segment of the posterior horn of the normal lateral meniscus, where it can simulate a meniscal tear (21). The magic angle effect is seen when the portions of the fibrocartilaginous menisci are oriented at approximately 55 degrees relative to the static magnetic field along the long axis of the magnet bore.

Exercise and Calcification

Increased meniscal signal intensity can occur as a transient reaction to recent stress. For example, this phenomenon has been documented in patients following recent

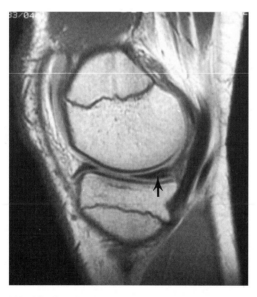

FIG. 30.6. Meniscal vascular pedicle. A sagittal proton density–weighted image through the medial meniscus demonstrates a linear area of increased signal intensity within the posterior horn *(arrow)* in a skeletally immature patient. This signal represents the meniscal vascular pedicle.

prolonged exercise, such as in long-distance runners. The above findings can occasionally simulate meniscal degeneration and/or tear (22,23).

Vascular Pedicle

The meniscal vascular pedicle is observed extending from the peripheral meniscocapsular junction into the meniscus in children and early adolescents. If one is not familiar with this entity, it can be confused with intrameniscal degeneration or an intrasubstance tear (Fig. 30.6). The characteristic location of the signal alteration and the age of the patient are clues to recognizing this entity. The vascular pedicle regresses in the adult and is poorly visualized (8).

Geniculate Artery

The lateral inferior geniculate artery can contribute to a pseudotear adjacent to the anterior horn of the lateral meniscus on sagittal images (24). In this situation, the apparent tear represents fibrofatty tissue that is interposed between the low signal intensity vessel and the adjacent meniscus. Identification of the vessel as separate from the meniscus on coronal images and the ability to track it as a tubular structure on successive sagittal images helps in recognition of this entity.

Intrameniscal Degenerative Changes

The normal meniscus demonstrates relatively homogeneous low signal intensity on T1-weighted, CSE and FSE T2-weighted, gradient echo, and short tau inversion recovery (STIR) images. Meniscal degeneration and tears result in increased meniscal signal intensity, which is usually most sensitively depicted on short TE images (25). To characterize the significance of intrameniscal signal changes, an MR grading system has been developed and has been correlated to histopathologic changes (26). Grade I signal abnormality refers to focal or globular increased signal intensity within the substance of the meniscus, without extension to an articular surface. This finding correlates histologically with foci of early mucinous degeneration and chondrocyte deficiency. Grade II changes refer to horizontal or linear intrasubstance signal abnormality that extends to the capsular periphery but does not communicate with the articular surface. Histologically, this grade correlates with mucinous degeneration of the meniscus. The posterior horn of the medial meniscus is the most common site for grade II signal abnormality (Fig. 30.7). Observation of such signal change does not serve as an effective prognostic indicator for temporal development of a tear (27). Grade II signal alterations have been further subdivided by some authors. Grade IIA changes refer to linear increased signal intensity that does not communicate with the articular surface of the meniscus on any image.

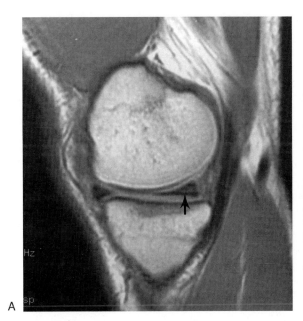
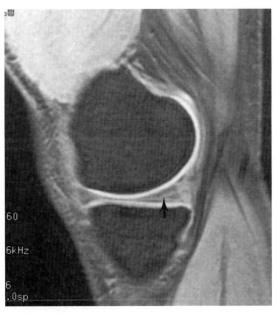

FIG. 30.7. Meniscal pseudotear. **A:** A sagittal proton density–weighted image demonstrates a small area of globular increased signal intensity within the posterior horn of the medial meniscus *(arrow)*. **B:** Gradient echo image accentuates the increased signal, causing it to appear to extend to the articular surface, simulating a tear *(arrow)*.

Grade IIB signal refers to increased signal intensity that extends to an articular surface on a single image, and is observed in only one imaging plane. At arthroscopy tears are seldom found in patients with such signal alterations. Grade IIC alterations indicate increased meniscal signal intensity that is wedge shaped and does not communicate with the articular surface. Approximately one-half of patients with these findings demonstrate a detectable tear at arthroscopy (28).

Grade III meniscal changes reliably indicate the presence of a meniscal tear (Fig. 30.8), and are diagnosed when increased meniscal signal intensity definitively extends either superiorly or inferiorly to the articular surface. Histopathologically, a meniscal tear corresponds to

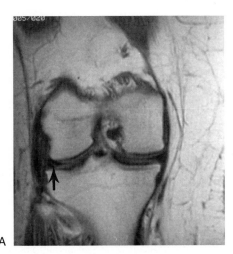
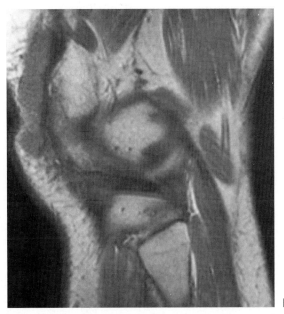

FIG. 30.8. Peripheral meniscal tear. **A:** A coronal T1-weighted image demonstrates a linear area of increased signal intensity within the peripheral portion of the lateral meniscus consistent with a tear *(arrow)*. **B:** Note that the peripheral tear is difficult to identify on the corresponding sagittal image.

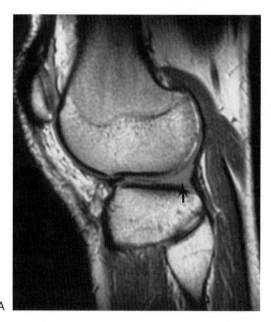 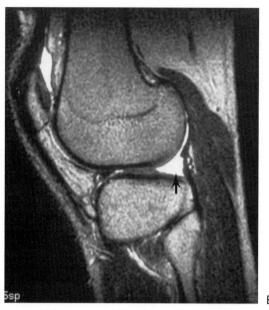

A   B

FIG. 30.9. Meniscectomy defect. **A:** A sagittal proton density–weighted image demonstrates an area of increased signal intensity in the expected location of the posterior horn of the lateral meniscus, consistent with the grade IIC signal abnormality *(arrow)*. **B:** A T2-weighted image confirms that the apparent area of increased signal represents fluid filling a meniscectomy defect *(arrow)*.

fibrocartilaginous separation. Less than 5% of meniscal tears are entirely intrasubstance tears, where disruption does not extend to an articular surface. Such tears are usually diagnosed on arthroscopy by probing the meniscus. In patients who have undergone previous meniscectomy, fluid that fills the meniscectomy space can simulate meniscal degeneration and tear on proton density–weighted images (Fig. 30.9).

In patients who have sustained a remote meniscal injury, high signal intensity may persist on follow-up MRI examinations. Therefore, MRI may not be reliable in differentiating acute from chronic meniscal tears.

MRI is considered to have yielded a false-positive result when the meniscal surface appears intact at arthroscopy despite the presence of an apparent meniscal tear on MRI. Although MRI may indeed overstage some meniscal abnormalities, the limitations of arthroscopy as a gold standard have also been recognized (18). For example, some areas of the menisci are poorly accessible at arthroscopy, such as the posterior and peripheral aspect of the medial meniscus and its capsular attachment.

Meniscocapsular Separation

Meniscocapsular separation indicates a peripheral meniscal tear that occurs near its attachment to the medial joint capsule. This tear is unique for two reasons. First, such a tear is capable of undergoing spontaneous healing, due to its proximity to the meniscal vascular supply. Second, this type of tear can be difficult to visualize at arthroscopy.

Meniscocapsular separation is recognized by the presence of vertical increased signal intensity at the meniscocapsular junction. Prominent fibrofatty tissue at the meniscocapsular junction can simulate such a tear. When distinction is difficult, the use of fat saturation images

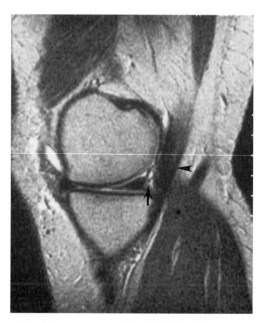

FIG. 30.10. Pseudo-meniscocapsular separation. A sagittal T2-weighted image demonstrates fluid within the meniscosynovial recess *(arrow)*, which should not be mistaken for meniscocapsular separation of the medial meniscus. Note the medial head of grastrocnemius *(*)* and the semimembranosus tendon *(arrowhead)*.

can be helpful. Fluid within the meniscosynovial recesses can also simulate a meniscocapsular separation (Fig. 30.10). However, the angular configuration of the meniscosynovial recess is a feature that usually allows differentiation.

Pseudo–Bucket Handle Tear

This pitfall is encountered on coronal MR images, particularly when the knee is relatively externally rotated. Posterior coronal images depict apparent separation between the posterior horn and a portion of the meniscal body, simulating a bucket-handle tear. Awareness of this entity and close correlation with sagittal images allows this pitfall to be avoided.

Pseudohypertrophy of the Anterior Horn

In patients with bucket-handle tears of the lateral meniscus, the posterior horn may become displaced anteriorly, so that it lies adjacent to the anterior horn. Thus, the anterior horn of the lateral meniscus appears unusually large. The primary clue to recognition of this entity is absence or truncation of the posterior horn of the lateral meniscus (29).

Meniscal Laxity

A lax, wavy, or buckled meniscus can be a normal variant unassociated with meniscal tear (3) (Figs. 30.11 and 30.12). This finding is most commonly encountered in the medial meniscus. It may be associated with joint lax-

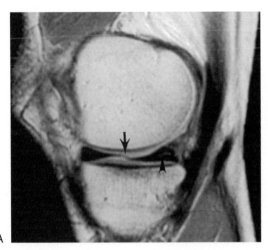
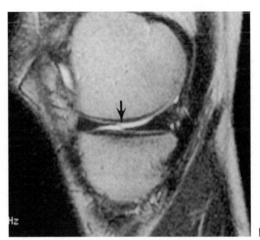

A   B

FIG. 30.11. Wavy meniscus. A proton density–weighted image **(A)** and corresponding T2-weighted image **(B)** demonstrate a linear area of increased signal intensity involving the posterior horn of the medial meniscus *(arrowhead).* Also note the wavy contour of the body of the medial meniscus *(arrows).* This normal variation is commonly seen in young patients.

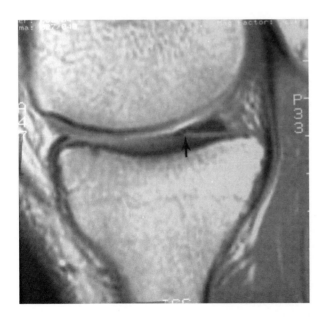

FIG. 30.12. Notch sign. A sagittal proton density–weighted image demonstrates a small notch *(arrow)* along the undersurface of the posterior horn of the medial meniscus, indicating a small undersurface tear. This finding must be differentiated from a normal variation of wavy meniscus. (From ref. 16, with permission.)

ity or ligamentous trauma. The lax or buckled meniscus may simulate a central or peripheral meniscal tear. This phenomenon may disappear with joint manipulation or subsequent imaging (3).

Meniscofemoral Ligaments

The meniscofemoral ligaments comprise the ligaments of Humphry and Wrisberg. These ligaments attach the medial portion of the lateral meniscus to the medial femoral condyle. The ligament of Humphry extends anterior to the posterior cruciate ligament (PCL). It is present in approximately one-third of anatomic dissections and is best visualized on sagittal images (Figs. 30.13 and 30.14). The ligament of Wrisberg is somewhat thicker, and is present in a higher percentage of anatomic dissections. It extends posterior to the PCL and is best visualized on posterior coronal images. MRI visualization of either ligament has been reported in one-third of patients in one series; both ligaments were observed in only 3% of MRI examinations (3,30). The meniscal insertion of the meniscofemoral ligament can simulate a vertical tear of the posterior horn of lateral meniscus (Fig. 30.15) (30). The apparent tear results from fibrofatty tissue that is interposed between the meniscal attachment and the meniscofemoral ligament.

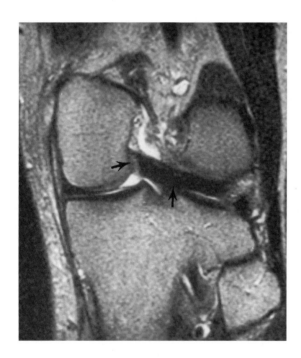

FIG. 30.13. Meniscofemoral ligament. A coronal fat-saturated proton density–weighted image demonstrates a prominent meniscofemoral ligament of Wrisberg *(arrows)*. The attachment of the ligament to the posterior horn of the lateral meniscus and the posterior medial femoral condyle are demonstrated.

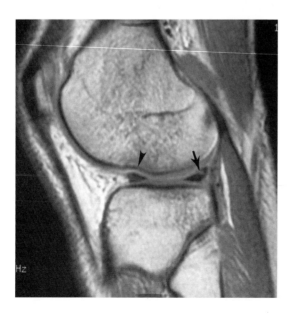

FIG. 30.14. Meniscofemoral ligament pseudotear. A sagittal proton density–weighted image demonstrates a focal area of increased signal intensity within the posterosuperior aspect of the lateral meniscus simulating a tear *(arrow)*. This finding is related to fibrofatty tissue surrounding a prominent Wrisberg ligament attachment to the lateral meniscus. Also note the normal notching contour waviness seen along the lateral femoral condyle *(arrowhead)*.

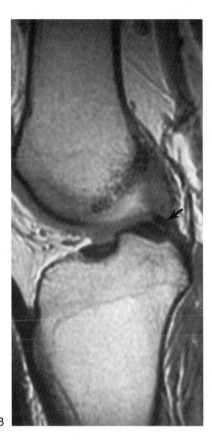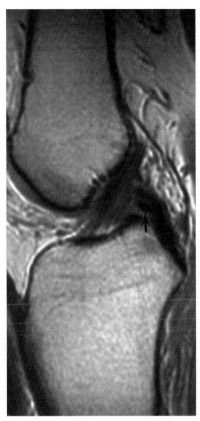

A,B

FIG. 30.15. Meniscofemoral ligament pseudo-tear. A and B: Sagittal proton density–weighted images demonstrate a prominent meniscofemoral ligament of Humphry *(arrow)*, with surrounding fibrofatty tissue simulating a meniscal tear *(arrow)* or a foreign body (B).

Transverse Ligament

The transverse intermeniscal ligament connects the anterior horns of the medial and lateral meniscus. It is observed in approximately one-third of patients on MRI (Fig. 30.16). Fibrofatty tissue surrounding this ligament

can simulate an oblique tear of the anterior horn of the lateral meniscus. Occasionally, fibrofatty tissue adjacent to the medial portion of the transverse ligament can also simulate a tear of the anterior horn of the medial meniscus. By tracing the low signal intensity transverse ligament across Hoffa's fat pad, one can usually differentiate

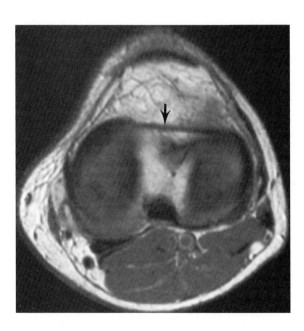

FIG. 30.16. Transverse intermeniscal ligament. Transaxial proton density–weighted image demonstrates the transverse intermeniscal ligament of the knee *(arrow)*. (From ref. 16, with permission.)

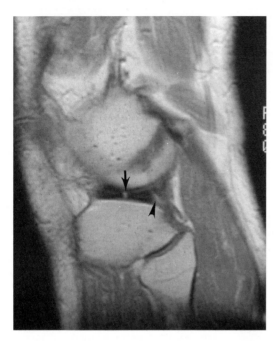

FIG. 30.17. Popliteal tendon pseudotear. A sagittal proton density–weighted image through the lateral meniscus demonstrates a focus of increased signal intensity *(arrow)*, representing a radial meniscal tear. Also noted is a linear area of increased signal intensity along the posterior aspect of the lateral meniscus *(arrowhead)*, representing fibrofatty tissue surrounding the popliteal tendon sheath.

this entity from an actual meniscal tear. The transverse ligament pseudotear should be considered when an apparent isolated tear of the anterior horn of the lateral meniscus is observed, since such tears are relatively uncommon (3).

Popliteus Tendon

Fluid contained within the popliteus tendon sheath can simulate a vertical tear of the posterior horn of the lateral meniscus. The popliteus tendon and its associated muscle can be followed on serial axial, sagittal, and coronal MR images (Fig. 30.17). The superior and inferior fascicle tear of the posterior horn of the lateral meniscus should not be confused with normal superior and inferior meniscocapsular defects, which allow the passage of the popliteal tendon through the popliteal hiatus.

Cruciate Ligaments

The anterior and posterior cruciate ligaments (ACL and PCL, respectively) are intracapsular and extrasynovial structures. The ACL is attached to the posteromedial aspect of the lateral femoral condyle. The distal portion of the ACL extends inferior and medial, attaching to the fossa anterior and lateral to the anterior tibial spine. The ACL is divided into two functional fiber bundles— the anterior medial bundle and the posterolateral bundle (31). The PCL originates in the lateral aspect of the

medial femoral condyle, crosses the ACL, and attaches to the posterior intercondylar fossa of the tibia.

Because the ACL has a relatively oblique course it is usually visualized segmentally, rather than being seen in its entirety on a single image. When ACL disruption is questioned, acquisition of sagittal oblique images oriented along the expected course of the ACL can be helpful. The PCL is usually visualized on a single sagittal image, as it is thicker, cord-like, and more closely aligned relative to the sagittal imaging plane.

Anatomic Variations

The cruciate ligaments may be congenitally absent. Accessory slips of the cruciate ligaments can be present (32). The PCL often has a relatively low insertion in children.

Signal Variations

The normal PCL displays uniformly low signal intensity on all pulse sequences and it has a well-defined morphology. However, the ACL typically is less well defined and exhibits mildly increased signal intensity on T1- and T2-weighted images (33). This is because the ACL is comprised of small fascicles of collagenous fibers; these fascicles are intertwined with fibrofatty tissue (34). Decreased ACL signal intensity with applied tension and reciprocal increased signal intensity with release of tension has been demonstrated (35). Hence, increased signal intensity of the ACL is more often seen on routine MR examination performed with the knee in relative flexion. The relative hyperintensity of the normal ACL should not be mistaken for edema and/or hemorrhage. Localized foci of relative increased signal intensity can occur in both cruciate ligaments secondary to eosinophilic degeneration. These findings are more prevalent in the elderly population and should not be mistaken for injury (36).

Joint Fluid

Intra-articular fluid commonly tracks along the synovial reflection of the ACL in patients with joint effusion. This must be differentiated from high signal intensity related to ACL injury (Fig. 30.18).

Imaging Planes

Because of the ACL's oblique course, it is usually not seen in its entirety on a single sagittal image. ACL depiction is improved when the knee is positioned in approximately 15 degrees of external rotation (2,37). If this cannot be achieved due to patient discomfort, sagittal oblique images can be acquired parallel to the expected course of the ACL. Correlation of findings observed on sagittal images to those on coronal images is also very helpful in reducing false-positive diagnosis for ACL injury.

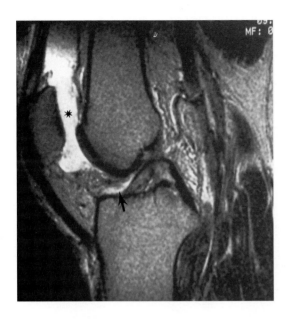

FIG. 30.18. Fluid around the anterior cruciate ligament (ACL). A sagittal T2-weighted image of the knee demonstrates synovial fluid tracking anterior to the ACL *(arrow)*. This is a common finding in patients with joint effusion **(*)** and should not be misinterpreted for ACL injury. Also noted is pretibial soft tissue edema in this patient with a history of trauma.

Partial Volume Effects

Partial volume averaging commonly occurs on sagittal images since the cruciate ligaments course obliquely through the intercondylar notch. The resultant apparent increased signal intensity due to averaging with adjacent fibrofatty tissue and synovial fluid can simulate a tear. The ACL can also undergo partial volume averaging with the lateral femoral condyle, with similar results (30).

Pulsation Artifacts

Pulsation of the popliteal artery results in phase errors (i.e., ghosting artifacts) that often project across the cruciate ligaments. The resultant increased signal intensity can simulate a cruciate ligament tear (Fig. 30.19). As with other motion artifacts, pulsation artifacts are displayed along the phase-encoding direction of the image. By default, the phase-encoding direction is usually prescribed along the shortest dimension of the relevant anatomy. This would be the anteroposterior direction for images acquired in the axial and sagittal planes. Because vascular pulsation artifact frequently interferes with evaluation of the cruciate ligaments and menisci, many centers employ gradient reorientation. With this approach, sagittal and axial images are acquired with phase encoding assigned along the superoinferior and mediolateral directions, respectively. Therefore, vascular pulsation artifacts are directed away from critical structures such as the cruciate ligaments or patellar articular cartilage, improving visualization of these structures. Pulsation artifact can also be reduced by applying spatially defined radiofrequency presaturation pulses above and below the imaging sections to reduce the signal intensity of inflowing blood.

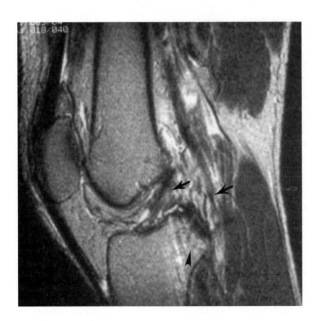

FIG. 30.19. Pulsation artifact. Popliteal artery pulsation artifacts *(arrows)* obscure the cruciate ligaments and can simulate injury. There is also a related apparent high signal intensity focus within the posterior tibia *(arrowhead)* that can be mistaken for marrow abnormality.

Postoperative Changes

Surgical reconstruction of the ACL can be extra-articular, intra-articular, or a combination of the two. Autogenous, allograft, xenograft, and synthetic tissues may be used to reconstruct the ACL (Fig. 30.20). Of these, the bone–patellar tendon–bone graft using the central one-third of the patellar tendon is the most common procedure for ACL reconstruction (38). Foci of relatively increased signal intensity with ill-defined margins and a

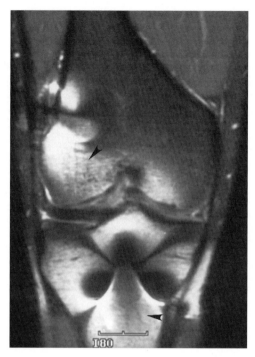

FIG. 30.21. Susceptibility artifact. A coronal proton density–weighted fat-saturated image demonstrates areas of artifactual increased and decreased signal intensity in the distal femur and proximal tibia in this patient with a reconstructed ACL. The hyperintense signal of the bone marrow *(arrowheads)* should not be mistaken for pathology.

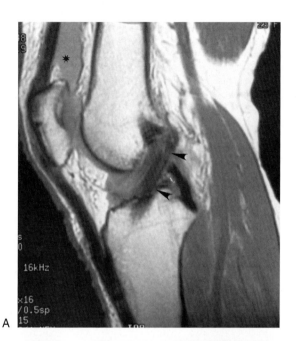

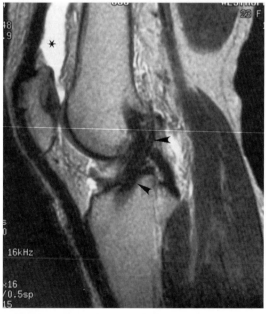

FIG. 30.20. Reconstructed ACL. Sagittal proton density **(A)** and T2-weighted **(B)** images of the knee demonstrate an intact reconstructed ACL *(arrowheads)*. The signal intensity and appearance of a reconstructed ACL can be variable. Also noted is a small joint effusion (*).

wavy contour are common observations with intact grafts. In some patients, intact grafts may not be discernible on MRI. In the series by Moeser et al. (38), the graft was not discernible in 11 of 27 patients. Metallic fixation devices placed during cruciate ligament reconstruction can result in susceptibility artifacts, which can obscure or simulate cruciate ligament or bone marrow abnormalities (Fig. 30.21).

Collateral Ligaments

The medial collateral ligament (MCL), also referred to as the tibial collateral ligament, has three layers (3). Layer 1 consists of deep fascia surrounding the sartorius and gastrocnemius muscles. The superficial MCL constitutes layer 2, with layer 3 representing the medial capsular ligament or true joint capsule. The MCL is typically 8 to 10 cm long, and extends from the medial epicondylar region superiorly to its attachment 4 to 5 cm inferior to the tibial plateau and posterior to the pes anserinus insertion.

The lateral aspect of the knee is divided into three structural layers (39). Layer 1 constitutes the iliotibial tract anteriorly, with the biceps femoris forming the posterior expansion. The quadriceps retinaculum anteriorly and patellofemoral ligaments posteriorly constitute layer 2. Layer 3, the deepest layer, consists of the lateral joint capsule and its attachments. The lateral collateral ligament (LCL) or fibular collateral ligament is 5 to 7 cm long, extracapsular, and free from meniscal attachment. The LCL extends from the lateral femoral epicondyle proximally to its conjoined distal insertion with the biceps femoris tendon on the fibular head. The LCL is located between the superficial and deep layers of layer 3.

Diagnostic Pitfalls

The collateral ligaments are a common site for injury during extreme valgus or varus stress. Injuries of the collateral ligaments are often associated with meniscal and ACL injuries. The MCL is injured with far greater frequency than is the LCL. The degree of injury to the collateral ligaments is often described on a graded scale. Grade I injury refers to edema surrounding the ligament. In grade II injury, focal increased signal intensity is observed within the substance of the ligament, and in patients with grade III injury the ligament is completely disrupted.

Collateral ligament injury is often best visualized on proton density– or T2-weighted images acquired in the coronal or axial planes. The use of fat suppression can be helpful in accentuating subtle signal alterations. LCL disruption is often well depicted on far lateral sagittal images.

Visualization of fluid immediately deep to the collateral ligaments should not be misinterpreted as evidence of injury, since such fluid may represent joint effusion. Collateral ligament injury also results in abnormal signal intensity along the nonarticular surface of the ligament. Fibrofatty tissue interposed between the collateral liga-

ment and joint capsule represents another potential pitfall. The use of fat-suppressed images allows for distinction of this normal variation from actual injury (Fig. 30.22). Bursal fluid collections along the collateral ligaments, such as those related to bursitis, can also simulate collateral ligament injury (34). The Pelligrini-Stieda condition refers to ossification of the proximal attachment of the medial collateral ligament; this can simulate ligamentous injury and hemorrhage. This pitfall is usually encountered on T1-weighted images. Close correlation of the MCL on proton density– and T2-weighted fat suppressed images is useful in excluding acute injury.

Extensor Mechanism

The quadriceps and patellar tendons constitute the extensor mechanism of the knee. The quadriceps muscle and tendon can be well visualized on axial and sagittal images. The patellar tendon is seen en face in the coronal plane, in profile in the sagittal plane, and in cross section in the axial plane. The normal patellar tendon increases in diameter as it progresses distally, with a normal diameter of under 7 mm (40).

Diagnostic Pitfalls

As with other ligaments and tendons, diagnosis of injury to the quadriceps and patellar tendons is diagnosed

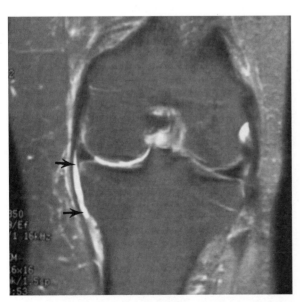

FIG. 30.22. Tibial collateral ligament bursa. A coronal fast spin echo (FSE) fat-saturated proton density–weighted image demonstrates fluid due to tibial collateral ligament bursitis *(arrows)*. This appearance should be differentiated from primary pathology of the medial collateral ligament.

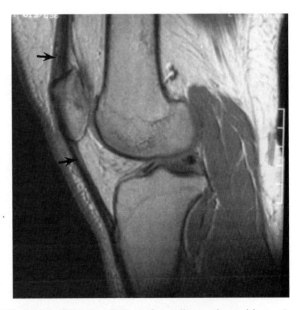

FIG. 30.23. Signal variation of patellar and quadriceps tendons. Sagittal proton density–weighted image demonstrates linear foci of increased signal intensity extending through the quadriceps and patellar tendons *(arrows)*. These represent fibrofatty tissue interposed between the laminae of the tendon complex and should not be mistaken for inflammatory and/or post-traumatic processes.

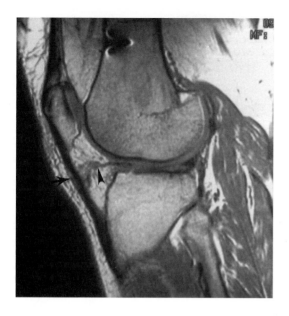

FIG. 30.24. Patellar tendon graft. A sagittal proton density–weighted image in a patient with ACL reconstruction demonstrates a linear area of increased signal intensity in the midportion of the patellar tendon *(arrows)*. This is a typical postoperative appearance in patients where the patellar tendon has been used for an ACL graft. Note the linear low signal intensity areas in the infrapatellar fat pad related to the arthroscopic tract. Also note a focal area of dephasing from metallic susceptibility in the distal femur.

on the basis of abnormal morphology and/or signal intensity. Morphologic changes may include thickening, irregularity, or disruption of tendinous fibers. Inflammatory changes can also produce focal thickening and increased signal intensity that simulates partial-thickness tears.

The normal gradual distal widening of the patellar tendon should not be mistaken as evidence of tendinitis or partial-thickness tear. Foci of increased signal intensity are frequently seen within the distal quadriceps tendon and at the proximal and distal insertions of the patellar tendon in normal individuals (41). These small foci of relative increased signal intensity are due to fibrofatty tissue that is interposed between tendinous laminae and should not be

interpreted as evidence of pathology (Fig. 30.23). A thin zone of relative increased signal intensity is also frequently present along the posterior aspect of the proximal patellar tendon. The consistent location of these signal changes and their lack of significant hyperintensity on T2-weighted images help to distinguish them from pathology.

Foci of ossification can occur within the patellar tendon as a normal variation. Fat-suppressed T2-weighted images help in distinguishing these foci of ossification from hemorrhage secondary to acute injury.

Surgical repair can result in focal thickening and altered signal intensity of the extensor tendons (Figs. 30.24 and 30.25). Following arthroscopy, foci of low sig-

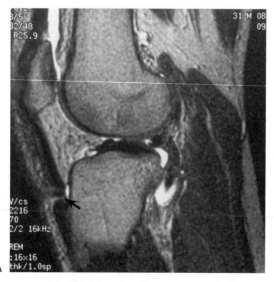
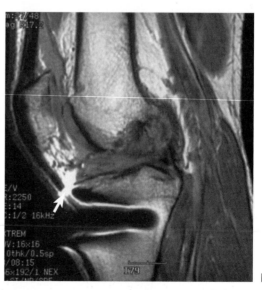

FIG. 30.25. Susceptibility artifact. **A:** A T2-weighted sagittal image through the patellar tendon demonstrates apparent disruption of this structure *(arrow)*, secondary to susceptibility artifact from a micrometallic fragment. **B:** Sagittal proton density–weighted image in another patient with ACL reconstruction also demonstrates apparent disruption of the patella tendon *(arrow)*.

nal intensity from micrometallic fragments and surgical staples are commonly observed.

Articular Cartilage

The articular surface of the knee joint is lined with hyaline cartilage. The junction between hyaline cartilage and subjacent marrow fat represents a fat–water interface where chemical shift misregistration artifact can arise. Such artifact leads to apparent displacement of signal intensity, causing potential alterations in the apparent thickness of hyaline cartilage.

Evaluation of the thickness of hyaline cartilage can be difficult when cartilage displays signal intensity similar to that of adjacent joint fluid. This is most likely to occur on conventional proton density– and T2-weighted images. The use of fat suppression helps to better delineate the cartilage thickness, since normal cartilage displays slightly less signal intensity than joint fluid. Three-dimensional spoiled gradient echo sequences with fat saturation also provide favorable depiction of hyaline cartilage (41). The depiction of early cartilage degeneration is frequently best shown on gradient echo and T2-weighted fat-saturated images (41).

Anatomic Variations

The hyaline cartilage can demonstrate a trilaminar appearance (8). This feature is most prominent in individuals with an immature skeleton and becomes less conspicuous with increasing age. Heterogeneous signal intensity is frequently observed within the hyaline cartilage overlying the medial tibial plateau. These changes are most conspicuous on fat-saturated images and can be observed in the absence of any documented cartilage abnormalities.

Diagnostic Pitfalls

Artifactual causes of heterogeneous signal intensity of hyaline cartilage include patient motion, vascular pulsation, or susceptibility artifacts due to the presence of air or metallic substances. When they involve the patellar cartilage, these artifacts can simulate chondromalacia. Magic angle phenomenon can also affect the hyaline cartilage when collagen bundles are oriented at approximately 55 degrees relative to the long axis of the magnet. The resultant increased cartilage signal intensity can simulate pathology (42). Increased thickness of the hyaline cartilage has been observed following meniscectomy, ACL transection, and in the very early stages of chondromalacia patellae. In the latter situation, these observations represent cartilage swelling and blistering (43).

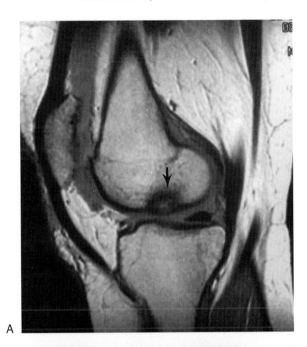

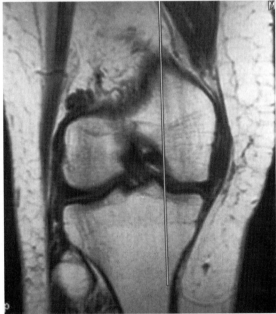

FIG. 30.26. Partial volume averaging. **A:** A sagittal proton density–weighted image demonstrates an apparent osteochondral lesion involving the medial femoral condyle *(arrow).* This finding is secondary to partial volume averaging of marrow with adjacent bone cortex notch and fibrofatty tissue. **B:** A coronal T1-weighted image in which the position of **A,** marked by a *vertical line,* confirms that this is secondary to partial volume averaging. (From ref. 16, with permission.)

Joint Space

Synovial Fluid

The knee joint normally contains approximately 1 cc of synovial fluid, which is detectable on MRI (44). Small amounts of fluid initially collect between the femoral

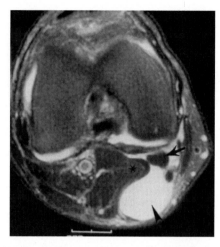

FIG. 30.27. Popliteal cyst. The posterior joint extension of the gastrocnemius-semimembranosus bursa arises between the medial head of the gastrocnemius muscle *(*)* and the more medial semimembranosus tendon *(arrow)*. This uncomplicated Baker's cyst demonstrates uniform bright signal on this transaxial T2-weighted image *(arrowhead)*.

condyles and the infrapatellar fat pad. With accumulation of slightly larger volumes, the fluid tends to distribute into the suprapatellar bursa and posteromedial to the PCL. Still larger volumes locate within the meniscosynovial recesses and popliteal tendon sheath. The "saddlebag" appearance of joint fluid along the lateral aspects of the joint space on coronal images indicates the presence of a significant joint effusion (16). Posterior extension of the joint space occurs between the medial head of the gastrocnemius muscle and the more medial semimembranosus tendon (Figs. 30.27 and 30.28). When such a posterior extension is prominent and symptomatic, it is often referred to as a Baker's cyst.

Delayed images following intravenous administration of gadolinium chelate contrast material can demonstrate enhancement of synovial fluid. This results in a mild arthrographic effect that can potentially assist in the detection of meniscal tears that are equivocal on standard examinations (45).

Synovial Tissue

The normal synovium is not well depicted on standard T1- and T2-weighted images because of the lack of contrast between the synovium and surrounding synovial fluid. Synovial hyperplasia can appear slightly higher in signal intensity than joint fluid on T1-weighted images and slightly lower in signal intensity than joint fluid on T2-weighted images. Images acquired following intravenous administration of gadolinium chelate contrast material best demonstrate synovitis, synovial hyperplasia, and other synovial pathology (46). On images acquired immediately after intravenous contrast material injection, rim-like enhancement can be observed along the periphery of the joint space. This reflects early diffusion of contrast material through the synovium and should not be misinterpreted as evidence of synovial inflammation (47).

Hemarthrosis

Hemorrhage into the joint space commonly occurs following direct trauma and in patients with bleeding diatheses. Hemarthrosis often appears as a fluid–fluid level on MRI, with the dependent portion being of relatively reduced signal intensity on T2-weighted images. Simple hemarthrosis must be differentiated from lipohemarthrosis, since the latter entity indicates an underlying fracture (48). This distinction may not always be straightforward,

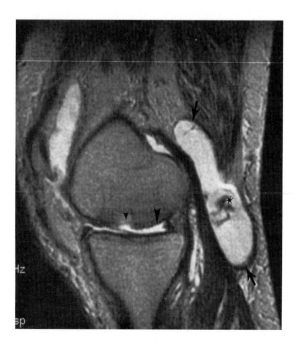

FIG. 30.28. Complicated popliteal cyst. Sagittal T2-weighted image demonstrates a large popliteal cyst *(arrows)* containing several low signal intensity areas *(*)*, which represent foci of hemorrhage. Osteochondral bodies can have a similar appearance. Also note the meniscectomy defect *(arrowhead)* and thinning of articular cartilage *(small arrowhead)* secondary to osteoarthritis.

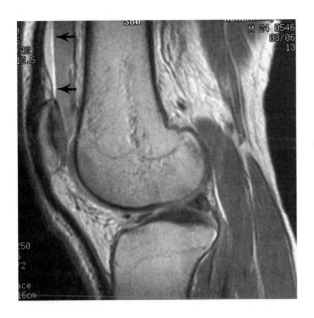

FIG. 30.29. Chemical shift misregistration artifact. A sagittal proton density–weighted image demonstrates lipohemarthrosis secondary to femoral condylar fracture. The differential signal intensity within the suprapatellar bursa and the chemical shift misregistration artifact (arrows) confirms the presence of intra-articular fat.

since both blood breakdown products and fat may produce similar high signal intensity on T1-weighted images. The presence of fat can be verified by suppression of high signal material on fat saturation images or by appreciating the sometimes subtle chemical shift misregistration artifact that typically occurs at fat–fluid interfaces (Fig. 30.29).

Intra-Articular Masses and Loose Bodies

Intra-articular blood clots can have low signal intensity on both T1- and T2-weighted images. Consequently, such clots can be mistaken for intra-articular loose bodies or other masses such as villonodular synovitis. The presence of relative increased signal intensity on T1-weighted images and the blooming effect from hemorrhage on gradient echo images helps in recognition of blood clots, although villonodular synovitis also frequently contains iron products. Other entities that can simulate osteochondral bodies or synovial hyperplasia include fat globules in patients with lipohemarthrosis, intra-articular air from joint aspiration or vacuum phenomenon, and metallic fragments.

Meniscal fragments, torn ACL fragments, and hypertrophied meniscofemoral ligaments are additional potential causes of simulation of intra-articular loose bodies (49). Actual intra-articular osteochondral fragments are common but are often difficult to diagnose on MRI. The search for intra-articular loose bodies is assisted by the presence of a joint effusion or intra-articular contrast material.

Osseous Structures and Soft Tissues

The evaluation of adjacent osseous structures for marrow edema, fractures, and other bone marrow lesions is

critical in the evaluation of patients presenting with knee pain.

Physis

The physeal cartilage remains unfused in patients with immature skeleton. Artifactual increased signal intensity of the physis can be observed due to chemical shift misregistration artifact at the interface between the cartilaginous physis and adjacent marrow fat. This should not be mistaken for abnormal increased signal and pathology (16) (Figs. 30.30–30.32).

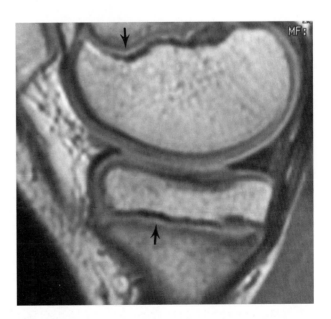

FIG. 30.30. Normal physis. Sagittal proton-density weighted image in a skeletally immature patient demonstrates the appearance of the normal physis. Note the mild hyperintense signal along the metaphyseal aspect of the proximal tibia, secondary to chemical shift misregistration artifact (arrows).

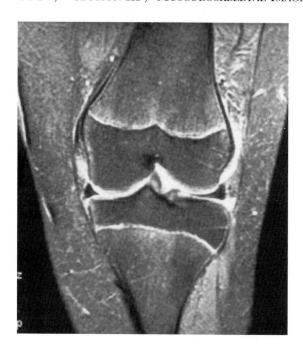

FIG. 30.31. Physeal line. Coronal fat-saturated proton density–weighted image demonstrates relative hyperintensity of marrow within the distal femur and the proximal tibia, secondary to residual hematopoietic marrow in a 14-year-old girl. Also seen is linear hyperintensity of the physeal plate.

Hematopoietic Marrow

Hematopoietic marrow is routinely observed within the distal femoral and proximal tibial metaphysis (50). The proportion of hematopoietic marrow generally decreases with age, as it is converted to fatty marrow. Reconversion of fatty marrow to hematopoietic marrow can occur in adults with anemia or marrow infiltration and in those who are tobacco smokers (51). Residual and/or reconverted hematopoietic marrow is more prevalent in females of reproductive age, probably representing a degree of physiologic anemia. Hematopoietic marrow is normally confined to the metaphyseal region, and it displays low signal intensity on both T1- and T2-weighted images relative to surrounding fatty marrow. However, the signal intensity of hematopoietic marrow may appear increased relative to fatty marrow on fat-saturated and short TI inversion recovery sequences.

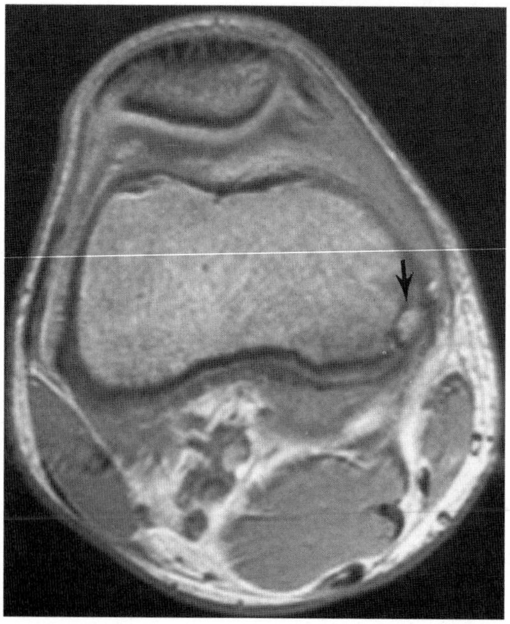

Other Entities

Reinforcement of weight-bearing trabeculae can result in a focus of decreased marrow signal intensity in the subchondral region of the medial tibia (16). Penetrating vessels commonly produce punctate foci of altered signal intensity in the distal femur and proximal tibia. Bone islands are a common entity, in which condensations of cortical bone produce foci of decreased marrow signal intensity on all pulse sequences (Fig. 30.33).

Vascular Pulsation Artifact

Ghosting artifacts attributable to pulsation of the popliteal artery can overlie the osseous structures. These artifacts can be of variable signal intensity and can simulate marrow pathology. They can be recognized as such by noting their alignment with the popliteal artery along the phase-encoding direction of the image and by observing that they extend beyond the anatomy. In such situations, it is also helpful to note that the apparent lesion maintains a size and shape concordant with that of the vessel from which it originates.

FIG. 30.32. Unfused tibial physis. A transaxial gradient echo image demonstrates an apparent cortical defect *(arrow)* along the medial aspect of the proximal tibia. This represents an unfused tibial physis and should not be mistaken for fracture.

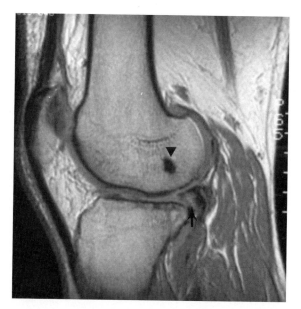

FIG. 30.33. Osteochondral body. A sagittal proton density–weighted image demonstrates the presence of an osteochondral body *(arrow)* within a meniscectomy defect, simulating meniscus with globular degenerative changes. Note the bone island in the femoral condyle *(arrowhead)*.

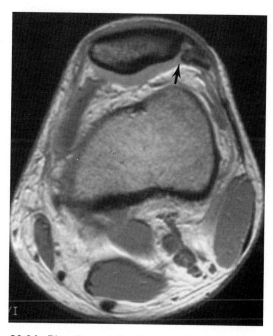

FIG. 30.34. Bipartite patella. Transaxial gradient echo T1-weighted image demonstrates a bipartite patella *(arrow)*, which should not be mistaken for patellar fracture.

Partial Volume Averaging

Partial volume averaging of marrow fat with adjacent cortical bone or other tissues frequently results in an area of apparent decreased marrow signal intensity in the vicinity of the intercondylar notch. These findings can closely simulate an osteochondral defect of the distal femur (Fig. 30.26). Similarly, volume averaging of marrow fat with the cartilaginous physis in a young patient can simulate an aggressive marrow lesion on transaxial images. In these situations, careful comparison of images acquired in multiple planes will usually permit recognition of the artifact.

Susceptibility Artifacts

Susceptibility artifacts from prostheses, fixation devices, or other sources of metal cause dephasing effects and resultant areas of low signal intensity that can interfere with evaluation of osseous structures. Such artifact is accentuated on fat-saturated images and frequently precludes complete evaluation of the marrow space.

Anatomic Variations

Congenital absence of the patella is among the various anatomic variations that may involve the osseous structures around the knee. More frequently, the patella may have a bipartite configuration, which can simulate a fracture (Fig. 30.34). The dorsal defect of the patella is usu-

ally observed along the superolateral aspect of the articular surface of the patella (3). This benign lesion usually displays sclerotic margins and intact articular cartilage, with the central defect having increased signal intensity on T2-weighted images.

Variations in the length of fibula are also common, and can alter the configuration of the tibiofibular joint. The patellocondylar notch refers to a normal shallow concavity along the anterior aspect of the lateral femoral condyle. Its major significance is that it must be differentiated from an osteochondral impaction fracture, which typically has a greater degree of depression.

The fabella is an accessory sesamoid bone within the lateral head of the gastrocnemius muscle. It appears as a focus of relative hyperintensity on T1-weighted images and corresponding decreased signal intensity on T2-weighted images, due to its contained fatty marrow. The fabella should not be mistaken for a soft tissue mass or other lesion.

Postoperative Soft Tissue Changes

In patients who have undergone previous arthroscopy, a linear area of decreased signal intensity is observed within the infrapatellar fat pad, corresponding to the arthroscope tract (Fig. 30.35). This finding should not be mistaken for inflammatory changes, such as those due to synovitis in a similar location. A corroborating finding indicating that previous arthroscopy has been performed is the presence of micrometallic fragments within the soft tissues.

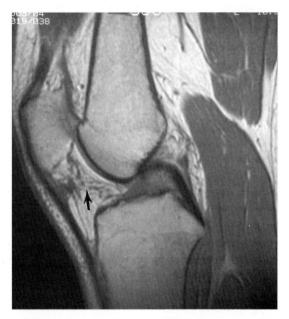

FIG. 30.35. Arthroscopic tract. Sagittal proton density–weighted image demonstrates a linear focus of low signal intensity in the infrapatellar fat pad *(arrow)*, representing scar along an arthroscopic tract.

REFERENCES

1. Crues JV, Mink JH, Levy TL, et al. Meniscal tears of the knee: accuracy of MR imaging. *Radiology* 1987;164:445.
2. Mink JH, Levy T, Crues JV. Tears of the anterior cruciate ligament and menisci of the knee: MR imaging evaluation. *Radiology* 1998;167:769.
3. Stoller DW. *Magnetic resonance imaging in orthopedics and sports medicine,* 2nd ed. New York: Lippincott-Raven 1997:203.
4. Escobedo EM, Hunter JC, Zink-Brody G, Wilson AJ, Harrison SD, Fisher DJ. Usefulness of turbo spin-echo MR imaging in the evaluation of meniscal tears: comparison with a conventional spin-echo sequence. *AJR* 1996;167:1223.
5. Arnoczky SP, Warren RF. The microvasculature of the human meniscus. *Am J Sports Med* 1982;10:90.
6. Silverman JM, Mink JH, Deutsch AL. Discoid menisci of the knee: MR imaging appearance. *Radiology* 1989;173:351.
7. Aochort PM, Patel D. Congenital discoid meniscus associations with bone changes in the tibia. *J Bone Joint Surg* 1974;56:171.
8. Semac MO Jr, Deutsch D, Bernstein BH, et al. MR imaging in juvenile rheumatoid arthritis. *AJR* 1988;150:873.
9. Heron CW, Calvert PT. Three dimensional gradient echo MR imaging of the knee: comparison with arthroscopy in 100 cases. *Radiology* 1992;183:839.
10. Quinn SF, Brown TR, Szumowski J. Menisci of the knee: radial MR imaging correlated with arthroscopy in 259 patients. *Radiology* 1992;185:577.
11. Buckwalter KA, Braunstein EM, Janizek DB, et al. MR imaging of meniscal tears: narrow versus conventional window width photography. *Radiology* 1990;187:827.
12. Mirowitz SA. Motion artifact as a pitfall in the diagnosis of meniscal tear on gradient reoriented MRI of the knee. *J Comput Assist Tomogr* 1994;18:279.
13. Levy LM, Di Chiro G, Brooks RA, et al. Spinal cord artifacts from truncation errors during MR imaging. *Radiology* 1998;166:479.
14. Turner DA, Rapoport MI, Erwin WD, et al. Truncation artifact: a potential pitfall in MR imaging of the menisci of the knee. *Radiology* 1991;179:629.
15. Elster AD. *Questions and answers in magnetic resonance imaging,* 1st ed. St. Louis: Mosby-Year Book, 1994:134.
16. Mirowitz SA. *Pitfalls, variants and artifacts in body MR imaging,* 1st ed. St. Louis: Mosby-Year Book, 1996:279.
17. Shogry MEC, Pope TL Jr. Vacuum phenomenon simulating meniscal or cartilaginous injury of the knee at MR imaging. *Radiology* 1991;180:513.
18. Quinn SF, Brown TF. Meniscal tears diagnosed with MR imaging versus arthroscopy: How reliable a standard is arthroscopy? *Radiology* 1991;181:843.
19. Herman LJ, Beltran J. Pitfalls in MR imaging of the knee. *Radiology* 1988;167:775.
20. Araki Y, Ootani F, Tsukkaguchi I, et al. MR diagnosis of meniscal tears of the knee: value of axial three dimensional Fourier transformation GRASS images. *AJR* 1992;158:587.
21. Peterfy CG, Janzen DL, Triman PF, VanDijke CF. Magic angle phenomenon. A cause for increased signal in the normal lateral meniscus on short TE MR images of the knee. *AJR* 1994;163:149.
22. Holder J, Haghigi P, Pathria MN, et al. Meniscal changes in the elderly: correlation of MR imaging and histological findings. *Radiology* 1992; 184:221.
23. Reinig JW, McDevitt ER, Ove PN. Progression of meniscal degenerative changes in college football players: evaluation with MR imaging. *Radiology* 1991;181:255.
24. Herman LJ, Beltran J. Pitfalls in MR imaging of the knee. *Radiology* 1988;167:775.
25. Crues JV, Stoller DW. The menisci. In: Mink JH, Reicher MA, Crues JV, Deutsch AL, eds. *MRI of the knee.* New York: Raven Press 1993:91.
26. Stoller DW, Martin C, Crues IV, Kaplan L, Mink JA. Meniscal tears: pathological correlation with MR imaging. *Radiology* 1987;731–735.
27. Kornick J, Trefelner E, McCarthy S, Lange R, Lynch K, Jokl P. Meniscal abnormalities in the asymptotic population at MR imaging. *Radiology* 1990;177;463–465.
28. Dillon EH, Pope CF, Jokl P, et al. The clinical significance of stage 2 meniscal abnormalities on magnetic resonance knee images. *Magn Reson Imaging* 1990;8:411.
29. Wright DH, DeSnet AA, Norris M. Bucket handle tears of the medial and lateral menisci of the knee: value of MR imaging in detecting displaced fragments. *AJR* 1995;165:621.
30. Vahey TN, Bennett HT, Arrington LE, et al. MR imaging of the knee: pseudo-tear of the lateral meniscus caused by the meniscofemoral ligament. *AJR* 1990;154:1237.
31. Dodds JA, Arnoczky SP. Anatomy of the anterior cruciate ligament: a blue print for repair and reconstruction. *Arthroscopy* 1994;10:132.
32. Bergman RA, Thompson SA, Afifi AK, et al. *Compendium of human anatomic variation: text, atlas and world literature.* Baltimore: Urban and Schwarzenberg, 1998.
33. Lee JK, Yao L, Phelps CT, et al. Anterior cruciate ligament tears: MR imaging compared with arthroscopy and clinical tests. *Radiology* 1988; 166:861.
34. Lee JK, Yao L. Tibial collateral ligament bursa: MR imaging. *Radiology* 1991;178:855.
35. Smith KL, Daniels LJ, Arnocky SP, Dodds JA. Effect of joint positioning and ligament tension on the MR signal intensity of the cruciate ligament of the knee. *J Magn Reson Imaging* 1994;4:819.
36. Hodler J, Haghighi P, Trudell D, et al. The cruciate ligaments of the knee: correlation between MR appearance and gross and histologic findings in cadaveric specimens. *AJR* 1992;159:357.
37. Mink JH, Deutsch AL. Occult cartilage and bone injuries of the knee: detection, classification, and assessment with MR imaging. *Radiology* 1989;170:823.
38. Moeser P, Bechtold RE, Clark T, et al. MR imaging of anterior cruciate ligament repair. *J Comput Assist Tomogr* 1989;13:105.
39. Seebacher J, Inglis A, Marshall J, et al. The structure of the posterolateral aspect of the knee. *J Bone Joint Surg* 1982;64:536.
40. Yu JS, Popp JE, Kaeding CC, et al. Correlation of MR imaging and pathologic findings in athletes undergoing surgery for chronic patellar tendinitis. *AJR* 1995;165:115.
41. Recht MP, Kramer J, Marcelis S, et al. Abnormalities of articular cartilage in the knee: analysis of available MR techniques. *Radiology* 1993; 187:473.
42. Rubenstein JD, Kim JK, Morava-Protzner I, et al. Effects of collagen orientation on MR characteristics of bovine articular cartilage. *Radiology* 1993;188:219.
43. Braunstein EM, Brandt KD, Albrecht M. MRI demonstration of hypertrophic articular cartilage repair in osteoarthritis. *Skeletal Radiol* 1990; 19:335.
44. Schweitzer ME, Falk A, Pathria M, et al. MR imaging of the knee: can changes in the intraarticular fat pads be used as a sign of synovial proliferation in the presence of an effusion? *AJR* 1993;160:823.

45. Drape JL, Thelen P, Gay-Depassier P, et al. Intraarticular diffusion of gadolinium-DOTA after intravenous injection in the knee: MR imaging evaluation. *Radiology* 1993;188:227.
46. Björkengren AG, Geborek P, Rydholm R, et al. MR imaging of the knee in acute rheumatoid arthritis: synovial uptake of gadolinium-DTPA. *AJR* 1990;155:329.
47. Winalsi CS, Aliabadi P, Wright RJ, et al. Enhancement of joint fluid with intravenously administered gadopentetate dimeglumine: technique, rationale and implications. *Radiology* 1993;187:179.
48. Kier R, McCarthy SM. Lipohemarthrosis of the knee: MR imaging. *J Comput Assist Tomogr* 1990;14:395.
49. Carpenter WA: Meniscofemoral ligament simulating tear of the lateral meniscus: MR features. *J Comput Assist Tomogr* 1990;14:1033.
50. Vogler JB III, Murphy WA. Bone marrow imaging. *Radiology* 1988;168:679.
51. Deutsch AL, Mink JH, Fox JM, et al. Peripheral meniscal tears: MR findings after conservative treatment or arthroscopic repair. *Radiology* 1990;176:485.

Variants and Pitfalls in Body Imaging,
edited by Ali Shirkhoda.
Lippincott Williams & Wilkins, Philadelphia, © 2000.

CHAPTER 31

The Foot and the Ankle: MRI

Zehava S. Rosenberg, Jose M. Mellado, and Jenny Bencardino

Distinction of normal anatomy on MRI from disease is one of the principal tenets in interpretation of MR imaging of the foot and ankle. Therefore, familiarity with normal anatomic variants and pitfalls in the foot and ankle is crucial for accurate diagnostic interpretation of MR images (1,2). In this chapter we describe the MR features of a number of tendinous, muscular, osseous, ligamentous, and other miscellaneous variants and pitfalls of the foot and ankle.

MAGNETIC RESONANCE IMAGING PROCOTOL

Routine MR imaging of the ankle and foot is obtained in three orthogonal planes: axial, coronal, and sagittal. For the ankle, the foot should be placed in neutral position or in slight plantar flexion in order to avoid the magic angle effect (which we discuss later) (Fig. 31.1). Transmit-receive extremity coils are used to enhance spatial resolution. The routine ankle MR protocol usually includes axial T1- (TR 600/TE 20) and T2-weighted (TR 2,000/TE 80) spin-echo images. We frequently utilize the fast spin-echo technique for T2-weighted images (TR 4,500/TE 90). Also performed are coronal T1-weighted and sagittal short-tau inversion recovery (STIR) images. Gradient-echo T2*-weighted images utilizing TR 700 to 900/TE 10 to 16 in the coronal or sagittal planes are useful for the assessment of articular cartilage when osteochondral lesions are suspected. In the evaluation of marrow abnormalities, fat suppression using STIR or frequency-selec-

Z. S. Rosenberg: Department of Radiology, New York University Medical School, and Orthopedic Institute, Hospital for Joint Diseases, New York, New York 10003.

J. M. Mellado: Rennonáncia Magnètica, Institut Diagnostic Per La Imaige, Hospital Joan XXIII, Tarragona, 43007 Spain.

J. Bencardino: Department of Radiology, Albert Einstein College of Medicine, Bronx, New York, and Long Island Jewish Medical Center, New Hyde Park, New York 11040.

tive techniques are indicated. Three-dimensional fourier transform (3DFT) data acquisition allows reconstruction of the ligaments in other planes. This technical capability may be of value for visualizing each ligament in its entirety. The slice thickness is 3 to 4 mm with an interslice gap of 1 mm. The acquisition matrix ranges from 256×192 to 512 with a field of view of 12 to 16 cm and one-signal excitation.

On MR imaging of the foot, the foot is also placed in neutral position. We obtain oblique axial images along the axis of the metatarsal shafts as well as oblique coronal images perpendicular to them. Sagittal images may be obtained in an oblique plane, depending on the metatarsals to be evaluated.

Tendons are best evaluated on axial images with the exception of Achilles tendon, where sagittal images are of great diagnostic value (Fig. 31.2). Ligaments are best evaluated on axial and coronal images using thin sections of 3 mm or less (Fig. 31.3).

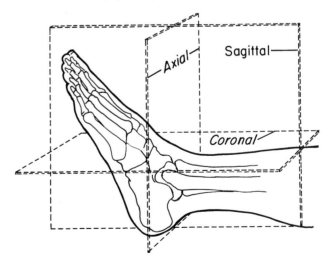

FIG. 31.1. Positioning and imaging planes for ankle MRI. The foot is placed in the neutral position or slight plantar flexion. Axial, coronal, and sagittal images are routinely obtained.

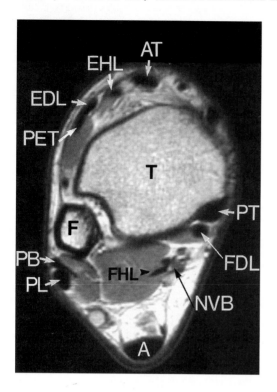

FIG. 31.2. Normal anatomy of ankle tendons. Axial T1-weighted (TR 600/TE 20) image through the tibial plafond demonstrates AT (anterior tibial tendon), EHL (extensor hallucis longus tendon), EDL (extensor digitorum longus tendon), PET (peroneus tertius tendon), PB (peroneus brevis tendon), PL (peroneus longus tendon), A (Achilles tendon), FHL (flexor hallucis longus tendon), FDL (flexor digitorum longus tendon), PT (posterior tibial tendon), and NVB (neurovascular bundle).

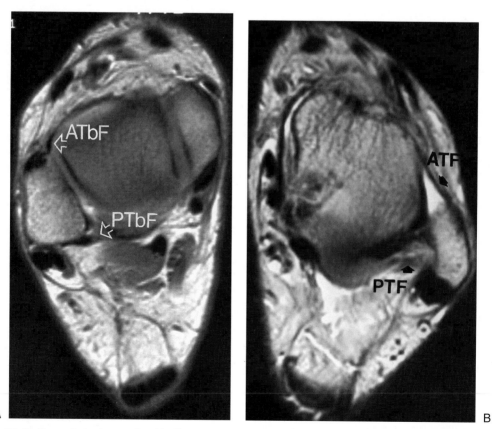

FIG. 31.3. Normal anatomy of ankle ligaments. **A:** Axial proton-density spin-echo (TR 2,900/TE 18) image at the level of ankle joint shows ATbF (anterior tibiofibular ligament) and PTbF (posterior tibiofibular ligament). **B:** Axial T2-weighted (TR 2,200/TE 90) image through the lateral malleolar tip demonstrates ATF (anterior talofibular ligament) and PTF (posterior talofibular ligament).

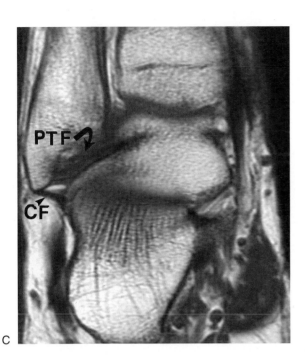

C

FIG. 31.3. *Continued.* **C:** Coronal T1-weighted (TR 650/TE 15) image depicts PTF (posterior talofibular ligament) and CF (calcaneofibular ligament).

SOURCES OF VARIATIONS

The Magic Angle Phenomenon

Tendons are typically low in signal on all pulse sequences. However, they can have an artifactual increased signal mimicking tendinosis or tear as a result of the magic angle effect (3). This manifests when the tendons form a 55-degree angle with the main magnetic vector, particularly when low T_{ES} of 10 to 20 milliseconds are utilized. The tendon's heterogeneity is usually focal, with absence of morphologic changes proximal and distal to it. Most of the ankle tendons are prone to the magic angle effect as they curve around the ankle (Fig. 31.4). The flexor hallucis longus tendon is also susceptible to this phenomena angle

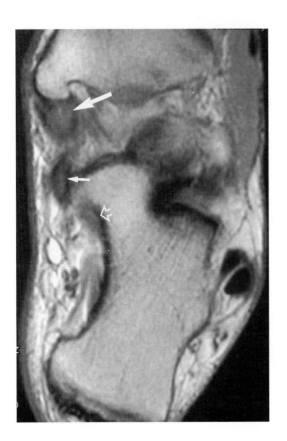

FIG. 31.4. Increased signal of normal tendons caused by the magic angle effect. Axial proton-density spin-echo (TR 2,000/TE 15) image obtained in dorsiflexion depicts marked increased signal of the posterior tibial *(long arrow),* flexor digitorum longus *(short arrow),* and flexor hallucis longus *(open arrow)* tendons in an asymptomatic individual.

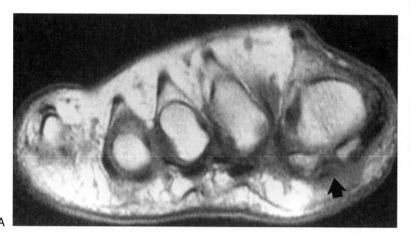

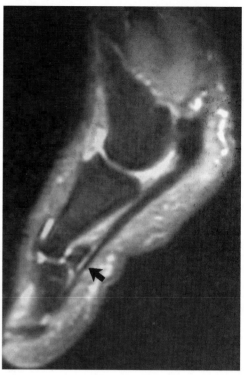

A

B

FIG. 31.5. Magic angle effect of flexor hallucis longus tendon in the foot. **A:** The tendon *(arrow)* is barely visualized in between the sesamoids and is suspected to be torn in this oblique coronal T1-weighted (TR 800/TE 18) image. **B:** On sagittal short-tau inversion recovery (STIR) image (TE 4,000/TE 11), the tendon *(arrow)* is normal.

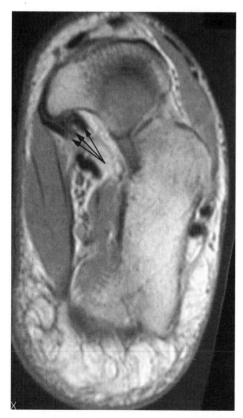

FIG. 31.6. Normal insertional bands *(arrows)* of posterior tibial tendon produce an apparent heterogeneity of the distal tendon at its insertion into the navicular as seen in this axial proton-density spin-echo (TR 2,950/TE 16) image.

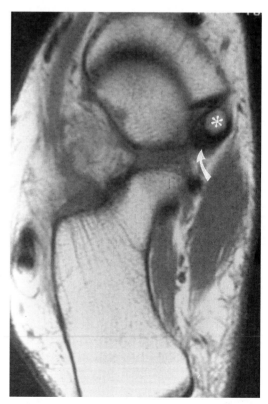

FIG. 31.7. The os tibiale externum *(asterisk)* is embedded within the posterior tibial tendon *(curved arrow)* producing an apparent heterogeneity on this axial T1-weighted (TR 800/TE 16) image.

effect between the first metatarsal sesamoids (Fig. 31.5). Imaging the ankle in plantar flexion, realigning the first toe in the magnet with the aid of pads, and increasing the TE will aid in decreasing the magic angle effect.

Normal Heterogeneity of the Distal Posterior Tibial Tendon

The posterior tibial tendon frequently displays heterogeneous signal at its insertion to the navicular tuberosity; this is often quite difficult to distinguish from a true tear of the tendon (1–3). The heterogeneity is related partly to the magic angle effect and also to fat interposed between the several insertion slips of the tendon (1–4) (Fig. 31.6). The os tibiale externum (type I accessory navicular bone) is a sesamoid bone embedded within the distal posterior tibial tendon. This ossicle can also contribute to the heterogeneity of the tendon at its insertion to the navicular tuberosity (Fig. 31.7).

Normal Heterogeneity of the Achilles Tendon

The Achilles tendon is not susceptible to the magic angle effect. Heterogeneity is, therefore, generally indica-

tive of pathology. Occasionally, however, increased signal of the Achilles tendon is related to variations in the confluence of the gastrocnemius and soleus tendons and should not be mistaken for disease. Rarely, far distal union and incomplete incorporation of the two tendons may produce heterogeneity as a result of persistence of fat planes between the tendon slips (Fig. 31.8) (5). An apparent increase in the AP diameter of the Achilles tendon may also be depicted. Careful scrutiny of the course of the soleus tendon relative to the gastrocnemius tendon on sequential axial images will avoid confusing these normal variations with disease.

Fluid Within Tendon Sheaths

A small amount of tendon sheath fluid is physiologic and is not consistent with disease. Conversely, a large amount of fluid within a tendon sheath is usually indicative of chronic tenosynovitis. Fluid within the tendon sheath of the flexor hallucis longus tendon, however, regardless of the amount, may be of no clinical significance (6). An asymptomatic extensive amount of fluid usually occurs in the presence of a large ankle joint effu-

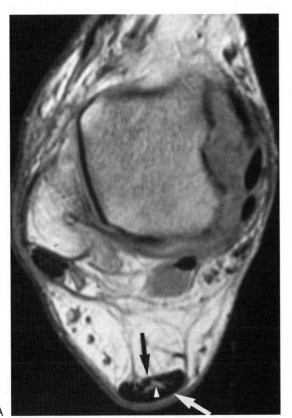
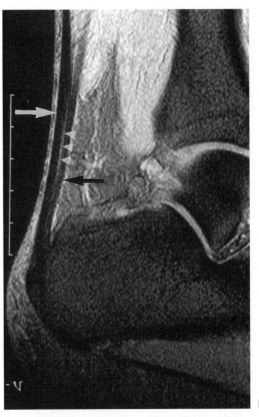

FIG. 31.8. Normal heterogeneity of the Achilles tendon caused by incomplete incorporation of the soleus into the gastrocnemius tendon as depicted on axial **(A)** proton-density spin-echo (TR 2,300/TE 15) image and sagittal **(B)** gradient echo image (TR 900/TE 10/flip angle 20). Fat planes *(arrowheads)* are maintained between the soleus *(black arrow)* and gastrocnemius *(white arrow)* tendons. This produces linear heterogenity and increased AP diameter of the conjoined Achilles tendon. (Reprinted with permission from reference 5.)

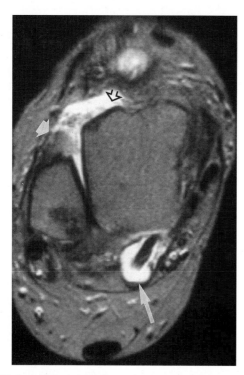

FIG. 31.9. Incidental finding of extensive fluid within the flexor hallucis longus tendon sheath *(long arrow),* in the presence of large joint effusion *(open arrow)* and a torn anterior tibiofibular ligament *(short arrow),* is depicted on an axial T2-weighted (TR 2,300/TE 90) image.

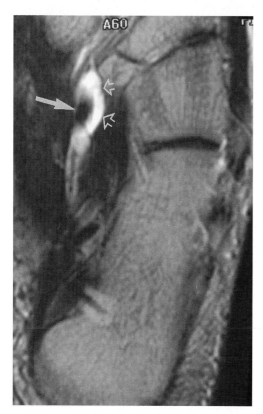

FIG. 31.10. Incidental finding of fluid *(open arrows)* at the intersection of the flexor hallucis longus and flexor digitorum longus tendons at Henry's knot *(arrow)* is noted on this axial T2-weighted (TR 2,300/TE 90) image.

sion and is produced by the occasional communication between the ankle joint and the flexor hallucis longus tendon (Fig. 31.9).

A large amount of tendon sheath fluid is also frequently seen in asymptomatic individuals at the intersection of the flexor digitorum longus and flexor hallucis longus tendons (Henry's knot) (Fig. 31.10).

PITFALLS

Pseudosubluxation of the Peroneus Brevis Tendon

The peroneal tendons are typically located within the retromalleolar groove posterior to the distal fibula. Occasionally, the peroneus brevis tendon is found medial to the tip of the fibula, simulating a medial subluxation of the tendon (Fig. 31.11). This normal finding reflects the slightly oblique course the tendon traverses from the fibula to the calcaneus. Supination of the foot during imaging may accentuate this finding. Additionally, at the groove, the peroneus brevis tendon is sometimes normally medial rather than anterior to the peroneus longus tendon. In those cases the medial pseudosubluxation may be more pronounced.

Accessory Muscles of the Posterior Ankle

Five accessory muscles have been reported in the posterior ankle: the accessory soleus, the accessory flexor digitorum longus, the tibiocalcaneus internus, the peroneocalcaneus internus, and the peroneus quartus muscles

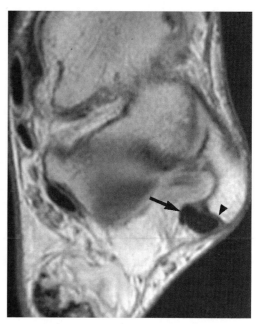

FIG. 31.11. Medial pseudosubluxation of the peroneus brevis tendon *(arrow)* relative to retromalleolar groove *(arrowhead)* is noted on this axial proton-density spin-echo (TR 2,000/TE 15) image.

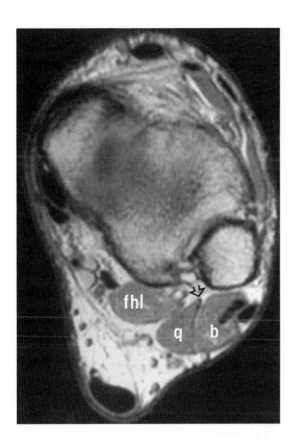

FIG. 31.12. Peroneus quartus muscle. An axial proton-density spin-echo (TR 2,000/TE 13) image depicts the peroneus quartus muscle as an additional mass (q) with a thin tendon *(open arrow)* between the muscles of the peroneus brevis (b) and the flexor hallucis longus (fhl).

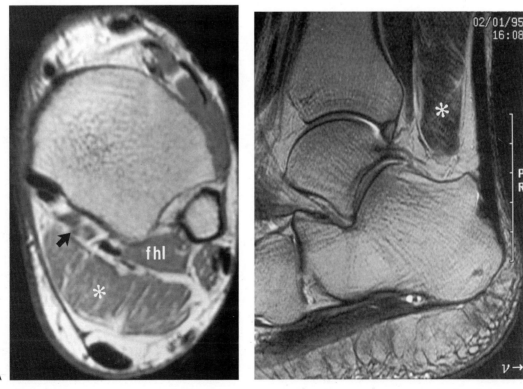

FIG. 31.13. Accessory soleus. **A:** The muscle *(asterisk)* displaces the neurovascular bundle *(arrow)* and the flexor hallucis longus muscle (fhl) anteriorly on this axial proton-density spin-echo (TR 2,000/TE 16) image. **B:** On a sagittal fast spin-echo (FSE) T2-weighted (TR 5,500/TE 96) image, the muscle *(asterisk)* descends within the pre-Achilles fat toward the calcaneus.

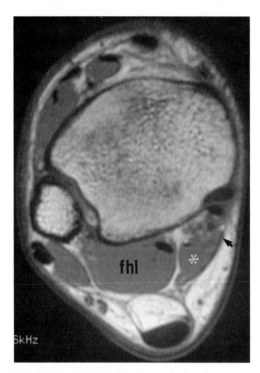

FIG. 31.14. Accessory flexor digitorum longus muscle. The muscle *(asterisk)* is located within the tarsal tunnel adjacent to the neurovascular bundle *(arrow)* and the flexor hallucis longus muscle (fhl) on this axial T1-weighted (TR 616/TE 14) image.

(7,8). Aside from the accessory soleus and peroneus quartus, all are located deep to the flexor retinaculum within the tarsal tunnel. These muscles are often clinically silent; however, they can present as painful soft tissue masses, overcrowd adjacent structures (particularly the neurovascular bundle) predispose to foot deformity, and may require surgical resection. The peroneus quartus originates from the lateral distal leg and most commonly inserts into the retrotrochlear eminence of the calcaneus (9,10). It descends along the lateral ankle and can predispose to overcrowding, dislocation, and tears of the peroneal tendons (Fig. 31.12). The accessory soleus descends posteriorly from the lower leg and inserts into the calcaneal tuberosity at or adjacent to the insertion of the Achilles tendon (11,12) (Fig. 31.13). The accessory flexor digitorum longus tendon originates from the lower leg and inserts onto the quadratus plantae or the flexor digitorum longus tendon (13) (Fig. 31.14). The peroneocalcaneus internus and tibiocalcaneus internus originate from the distal fibula and tibia, respectively, and insert into the undersurface of the sustentaculum tali in close proximity to the flexor hallucis longus tendon (Fig. 31.15) (14).

Symptomatic Accessory Navicular Bone

The type II accessory navicular bone is a secondary ossification center that is bridged to the tarsal navicular

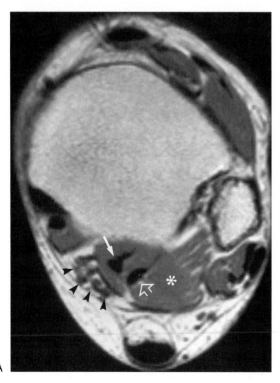

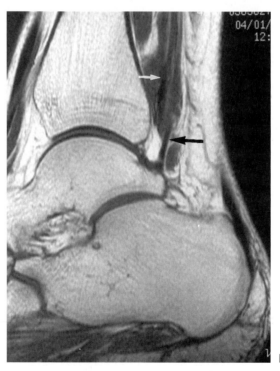

A   B

FIG. 31.15. Peroneocalcaneus muscle. **A:** Axial T1-weighted (TR 600/TE 15) image depicts the peroneocalcaneus muscle *(asterisk)* and its tendon *(open arrow)* lateral to the flexor hallucis longus muscle and tendon *(arrow)* and the neurovascular bundle *(arrowheads)*. **B:** Sagittal T1-weighted (TR 433/TE 22) image depicts the tendon of the flexor hallucis longus *(white arrow)* and the tendon of the peroneocalcaneus *(black arrow)* as they descend together in the posterior ankle.

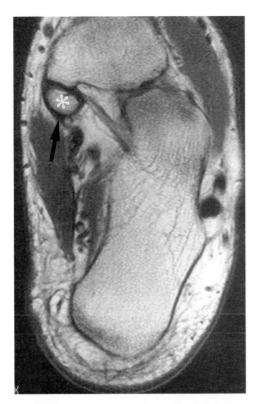

FIG. 31.16. Axial T1-weighted (TR 950/TE 22) image depicts an accessory navicular *(asterisk)* adjacent to the navicular bone. The posterior tibial tendon inserts into the ossicle.

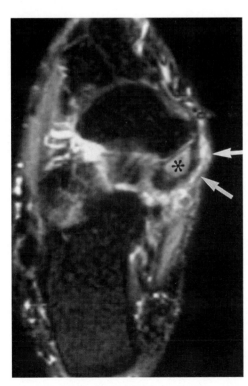

FIG. 31.17. A 40-year-old woman with a painful accessory navicular bone. A fat-suppressed proton-density spin-echo (TR 2,000/TE 28) axial image depicts increased signal in the accessory navicular *(asterisk)* as well as in the adjacent soft tissues *(arrows)*.

via a fibrous or cartilaginous interface (15) (Fig. 31.16). Shearing stress forces across the synchondrosis, transmitted by the repetitive pull of the posterior tibial tendon as it inserts onto the accessory ossicle, can generate pain and tenderness along the medial aspect of the midfoot. On MR images, edematous changes in the navicular, accessory navicular, synchondrosis, and adjacent soft tissues are diagnostic of this entity and are best detected on fat-suppressed or inversion-recovery (STIR) images (16) (Fig. 31.17).

Os Sustentaculi

The os sustentaculi is an accessory ossification center found medial to the sustentaculum tali in fewer than 1% of individuals. Stress forces at the attachment of the os to the calcaneus may produce pain along the medial subtalar joint. The os can be difficult to detect on routine radiographs of the ankle. Coronal, axial, and even sagittal MR images of the ankle depict the os sustentaculi as a distinct ossicle medial to the sustentaculum tali (17) (Fig. 31.18). The interface between the two bones may be irregular and

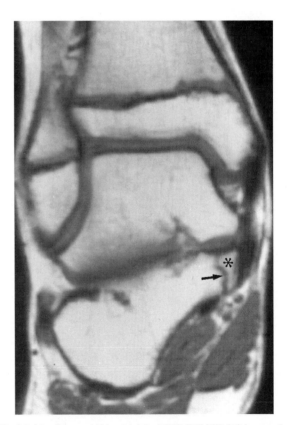

FIG. 31.18. Coronal T1-weighted (TR 650/TE 15) image in a 14-year-old with atraumatic medial foot pain. An os sustentaculi *(asterisk)* is separated from the rest of the sustentaculum tali by a low-signal irregular line *(arrow)*. (Reprinted with permission from Bencardino J, Rosenberg ZS, Beltran J, Sheskier S. The os sustentaculi: Depiction on MR images. *Skel Radiol* 1997;26:505–506.)

is low in signal intensity. The os should not be confused with a fracture of the sustentaculum tali.

Variations in the Fibular Groove

Normally the posterior surface of the fibula is round and convex at the distal leg. A shallow concavity in the posterior fibula develops about 1 cm above the ankle joint in 82% of the general population (18) (Fig. 31.19). This forms a retromalleolar groove, which accommodates the peroneal tendons as they course down the ankle. In the rest of individuals the posterior surface of the distal fibula remains flat (11%) or convex (7%). The latter configurations can predispose to dislocations and longi-

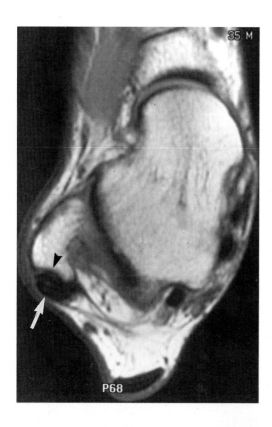

FIG. 31.19. A normal concave retromalleolar groove *(arrowhead)* accommodates the peroneal tendons *(arrow)* as seen on this axial T1-weighted (TR 600/TE 18) image.

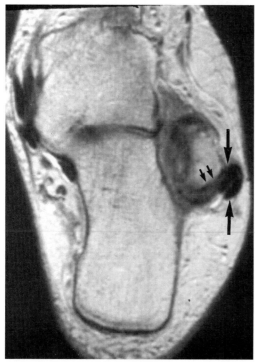

FIG. 31.20. A 34-year-old athlete with dislocation of the peroneal tendons associated with an absent retromalleolar groove. Axial FSE proton-density (TR 4,300/TE 21) image depicts the tendons *(long arrows)* lateral to the fibula. The posterior surface of the fibula is convex *(small arrows)* predisposing to the dislocation.

tudinal tears of the peroneal tendons (19) (Fig. 31.20). The integrity of the peroneal tendons and the superior retinaculum as well as the location of the tendons relative to the groove should therefore be scrutinized whenever a convex or flat retromalleolar groove is encountered on MR axial images.

True Coalition and Pseudocoalition at the Ankle

Frequently, the medial subtalar joint is not clearly seen on routine coronal MR studies of the hindfoot. Instead, an osseous "bar" between the talus and the calcaneus is traversed by a vague, low-signal, linear shadow that migrates from cranial to caudal location on sequential images (Fig. 31.21A). This reflects partial volume averaging generated by the obliquity of the medial subtalar joint relative to the orthogonal coronal plane and should not be confused with a true subtalar coalition. This partial volume averaging is not infrequently encountered on routine axial CT images and may be found on the axial MR plane.

The pseudocoalition is usually distinguishable from a true coalition on sagittal MR images, where the sustentaculum tali and medial subtalar joint are clearly visualized (Fig. 31.21B). In true coalition, however, morphologic changes of the sustentaculum tali and the medial talar facet, pseudoclefts or a complete osseous bridge at the medial subtalar joint, are found on all image planes (Fig. 31.22).

Sagittal T1-weighted images of the hindfoot can frequently simulate a bony coalition between the calcaneus and the navicular bone. This pitfall can easily be avoided by noting a normal relationship between the two bones on axial and coronal images. Also, in the absence of a true coalition, gradient-echo or STIR sagittal images will demonstrate bright signal between the calcaneus and navicular, precluding the existence of a calcaneonavicular bar.

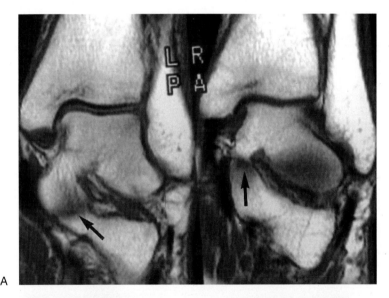

A

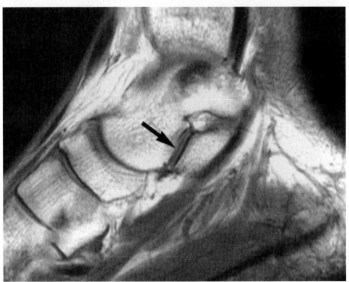

B

FIG. 31.21. Pseudocoalition of the medial subtalar joint. **A:** Consecutive, coronal T1-weighted (TR 500/TE 16) images depict "deformity" of the sustentaculum tali and the medial talus. A fleeting, poorly defined line *(arrows)* reflecting the true subtalar joint changes position relative to the bones. **B:** Sagittal T1-weighted (TR 500/TE 16) image in the same patient depicts a normal subtalar joint *(arrow).*

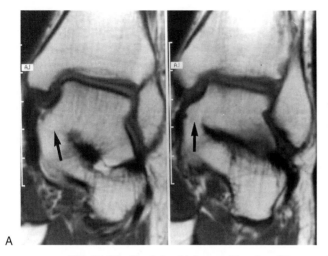
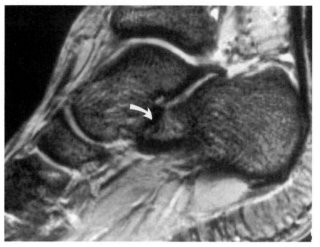

FIG. 31.22. Medial subtalar coalition in a 38-year-old woman. **A:** Consecutive, coronal T1-weighted (TR 600/TE 18) images demonstrate an osseous bridge *(arrows)* between the talus and the calcaneus. **B:** Sagittal gradient-echo T2*-weighted image (TR 700/TE 18, flip angle 20) confirms the osseous fusion *(curved arrow).*

Protuberances of the Lateral Wall of the Calcaneus

The peroneal tubercle (present in about 40% of people) arises from the lateral wall of the calcaneus and forms a sling between the peroneus brevis and peroneus longus tendons (18,19) (Fig. 31.23). The retrotrochlear eminence (present in about 98% of individuals) is located posterior to the peroneal tendons (Fig. 31.24). A hypertrophied retrotrochlear eminence is associated with the presence of the accessory peroneus quartus muscle (10,20).

Hypertrophy of either the peroneal tubercle or the retrotrochlear eminence can produce a deformity of the calcaneus on MR images and should not be interpreted as an osteochondroma or evidence of a healed fracture (Fig. 31.25). Both protuberances, particularly the peroneal tubercle, can irritate the sheath of the peroneus longus

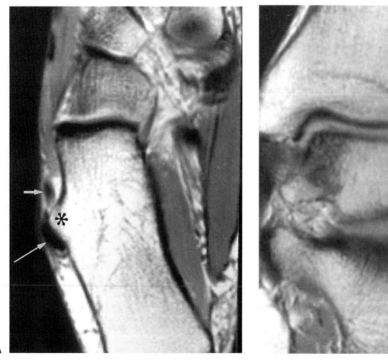

FIG. 31.23. A peroneal tubercle. Axial **(A)** and coronal **(B)** proton-density spin-echo (TR 2,000/TE 17) images depict a bony protuberance *(asterisk)* between the peroneus brevis tendon *(short arrow)* and peroneus longus tendon *(long arrow).*

tendon and predispose the tendon to tenosynovitis and tears (21).

Pseudo-osteochondral Defects

Occasionally an oval or linear focus of low signal intensity on far sagittal images simulates an osteochondritis desiccans defect of the posteromedial aspect of the talus (Fig. 31.26). Partial volume averaging of the obliquely inclined medial talar cortex with the insertion of the deltoid ligament accounts for this finding (22). A similar lesion is often simulated in the distal tibial subchondral bone on far posterior coronal images, where a focus of low signal intensity is occasionally seen (23) (Fig. 31.27).

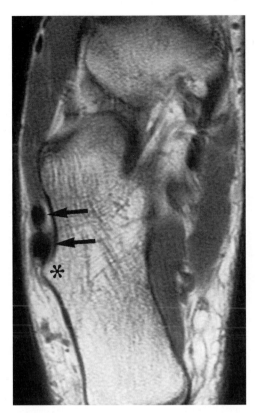

FIG. 31.24. Normal retrotrochlear eminence. An axial T1-weighted (TR 800/TE 14) image depicts the eminence *(asterisk)* posterior to the peroneal tendons *(arrows)*.

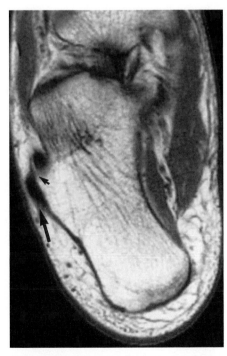

FIG. 31.25. Hypertrophied peroneal tubercle. An axial T1-weighted (TE 800/TE 14) image demonstrates displacement of the peroneus longus tendon *(long arrow)* as a result of a hypertrophied tubercle *(short arrow)*.

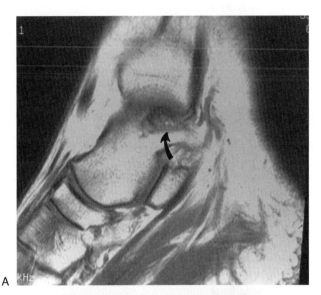

A

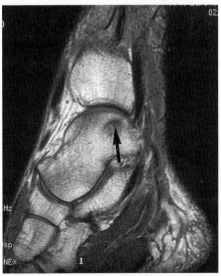

B

FIG. 31.26. Pseudo-osteochondral defects of the talus. Sagittal T1-weighted (TR 633/TE 22) images depict an oval **(A)** or linear **(B)** focus of low signal *(arrows)* in the posterior talar dome simulating an osteochondral defect or osteochondritis desiccans.

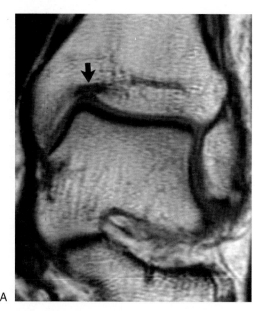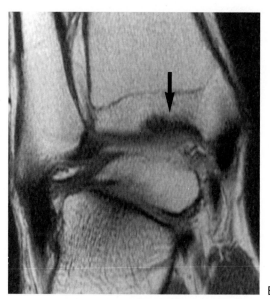

A   B

FIG. 31.27. Pseudo-osteochondral defect of the tibia. **A:** A coronal T1-weighted (TR 500/TE 16) image depicts a focus of low signal just above the tibial plafond. **B:** In another patient this pseudo-osteochondral defect *(arrow)* is more pronounced.

This reflects condensation of cortical trabeculae at a normal elevation in the posterior distal tibial articular surface. The typical peripheral location of the "lesions" and the absence of marrow abnormalities on other imaging planes testify to the innocuous nature of the findings.

Pseudocyst of Calcaneus

The calcaneus often demonstrates a radiolucency at the neutral triangle of the calcaneus on lateral plain radiographs, which may simulate a benign cyst (24). This normal rarefaction of trabeculae is produced by a paucity of trabeculae between the weight-bearing trabeculae of the calcaneus. It may be noted on MRI, particularly on sagittal images, as absence of normal trabecular pattern

and should not be mistaken for a true tumor of the calcaneus (Fig. 31.28).

Heterogeneity of the Ligaments of the Ankle

The ligaments of the ankle are frequently heterogeneous and striated (1,2). This phenomenon is particularly prominent in the posterior talofibular ligament and the posterior tibiotalar band of the deltoid ligament (Figs. 31.29 and 31.30). The anterior tibiofibular ligament may also manifest heterogeneity and even apparent fragmentation. The striation is most likely related to fat interposed between the fascicles of the ligaments and should not be misinterpreted as disease. Their characteristic appearance as well as absence of secondary changes associated with

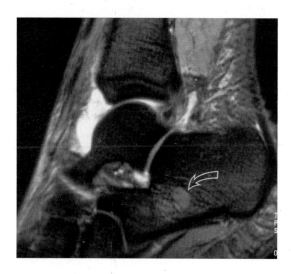

FIG. 31.28. Pseudocyst of the calcaneus. Normal rarefaction of the trabeculae at the neutral triangle can produce a "cyst" *(curved arrow)* in the calcaneus as seen on this STIR (TR 4,000/TE 11) sagittal image. Note fat suppression of bone marrow within the pseudocyst.

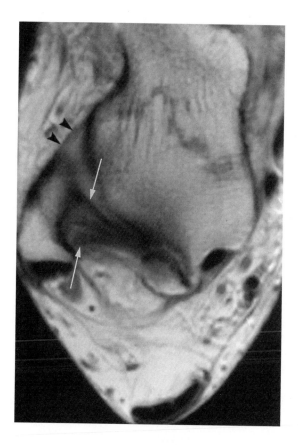

FIG. 31.29. Normal striation of the posterior talofibular ligament *(arrows)*. A slightly striated anterior talofibular ligament *(arrowheads)* is also depicted on this axial T1-weighted (TR 500/TE 15) image.

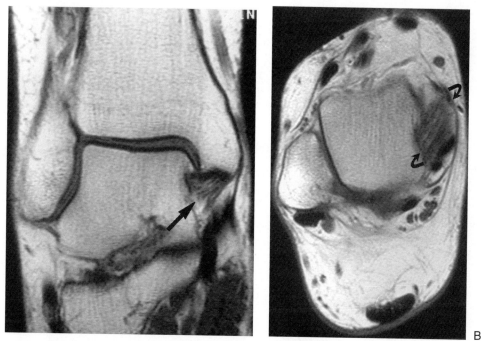

FIG. 31.30. Normal striation of the deep band of the tibiotalar component *(arrows)* of the deltoid ligament on coronal **(A)** and axial **(B)** T1-weighted (TR 800/TE 14) images.

ligamentous tears such as complete interruption, wavy appearance, thickening, attenuation, bone marrow, and soft tissue edema should obviate misinterpretation of the striation as disease (25).

Pseudo–Loose Bodies

On midline sagittal MR images the posterior tibiofibular and posterior talofibular ligaments are imaged in cross section and may appear as two low-signal-intensity oval structures suspicious for loose bodies posterior to the ankle joint (1,2). Occasionally they may even be partly surrounded by fluid because of their inti-

mate relationship with the joint capsule (Fig. 31.31). Similar pseudo–loose bodies may be seen anterior to the talus because of the anterior tibiofibular and anterior talofibular ligaments. Confusing the ligaments with loose bodies can easily be avoided by identifying the ligaments on sequential parasagittal images. Cross-sectional imaging of the calcaneofibular ligament on routine coronal images may also manifest as a low-signal round structure deep to the peroneal tendons and lateral to the calcaneus (Fig. 31.32). Familiarity with the normal structure will avoid potential pitfall and should aid in distinguishing it from a loose body or an avulsion fracture of the calcaneus.

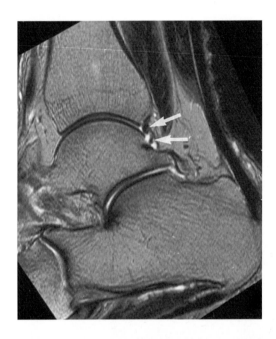

FIG. 31.31. On sagittal images the posterior tibiofibular and posterior talofibular ligaments *(arrows)* can simulate loose bodies.

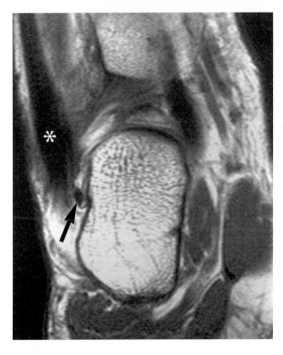

FIG. 31.32. The normal calcaneofibular ligament *(arrow)* can simulate an avulsion fragment when imaged in cross section on this coronal T1-weighted (TR 500/TE 22) image. *Asterisk* denotes the points to peroneal tendons.

Posterior Intermalleolar Ligament

The posterior intermalleolar ligament (also called the tibial slip of the posterior talofibular ligament) is occasionally found traversing from the medial to the lateral malleolus between the posterior tibiofibular and posterior talofibular ligaments (26). This accessory ligament can herniate into the ankle joint, undergo bucket-handle tears, and induce the posterior impingement syndrome (Fig. 31.33). It is best seen on coronal MR images as a thin low-signal-intensity band traversing between the medial and lateral malleoli.

Pseudosubluxation of Lisfranc Joint

On MR examination of the Lisfranc joint, the metatarsal bases are frequently aligned with the adjacent tarsal

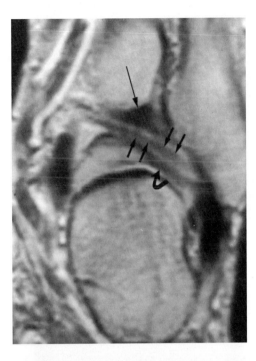

FIG. 31.33. The posterior intermalleolar ligament is manifested on this coronal FSE T2-weighted (TR 4,000/TE 23) image as an additional band *(short arrows)* between the posterior tibiofibular *(long arrow)* and posterior talofibular *(curved arrow)* ligaments. (Reprinted with permission from reference 25.)

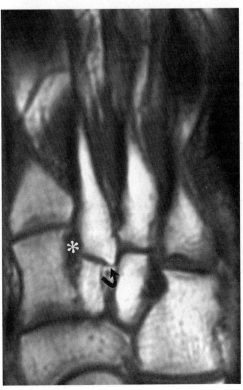

FIG. 31.34. Coronal T1-weighted (TR 600/TE 18) image of the forefoot demonstrates lateral pseudosubluxation *(arrow)* of the second tarsometatarsal joint in an asymptomatic volunteer. The Lisfranc *(asterisk)* and intermetatarsal ligaments are identified.

bones (27). The bases of the metatarsal bones are connected by intermetatarsal ligaments, except for the second metatarsal base, which is connected to the medial cuneiform by the oblique Lisfranc ligament. Incongruency of the Lisfranc joint has been described in normal individuals (28) (Fig. 31.34). Awareness of this normal variation prevents misinterpretation with tarsometatarsal joint subluxation. A negative history of trauma and absence of associated edematous changes confirm the benignity of this finding.

Fatty Pseudotumor

Focal areas of subcutaneous fat along the medial arch of the foot are often bordered by septa and fibrous bands simulating fatty tumors (Fig. 31.35). The high prevalence of this finding, the characteristic appearance, and typical location should obviate confusing it with a subcutaneous lipoma.

Prearticular Fat Pad Simulating Avulsion Fracture

A small prearticular fat pad hugs the medial surface of the talar neck. It is bordered medially by the anterior tibiotalar fascicle of the deltoid ligament. Occasionally this fat pad assumes a rounded shape on anterior coronal

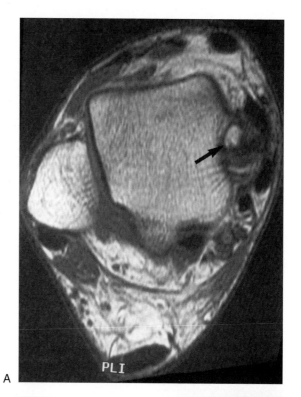

A

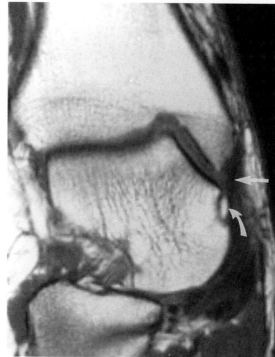

B

FIG. 31.36. Fat pad *(curved arrow)* bordered by the deltoid ligament *(straight arrow)* can simulate a talar avulsion fragment on **(A)** axial and **(B)** coronal T1-weighted (TR 566/TE 22) images.

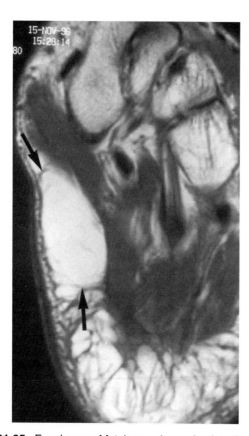

FIG. 31.35. Focal area of fat *(arrows)* can simulate lipoma in the subcutaneous fat of the foot on this axial T1-weighted (TR 750/TE 15) image.

or axial images and may simulate an avulsion fracture (Fig. 31.36). The characteristic location of the fat pad, absence of history of trauma to that location and normal plain films will indicate the benign nature of this finding.

REFERENCES

1. Noto AM, Cheung Y, Rosenberg ZS, et al. MR imaging of the ankle: Normal variants. *Radiology* 1989;170:121–124.
2. Link SC, Erickson SJ, Timins ME. MR imaging of the ankle and foot: Normal structures and anatomic variants that may simulate disease. *Am J Roentgenol* 1993;161:607–612.
3. Erickson SJ, Cox IH, Hyde JS, et al. Effect of tendon orientation on MR imaging signal intensity: A manifestation of the "magic angle" phenomenon. *Radiology* 1991;181:389–392.
4. Rosenberg ZS. Chronic rupture of the posterior tibial tendon. *MRI Clin North Am* 1994;2:79–87.
5. Mellado JM, Rosenberg ZS, Beltran J, Cheung YY. Low incorporation of the soleus tendon: MR interpretation pitfall. *Skel Radiol* 1998;27:222–224.
6. Schweitzer ME, Van Leersum M, Ehrlich SS, Wapner K. Fluid in normal and abnormal ankle joints: Amount and distribution as seen on MR Images. *Am J Roentgenol* 1994;162:111–114.
7. Sarrafian SK. *Anatomy of the foot and ankle. Descriptive, topographic, functional, 2nd ed.* Philadelphia: JB Lippincott, 1993;240–247.
8. Buschmann WR, Cheung Y, Jahss MH. Magnetic resonance imaging of anomalous leg muscles: Accessory soleus, peroneus quartus and the flexor digitorum longus accessorius. *Foot Ankle* 1991;12:109–116.
9. Sobel M, Levy ME, Bohne WHO. Congenital variations of the peroneus quartus muscle: An anatomic study. *Foot Ankle* 1990;11:81–89.
10. Cheung YY, Rosenberg ZS, Ramsinghani R, Beltran J, Jahss MH. Peroneus quartus muscle: MR imaging features. *Radiology* 1997;202:745–750.
11. Ekstrom JE, Shuman WP, Mack LA. MR imaging of accessory soleus muscle. *J Comput Assist Tomogr* 1990;14:239–242.
12. Yu JS, Resnick D. MR imaging of the accessory soleus muscle appearance in six patients and a review of the literature. *Skel Radiol* 1994;23:525–528.
13. Cheung YY, Rosenberg ZS, Colon E, Beltran J. MR imaging of the accessory flexor digitorum longus tendon. *Skel Radiol* 1999;28:130–137.
14. Mellado JM, Rosenberg ZS, Beltran J, Colon E. The peroneocalcaneus internus muscle: MRI features. *Am J Roentgenol* 1997;169:585.
15. Lawson JP. Not so normal variants. *Orthop Clin North Am* 1990;21:483–495.
16. Miller TT, Staron RB, Feldman F, et al. The symptomatic accessory tarsal navicular bone: assessment with MR imaging. *Radiology* 1995;195:849–853.
17. Bencardino J, Rosenberg ZS, Beltran J, et al. Dislocation of the posterior tibial tendon: MR imaging. *Am J Roentgenol* 1997;169:1109–1112.
18. Edwards ME. The relations of the peroneal tendons to the fibula, calcaneus, and cuboideum. *Am J Anat* 1928;42:213–253.
19. Rosenberg ZS, Beltran J, Cheung YY, Colon E, Herraiz F. MR features of longitudinal tears of the peroneus brevis tendon. *Am J Roentgenol* 1997;168:141–147.
20. Rosenberg ZS, Bencardino J, Cheung YY, Mellado JM, Beltran J. Normal muscle variants of the ankle. *Radiology* 1997;205P:645.
21. Thompson FM, Patterson AH. Rupture of the peroneus longus tendon. *J Bone Joint Surg [Am]* 1989;71:293–295.
22. Rosenberg ZS, Mellado JM. The central pseudodefect of the talus: A potential ankle MR interpretation pitfall. *J Comp Assis Tomog.* In press.
23. Pomerantz SJ, Kim TW. *Pitfalls and variations in neuro-orthopaedic MRI.* Cincinnati: MRI–EFI Publications, 1995;6.1–6.54.
24. Keats TE. *Atlas of normal roentgen variants that may simulate disease, 4th ed.* Chicago: Year Book Medical Publishers, 1988:699–700.
25. Schneck CD, Mesgarzadeh M, Bonakdarpour A. MR imaging of the most commonly injured ankle ligaments. Part 2. Ligament injuries. *Radiology* 1992;184:507–512.
26. Rosenberg ZS, Cheung Y, Beltran J, et al. Posterior intermalleolar ligament of the ankle: normal anatomy and MR imaging features. *Am J Roentgenol* 1995;165:387–390.
27. Preidler KW, Wang Y, Brossman J, Trudell D, Daenen B, Resnick D. Tarsometatarsal joint: Anatomic details on MR images. *Radiology* 1996;199:733–736.
28. Delfaut EM, Rosenberg ZS. Step Off and incongruities at Lisfranc joint in asymptomatic individuals: MR imaging features. *Radiology* 1998;209(p):345.

SECTION IV

Physical Aspects of Imaging Artifacts

Variants and Pitfalls in Body Imaging,
edited by Ali Shirkhoda.
Lippincott Williams & Wilkins, Philadelphia, © 2000.

CHAPTER 32

Physical Principles of CT Artifacts

Theodore Villafana and Harry G. Zegel

Computed tomography (CT) has artifacts that can be seen either as visible streaks, bands, and false image patterns or as inaccuracies in the resulting CT numbers. CT number inaccuracies can seriously affect quantitative CT number studies.

An image artifact, in general, can be defined as any discrepancy between what is really within the patient and what appears on the image. In CT, images are produced (or reconstructed) from attenuation data obtained over many angles around the patient and expressed as CT numbers. CT images, in fact, are just CT numbers displayed with some convenient gray scale. In CT scanning, therefore, one would define CT artifacts as a discrepancy between the reconstructed CT numbers and the true attenuation values within the patient. Regardless of how well defined they are, artifacts are obviously unwelcome. First, their presence may be confused with the presence or absence of important anatomic features. Second, their presence may visually obstruct the display of real features. In either case, inaccurate diagnosis can result. This is of particular concern in CT scanning, as this modality is particularly prone to artifacts due to the intricate reconstruction process involved.

In general, apart from calibration errors, artifacts in CT are caused by inconsistencies in the collected data. Unlike conventional radiography, where a projection is recorded from only one direction, the CT process requires gathering projections from many different angles around the patient and correlating them to form the final reconstructed images. Inconsistencies in these data may produce significant image artifacts. To further illustrate the

vulnerability of the CT process to artifacts, consider the filtered back projection algorithm, which is the algorithm of choice for CT reconstruction. This is described in many basic texts (1). Data from 1,000 or more projections through the patient are collected from different angles around the patient. Each of these angular projections contains readings from over 600 individual detectors. The accuracy of the final reconstruction depends on how positionally accurate each of these measurements are. The x-ray beam attenuation through any given picture element (pixel) in the patient must be the same regardless of the angle from which it is being viewed. Positional inaccuracy may, for instance, result from patient motion. Furthermore, CT numbers represent radiation attenuation occurring in various tissues. Attenuation, however, depends on x-ray beam energy. Beam energy, however, varies with depth within the patient. Energy, therefore, becomes even another factor affecting the image reconstruction results.

In general, the CT process is more likely to produce streaks if changes in the data vary abruptly from ray to ray or angular view to angular view. The CT process is much less likely to produce streaks for gradual changes and gradual errors from ray to ray or view to view (2). Streaks introduce angular sampling problems.

Categorization of artifacts is problematic since any one artifact can be due to different sources either individually or in combination. For example, streaks can be due to patient motion, partial volume effects, mechanical failure, aliasing, or scatter effects. Accordingly, there have been a number of different approaches to the classification of CT artifacts (Table 32.1). The most simplistic approach would be to consider artifacts as being related either to the patient or to the equipment. Joseph (2) classified the errors according to their type, Hsieh (3) classified them according to their appearance, Kreslel (4) clas-

_____

T. Villafana: Department of Radiology, MCP-Hahnemann University, Philadelphia, Pennsylvania 19129.

H. G. Zegel: Department of Radiology, MCP-Hahnemann University, Philadelphia, Pennsylvania 19129.

TABLE 32.1. *Classification of computed tomography artifacts*

Author	Breakdown by	Artifacts
Hsieh (3)	Appearance	Streaks, shading rings, bands, misc.
Joseph (2)	Type of error	Geometric errors
		Algorithm effects
		Attenuation measurement
		Photon spectrum error
Kreslel (4)	Cause of artifact	Physical causes
		Patient-related causes
		System-related causes
Villafana (1)	Effects on data	Data formation
		Data sampling
		Data detection
		Data processing
		Data recording and display

sified them according to their cause, and Villafana (1) classified them according to the process of events with the data. All approaches, however, have their relative merits. It will be the latter approach (1) that will be followed here. The entire spectrum of artifacts is beyond the scope of this text. These are related to CT angiography and to maximum intensity projection weighting functions. The interested reader is referred elsewhere for information about these types of artifacts (5–7).

We now describe each artifact, as classified in Table 32.2. First we look at the formation of the projection data. Factors determining quality of the data include patient motion, beam energy consistency, machine alignment, and x-ray output consistency. Then, one must sample the projection data, and there are many variables in the sampling process that must be understood. There are physical limitations in any sampling process, such as the Nyquist

TABLE 32.2. *Artifact sources*

Source area	Artifact
Data formation	Patient motion
	Polychromatic effects
	Clip artifact
	Noise artifact
	Mechanical imperfections
	Faulty x-ray source
Data sampling	Slice geometry
	Profile sampling
	Angular sampling
	Longitudinal sampling
	Out-of-field artifacts
Data detection	Detector imbalance
	Detector nonlinearity
	Scatter effects
Data processing	Algorithm effects
Data recording and display	Window level settings
	Pin-cushion distortions
	Video monitor linearity
	Chemical development
	Electrostatic discharges

limit, that if not adhered to can produce artifactual streaks. The sampling also directly affects the spatial resolution, low-contrast resolution, and noise performance of the system. Once the sampling process is decided upon, the data have to be detected and measured. Inconsistencies here can again lead to artifactual streaks. The efficiency of detection also affects the noise performance of the system. Once the data are detected, they must be processed and a suitable algorithm be chosen to reconstruct the final image. Finally, the reconstructed image has to be displayed and stored, which again may introduce image artifacts.

DATA FORMATION

As the x-rays travel through the body, attenuation occurs in various tissues that represent the basic data for image reconstruction. Attenuation within the patient along one view is linked to the attenuation from each of the other views obtained at different angles around the patient. Various factors affect the view-to-view consistency of projection data and can result in image artifacts, as follows.

Motion Artifacts

From the very beginning, motion has plagued CT scanning. The original scanners (EMI Mark I) took up to 6 minutes of scan time for each image. This resulted in significant patient motion, which often totally obliterated the image. Motion problems are responsible for much of the technologic developments in CT. Second-generation systems initially reduced scan times to just above 2 minutes and later to less than 1 minute per image. These systems were not fast enough, and CT wasn't fast enough until fan beam geometry was introduced with its pure rotary motion and hundreds of detectors, as used in third- and fourth-generation systems. The modern scanners could perform a scan within a second or two and thus minimize the motion problem (4).

The basis of the motion problem is seen in Fig. 32.1, which shows two different angular ray paths through a particular pixel within the scanner's field of view. Let ray path 1 pass through a pixel from one angle containing tissue A. At a later time, ray path 2 corresponding to the x-ray tube at a different angle around the patient passes through the same pixel position. If the original tissue has shifted to a new position and some other tissue B now occupies the original pixel position in question, then the projections of ray paths 1 and 2 are inconsistent. This inconsistency is manifested as a streak. The severity of the streak depends on the contrast of the moving structure and whether motion is abrupt or smoothly continuous (Fig. 32.2). Motion artifacts most commonly appear and are most prominent as large streaks parallel to air, bone, or other high-contrast interfaces. In the abdomen, the

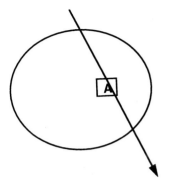
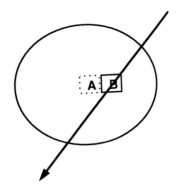

FIG. 32.1. The origin of the motion artifact. **A:** Ray path 1 intersecting a pixel at a particular position in patient, which contains tissue A. **B:** Ray path 2 intersecting same pixel position in patient from another angle around patient. Tissue A has moved and some other tissue B now occupies this position, and the attenuation between the two ray paths does not correlate. The resulting inconsistency is artifactual streaks.

most likely motion artifacts occur around and adjacent to diaphragmatic surfaces, or from bowel gas motion or barium contrast. In the pelvis, they can be from the various bony surfaces. Figure 32.3 shows an air/soft tissue interface image obtained on two different scanners from the same vendor but on separate patients. One scan was taken on an older scanner at 4.5 seconds, and the other on a more modern scanner at 2 seconds. Streaks are more apparent on the longer time scan than on the shorter time scan. This observation has been consistent for many different patient images when such comparisons are made. Motion streaks as well as aliasing and beam-hardening streaks are very similar and many times cannot be distinguished from one another except by an expert reader considering the surrounding structures. In general, motion, when present, will not only produce motion artifacts but will also worsen the aliasing and beam-hardening artifacts.

One important artifact is due to tissue motion associated with single-slice acquisition and is called misregistration artifact (Fig. 32.4A). That is, if a tissue structure

is adjacent to a given slice that has just been scanned, then that structure would be expected to be picked up on the subsequent scan of the level that contains that structure. However, if that tissue structure moves such that it is not within the adjacent slice when scanned, then that structure may not be detected at all. If only part of the

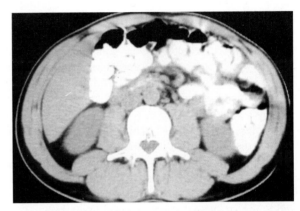

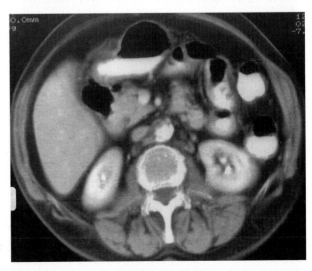

A

B

FIG. 32.3. Scan time effect. Comparison between typical scans taken at two different scan times. **A:** Scan taken at 2 seconds. **B:** Scan taken at 4.5 seconds. Bowel motion streaks are more evident on longer time scans. Shorter scan times would reduce streaks even further.

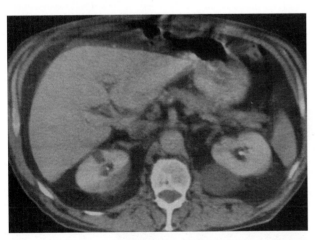

FIG. 32.2. Artifacts induced by motion. Notice streaks from the gastric air bubble and multiple contours in the right kidney and liver. As a result of breathing artifact, pseudo-subcapsular fluid collection is seen medial to the right kidney. Ascites is mimicked around the liver.

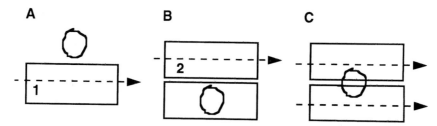

FIG. 32.4. Illustration of the misregistration artifact. **A:** Scan is obtained in plane 1. Adjacent structure of interest is missed. **B:** Scan later is obtained through plane 2. If structure of interest moves out of its original position, it will not be captured at all. **C:** If structure only moves partially out of slice, it will not contribute its full attenuation to either slice, and the image contrast will be reduced (partial-volume averaging effect).

structure is scanned, then there would result only a partial contrast on the image (partial volume effect). Note that in this latter case a streak need not be formed, but rather what has occurred is a loss of image contrast and the associated loss of ability to detect and clearly delineate anatomic structures (Fig. 32.5) (8). The misregistration artifact is minimized with faster scans especially if within a patient's breath hold. The advent of spiral scanning has also minimized this problem. This is true since x-ray beam is on continuously and every tissue structure in the spiral volume contributes to the image, and therefore structures are always captured and are not misregistered. Also in spiral scanning, one can arbitrarily choose the level to reconstruct and to assure that structure of interest is within the slice.

As in classic radiography, motion can also produce loss of spatial resolution, that is, an ability to see fine detail. In addition, motion affects low-contrast resolution, that is, the ability to visualize small differences in tissue densities. These losses, however, are usually minimal compared to the artifactual streaks caused by motion.

Sources of motion are many and include voluntary motion as well as involuntary motions such as peristalsis, blood vessel pulsations, and cardiac motion. Motion artifacts are particularly severe if sharp, high-contrast surfaces are present as well as radiography markers, tubes, catheters, clips, etc. Motion has also been associated with patient discomfort either due to the illness and or to the inability to remain stationary or hold one's breath (9). Discomfort and motion due to the effects of intravenous contrast material can produce artifacts (10) and has been demonstrated to produce significantly greater patient motion than when non-ionic contrast media is used (11,12). Motion streaks can potentially become important for spiral scanning since the scan area is more extended and patient cooperation more important. Table 32.3 summarizes these sources of motion artifacts as well as aggravating factors, and Table 32.4 lists the types of motion artifacts.

Double-fissure or double-contouring artifacts occur when a structure is at one position for a particular ray path and then at a second position when the opposing 180-degree view is obtained as seen in Fig. 32.6. This artifact is essentially the equivalent of an inplane misregistration and is usually found parallel to the long axis of the structure, as this ray path direction yields the greatest attenuation. A clinical example is shown in Fig. 32.7.

Motion artifacts can be minimized via a number of different approaches (Table 32.5). The most obvious is to reduce the scan time. As mentioned previously, this

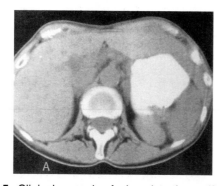
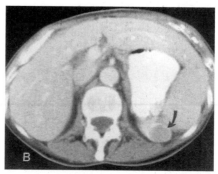

FIG. 32.5. Clinical example of misregistration artifact. **A:** Small renal cyst is missed. **B:** Small renal cyst visualized in absence of misregistration artifact after contrast injection (8).

TABLE 32.3. *Sources of motion artifacts*

Voluntary patient motion
Patient breathing
Bowel motion/peristalsis
Blood vessel pulsations
Cardiac motion
Patient discomfort (general or due to contrast injection)
Aggravating factors
    Radiopaque markers, tubes, catheters, bony structures,
      prostheses, etc.
    Sharp, high-contrast tissue interfaces
    Residual barium in bowel

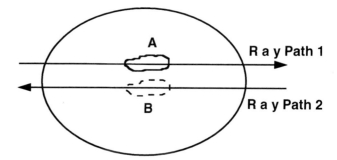

FIG. 32.6. Basis for the double-fissure or double-contouring artifact. Structure at position A is captured by ray path 1. When opposing 180-degree views are taken, a double image will occur if structure now has moved to position B, which intersects ray path 2.

approach dominated technologic advancements in CT from its inception. Once scanning times were reduced to a few seconds, scanning within a patient's breath hold became possible and the motion problem was greatly minimized. One cannot, however, just arbitrarily reduce scan times since one must be assured that enough photons have been collected to achieve a desired signal-to-noise ratio. Therefore, high-output x-ray tubes and highly efficient x-ray detector systems were required to achieve the current short scan times. A by-product of high-efficiency detection is reduced patient dose. Another obvious approach to minimizing the motion problem is to immobilize or sedate the patient.

One interesting approach to reduce the effects of motion artifacts involves the technique of overscanning. The idea in overscanning is that most of the motion discrepancy occurs between the beginning and the end of the scan. Overscanning beyond 360 to 400 degrees provides the same attenuation information as that from the initial angles (0–40 degrees). Any difference between these two data sets would be attributable to motion. If one then averages or feathers these data, then the motion artifacts will be minimized. This feathering procedure may not be productive for abrupt motion but is useful in the case of smooth, gradual motion. The need for overscanning is reduced as scan times are further reduced. Drawback to this technique are that patient dose is increased in the overlap region, and scan time is increased, which can therefore introduce even more motion blur. Alternatively, one can underscan, that is, take a shorter duration scan with perhaps fewer projections or the same number of projections but of shorter duration. In underscanning, fewer photons are collected and signal-to-noise ratio suffers, but this may be acceptable if objectionable streaks are minimized. Though motion inconsistencies and their

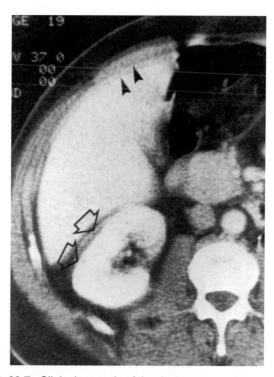

FIG. 32.7. Clinical example of the double-contouring artifact. Around the kidney *(open arrows)* the artifact mimics fluid collection, and around the liver *(arrowheads)* it mimics ascites (also see Fig. 32.2). (Adapted from ref. 44a.)

TABLE 32.4. *Types of motion artifacts*

Streaks
CT number inaccuracy
Misregistration artifacts
Double-contour artifacts

TABLE 32.5. *Approaches to minimize motion*

Reduce scan times further
Respiratory or cardiac gating
Patient immobilization/sedation/use of antiperistaltic agents
Overscanning/underscanning
Breath-hold scanning
    Obtain patient cooperation
    Hyperventilate patient for longer breath hold
Contrast injection parameters
    Ionic versus non-ionic media
    Injection rate
    Media temperature
Motion suppression algorithms
Center and window manipulation

resulting streaks are minimized via above approaches, classic blurring still occurs.

Motion artifacts can also be minimized by aligning the initial position of the x-ray source with the direction of motion (13). This is true since motion along the direction of the x-ray path does not affect adjacent ray paths and produces minimal projection discrepancy. Motion perpendicular to anatomic motion, however, immediately affects adjacent ray projections, and inconsistencies with their consequent streaks result. In practice for abdominal scanning, motion is most likely to occur up and down rather than left to right. One would then start the scan process at 12 or 6 o'clock positions rather than at the 3 or 9 o'clock position.

The use of antiperistaltic agents (e.g., glucagon or buscopan) can be of value in arresting motion artifacts arising from peristaltic motion. Bowel movement produces streak artifacts especially when the bowel contains air or dense contrast medium (see Fig. 32.2).

Respiratory and cardiac gating is another means by which motion can be compensated. For instance, in respiratory gating, data are collected during the quiescent period of respiration near the end of inspiration or expiration. One complicating problem in this approach is that the patient's breathing pattern may change during the scan. Adaptive predictive algorithms have been devised to compensate for this (14,15). This approach reduces not only motion-induced streaks but also classic motion blur.

Modern spiral CT scanners allow for three-dimensional (3D) volume acquisition and therefore have less potential for motion misregistration artifacts. Misregistration, as discussed previously, can lead to the possibility of missing a lesion between scans. Another problem minimized by spiral scanners is that of uneven breath holds by the patient. If the patient breathes deeper on one scan than another, the diaphragm could move the liver just enough between scans that nearby lesions could be missed. The 3D data acquisition capability of spiral scanning minimizes these problems since every point in the scanned volume contributes to the image, and structures cannot be misregistered. One also has the ability to postprocess any desired slice position to assure the best lesion contrast. During spiral scanning, one can also eliminate the interscan delay times that previously allowed motion between single-slice scans. For spiral CT, to assure a complete breath hold during data acquisition and minimize motion, one can also have the patient hyperventilate just before scanning begins.

An important innovation in spiral scanning that will even further reduce scan times is multidetector spiral scanning. With this technology, multiple detector arcs are used and more than one slice is acquired at the same time. This allows a greater table pitch (distance moved in one rotation), which results in either a shorter spiral time or greater anatomic coverage within the breath-hold time. If a dual-detector arc is used, then scan times are one-half or coverage is twice that with comparable image quality and patient dose. The fact is that one can go up to a pitch of

four and still maintain image quality as compared to a pitch of two for a single-slice system (16). It is expected that further innovations based on multidetector/multislice spiral acquisitions will follow.

Two important questions arise: Just how much does the patient move? Does this motion actually produce clinically significant image degradation? Stockberger and colleagues (17) devised an objective method of measuring patient motion undergoing spiral CT scans. Their method consisted of placing an acrylic rod on the patient such that each scan showed excursion of the rod during the scan, and then comparing the image quality with the measured degree of motion. They found that the magnitude of motion correlated with clinically perceived image degradation.

At present, due to the use of high output x-ray tubes and highly efficient detectors, modern scanners are capable of producing a CT image within 0.5 to 0.75 seconds. Such subsecond CT unit has been shown to reduce significantly motion artifacts for thoracic scanning (18). Presumably, faster scan times will also be beneficial in abdominal/pelvic scans not only for single-slice acquisition but also for spiral scanning.

Modern scanners can achieve an increase in longitudinal velocity and greater z-axis coverage for a given slice thickness and pitch. Alternatively, one can complete the volume acquisition in a shorter time for a given coverage and therefore reduce motion effects. If motion is a minimal problem (acquisition is within the breath hold of patient), one can reduce pitch or slice thickness and improve spatial resolution.

Finally, by manipulating the window and center level, one can differentiate between artifactual streaks and features from real anatomic structures. High-density artifacts are best seen with a narrow window at the high center level, while low-density artifacts are best seen at narrow windows at the low center level. One can thus alternate windows and mentally subtract artifactual features.

Polychromatic Effects

As described earlier, the CT process is based on the characterization of tissues by their attenuation values at each pixel position. The attenuation values, however, are dependent on the energy of the x-ray beam. For full consistency and accuracy in the data, any given pixel should therefore have received the same beam energy regardless of the angle of the x-ray beam or the attenuating structures surrounding that pixel. This could ideally be accomplished using a monochromatic beam. X-ray beams, however, are not monochromatic and have rather a polychromatic spectrum (e.g., many energies typical of Bremsstrahlung x-ray beams). Effective energies range between 60 and 70 keV, while the maximum energies can go up to 140 keV corresponding to a voltage of 140 kilovolt peak [KVP]. Given a spectrum of energies with each energy having different attenuating properties, we immediately have the problem of beam hardening. This problem results from preferential attenuation of low energies as compared to high energies, and therefore, as the beam travels through the patient, the average beam energy increases. Any given volume element (voxel) within the patient, however, is surrounded by varying thickness of tissues with different attenuation values ranging from air to bone. As a result, each voxel will see a different energy along different ray paths, and an inconsistency is immediately created with resulting streaks. This artifact is referred to as a polychromatic beam-hardening effect and is a significant factor in CT scan image quality.

The beam-hardening artifact results because the reconstruction program assumes a fixed monochromatic x-ray beam spectrum. It interprets any change in beam intensity as being due to different tissue attenuation properties of the patient along each ray path. It does not interpret such intensity change as being due to a shift in the effective beam energy. Beam-hardening artifacts are seen whenever highly absorbing structures are present, especially if multiple structures lie along the same ray paths.

In CT images of the head, three beam-hardening artifacts have been discussed (1): the apical, cupping, and interdense structure banding artifacts (Fig. 32.8). The apical and cupping artifacts, though present in head images, are not as clinically pronounced for body scanning. However, the interdense structure banding artifact is commonly seen, for instance, between femoral heads in pelvic views or around contrast media or behind ribs.

The apical artifact (Fig. 32.8A) is due to scanning two different slices of different cross-sectional diameters. As a result, the average energy of the thinner diameter section is lower since less attenuation has occurred and less

beam hardening has resulted. Each voxel then absorbs more of this lower energy, and the reconstruction process then assigns a higher CT number to the thinner diameter section than that assigned to the thicker diameter section. This occurs even though tissues may be exactly the same and their CT numbers would also be expected to be exactly the same. Again, the reconstruction process assumes a monochromatic beam and interprets the greater attenuation at each voxel in the thinner slice as having been due to a greater attenuation tissue CT number and not the fact that it was due to a lower average energy. Tissues will then, finally, have a greater CT number and appear lighter in the image. The apical effect does not result in streaks but does result in possible shading and has an adverse effect in the accuracy and reliability of the quantitative CT numbers. Furthermore, this effect is significant when one compares CT numbers between slices obtained for different patient diameters.

The cupping artifact (Fig. 32.8B) is due to the spherical or elliptical cross section of the patient, the result of which is the x-ray beam traveling through any given voxel and passing through different thicknesses from different angles. Voxels along x-ray paths at the periphery of the patient suffer less attenuation and therefore less beam hardening. These pixels will be traversed by softer radiation than pixels in the center of the patient. Therefore, the reconstruction process will interpret these tissues as having greater attenuation than at the patient center. The pixels in the periphery, as a consequence, will appear with a somewhat larger CT number as compared to pixels in the center of the patient. This artifact is most visible when uniform soft tissue sections with minimal bone structures are scanned.

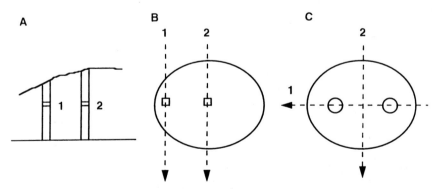

FIG. 32.8. Three manifestations of the beam-hardening artifacts. A: Apical artifact. Different body thicknesses are scanned. Tissues in thinner diameters suffer less overall absorption and average energy is lower, and therefore would then absorb relatively more. The reconstruction process interprets those tissues as having a higher CT number. B: Cupping artifact. Ray path 1 suffers less overall attenuation than ray path 2 due to shorter ray paths. Average energy along ray path 1 is lower, tissues absorb more, and again the reconstruction process interprets this as the tissues having a higher CT number in the periphery as compared to the center. Shading will therefore occur, yielding a darker region at the center of the patient. C: Interdense structure banding. Ray paths 1 and 2 undergo different degrees of beam hardening. Path 1 between the femoral heads produces greater beam hardening, and the average beam energy will be high. If beam energy is high, the tissues will attenuate less. CT numbers of these pixels will then be lower and tissues will appear having dark bands.

The interdense structure banding artifact (Fig. 32.8C), like the other polychromatic artifacts, again, involves the inconsistencies created by hardening of the x-ray beam. This time, hardening is caused by the presence of a highly absorbing structures such as bone. The problem is aggravated for regions between two very dense structures such as the femoral heads (Fig. 32.9A). Darker shading will result between and behind such structures since ray paths traveling across dense structures suffer more beam hardening and are therefore of greater average energy. Since they have greater energy, they suffer less attenuation and the reconstruction process assigns an artificially low CT number (darker gray).

Another beam-hardening effect is referred to as the environmental density artifact (19). This artifact has been described for situations where particular tissues are surrounded by contrast media. Specifically, the CT number of an avascular tissue such as a cystic lesion was observed to change following the arrival of contrast media in the surrounding capillary bed. This beam-hardening effect is in a manner very similar to the interdense structure effect, except here the dense structure surrounds the tissue of interest and the CT number is expected to decrease (20).

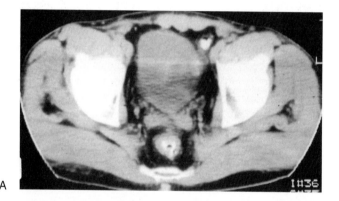

A

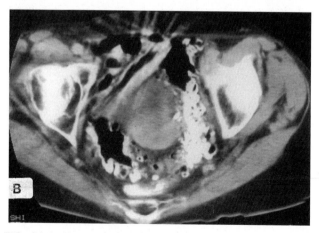

B

FIG. 32.9. Beam-hardening artifacts. **A:** Beam hardening between femoral heads. **B:** Beam-hardening streaks from barium in bowel aggravated by bowel motion as well as overt motion.

Various deviations from this expectation, possibly due to beam-hardening correction algorithms, have been noted.

Any dense structure can produce the polychromatic effect. Other examples are behind the ribs, in the vicinity of surgical clips, and prosthesis. One potentially confusing artifact seen on older units is the subcostal artifact beneath the ribs. Here, one sees regions of less attenuation with poorly defined borders over the normally homogeneous liver. Their characteristic location beneath the ribs and their symmetrical appearance help distinguish them from subcapsular lesions (21). Modern scanners with more sophisticated beam-hardening software have greatly diminished the frequency of this artifact.

In addition to bone, contrast media, whether barium or iodine, can cause the beam hardening artifact (Fig. 32.9B). The use of gadolinium-based contrast agents in CT has been shown to produce fewer beam-hardening artifacts than iodine (22). Beam-hardening artifacts occur around structures of low-attenuation properties since such structures will have less effective energy shift compared to the greater effective energy shift from the surrounding of more highly absorbing structures. Sharp and dense objects also produce beam-hardening artifacts. However, they are much more easily identified by the starburst-type streaks emanating from the location of such objects. These will be discussed in the next section.

To minimize the beam-hardening effect in the original EMI Mark I CT scanner, a separate water box was placed around the patient such that variable path lengths through asymmetrical patient heads could be equalized. The water box also helped minimize the overranging and ringing response of the limited dynamic range and adverse afterglow properties of the NaI radiation detectors which were originally used. With the water box in place, all ray path lengths through the patient were equal, resulting in less beam-hardening artifacts. The water box also eliminated the extremely large x-ray intensity difference at the air/tissue interface, which would have driven the original detectors well beyond their dynamic range.

There are a number of other ways to minimize the beam-hardening artifact; one of these is to prefilter the beam. The goal here would be to remove the low-energy components from the beam before it arrives at the patient. This, in effect, prehardens the beam and provides a more uniformly higher energy penetrating beam incident on the patient. Filtration can be accomplished with a flat filter, a bow-tie filter (23), or a combination of both. Bow-tie filters are shaped such that the thin part of the filter is at the center of field where patient thickness is expected to be greater and the filter is thicker toward the periphery where the patient is thinner. The idea here is to equalize the hardening of the beam over the full field much like the original Mark I head box. Less prehardening would be needed at the patient center, where the greatest attenuation and therefore greater hardening naturally occurs. More prehardening would be necessary toward the periphery, where the patient is thinner and therefore less attenuation takes place, resulting in less hardening. Bow-tie filters also help detectors stay within their linear range and avoid detector overranging effects. A potential problem for the bow-tie filter is that no one filter will match all patient shapes and sizes. Unfortunately, the bow-tie filters can also lead to inaccuracies in CT numbers depending on the position in the scan field and the shape of the object. This is of particular note if quantitative use of CT numbers is contemplated (24). While prefiltration can reduce beam-hardening artifacts as well as reduce patient radiation dose, the drawback is loss of x-ray intensity. This can lead to enhanced noise or longer scan time as well as lower image contrast.

Beam hardening can also be minimized via various software routines, which can be either water [e.g., single-pass corrections (25)] or bone [e.g., two-pass corrections (26)]. The correction process is relatively simple. For instance, one first determines the attenuation values of water (similar to soft tissue) as a function of thickness. Then one determines the attenuation values for the ideal monochromatic beam. For a given measured attenuation value, one then picks off the expected monochromatic value and makes the required correction. Essentially, one is just linearizing the detector signal. In practice, appropriate look-up tables or suitable approximation functions are used. This procedure is satisfactory for minimizing the cupping artifact from soft tissue. It will, however, break down in the presence of bone or any highly absorbing structures such as contrast material. As a consequence, water corrections will alleviate, though not necessarily eliminate, the interdense structure banding and streaks referred to earlier. The bone correction problem has also been addressed. Specifically, one can determine the amount of bone along each ray path and perform a second reconstruction with more accurate linearized data. Such beam-hardening corrections are referred to as second-pass reconstruction. They are usually applied in head scans. Recently, this correction technology has been extended to any number of distinct materials, especially the presence of iodinated contrast media (27). Since beam hardening and the linear partial-volume effect always appear together, the best strategy for any attempt to correct for beam hardening is to first scan at the thinnest clinically possible slices to minimize the partial-volume effect.

Beam-hardening artifacts would not exist if the incident beam were monoenergetic. There would then be just one energy that could not change. These artifacts, however, can also be eliminated if scans are done at two different energies (28–30). This approach, which depends on differential beam hardening between low- and high-energy x-ray beams, is considered clinically impractical at this time due to the need for specialized generators capable of very short time kV(p) switching, and/or to the extensive beam filtering that would be needed and that leaves the system x-ray photon starved and images very noisy. Instead, correction algorithms as discussed above are used to minimize polychromatic effects. Table 32.6 summarizes the various

TABLE 32.6. *Methods of minimizing beam hardening*

Thicker beam filtration
Beam-shaping filters (bow ties)
Software corrections
1st-pass algorithms (water correction)
2nd-pass algorithms (bone correction via postprocessing)
Use of monoenergetic beams (impractical)
Dual-energy scans (impractical)

approaches to minimizing beam-hardening artifacts. Finally, it must be stated that beam-hardening–type artifacts would be extremely difficult to totally remove since they are hardly distinguishable from partial volume and scatter effects, which can also be present.

Clip (Starburst) Artifacts

Whenever metallic objects are within the scan field, severe streaks are created. These streaks, which resemble a starburst, result primarily from missing projection data. Data are missing because of the near-total attenuation of the x-rays within the metallic object. It should be noted that streak artifacts are also contributed from nonlinear partial-volume effects and aliasing, since they all depend on the presence of highly attenuating structures. Additionally, they are all accentuated by patient motion. The partial volume and aliasing effects that are discussed below can be minimized by reducing slice thickness and increasing angular views. However, metallic objects with their high density and high atomic number very efficiently absorb radiation, and inconsistencies are introduced by the absence of data along ray paths intercepting that structure (data fallout). Reducing slice thickness, therefore, does not entirely eliminate these artifacts (Fig. 32.10). The dynamic range of the detectors is very important, since a limited dynamic range produces nonlinear effects, and streaks result even if data are not missing. Modern scanners have dynamic ranges up to a million to one, and the dynamic range problems, though still a factor, are not overwhelming. It is also possible to have similar artifacts produced by algorithm-related overshoot in the reconstruction process.

Often the center of the clip artifact is black, because the detectors range beyond their maximum CT values of 3,000 to 4,000 and cycle from these high CT values down to the other end of the scale to the negative CT number range. As a consequence, the computer interprets this cycling as tissues having greater transmission or lower CT number and thus assigns a relatively darker gray value. This feature was especially prevalent in older CT units having maximum CT values of 1,000.

To reduce these clip-induced artifacts (31), one can use smaller and less absorbing metallic implants. This then would help minimize the missing projection data problem. Increasing the beam energy by increasing the kVp

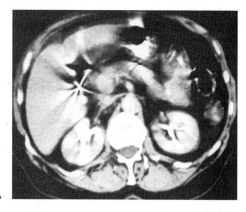

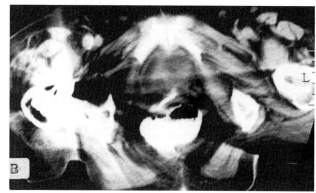

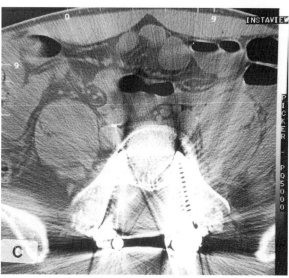

FIG. 32.10. Metal artifacts. **A:** Clip artifact at the gallbladder fossa. **B:** Right femoral prosthesis artifact. **C:** Spinal metallic screws in field.

will enhance the penetration ability of the beam and likewise reduce the missing data problem. Increasing beam energy, unfortunately, will also reduce the overall image contrast. More sophisticated approaches include reformatting images in other than the scan plane and averaging out the artifacts (32). Another approach is to artificially generate attenuation values for the missing projections before image reconstruction takes place (33). As can be expected, there is a wide variability in the degree to which metallic objects produce streaks, depending on the type of material. Tantalum and stainless steel as well as femoral prosthesis produce severe artifacts (Fig. 34.10B). Titanium and nonmetallic resorbable polydioxanione clips produce almost no artifacts (34).

It should be noted that the nonlinear partial-volume effect also produces similar streaks, since both effects are due to the presence of highly attenuating structures (35).

Noise-Induced Artifacts

We have mentioned that inconsistencies in the measured data lead to streak artifacts. Another possible inconsistency in the way data are formed is the result of quantum mottle or x-ray noise. X-ray noise is dependent on the number of x-ray photons (or signal) detected and utilized to make up the image. Noise itself is merely a statistical fluctuation in the number of x-ray photons. It represents a variation in the detected signal, that is, the lower the number of x-ray photons, the lower the signal-to-noise ratio and thus the greater the signal variation. But these signal variations, as they become greater, lead to significant inconsistencies and therefore streaks in the image. In addition to these streaks, one also expects classic noise variation in the image. Possible causes of noise are inadequately low milliamperage, loss of detector efficiency, scanning very thick or dense body parts, loss of gas pressure in ion chamber detection systems, parts of the patient lying outside the scanned field, or the characteristics of the reconstruction algorithm. Edge-enhancing algorithms tend to enhance noise, while smoothing algorithms decrease noise.

In addition, noise (σ) depends on a number of scan factors as follows:

$$\sigma = \frac{C}{D^{1/2}\, h^{1/2}\, L^{3/2}} \qquad [1]$$

where D is the radiation dose, h is the slice thickness, L is the pixel size, and C is a constant. As noted, noise increases as dose, slice thickness, or pixel size decreases.

Correcting for noise is very difficult since noise is random; however, nonlinear adaptive algorithms have been attempted (14). In spiral scanning it is very common to use 180-degree linear interpolation in algorithms. Such algorithms have been shown to minimally increase noise (15%) as compared to single-slice acquisition. Fourth-generation systems obtain ray projections by calculating differences between overlapping readings. This differencing procedure also produces noise running about 40% more.

Mechanical Imperfections

A variety of mechanical imperfections can cause inconsistencies in the data and therefore cause streak artifacts. Such inconsistencies can come from mechanical misalignment, from lack of rigidity in the gantry, or from x-ray tube rotor wobble. In all these cases, the actual x-ray beam position deviates from the ideal position assumed by the reconstruction algorithm. Streaks can radiate from any structure if that structure is not viewed consistently from the various projection angles around the patient. For example, one test for this is to scan a metal pin placed at the isocenter of the unit (at the axis of rotation). If the unit is not aligned exactly to the isocenter, streaks that are referred to as tuning-fork artifacts result. These were especially obvious for scanners with 180-degree rotation. In modern scanners, software corrections can be made for such isocenter misalignments as well as misalignments of the multiple detector array with respect to the target. In all cases, the best solution is to physically correct the mechanical problem or replace faulty components. Results vary from blurring of edges for only slight misalignments to objectionable streaks with significant misalignments.

In general, fourth-generation systems are less prone to mechanical problems since detectors are stationary. Likewise, spiral scanners avoid the sudden stopping and acceleration of the x-ray tube assembly with continuous rotary motion, and therefore reduce wear and tear on the equipment.

Faulty X-ray Source

If the x-ray output of a source varies, an inconsistency immediately occurs. The CT process will erroneously interpret an x-ray output variation as an attenuation variation along each ray path. The detectors cannot distinguish between increases or decreases in x-ray output as compared to attenuation changes along the various ray paths through the patient. The result is manifested as streaks crisscrossing the image field forming noise patterns (2,36). These streaks can be related, for instance, to variations in anode rotation. This so-called anode wobble

can become more pronounced toward the end of the useful life of the x-ray tube. Other factors producing x-ray output variations include momentary high-voltage arcs or electrical variations, leading to voltage and milliamperage variations.

Reference detectors incorporated within third-generation systems in a moving detector array under fixed geometry conditions with respect to the x-ray source are able to correct for the output variations for each particular angular view. Variations between angular views will still be present and will still lead to inconsistencies. Fourth-generation scanners with their fixed detector systems are significantly more sensitive to output fluctuations. This is due to the fact that they collect the data for each view over the whole scan time, while third-generation systems get each view essentially at an instant when each projection is made. In all cases, inconsistencies, faulty operation, or blocked reference detectors can lead to artifacts.

DATA SAMPLING

The previous section discussed what was happening to the data as it was being formed. This section discusses artifacts resulting from the manner in which data are sampled and collected. Since data will eventually be processed by a digital computer, they must first be sampled and then digitized. To sample the data, one breaks up the data field first into slices along the z-axis, and then each slice is divided into individual picture elements (pixels) along the x and y axes. Then, finally samples along x, y, and z are gathered at different angles around patient. Sampling along the z-xis leads to slice geometry effects, while sampling along x and y axes (profile sampling) leads to possible aliasing problems. Likewise, sampling along different angles around the patient (angular or view sampling) also leads to possible aliasing problem, which can result in visible streaks.

The slice thickness is determined by the collimator system defining the fan beam. These can be automatically adjusted to form slice thickness from about 1 to 10 mm. The thicker the slice, the more tissue coverage and the greater the number of x-ray photons arriving at the detectors. Any given detector will just integrate the total number of arriving photons to produce the output signal. The process is repeated at various angles around the patient to obtain a 360-degree data set to perform the final image reconstruction.

The number of pixels in the image is defined by the matrix size; a 256×256 matrix partitions a particular slice into 256 pixels in the vertical direction (x-axis) and 256 pixels in the horizontal direction (y-axis). The actual size of each pixel depends on both the field of view and the matrix size. The matrix size is merely the number of pixels in the particular direction of interest. The pixel size along any direction is given by the following equation:

$$\text{Pixel Size} = \frac{\text{FOV}}{\text{No. of pixels}} = \frac{\text{FOV}}{\text{Matrix size}} \quad [2]$$

Normally, pixels are square (256×256 or 512×512). Rectangular pixels, however, can also be utilized (512×256 matrix).

Pixel area along with the slice thickness form the voxel. Ideally, for greatest accuracy and spatial resolution this voxel should be as small as possible. To avoid noise problems, the smaller each individual voxel is, the longer it will take to collect the requisite number of x-ray photons over the entire patient volume of interest, and the greater the scan time and motion artifacts produced as well as the greater the radiation dose to the patient. Finally, there is the problem of the large amount of image data that are generated when small voxels are used. This affects the computer power needed, elongates reconstruction times, and requires more storage space for the final image data. Pixel size and slice thickness are of critical importance regarding artifacts. It is the voxel size that determines the partial-volume effect and the resulting artifacts.

The matrix size often refers to the display matrix. At a more fundamental level, we have to consider the measurement matrix, which refers to the method of profile sampling and view (or angular) sampling. We now turn to these latter two as well as the partial-volume effects as they relate to slice geometry.

Partial-Volume Averaging: Slice Geometry Effects

In general, the partial-volume effect refers to the situation where different tissues reside within the same voxel. This effect is normally present only in the z-axis since slice thicknesses are relatively large compared to pixel sizes. This can lead to inconsistencies and formation of artifacts. The partial-volume effect depends on a number of factors (Table 32.7). These factors include thickness of the slice and size of pixel. The greater these are, the greater the opportunity there is to have different tissues occupying the same volume. Likewise, the smaller the tissue structure and the sharper its features (abrupt edges), the more likely it will only partially intrude into any given voxel. Another factor is how different the attenuation coefficients (contrast difference) are between tissues residing in the voxel. The greater the difference, the greater the partial-volume effects and the greater the possibility of streaks. Slice sensitivity profile (SSP) effects define the detected response across the slice thickness dimension. Ideally, the SSP should be rectangular, defining a slice with sharp edges. In reality, such a profile is more gaussian shaped with blurry edges extending beyond the collimated thickness. This effect is dependent on the focal spot size and divergence of the beam, which is a function of distance from source to detectors. This produces a nonuniform intensity pattern over the slice width, which mimics variable tissue content within the slice.

There are a number of partial-volume artifacts; one of these is the Hounsfield partial-volume effect. This artifact is specific for first- and second-generation, 180-degree scanners and is seen when a structure is present within the beam on the 0-degree view but due to misalignment is not present on the 180-degree view. This inconsistency results in tuning fork–like artifact streaks emanating from small, high-contrast objects. Much more familiar, however, are the linear and nonlinear partial-volume artifacts. If different tissues occupy the same voxel, then the final CT number is the average attenuation value of those various tissues. This average could be a simple linear one if tissues are similar, and then only the CT number accuracy will be affected. If tissues are not similar, then nonlinear exponential attenuation predominates. The nonlinear partial-volume effect and the inconsistencies they produce result in streaks. These streaks can be seen from high-contrast structures with rapid changes in shape and size such as femoral heads, ribs, metallic structures, fluid/air interfaces, soft tissue bone interfaces, and contrast media–containing structures.

Figure 32.11 shows the simple linear averaging that can occur when two tissues each occupy half the voxel. One tissue has a CT number of 100 and another has a CT number of 200, and the average would then be 150. Of course, there is no such tissue within that voxel, but the average is what would be the final CT number reconstructed. Though no streaks appear in this case, the CT numbers would not accurately indicate the contents of voxel. This is of particular importance when relying on

TABLE 32.7. *Factors affecting partial-volume effect*

Factor	Effect
Slice thickness	Thin slices are more likely to contain one unique tissue
Pixel size	Small pixels are more likely to contain one unique tissue
Size and shape of tissue structure	The smaller and the more quickly changing the shape of structure, the less likely it will fill a voxel completely
Difference in attenuation between tissues residing in voxel	Simple linear averaging will occur; effect will be nonlinear streaks if larger CT number differences or abrupt boundaries exist
Slice sensitivity profile	Nonuniform x-ray intensity and detection over slice width mimics variable tissue content within slice

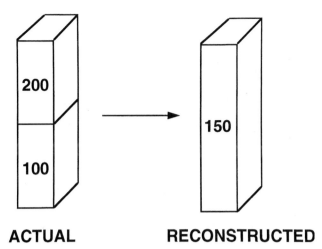

ACTUAL   **RECONSTRUCTED**

FIG. 32.11. Simple partial volume averaging affect. Two tissues residing in same volume element with equal volumes. One tissue has CT number of 100 and the other has CT number of 200. A CT number of 150 will result, as a simple average will appear in the final reconstruction.

actual CT values, such as in quantitative CT (24). Examples of the volume averaging are seen, for instance, when scanning a kidney containing a cyst. If the slice is occupied entirely by the cyst, then the CT number can accurately characterize it. If the slice contains both cyst and kidneys, the CT number by itself would make identification difficult.

The general equation governing the final CT number displayed (or final attenuation coefficient u) is as follows:

$$u = u_1 \frac{V_1 + u_2 V_2 + \ldots + u_n V_m}{V} \qquad [3]$$

where V_1, V_2, etc. are partial volume occupied by tissues with attenuation coefficient u_1, u_2, etc. V is the total volume of the voxel.

Volume averaging can also lead to loss of CT spatial resolution. For instance, a blood vessel or lesion can be entirely lost in a uniform tissue if its CT number contributes negligibly to the volume average of its voxel, in which case it will not be distinguishable from the surrounding tissues. For example, Fig. 32.12A shows both the pixel view of a nodule in the x,y plane and the view along the z-axis (slice thickness) direction. The nodule, if small enough and similar enough to background tissue, will not appreciably add to the CT number of the voxel it resides within to make its CT number distinguishable from surrounding pixels. Therefore, it may not be resolved. Figure 32.12B shows the case for a larger nodule, in which case the nodule will occupy a greater portion of the voxels it sits in and will become more distinguishable from its surroundings. The distinguishability, or better stated, the contrast of a structure depends on the slice thickness, the size of the nodule, the volume of the voxel occupied, and on how different the CT number (attenuation coefficient) of

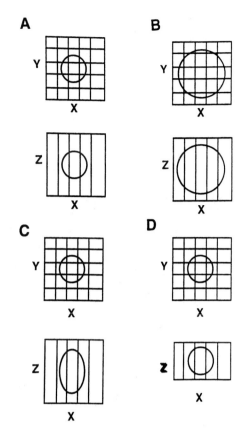

FIG. 32.12. Illustration of the partial-volume effect. **A:** Nodule occupying a group of pixels *(top)*. Same nodule viewed on longitudinal z-axis *(bottom)*. **B:** Large nodule occupies a larger volume of voxel and contributes more significantly to the volume average. **C:** Same-size nodule with thinner slice thickness allows a more significant contribution to each voxel, and the structure is more likely to be visible.

the nodule is compared to the background tissue. Figure 32.12C shows a nodule of the same size as in Figure 32.12A but thicker in the z-axis. Finally, Fig. 32.12D shows the result if nodule size remains constant but the slice thickness is reduced such that the nodule occupies a greater fraction of the voxel and does affect the volume average. In all cases, if a nodule or structure in a given voxel results in a sufficiently different CT number than the surrounding voxels, it will be displayed with a different shade of gray and be resolved. Similar effects are present when a tissue structure falls between two different slices and does not contribute its full attenuation to either slice, as seen in Fig. 32.13A. Only a partial attenuation is detected in either slice. Depending on how different the CT number is, that structure may not be detected. If a slice happens to fall exactly over the structure of interest (Fig. 32.13B), then contribution to the voxel average is more significant and visualization is more probable.

A compounding factor is that slices do not have distinct borders and are not entirely parallel, and the resulting slice geometry can also produce partial-volume averaging. Remember that the x-ray beam is diverging away

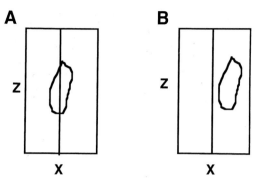

FIG. 32.13. Volume-averaging effect. **A:** Partial-volume effect occurring when structure falls between slices and does not contribute its full attenuation to either slice. **B:** Same structure as above, but fully within a given slice it contributes maximum attenuation to the slice and is more clearly delineated.

along the z-axis as it leaves the focal spot (along the fan beam the x-rays form a line source with minimal divergence). As the beam goes around patient, a biconcave slice geometry is formed (Fig. 32.14A). It is clear that the resulting slice thickness can vary from one end of the patient to another (dotted line) and that the intensity of radiation within the slice is not uniform over the dimensions of the patient. It is also clear that since the radiation profile is not uniform across the slice (z-axis) but rather biconcave in shape, there is a greater sensitivity at the center of the slice than at the edges. The biconcave geometry of the slice has a number of consequences. For instance, a given structure will suffer less volume averaging if it is at the isocenter as compared to a more peripheral position (Fig. 32.14B). A variation of this is seen in

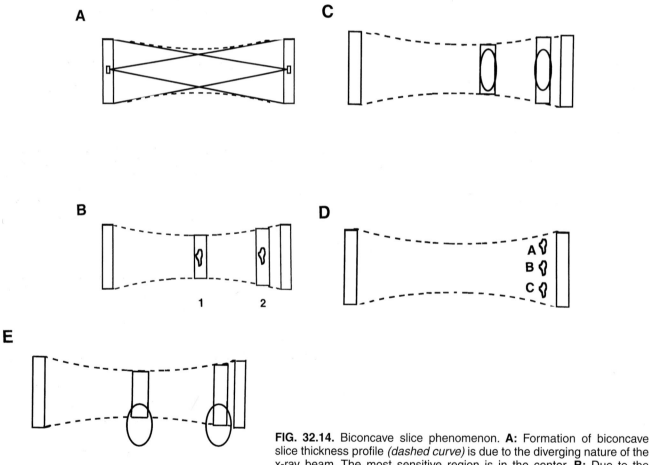

FIG. 32.14. Biconcave slice phenomenon. **A:** Formation of biconcave slice thickness profile *(dashed curve)* is due to the diverging nature of the x-ray beam. The most sensitive region is in the center. **B:** Due to the biconcave nature of the slice sensitivity profile, the structure in slice 1 will have less partial-volume averaging than structures in the more peripheral slice 2. **C:** The structure is completely within the slice along one ray path view, but may have more volume averaging when viewed along another ray path view. **D:** Structures A and C fall in less sensitive regions compared to structure B. This is due to the variation in sensitivity, which mimics variation in tissue content of voxel, and as a result variable partial-volume effects result. **E:** Structures intruding into a slice from one view may have a different degree of volume averaging as compared to another view. **F:** The possible loss of a structure if it falls in the dead zone between the biconcave slices.

Fig. 32.14C, which shows an object that is entirely within the slice thickness and contributes full attenuation to the voxel if it is located at the isocenter. That same structure occupies less than the slice thickness at a point more peripheral, and its attenuation will be mixed in with adjacent tissues. In all cases, volume-averaging effects increase as the distance between the source and the detector is reduced for points further from the isocenter. Due to divergence of the beam, a given structure lying at the center of the slice as compared to one at the bottom or on top of the slice will result in different CT numbers, and partial-volume artifacts result (Fig. 32.14D).

An additional consequence of the biconcave geometry is that an object can be intruding into a voxel from one view and intruding to a different magnitude from another view (Fig. 32.14E). The result here is that the partial-volume effect becomes angular dependent and further away from the isocenter (35).

Because of nonuniformity in slice sensitivity, there is also the problem of possibly missing a lesion in the region between slices (Fig. 32.14F), where sensitivity may be minimal or nonexistent. If a certain degree of overlap is programmed in scanning, then this problem is minimized. In that case, however, an increase in the patient dose in the region of overlap will result.

Volume averaging can result in the formation of vague and indistinct borders and margins, which may indicate that the edge of the structure is sloping within the thickness of the slice and does not necessarily represent an infiltration. An example of this is when the margins of the kidney are indistinct, which may be due to the small size of the kidney, and most likely the kidney margins are sloping within the CT slice. A repeat, thinner slice would improve visualization if this was critical to the interpretation of the scan. This can be seen in Fig. 32.15A, where sloping borders within the slice at pixel position 1 may hardly be intersecting any tissue. Pixel position 3 or 4 of the structure occupies nearly all of the slice and minimum volume averaging occurs. There has been a gradual variation of CT numbers across the structure, producing indistinct borders. Figure 32.15B is another situation yielding indistinct borders where structures overlap within the slice. Thinner slices is the obvious solution in this case. Yet another volume-averaging problem is seen in Fig. 32.15C, where a small structure is near a larger, more absorbing structure. If the two structures fall within the same slice thickness but different pixel positions, they will be distinguishable. If they fall within the same slice and the same pixel position, then the smaller structure may be averaged away by the larger structures with a different CT number. If thin slices are used (or thinner reconstruction intervals for spiral scanning), then each structure may fall within its own slice, producing less volume averaging, and be more distinguishable.

Figure 32.16 shows a clinical example of the partial-volume effect where the borders adjoining the liver and

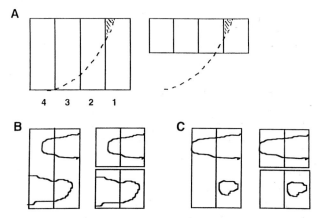

FIG. 32.15. Volume-averaging artifacts. **A:** Partial-volume artifacts and indistinct borders produced by a structure having a sloping surface in the slice thickness direction. Slice position 1 has the most volume averaging, and most likely its border may not appear in image *(shaded region)*. Pixel position 4 is essentially entirely within the slice and will have the full CT number characteristic of tissue content. There is a gradual variation between 1 and 4. Thinner slices, as seen on the *right*, yield less volume averaging at the same pixel position. **B:** Another example of indistinct borders due to volume averaging. Overlapping structure edges for A and B may not visualize edges distinctly. The thinner slice *(right)* clearly separates both structures and their respective borders. **C:** Overlapping structures, such that a structure can be lost if it lies entirely in the shadow of another, more attenuating structure. Thin slices again clearly separate and make structures more distinct. Similar results occur in spiral scanning by choosing smaller reconstruction intervals.

the stomach are entirely lost and one organ seems to merge with the other. A contributing factor in this case is the gastroesophageal junction and possibly the apex of the heart. In a somewhat related situation, if one desires the CT number of a tissue structure, one should measure

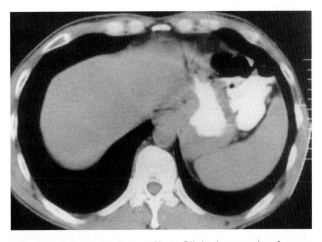

FIG. 32.16. Partial-volume effect. Clinical example of vague borders between the liver and the stomach produced by the partial-volume effect. Small hepatic lesions in this area may become difficult to recognize.

it at the center of the slice containing the structure and not at the top or bottom where sloping sides would lead to volume averaging and inaccurate CT numbers.

The partial-volume effect may also result in a size anomaly; that is, the diameter of small, low-contrast structures lying horizontally in or near the scan plane appear larger for thin slices than for thick slices, in that there is less volume averaging of the structure for thin slices. Thin slices more accurately portray the true dimensions of structures. This is also true for structures oriented obliquely within the slice plane. In a related effect, the appearance of blood vessels can appear nodular if only the short sequence of the vessels lies within the slice, which can be confusing. This is more pronounced with thinner slices. If a structure falls between two slices but is very different from the tissue otherwise residing in those voxels, then the structure will appear larger than it really is, since it could be detected in both slices. In general, the most reliable CT numbers are for voxels well away from tissue interfaces.

The partial-volume effects are reduced for systems having a greater distance between the x-ray source and the detectors as well as for systems having larger focal spots. Also, tight collimation will make slices be more parallel, and there will be less divergence of the beam over the dimensions of the patient. The focal spot size effect is due to the fact that point sources have the greatest divergence. Extended focal spot sizes act as line sources and have lesser divergence and form more parallel beams. For this reason, the large dimensions of the focal spot should be aligned along the z-axis of the gantry.

Spiral CT scanning has significantly affected the partial-volume averaging problem. Since one has a true 3D data set, there are no overlaps or missing segments. Every part of the volume is actually scanned. As a result, a lesion would not generally lie partly in one slice and partly in another. Reconstruction of a slice can be done at any given level, or one can choose a reconstruction interval and be assured that the lesion is entirely within the slice thickness or is suffering from minimal partial-volume artifacts (see Fig. 32.15C). The linear and nonlinear effects discussed above, however, will still be true even for spiral scanning since one still has a given slice thickness and pixel sizes.

In the above discussion, simple linear averaging has been emphasized. If the tissue contents of a given voxel include an abrupt edge of a highly absorbing, high-contrast material such as bone, metal, or contrast media, then the nonlinear volume-averaging effect occurs. The basis for this is that attenuation is exponential and nonlinear. When CT number differences are small, the exponential addition functions can be approximated linearly. When exponential attenuation inconsistencies along different ray paths become large enough, then visible streaks appear. This occurs for metal structures, high-contrast

interfaces, and bony structures. Nonlinear volume averaging streaks occur along with aliasing and beam-hardening streaks, and they can be hardly distinguished one from the other. They can be minimized most efficiently by decreasing slice thickness (36).

Partial-volume artifacts can also be reduced with computer algorithms (37); however, the simplest and most direct way to overcome the partial-volume effect is to scan thinner slices. An extension of this approach to minimize streaks is to scan multiple, thin slices and then average them into the larger, desired slice thickness. Presumably, the thinner slices will add linearly, and while the simple volume averaging is present, one overrides the nonlinear effect that produces the streaks (38). As an alternative, at least one CT vendor for a number of years configured a split-beam system wherein a dual-arc detector array is used that detects two thin slices simultaneously. These can either be reconstructed as individual thin slices or combined into a larger slice thickness. Again, the nonlinear effects and streaks generally can be minimized while having available short time scans free of noise problems when using dual-detector technology (39). The advantages of such an approach are multiple, and a number of other CT vendors have announced multidetector, multislice configurations for their future scanners. Tables 32.8 and 32.9 summarize partial-volume effects.

Profile Sampling

Figure 32.17 shows the intensity profile of the x-ray beam after it has emerged from the patient. The variations in intensity correspond to the variable transmission along each ray path. This profile, together with all the other profiles taken at different angles or views around the patient, represents the total information necessary for the reconstruction process. This intensity profile is incident on the detector array. Each detector intercepts and averages that portion of the profile that is incident over its face, which constitutes a sampling process. The sampled profile transmitted to the computer, therefore, is not the exact replica of the incident profile but only its degraded representation (dashed curve in Fig. 32.17). This degradation takes the final form of decreased spatial resolution (note that valleys and peaks tend to be flattened or smoothed out). Additionally, information is lost between detectors,

TABLE 32.8. *Partial-volume effect and missing structures*

Structure falls between two slice edges and does not contribute full contrast to either slice

Effect is aggravated if there are large space increments between slices

It may be lost in averaging effect if volume occupied is small

Effect is aggravated by low sensitivity slice edges

TABLE 32.9. *Partial-volume effects*

Type	Cause	Effect
Simple-volume averaging	Different tissues with similar CT numbers within slice	CT number discrepancies and spatial resolution loss
Profile-volume averaging	Different slice profile around isocenter	Same as above
Nonlinear-volume averaging	Very dissimilar tissues within slice	Streaks
Slice biconcavity	Diverging beam	Reduced sensitivity and/or missed tissue volume

Note: In all cases, the best cure is thinner slices. To reduce biconcavity effect, slices can be overlapped.

depending on how large the detectors are as well as the space between them. As either of these dimensions increases, progressive image degradation occurs.

As noted in Fig. 32.17, the sampled image has features that are not a true representation of the original profile. This by itself does not result in streak artifact and there will be only a loss of spatial resolution; however, another phenomenon occurs that does result in visible streaks. This latter effect is referred to as aliasing and can affect any digitizing and sampling systems. As seen on an image, aliasing along the profile appears as visible linear streaks or as a moiré pattern if linear streaks from different structures superimpose.

To understand aliasing effects, we use the concept of object or profile frequency, which refers to the rapidity with which x-ray intensity profiles change. High-frequency profiles, therefore, imply the presence of sharp-edged structures or relatively small structures where profiles are rapidly changing. Low frequencies represent larger, more diffuse and smooth profiles that are not as rapidly changing. A distinction has to be made between profile frequency (view sampling) and sampling frequency, which refers to how often a sample measurement is collected over the profile, that is, how closely samples are collected in time and space. The aliasing effect occurs when an object is not sampled at close enough intervals, that is, high-enough sampling frequency (Fig. 32.18). As noted, a simple sinusoidal profile has some particular frequency, and if the profile is sampled at a high sampling rate, that is, over very short intervals (Fig. 32.18A), then this frequency and amplitude of that profile can be completely and accurately determined. However, if sampling is coarse and the sampling distances are relatively large, that is, the sampling rate is low (less than two samples per cycle) (Fig. 32.18D), then the resulting pattern has totally different amplitudes and has a lower frequency than present in the original pattern, and therefore aliasing is present. If this had been a CT scan, aliasing would represent fictitious information, resulting in inconsistencies and streaks. If the signal pattern is sampled only once per cycle, then all frequency and all amplitude information is lost (Fig. 32.18C).

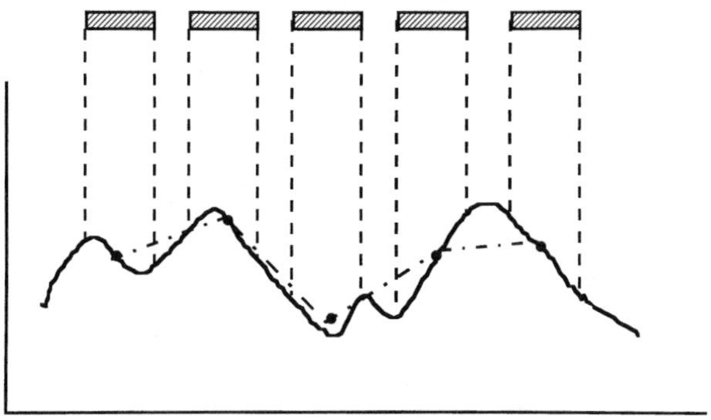

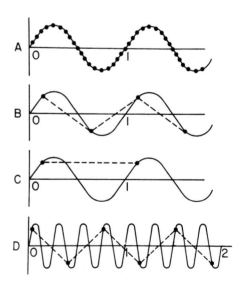

FIG. 32.18. Nyquist sampling. **A:** A pure sinusoidal signal sampled at many points very close to one another (high sampling rate) will reproduce signal very accurately. **B:** A signal sampled twice per cycle will yield accurate frequency information even though amplitude information may be in error. **C:** A signal sampled only once per cycle will lose all frequency and amplitude information. **D:** A sinusoidal signal sampled infrequently (less than twice per cycle) results in a bogus (aliased) curve *(dashed line)*. This inconsistency may result in streaks.

DISTANCE ALONG IMAGE

FIG. 32.17. Variation in intensity profile. Profile sampling of the intensities along the fan beam for one particular view or projection at a given angle. This intensity distribution falls on the detector bank. Detectors *(shaded)* average out the intensity over their face diameter. The detected profile is thus degraded *(line connecting dots)*, and loss of spatial resolution occurs (peaks and valleys are smoothed over), depending on the size of the detectors and the interdetector space.

When the pattern is sampled at least twice in a cycle, the recorded frequency is accurate and is identical to that of the original pattern (though amplitudes may be different) (Fig. 32.18B). We refer to this sampling frequency as the Nyquist frequency (f_n), which is the highest frequency that will be accurately sampled. As a consequence, if we are to preserve the full frequency information present in an image and avoid aliasing streaks we merely sample at twice the maximum frequency (f_m) present in the x-ray profile:

$$f_n = 2f_m = \frac{2}{d} \qquad [4]$$

The maximum frequency in the profile will be determined by the detector size. In this case, if the detector width is d, then an approximation to f_m is $1/d$. To sample at the Nyquist frequency, therefore, the profile must be sampled twice $1/d$ as is given in Eq. 4.

The important conclusion here is that one must obtain at least two samples per detector width. For third-generation systems this is accomplished with the quarter-offset method. Even then, two samples per detector width is a minimum, as there are, in fact, higher frequencies present in the image signals that go beyond the approximation of $1/d$ due to the sharp edges at the detector. In fact, it has been shown theoretically that up to four samples per detector width are needed to completely suppress aliasing (40). As a result, even the quarter-offset approach, which provides for only two samples per detector width, may not entirely eliminate aliasing. In practice, however, the problem of obtaining many samples per detector width is reduced due to the blurring produced by the finite focal spot size. The focal spot acts like a low-pass filter in that it blurs the higher frequencies produced by the detector sharp edges. Incorporating a low-pass (smoothing) filter into the detection process also removes the higher frequencies and reduces aliasing, but with the consequence of poorer spatial resolution. Unfortunately, then, such low-pass filtering regardless of source may also blur useful image information.

The requirement for at least two samples per detector width is easily accomplished with a fixed detector in fourth-generation systems. Here, one can sample the data at any arbitrary time and rate since the detectors are stationary and the beam slides across the detectors (Fig. 32.19C). The downside of this approach, however, is that fourth-generation systems have an x-ray scatter problem that occurs because scatter-suppressing collimators cannot be positioned in front of the detectors; the detectors must sample beam from all angles as the x-ray tube rotates around the patient. Scatter, when present, can lead to artifacts similar to beam hardening and the partial-volume effects. Another fourth-generation problem is that systems are more sensitive to x-ray output fluctuations. This is true since each view is acquired over an extended period of time.

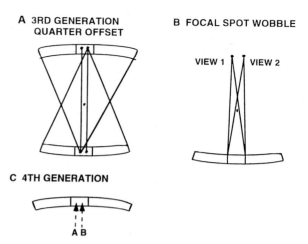

FIG. 32.19. Profile sampling schemes for third- and fourth-generation systems. **A:** Quarter offset method. Detectors are aligned one-quarter of their width to the side of the isocenter at opposing 0-degree and 180-degree views. This results in each detector receiving two distinct ray paths through the patient and aliasing is avoided since two samples per detector width are collected. **B:** Focal spot wobble. Once a view is taken (view 1) and the x-ray tube rotates one detector width, the focal spot of tube is deflected back to its previous position on the focal spot, and the detector sees a second view (view 2) through the patient onto the same detector, again avoiding aliasing problem. **C:** Fourth-generation systems have stationary detectors with the x-ray beam sweeping across each detector. Aliasing is avoided by taking multiple samples at each detector as the tube rotates around the patient. Here, the sample is taken at position A of the leading edge of the x-ray beam and then at position B. Therefore, two readings are obtained per detector, or even more if desired.

Third-generation systems present a different problem in that detectors are moving along with the x-ray beam and one cannot obtain two samples per detector width. The advantage, however, is that because of the fixed geometry between source and detectors, a collimator can be used to suppress x-ray scatter. To overcome the problem of obtaining two samples per beam width, the quarter-offset approach is used. Here the center of the detector array is offset by exactly one-fourth of a detector width. The central ray, therefore, will be displaced on either side of the isocenter by this amount. As a result, the 180-degree view would have sampled tissues along a ray displaced by one-half the detector width as compared to the 0-degree view. These two views will interleave each other and the requirement for two distinct samples per detector width is satisfied since, in effect, the sampling rate has been doubled (Fig. 32.19A). The quarter-offset approach relies on two sets of samples taken 180 degrees apart, separated by the time it takes the gantry to rotate between these two positions. As a result, any patient motion between these two times will significantly impair the alias-suppression feature. Notice that scans performed in less than 360 degrees (underscans) will leave some projections without their interleaved partner, and such scans will be more susceptible to aliasing streaks. Other limitations of the quarter-offset approach is that displacement of the interleaved samples increases for the peripheral detectors, which results in artifact reduction being location dependent.

Another approach for obtaining two samples per detector width is to wobble the focal spot (41,42). After a given projection is obtained, the detector/tube assembly rotates one-half of a detector width; then the focal spot is deflected back to the previous location and another projection obtained. The result is a slightly different view through the patient within the same detector sampling area, and the required two samples per detector width satisfy the conditions to suppress aliasing (Fig. 32.19B). One normally sees aliasing streaks at abrupt, high-contrast tissue interfaces, long structures, and metal objects. All third-generations systems, however, successfully implement either the quarter-offset or the focal spot wobble approach, and profile aliasing is not a major problem.

Angular Sampling

As a result of an inadequate number of angular view samples around the patient, streak artifacts can be formed. However, these streaks, although radiating from small, dense areas, always occur at some distance from the object. Streaks due to view undersampling usually lead to artifacts in the image emanating from the undersampled structure, but, as stated above, they first appear at some distance from that structure, because the sampling frequency near the high-density object may be high enough to satisfy the Nyquist criteria. Few, if any, streaks then occur near the object. The aliasing artifact becomes worse as the object is further from isocenter. Patient tables are designed such that their edges do not superimpose streaks over the image.

It has been shown that there is a relationship between the number of angular views (N) and the distance at which streaks will first appear (40). Ideally, one would choose N so that streaks would appear beyond the maximum patient diameter or expected field of view (FOV). The maximum resulting resolution obtainable in terms of the modulation transfer function (MTF), cutoff frequency MTF$_f$, and the fan angle (σ) is given by the following equations:

$$N = 2 \, (FOV) \, MTF_f/(1 - (\sin \sigma/2)) \qquad [5]$$

$$N = 3 \, (FOV) \, MTF_f \qquad [6]$$

These equations state that the number of views or projections needed to avoid view aliasing increase for a given spatial resolution as FOV increase. Likewise, resolution improves as the number of views increases. From Eq. 5, it is seen that the fan angle is also important. However, fan angles for most CT scanners are similar, and therefore the number of views depends on the FOV and MTF of the sys-

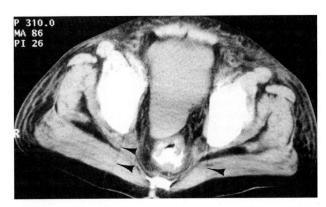

FIG. 32.20. Streak artifacts. Streaks from bone soft tissue interfaces *(arrowheads)*.

tem (Eq. 6). Typical fan angles are usually between 50 and 60 degrees, while the typical number of projections is well over 1,000. The maximum resolution (MTF$_f$) is usually determined by pixel size, detector width, and the smoothing function algorithm utilized in the reconstruction process. In general, the greater the number of views, the greater the spatial resolution (MTF) and the lesser the aliasing problem. Note also that the greater the fan angle, the greater the diameter at which streaks will appear and the lesser the aliasing problem. For a further discussion of MTF, the reader is referred elsewhere (43,44).

Whether due to profile or angular sampling, aliasing streaks combined with dynamic range problems are found around clips; biopsy probes; metallic high-contrast objects, such as prostheses; sharp, bony interfaces (Fig. 32.20); and air-fluid interfaces (Fig. 32.20). It should be noted that nonlinear partial-volume, scatter, and detector nonlinearities also produce similar artifacts.

Longitudinal Sampling

Another possible source of aliasing artifacts is longitudinal sampling, which is related to reconstruction intervals along the longitudinal z-axis of the patient in spiral scanning and is referred to as the stair-step artifact. It is seen on an image as a stair-step discontinuity for structures that have their long axis sloping along the longitudinal direction. Aliasing along the longitudinal direction occurs whenever the reconstruction interval is large and table increments are small. If spherical objects are imaged, the artifact manifests itself as concentric circles. If the reconstruction interval is small and the table increment is large, the artifact for spherical surfaces appears as spiraling circles (45). If linear or planar structures are scanned (such as in CT angiography), appearance is of an erratic or step-like nature.

The stair-step artifact can be virtually eliminated for short reconstruction intervals and small table increments. Table 32.10 lists the various approaches to minimizing aliasing streaks.

TABLE 32.10. *Minimizing aliasing effects*

Reduce slice thickness
Reduce detector sizes
Reduced pixel size
Increase number of projection views around patient
Decrease field of view (FOV)
Obtain two samples per detector width
  (third-generation systems)
Increase fan angle
For spiral scanning, reduce reconstruction intervals and
  reduce table increments

Out-of-Field Artifacts

The FOV scanned should be large enough to encompass the full patient size. Otherwise, attenuation data will be detected but not accounted for in the reconstruction process. This incomplete and inconsistent sampling will result in streaks and/or inaccurate CT numbers (Fig. 32.21). They arise not only from the patient's anatomy but also from any nearby scanned structures like patient life support lines and other objects.

Sometimes, one may opt to purposely scan a smaller FOV than the overall size of the anatomy in order to optimize spatial resolution. Under ideal conditions, the spatial resolution is given by the size of the pixel, which, in turn, depends on the FOV and matrix size as given by Eq. 2. The resolution increases (smaller sizes can be seen) as the FOV decreases, which is the justification for restricting the FOV. The best resolution obtainable for a system is given by the pixel size, which is expressed in terms of the FOV and matrix size as in Eq. 2. In practice, the focal spot size and other system limitations prevent the resolution's exceeding a certain value regardless of what FOV is used. For instance, a typical current system has an optimal FOV of 13 cm (46). In this case, further decreases in FOV need not improve spatial resolution.

DATA-DETECTION ARTIFACTS

After establishing how the attenuation data will be collected and sampled, the x-rays must be detected. Detectors either are placed on an arc that is moving along with the x-ray tube for third-generation systems, or are fixed in the gantry independent of x-ray tube motion for fourth-generation systems.

In the third-generation systems, each projection will yield the required ray profile and all data for one projection are collected in a very short period of time. However,

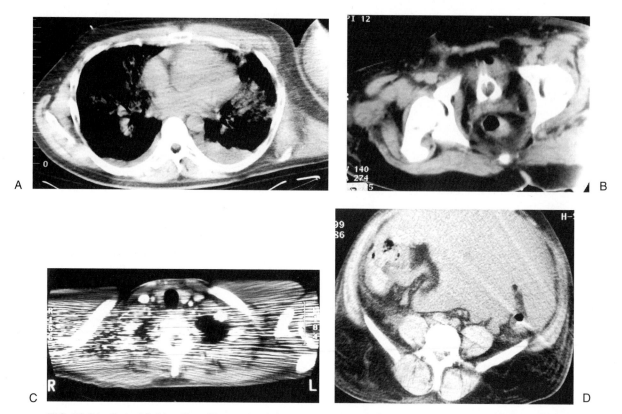

FIG. 32.21. Out-of-field artifact. The artifact occurs when part of the anatomy lies outside of the scanned field. **A:** The left arm is outside the scanning field. **B:** The entire left side of the image is distorted, and there is noise over the image. **C:** Patient support lines in the left side are out of field, resulting in streak artifacts. **D:** Both shoulders are out of the reconstruction field, resulting in extensive artifacts.

in the fourth-generation systems, the full profile of data for each angular view is obtained at the end of the full scan. In all cases, a fan beam of x-rays falls on an array of detectors. These detectors must be calibrated to yield equal sensitivities.

Detectors themselves can either be of the solid-state type or of the ion chamber type. Solid-state detectors are relatively small and very efficiently absorb the incident x-rays and therefore have a very high quantum efficiency ($\approx 99\%$). These detectors scintillate when they absorb x-ray energy. The light thus emitted is converted to an electrical signal via a photodiode. Scintillators include cadmium tungstate ($CdWO_4$) or combinations of ceramic yttrium (Y_3O_3) and gadolinium (Gd_2O_3).

Ion chamber detectors consist of a series of thin charged plates separated by a space filled with up to 20 or 30 atmospheres of pressurized xenon. Radiation produces ionization in the xenon, which is collected at the plates to produce the required signal. Since the active medium here is a gas, the quantum efficiency is inherently low. Pressurizing the gas increases the number of gas molecules available to absorb the x-rays, which increases sensitivity. Additionally, detectors are configured with depths of about 2 inches to increase the path length of the x-rays within the gas and therefore increase the probability of x-ray absorption. Gas detectors make up for their lower quantum efficiency, in part, by having less dead space between them.

The demand on CT detectors is very high (Table 32.11). They must have a wide and linear dynamic range to avoid overranging and the data dropout problem that contributes to the clip artifact. They must be very efficient to reduce patient dose, low image noise, and scan at relatively short times. They must also be configured in a very small space to preserve spatial resolution and to avoid aliasing affects. They must be very fast, that is, they must have very little afterglow or persistence. Minimal afterglow is necessary since samples are detected with only millisecond intervals between projections. In the

presence of afterglow, the signal from one projection affects the signal from a subsequent projection. The results from this would not be only classic blurring but also inconsistencies leading to streaks or shading and/or inaccurate CT numbers.

Finally, the signal from these detectors must be reproducible and capable of extremely little drift in their calibration. The calibration step is necessary to assure that each detector response is matched to all the other detectors to avoid artifactual streaks.

Third-Generation Ring Artifacts

If detectors do drift in their calibration, the resulting inconsistencies are manifested differently depending on whether detectors are fixed or moving. Third-generation systems with their moving detectors characteristically form rings, while fourth-generation systems are very tolerant of detector drifts.

In third-generation systems, each detector remains in a fixed geometry with respect to the x-ray tube. If any detector starts drifting, then data along each of the ray paths leading to that detector are changed as compared to the adjacent detector responses. Because of the back projection algorithm, a faint line or streak will occur depending on the magnitude of drift. As the tube/detector assembly rotates around the patient, a point such as P in Fig. 32.22 is affected only once. Points around the circle drawn, however, will have an error reinforced from the

TABLE 32.11. *Required detector characteristics*

Feature	Reason
Wide dynamic range	Avoid overranging and loss of data
Very efficient	Lower patient dose
	Shorter scan times
	(less motion problems)
	Low image noise
Very fast	Minimize:
(little afterglow)	CT number inaccuracies
	Shading
	Streaks
	Preserve spatial resolution
Small size	Preserve spatial resolution
	Minimize aliasing problem
Reproducible and	Avoid inconsistencies and
reliable	streaks

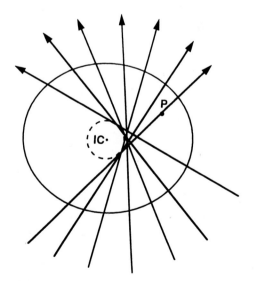

FIG. 32.22. Third-generation ring artifacts. The drifting detector will produce erroneous readings along each of its ray paths around the patient. A point such as P is sampled only once by that particular drifting detector. Points along the circle drawn *(dashed line)* is sampled many times, and erroneous values are reinforced along this circle centered around the isocenter (IC). Visible ring structures result for each drifting detector.

various intersecting view angles, and the locus of such points so intersected forms a circle around the isocenter of the unit. This is a result of the fact that each ray path measured at each detector is tangent to a circle whose radius is the distance from the isocenter to that particular detector. Drifts as small as 0.1% can cause these objectionable artifacts. If more than one detector is drifting, then a series of concentric circles will occur. If similar errors are experienced by a number of detectors simultaneously rather than single rings, we then get bands or a bull's eye–type pattern (Fig. 32.23A). It should be emphasized that detector malfunction or calibration drift produces ring artifacts in third-generation systems.

The system sensitivity to ring artifacts is not uniform across the detector arc. It is most severe and visible around the isocenter and less toward the periphery (Fig. 32.23B). The propensity to produce rings also depends on the particular algorithm. High-resolution algorithms tend to produce more prominent rings.

Detector calibration drift can be due to a number of reasons: a simple sensitivity drift, electronics dark current, noncompensated detector afterglow, and changes in or some radiation damage to the detector. In general, to the extent that these errors are predictable and characterized, they can be corrected.

To avoid these rings and bands, one needs a combination of very stable and reproducible detector elements as well as frequent detector calibration. In third-generation systems, if the patient is in place, then the detector is constantly behind the patient, and if the detector drifts, no calibration correction can be performed and the whole image suffers. This is very different for fourth-generation systems, in that detectors at the leading edge of the rotating fan can be calibrated just before it goes behind the patient. Historically, the first- and second-generation systems also provided opportunity for detector calibration before each data collection. Such calibrations assure that each detector and its electronic channel are responding with equal sensitivity.

If rings persist, even after drift correction, then the problem is either mechanical, due to rotation faults, or electronic, somewhere between the detector output and the computer, including the back projection array processor.

Both the solid-state and ion-chamber type of detectors are subject to calibration drift. The solid-state detectors, however, are somewhat more sensitive to this problem. Manufacturers usually recommend a calibration scan with no patient in place every few hours for solid-state systems.

Data collection for fourth-generation systems is such that errors are not reinforced for any one drifting detector and, therefore, detector problems are not as severe. Since each detector collects data over the full range of projection angles, detector drifts tend to average out over the full image. In fact, one can eliminate particular detectors

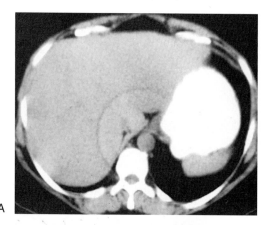

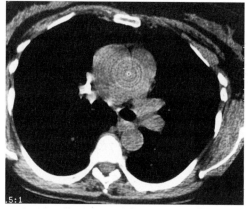

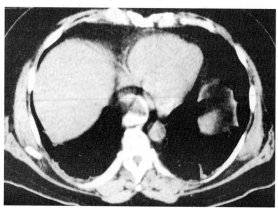

FIG. 32.23. A clinical example of third-generation ring artifacts. **A:** The example of a simple band. **B:** Multiple bands can occur if multiple detectors are drifting. **C:** An artifact suggestive of third-generation ring origin. The severity of the ring increases as the detector gets closer to the isocenter (seen here as a *solid band*).

without seriously affecting the image. If rings appear in fourth-generation systems, these are probably produced by a default in the back projection process rather than by faulty detectors.

Faulty detector channels can also be readily detected in scanograms (scout views). Since all scanograms are performed with a linear traverse across the patient, then the faulty channel will produce straight lines along the direction of the scanogram motion, regardless of gantry generation.

Detector Dynamic Range

Detectors must be linear over a very wide range of x-ray intensity values. The problem of nonlinearities due to limited dynamic range have already been discussed along with the associated problem of clip artifacts arising from data fallout. Dynamic range problems introduce nonlinearities similar to the beam-hardening effect.

The original EMI Mark I unit overcame the limited dynamic range of the original NaI scintillation crystals used at that time with a water-box fixture around the patient's head. This eliminated the large x-ray intensity difference resulting when x-rays pass either through air or through the patient's head. The water box eliminated the air, and the range of x-ray intensities was significantly reduced. Reduction of the incident x-ray intensity range to assure that it more closely falls within the dynamic range of the detectors can also be performed with a bow-tie filter.

Finally, software corrections for detector nonlinearities can be accomplished, to some extent, with simple linearization of the detector response, such as was done for the beam-hardening artifact effect minimization.

In summary, detectors play a vital part in the CT process and can introduce unwanted artifacts due to faulty measurements that are, consequently, used in the reconstruction process. Corrections for faulty x-ray measurements can take the form of frequent calibration of the detectors, reduction of incident range of x-ray intensities, or mathematical correction for nonlinearities (2).

Scatter

The effects of scatter are very much like the effects of beam hardening since both produce a cupping effect and dark bands between highly absorbing structures. Because the x-ray beam is collimated into a relatively thin fan beam, there is relatively little scatter in CT scanning. Scatter can have a significant impact on image quality (47).

Scatter directs photons to each detector. For ray paths through highly absorbing structures, there is relatively little primary radiation arriving at detectors and scatter becomes relatively more significant. Since additional photons (due to scatter) are detected along each ray path, the reconstruction process assumes that tissues along that ray path were not as dense as they really were, and a lower CT number is assigned in a nonlinear manner, which results in a darker

shade of gray, shading streaks, and inaccurate CT numbers. The scatter effect also depends on the size and composition of the patient being scanned. In essence, if rays pass through highly absorbing tissues or structures, then the detected intensity is low and the scatter contribution becomes increasingly important. The same situation exists if there is leakage current in the detector. Here again, if attenuation is high, the leakage current signal becomes significant compared to the detected signal, in which case the reconstruction process assumes that the greater amount of signal was due to lower attenuation in the tissues, and once again the CT numbers appear lower.

The scatter problem is of lesser importance in third-generation systems since antiscatter, predetector collimators can be utilized for each solid-state detector (Fig. 32.24A). If an ion chamber system is used, the depth of the chamber serves as a built-in collimation system (Fig. 32.24B). Fourth-generation systems, however, have to detect radiation from a wide range of angles, and collimation is impossible.

The scatter problem can be reduced by increasing the distance from the patient to the detector bank. This allows scattered rays to diverge away and not reach the detectors. Another factor that minimizes scatter is the use of bow-tie filters, which reduce radiation intensity incident on the periphery of the patient, where most scatter reaching the detectors is generated. The periphery produces more scatter than the center of the patient since there is less self-absorption of the scatter as compared to the thicker mid-regions of the patient.

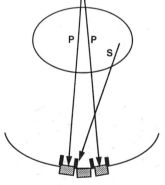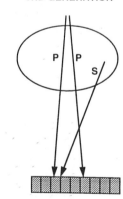

A. SOLID STATE DETECTORS 3RD GENERATION

B. GAS DETECTORS 3RD GENERATION

FIG. 32.24. Scatter collimation. **A:** Third-generation solid-state detectors are fixed relative to the moving fan beam and can be collimated effectively. Shown are primary rays (P) arriving at the detectors, and scattered rays (S) originating on the patient being collimated out. **B:** Third-generation gas detectors. The depth of the ion chamber serves as effective collimation. Shown are primary rays (P) and scattered rays (S). Primary rays having a long path length within the detector will yield a greater signal. Note: No collimation is possible since the detectors must detect rays from all angles. The scatter problem is more critical.

Finally, it is possible, in theory, to correct for scatter since it is approximately constant over the detector bank. It can also be corrected by measurement in a plane offset from the primary fan beam plane. However, this is not usually done in practice.

DATA PROCESSING

After the data are measured, the electrical signal created is digitized using an analog-to-digital converter and sent to the computer for processing. The data processing demands are great because of the many image points (pixels) involved as defined by the matrix size. To decrease processing time, data are sent through an array processor so that mathematical operations can be performed at each data point in parallel. The array processor can be a source of artifacts, as it can produce rings on fourth-generation systems where none are expected. Occasionally, the artifacts completely obliterate the image, which can be explained by a fault in the reconstruction process (Fig. 32.25). Regular maintenance and system calibration can reduce the occurrence of such artifacts.

In addition to the required back-projection algorithm used to perform the reconstruction, there are a number of software routines that are available to perform various imaging features. For instance, there are edge-enhancing and smoothing functions that can be applied to the data. Edge-enhancing systems in particular are prone to creating artifacts or to accentuating the appearance of artifacts that may already be present. This is particularly true when nonlinear effects are present such as the nonlinear partial-volume artifact, detector faults, and beam-hardening artifacts. As an example, third-generation rings are much more conspicuous using edge enhancement. Various software approaches to correct artifacts may in turn induce or accentuate artifacts of their own.

The nature of spiral scanning is such that unique planes have to be synthesized from spiral data. Various algorithms are available for this; however, the 180-degree linear interpolation algorithm produces the least effect on image quality and artifact formation, though slightly increasing the noise content as compared to the older 360-degree interpolation schemes. Other algorithms may introduce even more artifacts. The 180-degree linear interpolation is currently the preferred approach.

Finally, each manufacturer may incorporate proprietary software that may or may not make reconstructions prone to the various artifacts discussed here. Further discussion on algorithms and software induced artifacts are mathematically complex and beyond the scope of this text.

DATA DISPLAY AND CHEMICAL PROCESSING ARTIFACTS

A number of factors serve to introduce artifacts at the display stage. These include window/center level setting, pin cushion distortion of video displays, and adjusted vertical linearity of the video monitor, as well as the chemical processing yielding the final hard copy.

Window and Center Level Settings

Window/center level settings are used to optimize the gray scale display of CT images. The entire structure can be made to disappear depending on the window and levels chosen to view the images. Many units have 4,000 shades of gray available within the computer corresponding to the −1,000 to +3,000 range of CT numbers. No video monitor is capable of displaying all of these nor would it be advisable, since the human eye is incapable of appreciating all such gray steps. The window level control adjusts the available video gray scale to the specific tissues one desires to see. Specifically, the computer assigns the mid-gray density of the display device to the CT number corresponding to the chosen center level. The window determines the range of CT numbers that will be displayed within the given range of video grays around the chosen center level. Figure 32.26 shows what is happening for a particular window and center level of 0 (curve A). All tissues below −50 are assigned

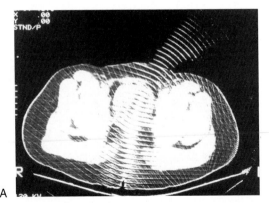 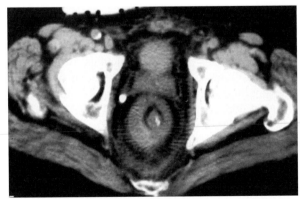

FIG. 32.25. Combination artifact. **A:** Criss-crossing artifact suggestive of reconstruction problems. **B:** Combinations of reconstruction and superimposition of streak patterns from an object on or near the patient in addition to beam hardening.

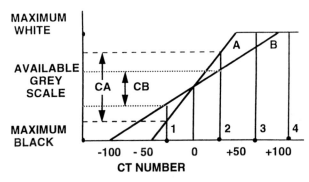

FIG. 32.26. Effects of window and level. Window level settings effect contrast of the image and visibility of specific tissues. Curve A with a level of 0 and window of 100 (±50) and curve B with level of 0 and window of 200 (±100). Curve A with a narrow window produces a larger contrast (difference in density) between tissue 1 and 2 as compared to curve B. Tissues falling in region 3 will be totally white with no contrast with the curve A window, and yet have some contrast and still be visible on the curve B window. Tissues falling in region 4 will not be visualized in either window as they will all be totally white.

black and all tissues above +50 are assigned the brightest value available. The tissues between −50 and +50 are assigned the grays in between, with the center level of 0 being the mid-gray. Notice from this figure that the window essentially defines the slope of the density curves. The resulting image contrast is the difference in display density between any two tissues. Along curve A the image contrast between tissues 1 and 2 is some value C_A. Curve B is for a level of 0 and a window of 200 (e.g., −100 to +100). It will result in image contrast C_B for the two displayed tissues. The narrower window of 100 (curve A), results in greater contrast C_A for the same two tissues when compared to C_B. The downside of the narrower window, however, is that all tissues above +50 will appear white and all tissues below -50 will appear black; fewer tissues will fall within the display range. The tissues falling outside the chosen window will not be visualized.

Pin-Cushion Distortion

Pin-cushion distortion is a nonlinear effect that is in part due to the curved face on a video monitor. The result is that linear structures will appear to be bowed inward, and all structures are distorted in size and shape. This looks further aggravated if an individual with astigmatism is observing the monitor display.

The best way to test for pin-cushion distortions is to image a wire grid composed of equally spaced crisscrossing linear wires or structures. The scan of such a phantom should show lines with equal spacing in all parts of the image. Figure 32.27A shows the possible pin cushion pattern when this artifact is present. Such distorted images bring into question any quantitative linear measurements that may be attempted (however, corrections are not that difficult).

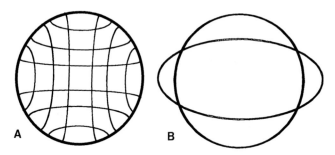

FIG. 32.27. Video display problems. **A:** The square grid phantom when scanned should have totally straight vertical and horizontal lines. Pin cushion artifacts result in bowing of the lines. **B:** A true circle scanned can appear elliptical *(dashed curve)* if vertical linearity of the monitor is not adjusted correctly.

Video Monitor Linearity

Another distortion that can occur is when vertical linearity on a monitor is not adjusted properly. Then circular bodies take on more elliptical shapes, such as in Fig. 32.27B. Again, such distortions affect accuracy of linear relationships on the image and their measurements.

Both of the above nonlinearity problems will result in erroneous information if measurements or judgments are made directly based on the video monitor. The approach for detecting this problem is to scan a known circular object and view the results on the video monitor, and then measure the horizontal diameters of the circle and compare it to the measured vertical diameter to be sure that they are the same.

Hard-Copy Processing

After the image is acquired and viewed, a hard copy is normally made. Historically, multiformat cameras have been used for this purpose. A multiformat camera exposes images of a video monitor. These cameras were limited by the video monitor spatial resolution. With laser printers, image information is directly converted into laser beam intensities. The laser directly exposes a film, and the video system is entirely bypassed. Image quality, therefore, is expected to exceed that available from multiformat cameras. In either case, the exposed film has to be chemically processed, and artifacts can result from such processing. Chemical variables and quality control programs for such systems are well documented in the literature (48). More recently, dry processing has been introduced, and similar quality control steps need to be taken.

One disconcerting processing artifact is attributable to static discharge on films, which may mimic lesions (49). These artifacts are usually round and are darker than the surrounding tissues. These types of artifacts are more likely to be seen under low humidity, mid-winter conditions, and may also occur due to the friction in automatic film-loading devices, or whenever films slide over surfaces or over each other. They may also appear from pressure marks when removing or loading the film from carriers and cassette.

Dirt on the cassette or in contact with film may also introduce artifactually low-density spots on image.

Dirt, dust, and lint on films and on cassettes not only can cause static discharges but also can increase the likelihood of their occurrence (49,50). Cleaning cassettes using antistatic solutions may eliminate these artifacts. To ensure that such images are indeed artifactual, one checks the image on the video monitor, as these artifacts appear only on hard copy and only after chemical processing. Alternately, one can refilm the image, since the chance of repeating an identical static discharge artifact is very low.

CONCLUSION

A variety of artifacts apply to abdominal and pelvic CT scanning. Some of these artifacts are rarely seen; others

TABLE 32.12. *Artifacts*

Image features	Artifact name	Cause	Remedy
Streaks and shading	Beam hardening	Differential attenuation In polychromatic beams (aggravated by motion)	Added filtration Bow-tie filter Software corrections
	Patient motion	Voluntary motion Breathing bowel motion Blood vessel pulsation Cardiac motion	Decrease scan time Overscan/underscan Software corrections Gating
	Nonlinear Partial volume	Beam divergence Abrupt high contrast in tissue thickness edges within voxel (aggravated by motion)	Decrease slice thickness Increase matrix size (decrease pixel size)
	Sampling deficiency	Insufficient sampling Profile sampling Angular sampling	Increase matrix size (decrease pixel size) Increase angular sampling Decrease size of detectors
	Clips and Metallic objects	Overranging of detectors Insufficient sampling of detectors Aggravated by motion	Use of wide dynamic range detectors Software corrections Minimize motion Thinner slices Large matrix size
	Out-of-field objects	Object or anatomy scanned but not within reconstructed field	Assure all anatomy within reconstructed field
	Equipment/ Misalignment	Equipment failures and malfunctions	Effective maintenance and calibration program
	Rotor wobble	Variable x-ray source output	Replace x-ray source
	Detector malfunction Circular rings Linear streaks	Calibration drift (third-generation ring artifact) Overranging (insufficient dynamic range)	Frequent calibration Choose wide dynamic range detectors
CT number inaccuracy	Beam hardening	Differential attenuation of polychromatic beam	Added filtration Bow-tie filters Software corrections Thinner slices
	Partial-volume effect Loss of resolution CT number errors		Larger matrix size (smaller pixels) Reconstructing FOV to be smaller Spiral scanning Decrease scan time
	Misregistration	Motion/breathing	Overlapping scans Spiral scanning
	Detector malfunctions/ calibration drifts	Detector system faults	Frequent calibrations Repairs and maintenance
	Generator kV(p) drifts		Frequent calibration
	Stair-step	Reconstruction intervals too short or too long relative to pitch	Short reconstruction intervals and short table increments
Structure disappearing, indistinct borders	Partial-volume effect	Tissue averaged out and/or indistinct borders within voxel Tissues very similar to surrounding	Reduce slice thickness
	Misregistration	Motion/breathing	Decrease scan time
	Wrong window/level settings	Tissues outside of window will not be seen	Assure correct window settings for tissues to be seen
Ghost structures	Double contouring	Tissues due to motion are recorded at opposing angles in duplicate	Decrease scan times

are quite common, such as the simple and nonlinear partial-volume and beam-hardening artifacts. Motion used to be the most severe streak artifact and still cannot be discounted; however, as scan speeds have increased, it has decreased in frequency and importance. Table 32.12 summarizes the more important feature of artifacts and how they are minimized.

With the rejuvenation of CT, continued technologic advances are to be expected. The most exciting of these currently is the advent of multidetector arc, multislice systems, which have the ability to scan with higher pitches in shorter scan times and minimal artifacts. Software and x-ray tube heat capacity advances are fully expected to take advantage of new imaging possibilities for the future, such as CT angiography, 3D techniques, and virtual imaging. If one collects a full 3D data set at relatively short scan times, the misregistration artifact is minimized, because there is no interscan delay time allowing the structure to move to new positions due to motion and not be scanned. Also, because of the ability to arbitrarily pick any level to reconstruct, we can ensure maximum lesion contrast and minimize the partial-volume effects. Dual-slice detector systems promise to minimize aliasing effects as well as nonlinear partial-volume effects, since relatively thin slices can be obtained and combined to give equivalent thicker slices with minimal artifacts.

Three-dimensional reconstructions are now also possible with minimal artifacts. Spiral scanning has also made CT angiography a more viable modality. As scan times and x-ray tube rotation times are reduced even further, one goal would be to accomplish real-time or near real-time CT fluoroscopy. Unfortunately, as these technologies mature, they will most likely introduce new artifacts, resulting in more diagnostic pitfalls and indicating that the artifact problem is not yet over.

REFERENCES

1. Villafana T. Physics and instrumentation: computed tomography. In: Lee SH, Rao KCVG, Zimmerman RA, eds. *Cranial MRI and CT.* New York: McGraw-Hill, 1992.
2. Joseph PM. Artifacts in computerized tomography in computed tomography. In: Newton TH, Potts DG, eds. *Radiology of the skull and brain, technical aspects of computed tomography.* St. Louis: CV Mosby, 1981.
3. Hsieh J. Image artifacts, causes and correction. In: Goldman LW, Fowlkes JB, eds. *Medical CT and ultrasound: current technology and applications.* Advanced Medical Publishing, Madison, Wisconsin 1995:487–518.
4. Krestal E. *Principles of computed tomography in imaging systems for medical diagnostics.* Siemens, Berlin, Germany 1990.
5. Kuszyk BS, Fishman EK. Technical aspects of CT angiograph. *Semin Ultrasound CT MRI* 1998;19:383.
6. Hsieh J. Non-stationary noise characteristics of the helical scan and its impact on image quality and artifacts. *Med Phys* 1997;24(9):1375.
7. Foley W, Oneson SR. Helical CT: clinical performance and imaging strategies. *Radiographics* 1994;14(4):894.
8. Wyatt S, Urban BA, Fishman EK. Spiral CT evaluation of the kidney. In: Fishman EK, Jeffrey RB Jr, eds. *Spiral CT principles: techniques and clinical applications.* New York: Raven Press, 1995.
9. Padhani AR, Watson CJE, Clements L, Calne RY, Dixon AK. Computed tomography in abdominal trauma: an audit of usage and image quality. *Br J Radiol* 1992;65:397.
10. Bernardino ME, Fishman EK, Jeffrey RB, Brown PC. Comparison of iohexal 300 and diatrizoate meglumine 60 for body CT: image quality, adverse reactions and aborted/repeated examinations. *AJR* 1992;158:665.
11. Stockberger SM, Hicklin JA, Liang Y, Wass JL, Ambrosius WT. Spiral CT with ionic and non-ionic contrast material: evaluation of patient motion and scan quality. *Radiology* 1998;206:631.
12. Vergara M, Sequel S. Adverse reactions to contrast media in CT: effects of temperature and ionic property. *Radiology* 1996;199:363.
13. Crawford CR, Pelc NJ. Method for reducing motion induced artifacts in projection imaging. U.S. patent 4,994,965. 1991.
14. Hsieh J, Gard MF, Ritchie CJ. Methods for reducing motion induced artifacts in a projection imaging system. U.S. patent 5,271,055. 1993.
15. Ritchie CJ, Hsieh J, Gard MF, Godwin JD, Kim Y, Crawford CR. Predictive respiratory gating: a new method to reduced motion artifacts on CT scans. *Radiology* 1994;190:847.
16. Liang Y, Kruger RA. Dual slice spiral scanning: comparison of the physical performance of two computer tomography scanners. *Med Phys* 1996;23:205.
17. Stockberger SM, Hicklin JA, Liang Y, Wass JL, Ambrosius WT, Kopecky KK. Objective measurements of motion in patients undergoing spiral CT examinations. *Radiology* 1998;206:625.
18. Rubin GD, Leung AN, Robertson VJ, Stark P. Thoracic spiral CT: influence of subsecond gantry rotation on image quality. *Radiology* 1998;208:771.
19. Rao PS, Alfidi RJ. The environmental density artifact: a beam hardening effect in computed tomography. *Radiology* 1981;141:223.
20. Young SW, Miller HH, Marshal WH. Computed tomography: beam hardening and environmental density artifact. *Radiology* 1983;148:279.
21. Haaga J, Reich NE. In: *Computed tomography of abdominal abnormalities.* St. Louis: CV Mosby, 1978.
22. Ruth C, Joseph PM. A comparison of beam hardening artifacts in x-ray computerized tomography with gadolinium and iodine contrast agents. *Med Phys* 1995;22:1977.
23. Jennings RJ. A method for comparing beam hardening filter materials for diagnostic radiology. *Med Phys* 1988;15(4):588.
24. Cann CE. Quantitative computed tomography. In: Moss AA, Gamgu, Genant HK, eds. *Computed tomography of the body.* Philadelphia: WB Saunders, 1983.
25. Kejewski PK, Bjorngard BE. Correction for beam hardening in computed tomography. *Med Phys* 1978;5:209.
26. Joseph PM, Spital RD. Method of correcting bone-induced artifacts in computerized tomography scanners. *J Comput Assist Tomogr* 1978;2:100.
27. Joseph PM, Ruth C. A method for simultaneous correction for spectrum hardening artifacts in CT images containing both bone and iodine. *Med Phys* 1997;24(10):1629.
28. Alvarez RL, Macovoski A. Energy selective reconstructions in x-ray computerized tomography. *Phys Med Biol* 1976;21:733.
29. Vetter JR, Holden JE. Corrections for scattered radiation and other background signals in dual-energy computed tomography material thickness measurements. *Med Phys* 1988;15:726.
30. Duerinckx AJ, Macorski A. Polychromatic streak artifacts in computed tomography images. *J Comput Assist Tomogr* 1978;2:481.
31. Robertson DD, Weiss PJ, Fishman EK, Magid D, Walker PS. Evaluation of CT techniques for reducing artifacts in the presence of metallic orthopedic implants. *J Comput Assist Tomogr* 1988;12(2):236.
32. Fishman EK, Magid D, Robertson DD, Brooker AF, Weiss P, Siegelman SS. Metallic hip implants—CT with multiplanar reconstruction. *Radiology* 1986;160:675.
33. Kalendar WA, Hebel R, Ebersberger J. Reduction of CT artifacts caused by metallic implants. *Radiology* 1987;164:576.
34. Gross SC, Kowalski JB, Lee SH, Terry B, Honickman SJ. Surgical ligation clip artifacts on CT scans. *Radiology* 1985;156:831.
35. Glover GH, Pelc NJ. Non-linear partial volume artifacts in x-ray computed tomography. *Med Phys* 1980;7(3):238.
36. Stockham CD. A simulation study of aliasing in computed tomography. *Radiology* 1979;132:721.
37. Henrich G. A simple computational method for reducing streak artifacts in CT images. *Comput Tomogr* 1980;4:67.
38. Hupke R. The advantage of fast and continuously rotating CT systems. In: Fuchs WA, ed. *Advances in CT.* New York: Springer-Verlag, 1990:3.
39. Hu H. Multi-slice helical CT: scan and reconstruction. *Med Phys* 1999;26(1):5.
40. Joseph PM, Schulz RA. View sampling requirements in fan beam computed tomography. *Med Phys* 1980;7:692.

41. Sohval AR, Fruendlich D. Plural source computed tomography device with improved resolution. U.S. patent 4,637,040. 1986.

42. Hsieh J, Gard MF, Gravelle S. A reconstruction technique for focal spot wobbling. In: *Proc SPIE Med Imaging,* vol 4. Newport Beach: 1992:175.

43. Villafana T. Advantages limitations and significance of the modulation transfer function in radiological practice. In: Moseley RD Jr. *Monograph in current problems in diagnostic radiology,* vol 8. Chicago: Yearbook Medical, 1978:3.

44. Barnes GT, Lakshminarayanan AV. Computed tomography: physical principles and image quality considerations. In: Lee JKT, Sagel SS, Stanley RJ, eds. *Computed body tomography with MRI correlation,* 2nd ed. New York: Raven Press, 1989.

44a. Berland LL. *Practical CT technology and techniques.* New York: Raven Press, 1987.

45. Wang G, Vannier MW. Stair-step artifacts in three-dimensional helical CT: an experimental study. *Radiology* 1994;79–83.

46. Mayo JR, Webb WR, Gould R, et al. High resolution CT of the lungs: an optimal approach. *Radiology* 1987;163:507.

47. Glover GH. Compton scatter effects in CT reconstructions. *Med Phys* 1982;9:860.

48. Haus AG. *Film processing in medical imaging.* Madison, WI: Medical Physics, 1993.

49. Wilbur AC, Kriz RJ. Round CT film static artifacts: simulation of focal pathology. *J Comput Assist Tomogr* 1989;13:730.

50. Spizarny DL, McCloud TC, Dedrick CG, Shepard JO. Pseudo-metastases secondary to film static artifact. *Comput Radiol* 1986;10:207.

Variants and Pitfalls in Body Imaging,
edited by Ali Shirkhoda.
Lippincott Williams & Wilkins, Philadelphia, © 2000.

CHAPTER 33

Physical Principles of Ultrasound Artifacts

Lance V. Hefner

PRINCIPLES OF ULTRASOUND

The modern ultrasound machine is a marvel of technology and is capable of producing exceptionally high-quality images. As technology has advanced, many earlier limitations have been overcome, but it behooves us, the operators of these wondrous machines, to understand their fundamental limitations. The ultrasound machine forms its images based on a number of assumptions that may or may not be correct. The machine does not have the judgment to differentiate between situations where those assumptions are correct and those in which they are inappropriate. This chapter discusses the assumptions that allow the ultrasound machine to construct an image, and the artifacts that can result from inappropriate assumptions.

The ultrasound machine operation is based on a series of premises:

1. The ultrasound transducer creates a series of small pulses of sound that travel in a straight line without deviation and at constant speed throughout the tissue.
2. The sound is reflected by structures within the patient, each reflector returning one echo along the same path as the initial sound pulse, with the return time indicating the reflector's depth.
3. The ultrasound energy does not spread, is uniformly attenuated in tissue, and the frequency is known and unchanging.
4. The listening time between pulses is sufficient for the deepest reflectors, and each succeeding sound pulse interrogates new tissue without overlap.
5. The echo energy accurately represents the reflectivity of tissue, its duration represents the tissue thickness, and the return time represents the reflector location. Therefore, the echo information represents the patient anatomy.

These premises provide a logical framework for the ultrasound machine operation (1,2). The ultrasound transducer is electrically pulsed and the transducer in turn produces a short pulse of sound. The sound travels into the patient until it interacts with a structure, which reflects some or all of the acoustic energy. The time required for the sound to travel and return allows the ultrasound machine to determine the total distance traveled, based on an assumed acoustic speed. When the total path length is divided by two, the result is the depth of the reflector. A period of time elapses between each pulse to provide time for the echoes from the most distant reflectors to return or the acoustic energy to dissipate. The position of the echoes is then mapped along a line, which represents depth within the patient. The amplitude of the echo determines the brightness of the line at that depth. A second pulse is then generated, which interrogates an adjacent area of tissue in a similar fashion. The second pulse is then followed by a third pulse, and so on. An image is built up based on the information acquired from a number of sound pulses interrogating a volume of tissue. In real-time ultrasound, the process will be repeated many times each second to show changes in the tissue over time.

We now examine these premises in some detail and discuss where the assumptions fail.

Pulse/Echo

The ultrasound transducer resonates when it receives an electrical impulse. Its behavior is similar to that of a tuning fork. When a tuning fork is struck, it will begin to vibrate and produce a tone. It will continue to give off the sound for a long period of time unless you stop the vibration by placing your hand or some other object over the tines of the fork (Fig. 33.1). It gives off acoustic energy in a series of wave fronts that continue for an extended period of time. If a sound-absorbing backing, called a damper, is attached to

---

L. V. Hefner: Department of Diagnostic Radiology, William Beaumont Hospital, Royal Oak, Michigan 48073-6769.

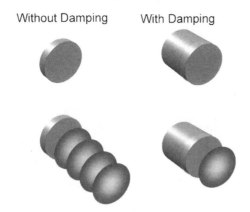

Without Damping   With Damping

FIG. 33.1. The transducer, before and after it is pulsed, produces sound like a tuning fork. Damping constrains the sound to a short pulse.

the back of the crystal, the resonance will be muffled and a much shorter sound pulse will be created. There are transducers that are designed without dampers. These are commonly used in continuous wave (CW) ultrasound. CW ultrasound is concerned with detecting the presence of flowing blood, which produces an audible frequency shift, rather than identifying a precise location.

Time/Distance Measurement

The ultrasound machine assumes that there is a direct relationship between the return time of an echo and the distance of a reflector. This assumption is based on the premise that sound has a finite velocity, and a period of time will elapse as the sound travels to a reflector and then returns to the transducer. If the distance is increased, then the period of time required for the sound to cover the distance will also increase. In Fig. 33.2, a transducer has produced a sound pulse. The sound pulse interacts with two reflectors. The distance to reflector 1 is d and the distance to reflector 2 is $d + x$. Reflector 2 is further away than reflector 1, by the additional distance x. The time it takes

for a sound pulse to travel to the reflectors is given by the following formula: time = distance divided by velocity. Therefore, the time an echo takes to return from reflector 2 should be larger than for reflector 1 by an amount proportional to the ratio of the distances or $(d + x)/d$.

Figure 33.3 shows a transducer and the resulting image. On the left the transducer has sent the sound pulse, and is waiting for the return of echoes from reflectors. The echo from the deeper reflector takes more time to reach the transducer. The first echo is displayed on the image as a closely positioned object. The second reflector is displayed in a more distance position on the image. The ultrasound unit constructs the image based on this simple model. The return time of an echo is proportional to the depth of the reflector in the field. This model works well as long as the acoustic energy takes a straight-line path, with no deviations, and the speed of sound remains constant.

Axial Resolution

The spatial pulse length determines the maximum axial (depth) resolution and the precision of depth location. The assumed speed of sound in tissue is 1.54 millimeters per microsecond (mm/μsec). A 7.5-megahertz (MHz) ultrasound wave will have a wavelength of 0.2 mm. The wavelength will be shorter at higher frequencies and longer at lower frequencies. A typical ultrasound pulse is 3 to 5 wavelengths in duration. This results in a spatial pulse length of 0.6 to 1.0 mm, at 7.5 MHz. The axial spatial resolution cannot be better than the spatial pulse length. This means that although objects smaller than 1 mm may return echoes, they will be presented as if they were 1 mm in size. This also places a practical limitation on our ability to visualize objects. In this case, objects separated by less than 1 mm, axially, will be merged into one larger object. Figure 33.4 shows two

Distance and Time

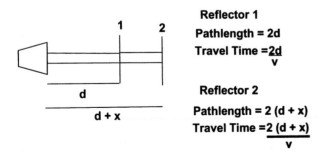

Reflector 1
Pathlength = 2d
Travel Time = $\dfrac{2d}{v}$

Reflector 2
Pathlength = 2 (d + x)
Travel Time = $\dfrac{2 (d + x)}{v}$

FIG. 33.2. Distance versus return echo time. The distance of a reflector is determined by the time required for a return echo.

Image Depth

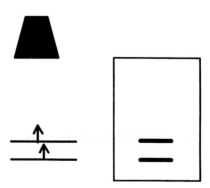

FIG. 33.3. Depth versus return echo time. The ultrasound image displays depth based on the return echo time.

Pulse Length

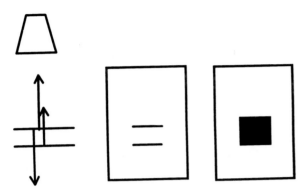

FIG. 33.4. Pulse length and axial resolution. The length of the ultrasound pulse determines axial (depth) resolution.

Beam Patterns

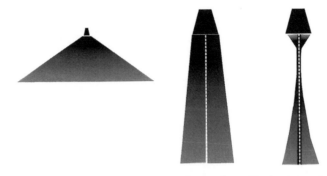

FIG. 33.5. Lateral (width) resolution varies with the type of transducer and reflector depth.

Beam Width Artifact

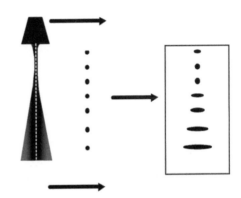

FIG. 33.6. Lateral resolution can result in errors. Changes in lateral resolution, with depth, can result in erroneous image width.

reflectors separated by a distance less than the spatial pulse length. These two reflections are merged into one larger reflection and appear on the image as a single reflector. This relationship between spatial pulse length, ultrasound frequency, and axial resolution explains why higher frequency transducers are often preferred for their increased ability to resolve detail.

A long sound pulse produces two serious problems:

1. It is impossible to accurately locate the reflectors, as the echoes continue as long as the sound pulse is ensonating the reflector.
2. It is impossible to separate superior and inferior reflectors, as the prolonged echoes may overlap, yielding one long echo with no separation between the reflectors.

Lateral Resolution

Ideally, the acoustic energy produced by the ultrasound transducer would travel only where desired. In reality, we have little control over the sound direction. There are several techniques that force most of the energy along the path we prefer, but there is always diffusion of the energy away from the ideal path. We call this distribution of the acoustic energy the beam pattern. Figure 33.5 shows several examples of beam patterns. On the left is the pattern from a small transducer. The small size of the transducer allows the sound to rapidly spread over a wide area. In the middle is a larger transducer with better focusing properties. At the right is a transducer that has been specially focused to concentrate the sound's energy in a narrow region. There are a number of methods to accomplish this focusing, both physical and electronic.

The width of the beam pattern determines the lateral resolution of the ultrasound image at a particular depth.

For example, if the width of the beam pattern changes as the depth increases, then the lateral resolution will also change with depth. Figure 33.6 shows a focused beam pattern. The energy is concentrated in a narrow focal zone and widens at depth. If this beam pattern is used to image a regularly spaced series of small reflectors, the image produced will closely match the width of the beam pattern at various depths. The lateral resolution is determined by the beam width, and even though reflectors smaller than the beam width are detected, they are displayed with a minimum size corresponding to the lateral resolution or beam width.

Speed of Sound

The speed of sound is different for various materials. It varies significantly dependent on the different types of human tissue. Table 33.1 lists the acoustic velocities of

TABLE 33.1. *Acoustic velocities*

Medium	Velocity (m/sec)
Air	348
Blood	1,570
Bone	3,360
Fat	1,500
Liver	1,550
Muscle	1,580
Soft tissue	1,540

several different materials. The average speed of sound for soft tissue is 1,540 meters per second.

The ultrasound unit cannot identify the type of tissue. It must assume that the average speed of sound in human tissue is a good estimate. In most cases, the errors this assumption produces are relatively minor and may be ignored. In less frequent cases the sound may transit a large section of tissue with an acoustic velocity significantly different from the average. In these cases, an artifactual error may arise.

Attenuation

A characteristic of ultrasound and sound, in general, is the attenuation of the acoustic energy with distance. This drop in amplitude is partially explained by distance, but in the case of ultrasound other processes play a more important role. These processes include reflection, scattering, and relaxation effects. These effects can result in the rapid diminishment of the ultrasound intensity. The attenuation of the ultrasound energy is described in terms of a unit called the decibel (one-tenth of a bel). This term is a ratio and is logarithmic. This means we may use it to compare the relative strengths of two ultrasound beams or the same ultrasound beam at varying depths in tissue. Because it is a logarithmic term, it is possible to easily describe large changes in strength. For example, a change of an order of magnitude (a factor of 10) can be described as a difference of 1 bel or 10 decibels. A change of two orders of magnitude (a factor of 100) is described as 2 bels or 20 decibels. This unit is useful in ultrasound as the acoustic energy attenuates on a logarithmic scale in tissue. At 1 MHz, ultrasound attenuates at 1 decibel per centimeter

of tissue. If the sound passes 5 cm (2 inches) into the body, and is completely reflected back from an object, it will travel 10 cm through tissue, round-trip. This results in a change of 10 decibels, or 90% of the initial energy has been lost. If this round-trip were of 20 cm (a depth of 4 inches), the change would be 20 decibels. The returning energy would have lost 99% of its strength compared to the starting signal.

To make matters worse, the rate of energy loss is proportional to the frequency. A 1-MHz signal loses energy at 1 dB/cm, while a 10-MHz signal loses energy at 10 dB/cm. This means every centimeter reduces the signal strength by a factor of 10. A round trip of 10 cm reduces the signal strength to one part in 10,000,000,000. Table 33.2 shows the attenuation in tissue for several different frequencies.

The ability of even the best ultrasound machine to detect returning echoes is limited. The limitation occurs when the returning echo is no larger than the level of background noise. The machine is unable to determine whether the echo is real or just noise. A good ultrasound machine can detect an echo that is 120 decibels weaker than the initial signal. The machine can pick up echoes that only have one part in 1,000 billion of the original signal. Table 33.2 shows signal losses much higher than 120 decibels. These high signal losses occur for the higher frequencies and at larger depths. This is why high-frequency transducers are often called shallow or near-field transducers. High-frequency transducers are unable to image deep tissue because of the high rate of attenuation of ultrasound at those frequencies. Figure 33.7 shows the drop in ultrasound intensity for four different frequencies at a range of depths.

Frequency

It is commonly assumed that the frequency label on the ultrasound transducer matches the frequency of the transducer. While this is generally true, it is also an oversimplification. The transducer may have a nominal frequency on its housing, but there will actually be a broad range of frequencies present. We call the range of frequencies the frequency spectrum of the transducer. Figure 33.8 shows a frequency spectrum for a typical transducer with the nominal frequency shown. Although, in this example, the transducer's peak energy

TABLE 33.2. *Changing attenuation with frequency*

Depth	1-MHz round-trip loss		5-MHz round-trip loss		10-MHz round-trip loss		20-MHz round-trip loss	
	dB	Reduction	dB	Reduction	dB	Reduction	dB	Reduction
5 cm	−10	0.1	−50	1.E−05	−100	1.E−10	−200	1.E−20
10 cm	−20	0.01	−100	1.E−10	−200	1.E−20	−400	1.E−40
20 cm	−40	0.0001	−200	1.E−20	−400	1.E−40	−800	1.E−80

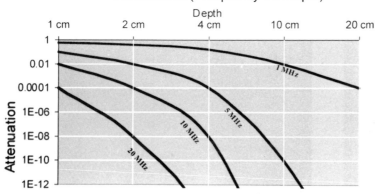

FIG. 33.7. Attenuation versus frequency and depth.

is at the nominal value, this is not always true. There is energy present over a range of frequencies, extending from frequencies lower than the nominal value to frequencies greater than the nominal value. The range of frequencies from the minimum to the maximum is called the bandwidth of the transducer. The purity of the transducer frequency is called the Q. The Q is defined as the nominal frequency divided by the bandwidth. For example, if the nominal frequency was 5 MHz and the bandwidth was 1 MHz (4.5 to 5.5 MHz), then the Q would equal 5 MHz/1 MHz, or 5.

In the discussion of attenuation we saw that the rate of attenuation of the ultrasonic energy is related to the frequency of the sound. Since the energy in the ultrasound pulse is not composed of a single frequency, we might expect the spectrum of the ultrasound to change as it travels through tissue. Higher frequencies are attenuated by the medium they pass through faster than lower frequencies. This results in a shift of the ultrasound spectrum as

the ultrasound beam travels through tissue. In Fig. 33.9, the solid line is the frequency spectrum of the original ultrasound beam. The dotted line is the spectrum of the return echo. The travel of the ultrasound energy through the tissue has resulted in a reduction of the energy at the higher frequencies. This results in an overall shift of the frequencies present in the return echo, and in the alteration of echoes from similar reflectors that are located at varying depths. A deeper object will appear to have been scanned with a lower frequency transducer than a shallow object. This effect is more pronounced for transducers with wide bandwidth, as there is greater range available for a shift. Higher Q transducers show less effects of a shift, but may exhibit less ability to penetrate into deeper tissue. Figure 33.10 presents two images produced from a series of identical reflectors. The left image shows a slight gradual increase in the apparent thickness of the reflectors, while the right image shows less increase in size but a fading of brightness with depth.

Frequency Spectrum

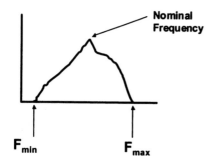

Bandwidth = F_{max} - F_{min}

FIG. 33.8. Transducer energy versus frequencies. A transducer's energy is spread over a range of frequencies.

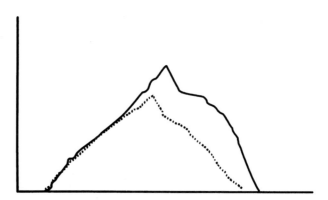

FIG. 33.9. Frequency versus energy absorption. High-frequency acoustic energy is absorbed faster than low-frequency information.

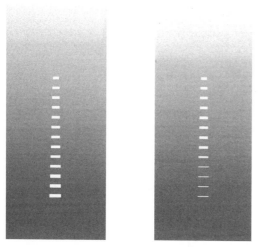

FIG. 33.10. Attenuation may alter a reflector's image. The variable attenuation of ultrasound frequencies may alter a reflector's image at different depths.

ULTRASOUND ARTIFACTS

The ultrasound machine bases the construction of the image on the information provided by the returning echoes. The processing of that data into the images is influenced by the application of a series of premises, which in general are valid. As we have already seen there are times when those premises may not be accurate. These inaccuracies can lead to inaccuracies in patient images. This section discusses some of the artifacts that result during ultrasonography (3).

Reverberation

The first artifact considered is reverberation. An assumption made by the ultrasound unit is that each reflector returns only one echo. There are conditions when this premise is untrue. When a strong reflector is located close to the transducer, and the ultrasound attenuation rate is low, the return echo may be of sufficient energy to reflect back from the transducer face. In this case a secondary pulse of reduced intensity will travel down into the patient. This secondary pulse is artifactual and any resulting echo will produce errors in the patient image. Figure 33.11 shows a reflector located close to the transducer. The acoustic energy is sufficiently strong for several reflections to occur, as the sound bounces back and forth between the reflector and the transducer face. A characteristic pattern results from this type of artifact. The right side of the figure shows a representation of the resulting ultrasound image. A series of diminishing echoes appear with equal spacing. The spacing is equal to the spacing between the transducer and the reflector because these echoes result from multiple transitions of the ultrasound energy across the distance between the transducer and reflector. The reflections gradually dimin-

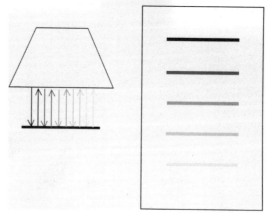

Reverberation

FIG. 33.11. Reverberation, which may occur between a reflector and the transducer face.

ish in intensity because the path length for each reverberation is longer than the preceding echo, and has experienced more tissue interaction resulting in increased attenuation.

Internal

A special case of reverberation may occur with a single strong reflector or when multiple strong reflectors are located near each other, and their orientation permits the ultrasound energy to bounce between the surfaces. As shown in Fig. 33.12, when the acoustic energy trapped between the reflectors bounces, sufficient energy may be transmitted through the reflector to return a detectable echo to the transducer. This is a case similar to general reverberation, but the spacing between the echoes may be

Internal Reverberation

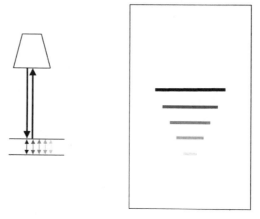

FIG. 33.12. Internal reverberation, which may occur between the front and back surface of a reflector.

very small. This artifact may assume an image similar to a comet tail (4).

Resonance: Tuning Fork

The concept of resonance was discussed earlier. Resonance is crucial to the production of the ultrasound pulse. It may also produce an artifact. A tuning fork is a precision instrument that is designed to vibrate at one particular frequency. As shown in the Fig. 33.13, if we strike the fork it begins to resonate, and while resonating it is a source of acoustic energy at its resonant frequency. Similarly, an ultrasound transducer is a source of sound at the frequencies characteristic of that transducer. A property of resonant objects is their ability to excite a matched resonant object into resonance. Figure 33.14 shows a resonating fork next to a quiescent fork. On the right, the forks are shown a moment later, after the acoustic energy from the first fork has arrived at the second fork. The second fork absorbs the energy arriving from the first fork, which matches its own resonant frequency, and begins to vibrate. The second fork becomes a secondary emitter of acoustic energy at that frequency. This effect only happens when the frequency of the sound energy impinging on the second fork matches the resonant frequency of the first fork. That is, if the energy hitting the second fork does not include energy at the resonant frequency, no secondary resonance occurs.

During ultrasound imaging, return echoes provide us with information about the position and nature of structures within the patient. We do not expect structures within the patient to exhibit resonant characteristics. We expect the structures to either transmit or reflect the sound. In a simple reflection, the returned reflection has a pulse width corresponding to the initial pulse width. The returned echo is smaller in amplitude than the initial pulse and this reduction increases with increased depth. However, the frequency spectrum of the returned echo

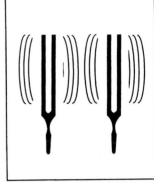
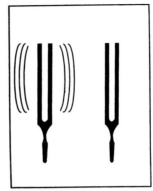

FIG. 33.14. A resonant object may be driven into resonance if bombarded by acoustic energy at its resonant frequency.

generally matches that of the initial pulse. In Fig. 33.15 reflectors are present at several depths, but there is no energy in the spectrum at the reflectors' resonant frequency. The returned energy is attenuated, but has a spectrum similar to that of the original pulse.

The image of a reflector when no resonance exists is an accurate representation of the thickness of the reflector. In Fig. 33.16 the reflector is ensonated and then displayed on the right. The general shape of the image closely matches the actual reflector.

If a resonance occurs, the reflector begins absorbing energy, at its resonant frequency. This energy, instead of being reflected back at the source or transmitted, now becomes the driving energy for a secondary source of acoustic energy. The returned reflection may show a sudden drop in amplitude at the resonant frequency. The energy, which would have been reflected back at that frequency, is being used to drive the resonance of the reflector. Subsequent reflections at greater depth may actually show an increase in energy at the resonant frequency. The

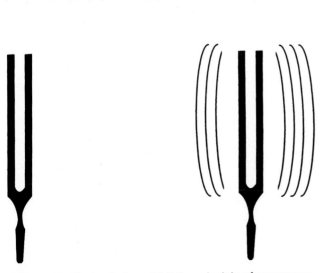

FIG. 33.13. Tuning forks exhibit the principle of resonance.

Resonance
OFF - FREQUENCY

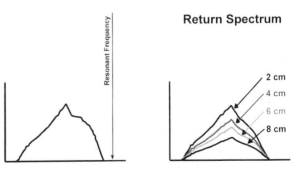

FIG. 33.15. When resonance is absent, the returned energy spectrum will lack discontinuous changes at a single frequency.

Resonance
OFF - FREQUENCY

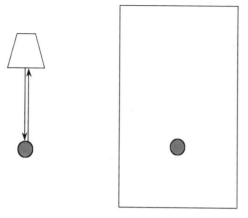

FIG. 33.16. Absence of resonance allows the image to accurately display the reflector, ignoring other possible artifacts.

Resonance
ON - FREQUENCY

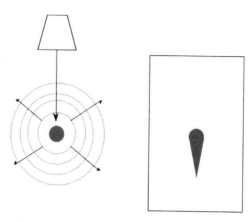

FIG. 33.18. Resonance will cause a reflector to display a long tail.

sound that was subtracted from the spectrum as it passed over the resonant object on its initial interaction is added back as the reflected energy is returning to the transducer. This is seen in Fig. 33.17; the resonant object is at a depth of 2 cm, and the frequency spectrum of the return energy shows a drop in energy at the resonant frequency. The spectra of deeper echoes shows an enhancement of energy at that frequency, as the resonator adds energy to the echoes returning from deeper in the tissue.

If the acoustic environment below the resonant reflector is relatively quiet, the energy being returned from the resonant object may be misinterpreted as increased thickness of the reflector. This occurs because the returned sound pulse may be much longer in duration than the initial pulse width. This increase in pulse width, as shown in Fig. 33.18, mimics what would actually happen if the sound were reflected from a thicker nonresonant object.

Resonance
ON - FREQUENCY

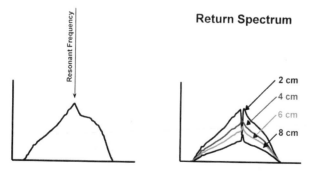

FIG. 33.17. Resonating reflectors cause artifacts. The presence of a resonating reflector will cause a discontinuity in the return energy spectrum at the resonant frequency.

Refraction

When we consider the position of a reflector in an ultrasound image, we make the assumption that the image of the object corresponds to its placement within the patient. This assumption is based on the belief that sound will travel in a straight line. We know from our earliest experiences as a child that this is not always true. Figure 33.19 illustrates a pencil in a glass of water. Either this photo is a cunning special effect, or the light hitting the

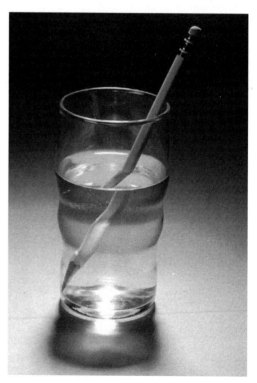

FIG. 33.19. An example of refraction. The illusion of a broken pencil is caused by refraction.

pencil and reflecting back does not travel in a straight line. From our own experience we know that energy, whether light or sound, is influenced by the medium in which it travels.

The concept of this directional distortion was discovered by Willebrod Snell (1591–1626) and is known as Snell's law (Fig. 33.20). It essentially states that a deflection occurs at the boundary between two different media, and the degree of deflection is determined by the difference in velocity of the two media.

The deflection predicted by Snell's law will be away from the perpendicular if the inferior medium has a faster acoustic velocity than the superior medium. The opposite deflection, toward the perpendicular, occurs if the inferior medium has a slower acoustic velocity than the superior medium (Fig. 33.21).

Refraction can give rise to several interesting and perplexing artifacts. In its simplest version, refraction may cause a simple shift in the position of an object. In Fig. 33.22, the ultrasound beam is directed straight down, but

Simple Refractive Error

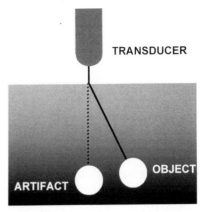

FIG. 33.22. Refractive error may result in artifacts, such as the misplacement of a reflector.

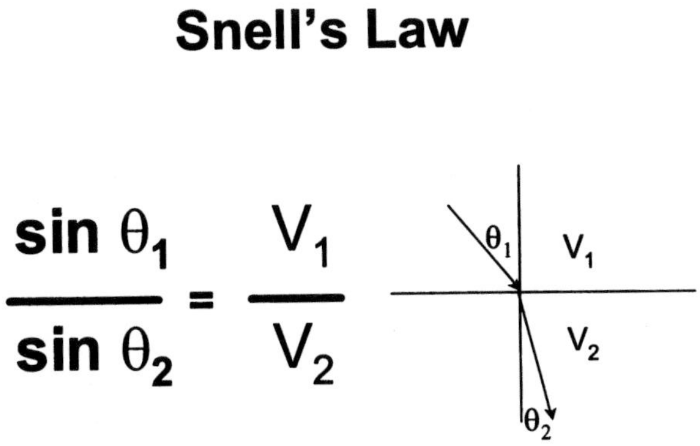

as the energy passes into another medium, the sound is deflected in a different direction. In this case, an object that actually exists to the side of the ultrasound beam may be misplaced to a position directly under the transducer.

A variation of this simple positional shift may occur as shown in Fig. 33.23, if the ultrasound beam passes through a layer of tissue with both a different acoustic velocity and a particular shape. An example of this is focusing. If the shape of the object has characteristics similar to a lens, it may behave similarly to an optical lens. The ultrasound beam may be focused as if it were a converging lens, and inferior objects may appear magnified, or, depending on the acoustic velocity, the tissue may behave as a diverging lens and inferior objects may appear to be smaller.

Snell's Law

$$\frac{\sin \theta_1}{\sin \theta_2} = \frac{V_1}{V_2}$$

FIG. 33.20. Snell's law, which is the mathematical description of refraction.

Refraction

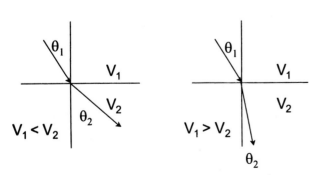

FIG. 33.21. Refraction. The sound's change in direction will be determined by the difference in acoustic velocity of the two media.

Focussing

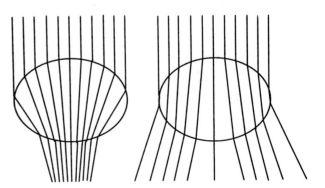

FIG. 33.23. Refraction may cause focusing. Refractive error may result in either the focusing or defocusing of the acoustic energy.

One of the most elegant ultrasound artifacts resulting from refraction is the ghost image (5), which results when an object is present in the acoustic field with the proper velocity and shape to act as a prism. We are familiar with the common optical prism (Fig. 33.24). When the pencil is seen through a prism, the pencil apparently splits into two completely separate pencils. In this figure the artifact is easy to detect, but if we were to see only the portion of the pencil covered by the prism and were unaware of the prism's presence, we might easily be misled into believing there were two pencils.

Figure 33.25 illustrates how this artifact may occur. The acoustic energy directed to the side of the actual object passes into the prismatic structure and is deflected to the center. As it passes out of the structure, the energy is once again deflected. The energy may strike an object and then be reflected to return through the two previous deflections, in reverse. The reflected energy appears to be coming from the sides rather than from directly beneath the transducer. In this fashion, the true object is invisible, while two false images appear to either side of its actual position (Fig. 33.26).

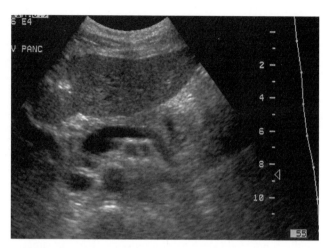

FIG. 33.26. A clinical example of double-image artifact of the superior mesenteric artery.

Reflection

The next major source of artifacts is the simple principle of reflection. Figure 33.27 gives examples of the two types of reflection, specular and diffuse. We are accustomed to reflection occurring from exceedingly smooth surfaces such as a mirror. Specular, or mirror-like, reflection occurs when the surface of the reflector is smooth in comparison to a wavelength of the reflected energy. The reflected light loses little energy and the reflected angle matches the incident angle. A specular light reflector must be exceedingly smooth, as the wavelength of light is very short. If the reflector surface is not smooth the reflector is said to be a diffuse reflector, and the reflected light travels in all directions, similar to a movie theater screen. The surfaces of organs are seldom sufficiently smooth to be specular reflectors of light, yet they may behave as good specular reflectors for ultrasound. The wavelength of ultrasound is significantly larger than the

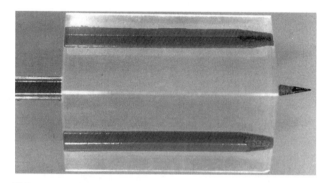

FIG. 33.24. An optical example of the ghost artifact is shown with a pencil and a prism.

GHOST (Double Image)

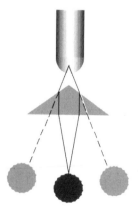

FIG. 33.25. The ghost artifact may create a double image from a single reflector.

Reflection

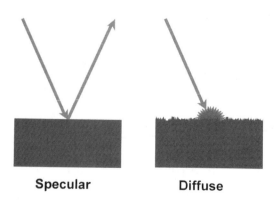

Specular   **Diffuse**

FIG. 33.27. Reflection may occur at a smooth surface (specular) or at a rough surface (diffuse).

wavelength of light, typically between 0.1 and 1 mm. Tissue surfaces smooth to within this range exhibit specular reflection of ultrasound. This is not a source of artifacts, in the special case where the surface of the reflector is perpendicular to the source of the ultrasound beam. More often, the acoustic energy may be redirected with little or no loss in energy in an entirely new direction.

When the ultrasound beam is redirected, a simple reflection artifact may occur. Figure 33.28 shows on the left the redirection of a portion of the ultrasound energy out of the expected area. Underneath the reflector is an area of shadow, which is not being examined by the ultrasound beam. On the right, the area on the image corresponding to this shadow area has been filled with echoes returning from an object outside the shadowed area. Figure 33.29 gives a clinical example of this artifact. This object may be inside the examined field, appearing as duplicate objects, or may be outside the examined area altogether. The misdirected sound has traveled from the mirror to the object and has been reflected. The reflected sound travels back to the mirror and bounces into the transducer, as if its path had not been altered. This misdirected energy fools the ultrasound machine into misplacing those echoes into the shadowed area inferior to the acoustic mirror.

Generally, this simple reflection artifact is easily detected by anyone with knowledge of the typical patient habitus. A slight tilt of the transducer alters the incident angle of the ultrasound beam and causes the artifact to change position or disappear altogether. More troubling is the case when the artifactual image is not clearly a recognizable anatomic feature that has been misplaced. In this case it may not be apparent that it is an artifact and the sonographer may not perform the simple tilt test to determine if reflection is present. This may occur if the specular reflector is not flat, but curved. In this case, as shown in Fig. 33.30, the shape and size of the artifact may

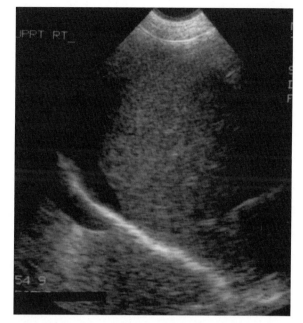

FIG. 33.29. Clinical example of reflection by the diaphragm. Image below the diaphragm is artifactual.

Complex Reflection Artifacts

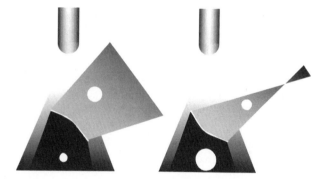

FIG. 33.30. Curved reflectors will cause artifacts, such as misplacing reflectors and distorting their shape.

Simple Reflection Artifact

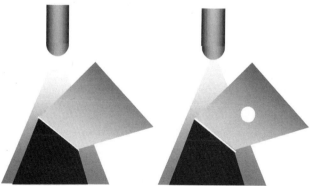

FIG. 33.28. Reflection may cause artifacts, such as sound energy directed in unexpected directions.

bear little relationship to the original object. The artifact may be larger, smaller, inverted, or appear like an object in a funhouse mirror.

Acoustic Shadowing

Another type of artifact may occur when a reflector is present in the examined field that is unusually bright; it returns most of the incident energy, with little energy remaining for transmittance. In this case (Fig. 33.31), inferior objects are cast in relative shadow, compared to adjacent objects. Objects located under a very bright reflector appear to be less reflective than similar anatomy, which is not shadowed by the superior reflector.

Acoustic Shadowing

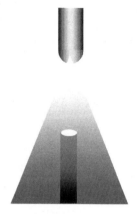

FIG. 33.31. Bright reflectors may cast acoustic shadows beneath them.

Acoustic Enhancement

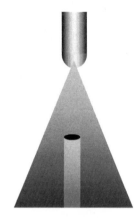

FIG. 33.32. Acoustic enhancement. Areas of low attenuation may cause inferior tissue to appear unusually bright.

Acoustic Enhancement

Acoustic enhancement is an artifact similar to acoustic shadowing. Ultrasound energy in the body is attenuated at a known rate. The amount of attenuation depends on the frequency of the ultrasound and the depth of penetration. Ideally, the ultrasound machine may be adjusted to compensate for this normal attenuation with a device called the time gain compensator (TGC). This device increases the amplification of returning echoes as the sound travels deeper to reduce the effect of attenuation and allow similar reflectors to appear equally bright in the image, regardless of their depth. The enhancement artifact occurs when an object is present in the field, which passes the ultrasound energy with no or little attenuation. In this case (Fig. 33.32), the TGC overamplifies the returning signals inferior to the low attenuation object, causing them to appear unusually bright.

Propagation Speed Error

The propagation speed artifact occurs because of the mistaken assumption that the speed of sound in tissue is constant. The ultrasound machine does not know the type of tissue under investigation and must therefore make an assumption about the acoustic velocity. If the material is uniform in terms of the velocity, then we may see some overall errors in size or position, but no errors in shape. If the acoustic velocity is greater than 1,540 meters per second, the image depth will be slightly reduced, because the echoes will return faster than expected. If the acoustic velocity is less than 1,540 meters per second, the image will be slightly increased, because the echoes will return slower than expected. This distance change occurs because the ultrasound machine relates return echo time to distance. Errors in shape occur when the object partially underlies an area of tissue with a velocity very different than the rest of the media. In Fig. 33.33 an organ

Propagation Speed Errors

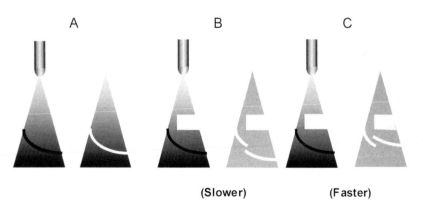

FIG. 33.33. Varying acoustic velocity may cause errors. The presence of tissue with an unexpected acoustic velocity may cause inferior reflectors to appear either too close or too far from the transducer.

boundary is shown that is inferior to an area of different acoustic velocity. The actual shape of the reflector is shown in Fig. 33.33A. The slower inclusion causes the boundary of the organ underlying it to be shifted away from the transducer in Fig. 33.33B. The faster inclusion causes the boundary of the organ underlying it to be shifted closer to the transducer in Fig. 33.33C.

Beam Width

We have already discussed details concerning the axial, or depth, resolution of an ultrasound transducer. The resolution in the lateral dimension will also influence the ultrasound image. As the ultrasound energy moves away from the transducer the energy spreads out. The actual pattern of the beam as it moves away from the transducer may be influenced by many factors that we will not cover here, but the shape often possesses a focal region with very good spatial resolution, and lower quality resolution, anterior and posterior to this focal region. We call this the beam pattern and it often has a classic hourglass shape. Figure 33.34 shows a beam pattern as it begins to sweep across a series of vertically placed point reflectors. On the far right is the resulting image. In the focal region, the lateral resolution is good, so the point reflectors are shown as points. Above and below this region, however, the point reflectors are imaged as line segments. The width of the line segment in the image is related to the width of the beam pattern at that depth. A clinical example is shown in Fig. 33.35. This can result in a filling artifact in the examination of cystic structures. Figure 33.36 shows a cyst that is being examined with a transducer. The walls of the cyst in the focal region are accurately represented. The walls posterior to the focal

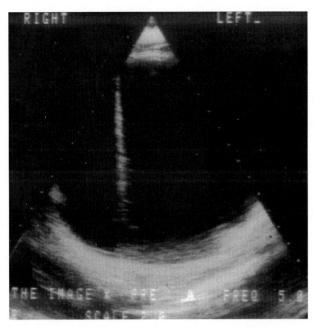

FIG. 33.35. Clinical example of artifact due to beam width. Artifactual thickening of the cerebral falx is due to changes in beam width.

region are imaged by the lower portion of the beam pattern and look excessively wide. This results in the appearance of debris within the cyst, although there may be no debris present. This artifact may be demonstrated by changing the interrogation angle of the cyst. If the wall thickening or the apparent debris rotates as the transducer is tilted, then this is an artifact.

Beam Width Artifact

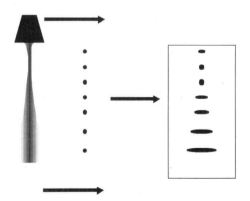

FIG. 33.34. Changes in lateral resolution with depth can result in erroneous image widths.

Beam Width Artifact

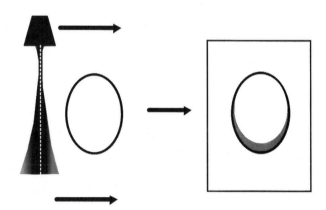

FIG. 33.36. Poor lateral resolution may result in errors. Scanning a cyst at a poor lateral resolution may result in erroneous wall thickening or filling.

Range Ambiguity

Range Ambiguity

The speed of ultrasound in tissue places a maximum limit on the thickness of tissue, which may be investigated each second. The average acoustic velocity in tissue is 1,540 meters per second. As the sound must both travel to a reflector and return, the maximum amount of material examined is no more than 770 meters each second. This may seem to be a very large number, but in actuality is barely enough for real-time ultrasound to be performed. Let us consider an abdominal examination, with a desired penetration of 20 cm. If we wish to obtain a good image, we may want the image to be composed of 500 separate lines, each line examining a different but adjacent section of tissue. When we combine all these lines we obtain a single ultrasound image (Fig. 33.37). To obtain this single image we may use five hundred 20-cm lines or 100 meters of our 770 meters of distance. If we desire to now examine this tissue in real time, we find that ten frames per second is impossible because that would require an acoustic velocity of 2,000 meters per second, and we are limited to 1,540 meters per second. We could, however, image at five frames per second, as that requires a velocity of only 500 meters per second. The seemingly large 770 meters of useful distance per second is rapidly used up when creating high-quality real-time images. In this example, we made an assumption that the sound will stop after 20 cm. This assumption is in error, and leads to the range ambiguity artifact. There is no fundamental reason that the sound will stop at 20 cm. The acoustic energy will continue until it is completely attenuated in the medium. The maximum depth of penetration may be greater than the assumed depth. If the sound strikes a strong reflector at a depth

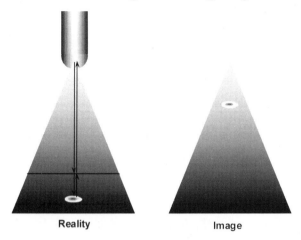

FIG. 33.38. The range ambiguity artifact, which may occur if the speed of sound is assumed to be infinite.

exceeding our arbitrary limit, a detectable echo may be returned. The ultrasound machine is producing a series of short pulses of sound and then waiting a period of time to listen for echoes before making the next pulse. If we have set up the machine, assuming a maximum depth of 20 cm, then an echo resulting from 21 cm will not arrive at the transducer in its appropriate interval. The echo from 21 cm will be imaged in the next interval as if it were at a depth of 1 cm (Fig. 33.38). There are several corrections for this artifact. The length of time between pulses may be increased, but this will require either fewer lines per image, reducing quality, or a lower frame rate. Another solution is to change to a higher frequency transducer. The attenuation rate is proportional to the frequency. If we increase the frequency of the transducer, the rate of attenuation may be increased until no echoes from the anatomy outside our area of interest are sufficiently large to be imaged.

Side Lobes

In our earlier discussion of the beam pattern, we indicated that the acoustic energy spreads out as it leaves the transducer. The majority of the energy is in a main central lobe, which travels directly out from the transducer face. The transducer also emits a smaller amount of energy at angles to the main lobe. We call this energy side lobes. Generally, the amount of energy present in a side lobe is so small that the much louder echoes from the main lobe obscure any echoes from the side lobe. On occasion, circumstances make it possible to discern echoes from a side lobe. This set of circumstances requires the presence of a nonechogenic object in the main lobe. This results in an area with no reflected energy to obscure side lobe echoes (Fig. 33.39). This can occur within a cystic structure. At these times the small echoes

The Sound Barrier

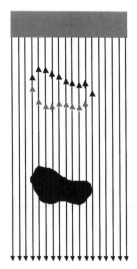

FIG. 33.37. The acoustic velocity of sound in tissue allows many projections to be made each second.

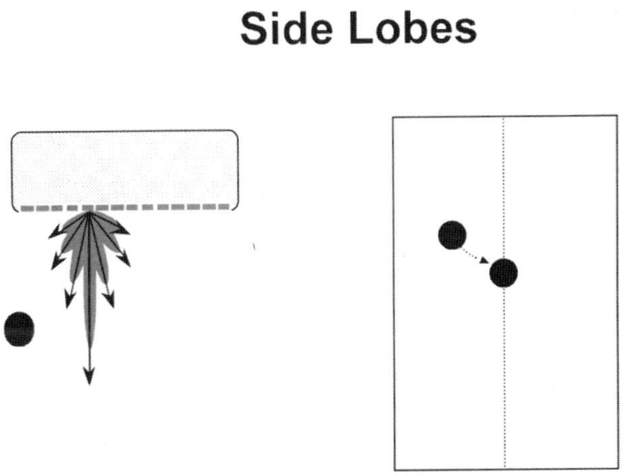

Side Lobes

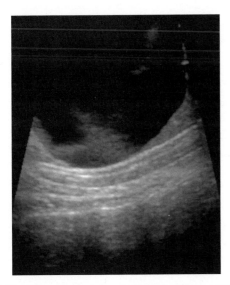

FIG. 33.39. Side lobes. Most acoustic energy is present in the central ray. The reduced energy in the side lobes may be visualized under special conditions.

FIG. 33.40. Clinical example of side lobe filling within a liver cyst.

from the side lobes may be imaged within the quiescent interior of the cyst, presenting an erroneous filling artifact (Fig. 33.40).

Aliasing

Aliasing occurs when there are insufficient samples to accurately determine the nature of an object. For exam-

Spatial Aliasing

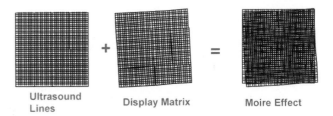

Ultrasound Lines + Display Matrix = Moire Effect

FIG. 33.41. Spatial aliasing (moiré effect) will result when imperfectly matched repeating patterns are superimposed.

ple, we take a high-speed photograph of a wheel once per second and it appears to be motionless in the photographs. What can be accurately said about the wheel? It may actually be stationary or it may be rotating at an integral number of turns per second. If it makes complete revolutions each second, it could be rotating once, twice, even ten times per second, but would appear motionless in our photographs. This phenomenon may occur in both the spatial and frequency domain. In the spatial domain, an ultrasound image composed of 500 lines may be mapped onto a television monitor of 525 lines. This can result in a spatial corollary of the spinning wheel example (Fig. 33.41). Spatial aliasing is known as the moiré effect. It is often seen on television as a spurious repeating pattern when the camera views a regular pattern, like a plaid or check. This effect is also present in the frequency domain in ultrasound, when the velocity of moving blood is being examined. If the rate of sampling is insufficient, the velocity of blood will be incorrectly calculated. This effect is called frequency aliasing.

REFERENCES

1. Zagzebski JA. *Essentials of ultrasound physics.* St. Louis: Mosby, 1996.
2. Merrit CRB. Physics of ultrasound. Rumack CM, ed. *Diagnostic ultrasound.* St. Louis: Mosby, 1998.
3. Kremkau FW. Artifacts in ultrasound imaging. *J Ultrasound Med* 1986;5:227.
4. Ziskin M. The comet-tail artifact. *J Ultrasound Med* 1982;1:1.
5. Muller N. Ultrasonic refraction by the rectus abdominus muscles: the double image artifact. *J Ultrasound Med* 1984;3:515.

Variants and Pitfalls in Body Imaging,
edited by Ali Shirkhoda.
Lippincott Williams & Wilkins, Philadelphia, © 2000.

CHAPTER 34

Physical Principles of MR Imaging Artifacts

Anil N. Shetty and John E. Kirsch

The artifacts seen on magnetic resonance (MR) images are truly a nonrepresentation of the object being imaged. Such artifacts can change the appearance of an image, and in some cases obscure the fine details of the anatomy. The origin of an artifact can be related to the coils, data acquisition, or image processing. In some instances, certain tissue produces undesirable artifacts when imaged with a certain type of pulse sequences. The image quality is dependent on how various anticipated artifacts can be removed from the final image. In some cases, these artifacts can be used to our advantage. Thus, to interpret MR images one should be knowledgeable and understand the origins of artifacts and be able to separate them from the anatomic structures. Artifacts are mainly classified as originating from the system or from tissue during the course of imaging (1–3). This chapter discusses each of the known artifacts, its origin, and the methods to remove or minimize its presence.

B1 INHOMOGENEITY

Virtually all magnetic resonance imaging (MRI) signals are based on the application of one or more radiofrequency (RF) bursts, or pulses. Tissue contrast will ultimately be defined by the time history of how a series of these RF pulses is applied.

The bulk magnetization in the body (M_0), created initially by the presence of a static main magnetic field (B0), is subsequently manipulated by the application of an RF field (B1) oriented perpendicular to B0. When the RF field is turned on, it will begin to rotate the directions of

A. N. Shetty: Department of Diagnostic Radiology, Wayne State University School of Medicine, Detroit, Michigan, and William Beaumont Hospital, Royal Oak, Michigan 48073-6769.

J. E. Kirsch: Siemens Medical Systems, Cary, North Carolina 27511.

the bulk magnetization. The direction will continue to evolve as long as the RF field is applied (4,5). Once the RF field is turned off, the orientation will cease to evolve and the total excursion will be based on the strength and duration of the pulsed RF field. The magnetization will then relax back toward the original state of equilibrium according to the characteristic tissue T1 and T2 relaxation times.

The total magnetization at any given time will always be equal to M_0, which is determined by the strength of B0. However, it is also composed of a longitudinal component M_L that lies parallel to the main field and a transverse component M_T that lies perpendicular to the main field. When the orientation of M_0 is changed due to an applied RF pulse, the amount of longitudinal and transverse components will change. Therefore, the magnitudes of M_L and M_T will depend on the time history of the RF pulsing.

Since the MRI signal is directly proportional to the magnitude of M_T, it therefore stands to reason that the MRI signal and tissue contrast will strongly depend on the accuracy of the RF pulsing. Two characteristics define RF pulse: phase and flip angle. The phase determines the precise direction of the B1 field when it is applied perpendicularly to B0. The flip angle, based on the strength and duration of the RF pulse, determines the extent of the excursion that is made by M_0 in its rotational direction. Both of these determine the end result of M_T in a series of RF pulsing, so their accuracy is crucial to the ultimate tissue contrast that is observed in the image.

In principle, therefore, for a consistent tissue contrast everywhere in the scan volume within magnet bore, the B1 field that is generated with each RF pulse must be uniform and homogeneous in both its phase and its strength throughout the duration of the pulse. Any RF inhomogeneity will in theory result in either a loss in regional signal or alteration in the local tissue contrast (6,7).

Most transmitting RF coils that are used in MRI are specifically designed and engineered to produce as uniform a B1 field as possible. However, similar to the main B0 magnetic field, the homogeneity begins to degrade away from the isocenter of the coil. Edge effects of distortion and overall field falloff are inevitable. This will occur to a greater extent with smaller volume coils such as those used for head and extremity scanning. A correctly operating transmission coil, however, should yield an adequately uniform B1 field in most regions of interest and applications designed for the specific coil type. If either the power amplifier that drives the coil or the coil itself malfunctions, global adverse effects on the RF homogeneity and image quality can result.

In addition to the inherent characteristics of the coil and general hardware operation, the presence of the human body can intrinsically distort the B1 field and may be a contributing factor to RF inhomogeneity. Due to the differences in chemical makeup and geometry of various aspects of the anatomy, the extent and behavior of the nonuniformity can vary greatly from patient to patient as well as from body part to body part (Fig. 34.1). Figure 34.1A is in an anatomic region of the body that created RF inhomogeneity, resulting in a relatively homogeneous image with uniform tissue contrast. However, Fig. 34.1B demonstrates a large degree of image nonuniformity caused by both coil- and body-induced B1 inhomogeneities taken from the same patient scan at a different anatomic region. The effect is primarily seen in posterior subcutaneous fatty tissue and adjacent muscles where bright signal is seen and fat suppression is significantly compromised. Note the characteristic diagonal behavior, which is quite common with certain RF coil designs.

Some MRI applications are more sensitive to B1 inhomogeneities than others. Different sequences of RF pulses with different flip angles are used to generate tissue contrasts that provide useful diagnostic information (8). Inhomogeneities can lead to either minor signal variations with little or no tissue contrast changes, or major alterations as drastic as complete tissue contrast reversal. In this example (Fig. 34.2), a slightly misadjusted transmitting body coil led to a global change in the RF uniformity that in most applications may not significantly affect the image quality. However, this particular MRI technique (inversion recovery) was more sensitive to such inhomogeneities (9).

The inversion recovery (IR) technique initially transmits a 180-degree flip angle RF pulse in order to invert the longitudinal magnetization M_L. After waiting a short period of time, another RF pulse is transmitted into the body, this time a 90-degree flip angle, to rotate the longitudinal magnetization into the transverse plane converting M_L to M_T, which can then be detected and processed. This type of technique accentuates intrinsic differences in the characteristic T1 relaxation of the tissues and is commonly used in certain body applications. However, the resulting tissue contrast with IR techniques is very dependent on the accuracy of the initial 180-degree RF pulse. If M_L does not get completely inverted, tissue contrast will be profoundly altered. Figure 34.2 is an example of changes that can occur due to spatial inaccuracies of the B1 field. Note the contrast reversal bilaterally in the muscle and fat.

Little can be done by the MRI technologist or physician to improve upon B1 inhomogeneities other than to use techniques or applications that are known to be less sensitive to these inaccuracies. Some improvements can be made by using RF transmission coils where particular care was taken to design a uniform B1 field. Primary efforts should be made to maintain a well-adjusted RF system in order to assure that the global inhomogeneities are kept to a minimum.

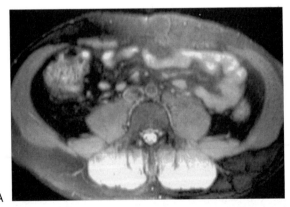
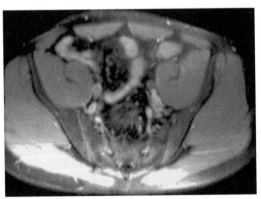

FIG. 34.1. B1 inhomogeneity. Axial proton-density weighted turbo spin echo fat suppressed image using a large homogeneous transmitting radiofrequency (RF) coil. **A, B:** Some anatomic regions are homogeneous (such as psoas and abdominal wall muscles). Others demonstrate inhomogeneous results (such as posterior gluteal muscles).

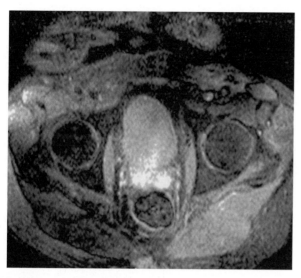

FIG. 34.2. B1 inhomogeneity. Axial inversion recovery scan demonstrating tissue contrast differences in each side due to global RF (B1) inhomogeneities.

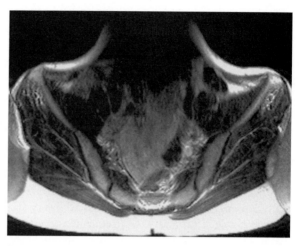

FIG. 34.3. B0 inhomogeneity. Local magnetic field inhomogeneity due to the presence of metallic object regional image distortions in the anterior portion of the abdomen caused by B0 inhomogeneity due to the presence of a belt buckle.

B0 INHOMOGENEITY

One of the principles of image formation in MRI lies in the presence of a strong static magnetic field B0 that creates and maintains a bulk magnetization in the body. In addition, B0 defines the characteristic resonant frequency of precession of the magnetization, ω_0, governed by Larmor's equation $-\omega_0 = \gamma B0$, where γ is the constant of proportionality called the gyromagnetic ratio and is unique to the nucleus (hydrogen, in the case of MRI). Under certain conditions when the magnetization can be detected, the signal will possess a given frequency determined by the strength of B0.

In MRI, it is crucial that all tissues being scanned in the volume of interest precess at the same initial reference frequency defined by B0. This then allows subsequent manipulations to be made in the magnetic field by the use of spatially varying gradient magnetic fields in order to volumetrically localize the signals in a predictable manner.

In reality, however, the scanning volume can never attain perfect uniformity of B0, meaning all parts will not experience precisely the same B0 field strength. Spatial inhomogeneity of the B0 field will give rise to different types of errors in MRI. One common consequence is a spatial distortion of the image. Unpredictable inhomogeneities of B0 will cause a spatial mismapping of the MRI signal coming from within the body. As a result, regional distortions could occur. Ferromagnetic objects that skew the magnetic field such as buckles, zippers, bra clips, hairpins, and dental fillings are common sources of localized B0 inhomogeneities (Fig. 34.3).

Careful screening of patients can avoid many unnecessary artifacts caused by metal on the body. However, image distortions from B0 inhomogeneity can also be either accentuated or minimized depending on the type of MRI pulse sequence technique that is used. For example, gradient echo imaging that relies on the free induction decay (FID) signal will inherently be sensitive to such inhomogeneities, while spin echo techniques that rephase them will be relatively robust. In addition, the extent to which the MRI signal is digitized, known as the reception bandwidth, determines the intrinsic field sensitivity of the spatial pixel mapping in the final image and can lead to large or small misregistrations of the distorted signal. Small bandwidths on the order of several hertz per pixel are favored for improving signal-to-noise ratios but will also lead to severe mismapping of pixels due to its sensitivity to B0 inhomogeneities. Large bandwidths, on the other hand, introduce noise into the image but have the advantage of being robust to field distortions.

Spatial distortion is only one effect of B0 inhomogeneities. Another consequence that alters the tissue contrast arises in fat suppression techniques, which are routinely employed in abdominal imaging to minimize the signal from fat that would otherwise obscure pathology. Different methods of reducing the fat signal exist, but one of the more widely used is known as spectral suppression, which is very sensitive to field nonuniformities.

It can only be assumed with this imaging technique that the fat resonant frequency is the same everywhere in the volume based on the assumption that B0 is perfectly uniform. In this ideal scenario, the narrow frequency band RF pulses will only suppress the fat. However, in a more realistic field that is not completely uniform, there will exist some regions where the fat magnetization will be precessing at a slightly lower or higher frequency than what is dictated by B0. In these cases, the narrow bandwidth RF pulses will no longer match the fat frequency and the suppression of the fat signal will become compromised in those areas (Fig. 34.4). Figure 34.4A shows a standard T1-weighted coronal pelvic scan. Note the high signal intensity from the subcutaneous fat and marrow of the femoral head. Figure 34.4B exhibits a corresponding T1-weighted fat-suppressed image of the same anatomic slice acquired in a relatively uniform B0 field. Other than in a few localized areas, the fat signal is low and of uniform intensity. Methods to maximize the uniformity of B0 involve the use of shim coils that generate slight spatially varying magnetic fields to shim the B0 field. Adjusting the shim field can aid in achieving a more uniform suppression of the fat signal from the body. Figure 34.4C demonstrates the effect of a poorly shimmed field. Owing to the very slight difference between fat and water frequencies, very little variation in B0 can severely compromise the outcome. In this specific example, the field varies diagonally resulting

in good fat suppression in some areas and little or no suppression in others.

Global variations in B0 can be effectively corrected with proper shimming procedures that should always be employed when using spectral fat-suppression techniques. However, more localized inhomogeneities caused for example by the presence of metal objects cannot be corrected by an external shim coil. Intrinsic differences in tissue magnetic susceptibility that lead to minute distortions at tissue boundaries are unavoidable and cannot be corrected.

RADIOFREQUENCY INTERFERENCE (SPIKES)

The RF antenna or coil that is used to detect the MRI signal is sensitive to other signals with outside origin.

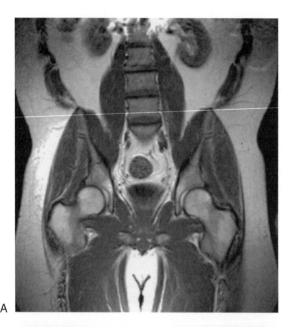

A

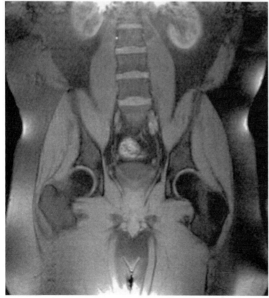

B

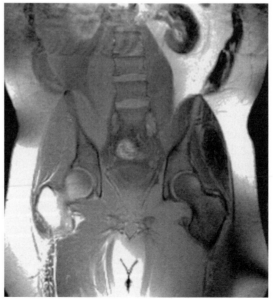

C

FIG. 34.4. Effects of shim on B0. **A:** Normal coronal T1-weighted spin echo pelvic scan. **B:** T1-weighted fat-suppressed spin echo scan of the same anatomic slice in a relatively uniform B0 field. **C:** A poorly shimmed field. Notice large areas of variations in fat suppression (areas of bright signal).

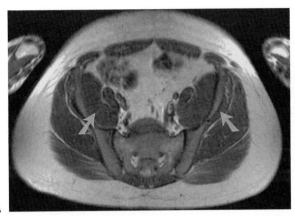 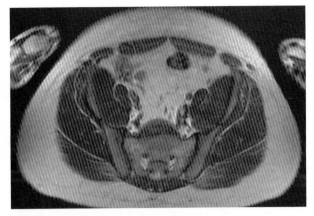

FIG. 34.5. RF interference (single spike). **A:** RF interference caused by a single spike event during the acquisition is demonstrated as fine stripes *(arrows)* within a normal, artifact-free image. **B:** The same anatomic region acquired with a spike event. The distinct banding pattern of frequency, intensity, and orientation depends on when the spike occurred during the acquisition.

One such source is a spike or electrical spark discharge in the environment, such as what could be generated by static electricity. A spike signal that is picked up by the coil in the time domain will reconstruct as parallel lines or bands in the image whose orientation, frequency, and intensity will depend on when it occurred during the acquisition and how strong it was relative to the MRI signal. Since the origin of the spike is independent of the MRI signal, this artifact will superimpose on the image (Fig. 34.5).

A more likely occurrence is multiple spikes within a given acquisition of an image. When this happens, each spike event will generate its own banding pattern in frequency and orientation in the image. These patterns will then cross-hatch with each other. If enough spikes create banding patterns in the image, a mottled appearance will become apparent along with elevating the overall noise level of the image (Fig. 34.6).

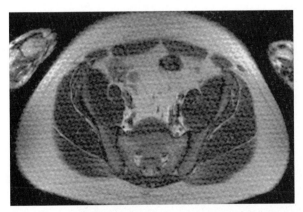

FIG. 34.6. RF interference (multiple spikes). Multiple spike events of the same anatomic position as seen in FIG. 34.5. Spiking that occurs at numerous times during an acquisition will cause banding patterns to crisscross in the image, leading to a mottled appearance.

Although the examples shown here are somewhat obvious, numerous low-level spikes during a scan can occasionally go undetected and simply yield overall poor image quality due to an elevated and noisy background. Many potential sources of spikes exist, such as lights, loose bolts, or parts in or around the magnet, and cabling and grounding connections. Qualified service personnel may be necessary to correct such a problem. However, one thing that can be done that substantially minimizes the occurrence of spiking is to maintain an appropriate humidity level in the scan room. If the air becomes too dry, it creates an ideal environment for static discharges to occur. By keeping a certain degree of moisture in the atmosphere, such events can be greatly reduced.

RADIOFREQUENCY INTERFERENCE (COHERENT)

The operating frequency of a MRI system typically falls in the megahertz (MHz) range. Hydrogen nuclei precess and emit signal at a characteristic frequency of approximately 63 MHz at a 1.5-T magnetic field strength. At these frequencies, many extraneous sources can potentially be found in the environment, coming from devices such as power supplies, radio stations, and other nearby medical equipment. It is a common practice to shield the MRI system from picking up these coherent signals by using either an RF tent that surrounds the vicinity of the magnet or an RF cabin that shields the entire exam room. However, if these preventative measures fail, such coherent sources of noise can be picked up and processed as an undesirable artifact in the MR image.

An image is composed of a matrix of pixels containing various MRI signal intensities representative of the tissues. In the majority of clinical practice, the pixel coordinates and positions are spatially defined by a unique phase and frequency of the signal. One direction of the

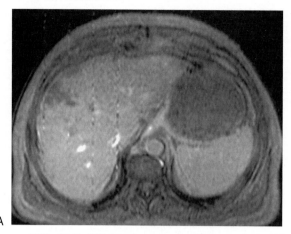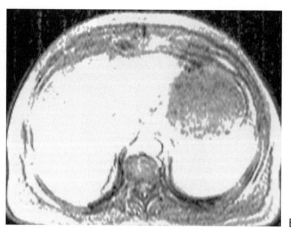

A

B

FIG. 34.7. RF interference (coherent noise). RF interference caused by constant frequency noise sources. Frequency encoding is left to right and phase encoding is front to back. Same interference lines are shown at normal windowing levels **(A)** and better depicted at high windowing levels **(B)**.

image will vary in phase while the other direction will vary in frequency. Extraneous coherent noise sources will typically possess a constant frequency of emission, but may have a random phase associated with it. If such signals get detected due to a leak in the RF shielding, they will become mapped in the image at a specific position in frequency and distributed across the phase direction. As a result, a line will be observed in the image (Fig. 34.7). In this example, the signal frequencies are mapped from left to right and the phases are mapped from front to back. If the extraneous noise has both a coherent frequency and phase, then the artifact would appear as a dot or star in some position within the image. However, this tends to be rare, and interference lines are more commonly observed.

This type of RF interference usually suggests that the RF shielding in the exam room may somehow be compromised. If the shield becomes damaged or the seal around the door becomes worn, RF leaks within the room can result. However, qualified service personnel should be consulted to systematically determine the source of the noise because it could also come from noisy electronic components within the MR system.

LOW SIGNAL COIL RECEPTION

Overall image quality is primarily governed by the inherent sensitivity and signal-to-noise ratio (SNR) of the receiver antenna or coil. Many aspects of the fundamen-

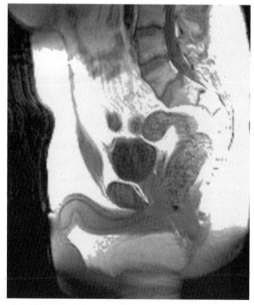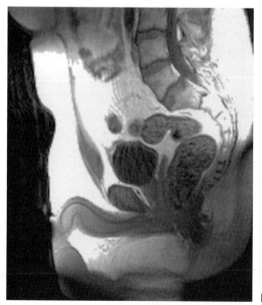

A

B

FIG. 34.8. Poor signal reception from coil sagittal scan of the lower abdominal region using a four element body array coil. **A:** When all four elements function properly, the image is of relatively uniform high intensity. Notice that dropout at upper and lower edges is due to the anatomy being outside the coil elements. **B:** Malfunctioning element yields a regional signal void in the buttock region.

tal coil design can influence this but are beyond the scope of this discussion. Nevertheless, if a properly operating coil was to malfunction in some way, the resulting SNR reduction will cause noticeable losses in overall image quality. Images will exhibit a type of graininess, making it difficult to evaluate, particularly in regions of low tissue contrast and small lesions.

In recent years, manufacturers have been designing coils with multiple elements and integrating them into MRI systems. These array coils provide greater anatomic coverage and higher inherent SNR as compared to single element coils. However, because they contain several individual elements, it is possible for one of them to malfunction while the others operate normally. When this occurs, the majority of the image may possess good image quality, but the vicinity of the specific coil element that is not picking up signal may show a localized signal loss.

When using a four-element body array coil, two elements are located anteriorly while the other two are positioned posteriorly. When all four are operating correctly, the scanned image will be relatively homogeneous with high SNR throughout the imaging volume (Fig. 34.8A). However, when one element is not picking up the correct level of signal, a regional void in the vicinity of that element will occur (Fig. 34.8B). At times, this may mimic localized signal losses due to the presence of metal, but can be distinguished by the lack of any geometric distortion associated with metal.

ANALOG-TO-DIGITAL CONVERTER (DIRECT CURRENT) OFFSET

The analog-to-digital converter (ADC) is responsible for digitizing the MRI signal. However, prior to doing so, the RF (MHz) signal becomes demodulated down to the audiofrequency (Hz–kHz) range so that accurate digitization can be achieved. Described in another way, the MRI signal that is detected in the laboratory frame of reference becomes processed in the rotating frame of reference where the frequency of reference is usually defined as the Larmor precessional frequency determined by the main field strength, B0.

Common with most electronic components, the ADC must be calibrated and adjusted so that it does not contain a nonzero direct current (DC) baseline. In other words, when the ADC samples the demodulated MRI signal, it should not superimpose a baseline offset value on top of that signal. If a DC offset in the ADC exists, it will generate a very characteristic artifact that is unique to this scenario.

In Fourier transform theory, where a time domain signal is transformed into its frequency domain counterpart, a constant or DC signal in time transforms to a spike or dot in frequency. Therefore, if an ADC offset exists, the image (which is simply the two-dimensional (2D) representation of the Fourier transform) will possess a dot artifact caused by the offset. This dot will be positioned in the center of the field of view (FOV) along the frequency encoding direction, but may not necessarily be positioned in the same way along the phase-encoding direction. This will depend on how the scan was acquired.

In the simplest case, the ADC samples the MRI signal the same way throughout the entire acquisition. The dot artifact will then be positioned centrally along phase encoding, thereby placing the dot in the middle of the 2D FOV. A more useful practice is to acquire the scan by a method called phase alternation. In this situation, each time the ADC samples the MRI signal, it alternates the phase by 180 degrees. In essence, it flip-flops the signal between positive and negative. By doing this, it causes any residual ADC offset that may exist to be reconstructed as a dot at the very edge of the FOV along the phase-encoding direction so it is away from regions of interest rather than in the middle where it can interfere.

If the FOV is freely shiftable from the isocenter of the magnet bore, then representation of the ADC offset artifact may not always be at the middle of the FOV or at the very edge (Fig. 34.9). In this example, the frequency-encoding direction is left to right, indicating an ADC offset artifact that is centered in that direction. Phase encoding is top to bottom and the artifact is neither centered nor at the edge of the FOV. It can be seen that there is a slight spread in the dot, which is typically caused by a drifting ADC baseline. Whatever the situation may be, the unique characteristic of the ADC offset artifact is that it will always be in the form of a dot in the image.

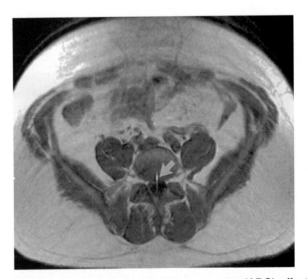

FIG. 34.9. Effect of analog-to-digital converter (ADC) offset axial MRI scan with an ADC offset artifact *(arrow)*. Frequency-encoding direction is left to right. Phase encoding is front to back. This type of artifact tends to exhibit itself as a dot that is centered along the frequency direction but may not necessarily be centered along the phase direction. If a drift in the ADC exists, there may be a slight spread to the dot in the phase direction as shown.

With a properly calibrated ADC and other components that can generate a nonzero signal baseline, this type of artifact should be negligible, although if present, little can be done by an operator during clinical scanning to avoid the artifact. Many MRI techniques are specifically programmed to make a measurement of the baseline prior to the scan that is then used to subtract whatever baseline may exist during the actual scan. In most cases, this can prevent the occurrence of this artifact.

ANALOG-TO-DIGITAL CONVERTER OVERFLOW

MRI is a digital imaging modality, and therefore the analog time domain signal must become digitized in magnitude in order for it to become processed as a final image. The ADC is an electronic component on the MRI system that performs this function. One characteristic of this device is that it has an upper limit to the signal magnitude that it can process. This threshold determines whether the signal can become accurately digitized. If the detected MR signal exceeds this limit, ADC overflow will occur and peculiar changes will be exhibited in the image. Improper signal gain adjustment of the receiver that leads to an excessive amplification of the signal entering the ADC can be caused by certain misadjustments in the MRI system.

With proper signal amplification, the expected tissue contrast is optimal and the background is uniformly dark (Fig. 34.10). Figure 34.11 depicts varying degrees of ADC overflow and the corresponding effects on the image. In Fig. 34.11A, the overall amplification of the signal was too high for digital processing, resulting in a clipped signal during the digital conversion. When the MR signal becomes clipped, the digital result is not a true representation of what really exists and the image can take on erroneous characteristics. In the case where the overflow is slight (Fig. 34.11A), it can typically

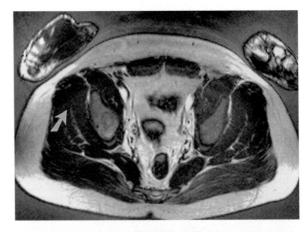

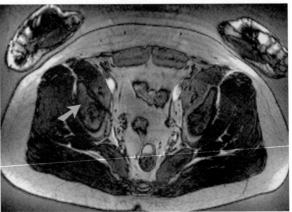

FIG. 34.11. Effects of ADC overflow. Axial MRI scan through the same region as in FIG. 34.10 at improper receiver gain settings depicting slight (A) and severe (B) ADC overflow and signal clipping (arrow).

result in only a minor increase in the intensity of the background, which is a direct consequence of the clipping. A halo effect around the body is very characteristic of ADC overflow. If the signal amplification is significantly above the ADC threshold for processing, then severe ADC overflow will result (Fig. 34.11B). Here, substantial edge enhancement occurs at tissue boundaries and a fundamental change in the tissue contrast can result. Normally bright tissue will become suppressed and darker tissues begin to enhance. Complete tissue contrast reversal has been known to happen in extreme cases. In any case, background air will always be increased, which is a telltale sign that ADC overflow occurred.

Incorrect signal gain amplification that leads to ADC overflow usually suggests an error in the MRI hardware. Manually overriding the receiver gain set by the system for the scan and reducing it so that the amplification no longer clips the ADC can avoid the problem, but may not be an option on the scanner. Little can be done to circumvent the occurrence until the system is serviced by qualified personnel.

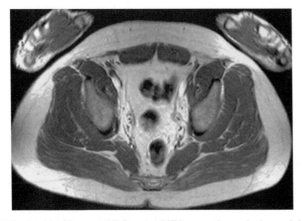

FIG. 34.10. Normal ADC axial MRI scan through the pelvis with proper signal amplification and normal ADC digitization and processing.

QUADRATURE RECEIVER ERRORS

As with all electromagnetic waves, the RF signal that is detected in MRI is actually composed of two components known by convention as the real (0-degree) part and the imaginary (90-degree) part. These two wave components are similar but perpendicular to each other as they travel in space, possessing a 90-degree phase shift between them. Once the receiver antenna picks up the signal, it can either be processed as one signal or separated into the two respective components. If the former is done, ambiguity will exist in the frequency of the signal. Therefore, in MRI it becomes split into two parts and converted into digital information for subsequent processing via two independent receiver channels. This is commonly known as quadrature, or phase sensitive, signal detection. The balance between these channels, however, is crucial so that the total signal does not become biased toward either of the two components. Usually such an imbalance can occur if the phase splitter does not separate the signals by exactly a 90-degree phase shift. If an imbalance exists, then an image artifact in the form of a very characteristic ghost will be generated (Fig. 34.12).

Unlike most ghost artifacts, which are randomly distributed and ill defined, quadrature ghosts will typically be extremely well defined and reflect the precise structures and contrast of the image if its intensity is strong enough. Additionally, they will be oriented upside down and mirrored relative to the primary image. This aspect is unique to quadrature ghost artifacts and no other ghost artifact possesses these characteristics. Therefore, quadrature receiver problems can usually be diagnosed relatively quickly and corrected by a qualified service engineer.

SYSTEM STABILITY

In a typical 2D MRI acquisition, a matrix of digital data is collected row by row for a given image. Each row will usually represent one MRI signal coming from the technique or experiment. To obtain the entire data set, the experiment must be repeated, each time filling in a row of the matrix. For example, the technique may be a conventional spin echo experiment. After pulsing a 90- to 180-degree RF pair, the spin echo is generated and the signal is picked up at an echo time, TE, digitized into 256 time samples, and processed as one row of 256 data points in the matrix. The experiment is repeated at a repetition time, TR, and is done 256 times, resulting in a complete data matrix of 256 × 256 points. This data set is then reconstructed into an image using the mathematical method of Fourier transformation (FT).

System stability is crucial to ensure an artifact free image. Each time a row of data is obtained, the MRI system must be stable and perform the exact same way every time. If it does not, then the rows of data will not align with one another and the reconstructed image will possess artifacts (Fig. 34.13A). In this specific example, the receiver antenna is electronically unstable and characteristics of the artifacts are typically randomized ghosting along the phase-encoded direction of the image, being top to bottom, while the frequency-encoded direction is left to right.

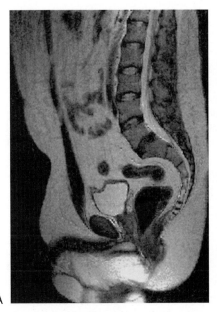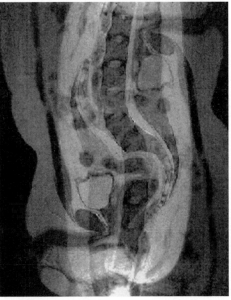

A   B

FIG. 34.12. Quadrature receiver errors. Sagittal whole-body scan through the lumbar spine and abdomen with a **(A)** balanced and **(B)** imbalanced quadrature receiver. Quadrature ghosts are characteristically upside down and mirrored relative to the primary image.

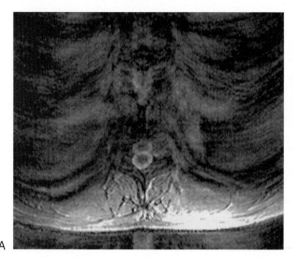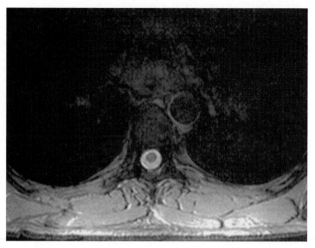

A B

FIG. 34.13. Effect of system instability ghosting artifacts caused by system instabilities in a study using an array coil with multiple antenna elements. **A:** An unstable element generated ghosts in one axial level. **B:** A stable element produced an artifact-free image at a different axial level.

System instabilities can frequently mimic bulk motion artifacts induced by the patient. Wholesale motion during the acquisition of a row of data will also cause a distortion or misalignment with respect to all the other rows. Upon reconstruction, randomized ghosting will occur that appears very similar to Fig. 34.13A. Because of these similarities, it can at times be very difficult to determine whether ghosting artifacts are caused by patient motion or system instabilities.

Although ghosting artifacts cannot be avoided when they are due to system instabilities, certain features of the ghosting can yield telltale signs of whether it is patient related or system related in order to determine whether a service engineer should be contacted. In the case shown here, for example, an array coil was used that contained multiple antenna elements at different anatomic locations along the long axis of the patient. If the patient was moving, then it would stand to reason that all slices in the study would show ghosting artifacts to a certain degree. System instabilities were suspected in this case, however, because at a different anatomic location containing a different coil element the images did not show ghosting artifacts (Fig. 34.13B).

Other clues to distinguish between the patient and the system exist. Physiologic ghosting will only follow the part of the anatomy that is actually moving. Rarely will there be a complete ghosting of the entire anatomic section caused by physiologic motion. Rather, one may find that the cerebrospinal fluid (CSF) shows ghosting from flow or the anterior portion of abdominal fat shows ghosting from breathing. On the other hand, if the system is unstable, it will not discriminate between anatomic parts and therefore will typically exhibit a wholesale ghosting of the entire slice (Fig. 34.13A).

ALIASING OR WRAPAROUND

Aliasing is a phenomenon routinely seen on MR images when inappropriate sampling conditions exist. A typical appearance in the final image would be when a part of the anatomy that is outside the intended FOV along one side reappears along the opposite side of the image (10,11). This is related to the fact that sometimes a region of high-frequency signal is inappropriately sampled, resulting in its mapping along the region of low frequency. Since this is fundamental to digital sampling of data points, in principle it can occur both along the phase- and frequency-encoding directions (11).

In MRI, once the imaging plane is established, the signal is sampled along either of the two remaining orthogonal directions during the presence of a gradient along that direction. The gradient amplitude and the FOV determine the range of frequency to be sampled along that direction. Thus, along the "read" direction, the FOV depends on the amplitude of the read gradient and the sampling interval. For example, the maximum precessional frequency (f_{max}) along the read direction is simply the product of gradient amplitude and the FOV/2 along the read direction and is given by the following equation (12):

$$f_{max}^{READ} = \gamma G_{READ} \left(\frac{FOV_{READ}}{2} \right) \quad [1]$$

This signal in turn is demodulated and converted into a digital form by sampling at a rate that is governed by the Nyquist criteria. The Nyquist condition for signal acquisition without aliasing states that for a signal that is periodic, with a precessional frequency f, then the sampling rate must be at least twice this precessional frequency. Although, one can sample at any high rate to avoid aliasing, it becomes impractical due to increased scan time when sampling points are increased. Increasing samples will also increase the bandwidth causing the SNR to decrease. Therefore, one must establish a minimum sampling frequency necessary to accurately recover and represent the signal. Such a sampling frequency is called the Nyquist frequency (13). For example, at a 2 mT/m gradient and for a FOV of 50 cm, the edge of FOV is at 25 cm and the frequency at that point is 2.0 mT/m × 63.72 MHz/T × 0.25 m = 31.86 kHz. The actual low-pass filter is set at 32.00 kHz. The sampling frequency or receiver bandwidth (BW) therefore is twice this frequency, 64.00 kHz, and the sampling interval is 16 microseconds. The low-pass filter is adjusted to receiver a BW of the frequency (from above) so that any frequency higher than the maximum is eliminated. The sampling frequency is established by sampling interval and the number of sampling points. For example, when sampled along the READ direction with 256 or 512 samples over a time during which the receiver is turned on, the receiver BW is given by the following equation (12,14);

$$\text{Receiver Bandwidth} = \frac{\text{Sampled points}}{\text{Sampling time}} = \frac{N}{T_s} = \frac{1}{\Delta T_s} \quad [2]$$

where ΔT_s is the sampling time between successive data points and T_s is the sampling interval. To image without aliasing, the receiver bandwidth should correspond to this Nyquist frequency, which should be at least twice the precessional frequency given by Eq. 1. For any sampling that is lower than this frequency, the object is said to be undersampled. In other words, signal frequency that is greater than one-half the Nyquist frequency is indistinguishable from those that are less than one-half the Nyquist frequency. A typical appearance of aliasing is shown in Fig. 34.14A, in which a reduced FOV was used. Most scanners are designed in such a way that all frequencies within the object are unambiguously sampled. A low-pass filter that filters frequencies above the Nyquist frequency does this. However, these filters never have ideal performance (Fig. 34.14B).

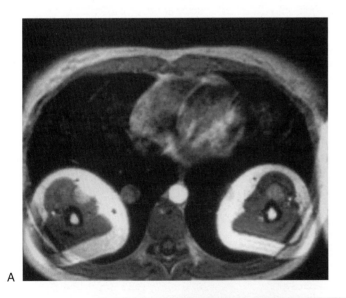

A

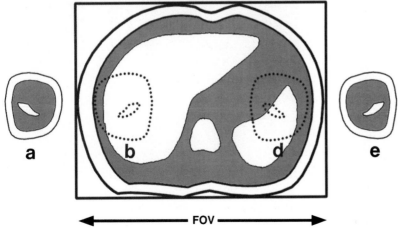

B

FIG. 34.14. Wraparound (aliasing) artifact. **A:** Aliasing artifact from arms presented when an axial imaging is performed with a small field of view (FOV). **B:** When the FOV is reduced, the signal arriving from regions *a* and *e* are very high and beyond the sampling range determined by the FOV. Under these conditions, the frequency corresponding to *a* is processed and presented as a frequency corresponding to region *d*. Similarly, the frequency corresponding to region *e* is processed as frequency from *b*. Since the fast Fourier transform (FFT) of data provides positional information from the frequency information, the aliasing is seen from the anatomic regions outside the FOV.

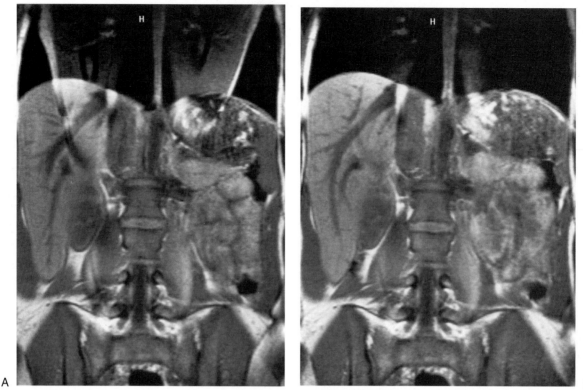

FIG. 34.15. Wraparound (aliasing) artifact—spatial presaturation. **A:** In a coronal orientation with a small FOV, aliasing artifacts are seen from both arms. **B:** Using spatial saturation pulses on either side on regions that are aliasing, the signal from those regions is considerably reduced.

Aliasing can occur in the phase and frequency direction and in addition along the slice direction when 3D imaging is performed. Fortunately, one can overcome aliasing along the READ direction by simply oversampling (doubling the sampling points) without time penalty. A familiar example describing aliasing arising from undersampling is the appearance of backward rotation of wagon wheels when watched on a movie or television screen. This is due to the same phenomenon in which the movie frames are sampled at the rate much

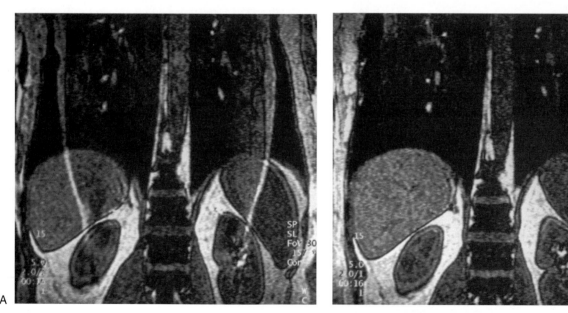

FIG. 34.16. Wraparound (aliasing) artifact—RF blanket. **A:** Without the use of RF blankets where aliasing is present. **B:** A repeat imaging with the same parameters but using an RF blanket to cover both arms.

smaller than actual rotational frequency of the wagon wheel.

Some other methods to remove aliasing artifacts include the following:

1. Extending the FOV along the direction where aliasing is present. Doubling the FOV samples twice as many points per TE for the same sampling interval. Sampling time being constant, the sampling interval is reduced to half. As a result, the fast Fourier transform (FFT) provides twice as many pixels from twice the number of sampled points. The objects are correctly represented in FFT with pixels covering the extended FOV. In the image domain, the extended portion of FOV is removed, and the final image is presented with correct FOV. Use of surface coils whose FOV is limited can also be useful in that the signal from tissues extending beyond the FOV is considerably reduced.

2. Use of saturation pulse to saturate the signal coming from the regions outside the intended FOV. This may increase the power deposition to the tissue and may reduce the number of slices for coverage (Fig. 34.15).

3. Use of an RF blanket greatly reduces the aliasing by simply generating no signal from the area over which the blanket is placed (Fig. 34.16). The blanket is in the form of a wrap around both arms, or one knee when the other is being imaged.

MOTION-RELATED ARTIFACTS

There are a variety of motions presented in different forms that ultimately tend to degrade the quality of the image (15–18). The motion that results in some sort of artifact in the final image can be from pulsation, cardiac motion, or respiration and classified as the invol-

untary type, or it can result from patient motion such as coughing or twitching while data are being sampled, and classified as the voluntary type. For example, gross patient motion that is aperiodic in any direction during data acquisition causes the signal to spread out spatially, thus producing blurring (19), whereas periodic motion will modulate signal spatially, creating alternating high- and low-intensity ghost-like images of the moving object (20). The signal intensity of the artifacts is proportional to the intensity of the moving source. For example, the artifacts in abdominal imaging have their origins in the motion of high-intensity structures, such as fat.

It is clear from the data collecting method that the sampling interval between two adjacent data points in the READ direction is in the order of a few tens of microseconds. Thus, from point to point along the READ direction the object appears stationary and the change due to gross motion is not apparent. However, along the phase direction the sampling interval between two points is the pulse repetition time, which can vary from a few hundred milliseconds to a few seconds. Any type of motion, therefore, will modulate the signal, creating repetitive ghosts of images along the PHASE direction. For example, if the motion is periodic, the ghosts will appear periodically with alternating signal intensity along the phase-encoding direction (Fig. 34.17).

The signal behavior in the presence of motion can be predicted knowing the nature of temporal variation in motion. Signal modulation can be described using the Bloch equation with components describing motion. To analyze the temporal variation in a spatial location, motion can be described in terms of the Fourier series. For simplicity, we assume a single frequency of motion. The displacement along any view direction is given by the following equation (21):

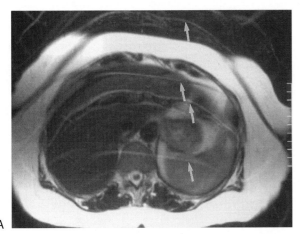
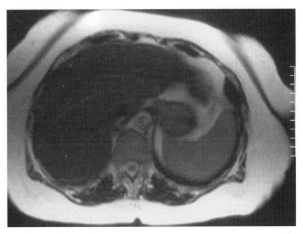

A   B

FIG. 34.17. Respiratory motion-related artifact. **A:** Conventional fast spin echo was performed when patient was asked to breath normally. Due to motion of diaphragm during respiration, the ghost artifacts are seen as repetitive bands extending along the anterior-posterior direction *(arrows)*. **B:** When the same patient was scanned during a breath hold, the resulting image is free from respiratory-related artifacts.

$$\delta\, r = \pm m \cdot f \cdot TR \cdot FOV \qquad [3]$$

where f is the fundamental frequency of motion, m is the harmonic component of particular frequency component, TR is the repetition time, and FOV is the view size. Along the frequency-encoding direction, the displacement of the ghost images is given by the following equation:

$$\delta\chi = \pm m \cdot \frac{\Delta f}{\gamma G \chi} \qquad [4]$$

The bandwidth of motional frequency Δf is much smaller than the bandwidth per pixel and therefore does not amount to much in terms of displacement along the frequency direction. This agrees well with our intuitive understanding based on sampling times along the frequency direction. However, along the phase direction they produce ghosts as described by Eq. 4. Amplitude of signal intensity of these ghosts is described by solving for signal variation in amplitude and position in terms of phase change.

There are various strategies available to eliminate or to reduce the artifacts resulting from motion.

Reorientation of Read and Phase Gradient Axes

One of the simplest methods to avoid artifacts masking the region of interest is to move the artifacts away from that region. This is achieved by swapping gradient axes between the phase and readout direction (22). In doing so, propagating motion artifacts will now be presented along the direction in which the phase gradient is rotated. For example, axial imaging of the abdomen will present a ghost-like artifact resulting from periodic motion of high-intensity fat as a result of respiration. Along with that, the abdominal aorta, due to pulsatile flow, also presents artifacts along the same direction, and the pancreas may be obscured by such artifacts. By swapping gradient axes, these artifacts will be presented left to right, which may be beneficial. It should also be noted that by swapping gradient axes, the chemical shift artifact would also rotate.

Respiratory Gating or Cardiac Triggering

In a conventional respiratory gating technique, a few lines of data are sampled during the deep inspiration or expiration period, during which the motion is at its minimum. This is achieved by observing normal respiratory waves using a nasal cannula and synchronizing data acquisition to coincide with a specific part of the cycle. However, the time required to acquire a complete image becomes prohibitively long, and during that time patient motion will likely create additional artifacts from motion. Also, data collected during the nonsteady part of the respiratory cycle is discarded (Fig. 34.17). Presently, most imaging can be performed in a breath-hold mode without the loss of tissue contrast. Cardiac triggering, on the other hand, requires the patient heart rate to control the scanning. The repetition time is controlled by patient's R-R interval (23). However, due to beat-to-beat variation, artifacts may not be completely eliminated (Fig 34.18). Recently, navigator echoes have been used to detect and use respiratory motion information to image the heart and abdomen (24). A 3D navigator echo technique along with cardiac triggering is used for imaging the coronary vessels. Another technique to compensate for respiratory-related motion artifact is to acquire phase-encoding steps and rearrange them to follow a smooth form, avoiding discontinuities. There are a few methods based on this technique such as centrally ordered phase encoding (COPE) (25) and respiratory-ordered phase encoding (ROPE) (26). The basic idea in these techniques is to monitor respiratory motion during the scan and rearrange phase-encoding steps or acquisition views so that the

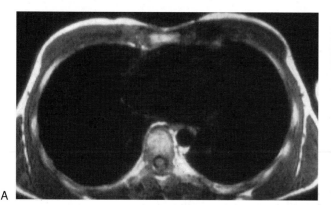
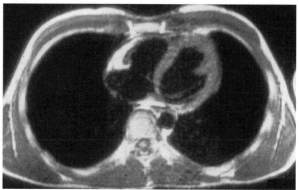

A

B

FIG. 34.18. Cardiac motion-related artifact. **A:** Spin echo imaging without cardiac or respiratory gating. Severe motion results in almost complete elimination of the signal from the heart. **B:** The same sequence is repeated with cardiac triggering. By synchronizing data acquisition to patients R-wave and restricting TR to fall within the patient's R-R interval, most of the motion artifact related to cardiac motion is eliminated.

component severely affected by motion is placed at the high end of the Fourier data set. These techniques substantially reduce scan times but are sensitive to random phase errors caused by within-view motion or aperiodic view-to-view motion. Within-view motion is a result of motion that occurs between excitation and data acquisition. This results in incomplete rephasing of the transverse magnetization at the time of data collection.

Gradient Moment Nulling

One method to improve phase inconsistency is to use a technique called gradient moment nulling, in which the phase of moving spins is made to coincide with that of stationary spins at the echo center (27,28). The method involves solving a set of simultaneous equations involving motion with linear, acceleration, and jerk terms. The results provide correct gradient profiles with timing, which are generally used along the slice and read directions in the gradient timing diagram, since the phase-encoding gradient is applied only briefly compared to slice and read gradients. The advantage of this type of technique is that it corrects for motions arising from linear, acceleration, and jerk terms. The drawback is the lengthening of echo time and the demand on the gradient electronics.

Spatial Presaturation Pulse

The spatial presaturation pulse is routinely used to eliminate signal from a region that would affect the imaging area (29). Due to motion, in a selected region of interest (ROI) signal from tissues of adjacent regions will overlap the ROI. A spatial presaturation will help eliminate the signal originating from unwanted regions entering the ROI. Spatial presaturation is accomplished by using a 90-degree RF pulse prior to imaging pulses and placed at the region whose signal is to be eliminated. Spatial presaturation is routinely used in abdominal imaging to reduce flow-related artifact and respiratory ghost artifact from adjacent tissues, and to eliminate the aliasing artifact. Typically a pair of parallel saturation pulses are applied superior and inferior to the slices. It can also be used in gradient echo imaging to suppress flow artifacts. In cardiac imaging with proper placement of presaturation pulse, the blood signal can be made to appear dark, thus, increasing adjacent myocardial contrast. The other uses of spatial presaturation pulses include selective imaging of arteries or veins, prevent aliasing from regions outside the FOV.

The technique of presaturation pulse requires no special hardware and has the advantage of being available on most scanners. One drawback in using spatial presaturation is the lengthening of pulse repetition time or the reduction in the number of imaging slices. Also, increasing the thickness of the saturation pulse requir-

ing additional RF power may increase total RF power deposition.

Pulse Sequence Parameters: TR and TE

The periodicity in ghost images is directly related to the respiratory cycle time T_{resp} (12). In a pulse sequence with a TR adjusted to T_{resp}, one can avoid a ghost artifact by moving it to the edge of the FOV. However, because of the wide variation in the tissue contrast, this approach is not recommended. The amount of dephasing and motion-related artifacts tend to worsen with the increase in TE. Reduction in TE, especially when performing magnetic resonance angiography (MRA) of the abdomen, helps in performing MRI as well as MRA in a breath-hold period. Spatial resolution can be improved by increasing the phase-encoding steps. The use of fast spin echo or turbo spin echo strategies reduces the concomitant increase in scan time.

With echo-planar MRI, one can perform rapid-acquisition spin echo, such as rapid acquisition with relaxation enhancement (RARE), which allows for imaging the complete liver in a single breath-hold period of 20 seconds. One can also use conventional gradients and perform turbo or fast spin echo sequences in a breath-hold period. The potential drawback with echo-planar imaging is the presence of other artifacts such as susceptibility artifact at the tissue-air interface and bright signal from fat in fast spin echo techniques.

One can also increase the signal averaging, resulting in reducing the intensity of ghosts. This will not displace ghosts completely. Also, signal averaging cannot improve the artifact from blurring that results from irregular motion. The improvement in SNR is by a factor of the square root of N, where N is the number of averages used for each phase-encoding step. Most routine spin echo imaging in the abdomen and other areas prone to motion uses turbo spin echo sequences performed in a single breath hold.

FLOW-RELATED ARTIFACTS

In conventional imaging of stationary tissues, gradients are structured to provide maximum amplitude echo signal. The maximum amplitude is a result of minimum cancellation of phases among spins in the transverse plane. With the introduction of flow, moving spins gain different amount of phases during gradient activity depending on where they lie on a flow profile. For example, in a laminar type of flow the flow velocity is maximal at the center and gradually decreases as one traverses to the vessel boundary. Thus, groups of spins that are close to the center have minimal shear, causing minimal phase loss and consequently attaining higher velocity, whereas spins along the edges experience maximal shear, resulting in minimum velocity. In MRI one uses a voxel (3D) or a pixel (2D) to define spatial resolution and SNR.

With a larger pixel or a voxel that encloses spins from edges, there will be severe phase loss, resulting in minimal signal, whereas those at the center will have maximal signal in the pixel or the voxel. As a result there is a variation in signal across the lumen of the vessel. This is a major contributor to flow effects in spin echo imaging. Another factor that influences phase cancellation is the prolonged TE in spin echo, in which the cancellation of random phases among spins results in black blood image.

Another type of flow void is also seen routinely on a spin echo that has a different origin. In a multislice spin echo study, with a constant flow there is magnetization washout between a selective 90-degree and a selective 180-degree RF pulse. The loss depends on the temporal spacing between selective RF pulses and the flow velocity. This effect is not present in gradient echo sequences due to absence of 180-degree RF pulse.

Reduction of Flow-Related Artifacts: Gradient Moment Nulling (GMN)

This technique is also known as flow compensation or motion artifact suppression technique (MAST) (30–32). During the presence of gradient activity, spin phase dispersion increases with flow velocity. This intravoxel phase dispersion would lead to loss of signal. GMN can be applied to reverse the effects of phase dispersion occurring at different flow velocities. Most scanners use techniques that include only first-order GMN. The technique has been very successful in gradient echo images (Fig. 34.19). In spin echo images the artifact from flow cannot be completely eliminated using GMN. This is due to the fact that during long echo time the flow artifacts normally seen on a spin echo image do not arise solely

from spin-phase dispersion. However, together with a presaturation pulse, GMN will improve image quality in a spin echo. The disadvantage in using GMN is that the minimum echo time is prolonged to accommodate additional gradient structures.

CHEMICAL SHIFT ARTIFACT

A routinely observed artifact when imaging an anatomic area that contains adipose and nonadipose components is chemical shift artifact (33–35). For example, along the frequency-encoding direction, the kidneys and bladder show this artifact as a dark boundary on one direction (Fig. 34.20). In 3D imaging, it is seen along the slice select direction when slice selection is used for frequency selection. MRI on commercial scanners is primarily based on protons as observable nuclei due to their natural abundance and high sensitivity. These protons may be found in a state such as attached to oxygen atom as in a water molecule or to carbon atoms as in a lipid hydrocarbon chain. In either state, protons are always surrounded by electrons, which shield them from the external magnetic field. Therefore, the presence of an electron cloud around protons makes protons experience a magnetic field slightly different from the main magnetic field, and as a result protons resonate at a slightly different frequency.

When atoms form chemical bonds, the electrons are shared between the atoms. The electrons spend much of their time near the atom, which has the most chemical affinity. Hydrogens are chemically bound to oxygen (as in water) and the electrons are pulled toward oxygen because of stronger affinity of oxygen to electrons than hydrogens. As a result, the hydrogen becomes less shielded from elec-

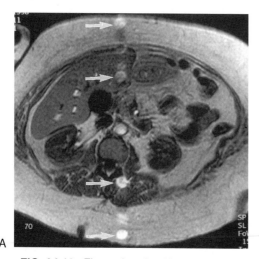
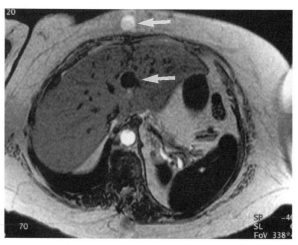

A   B

FIG. 34.19. Flow-related artifact. **A:** Standard gradient echo pulse sequence used without any type of compensation scheme in gradient structures. The pulsatile nature of flow presents a ghost-like artifact along the phase-encoding direction *(arrows).* **B:** Using a first-order gradient moment nulling (GMN), most of the artifacts from flow related to first-order motion are eliminated. However, artifacts due to higher-order motion such as acceleration and jerk motion are not removed *(arrows).*

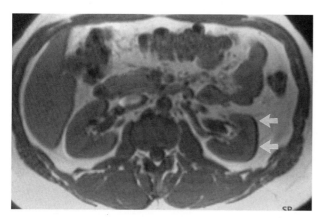

FIG. 34.20. Chemical shift artifact (CSA). Standard fast spin-echo with a bandwidth of 130 Hz per pixel shows chemical shift along the margins on the lateral side of the left kidney *(arrows).*

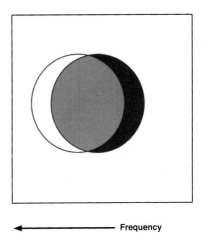

← Frequency

FIG. 34.21. CSA of the first kind. The frequency is increased from a right-to-left direction, and fat is seen along the low-frequency direction due to its slightly lower natural precessional frequency. This is indicated by the dark section of the circle.

trons, and therefore hydrogen protons resonate at a higher frequency when found in water molecules. In lipid molecules, the hydrogen is joined to carbon atoms, forming a hydrocarbon chain, and the carbon has lesser affinity for electrons; therefore, it does not strongly attract electrons. In this case, the electron cloud is pushed around hydrogens, forming a shield. As a result, hydrogens are shielded from the main magnetic field and protons of these hydrogens resonate at a slightly lower frequency. The shift in the resonance frequency of hydrocarbon protons such as in fat with respect to that of water protons is represented by chemical shift which is ≈ 3.5 ppm (parts per million) and amounts to 220 Hz in a 1.5-T system. Since the shift is directly related to the magnetic field, increasing the magnetic field inherently increases the shift between fat and water proton frequencies.

In MR images, the position of a pixel (signal) on the screen depends on the frequency of that signal. The frequency encoding is performed by placing a magnetic field gradient along one axis so those protons at different positions resonate at different frequencies. The position of a pixel on the screen is encoded based on the frequency of resonance of protons in that pixel at that position. Because lipid hydrocarbon (fat) and water protons resonate at different frequencies, they may appear at different spatial locations on MR images. This is called a chemical shift artifact (CSA) of the first kind (Fig. 34.21). The CSA gets worse at higher field strength systems. Since the position is determined by the frequency, we may compensate for the CSA by using a larger READ (frequency encoding) gradient to make the intended frequency range per pixel larger than the chemical shift.

The presence of CSA is detrimental to MRI when the area of interest involves fat, as in the abdomen. The presence or absence of CSA in an image can be determined based on pulse sequence parameters. For example, the sampling rate, together with the number of sampled

points along an axis, determines the total frequency difference across an image. A sampling time of 10 msec is equal to a frequency spread of 100 Hz per pixel. In a 256 × 256 image with each pixel 100 Hz wide, the total bandwidth of the image will be 100 × 256 = 25.6 kHz. In MRI, it is desirable to have the pixel frequency spread encompass both fat and water protons originating from the same location and be represented by a single pixel in an image domain. The relationship between bandwidth (gradient amplitude) and the frequency spread is illustrated in Fig. 34.22. In this example, the amount of misregistration

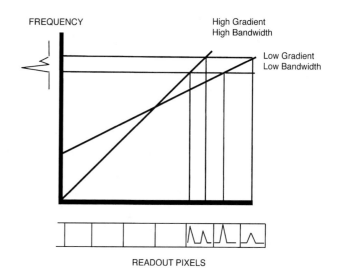

FIG. 34.22. CSA effect of bandwidth. The frequency bandwidth determines the extent of chemical shift misregistration. As the bandwidth decreases (gradient amplitude decreases), the separation between fat and water is indicated by two pixels. At a higher bandwidth, both fat and water will be represented by the same pixel. There exists a trade-off between bandwidth and the signal-to-noise ratio. The proper choice of bandwidth is determined by the nature of the imaging.

between fat and water protons is ≈ 2 pixels (220/100). When the bandwidth is reduced by one-half, which can be obtained by doubling the sample rate (increasing frequency sampling to 512 points) or by lowering the READ gradient amplitude and keeping the same number of sampling points, the same fat and water protons will now be represented by four pixels. When the bandwidth is reduced by another factor of 2, the shift between fat and water protons will be eight pixels. Although decreasing the bandwidth may provide an increase in SNR, it comes at the cost of severe CSA. Thus, in the abdomen where fat is a dominant part of the anatomy, careful consideration should be given to selecting the bandwidth to increase the SNR and at the same time reduce the undesired CSA.

There is another artifact, called CSA of the second kind, which is observed typically when gradient recalled echo (GRE) pulse sequences are used (36). Due to an absence of 180-degree refocusing RF pulse, fat and water proton spin populations precess such that they cycle in or out of phase with each other as TE is increased. For example, fat and water protons will be out of phase by 180 degrees in a particular time TE when the product of frequency difference (≈220 Hz) and TE is π radians. On substitution, we find that the corresponding TEs are 2.25 and 6.75 msec, whereas at TEs 4.5 and 9.0 msec they are in phase in the transverse plane. A consequence of selection of TE in GRE pulse sequences can be seen in abdominal imaging. At TEs where fat and water protons are out of phase, a dark boundary will be seen around anatomic regions surrounded by lipids (Fig. 34.23). MRI may be done with a TE that corresponds to in-phase imaging conditions; unlike CSA of the first kind, the artifact here will

extend along phase and frequency directions because of the result of phase cancellation in all directions (Fig. 34.24). This effect can be used to our advantage to differentiate lesions with high signal intensity such as hemorrhage from lipid-containing regions.

To increase the sensitivity of MRI for detection of pathology, a commonly used technique is to suppress the signal originating from fat protons prior to data acquisition (Figs. 34.25 and 34.26). Currently, there are a number of techniques available to effectively suppress the fat signal. One method is to use a frequency selective and spatially nonselective RF pulse, which is used prior to a spatially selective (slice selective) RF pulse (37). By using a frequency selective fat saturation pulse, due to unavoidable lengthening of TR the scan time is increased. Another method is to use a binomial pulse for selective excitation of fat signal and then crush the signal in the transverse plane. Yet another method uses a careful design of a spatially selective RF pulse with a sufficiently narrow bandwidth that will excite only water protons in a slice (38). This technique has advantages over the conventional fat-suppression technique in that the loop time is considerably shortened; thus, it can be performed in a breath hold. In the case illustrated in Fig. 34.27, water excitation imaging is done in a breath hold. Fat signal is fairly uniformly suppressed and the bladder appears isointense with bone marrow fat, suggesting that the pulse sequence is more like a T1-weighted sequence in which urine in the bladder appears dark due to its prolonged T1. The success of such a technique depends largely on the homogeneity of the main magnetic field. All frequency selective RF pulses assume that frequency of water protons is uniform across the FOV. A careful shimming of the magnet is a

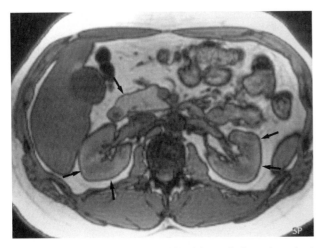

FIG. 34.23. CSA of the second kind (out-of-phase imaging). A gradient-echo pulse sequence in which TE is adjusted so that fat and water spins cancel their phase. Along the boundaries where they cancel each other and due to a relatively similar population of fat and water spins, a dark signal void *(arrows)* is presented.

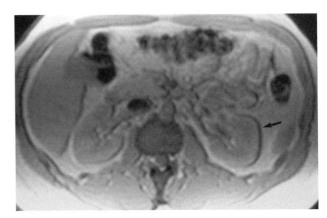

FIG. 34.24. CSA of the second kind (in-phase imaging). A gradient echo in which TE is adjusted so that the fat and water spin phases are same. In this case, phase addition takes place and the signal intensity at the boundary is slightly higher than either the fat or water spins alone. However, misregistration is still presented *(arrow)* due to an incorrect selection of bandwidth.

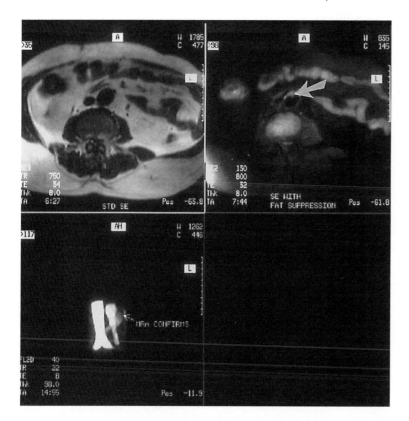

FIG. 34.25. Chemically selective fat-suppression imaging. Conventional spin echo without fat suppression is obtained to rule out the presence of aortic ulcer *(upper left)*. The same sequence when performed with fat suppression clearly demonstrates the presence of aortic ulcer *(upper right arrow)*. This was further confirmed by using the magnetic resonance angiography technique *(lower left)*.

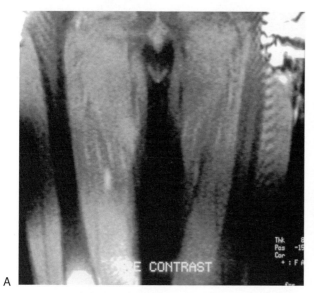
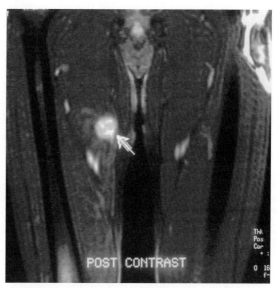

A   B

FIG. 34.26. Chemically selective fat suppression imaging. **A:** Standard gradient echo in coronal orientation prior to contrast injection. **B:** The same pulse sequence with fat suppression and contrast injection reveals the presence of tumor *(arrow)*.

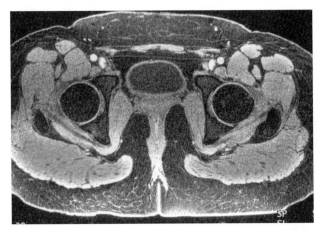

FIG. 34.27. Chemically selective—water excitation imaging. A 3D gradient echo imaging with water excitation. The selective RF pulse was designed to excite a narrow bandwidth comprised only of water spin protons. The imaging is performed in a single breath-hold period.

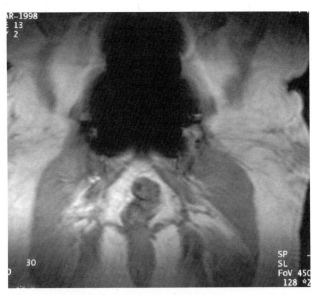

FIG. 34.29. Artifacts from ferromagnetic implants. The presence of a metallic implant causes a localized severe artifact. The large signal void is due to the presence of a metallic implant at the level of the lower spine.

necessary prerequisite to obtaining fairly good fat suppression in an image.

FERROMAGNETIC IMPLANTS

The presence of metal objects will distort the main magnetic field. Although metal objects are not a source of MR signal, they do create severe signal void at the location of the object (39). The distortion is localized and is based on the magnetic susceptibility of the material. Objects such as ferromagnetic materials will severely distort the field in regions close to the object. The outer edges show some unusual appearances based

on the magnetic lines of forces distributed by the presence of the object. For example, tissues near the edge of the object experience a strong magnetic field and it is dropped when we move farther from the object. Since the frequency encoding is based on spatial position, the change in frequency from magnetic field distortion will encode protons at different locations (Figs. 34.28 and 34.29).

ARTIFACTS FROM MAGNETIC SUSCEPTIBILITIES

The origin of susceptibility artifacts is the same as that described for the ferromagnetic objects (40–42). They are generally seen along the edges of tissues, which separates areas of different susceptibilities. A familiar example is the tissue-air interface. Ferromagnetic implants have the greatest susceptibility change at the edge of metal and tissue. The shape of the artifact from the susceptibility effects can change when the gradient axes between phase and frequency are swapped. The artifacts can be minimized by using a short TE to allow for minimum dephasing during TE. In terms of pulse sequences, gradient echo sequences produce pronounced artifacts followed by spin echo followed by fast spin echo. This is due to the absence of a 180-degree refocusing pulse on the gradient echo and to multiple refocusing 180-degree RF pulses on a fast spin echo sequence (Fig. 34.30).

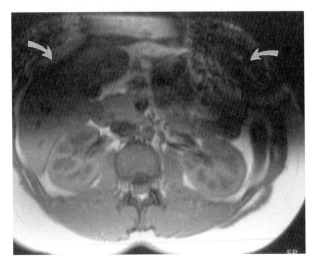

FIG. 34.28. Artifacts from ferromagnetic objects. Presence of a metal underwire in a bra results in field distortion and signal void (arrows) in a spin echo image.

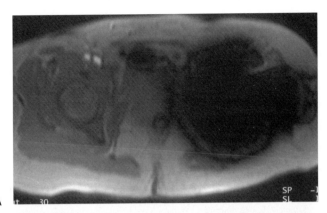

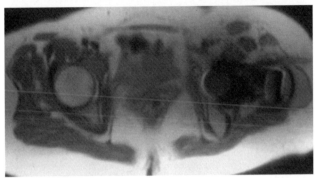

FIG. 34.30. Magnetic susceptibility induced artifacts from metallic implant. **A:** A gradient recalled echo in a patient with a metallic prosthetic left hip implant. The signal void is exaggerated with the gradient echo technique. **B:** In the same patient, the spin echo technique shows the artifact boundary.

GIBBS PHENOMENON

The Gibbs phenomenon, also known as truncation or edge ringing artifact, is routinely seen in an image obtained with a low-resolution data acquisition when displayed at a sufficiently high resolution (43,44). For exam-

ple, in a data acquisition size of 128×256, an abrupt drop in signal along the phase direction beyond 128 steps is like truncating data to 128 steps and zero filling the rest to form a 256-size grid. A series of curvilinear low-intensity bands may be seen on the edges both along the phase- and frequency-encoding directions. The most common occurrence is near the edges, where there is a sharp transition in signal in the tissue interface. Due to a smaller number of phase-encoding steps, which is a common practice to save time, the artifacts predominantly present along the phase-encoding direction. As illustrated in Fig. 34.31A, the image was obtained with a low-resolution matrix along the phase and frequency directions. The edges show overlapping bands parallel to the edge with high and low intensities. One method to avoid this artifact is to perform imaging with a sufficiently high resolution. By doubling the phase- and frequency-encoding steps, the sampling steps will increase and in turn they will reduce the spacing between ripples. However, the amplitude will remain the same. At present, this is the best approach for reducing the artifact by decreasing the spacing between lines. Other methods include extrapolation schemes in which the data are extended into the high-frequency region of the k-space. Methods such as constrained reconstruction (CORE), which uses different models for data extrapolation, are computer intensive (45).

THIRD-ARM ARTIFACT

The presence of gradients may result in deviation of matrix linearity, especially at the edges. The hardware for gradients is designed to provide perfect linear spatial mapping along the direction in which they are applied. However, when there is nonlinearity at the edges, there appears to be spatial mismapping of pixel positions such

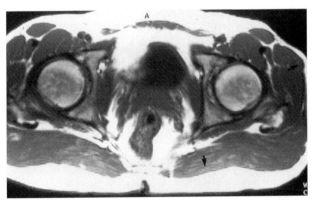

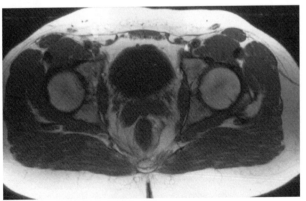

FIG. 34.31. Gibbs ringing artifacts from low-resolution imaging. **A:** Gibbs ringing artifacts or truncation artifacts are seen as low signal bands of alternating intensity at the edges (arrow). **B:** On increasing sampling points or decreasing sampling interval, the spacing between bands is considerably reduced; however, the amplitude of the band remains the same. Due to closeness in spacing the image looks smooth at the boundaries.

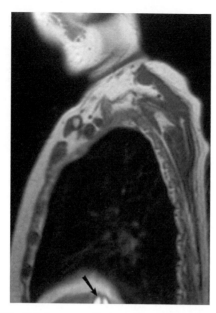

FIG. 34.32. Third-arm artifact sagittal imaging (spin echo pulse sequence) in which field of view along the head-to-feet direction is limited and the anatomy extends beyond the intended FOV. Due to spatial mismap of anatomy at the edges, the third-arm artifact is presented as a bright signal in the lower center *(arrow)*.

that slices obtained at the edges may produce bright artifact in the image. For example, when the slice selection is performed with an RF pulse and a gradient that is orthogonal to the plane of the slice, a predefined position and thickness is excited. With a gradient that is nonlinear at the edges or when the magnetic field outside of the imaging volume is nonuniform, intended excitation produces a number of unwanted excitations at locations outside the region of interest because of the resonance condition. If these excited areas fit into the frequency bandwidth during the signal reception, an image will be superimposed on the correct image based on its resonance frequency (Fig. 34.32).

REFERENCES

1. Bellon EM, Haacke EM, Coleman PE, et al. MR artifacts: a review. *AJR* 1986;147:1271.
2. Henkelman PM, Bronskill MJ. Artifacts in magnetic resonance imaging. *Rev Magn Reson* 1987;2:1.
3. Porter BA, Hastrup W, Richardson ML, et al. Classification and investigation of artifacts in magnetic resonance imaging. *Radiographics* 1987;7:271.
4. Hahn EL. Spin-echoes. *Physiol Rev* 1950;80:500.
5. Farrar TC, Becker ED. *Pulse and Fourier transform NMR*. New York: Academic Press, 1971 .
6. Bloom AL. Nuclear induction in inhomogeneous fields. *Physiol Rev* 1955;98:1105.
7. Young IR, Cox IJ, Bryant DJ, Bydder GM. The benefits of increasing spatial resolution as a means of reducing artifacts due to field inhomogeneities. *Magn Reson Imaging* 1988;6:585.
8. Mills TC, Ortendahl DA, Hylton NM, et al. Partial flip angle MR imaging. *Radiology* 1987;162:531.
9. Hearshen DO, Ellis J, Carson PL, Shreve P, Aisen AM. Boundary effects from opposed magnetization artifact in inversion recovery images. *Radiology* 1986;160:543–547.
10. Pusey E, Yoon C, Anselmo ML, Lufkin R. Aliasing artifacts in MR imaging. *Comput Med Imaging Graph* 1988;12:219.
11. Papoulis A. *The Fourier integral and its application*. New York: McGraw-Hill, 1962.
12. Haacke EM, Patrick JL. Reducing motion artifacts in two dimensional Fourier transform imaging. *Magn Reson Imaging* 1986;4:359–363.
13. Haacke EM. The effects of finite sampling in magnetic resonance imaging. *Magn Reson Med* 1987;4:407.
14. Bracewell RN. *The Fourier transform and its applications*. New York: McGraw-Hill, 1978.
15. Mitchell DG, Vinitski S, Burk DL Jr, et al. Multiple spin-echo MR imaging of the body: image contrast and motion-induced artifact. *Magn Reson Imaging* 1988;6:535.
16. Dixon WT, Brummer ME, Malko JA. Acquisition order and motional artifact reduction in spin warp images. *Magn Reson Med* 1988;6:74.
17. Haacke EM, Lenz GW. Improving MR image quality in the presence of motion by using rephasing gradients. *AJR* 1987;148:1251.
18. Silverman PM, Patt RH, Baum PA, Teitelbaum GP. Ghost artifact on gradient-echo imaging: a potential pitfall in hepatic imaging. *AJR* 1990;154:633.
19. Wehrli FW, Haacke EM. Principles of MR imaging. In: Potchen EJ, Haacke EM, Siebert JE, Gottschalk A, eds. *Magnetic resonance angiography: concepts and applications*. St. Louis: CV Mosby, 1993:9–34.
20. Wood ML, Henkelman RM. MR imaging artifacts from periodic motion. *Med Phys* 1985;12:143.
21. Duerk JL, Wendt RE III. Motion artifacts and motion compensation. In: Potchen EJ, Haacke EM, Siebert JE, Gottschalk A, eds. *Magnetic resonance angiography: concepts and applications*. St. Louis: CV Mosby, 1993:80–133.
22. Mirowitz SA. Motion artifact as a pitfall in diagnosis of meniscal tear on gradient reoriented MRI of the knee. *J Comput Assist Tomogr* 1994; 18:279.
23. Rogers WJ Jr, Shapiro EP. Effect of RR interval variation on image quality in gated, two-dimensional, Fourier MR imaging. *Radiology* 1993;186:883.
24. Wang Y, Rossman PJ, Grimm RC, Wilman AH, Riederer SJ, Ehman RL. 3D MR angiography of pulmonary arteries using real time navigator gating and magnetization preparation. *Magn Reson Med* 1996;36: 579.
25. Korin HW, Riederer SJ, Bampton AEH, Ehman RL. Altered phase-encoding order for reduced sensitivity to motion in three-dimensional MR imaging. *J Magn Reson Imaging* 1992;2:687.
26. Bailes DR, Gildendale DJ, Bydder GM, et al. Respiratory ordered phase encoding (ROPE): a method for reducing respiratory motion artifacts in MR imaging. *J Comput Assist Tomogr* 1985;9:835.
27. Mitchell DG, Vinitski S, Burk DL Jr, et al. Motion artifact reduction in MR imaging of the abdomen: gradient moment nulling versus respiratory-sorted phase encoding. *Radiology* 1988;169:155.
28. Hirohashi S, Otsuji H, Uchida H, et al. The usefulness of motion artifact suppression technic (MAST) in the MRI diagnosis of liver tumors. *Rinsho Hoshasen* 1989;34:591.
29. Felmlee JP, Ehman RL. Spatial presaturation: a method for suppressing flow artifacts and improving depiction of vascular anatomy in MR imaging. *Radiology* 1987;164:559.
30. Lipcamon JD, Chin LC. Phillips JJ, Pattany PM. NM of the upper abdomen using motion artifact suppression technique (MAST). *Radiol Technol* 1988;59:415.
31. Elster AD. Motion artifact suppression technique (MAST) for cranial MR imaging: superiority over cardiac gating for reducing phase-shift artifacts. *AJNR* 1988;9:671.
32. Zee CS, Boswell WD Jr, Norris SL, et al. The motion artifact suppression technique (MAST) in magnetic resonance imaging: clinical results. *Magn Reson Imaging* 1988;6:293.
33. Soila KP, Viamonte M, Starewicz PM. Chemical shift misregistration effect in MRI. *Radiology* 1984;153:819.
34. Smith RC, Lange RC, McCarthy SM. Chemical shift artifact: dependence on shape and orientation of the lipid-water interface. *Radiology* 1991;181:225.
35. Lufkin R, Anselmo M, Crues, et al. Magnetic field strength dependence of chemical shift artifacts. *Comput Med Imaging Graph* 1988;12:89.

36. Szumowski J, Eisen JK, Vinitski, et al. Hybrid methods of chemical shift imaging. *Magn Reson Med* 1989;9:379.
37. Anzai Y, Lufkin RB, Jabour BA, Hanafee WN. Fat suppression failure artifacts simulating pathology on frequency selective fat suppression MR images of head and neck. *AJNR* 1992;13:879.
38. Thomasson DM, Purdy DE, Finn JP. Fast spectrally selective excitation in 3D gradient echo imaging. *J Magn Reson Imaging* 1994;4(P):56(abst).
39. Shellok FG, Kanal E. Bioeffects and safety of MR procedures. In: Edelman RR, Hesselink JR, Zlatkin MB, eds. *Clinical magnetic resonance imaging,* vol 1. Philadelphia: WB Saunders, 1996.
40. Ludeke KM, Roschmann A, Tischler R. Susceptibility artifacts in NMR imaging. *Magn Reson lmaging* 1985;3:329.
41. Czervionke LF, Daniels DL, Wehrli FW, et al. Magnetic susceptibility artifacts in gradient-recalled echo MR imaging. *AJNR* 1988;9:1149.
42. Bach-Gansmo T, Ericsson A, Leander P, et al. Motion associated susceptibility artifacts. *Acta Radiol* 1992;33:606.
43. Constable RT, Henkelman RM. Data extrapolation for truncation artifact removal. *Magn Reson Med* 1991;17:108.
44. Amartur S, Haacke EM. Modified iterative model based on data extrapolation method to reduce Gibbs ringing. *J Magn Reson Imaging* 1991;1:307.
45. Haacke EM, Liang ZP, Izen SH. Constrained reconstruction: a super-resolution optimal signal-to-noise alternative to the Fourier transform in magnetic resonance imaging. *Med Phys* 1989;16:388.

SUGGESTED READINGS

Fukushima E, Roeder SBW. *Experimental pulse NMR.* Reading, MA: Addison-Wesley, 1981.
Hendrick RE, Russ PD, Simons JH, eds. *MRI: principles and artifacts.* New York: Raven Press, 1993.
Henkelman RM, Bronskill MJ. Artifacts in Magnetic Resonance Imaging. *Raves Magn Reson Med* 1987;2:1.
Wesbey G, Edelman RR, Harris R. Artifacts in MR imaging: description, causes and solutions. In: Edelman RR, Hesselink JR, Zlatkin MB, eds. *Clinical magnetic resonance imaging.* Philadelphia: WB Saunders, 1990:88–144.

Subject Index

Note: Page numbers in *italics* indicate figures; page numbers followed by t indicate tables.